Comprehensive

Vascular and Endovascular Surgery

ELSEVIER CD-ROM LICENCE AGREEMENT

Comprehensive

Vascular and Endovascular Surgery

Edited by
John W Hallett Jr MD FACS
Clinical Professor of Surgery
Tufts Medical School
Boston, Massachusetts, USA
Director of Vascular Care of Maine
Eastern Maine Medical Center
Bangor, Maine, USA

Joseph L Mills MD
Professor of Surgery and Chief
Division of Vascular Surgery
University of Arizona
Tucson, Arizona, USA

Jonothan J Earnshaw DM FRCS
Consultant Surgeon
Department of Vascular Surgery
Gloucestershire Royal Hospital
Gloucester, UK

Jim A Reekers MD PhD
Professor of Interventional Radiology
Department of Radiology
Academic Medical Center
University of Amsterdam
Amsterdam, The Netherlands

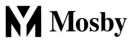 **Mosby**

Edinburgh • London • New York • Oxford • Philadelphia • St Louis • Sydney • Toronto 2004

MOSBY An affiliate of Elsevier Limited

First published 2004

ISBN 0 7234 3232 5

British Library Cataloguing in Publication Data
A catalogue record for this book is available from the British Library

Library of Congress Cataloging in Publication Data
A catalog record for this book is available from the Library of Congress

Notice
Medical knowledge is constantly changing. Standard safety precautions must be followed, but as new research and clinical experience broaden our knowledge, changes in treatment and drug therapy may become necessary or appropriate. Readers are advised to check the most current product information provided by the manufacturer of each drug to be administered to verify the recommended dose, the method and duration of administration, and contraindications. It is the responsibility of the practitioner, relying on experience and knowledge of the patient, to determine dosages and the best treatment for each individual patient. Neither the Publisher nor the editors or contributors assume any liability for any injury and/or damage to persons or property arising from this publication.

your source for books,
journals and multimedia
in the health sciences
www.elsevierhealth.com

The
publisher's
policy is to use
**paper manufactured
from sustainable forests**

Printed in Spain

Commissioning Editor: *Joe Rusko*
Project Development Manager: *Hilary Hewitt/Charlotte Mossop*
Project Manager: *Glenys Norquay*
Illustration Manager: *Mick Ruddy*
Designer: *Andy Chapman*
Illustrator: *Lynda Payne*

Contents

List of Contributors

Rainier V Aquino MD
Vascular Fellow
University of Pittsburgh Medical Center
Pittsburgh, Pennsylvania, USA

Ginger Barthel RN MA
Vice President
Clinical Operations
Advocate-Lutheran General Hospital
Park Ridge, Illinois, USA

Jonathan D Beard ChM FRCS
Consultant Vascular Surgeon
Sheffield Vascular Institute
Northern General Hospital
Sheffield, UK

Jean-Pierre Becquemin MD FRCS
Professor of Vascular Surgery
Head of Department of Vascular Surgery
Henri Mondor Hospital
Paris, France

Michael Belkin MD
Chief
Division of Vascular Surgery
Brigham & Women's Hospital
Harvard Medical School
Boston, Massachusetts, USA

Tamer N Boules MD
Resident in General Surgery
Section of Vascular Surgery
University of Michigan Medical School
Ann Arbor, Michigan, USA

Thomas C Bower MD
Professor of Surgery
Consultant in Vascular Surgery
Division of Vascular Surgery
Mayo Clinic
Rochester, Minnesota, USA

Kevin G Burnand MBBS MS FRCS
Professor of Surgery
Department of Academic Surgery
King's College London
St Thomas' Hospital
London, UK

John Byrne MCh FRCSI(Gen)
Consultant Vascular Surgeon
Cardiff Vascular Unit
University Hospital of Wales
Cardiff, UK

Richard P Cambria MD
Professor of Surgery
Harvard Medical School
Division of Vascular Surgery
Massachusetts General Hospital
Boston, Massachusetts, USA

Christopher G Carsten III MD FACS
Attending Vascular Surgeon
Academic Department of Surgery
Greenville Hospital System
Greenville, South Carolina, USA

Elliot L Chaikof MD PhD
John E Skandalakis Professor of Surgery
Chief, Division of Vascular Surgery
Emory University
Atlanta, Georgia, USA

Gregory S Cherr MD
Vascular Fellow
Department of General Surgery
Wake Forest University School of Medicine
Winston-Salem, North Carolina, USA

Kenneth J Cherry Jr MD
Professor of Surgery
Division of Vascular Surgery
Mayo Clinic
Rochester, Minnesota, USA

W Darrin Clouse MD
Assistant Professor of Surgery
F Edward Hébert School of Medicine
Uniformed Services University of Health Sciences
Bethesda, Maryland, USA
Wilford Hall Medical Center
Lackland Airforce Base, Texas, USA

David L Cull MD FACS
Attending Vascular Surgeon
Academic Department of Surgery
Greenville Hospital System
Greenville, South Carolina, USA

Alun H Davies MA DM FRCS ILTM
Reader and Honorary Consultant
Department of Vascular Surgery
Imperial College
Charing Cross Hospital
London, UK

Christoph Domenig MD
Research Fellow in Vascular Surgery
Division of Vascular Surgery
Harvard Medical School
Boston, Massachusetts, USA

Magruder C Donaldson MD
Associate Professor of Surgery
Harvard Medical School
Department of Surgery
Brigham & Women's Hospital
Boston, Massachusetts, USA

Josée Dubois MD
Professor of Radiology
Department of Radiology
Ste-Justine Hospital
Montreal, Quebec, Canada

Walter N Durán PhD
Professor of Physiology and Surgery
Department of Pharmacology and Physiology
New Jersey Medical School
University of Medicine and Dentistry of New Jersey
Newark, New Jersey, USA

Jonothan J Earnshaw DM FRCS
Consultant Surgeon
Department of Vascular Surgery
Gloucestershire Royal Hospital
Gloucester, UK

James M Edwards MD
Chief of Surgery, Portland VAMC
Associate Professor of Surgery
Oregon Health and Science University
Portland, Oregon, USA

Matthew S Edwards MD
Vascular Fellow
Department of General Surgery
Wake Forest University School of Medicine
Winston-Salem, North Carolina, USA

Julie A Freischlag MD
Professor of Surgery and Chair
Department of Surgery
Johns Hopkins Medical Institutions
Baltimore, Maryland, USA

Andrew T Gentile MD RVT
Vascular Surgeon
Tucson Vascular Surgery
Tucson, Arizona, USA

Richard G J Gibbs MD FRCS
Specialist Registrar in Vascular Surgery
Department of Surgery
Charing Cross Hospital
London, UK

Mary E Giswold MD
Surgical Resident
Division of Vascular Surgery
Oregon Health and Science University
Portland, Oregon, USA

Peter Gloviczki MD FACS
Professor of Surgery, Mayo Medical School
Chair, Division of Vascular Surgery
Director, Gonda Vascular Center
Mayo Clinic
Rochester, Minnesota, USA

Bruce H Gray DO
Director of Endovascular Services
Greenville Hospital System
Greenville, South Carolina, USA

John W Hallett Jr MD FACS
Clinical Professor of Surgery
Tufts Medical School
Boston, Massachusetts, USA
Director of Vascular Care of Maine
Eastern Maine Medical Center
Bangor, Maine, USA

Kimberley J Hansen MD
Professor of Surgery
Department of General Surgery
Wake Forest University School of Medicine
Winston-Salem, North Carolina, USA

Paul N Harden BSc (Hons) MB ChB FRCP
Consultant Nephrologist
Oxford Kidney Unit
The Churchill Hospital
Oxford, UK

E John Harris Jr MD
Associate Professor of Surgery
Medical Director, Stanford Vascular Laboratory
Division of Vascular Surgery
Stanford University School of Medicine
Stanford, California, USA

Johanna M Hendriks MD
Consultant Vascular Surgeon
Department of Vascular Surgery
Erasmus University Medical Center
Rotterdam, The Netherlands

Robert W Hobson II MD
Professor of Surgery and Physiology
Department of Surgery
New Jersey Medical School
University of Medicine and Dentistry of New Jersey
Newark, New Jersey, USA

Andrew W Hoel MD
Resident
Harvard Medical School
Department of General Surgery
Brigham and Women's Hospital
Boston, Massachusetts, USA

Manju Kalra MBBS
Instructor in Surgery, Mayo Medical School
Senior Association Consultant
Division of Vascular Surgery
Mayo Clinic
Rochester, Minnesota, USA

Edouard Kieffer MD
Professor of Vascular Surgery and Chief
Department of Vascular Surgery
Pitié-Salpêtrière University Hospital
Paris, France

Constantinos Kyriakides MD FRCS (Eng, Ed)
FRCS (Gen Surg)
Consultant Vascular Surgeon
Department of Vascular Surgery
The Royal London Hospital
London, UK

Frank A Lederle MD
Professor of Medicine
Veterans Affairs Medical Center
Minneapolis, Minnesota, USA

Nicholas J M London MBChB FRCS MD
FRCP(Edin)
Professor of Surgery
Department of Surgery
University of Leicester
Leicester Royal Infirmary
Leicester, UK

William C Mackey MD
Professor and Chairman
Department of Surgery
Tufts University School of Medicine
Boston, Massachusetts, USA

Peter J Mackrell MD
Fellow in Vascular Surgery
Academic Department of Surgery
Greenville Hospital System
Greenville, South Carolina, USA

Catharine L McGuinness MB BS MS
FRCS (Gen Surg)
Senior Lecturer and Consultant Vascular Surgeon
Surgical Unit
St Thomas' Hospital
London, UK

Mark H Meissner MD
Associate Professor
Department of Surgery
University of Washington School of Medicine
Seattle, Washington, USA

Matthew T Menard MD
Instructor in Surgery
Division of Vascular Surgery
Brigham and Women's Hospital
Harvard Medical School
Boston, Massachusetts, USA

Joseph L Mills MD
Professor of Surgery and Chief
Division of Vascular Surgery
University of Arizona
Tucson, Arizona, USA

Gregory L Moneta MD
Professor of Surgery
Division of Vascular Surgery
Oregon Health and Science University
Portland, Oregon, USA

Jonathan G Moss MDChB FRCS(Ed) FRCR
Consultant Interventional Radiologist
Department of Radiology
Gartnavel General Hospital
North Glasgow Hospitals University NHS Trust
Glasgow, UK

Scott Musicant MD
Research Fellow in Vascular Surgery
Division of Vascular Surgery
Oregon Health and Science University
Portland, Oregon, USA

A Ross Naylor MBChB MD FRCS
Professor in Vascular Surgery
Department of Surgery
Leicester Royal Infirmary
Leicester, UK

Mark R Nehler MD
Assistant Professor and Program Director
Division of Vascular Surgery
Department of Surgery
University of Colorado Health Sciences Center
Denver, Colorado, USA

Thelinh Nguyen MD
Attending Physician
The Vascular Center
Mary Black Health System
Spartanburg, South Carolina, USA

Patrick J O'Hara MD
Staff Surgeon
Department of Vascular Surgery
Cleveland Clinic Foundation
Cleveland, Ohio, USA

Vincent L Oliva MD
Associate Professor of Radiology
Department of Radiology
CHUM – Notre-Dame Hospital
Montreal, Quebec, Canada

Matthijs Oudkerk MD PhD
Professor of Radiology
Department of Radiology
Academisch Ziekenhuis Groningen
Groningen, The Netherlands

Kenneth Ouriel MD
Professor of Surgery
Department of Vascular Surgery
The Cleveland Clinic Foundation
Cleveland, Ohio, USA

Frank T Padberg Jr MD
Professor of Surgery
Department of Surgery
New Jersey Medical School
University of Medicine and Dentistry of New Jersey
Newark, New Jersey, USA

Frank B Pomposelli Jr MD
Associate Professor of Surgery
Harvard Medical School
Boston, Massachusetts, USA

Janet Powell MD PhD
Medical Director
University Hospitals Coventry &
Warwickshire NHS Trust
Coventry, UK

Todd E Rasmussen MD
Assistant Professor of Surgery
Malcolm Grow United States Air Force
Medical Center
Andrews Air Force Base, Maryland, USA

Amy B Reed MD
Assistant Professor of Surgery
Division of Vascular Surgery
University of Cincinnati College of Medicine
Cincinnati, Ohio, USA

Jim A Reekers MD PhD
Professor of Interventional Radiology
Department of Radiology
Academic Medical Center
University of Amsterdam
Amsterdam, The Netherlands

Robert Y Rhee MD
Associate Professor of Surgery
Division of Vascular Surgery
UPP Vascular Surgery
Pittsburgh, Pennsylvania, USA

Jeffrey M Rhodes MD
Assistant Professor of Surgery
Division of Vascular Surgery
University of Rochester Medical Center
Rochester, New York, USA

David A Rigberg MD
Assistant Professor of Surgery
Division of Vascular Surgery
University of California, Los Angeles
Los Angeles, California, USA

Frank C T Smith BSc MD FRCS (Eng) FRCS (Ed)
FRCS (Glas)
Consultant Senior Lecturer in Vascular Surgery
University Department of Surgery
Bristol Royal Infirmary
Bristol, UK

Gilles Soulez MD MSc
Associate Professor of Radiology
Department of Radiology
CHUM – Notre-Dame Hospital
Montreal, Quebec, Canada

Soni Soumian FRCS
Research Fellow in Vascular Surgery
Department of Vascular Surgery
Imperial College
Charing Cross Hospital
London, UK

Kong Teng Tan MD FRCR
Radiologist
Department of Radiology
Royal Hallamshire Hospital
Sheffield, UK

Thomas T Terramani MD
Resident in Vascular Surgery
Division of Vascular Surgery
Emory University
Atlanta, Georgia, USA

Stephen C Textor MD
Professor of Medicine and Consultant
Divisions of Hypertension and Nephrology
Mayo Clinic Foundation
Rochester, Minnesota, USA

Robert W Thompson MD
Professor of Surgery, Radiology, Cell Biology and
   Physiology
Department of Surgery
Washington University School of Medicine
St Louis, Missouri, USA

Edwin J R van Beek MD PhD FRCR
Senior Clinical Lecturer in Radiology
Unit of Academic Radiology
Royal Hallamshire Hospital
Sheffield, UK

Lukas C van Dijk MD PhD
Consultant Radiologist
Department of Radiology
Erasmus University Medical Center
Rotterdam, The Netherlands

Marc R H M van Sambeek MD PhD
Consultant Vascular Surgeon
Department of Vascular Surgery
Erasmus University Medical Center
Rotterdam, The Netherlands

Shubha Varma MD
Fellow in Vascular Surgery
Department of Surgery
New Jersey Medical School
University of Medicine and Dentistry of New Jersey
Newark, New Jersey, USA

Dierk Vorwerk MD
Professor of Radiology and Chairman
Department of Radiology
Klinikum Ingolstadt
Ingolstadt, Germany

Thomas W Wakefield MD
S Martin Lindenauer Professor of Surgery
Section of Vascular Surgery
University of Michigan Medical School
Ann Arbor, Michigan, USA

John V White MD
Clinical Professor of Surgery
University of Illinois School of Medicine
Chair, Department of Surgery
Advocate-Lutheran General Hospital
Park Ridge, Illinois, USA

Christopher L Wixon MD
Assistant Professor of Surgery
Mercer University School of Medicine
Savannah, Georgia, USA

John H N Wolfe MS FRCS
Consultant Vascular Surgeon
Regional Vascular Unit
St Mary's Hospital
London, UK

Foreword

When asked to write this foreword, I asked myself 'Why another text on vascular surgery? Don't we have enough or maybe too many already?' However, as soon as I began the review process, I began to understand what was new and compelling about this textbook. This text is truly a good one for the early 21st century.

In an extraordinarily presentable style, Drs Hallett, Mills, Earnshaw, and Reekers have outlined the facts and fundamentals of vascular surgery and newer catheter-based interventions. My bias is not to separate vascular and endovascular surgery, for both are parts of modern vascular surgery. Less invasive interventions encompass alternative therapies to open surgery and are increasingly successful (e.g. structured exercise programs, cilostazol, and balloon/stent angioplasty for claudication).

However, the separation of open and endovascular therapies in the new textbook works. This text highlights the traditional open methods alongside the endovascular challenger. But what is so compelling about this book is that it puts those various therapies side by side and lets the reader decide what is best for the patient. This is what *Comprehensive Vascular and Endovascular Surgery* is written to do. We don't have perfect answers to some of these controversies. But, if we don't have the alternative facts laid out before us in a concise and cogent way, we will never make progress in reaching a consensus based on outcomes analysis.

Comprehensive Vascular and Endovascular Surgery is evidence-based. Reasonably short, readable, and extremely well supported with excellent graphics and tables, each chapter has an introductory section of 'talking points.' There are up-to-date references, which make this book remarkably current.

Endovascular surgery is still an unproven option – even for AAA, where success is widely touted and also increasingly offered for occlusive disease. We must remember that occlusive disease has proven to be a wily and competent opponent. Witness all of the failure of therapies for disease below the inguinal ligament: endarterectomy - open and closed even with long vein patches, synthetic bypass, homografts, laser burning, catheter reaming or boring or blasting. Vein bypass has been the standard. There are still concerns that balloons and stents (even those with drugs eluting) may not be durable or excessively expensive when health-care resources are already stressed. But, the controversies of open and endovascular therapies continue, and we must address them. And we will.

All textbooks should be read with healthy scientific criticism, including this one. But *Comprehensive Vascular and Endovascular Surgery* addresses current controversies in a factual and remarkably readable way. Appropriate for both experienced surgeons preparing for recertification and as a primer for vascular trainees, it is a new compass to help us keep our sights on the welfare of our patients.

William M Abbott MD
Department of Vascular Surgery
Massachusetts General Hospital
Boston, Massachusetts, USA

September 2003

Preface

For years, futuristic medical writers have predicted the burgeoning impact of heart and vascular diseases on our aging population. By 2010, the 'baby boomer' generation will add millions of patients who need evaluation and management. The challenges on healthcare resources will be daunting.

How do we evaluate efficiently the amazing spectrum of arterial, venous and lymphatic diseases? How do we effectively manage them – and do it at an affordable cost? Basic and clinical research will provide some of the answers. But just as important will be the collaboration and communication that occurs among specialists who specialize in vascular care.

This new textbook links specialists in vascular surgery, interventional radiology and vascular medicine across the Atlantic Ocean, from North America to Great Britain and on to Europe. We have selected authors who are experienced enough to know what works but still have the energy and courage to evaluate new techniques. The textbook format emphasizes key concepts, uses color illustrations to enhance understanding of techniques, tabulates the best clinical trials, and includes important contributions from the literature as references. Of course, acquisition of new knowledge is so rapid today that our readers must supplement our suggested references with information from recent meetings, journals and the Internet.

We hope that this first edition of *Comprehensive Vascular and Endovascular Surgery* provides a practical and user-friendly reference for healthcare providers specializing in vascular diseases. We also request that you send us suggestions that could be used to improve future editions. Stay in touch. Do good work, and share your experience and knowledge with those around you who are dedicated to vascular care.

John W Hallett Jr
Joseph L Mills
Jonathan J Earnshaw
Jim A Reekers

September 2003

CHAPTER 1

Historical Perspectives in Vascular Surgery: The Evolution of Modern Trends

Todd E Rasmussen and Kenneth J Cherry Jr

A comprehensive history of vascular surgery is beyond the scope of this chapter for several reasons. Foremost, attempts to account for all of the contributions of Antyllus, Paré, Lambert, Eck, Murphy, the Hunters, Cooper, Mott, Matas, Halstead, Carrel, Exner, Goyanes, and other pioneers of surgery and medicine would fail to do them justice. Furthermore a comprehensive and modern historical account would incorporate the contributions of transplant and cardiovascular surgery, venous surgery, vascular medicine and pharmacology, diagnostic and therapeutic radiology and non-invasive vascular testing. Such breadth would surely require more text than the editors are willing to spare.

This chapter will therefore not represent a complete history of vascular surgery but rather a perspective – a perspective of those people and advances of the modern era which have sparked or perpetuated an evolution of patient care that has made our practices what they are today. The omission of certain surgeons and reports may dismay some readers, and the inclusion of others will undoubtedly cause similar discord. Other interpretations and appraisals of our history are as valid as this one; therefore this effort can be seen as a starting point for collegial discussion.

THE BEGINNINGS OF AORTIC SURGERY

The first operations on the aorta took place in the early 1800s and were for aneurysmal disease, invariably due to syphilis, in young to middle-aged men. In 1817, Sir Astley Cooper, a student of John Hunter, ligated the aortic bifurcation in a 38-year-old man who had suffered a ruptured iliac artery aneurysm.[1] The patient died soon after the operation. Keen, Tillaux, Morris, and Halstead reported similar attempts to ligate aortic and iliac artery aneurysms without patient survival in the 100 years following Cooper's initial report.

In 1888, during the era of arterial ligation for aneurysmal disease, Rudolph Matas revived the dormant but centuries-old concept of endoaneurysmorrhaphy for the treatment of arterial aneurysms. Matas successfully performed the technique on a brachial artery aneurysm, after an initial attempt at proximal ligation had failed, in a patient named Manuel Harris, who had a traumatic aneurysm following a shotgun injury to his arm.[2] The concept of opening and evacuating the contents of the arterial aneurysm sac had been introduced by Antyllus nearly 16 centuries prior. Although in this instance the technique was successful, Matas was reluctant to apply this method broadly during the era when aneurysm ligation was the prevailing dogma. The technique of open endoaneurysmorrhaphy was not used for more than a decade following Matas's original description.

In 1923, while Professor of Surgery and the Chief of the Department of Surgery at Tulane University, Matas was the first to ligate successfully the abdominal aorta for aneurysmal disease

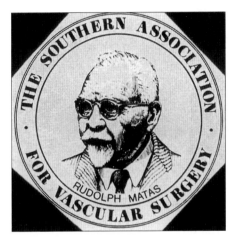

Figure 1.1 Official seal of the Southern Association for Vascular Surgery. (Reproduced with permission from Ochsner J. J Vasc Surg 2001;34:387–92.)

with survival of his patient.[3] He reported this technique again in the *Annals of Surgery* in 1940.[4] Matas eventually improved and refined the technique of open endoaneurysmorrhaphy, described in three forms: obliterative, restorative, and reconstructive. The reconstructive form of endoaneurysmorrhaphy allowed for maintenance of arterial patency. In all, Matas operated on more than 600 abdominal aortic aneurysms, with remarkably low morbidity and mortality rates. In 1940, at the age of 80 years, he presented to the American Surgical Association his experience with the operative treatment of abdominal aortic aneurysms.[5] Through his success and pioneering techniques, Matas demonstrated the efficacy of a direct operative approach to the aorta and began the era of aortic reconstruction. In 1977, during the organization of the Southern Association for Vascular Surgery, a likeness of Matas was chosen as the new society's logo (**Fig. 1.1**).[6] Matas is widely held as the father of American vascular surgery and in one of his most significant addresses, 'The soul of the surgeon', he established and emphasized the qualities of a surgeon to which we all should aspire.[7]

PERIPHERAL ARTERIAL RECONSTRUCTION

During this same era, vascular reconstruction of the peripheral arteries was developing rapidly. The first attempts to place venous autografts into the peripheral circulation were described by Alfred Exner in Austria and Alexis Carrel in France at the beginning of the 20th century.[8] Separately, these two individuals pioneered the vascular anastomosis; Exner using techniques with Erwin Payr's magnesium tubes and Carrel using segments of vein. Carrel and Charles Guthrie developed the model of the arterial anastomosis in dogs at the Hull Physiological Laboratory in Chicago.[9] In 1912, Carrel was awarded the Nobel prize in Physiology and Medicine in 'recognition of his work on vascular

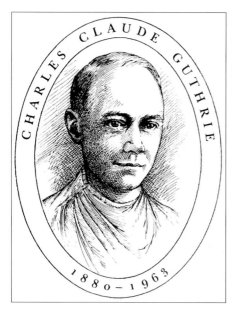

Figure 1.2
Charles C Guthrie,
as illustrated in the
official logo of the
Midwestern Vascular
Surgical Society.
(Reproduced with
permission from
Pfeifer JR, et al.[10])

suture and the transplantation of blood vessels and organs'. Guthrie, who was born in Missouri, returned to Washington University in St Louis as Professor. He eventually joined the faculty at the University of Pittsburgh as the Chair of Physiology and Pharmacology. A likeness of Guthrie was designated as the logo for the Midwestern Vascular Surgical Society during its first annual meeting at the Drake Hotel in Chicago in 1977 (**Fig. 1.2**).[10] The first use of a venous autograft in the human arterial circulation was performed by the Spanish surgeon José Goyanes in 1906, following resection of a syphilitic popliteal aneurysm. One year later, a German surgeon, Erich Lexer, used a reversed greater saphenous vein as an interposition graft in the axillary position of the arm.[8]

The modern technique of venous grafting fell out of favor following these initial reports until revived by Jean Kunlin with dramatic success in 1948 in Paris. One of Kunlin's first patients was initially under the care of his close associate René Leriche. The patient had persistent ischemic gangrene following symphathectomy and femoral arteriectomy. Kunlin performed a greater saphenous vein bypass from the femoral to the popliteal artery in his patient, employing end-to-side anastomotic techniques at the proximal and distal aspects of the bypass. The concept of end-to-side anastomosis was important as it allowed for preservation of side branches, and in 1951, Kunlin reported his results of 17 such bypass operations.[11] In 1955, Robert Linton, from the Massachusetts General Hospital, popularized use of the reversed greater saphenous as a bypass conduit in the leg, when he reported his experience in *Surgery*.[12]

Heparin was first discovered in 1916 by Jay Maclean and reported in 1918.[13] However, heparin remained too toxic for clinical use until Best and Scott reported the purification of heparin in 1933.[14] Four years later, in 1937, Murray demonstrated that heparin could prevent thrombosis in venous bypass grafts and reported its use in the *Annals of Surgery*.[15] Murray and Best noted that the use of this novel anticoagulant was important not only during repair of blood vessels but also in the treatment of venous thrombosis.[15,16] The availability of heparin emboldened surgeons to attempt vascular reconstructions that had previously been occasioned by high rates of thrombosis.

AORTIC THROMBOENDARTERECTOMY

Attempts at thromboendarterectomy were first described by Severeanu, Jianu, and Delbet in the early 1900s. These were prior to the discovery of heparin and generally resulted in failure due to early thrombosis.[8] Subsequently, the technique was abandoned until the mid-1940s when John Cid Dos Santos performed the first successful thromboendarterectomy of the aortoiliac segment using an ophthalmic spatula and a gallstone scoop.[8] Edwin J Wylie in San Francisco and others soon took up and perfected the technique of aortic thromboendarterectomy in the USA.[17,18] Wylie and colleagues developed and extended endarterectomy techniques to the great vessels, mesenteric arteries, and the renal arteries as well as the aorta. The technique of thromboendarterectomy was also used briefly for the management of some abdominal aortic aneurysms, as described by Wylie, who reported the use of fascia lata to wrap an aneurysmal aorta following thromboendarterectomy and tailoring of the vessel.[19] The techniques of transaortic renal endarterectomy pioneered by Wylie, Stoney, and Erhenfeld are still the most commonly employed reconstructive techniques of these vessels at the University of California, San Francisco, the Mayo Clinic in Rochester, and Wake Forest University.

DEVELOPMENT OF AORTIC PROSTHESES

Successful operations for aortic coarctation in the 1940s by Clarence Crafoord in Sweden and Robert Gross in the USA stimulated interest in arterial homografts that might be used in instances where primary aortic repair could not be accomplished.[20,21] In 1948, Gross and colleagues reported the use of preserved arterial grafts in humans with cyanotic heart disease and aortic coarctation.[22] Initial successes with arterial homografts in pediatric and cardiac surgery led to their use in the operative treatment of aortoiliac occlusive disease and aortic aneurysms. Jacques Oudot in 1950 replaced a thrombosed aortic bifurcation with an arterial homograft, and 1 year later, another French vascular surgeon, Charles Dubost (**Fig. 1.3**), did the same

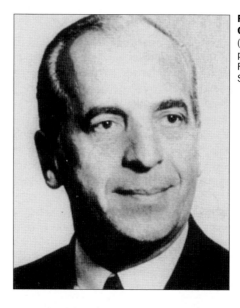

Figure 1.3
Charles Dubost.
(Reproduced with
permission from
Friedman SG. J Vasc
Surg 2001;33:895–8.)

following resection of an abdominal aortic aneurysm.[23,24] Arterial homografts seemed initially to be an efficacious substitute for the thoracic and abdominal aorta. At first, fresh grafts were used; then, Tyrode's solution, a preservative, was used to preserve grafts for short periods of time.[22] Development of the techniques of freezing then lyophilization allowed for the establishment of artery banks.[25,26] Despite early successes, arterial homografts did not provide a durable bypass conduit for the aorta and a satisfactory aortic substitute was still lacking.

The eventual development of synthetic grafts propelled aortic surgery to its present day maturity. As a surgical research fellow at Columbia University under the mentorship of Arthur Blakemore, Arthur Voorhees made a fortuitous observation in 1947. Voorhees recognized that a silk suture inadvertently placed in the ventricle of the dog became 'coated in endocardium' after a period of time *in vivo*. His observation caused him to speculate that a 'cloth tube acting as a lattice work of threads might indeed serve as an arterial prosthesis'.[8]

In 1948, during an assignment to Brooke Army Medical Center in San Antonio, Voorhees fashioned synthetic grafts from parachute material and placed them in the aortic position of the dog. Although few of the initial prostheses lasted for more than a week, Voorhees remained optimistic and returned to Columbia in 1950 to resume his surgical residency. Alfred Jaretzki joined Voorhees and Blakemore in 1951 and their collaboration resulted in a report in the *Annals of Surgery* in 1952 of cloth prostheses in the animal aortic position.[8,27] Having established the efficacy of such in the animal model, the group reported in 1954 the use of vinyon-N cloth tubes used to replace the abdominal aorta in 17 patients with abdominal aortic aneurysms.[8,28] Unfortunately, the early synthetic fabrics available were subject to degenerative problems as well as failure to be incorporated.

Michael DeBakey's (**Fig. 1.4**) introduction of knitted Dacron in 1957 allowed widespread application of the prosthetic graft replacement technique for large and medium-sized arteries, and modern conventional aortic surgery began in earnest.[29] Modifications of the knitted Dacron graft were provided initially by Cooley and Savauge and later by others, which improved the original knitted Dacron that DeBakey provided.[30]

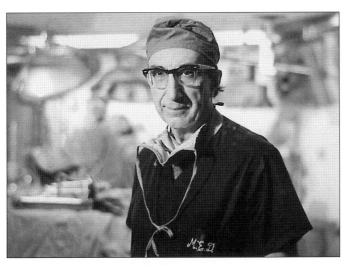

Figure 1.4 Michael E DeBakey, MD. (Reproduced with permission from McCollum CH. J Vasc Surg 2000;31:406–9.)

THORACOABDOMINAL AORTIC ANEURYSMS

Samuel N Etheredge performed the first successful repair of a thoracoabdominal aortic aneurysm in 1954.[31] Etheredge used a plastic tube or shunt, first proposed by Schaffer in 1951, to maintain distal aortic perfusion as he moved the clamp down the graft after each successive visceral anastomosis had been completed. DeBakey and colleagues used modifications of Etheredge's technique and extended the use of graft replacement and bypass to visceral arteries in patients with thoracoabdominal aortic aneurysms. In 1956, DeBakey, Creech, and Morris reported a series of complicated thoracoabdominal aneurysm repairs involving the renal and mesenteric arteries.[32]

In the late 1960s and early 1970s, Edwin J Wylie and Ronald J Stoney in San Francisco popularized the long spiral thoracoabdominal incision for the approach of thoracoabdominal aortic aneurysms and presented their results at the Annual Meeting of the Pacific Coast Surgical Association in 1973.[33] In his discussion of Wylie and Stoney's paper, Etheredge made reference to the polyethylene bypass tube that he had used as a shunt during his original aneurysm resection. Etheredge noted that he had 'fashioned the tube over his gas kitchen stove with a spoon for shaping'. Also during the discussion Etheredge showed pictures of the original thoracoabdominal aortic aneurysm repair, including a picture of the patient 18 years after operation.[33]

Extending the work of Matas and Carrel, DeBakey's younger partner, E Stanley Crawford, provided the greatest advancement in the operative management of thoracoabdominal aortic aneurysms. Crawford introduced a direct approach to the aneurysm, where the aorta was clamped above and below the aneurysm and then opened longitudinally throughout the aneurysm's length.[34,35] A fabric graft was then sewn into the lumen of the proximal and distal aorta into non-aneurysmal artery. Inclusion of major groups of intercostal or visceral vessels were then sewn into the wall of the fabric graft using modifications of Carrell's patch method of anastomosis, sometimes referred to as a 'Crawford window'.[34,35] Currently, combinations of the separate graft replacement technique and the inclusion technique are used and provide better results for repair of thoracoabdominal aortic aneurysms than thought possible even 10–15 years ago. The ability to handle aortic dissections operatively was first reported by DeBakey with primary resection as well as fenestration. Grafting has largely supplanted these other techniques, but fenestration, both operative and endovascular, is still of great utility in treating some of these patients.

MESENTERIC OCCLUSIVE DISEASE

Chronic mesenteric ischemia was first recognized by Dunphy in 1936. He reviewed autopsy results of patients dying of gut infarction and documented that most patients had the prodrome of abdominal pain and weight loss associated with this syndrome.[36] RS Shaw and EP Maynard, III, from the Massachusetts General Hospital, first reported, in 1958, thromboendarterectomy of the paravisceral aorta and superior mesenteric artery for treatment of chronic intestinal ischemia.[37] Following this report, Morris, Crawford, Cooley, and DeBakey described the use of a retrograde aortomesenteric bypass using knitted Dacron in the treatment of chronic mesenteric ischemia.[38] Although this technique avoided exposure of the mid-aorta, it was associated with tortuosity and kinking of the retrograde grafts.

The early experience with retrograde grafts and the problem with tortuosity led Wylie and Stoney to develop other techniques to establish visceral flow.[39,40] Wylie's technique evolved from experience doing renal endarterectomy and was facilitated by the thoracoretroperitoneal approach that he had championed for the exposure of thoracoabdominal aortic aneurysms.[39,40] Trans-aortic endarterectomy was accomplished through a trap-door aortotomy and eversion endarterectomy of the mesenteric vessels. This technique is now applied transabdominally after medial visceral rotation to avoid the morbidity of the thoraco-abdominal incision.

CAROTID ARTERIAL RECONSTRUCTION

The prevailing thought at the turn of the 20th century was that the major cause of stroke was intracranial vascular disease. A neurologist, Ramsay Hunt, was one of the first to assert that the extracranial carotid circulation was a potential source of cerebral infarcts. In an address to the American Neurological Association in 1913, he recommended the routine examination of the carotid arteries in patients with cerebral symptoms.[41] Egas Moniz described the first cerebral arteriography in 1927, originally as a technique to diagnose cerebral tumors.[8] In 1950, a neurologist from the Massachusetts General Hospital, Miller Fisher, reported the results of postmortem examinations of the brains of patients who had died from cerebral vascular occlusive disease. In his observations, Fisher found that a minority of strokes were caused by primary hemorrhagic disease and he concluded that the majority of strokes were in fact caused by embolic disease.[42,43]

Three years after Fisher proclaimed that 'it is conceivable that some day vascular surgery will find a way to bypass the occluded portion of the artery', DeBakey performed the first carotid endarterectomy in the USA. He performed a thromboendarter-ectomy on the patient – a 53-year-old man with a symptomatic carotid stenosis – closed the artery primarily, and confirmed patency with an intraoperative arteriogram.[44] Nine months later, Eascott, Pickering, and Rob (**Fig. 1.5**) successfully treated a patient with a symptomatic carotid stenosis by means of a carotid bulb resection and primary end-to-end anastomosis of the internal and common carotid arteries.[45]

A 1961 report by Yates and Hutchinson to the National Research Council of Great Britain further emphasized the importance of extracranial carotid occlusive disease as a cause of stroke.[46] Whisnant, from the Mayo Clinic, further identified the risk of stroke in the presence of transient ischemic attacks and provided additional basis for operation on symptomatic disease of the carotid arteries and great vessels, which was becoming widely accepted.[47] Endarterectomy or 'disobliteration' of not only symptomatic carotid lesions but also lesions of the subclavian and innominate arteries was advanced by investigators such as Thompson in Dallas, Wylie in San Francisco, and Inaharna in Portland. These investigators, as well as others, refined techniques, determined the range of uses, and clarified indications and contraindications. The origins of prophylactic carotid endarter-ectomy for asymptomatic disease, a topic of debate today, can be traced to Jesse Thompson and colleagues in Dallas in the mid-1970s.[48]

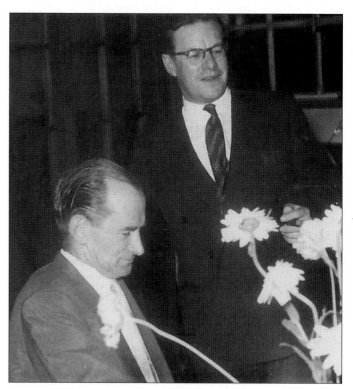

Figure 1.5 Charles Rob and Felix Eascott, 1960. (Reproduced with permission from Rosenthal D. J Vasc Surg 2002;36:430–6.)

MILITARY VASCULAR SURGERY

Hippocrates was credited with the phrase 'He who wishes to be a surgeon should go to war'. This notion remains valid and no history of vascular surgery would be complete without examination of the contributions made by military vascular surgeons. Claudius Galen, regarded as one of the greatest surgeons of antiquity, was known for his treatment of traumatic wounds.[8] As a surgeon to the gladiators in the 2nd century AD, he cared for orthopedic, abdominal, and vascular injuries using sutures, dressings, and splints. The use of cautery was paramount in the treatment of bleeding at the time. It was not until the 16th century that the French physician Ambrose Paré advocated a method other than boiling oil or cautery to control hemorrhage. Paré introduced the concept of ligature for control of bleeding in a battle in which he had exhausted the supply of boiling oil.[49] Ligation of vascular injuries as first documented by Paré would remain the treatment of choice until 1952.

The English Surgeon General during World War I, George Makins, reported a large experience with the treatment of vascular injuries in his paper 'On Gunshot Injuries of the Blood Vessels'.[50] In this report, Makins reviewed over 1000 vascular injuries treated during World War I and described the preferred treatment of such at the time, ligation. It may be that the first attempts at vascular repair in the battlefield were by German surgeons in World War I, specifically a surgeon by the name of Jaeger.[8,51] Reports of successful vascular repairs appeared in the German literature during and following World War I but these were largely ignored and enthusiasm for this concept waned.

Despite improvements in mobile hospitals and surgical units, and the availability of antibiotics and whole blood, World War

II did little to advance the treatment of battlefield vascular injuries beyond the principle of ligation. In their classic review of nearly 2500 cases of arterial wounds treated in the Second World War, DeBakey and Simeone found only 81 instances of suture repair.[52] The amputation rate in this 'highly selective group' of patients with 'minimal wounds' was 36%, as compared with an amputation rate of 49% following ligation. The major obstacle to vascular repair during the Second World War was prolonged evacuation time, which averaged more than 10 hours, practically precluding successful arterial repair and limb salvage.[51,52] Although the concept of bringing the surgeon close to the battlefield was explored, it was considered unworkable to provide definitive operative care of vascular injuries at forward echelons.

To explore the possibility of vascular repair in the wartime setting, a program was initiated at Walter Reed Army Hospital in 1949. The program was designed to study blood vessel reconstruction as well as to assess the effects of ischemia on muscle viability. Soon after the initiation of this program, the Korean Conflict began and Walter Reed was designated the vascular specialty center. Initially, treatment of vascular injuries followed guidelines established in World War II, consisting mainly of ligation. Critical assessment of this practice revealed high rates of arterial and venous insufficiency and amputation. A new policy of vascular reconstruction to restore or maintain perfusion was begun in 1951 under the guidance of Carl Hughes, Edward Janke, and SF Seeley.[8,51] This program represented the first formal deviation from the practice of ligation started by Paré. By using the techniques of direct anastomosis, lateral repair, and interposition graft placement, the initial limb salvage rates were encouraging.[53,54] A contingent of Army Surgical Researchers went to Korea armed with this new information plus perhaps the most important advance in the care of battlefield vascular injuries, the medical evacuation helicopter. Time from injury to surgical care was reduced to 1 or 2 hours in most cases with the use of air evacuation maneuvers. With the arrival of these vascular surgery repair teams, vascular repair was begun in earnest in the Mobile Army Surgical Hospitals (MASH).[51] Subsequently, limb salvage rates associated with battlefield vascular injuries nearly doubled. In his sentinel review of more than 300 major arterial repairs performed during the Korean War, Hughes reported a 13% amputation rate.[55,56]

The lessons learned in Korea were advanced in the Vietnam Conflict. Foremost, the importance of rapid transport of the wounded soldier to surgical care was realized; in one report, 95% of wounded patients reached surgical attention by helicopter.[57] Recognizing the opportunity, Norman Rich and Carl Hughes initiated the Vietnam Vascular Registry in 1966 to document and analyze vascular injuries.[58] In a landmark review of more than 1000 arterial injuries treated during the Vietnam War, Rich and Hughes reported a limb salvage rate of 87%.[59] The Vietnam Vascular Registry also provided important information related to management of venous injuries, missile emboli, and the management of concomitant bony and vascular injuries.[60–62]

EVOLUTION OF ENDOVASCULAR PROCEDURES

A Swedish radiologist, Sven-Ivar Seldinger (1921–1998), described a minimally invasive access technique to the artery in 1953.[63]

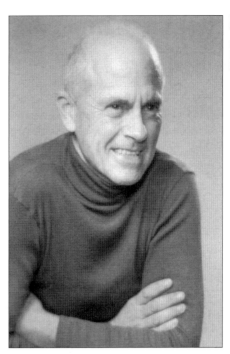

Figure 1.6 Charles Theodore Dotter. (Courtesy of The Dotter Interventional Institute, Portland.)

Seldinger's technique used a catheter passed over a wire that in turn was introduced through the primary arterial puncture site. The wire was advanced to the desired site and then the appropriate catheter was advanced over the wire. Previous to Seldinger's technique, arteriography was limited and performed using a single needle at the puncture site in the artery for the injection of contrast material.

One decade after Seldinger's technique had been described, Thomas Fogarty and colleagues reported the use of the thrombo-embolectomy catheter. That report in 1963, while Fogarty was a surgical resident, detailed the use of a balloon-tipped catheter to extract thrombus and/or embolus from a vessel lumen without having to open the vessel.[64] A year later, Charles Theodore Dotter (**Fig. 1.6**) reported the use of a rigid Teflon dilator passed through a large radiopaque catheter-sheath to perform the first transluminal treatment of diseased arteries.[65] Five years after his original report, Dotter elaborated on a technique for percutaneous transluminal placement of tubes within arteries to relieve obstructed arteries and restore blood flow.[66] Together, the work of Fogarty and Dotter in the early to mid 1960s heralded an evolution from diagnostic to diagnostic *and* therapeutic endovascular procedures.

Silastic balloons were later introduced by a Swiss radiologist, Andreas R Gruntzig. Gruntzig extended the work of Fogarty and Dotter and in 1974 reported that percutaneous transluminal angioplasty with a silastic balloon could be performed in different vascular beds, including coronary, renal, iliac, and femoral.[67] Metallic stents in a variety of designs followed percutaneous balloon angioplasty, beginning with the stent developed by Julio Palmaz in 1985.[68] Arguably the greatest advance in transluminal endovascular interventions came when Juan Parodi performed the first endovascular abdominal aortic aneurysm repair.[69] His repair merged the old and the new by attaching a woven Dacron graft to a Palmaz stent and delivering it through a large-bore sheath placed via surgical exposure of the femoral artery.

CLOSING COMMENT

The management of patients with peripheral vascular disease has evolved such that effective treatments often can be performed not only with minimal morbidity but also with short – and, in many cases, no – hospital stay. We have evolved such that the effectiveness of a procedure or treatment is critically assessed in clinical research studies in thousands of patients and measured by single-digit percentages. The pathophysiology and sometimes-genetic basis of vascular disease is understood so well in some cases that disease processes are managed effectively with non-operative means. The rapidness with which the treatment of peripheral vascular disease has evolved over the past century is remarkable and one can only imagine how the practice of vascular surgery will look during the next 50 years if such great progress continues apace.

REFERENCES

1. Brock RC. The life and work of Sir Astley Cooper. Ann R Coll Surg Engl 1969;44:1–2.
2. Matas R. Traumatic aneurism of the left brachial artery. Med News 1888;53:462.
3. Matas R. Ligation of the abdominal aorta: report of the ultimate result, one year, five months and nine days after ligation of the abdominal aorta for aneurysm of the bifurcation. Ann Surg 1925;81:457.
4. Matas R. Aneurysm of the abdominal aorta at its bifurcation into the common iliac arteries. Ann Surg 1940;112:909.
5. Matas R. Personal experiences in vascular surgery. A statistical synopsis. Ann Surg 1940;112:802.
6. Ernst CB. The Southern Association for Vascular Surgery: the beginning. J Vasc Surg 2001;34:381–3.
7. Matas R. The soul of the surgeon. Tr Miss M Assoc 1915;48:149.
8. Friedman SG. A history of vascular surgery. New York:Futura; 1989.
9. Carrel A, Guthrie CC. Results of biterminal transplantation of veins. Am J Med Sci 1906;132:415.
10. Pfeifer JR, Stanley JC. The Midwestern Vascular Surgical Society: the formative years, 1976 to 1981. J Vasc Surg 2002;35:837–40.
11. Kunlin J. Le traitement de l'ischemie arteritique par la greffe veineuse longeu. Rev Chir 1951;70:206.
12. Linton RR. Some practical considerations in surgery of blood vessels. Surgery 1955;38:817.
13. Howell WH. Two new factors in blood coagulation – heparin and proantithrombin. Am J Physiol 1918;47:328–41.
14. Best CH, Scott C. The purification of heparin. J Biol Chem 1933; 102:425.
15. Murray DWG, Best CH. The use of heparin in thrombosis. Ann Surg 1938;108:163.
16. Murray DWG. Heparin in surgical treatment of blood vessels. Arch Surg 1940;40:307.
17. Wylie EJ. Thromboendarterectomy for atherosclerotic thrombosis of major arteries. Surgery 1952;32:275.
18. Freeman NE, Gilfillan RS. Regional heparinization after thromboendarterectomy in the treatment of obliterative arterial disease: preliminary report based on 12 cases. Surgery 1952; 31:115.
19. Wylie EJ Jr, Kerr E, Davies O. Experimental and clinical experience with the use of fascia lata applied as a graft about major arteries after thromboendarterectomy and aneurysmorrhaphy. Surg Gynecol Obstet 1951;93:257.
20. Crafoord C, Nylin G. Congenital coarctation of the aorta and its surgical treatment. J Thorac Surg 1945;14:347–61.
21. Gross RE. Treatment of certain aortic coarctations by homologous grafts: a report of nineteen cases. Ann Surg 1951;134:753.
22. Gross RE, Hurwitt ES, Bill AH Jr, et al. Preliminary observations on the use of human arterial grafts in the treatment of certain cardiovascular defects. N Engl J Med 1948;239:578–9.
23. Oudot J, Beaconsfield P. Thrombosis of the aortic bifurcation treated by resection and homograft replacement: report of five cases. Arch Surg 1953;66:365–70.
24. Dubost C, Allary M, Oeconomos N. Resection of an aneurysm of the abdominal aorta: re-establishment of the continuity by a preserved human arterial graft, with results after five months. Arch Surg 1952;64:405–8.
25. Deterling RA Jr, Coleman CC, Parshley MS. Experimental studies on the frozen homologous aortic graft. Surgery 1951;29:419.
26. Marangoni AG, Cecchini LP. Homotransplantation of arterial segments by the freeze-drying method. Ann Surg 1951;134:977.
27. Voorhees AB Jr, Jaretzki A III, Blakemore AH. Use of tubes constructed from Vinyon-N cloth bridging arterial defects. Ann Surg 1952;135:332.
28. Blakemore A, Voorhees AB Jr. The use of tubes constructed from Vinyon-N cloth in bridging arterial defects: experimental and clinical. Ann Surg 1954;140:324–34.
29. DeBakey ME, Cooley DA, Crawford ES, Morris GC Jr. Clinical application of a new flexible knitted Dacron arterial substitute. Arch Surg 1958;77:713.
30. Sauvage G, Berger KE, Wood SJ, et al. An external velour surface for porous arterial prosthesis. Surgery 1971;70:940–53.
31. Etheredge SN, Yee JY, Smith JV, et al. Successful resection of a large aneurysm of the upper abdominal aorta and replacement with homograft. Surgery 1955;38:1071.
32. DeBakey ME, Creech O, Morris GC. Aneurysm of the thoracoabdominal aorta involving the celiac, mesenteric and renal arteries. Report of four cases treated by resection and homograft replacement. Ann Surg 1956; 144:549–73.
33. Stoney RJ, Wylie EJ. Surgical management of arterial lesions of the thoracoabdominal aorta. Am J Surg 1973;126:157–64.
34. DeBakey ME, Crawford ES, Garrett HE, Beall AC, Howell JF. Surgical considerations in the treatment of aneurysms of the thoracoabdominal aorta. Ann Surg 1965;162:350–62.
35. Crawford ES. Thoraco-abdominal aortic aneurysms involving renal, superior mesenteric and celiac arteries. Ann Surg 1974;179:763–72.
36. Dunphy JE. Abdominal pains of vascular origins. Am J Med Sci 1936;192:109.
37. Shaw RS, Maynard EP. Acute and chronic thrombosis of the mesenteric arteries associated with malabsorption. N Engl J Med 1958;258:874.
38. Morris GC, Crawford ES, Cooley DA, DeBakey MA. Revascularization of the celiac and superior mesenteric arteries. Arch Surg 1962;84:95–107.
39. Stoney RJ, Wylie EJ. Surgical management of arterial lesions of the thoracoabdominal aorta. Am J Surg 1973;126:157–63.
40. Stoney RJ, Ehrenfeld WK, Wylie EJ. Revascularization methods in chronic visceral ischemia. Ann Surg 1977;186:468–76.
41. Hunt JR. The role of the carotid arteries in the causation of vascular lesions of the brain with remarks on certain special features of the symptomatology. Am J Med Sci 1914;147:704–13.
42. Fisher M. Occlusion of the internal carotid artery. Arch Neurol Psychiat 1951;65:346–77.
43. Fisher M, Adams RD. Observation on brain embolism with special reference to the mechanism of hemorrhagic infarction. J Neuropath Exp Neurol 1951;10:92.
44. DeBakey ME. Successful carotid endarterectomy for cerebral vascular insufficiency: nineteen year follow up. JAMA 1975;233:1083–5.
45. Eascott HHG, Pickering GW, Rob C. Reconstruction of internal carotid artery in a patient with intermittent attacks of hemiplegia. Lancet 1954;2:994–6.
46. Yates PO, Hutchinson EC. Cerebral infarction: the role of stenosis of the extracranial arteries. Med Res Council Spec Report (London) 1961;300:1.
47. Whisnant JP, Matsumoto N, Elveback LR. Transient cerebral ischemic attacks in a community: Rochester, Minnesota, 1955 through 1969. Mayo Clin Proc 1973;48:194–8.

48. Thompson JE, Patman RD, Talkington CM. Asymptomatic carotid bruit. Ann Surg 1978;188:308–16.
49. Wangensteen WO, Wangensteen SD, Klinger CF. Wound management of Ambrose Paré and Dominique Larrey, great French military surgeons of the 16th and 19th centuries. Bull Hist Med 1972;46:207.
50. Makins GH. On gunshot injuries to the blood vessels. Bristol:John Wright & Sons; 1919.
51. Rich NM, Rhee P. An historical tour of vascular injury management: from its inception to the new millennium. Surg Clin North Am 2001; 81:1199–215.
52. DeBakey ME, Simeone FA. Battle injuries of arteries in World War II. An analysis of 2471 cases. Ann Surg 1946;123:534–79.
53. Jahnke EJ, Seeley SF. Acute vascular injuries in the Korean War: an analysis of 77 consecutive cases. Ann Surg 1953;138:158.
54. Hughes CW. The primary repair of wounds of major arteries. Ann Surg 1955;141:297.
55. Hughes CW. Arterial repair during the Korean War. Ann Surg 1958; 147:155.
56. Jahnke EJ. Late structural and functional results of arterial injuries primarily repaired. Surgery 1958;43:175.
57. Rich NM. Vietnam missile wound evacuation in 750 patients. Mil Med 1968;133:9.
58. Rich NM, Hughes CW. Vietnam vascular registry: a preliminary report. Surgery 1969;65:218.
59. Rich NM, Baugh JH, Hughes CW. Acute arterial injuries in Vietnam: 1000 cases. J Trauma 1970;10:359–69.
60. Rich NM, Hughes CW, Baugh JH. Management of venous injuries. Ann Surg 1970;171:724–30.
61. Rich NM. Vascular trauma. Surg Clin North Am 1973;53:1367–92.
62. Rich NM, Collins GJ Jr, Anderson CA, et al. Missile emboli. J Trauma 1978;18:236–9.
63. Seldinger S. Catheter placement of the needle in percutaneous arteriography, a new technique. Acta Radiol 1953;39:368.
64. Fogarty T, Cranley J, Krause R, et al. A method for extraction of arterial emboli and thrombi. Surg Gynecol Obstet 1963;116:241.
65. Dotter CT, Judkins MP. Transluminal treatment of arteriosclerotic obstruction. Circulation 1964;30:654–70.
66. Dotter CT. Transluminally-placed coilspring endarterial tube grafts: long-term patency in canine popliteal artery. Invest Radiol 1969;4:329–32.
67. Gruntzig A, Hopff H. Perkutane rekanalisation chronischer arterieller verschlusse mit einem neuen dilatationskatheter. Modifikation der Dotter-technik. Dtsch Med Wochenschr 1974;99:2502–10.
68. Palmaz J, Sibbitt R, Reuter S, et al. Expandable intraluminal graft: a preliminary study. Radiology 1985;156:72–7.
69. Parodi JC, Palmaz JC, Barone HD. Transfemoral intraluminal graft implantation for abdominal aortic aneurysms. Ann Vasc Surg 1991; 5:491–9.

CHAPTER
2

Vascular Biology

Janet Powell

KEY POINTS

- Endovascular and vascular surgeons are largely concerned with correction of degenerative vascular disease, explained by the abnormal biology (or pathology) of blood vessels.

- Biologic responses of blood vessels to vascular and endovascular procedures limit the long-term success of surgical intervention.

- Understanding vascular biology may lead to new medical and interventional techniques being developed.

- Nitric oxide is one of the pivotal molecules coordinating vascular function.

- The vessel wall responds to injury with atherosclerosis and intimal hyperplasia, often exacerbated by blood elements.

- The vessel wall remodels in response to hemodynamic changes.

- Monogenic vascular disorders are uncommon, but provide valuable insight into mechanisms of vascular disease.

- Growth factors, together with extracellular matrix cues, regulate the growth of new blood vessels. Growth factors can be used as adjuncts for revascularization and recovery of tissue loss.

Many of the contemporary challenges faced by vascular and endovascular surgeons have their basis in vascular pathology, or abnormal vascular biology. The success of endovascular aneurysm repair depends, in part, on the absence of endoleak through lumbar and other vessels and arresting the process of aortic dilatation at the aneurysm neck. The success of peripheral bypass surgery depends on the limitation of anastomotic hyperplasia and controlling the progression of atherosclerosis in inflow and outflow vessels. Intimal hyperplasia with recurrent stenosis is a common consequence of femoral angioplasty. In other cases, tissue loss and absence of vessels for reconstruction lead to amputation being the treatment offered. Advances in vascular biology can be harnessed by vascular and endovascular specialists to improve the results of their intervention.

RESPONSE OF THE VESSEL WALL TO INJURY: THE ROLE OF NITRIC OXIDE

The classic theory of atherosclerosis as an arterial response to injury was enunciated by Russell Ross.[1,2] The endothelium is the guardian of the vessel wall, providing an antithrombotic non-sticky surface for blood flow, synthesizing molecules that regulate vessel tone and diameter, and allowing nutrients to pass from the blood to the underlying smooth muscle. The endothelium can be damaged by physical forces or blood components, the combination of the two leading to the development of atherosclerosis in large arteries. The endothelium is fragile: even the most careful dissection of the saphenous vein for bypass grafting will cause some damage to the endothelium. In the arterial circulation, smoking metabolites, oxidants, and oxidized lipids are probably the most common chemicals that damage the endothelium. All of these chemicals cause alterations in the endothelial surface, activating the endothelium to facilitate leukocyte and platelet adhesion, and damage the metabolism of endothelium, with reduction of nitric oxide (NO) synthesis.

Nitric oxide (previously known as endothelium-derived relaxing factor) is one of the pivotal molecules coordinating vascular function.[3] This molecule is very chemically reactive and it has a short biologic half-life, with an intravascular half-life of about 2ms and an extravascular half-life of less than 2s. Therefore, it is not surprising that it took several years to identify the substance, produced by endothelium, that caused the relaxation of blood vessels. Increased blood flow and many agonists that bind to endothelial cell receptors lead to an influx of calcium into the endothelium, which results in increased production of NO. Secretion of NO into the vessel lumen results in reduction of the adhesive properties of platelets and leukocytes. Increased levels of NO within endothelial cells dampens metabolic pathways leading to endothelial cell activation. Secretion of NO into the smooth muscle cells of the media causes vasorelaxation (via the interaction of NO with the enzyme guanylate cyclase). These coordinating and protective roles of NO are shown in **Figure 2.1**.

Nitric oxide is synthesized from L-arginine and molecular oxygen by the enzyme nitric oxide synthase. To effect this complex chemistry, the enzyme depends on several cofactors, including tetrahydrobiopterin. Smoking appears to impair the synthesis and/or bioavailability of tetrahydrobiopterin. Not surprisingly, endothelium-dependent relaxation and endothelial NO synthesis are impaired in smokers. This effect of smoking is observed even in healthy young persons (20–30 years old), with endothelium-dependent relaxation of the femoral artery being almost absent. Such altered vasoreactivity is probably the earliest sign of vascular dysfunction.

Physical or chemical injury to the endothelium facilitates the adhesion of platelets, leukocytes, and monocytes to the vessel wall. The adherent monocytes secrete enzymes and growth factors, which facilitate their migration into the vessel wall, with damage to the subendothelium. Once resident in the endothelium, these cells (macrophages) alter their phenotype, a process accelerated by oxidant stress. The expression of specific

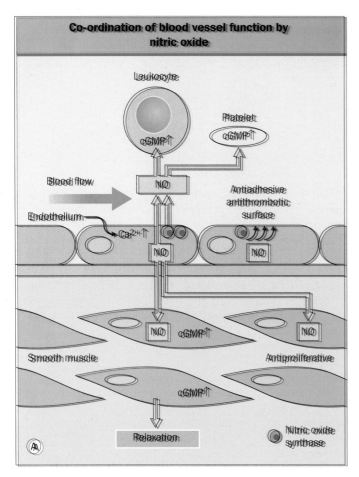

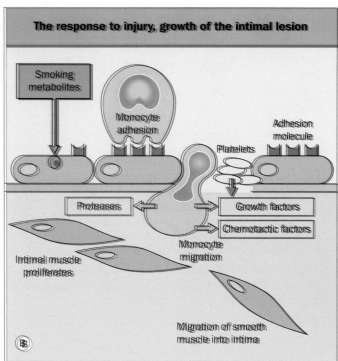

Figure 2.1 The coordinating and protective roles of nitric oxide. (A) Coordination of blood vessel function by nitric oxide. (B) The response to injury, growth of the intimal lesion.

cell surface receptors permits the uptake of oxidized lipids and cholesterol, particularly oxidized low-density lipoproteins. The altered pattern of gene expression of growth factors, chemoattractants, and proteases causes the proliferation and migration of underlying smooth muscle cells into the intima. The stage is set for the development of intimal pathology: atherosclerosis and intimal hyperplasia (Fig. 2.1). Blood-borne factors such as fibrinogen and homocysteine accelerate such processes.

VESSEL REMODELING: HEMODYNAMIC STRESS

Hemodynamic stress has critical effects on the biology of the cells in blood vessels. The normal hemodynamic stress is related to blood flow and how this flow and components of the blood interact with the vascular endothelium. Abnormal hemodynamic stresses occur during angioplasty, in the fashioning of vein grafts and other endovascular and vascular interventions. The hemodynamic forces can be resolved into two principal forces: shear stress and pressure. Shear stress is the frictional force acting at the interface between the circulating blood and the endothelium of the vessel wall. Pressure which acts perpendicular to the vessel wall also imposes circumferential deformation on blood vessels. Therefore, it becomes convenient to address the vascular biology of hemodynamic forces in two parts: the effect of shear stress, where the endothelial monolayer transduces mechanical signals into biologic responses, and circumferential stretch and deformation, which impose different, usually pathologic, biologic responses.

Within the vascular tree, there are gradients of shear stress that typically occur near vessel bifurcations and branches, in regions of arterial narrowing and in areas of extreme curvature such as in the carotid bulb. The regions of disturbed blood flow correlate well with the distribution of atherosclerotic lesions. The carotid bulb provides a good example, where the medial wall experiences high shear stress with the lateral wall experiencing recirculation vortexes that vary with the cardiac cycle, resulting in flow reversal and low mean shear stress: the lateral wall usually has more extensive atherosclerotic lesions. These different types of blood flow have important effects on the biology of the endothelium. Steady laminar blood flow tends to have effects that are antithrombotic, anti-adhesive, and growth inhibitory to the underlying smooth muscle cells, activated through the release of NO and other mechanisms. In contrast, in situations of flow reversal, changes in the endothelium promote thrombosis and the recruitment and adhesion of monocytes. Clearly, this mechanotransduction at the endothelial surface underpins the focal development of atherosclerosis.

The mechanosensors on the endothelium that sense changes in blood flow and shear stress are poorly defined at the molecular level, but at the cellular level a timescale of cell-signaling pathways has been carefully described. One of the important molecules involved in the regulation of blood vessels in response to altered flow is NO, and reactive hyperemia on release of a tourniquet provides an elegant physiologic example of this phenomenon. After release of a limb tourniquet, there is a sudden increase in blood flow. This stimulates both the synthesis and release of NO and causes the dilatation of

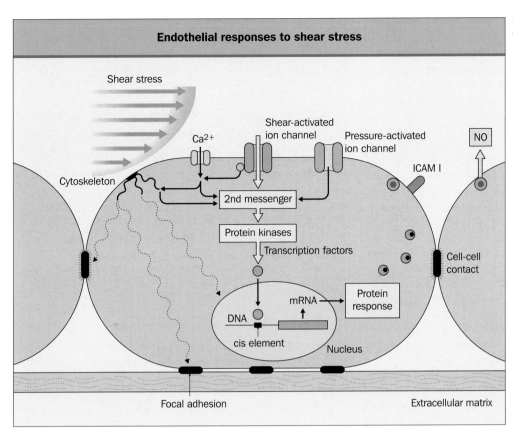

Figure 2.2 **Endothelial responses to shear stress.**

numerous blood vessels, resulting in the hyperemia of the limb. The endothelium responds to sudden increases in shear stress within milliseconds, with changes in membrane potential and an increase in intracellular calcium concentration, probably achieved through calcium influx. These changes in intracellular calcium concentration drive changes in potassium channel activation, the generation of inositol triphosphate and diacylglycerol, and changes in G-protein activation, to inform the cell-signaling cascades within the endothelial cells. These signaling cascades within the endothelial cell are activated within a period of several minutes up to one hour and include activation of the mitogen-activated protein kinase (MAP kinase) signaling cascade and the trans-location of the transcription factor NFκB from the cytosol into the nucleus.[4] These changes are shown in **Figure 2.2**. There are also changes within the cytoskeleton of the cell and the cell membrane, both of which are likely to facilitate the release of NO and other vasodilators, including prostacyclin. These imme-diate changes in response to dramatic changes in shear stress are followed within a few hours by changes in the regulation of a subset of genes comprising up to 3% of the repertoire of expressed genes within the endothelium.[5] Specific examples include the increased synthesis of nitric oxide synthase and tissue plasminogen activator, intercellular adhesion molecule-1, monocyte chemoattractant protein-1, and platelet-derived growth factor (PDGF)-B. Some of these genes have a particular consensus of nucleotides in the 5′ (promoter) region of the gene, which is known as the shear stress responsive element. Mutation of this limited cassette of bases can result in the loss of sensitivity of gene expression in response to shear stress. Genes may be downregulated as well as upregulated. The genes which are downregulated in response to increased shear stress include

thrombomodulin and the vasoconstrictor endothelin-1. Later, within a timeframe of several hours, there are further changes to the cytoskeleton and focal adhesion sites, so that the cells become aligned or more aligned to blood flow.

The totality of these changes impact upon the anticoagulant and anti-adhesive nature of the endothelial cell surface. While these changes may explain much of the pathology observed by the vascular surgeon, it is also these same responses of the endothelium to shear stress that in part control the adaptation of a vein graft to arterial flow. However, for the vein graft, one has to consider not only the primary hemodynamic force of shear stress but also circumferential deformation.[6] Some of the changes observed in vein grafts or dialysis fistulae, particularly some of the proadhesive changes, might occur more rapidly in response to changes in pressure and circumferential deformation, rather than changes in shear stress. These changes in pressure or circumferential deformation also control the cytoskeletal biology of the underlying smooth muscle cell. Permeability changes resulting from pressure are thought to permit an increased exposure to oxygen radicals such as superoxide. The oxidation of lipids results in changes of smooth muscle cell gene expression, with increased secretion of the growth factors and proteases that predispose to intimal hyperplasia (the migration of proliferative smooth muscle cells into the intima).

These changes, too, are likely to be influenced by early changes in cellular calcium concentration and the activity of cation channels in the cell membrane. The earliest responses that have been observed include: increases in the C-fos gene, an increase of apoptopic markers, and changes in the expression of genes associated with the reorganization of actin filaments. These changes have been much more difficult to elucidate than the changes in the endothelium, since, for endothelium, one has had access to numerous experiments using cultured endothelial cells, which retain a phenotype similar to that of the native endothelium. In contrast, in culture, smooth muscle cells rapidly lose the contractile phenotype they have in the arterial wall and acquire the synthetic phenotype of the smooth muscle cells observed in intimal lesions.

Because much of the pathology of vein grafts has been associated with abnormal smooth muscle cell proliferation and the elaboration of a dense extracellular matrix, there has been considerable focus on how pressure or circumferential deformation alters the replicative activity of the smooth muscle cell. Most of this work has explored how the pressure of angioplasty alters the replicative activity of the smooth muscle cell, in experimental models. However, there seems to be a wide gap between the response of the normal vessel in an experimental model to pressure, and the response of the atherosclerotic artery to pressure at angioplasty, and the biology of this pressure response in diseased vascular tissue remains largely uncharted. Although the response in humans is largely unexplored, it has not prevented the advent of gene-based therapies, developed in animals, to try to prevent intimal hyperplasia by targeting elements of the cell replicative machinery.

The PREVENT Trial[7] has explored the possibility of cell cycle blockade by the ex-vivo gene therapy of vein grafts being prepared for implantation into patients with peripheral limb ischemia. This used the pivotal cell cycle transcription factor E2F to repress smooth muscle replication. The response of vascular smooth muscle cells to pressure and circumferential deformation remains an important and largely uncharted area of vascular biology research.

GENETIC INSIGHTS INTO ANEURYSMAL DISEASE: MATRIX AND METALLOPROTEINASES

There are at least two rare monogenic disorders associated with the development of aortic and/or arterial aneurysms before the onset of 'middle age'. In both Marfan syndrome and Ehlers–Danlos syndrome type IV, there are deletions and/or mutations in genes encoding the extracellular matrix proteins essential for coordinating cellular metabolism and directly contributing to the mechanical and elastic properties of arteries. The Marfan gene is fibrillin, a key component of microfibrils forming the elastic scaffold, while the Ehlers–Danlos type IV gene is type III collagen. Mutations in these genes are not associated with the common form of 'atherosclerotic' abdominal aortic aneurysm (AAA), which has a prevalence of about 5% in men over 60 years of age. However, many AAAs are found in familial clusters, and 20–30% of the brothers of patients with AAA also will develop an AAA. This has directed attention at the genes of other major extracellular matrix components in aorta, including elastin and type I collagen. Interestingly, elastin gene mutations give rise to a rare form of stenosing arterial disease, supravalvular aortic stenosis, rather than aneurysms. There is no evidence to link mutations in the type I collagen gene to AAA. Nevertheless, aneurysmal disease is characterized by thinning of the extracellular matrix in the aortic media, with elastin destruction, loss of smooth muscle cells, and a transmural ingress of inflammatory cells (**Fig. 2.3**). This has focused attention on a family

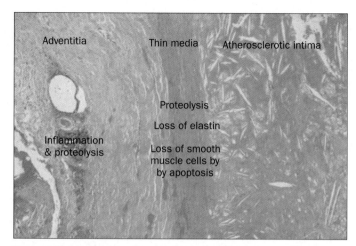

Figure 2.3 Section through an abdominal aortic aneurysm. There are numerous inflammatory cells in the adventitia and some in the media. The media is very thin, with loss of elastic tissue through proteolysis and loss of smooth muscle cells by apoptosis.

of enzymes, the matrix metalloproteinases (MMPs), which have the ability to break down the extracellular matrix of the arterial wall.

Matrix metalloproteinases have their activity regulated at several different levels, including transcription (how much mRNA is produced), activation (proteolytic processing of the inactive form or zymogen produced in cells), and inhibition (principally by tissue inhibitors of MMPs). One of the members of this MMP family, MMP-9, with the ability to degrade elastin, denatured collagen, type IV collagen, fibronectin, and other matrix components, has been specifically linked with AAA disease (**Fig. 2.4**). MMP-9 is an enzyme produced by macrophages and other cells in the aneurysm wall. To investigate the role of this enzyme in aneurysmal disease, Robert Thompson and colleagues have manipulated the genes of mice, producing animals where the MMP-9 gene has been knocked out.[8] The mice mature normally. Mice are not men, do not smoke, and usually do not develop aortic aneurysms: rare blotchy mice with defective genes for lysyloxidase (an enzyme needed to cross-link and stabilize collagen fibers) do develop aortic aneurysms in males. However, normal mice, most other small animals, and excised human arteries will develop aneurysms if a powerful elastin-degrading enzyme (elastase) is infused into the aorta. The degradation of aortic elastin is associated with inflammation, weakening, and dilatation of the aortic wall. Importantly, aneurysms were suppressed after elastase was instilled into the aorta of MMP-9 knockout mice, although inflammation was still evident. Hence, experimental genetics indicate an important role for the degradation of elastin by MMP-9 in the formation of aneurysms.

Knockout mice are being used widely to provide information about the possible involvement of a variety of genes, mainly associated with proteolysis or lipid metabolism, in aneurysm development. The knockout approach can be complemented by the overexpression of genes in mice. Such experiments have indicated an important role for the plasminogen system. Plasmin can activate MMPs and degrade laminin, fibronectin, and other matrix components. The likely cooperation of plasminogen and MMP systems in stimulating experimental aneurysms (**Fig. 2.4**) suggests that proteinases will be important future targets for

Proteases and the formation of experimental aneurysms

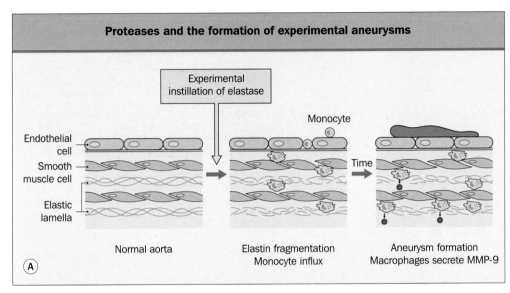

Figure 2.4 Proteases and inflammatory cells in aneurysmal disease. (A) Proteases and the formation of experimental aneurysms. (B) Role of macrophages and other inflammatory cells. MMP-9, matrix metalloproteinase-9; uPA, urokinase-type plasminogen activator 4; PAI-1, plasminogen activator inhibitor-1; TIMP, tissue inhibitor of metalloproteinases.

Role of macrophages and other inflammatory cells

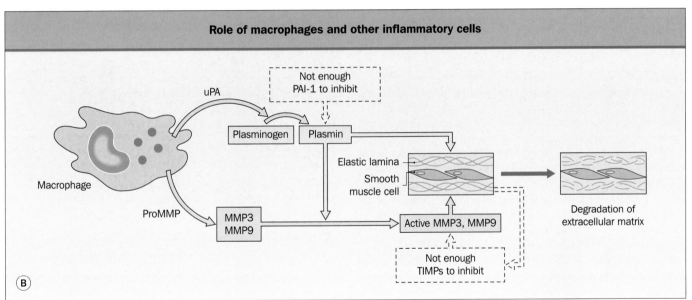

pharmaceutical intervention. Similar proteolytic interactions also may underlie the destruction of stabilizing fibrous caps on atherosclerotic plaques, leading to plaque rupture.

So much for mice: what of men? The amount of MMP-9 that is synthesized by a cell depends on the binding of regulatory transcription factors to the 5′-non-coding sequence (promoter) of the gene (**Fig. 2.4**). A single nucleotide polymorphism 1562 bases away from the start of the MMP-9 gene (–1562 C>T) influences the rate of MMP-9 mRNA transcription.[9] This is known as a functional polymorphism and can be used to gain insight into mechanisms of disease. The functionality of promoter polymorphisms usually are investigated in cultured cells, using hybrid gene constructs where the MMP-9 gene promoter is linked to a gene that is easy to measure, such as firefly luciferase. Such approaches show that the –1562T allele supports a 30% increase in luciferase activity compared with the –1562C allele. This difference is likely to result from the fact that the –1567 to –1559 region supports the binding of a transcription factor (**Fig. 2.5**). These are laboratory bench experiments: what

happens at the bedside? Patients with the –1562T allele appear to be more likely to have severe coronary artery atherosclerosis.[9] A separate length polymorphism of the MMP-9 gene also has been shown to have functional effects on MMP-9 transcription and has been linked to intracranial aneurysms.[10] The investigation of functional polymorphisms is likely to be one of the most useful approaches to complex genetic traits such as AAA.

CREATING BLOOD VESSELS: GROWTH FACTORS

New blood vessels can develop by sprouting of existing vessels, in response to growth factor stimuli or through maturation of bone-marrow-derived endothelial cell progenitors (angioblasts). In addition, growth factors facilitate the development of arteries from arterioles, a novel approach for the treatment of critical coronary or limb ischemia. These three forms of vessel growth are known as angiogenesis, vasculogenesis, and arteriogenesis.[11] A variety of growth factors (and cytokines) coordinate the

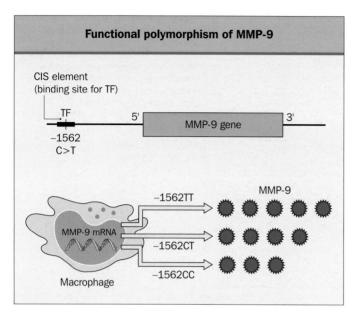

Figure 2.5 Functional polymorphism of matrix metalloproteinase-9 (MMP-9). The –1562T allele is associated with increased MMP-9 production. TF, transcription factor.

Process		Example factors involved
Angiogenesis	New capillaries	VEGF, bFGF, PDGF
Vasculogenesis	Primary plexus	VEGF, GM-CSF
Arteriogenesis	Arterioles → collateral arteries	MCP-1, TGF-β, GM-CSF

Table 2.1 Growth factors, chemokines and new blood vessels. VEGF, vascular endothelial growth factor; bFGF, basic fibroblast growth factor; PDGF, platelet-derived growth factor; GM-CSF, granulocyte–monocyte colony-stimulating factor; TGF-β, transforming growth factor β; MCP-1, monocyte chemoattractant protein-1.

reprogramming of endothelial cells, mesenchymal cells, and monocytes associated with new vessel formation (**Table 2.1**).

Growth factors interact with specific cell surface receptors. Binding of the growth factor to the receptor results in changes in the shape and/or phosphorylation of the receptor tail on the inside of the cell. This in turn leads to the recruitment of a variety of adaptor proteins or a sequence of enzyme phosphorylations. Both processes eventually lead to the altered transcription of the cellular genes, permitting the cell to migrate, proliferate, or change its phenotype. Cues from fibrin or the extracellular matrix often are necessary to facilitate these processes (**Fig. 2.6**).

Both angiogenesis and arteriogenesis have been manipulated using growth factors in human studies. The idea that bone-marrow-derived stem cells contribute to vessel development in adults is a much newer concept. Vascular endothelial growth factor (VEGF; protein and DNA encoding VEGF) has been used to promote capillary development in critical limb ischemia, with mixed results.[12] A single bolus of basic fibroblast growth factor at coronary angioplasty did not alter exercise duration during follow-up. However, granulocyte–macrophage colony-stimulating factor appears to promote collateral growth in patients with coronary artery disease. These studies are in their infancy, but application of growth factor biology promises new treatments for critical limb ischemia.

One of the growth factors involved in angiogenesis, PDGF, stimulates the proliferation of smooth cells and fibroblasts. With this latter effect on fibroblasts, it is not surprising that topical PDGF is reported to facilitate the healing of diabetic foot ulcers.[13] There is enormous potential for the therapeutic use of growth factors in a vascular surgical practice.

In conclusion, this chapter has highlighted four areas of vascular biology of relevance to the vascular or endovascular

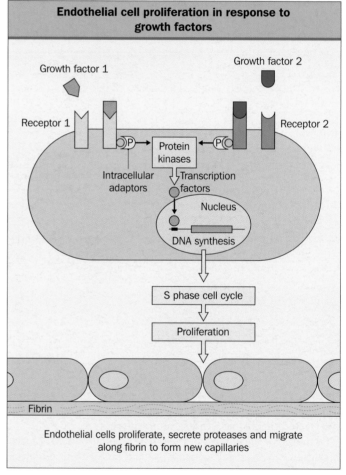

Figure 2.6 Endothelial cell proliferation in response to growth factors.

surgeon. The crucial role of the vasculature in cancer and in the inflammatory joint widens the interest in vascular biology. In the future, knowledge of how tumors control vascular invasion and how inflammatory cell migration can be controlled may bring new treatments that impinge on the practice of vascular surgery.

REFERENCES

1. Ross R. The pathogenesis of atherosclerosis – an update. N Engl J Med 1986;314:488–500.
2. Ross R. The pathogenesis of atherosclerosis: a perspective for the 1990s. Nature 1993;362:801–9.
3. Verma S, Anderson TJ. Fundamentals of endothelial function for the clinical cardiologist. Circulation 2002;105:546–9.
4. Traub O, Berk BC. Laminar shear stress: mechanisms by which endothelial cells transduce an atheroprotective force. Arterioscler Thromb Vasc Biol 1998;18:677–85.
5. Garcia-Cardeña G, Comander J, Anderson KR, et al. Biomechanical activation of vascular endothelium as a determinant of its functional phenotype. Proc Natl Acad Sci USA 2001;98:4478–85.
6. Seiler C, Pohl T, Wustmann K, et al. Promotion of collateral growth by granuloctye-macrophage colony-stimulating factor in patients with coronary artery disease: a randomized, double-blind, placebo-controlled study. Circulation 2001;104:2012–7.
7. Mann MJ, Whittemore AD, Donaldson MC, et al. Ex-vivo gene therapy of human vascular bypass grafts with E2F decoy: the PREVENT single-centre, randomised, controlled trial. Lancet 1999;354:1493–8.
8. Pyo R, Lee JK, Shipley M, et al. Targeted gene disruption of matrix metalloproteinase-9 (gelatinase B) suppresses development of experimental abdominal aortic aneurysms. J Clin Invest 2000;105:1641–9.
9. Zhang B, Ye S, Herrmann S-M, et al. Functional polymorphism in the regulatory region of gelatinase B gene in relation to severity of coronary atherosclerosis. Circulation 1999;99:1788–94.
10. Peters DG, Kassam A, St Jean PL, et al. Functional polymorphism in the matrix metalloproteinase-9 promoter as a potential risk factor for intracranial aneurysm. Stroke 1999;30:2612–6.
11. Van Royen N, Piek JJ, Buschmann I, et al. Stimulation of arteriogenesis: a new concept for the treatment of arterial occlusive disease. Cardiovasc Res 2001;49:543–53.
12. Morishita R, Aoki M, Kaneda Y, Ogihara T. Gene therapy in vascular medicine: recent advances and future perspectives. Pharmacol Ther 2001;91:105–14.
13. Gough A, Clapperton M, Rolando N, et al. Randomised placebo-controlled trial of granulocyte-colony stimulating factor in diabetic foot infection. Lancet 1997;350:855–9.

CHAPTER

3

Thrombosis and Hemostasis

Tamer N Boules and Thomas W Wakefield

KEY POINTS

- Hemostasis requires the interaction of platelets, coagulation and fibrinolytic factors, endothelium, proinflammatory and anti-inflammatory mediators, and leukocytes.

- Clot formation is typically initiated by vascular injury, in which a platelet plug forms and is reinforced with fibrin produced via the extrinsic pathway.

- Physiologic anticoagulants such as antithrombin III and activated protein C oppose thrombosis, serving to localize it to sites of vascular injury.

- Under normal conditions, clot formation is balanced by plasmin-mediated fibrinolysis, resulting in the formation of D-dimers and other fibrin degradation products.

- Endothelium normally sustains an antithrombotic environment, but during states of injury or dysfunction, produces various prothrombotic and proinflammatory agents that augment clot formation.

- Thrombosis and inflammation are interrelated processes; during thrombosis, leukocytes as well as platelets and endothelial cells are activated, and subsequently release tissue-factor-rich procoagulant microparticles, further augmenting thrombosis.

- Arterial thrombosis may be the result of plaque rupture and release of thrombogenic material into the bloodstream, as well as platelet accumulation along points of high shear forces at stenoses.

- Hypercoagulability, stasis, and endothelial injury contribute to venous thrombosis.

- Factor V Leiden, elevated levels of factor VIII, prothrombin 20210A, and hyperhomocystinemia are the most common causes of primary venous thrombosis.

- Von Willebrand disease is the most common inherited bleeding disorder. Congenital hemophilias, platelet defects, and disorders of fibrinolysis are less common.

INTRODUCTION

Normal hemostasis relies on the balanced interaction of multiple components of blood. These include the coagulation factors critical to the production of cross-linked fibrin as an end product of the clotting cascade, as well as the physiologic anticoagulant and fibrinolytic mechanisms necessary to keep the thrombotic process localized to the area of injury. Also central to normal thrombosis are platelets, necessary not only for the formation of the initial hemostatic 'plug' through aggregation at sites of vessel wall injury, but also providing a phospholipid surface for enzymatic reactions of the coagulation cascade.

Other factors are also important in hemostasis. Depending on their state of activation, endothelial cells have been shown to express procoagulant and anticoagulant activity, platelet pro-aggregation factors, vasoconstrictor and vasodilatory substances, as well as adhesion molecules important in the trafficking of leukocytes, facilitating the inflammatory response. It is through this mechanism and others that thrombosis and inflammation are closely linked, especially in the venous circulation. Thrombosis is known to directly elicit an inflammatory response. However, only recently have the molecular and cellular events occurring at the thrombus–vessel wall interface been elucidated. A host of cytokines including tumor necrosis factor (TNF), interleukin (IL)-6, IL-8, and IL-10, have been identified as not only amplifiers of inflammation but also promoters of thrombosis.

COAGULATION MECHANISMS

Hemostasis is typically initiated by damage to the vessel wall and disruption of the endothelium, although it may originate also in the absence of vessel wall damage. This injury results in the exposure of subendothelial collagen to circulating platelets. Ultimately, platelets bind to these exposed sites and are activated. Vessel wall damage simultaneously results in release of tissue factor (TF), a cell membrane protein, from injured cells and the activation of the extrinsic pathway of the coagulation cascade. These two events are critical to the activation and acceleration of thrombosis.

The adhesion of platelets to exposed collagen is the first step in the formation of an effective hemostatic 'platelet plug', resulting in platelet activation. This interaction is mediated by von Willebrand factor (vWF), whose platelet receptor is glycoprotein (Gp) Ib.[1] Similarly, fibrinogen forms bridges between platelets by binding to the GpIIb/IIIa receptor on adjacent platelets, resulting in platelet aggregation.[2,3] Activation of platelets leads to the 'release reaction' in which the prothrombotic contents of platelet granules (dense bodies and alpha granules) are secreted in response to transmembrane signals and a subsequent influx of calcium.[4] These granules are rich in receptors for coagulation factors Va and VIIIa,[5,6] as well as fibrinogen, vWF, and adenosine diphosphate (ADP), a potent activator of other platelets. Platelet activation also leads to the elaboration of arachidonic acid metabolites such as thromboxane A_2, a powerful initiator of platelet aggregation.[4] Simultaneous contraction of platelets during activation results in a dramatic shape change from one that is initially discoid to that of a 'spiny' sphere with long pseudopodia.[4] This shape change leads to the externalization of negatively charged procoagulant phospholipids (phosphatidylserine and phosphatidylinositol), normally located within the inner leaflet of the platelet membrane.[7] This special surface facilitates the assembly of the coagulation factors, accelerating their reactions.[8] Platelets also release microparticles, rich in TF and other procoagulants.

Fibrin is critical in stabilizing the initial platelet plug. The formation of fibrin involves several enzymatic steps leading to the formation of thrombin, which converts fibrinogen to fibrin (**Fig. 3.1**).[9] Coagulation is initiated through the *extrinsic pathway* by the release of TF into blood, where it complexes with and activates factor VII to activated VII (VIIa). The TF–VIIa complex then activates factors IX and X to IXa and Xa in the presence of calcium (Ca^{2+}).[10] Feedback amplification is achieved as factors VIIa, IXa, and Xa are all capable of activating factor VII to VIIa, especially when bound to TF.[11] Factor Xa is also capable of activating factor V to Va (on the platelet phospholipid surface).[11] Factors Xa, Va, and II (prothrombin) form on the platelet phospholipid surface in the presence of Ca^{2+} to initiate the *prothrombinase complex*, which catalyzes the formation of thrombin from prothrombin.[8] Thrombin feedback amplifies the

system by activating not only factor V to Va but also factor VIII (normally circulating bound to vWF) to VIIIa and factor XI to XIa. After activation, factor VIIIa dissociates from vWF and assembles with factors IXa and X on the platelet surface in the presence of Ca^{2+} to form a complex called the *Xase complex*, which catalyzes the activation of factor X to Xa.[8] This further facilitates thrombin production through amplified activity of the prothrombinase complex.

Thrombin is central to all of coagulation. Its action occurs through the cleavage and release of fibrinopeptide A (FPA) from the α chain of fibrinogen, and fibrinopeptide B (FPB) from the β chain of fibrinogen.[12] This leaves newly formed fibrin monomers which then covalently cross-link, leading to fibrin polymerization. This cross-linking strengthens and stabilizes the clot. Thrombin also activates factor XIII to XIIIa, which catalyzes this cross-linking of fibrin as well as that of other plasma proteins, such as fibronectin and α₂-antitrypsin, resulting in their incorporation into the clot and the formation of a 'stronger' clot, less likely to undergo thrombolysis.[13] In addition, factor XIIIa activates platelets as well as factors V and VIII, further amplifying thrombin production.[8]

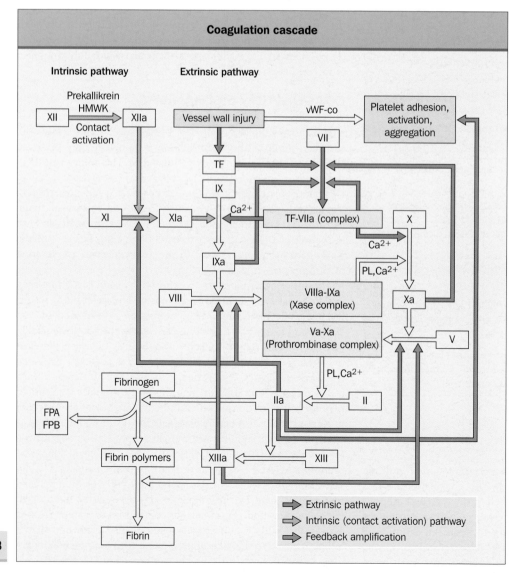

Figure 3.1 Coagulation cascade. Coagulation is initiated by formation of a platelet plug and release of tissue factor (TF) from injured cells, resulting in fibrin production through the extrinsic pathway. Alternatively, activation of factor XII on negatively charged surfaces leads to clot production via the intrinsic pathway. Thrombin (IIa) and other activated factors (VIIa, IXa, Xa, and XIIIa) are capable of amplifying coagulation through multiple positive feedback pathways. co, collagen; FPA, fibrinopeptide A; FPB, fibrinopeptide B; HMWK, high-molecular-weight kininogen; PL, phospholipid; vWF, von Willebrand factor.

The extrinsic pathway, via TF exposure, is the main mechanism by which coagulation is initiated *in vivo* in response to trauma or tissue damage. Alternatively, coagulation can be activated through the *intrinsic pathway*, whose true physiologic role remains to be clarified. This route requires activation of factor XI to XIa, which subsequently converts factor IX to IXa,[14] promoting formation of the Xase complex and ultimately thrombin (**Fig. 3.1**). One mechanism by which this occurs *in vitro* is through the *contact activation system*, in which factor XII (Hageman factor) is activated to XIIa when complexed to prekallikrein and high-molecular-weight kininogen (HMWK) on a negatively charged surface; factor XIIa then activates factor XI to XIa. Both thrombin and factor XIa (in an autocatalytic manner) are also capable of activating factor XI.[15] The physiologic importance of the intrinsic pathway is not completely clear, as patients deficient in factor XII, prekallikrein, or HMWK, usually have no difficulties with bleeding, whereas deficiency of factor XI leads to a moderately severe bleeding disorder.[13] The contact activation system is most important in extracorporeal bypass circuits, such as cardiopulmonary bypass and extracorporeal membrane oxygenation (ECMO).

PHYSIOLOGIC ANTICOAGULANT MECHANISMS

Physiologic anticoagulants oppose further thrombin formation and serve to localize thrombotic activity to sites of vascular injury, therefore maintaining hemostatic balance. Just as thrombin is essential to normal coagulation, *antithrombin III* (ATIII) is the central anticoagulant protein. ATIII acts by binding to and 'trapping' thrombin. This interferes with coagulation by three major mechanisms (**Fig. 3.2**). First, inhibition of thrombin prevents the removal of FPA and FPB from fibrinogen, a thrombin substrate, thus limiting fibrin formation.[16] Secondly, thrombin becomes unavailable for factor V and VIII activation, slowing the coagulation cascade. Thirdly, thrombin-mediated platelet activation and aggregation is inhibited. In the presence of heparin, this inhibition of thrombin by ATIII is markedly accelerated, resulting in systemic anticoagulation. ATIII also has been shown to directly inhibit factors VIIa, IXa, Xa, XIa, and XIIa.[9,17,18]

A second natural anticoagulant is *activated protein C (APC)*. It is produced on the surface of intact endothelium when thrombin binds to its receptor, thrombomodulin (**Fig. 3.3**). This

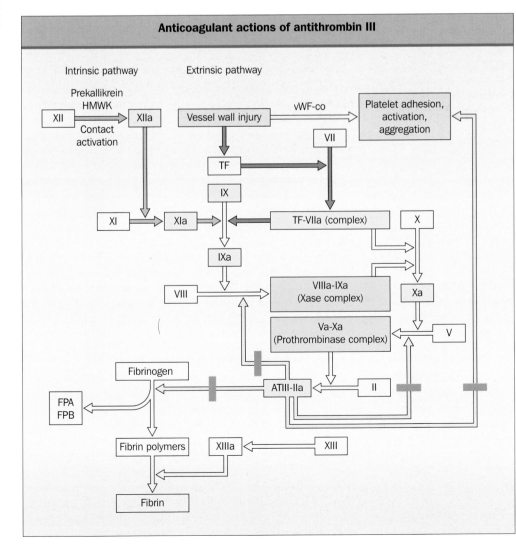

Anticoagulant actions of antithrombin III

Figure 3.2 Anticoagulant actions of antithrombin III. Antithrombin III (ATIII) acts by binding to and 'trapping' thrombin. This not only prevents the formation of fibrin from fibrinogen, but also inhibits multiple positive feedback pathways that normally amplify coagulation, including platelet aggregation. ATIII also directly inhibits factors VIIa, IXa, Xa, XIa, and XIIa. The actions of ATIII are accelerated by heparin. FPA, fibrinopeptide A; FPB, fibrinopeptide B, TF, tissue factor.

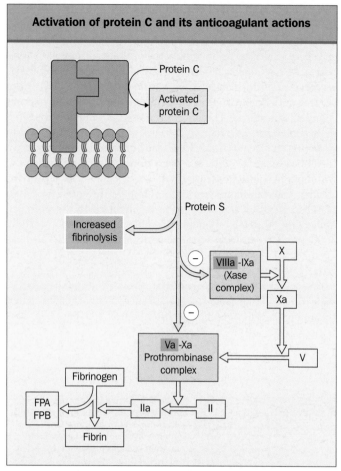

Figure 3.3 Activation of protein C and its anticoagulant actions.
Protein C is activated by the thrombin–thrombomodulin complex on the surface of endothelium. In the presence of protein S, activated protein C inactivates factors Va and VIIIa. It also inhibits plasminogen activator inhibitor-1 (PAI-1), therefore increasing fibrinolysis. FPA, fibrinopeptide A; FPB, fibrinopeptide B.

thrombin–thrombomodulin complex not only inhibits the actions of thrombin, but also activates protein C to APC.[19–21] APC, in the presence of its cofactor, protein S, inactivates factors Va and VIIIa, therefore reducing Xase and prothrombinase activity.[22–24] APC also increases fibrinolysis by inactivation of an inhibitor of tissue plasminogen activator (tPA).[25]

Another innate anticoagulant is *tissue factor pathway inhibitor (TFPI)*. As it is mostly bound to low-density lipoproteins (LDL) in plasma, it has also been termed *lipoprotein-associated coagulation inhibitor*. This protein binds the TF–VIIa complex, thus inhibiting the activation of factor X to Xa and formation of the prothrombinase complex.[13] Interestingly, factor IX activation is not inhibited. Finally, heparin cofactor II is another inhibitor of thrombin[26] whose action appears to be focused in the extravascular compartment. The activity of heparin cofactor II is augmented by both heparin (in a manner analogous to ATIII) and dermatan sulfate.[27] Its role in physiologic hemostasis is not yet fully understood.

FIBRINOLYTIC MECHANISMS

In addition to these natural anticoagulants, physiologic clot formation is balanced by a constant process of thrombolysis in order to prevent pathologic intravascular thrombosis. The central fibrinolytic enzyme is plasmin, a serine protease generated by the proteolytic cleavage of the proenzyme plasminogen. Its main substrates include fibrin, fibrinogen, and other coagulation factors. Plasmin also interferes with vWF-mediated platelet adhesion by proteolysis of GpIb.[28]

Activation of plasminogen occurs through four major mechanisms. In the presence of thrombin, vascular endothelial cells produce and release tPA as well as α_2-antiplasmin, a natural inhibitor of excess fibrin-bound plasmin. As clot is formed, plasminogen, tPA, and α_2-antiplasmin become incorporated into the fibrin clot.[8] In contrast to free circulating tPA, fibrin-bound tPA is an efficient activator of plasminogen. A second endogenous pathway leading to the activation of plasminogen is through the urokinase-type plasminogen activator (uPA), also produced by endothelial cells but with less affinity for fibrin.[29] The activation of uPA *in vivo* is not completely understood. However, it is hypothesized that plasmin, in small amounts (produced through tPA), activates uPA, leading to further plasminogen activation and amplification of fibrinolysis.[30] The third mechanism of plasminogen activation involves factors of the contact activation system; activated forms of factor XII, kallikrein, and factor XI can each independently convert plasminogen to plasmin.[31] These activated factors may also catalyze the release of bradykinin from HMWK, which further augments tPA secretion. Finally, APC has been found to proteolytically inactivate plasminogen activator inhibitor type-1 (PAI-1), an inhibitor of tPA released by endothelial cells in the presence of thrombin, thus promoting tPA activity and fibrinolysis.[32]

The degradation of fibrin polymers by plasmin ultimately results in the creation of fragment E and two molecules of fragment D, which, during physiologic thrombolysis, are released as a covalently linked dimer (D-dimer).[8] Clinically, detection of D-dimer in the circulation is a marker for ongoing clot formation and fibrinolysis. In contrast, during therapeutic administration of thrombolytics and other systemic fibrinolytic states, circulating fibrinogen becomes a second target for plasmin in addition to clot-associated fibrin (**Fig. 3.4**). This circulating plasmin is not inhibited by α_2-antiplasmin. Furthermore, in *fibrinogenolysis*, circulating fibrinogen is degraded by plasmin through the removal of FPB as well as the carboxy-terminal portion of its α-chain, producing fragment X.[33] Fragment X is then further broken down to one molecule of fragment D and fragment Y. Finally, fragment Y is degraded to one molecule of fragment E and two molecules of fragment D, as monomers;[8] no D-dimer is formed. Of note, fragments Y and D are potent inhibitors of fibrin formation.

ENDOTHELIUM AND HEMOSTASIS

Through its ability to express procoagulants and anticoagulants, vasoconstrictors and vasodilators, as well as key cell adhesion molecules and cytokines, the endothelial cell has emerged as one of the pivotal regulators of hemostasis. Under normal conditions, vascular endothelium sustains a vasodilatory and local fibrinolytic state in which coagulation, platelet adhesion and activation, as well as inflammation and leukocyte activation, are suppressed (**Fig. 3.5**). Vasodilatory endothelial products include adenosine, nitric oxide (NO), and prostacyclin (PGI$_2$).[34] A non-thrombogenic endothelial surface is maintained through four main mechanisms:

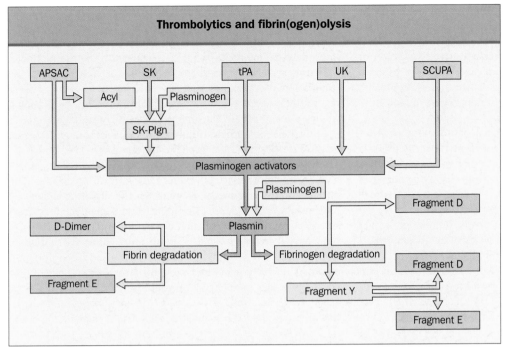

Thrombolytics and fibrin(ogen)olysis

Figure 3.4 Thrombolytics and fibrin(ogen)olysis. Thrombolytics are activators of plasminogen. The three main agents are streptokinase (SK), tissue plasminogen activator (tPA), and urokinase (UK). SK must complex with plasminogen prior to activating other plasminogen molecules, while the other agents act directly. Single-chain UK-type plasminogen activator (SCUPA) and anisoylated plasminogen–SK activator complex (APSAC) are fibrin-selective forms of UK and SK, respectively. APSAC requires in-vivo deacylation prior to acquiring activity. As opposed to fibrinogenolysis, fibrinolysis results in the production of D-dimers.

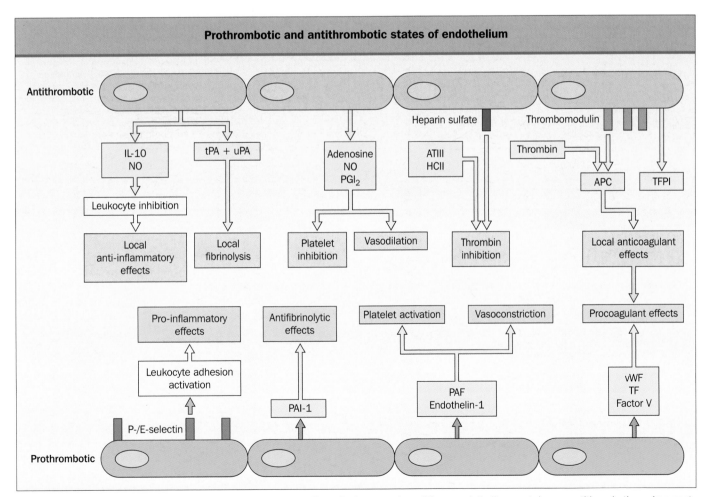

Prothrombotic and antithrombotic states of endothelium

Figure 3.5 Prothrombotic and antithrombotic states of endothelium. Under normal conditions, endothelium sustains an antithrombotic environment through the local production of certain cytokines, thrombolytics, platelet inhibitors, and anticoagulants. However, during states of endothelial injury or dysfunction, a prothrombotic and proinflammatory state is created in which leukocytes and platelets are activated, thrombolysis is inhibited, and procoagulants are released. APC, activated protein C; ATIII, antithrombin III; HCII, heparin cofactor II; IL-10, interleukin-10; NO, nitric oxide; PAF, platelet activating factor; PAI-1, plasminogen activator inhibitor-1; PGI_2, prostacyclin; TF, tissue factor; TFPI, tissue factor pathway inhibitor; tPA, tissue plasminogen activator; uPA, urokinase-type plasminogen activator; vWF, von Willebrand factor.

(1) endothelial production of thrombomodulin and subsequent activation of protein C; (2) endothelial expression of surface heparin sulfate and dermatan sulfate, with acceleration of ATIII and heparin cofactor II activity; (3) constitutive expression of TFPI by endothelium (which is markedly accelerated in response to heparin); and (4) local production of tPA and uPA. Finally, the elaboration of NO and IL-10 by endothelium inhibits the adhesion and activation of leukocytes.[34]

In contrast, during states of endothelial disturbances, whether physical (e.g. vascular trauma) or functional (e.g. sepsis), a prothrombotic and proinflammatory state of vasoconstriction is supported by the endothelial surface (**Fig. 3.5**).[34] Endothelial release of platelet activating factor (PAF) and endothelin-1 promotes vasoconstriction.[35] Furthermore, during prothrombotic conditions, endothelial cells increase production of vWF, TF, PAI-1, as well as factor V, in order to augment thrombosis.[34] Lastly, in response to endothelial injury, endothelial cells are 'activated', resulting in increased surface expression of certain cell adhesion molecules (such as P-selectin or E-selectin), promoting the adhesion and activation of leukocytes. This initiates and amplifies inflammation and thrombosis.

THROMBOSIS AND INFLAMMATION

There is growing evidence that thrombosis and inflammation are interrelated. This relationship now appears to be bidirectional. States of systemic inflammation, such as sepsis, result in the elaboration of cytokines that also activate coagulation. More recently, however, the inflammatory response has been shown to play a major role in the amplification of thrombosis.

In response to a toxic stimulus, such as endotoxin in the case of sepsis, stimulated macrophages release both TNF and IL-1. These cytokines are well known for their ability to stimulate leukocyte–endothelial adhesion and activation through the upregulation of adherence proteins on the endothelial surface. This results in the production of several secondary mediators and the amplification of the classic inflammatory response. However, it is now known that these cytokines also stimulate the release of TF from both macrophages and endothelium, resulting ultimately in formation of thrombin and fibrin clot via the extrinsic pathway. TNF promotes thrombosis in several other ways as well. First, TNF downregulates endothelial thrombomodulin expression and promotes its degradation at the

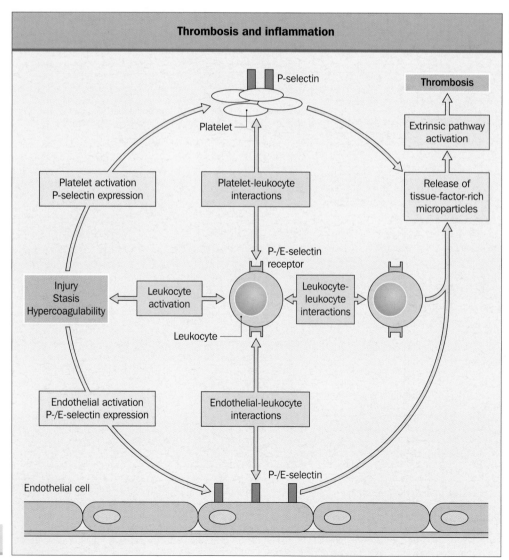

Figure 3.6 Thrombosis and inflammation. In response to vascular injury, stasis, or hypercoagulability, leukocytes, platelets, and endothelial cells are activated. This results in expression of surface P-selectin and E-selectin on platelets and endothelium, which not only increases local inflammation, but also leads to the release of tissue-factor-rich procoagulant microparticles, thus augmenting thrombosis.

endothelial cell surface.[36] Secondly, TNF increases C4b-binding protein (C4b-BP) levels; since circulating C4b-BP binds protein S, this reduces the amount of free protein S available as the protein C cofactor.[37] Thirdly, TNF inhibits fibrinolysis by suppressing the release of tPA and inducing expression of tPA inhibitors such as PAI-1.[38–43] Lastly, TNF further inhibits fibrinolysis by decreasing the production of protein C, an inhibitor of PAI-1.

The local inflammatory response to thrombosis has also been well established. In the setting of vascular wall injury, activated platelets aggregate to form a platelet plug and fibrin clot formation occurs in response to the release of TF. Circulating neutrophils and monocytes then interact with these platelets through P-selectin, and with the endothelium through P-selectin and E-selectin, together with other cell adhesion molecules, becoming well incorporated into the clot at the thrombus–vessel wall interface (**Fig. 3.6**). This not only generates a local inflammatory response, but also amplifies thrombosis through further monocyte TF expression and induction of endothelial TF expression. Activated platelets also release certain chemoattractants such as platelet factor 4 (PF4) and neutrophil activating peptide-2 (NAP-2) that increase leukocyte recruitment.[34,37]

ARTERIAL VERSUS VENOUS THROMBOSIS

Classically, the elements required for the initiation of thrombosis were described by Virchow more than a century ago as the triad of stasis, endothelial injury, and hypercoagulability of the blood. In the arterial circulation, endothelial injury (whether acute or chronic) is central to thrombosis. This is most clearly demonstrated by the typical atherosclerotic plaque, often the result of long-term intimal injury. In advanced lesions, the lipid core of the plaque is rich in inflammatory cells (often apoptotic), cholesterol crystals, and TF (generated by activated macrophages within the plaque). Ulceration or fissuring of the plaque, as in acute coronary syndromes, results in exposure of the highly thrombogenic lipid core to the bloodstream, with activation of the coagulation cascade, platelet aggregation and activation, and deposition of clot (**Fig. 3.7**).[44] Contributing to this is the increased platelet deposition that occurs at the apex of stenoses, the points of maximal shear forces. Thrombosis in the venous circulation differs significantly. Although direct endothelial injury, blood stasis, and changes in its composition leading to hypercoagulable states are known risk factors in venous thrombosis, the inciting event involves the formation of thrombus from local procoagulant events, such as small endothelial

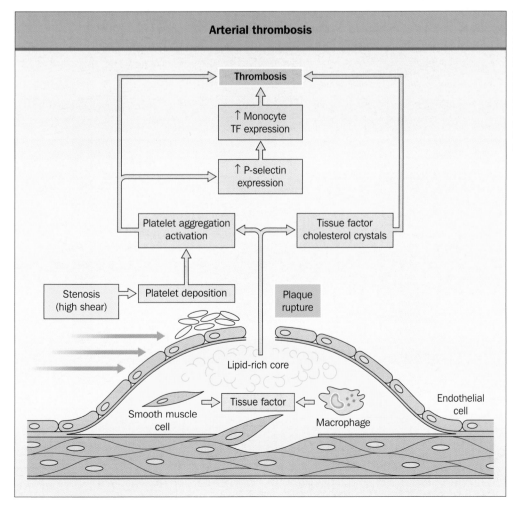

Figure 3.7 Arterial thrombosis. Rupture of atherosclerotic plaques results in exposure of their highly thrombogenic lipid contents to the bloodstream. This leads to platelet aggregation and P-selectin expression, further monocyte tissue-factor expression, and amplification of thrombosis. In addition, arterial flow across the stenosis results in platelet deposition at its apex, the point of maximal shear force.

disruptions at venous confluences, saccules, and valve pockets. In the second stage, neutrophils and platelets adherent to this thrombus become activated, generating inflammatory and procoagulant mediators that amplify thrombosis further.[45] With progression, leukocytes (initially neutrophils and subsequently monocytes) extravasate into the vein wall in response to the chemokine gradient generated by the initial thrombotic event, ultimately resulting in transmural venous inflammation. A balance between proinflammatory and anti-inflammatory cytokines and chemokines determines the ultimate vein wall response. The earliest elevated glycoprotein on endothelial cells and platelets, P-selectin, plays an essential role in thrombogenesis. In models of venous thrombosis in the primate, P-selectin inhibition, given prophylactically, decreases thrombosis in a dose-dependent fashion. Additionally, P-selectin inhibitors can treat established venous thrombosis as effectively as heparin, without anticoagulation.[46,47] It is hypothesized that selectins, expressed after a thrombogenic stimulus, facilitate interactions between leukocytes and endothelial cells, leukocytes and leukocytes, and leukocytes and platelets (**Fig. 3.6**). TF-rich procoagulant microparticles are released from leukocytes, platelets, and endothelium, further amplifying coagulation.

TESTS OF THROMBOSIS

Tests of thrombosis are designed to evaluate platelet function, coagulation, and fibrinolysis (**Table 3.1**). Platelet function abnormalities are manifested by mucocutaneous bleeding or excessive hemorrhage after surgery or trauma.[9] Usually, a platelet count of 50 000/μL or more ensures adequate hemostasis, while a count of less than 10 000/μL risks spontaneous bleeding. The bleeding time measures the ability and speed with which a platelet plug is formed *in vivo* at sites of vascular injury.[48] Unfortunately, since it is operator-dependent and often abnormal in other disorders, it is considered relatively insensitive and non-specific.[49] Platelet aggregation tests are not widely available.

Tests of coagulation include the activated partial thromboplastin time (aPTT), prothrombin time (PT), thrombin clotting time (TCT), and activated clotting time (ACT). The aPTT evaluates the intrinsic and contact activation pathways of coagulation – specifically, the function of all the factors except factors VII and XIII – and is important in the monitoring of heparin therapy. The PT/INR (international normalized ratio) evaluates the extrinsic pathway: factors VII, X, V, II, and

Laboratory tests of thrombosis.		
Test	Description	Normal values*
Platelet function		
Platelet count	Increased in some myeloproliferative disorders; decreased in autoimmune disorders, in response to drugs, and during extracorporeal circulation	150–450,000/μL
Peripheral smear	Assesses platelet and blood cell morphology	Requires interpretation
Bleeding time	Measures the ability and speed of platelet-plug formation *in vivo* at sites of vascular injury	2.5–9.5min
Aggregation	Measures response to agonists that cause aggregation	Requires interpretation
Coagulation		
aPTT	Evaluation of intrinsic coagulation system; used to monitor heparin	21–34s
PT	Evaluation of extrinsic coagulation system; used to monitor warfarin	9–11s
INR	Standardizes PT values between laboratories	1.0
TCT	Time necessary for conversion of fibrinogen to fibrin by exogenous thrombin; specific for fibrinogen deficiencies and monitoring heparin	7.7–9.3s
ACT	Whole blood clotting following activation of contact pathway	70–120s
Fibrinolysis		
Fibrin(ogen) degradation products	Identifies conditions of fibrinolysis and fibrinogenolysis	>8μg/dL
D-dimer	Detects circulating cross-linked fibrin fragments; marker for clot production and lysis, and DIC	<0.20μg/mL
Plasminogen activity	Measures plasma plasminogen function; plasminogen antigen levels may also be measured	81–151%
*Normal values based on University of Michigan Laboratory reference ranges		

Table 3.1 Laboratory tests of thrombosis. ACT, activated clotting time; aPTT, activated partial thromboplastin time; DIC, disseminated intravascular coagulation; INR, international normalized ratio; PT, prothrombin time; TCT, thrombin clotting time.

fibrinogen. This test remains the most common mode of monitoring patients on the oral anticoagulant, warfarin. The ACT measures the ability of the whole blood to clot, and therefore is an indicator of platelet function and the coagulation cascade together. It is frequently used to monitor heparin-based anticoagulation intraoperatively during peripheral vascular procedures and while on cardiopulmonary bypass. In terms of fibrinolysis, fibrin and fibrinogen degradation products result from the proteolytic effects of plasmin. During states of fibrinolysis, the D-dimer fragment is formed and serves as a marker for ongoing clot formation and plasmin-mediated breakdown. During fibrinogenolysis, no D-dimer is formed; rather, fragment E and two fragment D monomers are formed. Other tests of fibrinolysis are less well characterized. Plasminogen, plasminogen activator, and antiplasmin levels can be measured and are often useful in evaluating patients with recurrent thrombosis and suspected fibrinolytic abnormalities.

HYPERCOAGULABLE STATES

Several conditions can result in a hypercoagulable state and subsequent vascular thrombosis. Our understanding of these conditions has recently expanded substantially, with the three most common causes for thrombosis being recognized within the past few years. These disorders can be classified according to their severity (**Table 3.2**). Components of the appropriate hypercoagulable screen are listed in **Table 3.3**. Not every patient with a thrombotic event should be screened, but patients with strong family histories, young patients with arterial and venous thrombosis of unclear cause, and patients with multiple episodes of thrombosis should undergo such. Although anticoagulation with heparin and warfarin is used most often as treatment for these conditions, novel antithrombotic agents that target specific points in the coagulation cascade, platelets, and the inflammatory component of thrombosis are currently in development (**Table 3.4, Figs 3.8 and 3.9**).

Defects with high risk for thrombosis

Antithrombin III deficiency exists on both a congenital and acquired basis, and accounts for 1–2% of venous thromboses.[50] Produced in the liver, ATIII inhibits thrombin plus factors VIIa, IXa, Xa, XIa, and XIIa. The congenital syndrome usually occurs by age 50. The diagnosis should be suspected in a patient who can not be adequately anticoagulated with heparin or who develops a thrombosis while on heparin. Episodes of native arterial and arterial graft thrombosis have also been described with this deficiency.[51] The diagnosis is made by measuring ATIII antigen and activity levels while off anticoagulation, as heparin may decrease levels by 30% for up to 10 days following its cessation and warfarin increases ATIII levels. Homozygote individuals usually die *in utero*, while heterozygotes usually have ATIII levels of less than 70%. Treatment requires administration of fresh frozen plasma (containing ATIII) with heparin, followed by oral anticoagulation. ATIII concentrates are also available.[52] Additional acquired causes of ATIII deficiency (as a result of protein loss, consumption, or decreased production) include liver disease, disseminated intravascular coagulation (DIC), malnutrition, and nephrotic syndrome.

Protein C deficiency accounts for 3–5% of venous thromboses.[50] Protein C with its cofactor protein S inactivates

Hypercoagulable disorders.		
Severity	*Frequency (%)*	*Sites of thrombosis*
High risk for thrombosis		
Antithrombin III deficiency	1–2	Venous > arterial
Protein C deficiency	3–5	Venous > arterial
Protein S deficiency	2–3	Venous > arterial
Lower risk for thrombosis		
Factor V Leiden	20–60	Venous > arterial
Hyperhomocystinemia	10	Venous and arterial
Prothrombin 20210A	4–5	Venous
Dysplasminogenemia	<1	Venous and arterial
Dysfibrinogenemia	1–3	Venous and arterial
Variable risk for thrombosis		
Elevated factor VIII level	20	Venous
HIT/HITTS	1–30*	Venous and arterial
Lupus anticoagulant	8–12	Venous and arterial
Abnormal platelet aggregation	Not known	Arterial > venous
*Frequency of patients who develop HIT/HITTS among patients in whom heparin administered		

Table 3.2 Hypercoagulable disorders. HIT/HITTS, heparin-induced thrombocytopenia/heparin-induced thrombocytopenia and thrombosis syndrome.

Components of the hypercoagulable screen.
Standard coagulation tests (i.e. aPTT, TCT, ACT)
Mixing studies (if aPTT elevated)
Antithrombin III antigen level and activity assay
Protein C antigen level and activity assay
Protein S antigen level
APC resistance assay and factor V Leiden genetic analysis
Prothrombin 20210A gene analysis
Homocysteine level
Factor VIII level
Antiphospholipid and anticardiolipin antibody screen
Platelet count, platelet aggregation tests (if available)
Functional plasminogen assay (or some test of fibrinolysis)

Table 3.3 Components of the hypercoagulable screen. ACT, activated clotting time; APC, activated protein C; aPTT, activated partial thromboplastin time; TCT, thrombin clotting time.

Future antithrombotic agents.

Drug	Mechanism of action
Oral heparins	
SNAC-UFH SNAD-LMWH	Heparin is bound non-covalently to carrier proteins, enabling passage through GI mucosa
Direct thrombin inhibitors	

Recombinant hirudin and analogs
  Desirudin
  Lepirudin
  Bivalirudin
  Argatroban
  H376/95 (Melagatran)
	Bind to thrombin and inhibit its activity directly without need for cofactors (e.g. ATIII); Melagatran administered orally, while other agents are given intravenously

Ancrod (defibrination agent)	Serine protease that cleaves fibrinopeptide A from fibrinogen, resulting in less stable fibrin clot more easily degraded by plasmin
P-selectin inhibitors (rPSGL-Ig)	Decrease amplification of thrombosis by reducing inflammatory response
Factor VIIa inhibitors	Compete with factor VIIa for TF binding
Tissue factor pathway inhibitor	Inhibits the factor VIIa–TF complex
Activated protein C	Inactivates factors Va, VIIIa, as well as inhibitors of tPA
Fondaparinux (synthetic pentasaccharide)	Augments ATIII inhibition of factor Xa without inhibiting thrombin

Table 3.4 Future antithrombotic agents. ATIII, antithrombin III; GI, gastrointestinal; rPSGL, recombinant P-selectin glycoprotein ligand-1; SNAC–UFH, N-[8-(2-hydroxybenzoyl)amino]caprylate unfractionated heparin; SNAD–LMWH, sodium N-[10-(2-hydroxybenzoyl)amino]decanoate low-molecular-weight heparin; TF, tissue factor; tPA, tissue plasminogen activator.

factors Va and VIIIa, and promotes fibrinolysis. Both protein C and S are made in the liver. Although venous thrombosis is most common in protein C deficiency, arterial thrombosis has also been described, especially in patients aged 50 years or younger.[53] Thrombosis usually occurs between 15 and 30 years of age. When homozygous, patients usually die in infancy from a DIC-like state termed *purpura fulminans*. The diagnosis is made by measuring protein C antigen and activity levels. Heterozygotes usually have antigenic levels less than 60%.[8] Acquired deficiency may also result from liver disease, DIC, and nephrotic syndrome. Protein S deficiency accounts for 2–3% of venous thromboses and clinically presents and behaves like protein C deficiency. However, in addition to the already mentioned acquired causes, inflammatory diseases such as systemic lupus erythematosus (SLE) that result in elevated levels of C4b-BP can lead to a relative protein S deficiency by depleting the free protein S supply. Protein S deficiency can be diagnosed by measuring *free* protein S antigen levels. Treatment of both protein S and C deficiency is heparin followed by lifelong oral anticoagulation. However, in both deficiencies, treatment should be instituted

only after the first episode of thrombosis, as many heterozygotes remain asymptomatic.[50] Since protein C and S are vitamin-K-dependent factors with short half-lives relative to other liver-produced factors (II, IX, X), initiation of warfarin prior to complete anticoagulation with heparin may result in an initial hypercoagulable state, microcirculatory thrombosis, and the syndrome of warfarin-induced skin necrosis, in patients diagnosed with venous thromboembolism.[54]

Defects with lower risk for thrombosis

Resistance to APC (factor V Leiden) has been reported to be present in 20–60% of all cases of venous thrombosis.[55] The defect is due to resistance to inactivation of factor Va by APC, most commonly secondary to a mutation resulting in a Glu→Arg amino acid substitution at position 506 of the factor V gene.[56] Thrombotic manifestations have been found in both the arterial and venous circulation, although the latter predominate. Both homozygous and heterozygous forms exist. Although the homozygous form is not lethal in infancy, the relative risk for thrombosis is increased 80-fold.[57] In the heterozygous form, the relative risk is increased only sevenfold, but in the setting of other risk factors, such as oral contraceptive use or the presence of other hypercoagulable defects (such as protein C or S deficiency), this risk increases markedly. The diagnosis of factor V Leiden is made by genetic analysis as well as by a functional assay in which exogenous APC is added to the plasma; if the aPTT is not prolonged, factor V may be abnormal, suggesting the Leiden mutation.[50] However, the genetic analysis is critical to differentiate homozygous from heterozygous forms. Although treatment for this disorder involves heparin and warfarin anticoagulation, the relatively low risk for recurrent thrombosis in heterozygotes suggests that not all patients require long-term anticoagulation after the first episode.

Hyperhomocystinemia, a known risk factor for atherosclerosis, has also been found to be a risk factor for venous thrombosis, accounting for 10% of venous thromboses overall. As with other hypercoagulable states, the combination of hyperhomocystinemia with other disorders such as factor V Leiden increases the risk of thrombosis further. The mechanism of thrombosis may relate to decreased availability or production of nitric oxide (hindering vasodilation), a direct toxic effect on vascular endothelium, as well as reduced protein C and plasminogen activation.[58–63] Treatment is directed to reducing homocysteine levels using folic acid, vitamin B_6, and vitamin B_{12}.

The recently identified prothrombin 20210A polymorphism, in which the prothrombin gene is altered at position 20210 by a Glu→Arg substitution, results in a hypercoagulable state that accounts for 4–5% of venous thromboses and increases the risk of thrombosis by 5.4 times.[64] Interestingly, this abnormality is associated with myocardial infarction in younger women. However, the polymorphism has not been found to be increased in those with arterial disease.

Known defects in fibrinolysis, such as dysplasminogenemia, are quite rare, accounting for less than 1% of venous thromboses. Other fibrinolytic abnormalities are less well defined, but may affect up to 10% of the population.[65] Although most of these conditions are congenital, an acquired state of impaired fibrinolysis caused by increased levels of tPA inhibitors may account for the temporarily heightened risk of deep venous thrombosis (DVT) in the postoperative patient. Abnormal

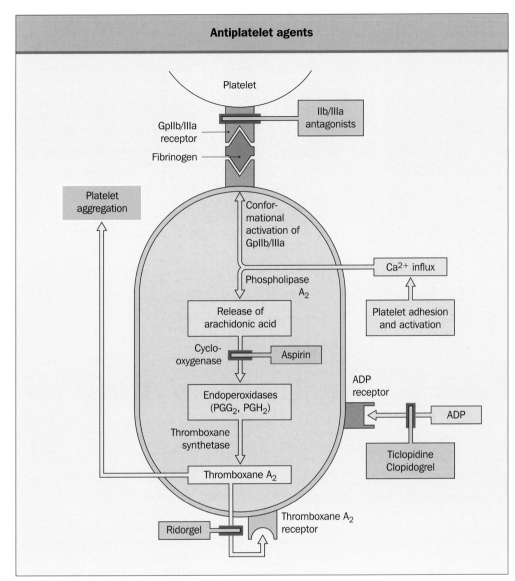

Antiplatelet agents

Figure 3.8 Antiplatelet agents.
Antiplatelet agents include inhibitors of cyclo-oxygenase (e.g. aspirin), which inhibit the production of thromboxane A_2, a potent platelet activator and vasoconstrictor. ADP, thromboxane A_2, and glycoprotein (Gp) IIb/IIIa receptor antagonists have also been developed. PGG_2, prostaglandin G_2; PGH_2, prostaglandin H_2.

fibrinogens (dysfibrinogenemias) may be responsible for 1–3% of episodes of venous thrombosis.

Defects associated with variable risk for thrombosis

Elevated factor VIII levels have recently been identified as a risk factor for both primary and recurrent venous thrombosis.[66] Elevated factor VIII levels are found in approximately 20% of patients with venous thrombosis. The risk of thrombosis appears to increase in a 'dose-dependent' fashion; that is, with progressive increases in factor VIII levels (especially above the 90th percentile), the incidence of thrombosis rises. Furthermore, there is evidence that this abnormality may be genetically inherited.[67] The exact mechanism by which high factor VIII levels result in thrombosis is still not completely clear. Treatment includes oral anticoagulation following the first episode of thrombosis. The optimal duration of anticoagulation remains to be determined, although the high risk of recurrence (37% at 2 years) argues for extended prophylaxis with warfarin.[66]

Heparin-induced thrombocytopenia (HIT) occurs in 1–30% of patients on heparin.[50] A more severe form of HIT associated with thrombosis – heparin-induced thrombocytopenia and

thrombosis syndrome (HITTS) – is much less frequent. This syndrome is caused by a heparin-dependent IgG antibody that results in platelet aggregation during heparin administration. This antibody binds to the heparin–PF4 complex. It then binds by its Fc portion to a platelet Fc receptor. This results in platelet activation, aggregation, and the release of cytokines, catecholamines, and microparticles. This also leads to the deposition of complement and immunoglobulins on the endothelial surface, stimulating the release of TF and resulting arterial/venous thrombosis.[68] The syndrome should be suspected in patients who develop thrombosis while on heparin, as well as when there is a fall in the platelet count to less than 100 000/μL or by 50% from its baseline pre-heparin level. It usually begins 3 to 14 days after heparin exposure. The illness may vary from isolated thrombocytopenia to thrombosis, embolic episodes, and death. Both standard unfractionated heparin as well as low-molecular-weight heparin (LMWH) may cause HIT. The diagnosis can be made by the serotonin release assay, a platelet aggregation assay, fluorescence-activated cell sorter (FACS) analysis for platelet microparticles, and, more recently, by an enzyme-linked immunosorbent assay (ELISA) to detect the antibody.[69–71]

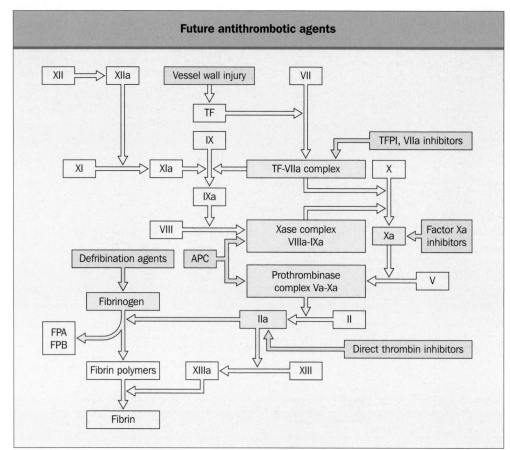

Figure 3.9 Future antithrombotic agents. Agents that target various points in the coagulation cascade are in development. Indications for their use include intolerance to conventional anticoagulants (e.g. in heparin-induced thrombocytopenia), and, in certain settings, as prophylaxis and treatment of venous thromboembolic disease. APC, activated protein C; FPA, fibrinopeptide A; FPB, fibrinopeptide B; TF, tissue factor; TFPI, tissue factor pathway inhibitor.

Treatment involves stopping heparin, initiating an alternative anticoagulant (such as hirudin or argatroban), and, under its protection, initiating warfarin.

Presence of lupus anticoagulant with antiphospholipid antibodies, usually IgG, results in a hypercoagulable state.[72] This syndrome consists of the presence of an antiphospholipid antibody in association with arterial or venous thrombosis, recurrent fetal loss, thrombocytopenia, and livedo reticularis. Strokes, myocardial and visceral infarctions, and extremity gangrene may occur. Arterial vascular bypass grafts are especially susceptible to failure, with a 50% thrombosis rate in one series.[73] The diagnosis is suggested by a prolonged aPTT, while other coagulation tests remain normal. This finding is artifactual, accounting for the misleading syndrome name, since, during the test, the necessary phospholipids are antagonized by the antibody, making them unavailable for in-vitro clotting. In addition, the aPTT remains prolonged despite mixing the patient's plasma with normal plasma. The diagnosis can made on clinical grounds with either an abnormal clot-based functional assay off anticoagulants or by direct ELISA measurement of the antiphospholipid antibody. Although 80% of patients with a positive aPTT test (lupus anticoagulant) have the antibody by ELISA, only 10–50% of those with the antibody have a positive aPTT test. The prolonged aPTT is a better predictor of thrombotic events, while high titers of antibody are more predictive of recurrent fetal loss.[74] Although the lupus anticoagulant has been reported in 5–40% of SLE patients, it can exist in patients without SLE and can also be induced in patients by infection, drugs, and cancer. Possible mechanisms responsible for the

thrombotic effects of this syndrome include inhibition of endothelial prostacyclin production, inhibition of protein C activation, increased PAI-1 levels, direct platelet activation, direct endothelial activation by antiphospholipid antibodies, increased monocyte TF expression, and decreased free protein S levels.[75–80] No one dominant mechanism has emerged, suggesting a multifactorial cause of thrombosis. Treatment consists of anticoagulation with a goal INR of 3 to 4 once warfarin is initiated. As the aPTT is artifactually prolonged, heparin therapy should be monitored with the TCT or anti-factor Xa level.

Abnormal platelet aggregation has been associated with thrombosis in the setting of advanced malignancy of the lung and uterus, and after carotid endarterectomy. 'Hyperactive' platelets have also been seen in the setting of graft thrombosis following peripheral vascular reconstructions. Diabetes mellitus, known to be associated with hyperactive platelets, may contribute to these conditions. Sophisticated tests of platelet function, and specifically aggregation, are not uniformly available. Thus, relatively little is known about the influence of platelet aggregation on hypercoagulable states.

BLEEDING DISORDERS

Coagulation factor deficiency
Von Willebrand disease (VWD), a deficiency of vWF, is the most common inherited coagulation disorder.[81] Normally, vWF is produced by endothelial cells and megakaryocytes but is complexed to factor VIII in the blood. Symptoms include easy bruising, epistaxis, and prolonged bleeding following surgery,

but in females, menorrhagia is common.[82] VWD has subtypes which are transmitted in both autosomal dominant and autosomal recessive forms. Laboratory tests reveal a prolonged aPTT and bleeding time, decreased factor VIII activity, decreased vWF levels by ELISA, and abnormal platelet aggregation in response to ristocetin. Treatment depends on severity. In mild cases, desmopressin acetate (DDAVP) may be used to manage epistaxis or as prophylaxis for minor surgeries. More severe bleeding requires replacement with cryoprecipitate. Recently, recombinant factor VIII/vWF concentrates that avoid the infectious risks of transfusion are available.[83]

Hemophilia A is a sex-linked recessive deficiency of factor VIII, occurring in 1/10 000 births.[37] Epistaxis and hematuria are common. Findings in severe forms include joint, intramuscular, and retroperitoneal bleeding. The aPTT is prolonged and factor VIII levels are decreased. The minimum level required for hemostasis is 30%, and spontaneous bleeding is uncommon with levels greater than 5–10%.[84] Treatment originally consisted of factor VIII concentrates and cryoprecipitate, but this resulted in widespread transmission of HIV in the 1980s. Introduction of recombinant factor VIII has eliminated this risk. However, development of neutralizing anti-factor-VIII antibodies, occurring in 10–15% of patients, remains a problem. To combat this, new forms of factor VIII are being investigated. Hemophilia B is a similar sex-linked recessive deficiency of factor IX. Clinically indistinguishable from hemophilia A, it also presents with a prolonged aPTT. Treatment consists of factor IX concentrates and vitamin K.[84] Other factor deficiencies are much rarer. Most are autosomal recessive, and may be treated with fresh frozen plasma, specific factor concentrates, or vitamin K when appropriate.

Inherited platelet and fibrinolytic disorders are much less common. Platelet disorders present with mucosal bleeding (e.g. epistaxis or gastrointestinal), easy bruising, petechiae, purpura, and menorrhagia, associated with an elevated bleeding time. Inherited platelet defects include those involving the GpIIb/IIIa receptor and the GpIb receptor. Fibrinolytic abnormalities leading to bleeding include α_2-antiplasmin deficiency as well as PAI-1 deficiency. Patients may present with bleeding after trauma or surgery, which may even be delayed, presenting 24 to 36 hours later.

SUMMARY

Normal hemostasis requires the interaction of platelets, coagulation and fibrinolysis factors, endothelium, proinflammatory and anti-inflammatory mediators, and leukocytes. Clot formation is typically initiated by vascular injury, in which a platelet plug forms and is reinforced with fibrin. Clot formation is balanced by plasmin-mediated fibrinolysis and the action of physiologic anticoagulants. Endothelium is capable of sustaining either a prothrombotic or antithrombotic environment in response to various local factors. Arterial thrombosis may be the result of plaque rupture and release of thrombogenic material into the bloodstream, as well as platelet accumulation along points of high shear forces at stenoses. Hypercoagulability, stasis, and endothelial injury contribute to venous thrombosis. Factor V Leiden, elevated levels of factor VIII, prothrombin 20210A, and hyperhomocystinemia are the most common causes of primary venous thrombosis. Von Willebrand disease is the most common inherited bleeding disorder. Congenital hemophilias, platelet defects, and disorders of fibrinolysis are less common.

REFERENCES

1. Hickey MJ, Williams SA, Roth GA. Human platelet glycoprotein IX: an adhesive prototype of leucine rich glycoproteins with flank-center-flank structures. Proc Natl Acad Sci USA 1989;86:6773–7.
2. Bennett JS, Vilaire G, Cines DB. Identification of the fibrinogen receptor on human platelets by photoaffinity labeling. J Biol Chem 1982;257:8049–54.
3. Savage B, Ruggeri ZM. Selective recognition of adhesive sites in surface-bound fibrinogen by glycoprotein IIb/IIIa on nonactivated platelets. J Biol Chem 1991;266:11227–33.
4. Shapiro AD. Platelet function disorders. Haemophilia 2000;6(Suppl 1) 120–7.
5. Sims PJ, Faioni EM, Wiedmer T, et al. Complement proteins C5b-9 cause release of membrane vesicles from the platelet surface that are enriched in the membrane receptor for coagulation factor Va and express prothrombinase activity. J Biol Chem 1988;263:18205–12.
6. Gilbert GE, Sims PJ, Wiedmer T, et al. Platelet-derived microparticles express high affinity receptors for factor VIII. J Biol Chem 1991;266:17261–8.
7. Ferguson JJ, Waly HM, Wilson JM. Fundamentals of coagulation and glycoprotein IIb/IIIa receptor inhibition. Eur Heart J 1998;19(Suppl D):D3–9.
8. Hassouna HI. Laboratory evaluation of hemostatic disorders. Hematol Oncol Clin North Am 1993;7:1161–249.
9. Triplett DA. Coagulation and bleeding disorders: review and update. Clin Chem 2000;46:1260–9.
10. Zur M, Radcliffe RD, Oberdick J, et al. The dual role of factor VII in blood coagulation: initiation and inhibition of a proteolytic system by a zymogen. J Biol Chem 1982;257:5623–31.
11. Dahlbäck B. Blood coagulation. Lancet 2000;355:1627–32.
12. Blomback B, Blomback M. The molecular structure of fibrinogen. Ann NY Acad Sci 1972;202:77–97.
13. Davie EW, Fujikawa K, Kisiel W. The coagulation cascade: initiation, maintenance, and regulation. Biochemistry 1991;30:10363–70.
14. DiScipio RG, Kurachi K, Davie EW. Activation of human factor IX (Christmas factor). J Clin Invest 1978;61:1528–38.
15. Naito K, Fujikawa K. Activation of human blood coagulation factor XI independent of factor XII: factor XI is activated by thrombin and factor XIa in the presence of negatively charged surfaces. J Biol Chem 1991; 266:7353–8.
16. Rosenberg RD, Damus PS. The purification and mechanism of action of human antithrombin-heparin cofactor. J Biol Chem 1973;248:6490–505.
17. Kurachi K, Fujikawa K, Schmer G, et al. Inhibition of bovine factor IXa and factor Xab by antithrombin III. Biochemistry 1976;15:373–7.
18. Kurachi K, Davie EW. Activation of factor XI (plasma thromboplastin antecedent) by factor XIIa (activated Hageman factor). Biochemistry 1977;16:5831–9.
19. Esmon CT, Owen WG. Identification of an endothelial cell cofactor for thrombin-catalyzed activation of protein C. Proc Natl Acad Sci USA 1981;78:2249–52.
20. Owen WG, Esmon CT. Functional properties of an endothelial cell cofactor for thrombin-catalyzed activation of protein C. J Biol Chem 1981;256:5532–5.
21. Esmon NL, Owen WG, Esmon CT. Isolation of a membrane-bound cofactor for thrombin-catalyzed activation of protein C. J Biol Chem 1982;257:859–64.
22. Kisiel W, Canfield WM, Ericsson LH, et al. Anticoagulant properties of bovine plasma protein C following activation by thrombin. Biochemistry 1977;16:5824–31.

23. Marlar RA, Kleiss AJ, Griffin JH. Mechanism of action of human activated protein C, a thrombin dependent anticoagulant enzyme. Blood 1982;59:1067–72.

24. Vehar GA, Davie EW. Preparation and properties of bovine factor VIII (antihemophilic factor). Biochemistry 1980;19:401–10.

25. Greenfield LJ, Proctor MC, Wakefield TW. Coagulation cascade and thrombosis. In: Ernst CB, Stanley JC, eds. Current therapy in vascular surgery, 4th edn. St Louis:Mosby; 2001:813–7.

26. Tollefsen DM, Majerus PW, Blank MK. Heparin cofactor II: purification and properties of a heparin-dependent inhibitor of thrombin in human plasma. J Biol Chem 1982;257:2162–9.

27. Geiger M, Krebs M, Jerabek I, et al. Protein C inhibitor (PCI) and heparin cofactor II (HCII): possible alternative roles of these heparin-binding serpins outside the hemostatic system. Immunopharmacology 1997;36:279–84.

28. Adelman B, Michelson AD, Loscalzo J, et al. Plasmin effect on platelet glycoprotein Ib–von Willebrand factor interactions. Blood 1985;65:32–40.

29. Gurewich V, Pannell R. Fibrin binding and zymogenic properties of single-chain urokinase (pro-urokinase). Semin Thromb Hemost 1987;13:146–51.

30. Sidelmann JJ, Gram J, Jesperson J, et al. Fibrin clot formation and lysis: basic mechanisms. Semin Thromb Hemost 2000;26:605–18.

31. Hajjar KA, Nachman RL. Endothelial cell-mediated conversion of Glu-plasminogen to Lys-plasminogen: further evidence for assembly of the fibrinolytic system on the endothelial cell surface. J Clin Invest 1988;82:1769–78.

32. Esmon CT. The regulation of natural anticoagulant pathways. Science 1987;235:1348–52.

33. Schmaier AH. Disseminated intravascular coagulation: pathogenesis and management. J Intensive Care Med 1991;6:209–228.

34. Becker BF, Heindl B, Kupatt C, et al. Endothelial function and hemostasis. Z Kardiol 2000;89:160–7.

35. Gross PL, Aird WC. The endothelium and thrombosis. Semin Thromb Hemost 2000;26:463–78.

36. Esmon NL, Esmon CT. Protein C and the endothelium. Semin Thromb Hemost 1988;14:210–5.

37. Wakefield TW. Hemostasis. In: Greenfield LJ, Mulholland MW, Oldham KT, et al, eds. Surgery: scientific principles and practice, 3rd edn. Philadelphia:Lippincott Williams & Wilkins; 2001:86–111.

38. Nawroth PP, Stern DM. Modulation of endothelial cell hemostatic properties by tumor necrosis factor. J Exp Med 1986;163:740–5.

39. Bevilacqua MP, Pober JS, Majeau GR, et al. Recombinant tumor necrosis factor induces procoagulant activity in cultured human vascular endothelium: characterization and comparison with the actions of interleukin-1. Proc Natl Acad Sci USA 1986;83:4533–7.

40. Conway EM, Bach R, Rosenberg RD, et al. Tumor necrosis factor enhances expression of tissue factor mRNA in endothelial cells. Thromb Res 1989;53:231–41.

41. Schleef RR, Bevilacqua MP, Sawdey M, et al. Cytokine activation of vascular endothelium: effects on tissue-type plasminogen activator and type I plasminogen inhibitor. J Biol Chem 1988;263:5797–803.

42. Van Hinsbergh VW, Kooistra T, van den Berg EA, et al. Tumor necrosis factor increases production of plasminogen activator inhibitor in human endothelial cells in vitro and rats in vivo. Blood 1988;72:1467–73.

43. Medina R, Schocher SH, Han JH. Interleukin-1, endotoxin, or tumor necrosis factor/cachectin enhance the level of plasminogen activator messenger RNA in bovine aortic endothelial cells. Thromb Res 1989;54:41–52.

44. Rauch U, Osende JI, Fuster V, et al. Thrombus formation on athero-sclerotic plaques: pathogenesis and clinical consequences. Ann Intern Med 2001;134:224–38.

45. Stewart GJ. Neutrophils and deep venous thrombosis. Haemostasis 1993;23:127–40.

46. Myers DD Jr, Schaub R, Wrobleski SK, et al. P-Selectin antagonism causes dose-dependent venous thrombosis inhibition. Thromb Haemost 2001;85:423–9.

47. Myers D, Wrobleski S, Londy F, et al. New and effective treatment of experimentally induced venous thrombosis with anti-inflammatory rPSGL-Ig. Thromb Haemost 2002;87:374–82.

48. Mielke CH. Measurement of the bleeding time. Thromb Haemost 1984;52:210–1.

49. Rodgers RP, Levin J. A critical reappraisal of the bleeding time. Semin Thromb Haemost 1990;16:1–20.

50. Wakefield TW, Schmaier AH. Vascular thrombosis due to hypercoagulable states. In Rutherford RB, ed. Vascular surgery, 5th ed. Philadelphia: WB Saunders; 2000:726–32.

51. Towne JB, Bandyk DF, Hussey CV, et al. Antithrombin deficiency – a cause of unexplained thrombosis in vascular surgery. Surgery 1981;89:735–42.

52. Menache D. Antithrombin III concentrates. Hematol Oncol Clin North Am 1992;6:1115–20.

53. Eldrup-Jorgensen J, Flanigan DP, Brace L, et al. Hypercoagulable states and lower limb ischemia in young adults. J Vasc Surg 1989;9:334–41.

54. Cole MS, Minifee PK, Wolma FJ. Coumadin necrosis: a review of the literature. Surgery 1988;103:271–7.

55. Svensson PJ, Dahlback B. Resistance to activated protein C as a basis for venous thrombosis. N Engl J Med 1994;330:517–22.

56. Kalafatis M, Mann KG. Factor V Leiden and thrombophilia. Arterioscler Thromb Vasc Biol 1997;17:620–7.

57. Rosendaal FR, Koster T, Vandenbroucke JP, et al. High risk of thrombosis in patients homozygous for factor V Leiden (activated protein C resistance). Blood 1995;85:1504–8.

58. Loscalzo J. The oxidant stress of hyperhomocyst(e)inemia. J Clin Invest 1996;98:5–7.

59. Tawakol A, Omland T, Gerhard M, et al. Hyperhomocyst(e)inemia is associated with impaired endothelium-dependent vasodilation in humans. Circulation 1997;95:1119–21.

60. Upchurch GR, Welch GN, Randev N, et al. The effect of homocysteine on endothelial nitric oxide production (abstract). FASEB J 1995;9:A876.

61. Starkebaum G, Harlan JM. Endothelial cell injury due to copper-catalyzed hydrogen peroxide generation from homocysteine. J Clin Invest 1986;77:1370–6.

62. Graeber JE, Slott JH, Ulane RE, et al. Effect of homocysteine and homocystine on platelet and vascular arachidonic acid metabolism. Pediatr Res 1982;16:490–3.

63. Nehler MR, Taylor LM Jr, Porter JM. Homocysteinemia as a risk factor for atherosclerosis: a review. Cardiovasc Surg 1997;5:559–67.

64. Cumming AM, Keeney S, Salden A, et al. The prothrombin gene G20210A variant: prevalence in a UK anticoagulant clinic population. Br J Haematol 1997;98:353–5.

65. Towne JB, Bandyk DF, Hussey CV, et al. Abnormal plasminogen: a genetically determined cause of hypercoagulability. J Vasc Surg 1984;1:896–902.

66. Kyrle PA, Minar E, Hirschl M, et al. High plasma levels of factor VIII and the risk of recurrent venous thromboembolism. N Engl J Med 2000;343:457–62.

67. Kraaijenhagen RA, in't Anker PS, Koopman MMW, et al. High plasma concentration of factor VIIIc is a major risk factor for venous thromboembolism. Thromb Haemost 2000;83:5–9.

68. Cancio LC, Cohen DJ. Heparin-induced thrombocytopenia and thrombosis. J Am Coll Surg 1998;186:76–91.

69. Sheridan D, Carter C, Kelton JG. A diagnostic test for heparin-induced thrombocytopenia. Blood 1986;67:27–30.

70. Jackson MR, Krishnamurti C, Aylesworth CA, et al. Diagnosis of heparin-induced thrombocytopenia in the vascular surgery patient. Surgery 1997;121:419–24.

71. Lee DH, Warkentin TE, Hayward CP, et al. The development and evaluation of a novel test for heparin induced thrombocytopenia (abstract). Blood 1994;84:188a.

72. Greenfield LJ. Lupus-like anticoagulants and thrombosis. J Vasc Surg 1988;7:818–9.

73. Ahn SS, Kalunian K, Rosove M, et al. Postoperative thrombotic complications in patients with the lupus anticoagulant: increased risk after vascular procedures. J Vasc Surg 1988;7:749–56.

74. Lynch A, Marlar R, Murphy J, et al. Antiphospholipid antibodies in predicting adverse pregnancy outcome: a prospective study. Ann Intern Med 1994;120:470–5.

75. Carreras LO, Defreyn G, Machin SJ, et al. Arterial thrombosis, intra-uterine death, and "lupus" anticoagulant: detection of immunoglobulin interfering with prostacyclin formation. Lancet 1981;1:244–6.

76. Comp PC, DeBault LE, Esmon NL, et al. Human thrombomodulin is inhibited by IgG from two patients with non-specific anticoagulants (abstract). Blood 1983;62 (Suppl 1):299a.

77. Violi F, Ferro D, Valesini G, et al. Tissue plasminogen activator inhibitor in patients with systemic lupus erythematosus and thrombosis. BMJ 1990;300:1099–102.

78. Vermylen J, Blockmans D, Spitz B, et al. Thrombosis and immune disorders. Clin Haematol 1986;15:393–412.

79. Ferro D, Pittoni V, Quintarelli C, et al. Coexistence of antiphospholipid antibodies and endothelial perturbation in systemic lupus erythematosus patients with ongoing prothrombotic state. Circulation 1997;95:1425–32.

80. Reverter JC, Tassies D, Font J, et al. Hypercoagulable state in patients with antiphospholipid syndrome is related to high induced tissue factor expression on monocytes and to low free protein S. Arterioscler Thromb Vasc Biol 1996;16:1319–26.

81. Murray EW, Lillicrap D. von Willebrand disease: pathogenesis, classification, and management. Transfus Med Rev 1996;10:93–110.

82. Werner EJ. von Willebrand disease in children and adolescents. Pediatr Clin N Am 1996;43:683–707.

83. Phillips MD, Santhouse A. von Willebrand disease: recent advances in pathophysiology and treatment. Am J Med Sci 1998;316:77–86.

84. Collins JA. Blood transfusion and disorders of surgical bleeding. In: Sabiston DC, ed. Textbook of surgery, 14th edn. Philadelphia:WB Saunders; 1991:85–102.

CHAPTER
4

Hemodynamics

Christopher L Wixon

KEY POINTS

- Although a patient may exhibit a constellation of vascular lesions, which is unique to the individual, each lesion must obey the principles of physics and fluid mechanics.

- An individual's response to a change in the hemodynamic pattern should occur in an orderly and predictable manner.

- Understanding hemodynamics provides artistic dimension to the technical exercise of creating vascular anastomoses.

- Poor comprehension of vascular hemodynamics will result in ill-advised interventions within a fragile patient population, the result of which may be devastating.

INTRODUCTION

Hemodynamics pervade nearly all aspects of vascular surgery: they govern distribution patterns of atherosclerotic plaque and myointimal hyperplasia, the development and growth of abdominal aortic aneurysms, and the degree of ischemia distal to an area of stenosis or occlusion, and serve as a basis for the correct interpretation of non-invasive evaluation. For vascular surgeons, a basic understanding of hemodynamics can be compared to the musician's fundamental knowledge of the scale. Without a broad comprehension of the essentials, one is simply imitating the score that has been composed by another. Failure to grasp these tenets prevents one from venturing off the narrow path – it is an operation performed in darkness. Accordingly, it is no coincidence that many of the innovators who have contributed significantly to the field of vascular surgery have possessed a considerable background in physics and engineering.

The importance of the pulse as a means of state of health is attributed to Galen, who postulated that blood flows freely through the body – without conduit – in an ebb-and-tide fashion.[1] Galen's tenets were defended by the Church with such tenacity that they remained doctrine for nearly 14 centuries and little progress was made from the standpoint of vascular physiology. How strange it must have been for those early surgeons who were called upon to stem the tide of a life-threatening laceration.

It was not until the Renaissance, that a correct understanding of circulation was offered by William Harvey.[2] Shortly thereafter, the basis to understand fluid dynamics was provided by Sir Isaac Newton, who provided concepts of mass, acceleration, and viscosity in his magnum opus, *The Principia Mathematica*.[3] These concepts continue to serve as a basis in the modern description of blood flow in vessels.

Hemodynamics is defined as the physics of blood in circulation and is described in terms of pressures and velocities within the blood vessels. In the most simple terms, blood flow through the vascular system occurs from an area of high energy to an area of lower energy. Obviously, the heart serves as the source of energy, delivering discrete quanta of energy (the left ventricular stroke volume) with each systole. Under most circumstances, the majority of the energy exists in the form of pressure, and the difference in energy between any two points can usually be expressed as the pressure gradient.

The purpose of this chapter is to review the tenets of fluid dynamics, vessel wall mechanics, and shear stress from a conceptual basis as they pertain to the daily working of the clinical vascular surgeon. Emphasis will be placed upon qualitative assessment, rather than quantitative formulations. These considerations are helpful in understanding normal physiology of the arterial system and the expected consequence of circulatory perturbations. For a complete discussion regarding quantitative assessment, the author defers to more comprehensive texts.[4-7]

VESSEL WALL MECHANICS

In contradistinction to Galen's belief that blood flows freely throughout the vascular system, one now recognizes a well-organized arterial system whose purpose is to confine, store, and channel energy to areas of relative need. In a way, the blood vessels can be likened to a highly complex and dynamic network, constructed in both parallel and series configurations. In this system, the vessel wall serves as an insulator, which prevents the dissipation of energy while en route to its desired location. Additionally, many of the blood vessels within the vascular system have the unique ability to provide capacitance – that is, they maintain the ability to store energy during the systolic phase. This stored energy may later be released to the system during the diastolic phase. In this manner, the oscillating cardiac output can be converted to a more continuous flow of energy throughout the cardiac cycle.

Capacitance – the ability of a blood vessel to store energy during the systolic phase and dissipate energy during the diastolic phase – remains a function of vessel wall composition. With each systole, the left ventricular stroke volume is transmitted to the ascending aorta with a uniquely shaped pressure waveform, which then changes based upon the compliance characteristics of the blood vessel through which it traverses and upon the peripheral vascular resistance. These characteristics not only influence the pressure and flow velocity within each of the vessels, but also may influence the direction of blood flow within the vessel.

In general, when a vessel is subjected to a transmural pressure, it will distend. The resultant change in blood vessel diameter

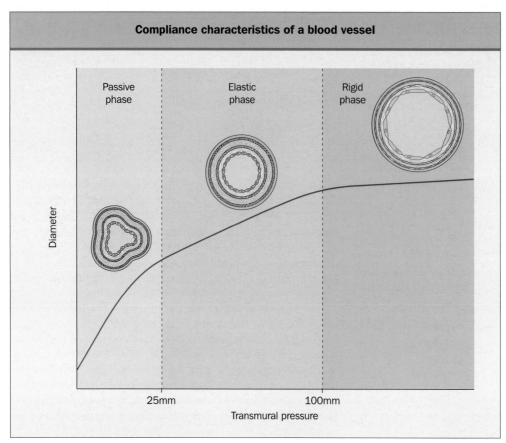

Compliance characteristics of a blood vessel

Passive phase

Elastic phase

Rigid phase

Diameter

25mm

100mm

Transmural pressure

Figure 4.1 Compliance characteristics of a blood vessel. At low transmural pressures, the artery is passively collapsed and both elastin and collagen fibers remain in a resting, fully contracted state (left panel). As the intravascular pressure distends the blood vessel, the elastin fibers straighten, conferring their elastic modulus to the artery (middle panel). At higher pressures, the tightly bound collagen fibers prevent significant dilation, creating a relatively rigid state in which large changes in pressure generate small changes in radius (right panel).

is a function of the blood vessel compliance and is determined by the relative contribution of elastin and collagen fibers within the blood vessel wall. It has been shown that individual elastin fibers may be stretched to an additional 50–70% of their resting length, while the more tightly bound cross-links of the collagen fibers restrict their extensibility to only 2–4%.[8,9] When transmural pressures are sufficiently low (<25mmHg), the artery is passively collapsed and remains very distensible (**Fig. 4.1**, left panel). At intermediate pressures (25–100mmHg), the elastic lamellae within the vessel wall media begin to straighten and confer their elastic modulus to the vessel wall (**Fig. 4.1**, middle panel). At pressures greater than 100mmHg, arteries become increasingly stiff as the elastic lamellae approach their fully distended state and recruitment of the relatively non-distensible collagen fibers occurs (**Fig. 4.1**, right panel).

When the architecture of the blood vessel is evaluated with regard to anatomical location, a relative change in the number of elastic lamellae and of collagen fibers is noted. These structural features confer unique compliance characteristics. In the proximal vessels, the high elastin-to-collagen ratio permits pressure energy to be stored as potential energy as the elastin fibers become distended.[10] After closure of the aortic valve this stored energy is then transmitted to the more distal vessels and permits continued flow during the diastolic phase. As one examines the arteries more distally, the elastin/collagen ratio gradually decreases, creating arteries that are increasingly stiff (**Fig. 4.2**). Because of the relative decrease in elastin, the more distal arteries fail to store significant amounts of energy, and the energy that is received is manifest as pure pressure energy.

Factors that increase the amplitude of the pressure wave include increasing left ventricular contractility, increasing stiffness of the arterial wall, and increasing the resistance of the more peripheral circulation. Because only small quantities of energy dissipate in large arteries (frictional energy losses), the mean pressure within the more proximal circulation diminishes only slightly (**Fig. 4.2**). Likewise, the diastolic pressure changes only a minor degree. However, the increasing stiffness of the more peripheral arteries generates increased amplitude of the systolic waveform as one proceeds more peripherally, a phenomenon known as *systolic amplification*.

The consequence of storage of relatively small amounts of potential energy in the more peripheral arteries permits higher pressures in these arteries at end-systole and provides the physiologic explanation for the resting ankle brachial index of greater than 1.0. Additionally, the transiently higher pressure in the more peripheral arteries, coupled with the relatively high peripheral vascular resistance at the level of the arterioles, provides the opportunity for blood to transiently flow retrograde in early diastole. However, owing to the small capacitance of the more peripheral arteries, the early diastolic pressure diminishes more rapidly than in the proximal arteries and retrograde flow yields to the sustained pressure in the more proximal arteries in the later phases of diastole. Thus, an understanding of vessel wall mechanics serves as a basis for the understanding of the Doppler-derived triphasic waveform and provides a basis for correct interpretation of non-invasive examination.

As a person ages, several developments occur that cause the arteries to become significantly more rigid at smaller pressures

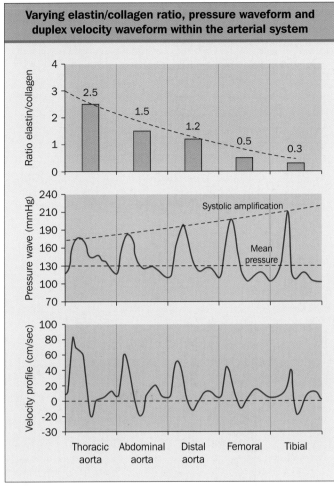

Figure 4.2 Varying elastin/collagen ratio, pressure waveform, and duplex velocity waveform as a function of location within the arterial system. Although mean pressure does not significantly change throughout the vascular system, the decreased elastin/collagen ratio in the periphery creates relatively non-compliant vessels and generates higher pressures in the peripheral arteries in end-systole, a phenomenon known as systolic amplification. The higher pressure in the periphery generates the brief opportunity for reversal of flow in early diastole.

(**Fig. 4.3**). The increasing calcification and loss of elastin that accompanies aging, generally increases the stiffness of the blood vessel walls and increases arterial pressure in systole. Conversely, gradual blood vessel dilation causes the collagen fibers to become load-bearing at progressively lower pressures. Hence, there is a tendency to gravitate toward hypertension as one ages. Accordingly, given the relatively high ratio of elastin to collagen in a child, the presence of hypertension in childhood is indeed rare, and should be cause for further investigation.

An understanding of vessel wall mechanics is most useful to the vascular surgeon when one contemplates the formation, growth, and risk of rupture associated with an aneurysm. In order to understand how these relate to potential changes in aneurysm morphology, one must first examine the mechanical properties of the blood vessel. For any discrete point in time, the distending force within the tube must be at equilibrium with the retractile forces of the blood vessel. When the blood vessel is exposed to a transmural pressure gradient, the vessel distends in the longitudinal and circumferential direction as the pressure energy is distributed to the underlying collagen and elastin

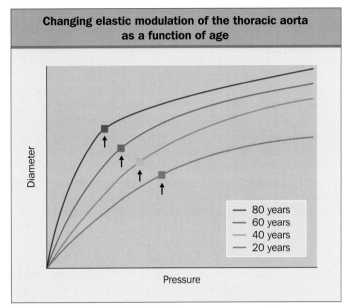

Figure 4.3 Changing elastic modulation of the thoracic aorta as a function of age. The gradual loss of elastin and generalized dilation of arteries cause collagen fibers to be load-bearing at progressively lower pressures (arrow).

fibers. From a practical standpoint, the changes that occur in a longitudinal direction are negligible compared with the changes that occur in a radial direction. The circumferential distending force within the tube is simply the product of the transmural pressure gradient and the area over which the force is exerted:

$$F_{distending} = P_t \times A$$

or

$$F_{distending} = P_t \times (D_i \times L)$$

Where: P_t is the transmural pressure gradient
D_i is the internal diameter
L is the length of the tube

Given the cylindrical morphology of most blood vessels, the two walls of the vessel exert an opposing retractile force in the circumferential direction:

$$F_{retractile} = \sigma \times 2 \times (h \times L)$$

Where: σ is the wall circumferential wall stress
h is the thickness of the tube
L is the length of the tube

In the steady state, the distending force and the retractile forces are equal, and one may set the two equations equal and solve algebraically for wall stress:

$$\sigma = P_t \times D_i /2h$$

or

$$\sigma = P_t \times r_i /h$$

This calculation yields the force percent area for the vessel wall at rest. For a vessel of infinitely thin wall, this becomes the well-known Law of Laplace:

$$T = P_t \times r$$

Where T is the wall tension and r is the radius

In fact, it is wall tension that should be our primary focus. Wall tension is the driving force behind conformation changes in aneurysm morphology, and ultimately, when the wall tension exceeds the bursting strength of the aneurysm wall, rupture occurs.

An understanding of these factors has a direct involvement in understanding the behavior of abdominal aortic aneurysms, as degradation of collagen fibers causes aneurysmal degeneration and rupture of vessels. Although aneurysmal degeneration occurs with loss of elastic fiber content, rupture does not generally occur, owing to the preservation of normal vessel wall bursting-strength characteristics.[11] Studies have demonstrated that although disruption of elastin may be an early event in the formation of aneurysms, collagen is the critical element that prevents aneurysm rupture.[11]

Examining the derivation of the Law of Laplace provides an interesting geometric detail – that is, the protective effect of aneurysm formation. Because an aneurysm is spherical, rather than cylindrical, the retractile forces that the aneurysm provides must reflect its spherical geometry. In other terms, as the vessel degenerates from a cylindrical to a spherical shape, the wall stress becomes distributed over a longitudinal as well as a transverse direction, such that wall tension is reduced at any given diameter (**Fig. 4.4**).

Another factor that has been suggested is the protective effect of laminated thrombus within the aneurysm sac. That is, if the wall stress (ω) is proportional to the inverse of the wall thickness, to what degree does the thrombus provide a protective effect by reducing wall stress? Returning to the basic principles of vessel compliance, one remembers that compliance remains a strict function of the structural content, based upon relative contributions of elastin and collagen. Taken alone, the thrombus that lines the aneurysm sac is a poorly organized semi-solid and offers little resistance to intraluminal changes in pressure. Although specific determination of intra-aortic thrombus compliance characteristics does not exist, it seems likely the intra-aortic thrombus would offer precious little resistance to intraluminal pressure and demonstrate low bursting strength. Based upon these mechanical properties, we are inclined to believe that the thrombus readily transmits pressure out to the aortic wall and offers little protective effect. Alternatively, the increased proteolytic effect of the thrombus against the vessel wall may actually increase the rate at which the aortic wall degenerates.[12,13]

Perhaps the most germane topic to which vessel wall mechanics may be applied relates to concepts of aneurysm growth or shrinkage after endoluminal exclusion. There is little doubt that abdominal aortic aneurysm growth after endoluminal exclusion is related to persistent pressure in the aneurysm sac. Such a situation represents non-satisfactory exclusion of the sac and a failure of endovascular aortic techniques. Failure to acknowledge the relationship between intramural pressure and sac volume is a rejection of the fundamental relationship of pressure and radius as established by Laplace. It is less clear, however, whether persistence in size (lack of sac shrinkage) represents an intermediate pressure that is acceptable. In any case, owing to the spherical configuration of abdominal aortic aneurysms and the expected conformational changes in aneurysm morphology, we favor volumetric analysis as a measure of post-operative success.

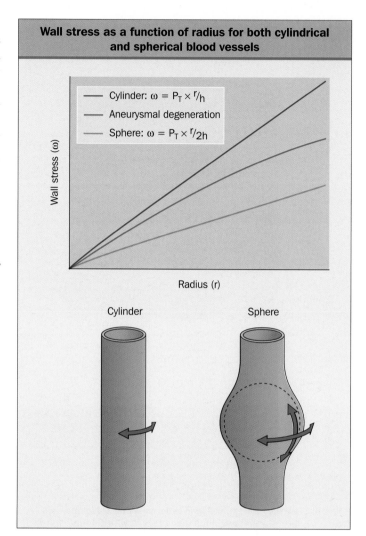

Figure 4.4 Wall stress (ω) as a function of radius for both cylindrical and spherical blood vessels. The spherical form distributes wall tension in both the longitudinal and circumferential directions, reducing the wall stress by 50%.

FLUID MECHANICS

Fundamental to understanding fluid mechanics is the basic principle of conservation of energy, as first noted by the Swiss physician Daniel Bernoulli. In his book *Hemodynamica*, published in 1738, he formulated the principles of conservation of energy as it pertains to fluids in motion. In the most simple terms, the sum of the energies of a flowing fluid (pressure + kinetic + gravitational) at any two points must be equal. Of note, Bernoulli failed to identify the significance of frictional energy losses and, therefore, did not recognize the importance of viscous forces as they relate to pressure gradient or shear stress.

Accordingly, it is important to understand all forms of energy, as they exist. For simplicity, we will assume that the conditions of an ideal flow apply – that is, a Newtonian fluid at constant, laminar flow within the confines of a rigid tube of uniform bore.

Pressure energy

The primary form of energy within the vascular system is pressure, which is generated by the left ventricle and conferred

Correlating units by which pressure may be expressed.			
	cm H_2O	psi	atm
50	68	0.9	0.066
100	136	1.9	0.131
200	272	3.8	0.261
760	1033	14.4	1.0

Table 4.1 Correlating units by which pressure may be expressed.

to the blood vessels. Remarkably, the first direct measurement of blood pressure was not performed until 1733, when Steven Hales (an ordained minister) attached a long glass tube directly to the left carotid artery of a horse and measured the height of blood of the column of blood (9ft 6in).[14]

In clinical practice, we continue to express pressure in millimeters of mercury. Despite the pervasive use of such parameters, the relationship between millimeters of mercury and other standard measures of pressures remains poorly understood. Briefly, pressure can be stated in terms of height of a column of fluid based upon the fluid density and the gravitational force which acts upon it:

Pressure = ρgh

Where: ρ is the density of the fluid
g is the gravitational force
h is the height of the fluid column

Such measures may be correlated with other units of pressure and may be more familiar in the setting of bioengineering (**Table 4.1**).

Pressure energy has the ability to do work, which is largely accomplished during the systolic phase as the elastic and collagen fibers are stretched and the blood vessel distends. After the aortic valve closes, the transfer of energy from the myocardium ceases and the energy that was previously stored in the blood vessel wall is released back to the lumen in the form of diastolic pressure. Although pressure is the primary form of energy conferred to the blood vessels, pressure may be converted into, or restored from, other forms of energy.

Gravitational energy

No one is more familiar with the energy changes that accompany gravitational changes than the patient with ischemic rest pain. As the individual lays supine, the benefit of gravitational pressure energy is lost in the lower extremity, reducing peripheral perfusion pressure to the point such that the tissue's resting metabolic needs cannot be satisfied. In order to restore perfusion pressure to peripheral vascular beds, the ischemic extremity is simply dangled in a dependent position, which converts potential gravitational energy (ρgh; where ρ = the fluid density, g = the gravitational acceleration force, and h = the height of the column of fluid) to hydrostatic pressure. These pressures can be augmented even further by shaking the limb, which creates additional centripetal forces that supplement gravitational acceleration forces, thereby increasing the hydrostatic pressure

to an even greater degree. The net effect of converting potential gravitational energy to hydrostatic pressure, however, does not change the overall energy of the system. It is for this reason that proper non-invasive evaluation of the ankle brachial index be performed in the supine position.

For the purposes of simplicity, for the remainder of the discussion it will be assumed that a 'gravitational neutral' state applies, such that net pressure energy is neither lost nor gained to changes in potential energy.

Frictional energy

As blood flows throughout the vascular system, frictional energy losses occur continuously, converting a small portion of the total energy supplied by the left ventricle into heat. Therefore, as the blood travels along the circulatory pathway, the sum total of energy continuously diminishes from the point at which it leaves the heart until it reaches the low-energy, high-volume venous pool.

One aspect of frictional energy losses occurs from the interaction of moving blood particles along a stationary vessel wall. The expression of endothelial adhesion molecules generates a covalent attraction between the vessel wall and the blood particles. Theoretically, those particles that are immediately adjacent to the wall experience the greatest degree of attraction and travel at infinitely slow velocities.

In addition, frictional energy loss occurs secondary to particle–particle interactions (**Fig. 4.5**). Under normal conditions when blood flow occurs below a critical velocity, blood flow is both orderly and laminar. Each concentric lamina of blood that

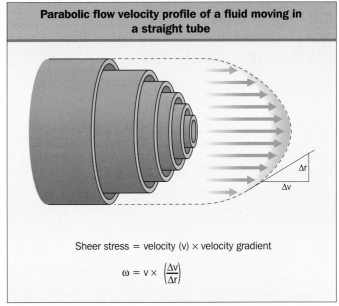

Parabolic flow velocity profile of a fluid moving in a straight tube

Sheer stress = velocity (v) × velocity gradient

$$\omega = v \times \left(\frac{\Delta v}{\Delta r}\right)$$

Figure 4.5 Parabolic flow velocity profile of a fluid moving in a straight tube. Blood flow can be thought to occur in concentric lamellae of different velocities, creating frictional losses through particle-to-particle interactions. Given the relationship of sheer stress (ω), velocity (v), and radius (r), it is noted that the tangential sheer stress becomes small at any point along the center of the vessel as Δv/Δr becomes infinitely small. That is, because adjacent lamellae that are situated most centrally possess low velocity gradients, both shear stress and frictional energy losses are very small within the center of a vessel. Accordingly, blood vessels of large diameter are most efficient at transmitting flow with relatively small frictional losses.

lies more central within the blood vessel is attracted to the blood vessel wall by a slightly smaller amount and, therefore, travels at a slightly higher velocity. Such a relationship permits a velocity profile within the blood vessel which is parabolic in contour and allows each infinitesimal layer to travel with a unique velocity vector, permitting particle-to-particle interactive forces between layers. These interactions are greatest along the circumference of the blood vessel, where velocity gradients between lamina are the greatest, because the particles that flow in the central portion of the lumen are influenced by frictional energy losses to the smallest degree. Accordingly, those blood vessels with diameters that are relatively large transmit blood flow with relatively small frictional energy losses.

While frictional energy losses within large blood vessels are relatively negligible, the smaller-diameter blood vessels in the microcirculation create frictional energy losses that become quite significant, such that the majority of the intraluminal energy (pressure) is dissipated at the level of the arteriole. Poiseuille first noted this phenomenon in the late 1840s. From his observations, he correctly predicted that the pressure gradient that occurs across a vessel varies directly with the flow of blood, the viscosity of the blood, and the length of the tube, and varies inversely with the radius of the vessel. He also noted that the relationship with the radius was non-linear.

Mathematically, this was not solved until 1860, by Haganbach, who correctly expressed the relationship of a pressure gradient to blood flow, fluid viscosity, length of the conduit, and radius of the conduit:

$$\Delta P = 8QL\mu/\pi r^4$$

Where: Q = flow
L = length
μ = viscosity
r = radius

Stated otherwise:

$$\Delta P = Q R$$

Where R = resistance = $8L\mu/\pi r^4$

It should be noted that the Poiseuille–Haganbach equation holds true for an ideal fluid traveling at constant laminar flow in a rigid tube of uniform bore. While blood does indeed function as an ideal fluid in vessels of diameter greater than 100 microns, predicting energy losses during conditions of dynamic flow and within vessels of changing diameter and direction is much more difficult.[15] Predicting frictional losses under these circumstances require the application of differential equations and computational analysis.

From a clinical standpoint, the importance of defining a critical stenosis – that is, a lesion that produces a reduction of perfusion pressure beyond the stenosis – is evident. Previous studies have demonstrated that a lesion of the abdominal aorta does not become hemodynamically significant until 90% cross-sectional luminal narrowing exists. For smaller arteries, such as the iliac, renal, or carotid, hemodynamic significance occurs at smaller cross-sectional luminal narrowing (70–90%). Of particular importance is differentiation between cross-sectional luminal narrowing and percent diameter narrowing. In general, a 50% reduction in diameter narrowing produces a 75% cross-sectional narrowing, and a 66% diameter reduction produces a

90% cross-sectional luminal narrowing. Accordingly, traditional parameters of hemodynamic significance have generally been set at a greater than 60% diameter reduction.

While these parameters provide useful guidelines in predicting hemodynamic consequence, such a definition, based solely upon diameter reduction, is an oversimplification. Additional factors that must be considered include the length of the stenosis, the roughness of the endothelial surface, the flow velocity, and the viscosity of the blood (largely a function of the hemoglobin concentration).

The importance of a conceptual understanding of the Poiseuille–Haganbach equation is evident when contemplating the hemodynamic significance of a stenosis within the dynamics of the circulatory system. The phenomenon of the 'disappearing pulse' is one such example which exists in an individual with classic symptoms of vasculogenic claudication, but who exhibits palpable pulses at rest. In this situation, a brief period of exercise reduces peripheral vascular resistance in the extremity and creates a reactive hyperemia such that the increased velocity across the lesion produces a significant pressure gradient across a previously non-critical lesion, rendering the previously palpable pulse non-palpable. The principle serves as a basis for correct interpretation of the post-exercise ankle brachial index measurement and for intravascular pressure monitoring before and after hyperemic challenge (**Fig. 4.6**).

Approximately 50 years have passed since Dr Leriche described the syndrome that bears his name, for individuals with aortoiliac disease: diminished femoral pulses, buttock claudication, and impotence. However, the clinical distinction between vasculogenic and neurogenic claudication frequently remains difficult. Although one seldom considers numbness of the extremity to be a symptom consistent with vasculogenic claudication, this author has been impressed by the atypical nature of symptoms experienced by individuals who present with focal iliac artery stenoses. A potential explanation for this observation is the change in *distribution of available blood flow* which accompanies periods of exercise in these individuals. That is, during periods of exercise, flow is generally increased to the skeletal muscle through the vasodilatory effect created by the relative muscle ischemia. If such a process occurs distal to a flow-limiting stenosis, the muscle group may *steal* blood both from peripheral nerves and from skin, and produce a transient, ischemic neuropathy which is expressed as numbness or burning of the extremity (**Fig. 4.7**). These symptoms may precede or occur completely independent of classic muscle claudication. These symptoms frequently resolve with either catheter-based or surgical intervention.

While traditional standards that utilize percent of diameter narrowing (>60%) are sufficient in most circumstances, several clinical situations exist in which traditional parameters of hemodynamic significance may not apply. These include conditions in which velocity profiles within the area of stenosis are elevated, and encompass the condition of a moderate-grade iliac stenosis proximal to a femoral-to-femoral bypass and a subclavian stenosis proximal to a patent arteriovenous fistula.[16] In these situations, traditional parameters of hemodynamic significance may not be applicable to lesions of less than 50% diameter reduction. In these cases, we generally rely upon more physiologic measurements of systolic pressure gradients across the lesion rather than angiographic measures of percent luminal narrowing.

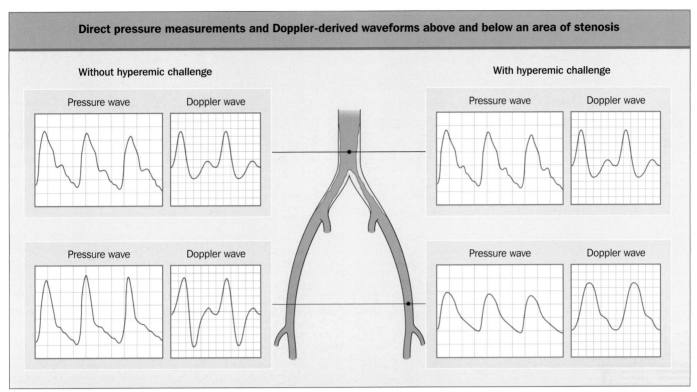

Direct pressure measurements and Doppler-derived waveforms above and below an area of stenosis

Without hyperemic challenge

Pressure wave   Doppler wave

Pressure wave   Doppler wave

With hyperemic challenge

Pressure wave   Doppler wave

Pressure wave   Doppler wave

Figure 4.6 Direct pressure measurements and Doppler-derived waveforms above and below an area of stenosis, with and without hyperemic challenge. Prior to hyperemic challenge, systolic amplification is noted at the level of the femoral artery with attendant retrograde flow in early diastole by Doppler evaluation. After hyperemic challenge, the increased velocity across the stenosis generates a significant pressure gradient that was not previously present. Reduction of systolic amplitude and loss of diastolic notch is evident upon pressure analysis. On duplex ultrasound, prolongation of acceleration time and loss of triphasic waveform are noted.

Frictional energy losses may become more pronounced when blood flow is heterogeneous, creating greater velocity gradients between adjacent lamellae. Such a transition, from laminar to non-laminar flow, occurs as a function of the dimensionless Reynold's number (Re):

Reynold's Number (Re) = $v\rho 2r/\eta$

Where: v = velocity
ρ = density of the fluid
r = radius of the tube
η = fluid viscosity

Turbulent flow occurs when Re exceeds 2000, and produces the physical findings of a bruit or thrill, or the Doppler findings of spectral broadening. In general, the viscosity of blood is approximately 3.5 times that of water and the density of blood is approximately 1.035 times that of water. Because the density and viscosity of blood do not change significantly, the diameter of the blood vessel and the velocity of blood largely dictate the degree of turbulence. From the standpoint of energy conservation, turbulent flow is important because the loss of energy (pressure) that occurs between two points exceeds that which would be expected from the Poiseuille–Haganbach equation. (**Fig. 4.8**).

Within the complexities and dynamics of the circulatory system, additional factors predispose to turbulent flow and turbulence likely occurs at lower Reynold's number values. These include conditions of pulsatile flow, changes in vessel diameter, and changes in vessel direction. Clinical conditions associated with turbulent flow occur at the aortic root after periods of exercise or severe anemia, at the carotid bifurcation, and at the level of an arteriovenous fistula anastomosis. More commonly, flow may become turbulent during only a portion of the cardiac cycle; for example, with blood flow acceleration during the systolic phase.

The area distal to a stenosis is another condition that is predisposed to turbulent flow. As the blood traverses the stenosis, the velocity within the stenosis increases by a factor of the square of the change in radius (e.g. a 50% reduction in diameter produces a fourfold increase in velocity). Beyond the stenosis, the velocity jet enters a blood vessel of normal diameter. The combination of a vessel of large diameter and changing velocity profiles provides circumstances that satisfy Reynold's conditions and results in turbulent flow beyond the area of stenosis (**Fig. 4.9**). This is manifest clinically as a bruit or thrill. The vibrations and energy released from the enhanced particle-to-particle interaction may contribute to the development of post-stenotic dilation.

Kinetic energy

The formula to calculate the kinetic energy of a particle was first described by Newton and is well known. Newton's Law states that kinetic energy is a function of both the mass and the velocity by which the mass travels:

KE = $\frac{1}{2} mv^2$

Under most circumstances, the kinetic energy component of the total energy is relatively small, equivalent to a few millimeters

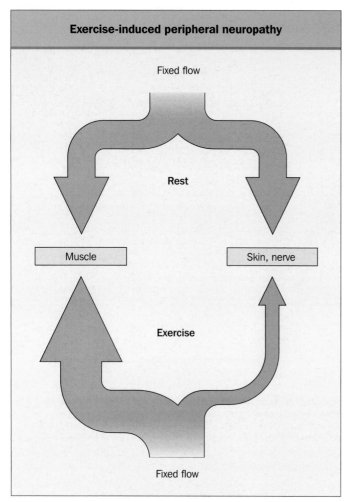

Figure 4.7 **Exercise-induced peripheral neuropathy.** The presence of an inflow stenosis creates a fixed blood flow which is available for distribution to the various components of the extremity. At rest, the metabolic requirements of all organs are satisfied. However, during periods of exercise, the combination of a fixed inflow and a greatly reduced resistance within the muscle creates a steal which temporarily deprives the peripheral nerves from resting metabolic requirements. This scenario is most frequently observed in a person with an iliac stenosis, owing to the large muscle mass supplied by the diseased iliac artery. Patients who suffer this form of claudication experience numbness and burning sensations, and it is frequently confused with nerve-root compression syndromes.

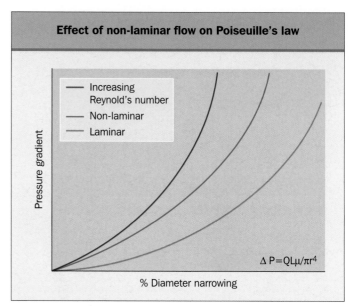

Figure 4.8 **Effect of non-laminar flow on Poiseuille's Law.** The increased heterogeneity of flow increases the hemodynamic significance of a lesion, generating pressure gradients which exceed those that would have otherwise been predicted.

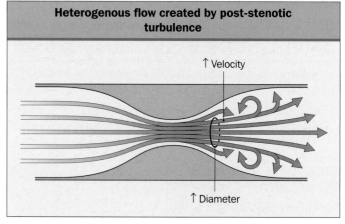

Figure 4.9 **Heterogenous flow created by post-stenotic turbulence.** Immediately beyond the stenosis, the relatively large velocity vectors which emerge from the stenosis occur within the confines of a normal blood vessel diameter and satisfies Reynold's criteria for turbulence.

of mercury. The density, or mass of the blood, does not vary, and, therefore, all changes in kinetic energy can be attributed to changes in blood flow velocity.

Returning to Bernoulli's principle of conservation of energy, it is noted that during conditions of constant flow, as blood enters an area of stenosis, the velocity must increase by the square of the inverse change of the radius.

$$\Delta v = (1/\Delta r)^2$$

In such a case, even relatively small changes in radius generate significant changes in velocity. Assuming no changes in gravitational or frictional energies occur, Bernoulli's Law implies that the hydrostatic pressure in the region of the stenosis must be smaller than the pressure in the more proximal portion (**Fig. 4.10**).

Bernoulli's principle provides the basis for understanding the Venturi effect, the airfoil, and has supplied an explanation for

the measure of negative pressures within the anastomosis of arteriovenous fistula.[17]

In terms of application of Bernoulli's principle to vascular surgery, the most pertinent area relates to that of the natural history of aortic dissection. In most patients, a discrete entry point generates a false lumen between the inner two-thirds and the outer third of the media. In cases in which the false lumen fails to re-enter the true lumen, a blind cul-de-sac is formed, which promotes the propagation of the dissection. To be more specific, although both the true lumen and false lumen are presented with systemic pressures in early systole, the higher blood flow velocity in the true lumen (compared with that in the false lumen) generates a transmural pressure gradient between the true and false lumens (as defined by Bernoulli's principle of conservation of energy). The lower pressure in the true lumen causes it to collapse in deference to the sustained pressures in

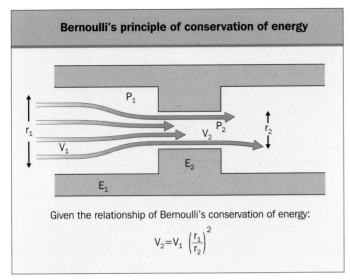

Bernoulli's principle of conservation of energy

Given the relationship of Bernoulli's conservation of energy:

$$V_2 = V_1 \left(\frac{r_1}{r_2}\right)^2$$

Figure 4.10 Bernoulli's principle of conservation of energy. Due to the increased velocity and increase in kinetic energy within an area of stenosis, Bernoulli's Law dictates that the pressure within the area of stenosis must decrease relative to that in the area of larger diameter.

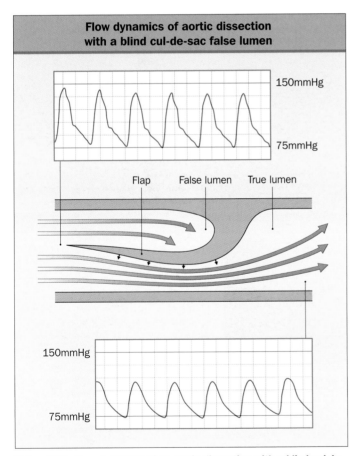

Flow dynamics of aortic dissection with a blind cul-de-sac false lumen

Figure 4.11 Flow dynamics of an aortic dissection with a blind cul-de-sac false lumen. The increased flow velocity through the true lumen generates significant kinetic energy that does not exist within the false lumen. Bernoulli's Law dictates that the loss of kinetic energy in the false lumen must create a higher pressure in order to preserve total energy. The resultant pressure gradient that develops between the true lumen and the false lumen further 'draws' the dissection flap into the true lumen, thereby reducing the distal perfusion. From a physiologic standpoint, the true lumen is generally the smaller of the two lumens and possesses a lower pressure.

the false lumen (**Fig. 4.11**). As the problem progresses, the true lumen collapses further, generating abnormally higher velocities in the true lumen and exacerbating the gradient further. At some point, the true lumen becomes compromised to the degree that distal ischemia ensues. In these cases, we favor early fenestration of the false channel to normalize pressure gradients between the two lumens.

In cases in which re-entry of the false lumen has occurred, and post fenestration, the distal ischemic symptoms are generally relieved, but the individual is left with a double-barrel aorta. The outer wall of the false lumen contains only the outer third of the media and the adventitia. If one recalls the vessel wall mechanics discussed earlier, the greatly reduced vessel wall thickness requires that the wall must expand along its new compliance curve until it reaches a diameter which generates sufficient wall tension to oppose the intramural pressure. Hence, strict control of intravascular pressure remains paramount in preventing chronic aneurysmal degeneration of the false lumen.

Shear stress and atherosclerosis

The distinctive pattern of atherosclerotic plaque distribution is well known to practicing vascular surgeons. These areas include, among others, the carotid bifurcation, the terminal aorta, and the superficial femoral artery. Remarkably, despite the marked extent of disease that afflicts these areas, the more distal blood vessel is often paradoxically free of disease. Of particular note is the dramatically focal distribution of atherosclerosis in the region of the carotid bifurcation and the predictable absence of disease in the more distal internal carotid artery.[18] Recognizing such a focal pattern of disease has permitted vascular surgeons to safely offer patients surgical endarterectomy of such lesions without prior invasive imaging of the more distal circulation.[19]

Although systemic risk factors are involved in the development of arterial diseases, local flow-induced arterial wall forces also play a major role. While multiple hypotheses have been proposed to account for these unique distribution patterns, knowledge of blood flow shear stress on blood vessel walls has led to the hypothesis that fluid dynamics significantly contribute to localizing atherosclerotic factors.

Shear stress is defined as the cumulative tangential drag generated upon the blood vessel wall as blood flows over the endothelial surface. It may be calculated by the Poiseuille equation:[20]

$$\omega = 4\eta Q / \pi r^3$$

Where: ω = shear stress
η = blood viscosity
Q = blood flow
r = radius of the vessel

Thus, for a given rate of blood flow, the most significant contribution to change in shear stress is related to changes in vessel radius.

The effect of fluid shear forces upon the blood vessel wall was first noted by Donald Fry, who demonstrated an increased permeability within endothelial cells that are subjected to varying shear stress.[21] When pulsatile flow in an arterial segment is smooth and undisturbed, the probability of platelet activation, the development of intimal hyperplasia, or the deposition of atherosclerosis remains small. However, varying blood vessel diameter, blood vessel tortuosity, and points of bifurcation produce changes in mural blood flow velocity, which generate abnormal and altering shear stress values. Recently, it has been noted that this varying shear stress triggers the endothelial cell to release prostaglandins, which stimulate the underlying smooth muscle cells.[22]

While investigators initially proposed that areas of high shear stress were thought to be injurious, it was later proven that under conditions of *abnormally low shear stress* or in *regions of high shear stress gradients*, arteries were predisposed to the development of myointimal hyperplasia and accelerated arteriosclerosis.[23] Such conditions are caused by low-amplitude velocity oscillations of fluid adjacent to the blood vessel wall. These locations exist in regions of flow separation, with down-stream vortex formation, and predispose to prolonged particle residence times, exposing the luminal surface to circulating atherogenic agents for prolonged intervals (**Fig. 4.12**). Accordingly, anatomic conditions that predispose to abnormal shear stress exist in areas of blood vessel bifurcations or branch points, and in regions of blood vessel anastomoses.

The infrarenal abdominal aorta may be particularly prone to the development of atherosclerosis based upon relatively low shear stress values. Because a high percentage of blood delivered to the abdominal aorta is diverted to the visceral and the renal arteries, the volume of blood flow delivered to the infrarenal aorta is significantly diminished. Additionally, because the blood flow velocity of the infrarenal segment is dependent upon the muscular activity of the lower extremities, an increasingly sedentary lifestyle may further predispose one to low shear stress and accelerated atherosclerosis in this segment of artery. Finally, the slowly degenerative process of both collagen and elastin fibers within the wall of the aorta predispose this segment

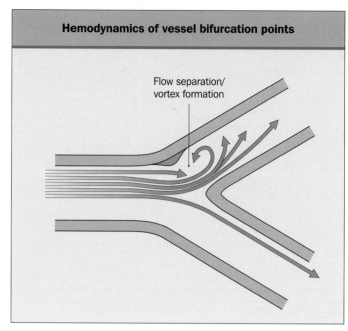

Figure 4.12 Hemodynamics of vessel bifurcation points. A branch point or bifurcation of a blood vessel creates areas of flow separation and vortex formation in the area distal to the bifurcation. The oscillating and low-amplitude shear stress in these regions predispose to increased particle residence times, which may result in more substantial platelet–endothelial interaction and, ultimately, accelerated atherosclerosis.

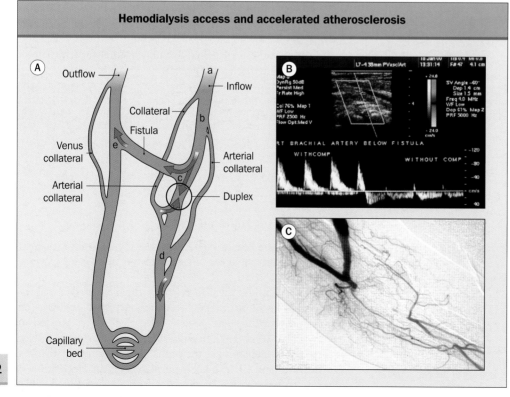

Figure 4.13 Hemodialysis access and accelerated atherosclerosis. The unique flow characteristics of the artery distal to a patent arteriovenous fistula create flow dynamics that may predispose the artery to accelerated atherosclerosis (A). As noted in the duplex ultrasound of the artery distal to the fistula (B), flow may be antegrade in systole, and largely retrograde in diastole. The to-and-fro blood flow may predispose to accelerated atherosclerosis in this segment of artery. In persons who develop the ischemic steal syndrome after hemodialysis access, this area seems to be a favorite location for progression of disease (C). Because the symptoms tend to be progressive in those who develop the chronic form of the ischemic steal syndrome, early intervention is warranted.

to increase in diameter, and, in many cases, permit aneurysmal degeneration. This increase in luminal diameter further diminishes mural shear stress to levels that provide further opportunity for accelerated atherogenesis. Thus, although the etiology of aneurysm genesis is frequently quoted as secondary to atherosclerosis, the above provides us a more plausible relationship that atherosclerosis is likely a secondary phenomenon that ensues aneurysm formation.

Additionally, shear forces appear to be important in the maintenance of blood vessel luminal diameter.[20] For example, adaptation occurs in a blood vessel upstream from an arteriovenous fistula. The decreased resistance generated by the arteriovenous fistula dramatically increases blood flow velocity in the donor artery, which increases the mural shear stress. Such an increase in mural shear stress is sensed by the endothelial cell and causes the blood vessel to dilate in attempt to normalize its shear stress.[24] Due to the conditions defined by the Poiseuille–Hagenbach equation, shear stress (ω) varies directly with an increase in blood flow, and inversely to the third power with change of radius. Thus, under conditions of constant flow, a twofold increase in blood vessel diameter would accommodate an increased blood flow of eightfold. A similar situation arises in positions of increased flow in a collateral vessel which dilates in attempt to compensate for increased flow around an obstructed artery.

Conversely, reduction in shear stress secondary to reduced blood flow has been noted to stimulate reduction in arterial diameter in an attempt to normalize the shear stress. One example of such a process involves an artery distal to an arteriovenous fistula, which has been noted to chronically reduce luminal diameter. Even in the face of reduced distal perfusion pressure, such as in the case of persons with the ischemic steal syndrome, the oscillating shear stress in the artery distal to the fistula may predispose to accelerated atherosclerosis and may exacerbate the ischemic steal syndrome after hemodialysis access procedures (**Fig. 4.13**).[25] Likewise, donor arteries to amputated or atrophic limbs have been noted to have a reduced diameter when compared with those supplying a normal contralateral limb.

REFERENCES

1. Pearcy L. Galen's pergamum. Archaeology 1985;38:33–9.
2. Harrison WC. Dr. William Harvey and the discovery of circulation. New York:MacMillan; 1967.
3. Newton I. The principia. Motte A, translator. New York:Prometheus; 1995.
4. Strandness DE, Sumner DS. Hemodynamics for surgeons. New York:Grune & Statton; 1975.
5. McDonald DA. Blood flow in arteries, 2nd edn. Baltimore, MD:Williams & Wilkins; 1974.
6. Nichols WW, O'Rourke MF. McDonald's blood flow in arteries. Philadelphia, PA:Lua & Febiger; 1990.
7. Lee BY, Trainor FS. Peripheral vascular surgery: hemodynamics of arterial pulsatile blood flow. New York:Meredith Corporation; 1973.
8. Krafka JJ. Comparative study of the histo-physics of the aorta. Am J Physiol 1939;125:1–14.
9. Ayer JP, Hass GM, Philpott DE. Aortic elastic tissue: isolation with use of formic acid and discussion of some of its properties. AMA Arch Pathol 1958;65:519–44.
10. Fischer GM, Llaurado JG. Collagen and elastin content in canine arteries selected from functionally different vascular beds. Circ Res 1966;19:394–9.
11. Dobrin PB, Baker WH, Gley WC. Elastolytic and collagenolytic studies of arteries: implications for the mechanical properties of aneurysms. Arch Surg 1984;119:405–9.
12. Tromholt N, Jorgensen SJ, Hesse B, et al. In vivo demonstration of focal fibrinolytic activity in abdominal aortic aneurysms. Eur J Vasc Surg 1993;7:675–9.
13. Wolf YG, Thomas WS, Brennan RJ, et al. CT findings associated with rapid expansion of abdominal aortic aneurysms. J Vasc Surg 1994; 20:529–35; discussion 596–7.
14. Fishman AP, Richards DW. Circulation of the blood: men and ideas. New York:Oxford University Press; 1964.
15. Wormersley JR. Method for the calculation of velocity, rate of flow and viscous drag in arteries when the pressure gradient is known. J Physiol 1955;127:553–62.
16. Wixon CL, Mills JL, Berman SS. Distal revascularization-interval ligation for maintenance of dialysis access in ischemic steal syndrome. Semin Vasc Surg 2000;13:77–82.
17. Holman E. The anatomic and physiologic effects of an arteriovenous fistula. Surgery 1940;8:362–5.
18. Zarins CK, Giddens DP, Bharadvaj BK, et al. Carotid bifurcation atherosclerosis: quantitative correlation of plaque localization with flow velocity profiles and wall shear stress. Circ Res 1983;53:502–14.
19. Golledge J, Ellis M, Sabharwal T, et al. Selection of patients for carotid endarterectomy. J Vasc Surg 1999;30:122–30.
20. Zarins CK, Zatina MA, Giddens DP, et al. Shear stress regulation of artery lumen diameter in experimental atherogenesis. J Vasc Surg 1987; 5:413–20.
21. Fry DL. Acute vascular endothelial changes associated with the increased blood velocity gradients. Circ Res 1967;22:165–97.
22. Koller A, Sun D, Kaley G. Role of shear stress and endothelial prostaglandins in flow- and viscosity-induced dilation of arterioles in vitro. Circ Res 1993;70:123–30.
23. Friedman MH, Hutchins GM, Borgesson C, et al. Correlation of human arterial morphology with hemodynamic measurements in arterial casts. Atherosclerosis 1981;39:425–36.
24. Schumacker HB. Aneurysm development and degenerative changes in dilated artery proximal to arteriovenous fistulae. Surg Gynecol Obstet 1970;130:636–40.
25. Wixon CL, Hughes JD, Mills JL. Understanding strategies for the treatment of vascular steal syndromes. J Am Coll Surg 2000;191:301–10.

CHAPTER
5
Evidence-Based Medicine: Basic Concepts, Population Dynamics, Outcomes Analysis

John V White and Ginger Barthel

KEY POINTS

- Despite the use of rigorous methodologies, the value of trials may be limited if results are applied inappropriately.

- The case report, as a method for communicating outcomes, has limitations due to lack of an established research protocol and the high likelihood of investigator bias.

- Case control studies provide well-defined inclusion/exclusion criteria as well as consecutive patients with matches criteria, yielding information which can be applied to the community at large.

- Randomized, prospective, blinded clinical trials provide the strongest link between cause and effect and the presence or absence of differences produced by the treatment modality.

- Meta-analysis utilizes data from carefully selected, previously published studies to produce a rigorous systematic, and quantitative review of available information.

- Markov analysis is a computer-based analytic tool used to determine whether, in a sequence of events, one event is related to another, such as treatment to outcome.

- Monte Carlo simulation is a computer tool that attempts to use probabilities for the occurrence of events to predict outcomes.

- Validated generic quality of life survey instruments have value in assessing overall health status.

- Disease-specific questionnaires are focused upon the patient's underlying disease, its impact on general health, and the benefit and adverse effects of the treatment.

- Not all published data is equivalent and it is essential for the surgeon to recognize the strength of the evidence presented in a report prior to incorporating that diagnostic or therapeutic modality in the realm of patient care.

"Every hospital should follow every patient it treats long enough to determine whether the treatment has been successful, and then to inquire 'if not why not' with a view to preventing similar failures in the future."

Ernest Codman, MD, 1914

INTRODUCTION

Surgery is a specialty of inherent complexities. It represents an attempt to alter anatomy in order to effect a change in physiology. Among the many surgical specialties, vascular surgery is a relatively young field. Born slightly more than 50 years ago with the development of the synthetic vascular graft by Voorhees and colleagues, it evolved almost coincident with the vascular laboratory.[1,2] This conjoined progression has provided a scientific basis for vascular diagnosis and treatment. Vascular surgery, however, is a dynamic field. The productivity of clinical and basic research programs continues to increase and breakthroughs are reported on a daily basis. As such, appropriate patient care practice requires that all surgeons continually renew and refine both their cognitive and technical skills. Outdated diagnostic and therapeutic endeavors must be eliminated and new modalities must be embraced, even at the expense of requiring the mastery of additional skills.

The bigger challenge, however, is for outcomes to report not only the technical results but also the patient benefits derived from the intervention. Proceeding on the basis of sound scientific evidence assures both the surgeon and patient of the potential value of any diagnostic or therapeutic intervention. This is the goal of evidence-based medicine; and while the concept is not new, it is increasingly important.[3]

The current system of evidence-based medicine is the result of the convictions of Ernest Codman, MD, who served as the catalyst of these efforts most effectively at the start of the last century.[4] A graduate of Harvard Medical School in 1885, Dr Codman became a member of the Harvard Medical School faculty and a surgeon at the Massachusetts General Hospital after graduation. Shortly thereafter, he became concerned about the results of surgical procedures and pushed for a system that analyzed patient outcomes and surgeon competency. While this effort, unfortunately, cost him his position on the Harvard faculty, it did initiate a groundswell of activity that has led to the formation of numerous organizations to ensure higher standards of care. Agencies such as the Joint Commission on Accreditation of Healthcare Organizations (JCAHO), specialty societies, and the Agency for Healthcare Research and Quality (AHRQ) all function as oversight bodies and are able to facilitate the dissemination of evidence-based recommendations, as has been done through clinical guidelines.[5]

These types of agencies are not, however, in a position to bring about the transition needed to obtain the highest level of medical practice that these guidelines recommend.[6] The actual practice of evidence-based medicine must be derived from a widespread effort among practitioners. To accomplish this, physicians need to become familiar with the process of evidence-based practice.

RESEARCH METHODOLOGIES AND DATA COLLECTION

The process of delivering evidence-based medical care requires that the physician continuously seek the most appropriate diagnostic and therapeutic interventions for a given patient. Utilizing the best available literature, data regarding diagnosis and treatment are gathered and critically evaluated. Conclusions about the best approach to patient care are developed and applied to the care of the patient. The process is one of continuous learning and quality improvement. In order to incorporate evidence-based practice into patient care, surgeons must be familiar not only with current data but also with the strength of the data and the manner in which it can be appropriately applied.

There are both primary and secondary types of studies that provide appropriate clinical data applicable to the care of patients (**Table 5.1**). Primary studies are largely observational or experimental studies that directly involve patients. *Observational studies* provide insight into the natural history of a disease process and may suggest potential causative factors or diagnostic or therapeutic targets. *Experimental studies* involve a collaborative effort between patients and investigators, either prospectively or retrospectively. *Secondary studies* reassess appropriate published data through rigorous systematic processes, such as meta-analysis or computer simulation.

Though frequently disputed, each of these forms of clinical research can be of significant value to the surgeon when the information reported is clearly understood and appropriately applied. In surgery, the need for a wider variety of research methodology stems from the fact that surgical specialties have the added dimension of surgical skills, which impact directly upon diagnostic and therapeutic modalities.

The act of surgery creates inherent difficulties in the performance of surgical clinical research. Pharmacologic studies, for example, are designed to evaluate a new treatment that is generally well matched to the disease. The response to the treatment may be directly assessed and compared with a control group in a randomized, blinded, and prospective manner. Drug administration procedures are well defined and expected blood levels of the target medication are often achieved. The specific outcomes of the study are related to the effectiveness of the drug. The evaluation of vascular surgical technology and techniques, however, is based upon not only the patient's pathophysiology and co-morbid conditions but also upon numerous other variables. These include patient collaboration, surgical judgment, and unquantified physiologic modifiers.[7]

Patient collaboration may be difficult in studies comparing open vascular surgery to less invasive treatments. Surgical judgment may impact upon the interpretation of inclusion and exclusion criteria. Unquantified physiologic modifiers, such as anatomic variation, distal vasculature, differences of vascular wall architecture and biology, and hemostatic mechanisms, may alter the conduct of a vascular intervention. Each of these can independently change the outcome of a surgical procedure and make the performance of surgical research more challenging than that in non-surgical specialties.[8]

Case reports

Surgeons utilize case reports as one of the basic methods of communication for outcomes. This may be due to the great spectrum of patient physiologic states that must be considered when applying a surgical intervention. The case report generally consists of selective retrospective information regarding the diagnosis and/or treatment of a small group of patients. Inclusion and exclusion criteria for the study group are infrequently established. There is no control group provided for comparison. The report focuses on a small aspect of the course of the patient's illness and treatment. The brief communication is often coupled with an overview of available literature to place the patient information into the appropriate context. There is often a significant amount of investigator bias present in these reports as a result of limitations in the amount and type of patient information set forth in a small group of patients. It is now recognized that the opinion of recognized clinical experts, once considered the most valuable form of scientific information, may be misleading by preventing alternative interpretations of data.[9] Therefore, the utility of case reports in assisting a surgeon to develop appropriate evidence-based patient care plans is quite limited.

The case report, however, has not been rendered useless. Its value lies in the communication of a surgical technique or a benefit or adverse effect of a treatment not well detailed in previous studies. It also serves to identify unquantified physiologic modifiers that may impact upon outcome. In light of inherent biases, however, the conclusion of a case report should not be directly applied to patient care. It should serve only to stimulate the development of questions or hypotheses regarding a given diagnostic or therapeutic modality and lead to greater data collection or the organization of appropriate clinical trials.

Case-control study

A second form of observational study methodology is the case-control study. This form of study methodology provides insight into a disease by comparing patients with the disorder to matched controls from the same population of patients. In case-control investigations, the criteria for inclusion into the study group are well defined and consecutive patients meeting those criteria are entered. This is true whether the study is prospective or retro-

Types and characteristics of commonly used clinical research methods.		
	Controls	*Likelihood of bias*
Observational studies:		
Case reports	No	High
Case-control study	Yes	Moderate
Cohort study	Yes	Moderate
Experimental studies:		
Non-randomized clinical trials	Yes	Moderate
Randomized, prospective clinical trials	Yes	Low
Secondary (computer-based) studies:		
Meta-analysis	Yes	Low*
Markov analysis	Yes	Low*
Monte Carlo simulation	Yes	Low*
*Dependent upon data selection criteria.		

Table 5.1 Types and characteristics of commonly used clinical research methods.

spective, using large databases such as hospital logs. Controls are selected from a pool of candidates, according to the match parameters, and, therefore, are not consecutive or randomized for inclusion into the protocol. The specific parameters used to create the match are based upon the control variables of the disease. The match should use patient characteristics or descriptors that need to be controlled but are not the subject of the study.[10] Age, gender, ethnic background, and race are often used as matching criteria. For example, to study the impact of diabetes upon lower extremity arterial occlusive disease in men, a group of age-matched men might be used as the control group. The target group and the controls may be selected from a hospital log that has been chronologically defined. The use of hospital logs is an acceptable method for identifying patients and controls because it can be assumed that the two groups were derived from the same general community and the quality of information is equivalent. Therefore, observations made regarding this group of patients should apply to the community at large. The study methodology is somewhat limited by the fact that the controls are selected by specific variables, as interpreted by the investigators, and this may bias the results.

Cohort study

The cohort study is another form of investigation based upon observation and is a useful epidemiological tool. The goal of this methodology is to describe the natural history of a disease or its treatment over time, or to analyze the relationships between risk factors and the disease or its response to some intervention.[11] The Framingham study of coronary disease represents a large cohort study designed to examine the natural history of coronary artery disease and its associated risk factors.[12] This methodology differs from the case-control study in that a target group of patients is compared to equivalently evaluated controls. One of the advantages of a *retrospective cohort study* is that the time course of significant events in the natural history of the disease can be easily identified. The weakness of the retrospective study, however, is that the acquisition of data is limited to that which is available from the database. No additional information of interest can be collected. The *prospective cohort study* provides a powerful tool for observation of a disease or its response to treatment. The control population is selected by the same specific inclusion and exclusion criteria used to identify the target population so that there is less likelihood of investigator bias than in case-control studies.

Randomized clinical trial

The randomized prospective clinical trial has long been considered the optimal method for detecting the presence or absence of differences produced by a new diagnostic or therapeutic modality.[13] A randomized clinical trial provides the strongest link between cause and effect. The most effective methodology for this type of study is the prospective, randomized, double-blinded study.[14] Randomization helps to ensure that the groups of patients allocated to different diagnostic or therapeutic regimens are comparable, and can most effectively limit the impact of investigator bias on the results of the study. Ideally, the study is conducted so that neither the investigators nor the patients are aware of which group contains which patients. While this is possible for some diagnostic and some pharmaceutical studies, it is difficult for many studies comparing new therapeutic

technology or techniques, especially those that compare open with less invasive procedures for the treatment of patients with vascular disease.

Despite the statistical power of the large, randomized, prospective study, there are many well-recognized limitations.[15] The inclusion of only specialized sites of treatment may yield clear results on efficacy but not on effectiveness. Efficacy is defined as the performance of a diagnostic or therapeutic endeavor under carefully controlled conditions, such as FDA trials, while effectiveness is the performance of that test or intervention when broadly applied to the community at large.[16] There may be significant differences in the two parameters. Though a retrospective, large database study and not a randomized, prospective trial, Kempczinski and colleagues clearly demonstrated the differences in these two concepts. Evaluating the performance of carotid endarterectomy in the community, they found that the combined morbidity and mortality of this procedure was significantly different in community hospitals (effectiveness) compared with university centers (efficacy).[17]

Large randomized experimental studies are quite time-consuming and costly. The development of a detailed protocol for the conduct of the study and the collection of data may require years. During this time, improved diagnostic and therapeutic regimens may be developed which render the impact of the study limited. This was true, for example, with the Asymptomatic Carotid Atherosclerosis Study.[18,19] The study randomized patients with a 50% or greater stenosis of the carotid artery to surgery or medical therapy. No stratification of degree of stenosis was made. After the onset of data collection in this randomized study, methods for the improved non-invasive detection and quantification of carotid artery stenoses were developed and subsets of patients with differing degrees of stenosis could more easily be identified. Since the methodology of the study was set and could not be changed, the study was conducted with less than ideal diagnostic criteria, limiting the value of the study. Though the surgical group demonstrated a reduction in ipsilateral neurologic events, there was no reduction in the combined endpoint of stroke and death.

Inclusion and exclusion criteria for patient enrollment in a randomized study can also be controversial.[20] Broad inclusion criteria permit the rapid enrollment of large numbers of patients who may be dissimilar, whereas definitive exclusion criteria may slow enrollment but can endure the comparability of the patients. Additionally, patient cooperation may decrease over time. Many patients prefer the option to choose their own form of treatment even if the scientific basis for that treatment may not be solidly established.

Secondary study design

Meta-analysis is an analytical tool that permits the evaluation of a diagnostic or therapeutic modality through the appropriate use of previously published smaller studies.[21] Meta-analysis is *not* the simple pooling of data reported in numerous small studies, a notion that has caused frequent investigational errors. The simple pooling of data from multiple small studies often compounds biases and may further reduce the ability to detect important differences between study groups.[22] A meta-analysis of available data is a rigorous, systematic, and quantitative review. In order to undertake a meta-analysis to address a research question or hypothesis, the investigator must first define the appropriate study population and methodology criteria. The literature is then exhaustively reviewed for the identification of all relevant studies that meet the established criteria. These studies are then critically evaluated to determine and correct for possible bias in data collection. Reports in which data collection did not adhere to the established meta-analysis criteria or in which an unquantified bias was introduced are not included. The raw data from the selected smaller studies are then combined and analyzed. This methodology permits the detection of statistically significant differences between study groups that may not have been possible in the individual reports due to the enrollment of a small number of patients.

Computer analysis and simulation

A *Markov analysis* is a computer-based analysis designed to determine whether one event is related to another in a sequence of events. It can analyze the likelihood of future changes in health states of a person or population.[23] A state transition diagram is created which lists all of the possible health state transitions after an event.[24] The probability of each health state transition is entered into the computer. Though it would be possible to hand calculate the health state transitions after a single event, calculations become more complex with each change in health state. The Markov analysis will identify the likelihood of future changes in health states. For example, the possible health states after lower extremity bypass include an improvement in health, a worsening of health, or death. It may be possible to predict the likelihood after a bypass through manual calculations. Adding another event, such as angioplasty after failure of a bypass, will add another series of outcomes and probabilities in health state transitions. The incremental complexities are easily handled through Markov analysis. A well-performed analysis provides excellent insight into outcomes and is a valuable tool for extending the impact of available data. For example, Michaels & Galland used Markov analysis to determine the best approach for treatment of patients with popliteal aneurysms.[25] The study concluded that the best therapeutic plan is elective resection, which produces better results 1–2 years after presentation than does conservative management. The authors noted that the values of the rate of development of symptoms, limb loss, and mortality were crucial in determining the outcome of the analysis.

A *Monte Carlo simulation* is a computer tool that attempts to simulate possible real-life outcomes by randomly selecting from a range of acceptable values for several variables and predicting final outcomes.[26] The simulation calculates numerous outcome scenarios, rather than just one, and the probabilities of obtaining that outcome. The use of multiple probabilities makes simple hand calculations difficult or impossible. Because this computer analytical tool and Markov analysis use probabilities obtained from acceptable studies reported in the literature, they provide excellent methods for evaluating treatments and technologies.

LEVELS OF EVIDENCE AND DATA ANALYSIS

In order to ensure that patient care decisions are made based upon the strongest available evidence, physicians must be able to identify the best studies. This is, perhaps, the greatest challenge of evidence-based medicine. The escalating volume of literature has made the acquisition of needed information more difficult. Important and vital advances in patient care can become buried

	Table 5.2 Levels of evidence.	
I	Evidence obtained from at least one properly randomized controlled trial
II-1	Evidence obtained from well-designed controlled trials without randomization
II-2	Evidence obtained from well-designed cohort or case-control analytic studies, preferably from more than one center or research group
II-3	Evidence obtained from comparisons between times or places with or without the intervention; dramatic results in uncontrolled experiments could also be included in this category
III	Opinions of respected authorities, based on clinical experience, descriptive studies, or reports of expert committees

Table 5.2 Levels of evidence.

in mounds of literature that are of limited value, if any at all. This has led to a significant effort to evaluate scientific publications on the strength of their hypothesis, methodology, data analysis, and conclusions.[27] Though there remains considerable controversy about optimal methods for establishing the strength of data contained in a publication, most have adopted some variation of the levels of evidence set forth by the Canadian Task Force on the Periodic Health Examination (**Table 5.2**).[28]

It has generally been accepted that the randomized, controlled trial is the best method for identifying the presence or absence of differences between treatment effects with least investigator bias. This concept stems from a landmark publication by Sacks and colleagues, which reported that observational studies were far more likely to identify the new or target treatment to be effective than were randomized, controlled studies.[29] There is more recent evidence, however, that this may not be true. Comparisons between the findings of observational (case-control and cohort) and randomized trials evaluating the type of anesthesia used for carotid endarterectomy, for example, have demonstrated that observational studies do not overestimate the treatment effect.[30]

The findings of these studies are important to the future of evidence-based surgery. Many surgical techniques cannot be appropriately tested in randomized clinical trials.[31] Observational studies may be more suitable for emergency treatments or those comparing disparate therapies, such as aortic stent-grafting versus open aneurysm repair. Therefore, the evaluation of a diagnostic test or the indications for treatment may best be tested in large, randomized, prospective studies. Surgical technology and techniques may be better assessed through large observational studies, such as case-cohort studies.

Vascular surgeons must be aware of the available evidence, its strength, and the appropriate application of the evidence, to care for the individual patient. Even with the use of rigorous methodologies, the value of trials may be limited if physicians inappropriately apply the results. Carotid endarterectomy has been one of the most rigorously evaluated vascular surgical interventions. As the technique of endarterectomy became standardized and results improved, the procedure was performed with increasing frequency. Nevertheless, after the results of the randomized, prospective trial on extracranial-intracranial bypass

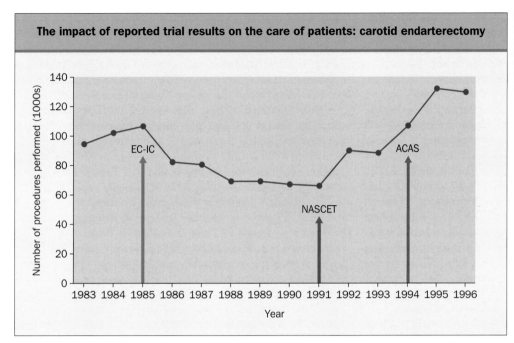

Figure 5.1 The impact of reported trial results on the care of patients: carotid endarterectomy. ACAS, Asymptomatic Carotid Atherosclerosis Study; EC-IC, extracranial-intracranial bypass study; NASCET, North American Symptomatic Carotid Endarterectomy Trial.

failed to demonstrate benefit to that procedure, physicians too referred fewer patients for extracranial carotid endarterectomy.[32,33] This represents the inappropriate extrapolation of the results of the study. To more directly evaluate carotid endarterectomy, vascular surgeons and neurologists organized the North American Symptomatic Carotid Endarterectomy Trial.[34] This well-designed and well-executed trial clearly demonstrated the benefit of the surgical procedure in a subset of patients. This resulted in an increase in referrals of patients for carotid endarterectomy, with procedures increasing 3.4% per month for the first 6 months after the release of the data (**Fig. 5.1**).[35] After the release of the Asymptomatic Carotid Atherosclerosis Study data, the endarterectomy rate increased 7.3% over the first 7 months.

Despite the completion of more than seven major trials, the indications for carotid endarterectomy remain somewhat controversial (**Table 5.3**).[36] This may be due to the fact that no trial is flawless and no data analysis and interpretation beyond question. The application of evidence is rarely uniform among all practitioners. This may be the result of regional differences in patient populations, the availability of services or specialists.[37] Finally, the results of the major trials indicate that validity of the data is dependent upon the achievement of a low morbidity and mortality rate. This suggests that each surgeon must assess his or her own skills when applying such information to specific patients.

Outcomes assessment

The performance of large clinical trials or epidemiological studies and significant levels of evidence will not provide an accurate assessment of appropriate patient care. Perhaps as important as the type of clinical trial is the recording of meaningful outcomes. The adequacy of patient treatment cannot be described only in terms of graft patency, morbidity, and mortality. The ultimate value of a therapeutic intervention is its ability to improve a patient's quality of life and personal productivity. Though it is generally presumed that complete cure of the patient's disease

Indications for carotid endarterectomy.
Best indications
• Stenosis ≥70%
• Overall good general health
• Hemispheric transient ischemic attacks
• Tandem extracranial and intracranial occlusive lesions
• Evidence for lack of collateral vessels
Acceptable indications but with higher risk
• Widespread leukoaraiosis
• Contralateral internal carotid artery occlusion
• Intraluminal thrombus
Acceptable indications but with lesser benefit
• Lacunar stroke
• Nearly occluded internal carotid artery

Table 5.3 Indications for carotid endarterectomy. Leukoaraiosis: bilateral patchy or diffuse areas of low attenuation on CT or hyperintense T2 MR areas.[77]

will do this, few vascular procedures directly impact the underlying arterial occlusive or aneurysmal process. Endarterectomy, reconstruction, and revascularization procedures do little to reduce the progress of the underlying atherosclerotic occlusive disease. Both recurrent and progressive distal atherosclerosis can reduce the hemodynamic benefit of vascular intervention.[38–40] Life expectancy of patients with lower extremity ischemia remains severely reduced despite successful revascularization and the maintenance of a patent graft.[41,42] Similarly, aneurysm repair does not alter the metabolic pathways that weaken the aortic wall. Growth of the aneurysm neck and recurrent aneurysm formation has been demonstrated for patients treated with either open surgery or aortic stent-graft placement.[43,44]

Vascular procedures, then, are designed to reduce the complications of arterial and venous diseases and to improve the quality of the patient's life rather than directly impact upon the disease processes. Appropriate assessment of vascular interventions and proof of their benefit, therefore, requires evaluation of not only the technical outcomes but also the impact upon the patient's quality of life. This perspective was stressed by the United States Congress when it created the Agency for Health Care Policy and Research, now known as the Agency for Healthcare Research and Quality (AHRQ), in 1989.[45] Since that time, a significant effort has been devoted to developing methods to better assess the outcomes of diagnostic and therapeutic interventions. The AHRQ emphasizes that treatments should be evaluated on the basis of outcomes that directly affect the patient, such as physical functioning, pain, and psychological well-being, rather than on the basis of intermediate parameters, such as laboratory tests.[46]

The need for more complete outcomes assessment is clear. There is a mounting body of evidence that vascular laboratory values do not accurately describe the impact of the disease upon the patient. Feinglass and associates assessed the ankle–brachial index (ABI) and patient-reported limitations in 555 patients with lower limb ischemia.[47] They noted only a modest correlation between these two sets of data. Many patients with significant reductions in ABI to the range of 0.4–0.6 experienced minimal limitations on their daily activities whereas many patients with ABI values in the range of 0.8–0.9 felt they were very limited. Similar findings were reported by Chetter and colleagues, who evaluated 235 patients with lower limb ischemia by means of ABI measurement, treadmill walking distance, and a survey on quality of life.[48] They found that increasing ischemia was associated with worsening quality of life but that the correlation of laboratory values and quality-of-life scores was tenuous. Barletta and associates evaluated 251 claudicants and 89 age-matched controls with treadmill walking distance and quality of life as reported on a general health survey.[49] They noted a reduction in physical, emotional, and social functioning in claudicants compared with the controls but the level of reduction of these quality-of-life parameters did not correlate with walking distance. Thus, while the vascular laboratory can provide the physician with a quantitative assessment of blood flow, it does not indicate the degree of impairment experienced by the patient because of the vascular disease.

Anatomic and vascular laboratory studies also fail to effectively assess the complete impact of vascular intervention upon the patient. This has been demonstrated by numerous investigators. Currie and colleagues noted significant improvements in physical function and pain assessed by a general health survey in 34 patients undergoing surgery and 74 patients undergoing angioplasty for claudication.[50] The improvements reported by the patients, however, did not correlate with increases in ABI. In another study, 150 consecutive patients with limb-threatening ischemia who underwent vascular intervention were evaluated pre- and postoperatively with regard to surgical outcome and quality of life by Johnson and associates.[51] There were six treatment subgroups: angioplasty, thrombolysis/thrombectomy, bypass, primary amputation, amputation after failed revascularization, and primary bilateral amputation. These investigators found that reconstructive surgery significantly improved mobility, pain, anxiety, depression, lifestyle, and self-care ability. The benefits of angioplasty were similar but this treatment modality did not reduce anxiety or depression. The other interventions demonstrated even less positive impact upon the patient's general health.

Several investigators have also noted discrepancy between an excellent clinical outcome and patient-reported improvement. Gibbons and colleagues evaluated the activities of daily living, mental well-being, and symptoms of vascular disease in 156 patients with limb-threatening ischemia.[52] Though limb salvage was 97% at 6 months, only 45% of patients reported feeling 'back to normal'. Nicoloff and colleagues evaluated the functional status in 112 patients who had undergone infrainguinal bypass 5–7 years previously.[53] These investigators found that 30% of patients who were ambulatory preoperatively were not ambulatory at the time of evaluation postoperatively. Only 14.3% of the patients experienced an 'ideal' surgical result of an uncomplicated operation with long-term symptom relief, maintenance of functional status, and no repeat or recurrent operations.

Even an aggressive policy of graft patency maintenance may have a variable impact upon the patient. Ronayne documented greater anxieties and less satisfaction among patients requiring repeat vascular surgical interventions compared with those undergoing their first procedure.[54] Seabrook and colleagues reported a persistently decreased ability to perform activities of daily living, such as walking distances, performing household chores, bathing, and participating in social activities, in patients who had undergone successful revascularization.[55] Despite this, those with a patent graft did experience an improvement in their sense of well-being. The benefits and adverse effects of vascular surgical interventions, then, must be clearly and completely defined by the impact upon the patient's quality and quantity of life, not simply by clinical parameters. To accomplish this, both generic and disease-specific evaluative instruments must be used.

The TransAtlantic Inter-Society Consensus (TASC) group, comprised of representatives from the major vascular societies of North America and Europe, attempted to embrace this concept and address the need for more complete assessment of vascular therapy for arterial occlusive disease of the lower extremity.[56] The group recommended that the outcome of vascular treatment of the lower extremity be based upon a combination of hemodynamic, anatomic, and patient-reported assessment of symptomatic improvement and quality of life. The multiple components provide a complete evaluation of not only the underlying disease process but also the impact of the disease on the patient's quality of life and the potential benefits and adverse effects of treatment (**Table 5.4**). For assessment of improvements in quality of life, the use of both generic health and disease-specific patient survey tools are recommended.

Generic quality-of-life survey instruments

Several generic health surveys which assess a patient's overall health status have been developed and standardized in large populations of patients (**Table 5.5**).[57–61] These instruments obtain important data directly from patients in four major categories:

- functional status;
- perceived health;
- psychological well-being; and
- role function.

Recommended outcomes measures in peripheral arterial disease.
• Objective/hemodynamic assessment of the limb
• Patency of the treated segment
• Symptomatic status of the limb
• General quality of life of the patient
• Value assessment of quality of life of the patient

Table 5.4 Recommended outcomes measures in peripheral arterial disease. (From Dormandy et al.[56])

Generic quality-of-life survey instruments.
• Nottingham Health Profile[57]
• EuroQol[58]
• Sickness Impact Profile[59]
• Medical Outcomes Study SF-36[60]
• Quality of Well-Being Scale[61]

Table 5.5 Generic quality-of-life survey instruments.

Domains of the SF-36 survey.
• Perception of health
• Psychological well-being
• Role limitations due to physical health problems
• Role limitations due to mental health problems
• Physical function
• Social relations
• Pain
• Fatigue

Table 5.6 Domains of the SF-36 survey.

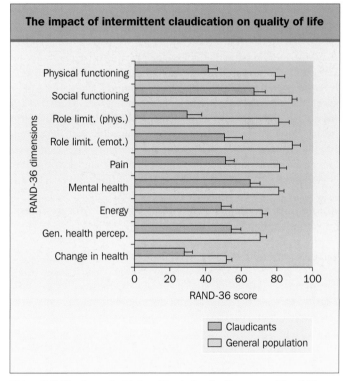

Figure 5.2 The impact of intermittent claudication on quality of life as indicated by the SF-36 survey. Note the differences in domain scores and overall change in health of patients with intermittent claudication compared with the general population.

Functional status provides insight into how well the patient performs basic physical tasks important in the activities of daily living. Perceived health indicates how healthy or ill the patient believes he or she is. Psychological well-being reveals the degree to which the patient is distressed, anxious, or depressed about the illness. Role function demonstrates the extent to which the disease impacts upon the patient's ability to work and to care for family or resources.

Each of the listed instruments has proven reliability and validity.[62] Reliability indicates that each person with the same overall health condition will interpret and answer the questions in the survey in the same way. Validity indicates that each question actually measures what is intended and that the answers given by a patient to similar questions are consistent within a survey and over time if there has been no change in general health status. These demonstrated characteristics of a survey tool are crucial to the value of its data. Therefore, quickly constructed questionnaires that have not been subjected to rigorous reliability and validity testing should not be used and the results of such in publications should be taken with a strong measure of skepticism.

In the USA, efforts to better describe a patient's health status and the outcomes of that patient's interaction with the health-care system began to coalesce in the 1980s with the Medical Outcomes Study.[60] The study undertook the development of a patient assessment tool that could determine:

• how patients with the same health problem fare over time despite different treatments;
• how the lives of patients with different health problems are affected by those conditions; and
• how the benefits on the patients' lives of treatments compare across conditions.

The end result of the study was the development of a general health outcomes assessment tool, the Short Form-36 (SF-36). This survey tool, which is completed by the patient, obtains information about eight areas of the patient's life (**Table 5.6**). An overall general health score can be calculated and each of the domains can be individually scored and tracked as well.

The value of survey tools such as the SF-36 lies in the fact that they have been standardized in large populations of patients over time in a manner similar to laboratory studies. They are capable of demonstrating the impact of disease that may extend far beyond physiologic parameters, especially for chronic illnesses such as diabetes, hypertension, and angina. This is certainly true of claudication as assessed by the SF-36 (**Fig. 5.2**).[63]

51

Generic quality-of-life instruments may also serve as a guide to the establishment of appropriate treatment goals. Johnson and colleagues studied the quality of life in patients who had either revascularization or amputation for limb-threatening ischemia.[64] They noted that successful revascularization resulted in greater mobility, self-care, and lifestyle than amputation. There was, however, a 22% subset of patients undergoing amputation who had scores equivalent to those who were grafted. Treatment goals, therefore, may be different.

Because generic quality-of-life instruments are not disease-specific, they reflect only changes in the overall health status of the patient. Perception of health may not be significantly altered by the treatment of only one of several co-morbid condition, as noted by Duggan and colleagues, who studied 17 patients with patent lower extremity bypasses and found continued decline in perceived health over an 18-month interval.[65] Cook & Galland identified a reduction in perceived health of 24 claudicants despite an improvement in walking distance maintained for 1 year after angioplasty.[66] This reduction was due to the development or worsening of co-morbid conditions. Similar data have been demonstrated in patients undergoing carotid endarterectomy for symptomatic disease. Dardik and colleagues noted an improvement in overall general health scores 3 months after a successful surgical endeavor but not when complications occurred.[67] When used with objective and hemodynamic assessments, the generic health surveys provide the vascular specialist with invaluable insight into the specific effects of the patient's vascular disease and co-morbid conditions on the patient's life and the impact of therapy upon the patient's life and level of functioning. They do not, however, provide information upon the impact of a specific disease on the patient's quality of life. For this, disease-specific survey instruments must be used.

Disease-specific survey instruments

The quest for disease-specific instruments has focused upon symptomatic arterial occlusive disease of the lower extremity. Ideally, such a tool would permit documentation of the presence of peripheral arterial disease, its impact upon the patient's general health, and the response to treatment. The tool should be able to detect improvement or deterioration in health caused by the disease and its treatment independent from that caused by co-morbid conditions. Just over four decades ago, Rose and colleagues developed one of the first questionnaires to identify patients with claudication.[68] However, this questionnaire, though widely used, lacks sensitivity. Subsequently, Hiatt and Regensteiner developed the Walking Impairment Questionnaire (WIQ) to more clearly define the presence and impact of claudication upon the patient.[69] It attempts to assess the reason for difficulty walking, degree of pain, walking distance and speed, and stair-climbing. It also is useful for the documentation of the benefits of treatment. Unlike the tenuous relationship between patient-reported improvement and ABI, the WIQ scores do improve with increased walking distance. This was demonstrated by Regensteiner and colleagues, who noted that after a 24-week supervised exercise therapy program, claudicants had WIQ score improvement which paralleled increases in treadmill walking distances.[69]

There are several other disease-specific questionnaires which have been developed for the assessment of patients with lower extremity arterial occlusive disease (**Table 5.7**).[70–72] Significant progress is being made toward evaluating these instruments in

Disease-specific survey instruments for leg ischemia.
• Rose Questionnaire[68]
• Walking Impairment Questionnaire[69]
• King's College Hospital Vascular Quality of Life Questionnaire[70]
• Intermittent claudication questionnaire[71]
• Claudication Scale (CLAU-S) quality-of-life questionnaire[72]

Table 5.7 Disease-specific survey instruments for leg ischemia.

large populations in the setting of various co-morbid conditions. Continued evaluation of these tools is essential for improved assessments of the benefits and adverse effects of treatment of arterial occlusive disease of the leg.

Challenges for the future

Quality-of-life and disease-specific instruments to more clearly identify the patient's underlying disease, its impact upon the patient's general health, and the outcomes of treatment have demonstrated their value in assessing symptomatic disease. The SF-36 has established the adverse effects of a wide variety of symptomatic disorders on a patient's general health. Disease-specific instruments such as the WIQ have been proven useful for the assessment of the impact of symptomatic arterial occlusive disease and its treatment on the patient, independent of co-morbid conditions. There are, however, several vascular disorders which are life threatening but without significant symptoms. These include asymptomatic aortic aneurysms and asymptomatic critical carotid artery stenoses. Appropriate tools are needed to better describe the disease and its treatment in asymptomatic patients.

Current instruments such as the SF-36 have been used to assess small groups of patients with asymptomatic infrarenal aortic aneurysms. Perkins and colleagues used the SF-36 to study changes in quality of life in 59 consecutive patients undergoing elective aneurysm repair.[73] They noted improvement in quality-of-life scores between 6 weeks and 3 months postoperatively. Using the SF-36, Lloyd and associates evaluated the quality of life in 82 patients 6 months after undergoing elective aneurysm repair by either open or endovascular methods.[74] They noted that physical function and vitality scores were still lower than preoperative levels. In similar studies, patients have been noted to have overall scores return to baseline levels by 8 weeks or to exceed baseline levels by 3 months.[75,76] The discrepancy in the results of these studies most likely lies in the fact that the SF-36 does not discriminate between the impact of the target disease or co-morbid conditions. Therefore, more disease-specific instruments, especially those with sensitivity to asymptomatic conditions, must be developed.

As the economic burden of healthcare continues to escalate, there must be a greater effort to identify those diagnostic and therapeutic modalities that are of greatest benefit in improving patients' quality of life and productivity. For vascular surgery, this will require the development and utilization of both generic and disease-specific survey tools that clearly demonstrate the impact of vascular disease upon the patient and document the benefits of therapy.

REFERENCES

1. Blakemore AH, Voorhees AB Jr. Use of tubes constructed from Vinyon "N" cloth in bridging arterial defects. Experimental and clinical results. Ann Surg 1954;140:324–34.

2. Baker JD. The vascular laboratory. In: Rutherford RB, ed. Vascular surgery, 5th edn. Philadelphia:WB Saunders; 2000:127–39.

3. Evidence-based Medicine Working Group. Evidence-based medicine. JAMA 1992;268:2420–5.

4. Passaro E Jr, Organ CH Jr, Ernest A. Codman: the improper Bostonian. Bull Am Coll Surg 1999;84:16–22.

5. US Congress, Office of Technology Assessment. The development of clinical practice guidelines. In: Identifying health technologies that work: searching for evidence. Washington:US Government Printing Office; 1994;OTA-H-608:145–71.

6. US Congress, Office of Technology Assessment. The impact of clinical guidelines on practice. In: Identifying health technologies that work: searching for evidence. Washington:US Government Printing Office; 1994;OTA-H-608:173–98.

7. Fung EK, Lore JM Jr. Randomized controlled trials for evaluating surgical questions. Arch Otolaryngol Head Neck Surg 2002;128:631–4.

8. Solomon MJ, McLeod RS. Should we be performing more randomized controlled trials evaluating surgical operations? Surgery 1995;118:459–67.

9. US Congress, Office of Technology Assessment. Identifying health technologies that work: searching for evidence. Washington:US Government Printing Office; 1994;OTA-H-608:1.

10. Wacholder S, Silverman DT, McLaughlin JK, Mandel JS. Selection of controls in case-control studies. Am J Epidemiol 1992;135:1042–50.

11. White E, Hunt JR, Casso D. Exposure measurement in cohort studies: the challenges of prospective data collection. Epidemiol Rev 1998; 20:43–56.

12. Kannel WB. The Framingham study: historical insight on the impact of cardiovascular risk factors in men versus women. J Gend Specif Med 2002;5:27–37.

13. Sacks H, Chalmers TC, Smith H Jr. Randomized versus historical controls for clinical trials. Am J Med 1982;72:233–40.

14. Chalmers TC, Smith H Jr, Blackburn B, et al. A method for assessing the quality of a randomized control trial. Control Clin Trials 1981;2:31–49.

15. Buring JE, Jonas MA, Hennekens CH. Large and simple randomized trials. In: Tools for evaluating health technologies. Washington:US Government Printing Office; 1995:83–7.

16. US Congress, Office of Technology Assessment. Identifying health technologies that work: searching for evidence. Washington:US Government Printing Office; 1994;OTA-H-608:4.

17. Kempczinski RF, Brott TG, Labutta RJ. The influence of surgical specialty and caseload on the results of carotid endarterectomy. J Vasc Surg 1986;3:911–6.

18. Asymptomatic Carotid Atherosclerosis Study Group. Study design for randomized prospective trial of carotid endarterectomy for asymptomatic atherosclerosis. Stroke 1989;20:844–9.

19. Hobson RW 2nd, Weiss DG, Fields WS, et al. Efficacy of carotid endarterectomy for asymptomatic carotid stenosis. The Veterans Affairs cooperative study group. N Engl J Med 1993;328:221–7.

20. Buring JE, Jonas MA, Hennekens CH. Large and simple randomized trials. In: Tools for evaluating health technologies. Washington:US Government Printing Office; 1995:72–3.

21. L'Abbe KA, Detsky AS, O'Rourke K. Meta-analysis in clinical research. Ann Intern Med 1987;107:224–33.

22. Jones DR. Meta-analysis: weighing the evidence. Stat Med 1995; 14:137–49.

23. Sonnenberg FA, Beck JR. Markov models in medical decision making: a practical guide. Med Decis Making 1993;13:322–38.

24. Detsky AS, Naglie G, Krahn MD, et al. Primer on medical decision analysis: Part 2 – Building a tree. Med Decis Making 1998;17:126–35.

25. Michaels JA, Galland RB. Management of asymptomatic popliteal aneurysms: the use of a Markov decision tree to determine the criteria for a conservative approach. Eur J Vasc Surg 1993;7:136–43.

26. Concato J, Feinstein AR. Monte Carlo methods in clinical research: applications in multivariable analysis. J Investig Med 1997;45:394–400.

27. Meakins JL. Innovations in surgery: the rules of evidence. Am J Surg 2002;183:399–405.

28. Canadian Task Force on Periodic Health Examination. The periodic health examination. Can Med Assoc J 1979;121:1193–1254.

29. Sacks H, Chalmers TC, Smith H Jr. Randomized versus historical controls for clinical trials. Am J Med 1982;72:233–40.

30. Benson K, Hartz AJ. A comparison of observational studies and randomized, controlled trials. N Engl J Med 2000;342:1878–86.

31. Solomon MJ, McLeod RS. Should we be performing more randomized controlled trials evaluating surgical operations? Surgery 1995;118:459–67.

32. The EC/IC Bypass Study Group. Failure of extracranial-intracranial arterial bypass to reduce the risk of ischemic stroke. Results of an international randomized trial. N Engl J Med 1985;313:1191–2000.

33. Cronenwett JL, Birkmeyer JD, eds. The Dartmouth atlas of vascular health care. Chicago:AHA Press; 2000:42–3.

34. Executive Committee for the Asymptomatic Carotid Atherosclerosis Study. Endarterectomy for asymptomatic carotid artery stenosis. JAMA 1995;273:1421–8.

35. Gross CP, Steiner CA, Bass EB, Powe NR. Relation between prepublication release of clinical trial results and the practice of carotid endarterectomy. JAMA 2000;284:2886–93.

36. Barnett HJ, Meldrum HE, Eliasziw M, et al. The appropriate use of carotid endarterectomy. CMAJ 2002;166:1169–79.

37. Glasziou PP, Irwig LM. An evidence based approach to individualizing treatment. BMJ 1995;311:1356–9.

38. Robb JV, Wylie EJ. Factors contributing to recurrent lower limb ischemia following bypass surgery for aortoiliac occlusive disease, and their management. Ann Surg 1981;193:346–52.

39. Valentine RJ, Myers SI, Hagino RT, Clagett GP. Late outcome of patients with premature carotid atherosclerosis after carotid endarterectomy. Stroke 1996;27:1502–6.

40. Dawson I, van Bockel JH. Reintervention and mortality after infrainguinal reconstructive surgery for leg ischaemia. Br J Surg 1999;86:38–44.

41. Dawson I, Keller BP, Brand R, et al. Late outcomes of limb loss after failed infrainguinal bypass. J Vasc Surg 1995;21:613–22.

42. Abou-Zamzam AM, Lee RW, Moneta GL, et al. Functional outcome after infrainguinal bypass for limb salvage. J Vasc Surg 1997;25:287–95.

43. Plate G, Hollier LA, O'Brien P, et al. Recurrent aneurysms and late vascular complications following repair of abdominal aortic aneurysms. Arch Surg 1985;120:590–4.

44. Matsumura JS, Pearce WH, Cabellon A, et al. Reoperative aortic surgery. Cardiovasc Surg 1999;7:614–21.

45. US Congress, Office of Technology Assessment. Identifying health technologies that work: searching for evidence. Washington:US Government Printing Office; 1994;OTA-H-608:33.

46. US Congress, Office of Technology Assessment. Identifying health technologies that work: searching for evidence. Washington:US Government Printing Office; 1994; OTA-H-608:34.

47. Feinglass J, McCarthy WJ, Slavensky R, et al. Effect of lower extremity blood pressure on physical functioning in patients who have intermittent claudication. J Vasc Surg 1996;24:503–12.

48. Chetter IC, Dolan P, Spark JI, et al. Correlating clinical indicators of lower-limb ischaemia with quality of life. Cardiovasc Surg 1997;5:361–6.

49. Barletta G, Brevetti G, O'Boyle C, et al. Quality of life in patients with intermittent claudication: relationship with laboratory exercise performance. Vasc Med 1996;1:1–3.

50. Currie IC, Lamont PM, Baird RN, Wilson YG. Treatment of intermittent claudication: the impact on quality of life. Eur J Vasc Endovasc Surg 1995;10:356–61.

51. Johnson BF, Singh S, Evans L, et al. A prospective study of the effect of limb-threatening ischaemia and its surgical treatment on the quality of life. Eur J Vasc Endovasc Surg 1997;13:306–14.

52. Gibbons GW, Burgess AM, Guadagnoli E, et al. Return to well-being and function after infrainguinal revascularization. J Vasc Surg 1995;21:35–44.

53. Nicoloff AD, Taylor LM, McLafferty RB, et al. Patient recovery after infrainguinal bypass grafting for limb salvage. J Vasc Surg 1998; 27:256–63.

54. Ronayne R. Feelings and attitudes during early convalescence following vascular surgery. J Adv Nurs 1985;10:435–41.

55. Seabrook GR, Cambria RA, Freischlag JA, Towne JB. Health-related quality of life and functional outcome following arterial reconstruction for limb salvage. Cardiovasc Surg 1999;7:279–86.

56. Dormandy JA, Rutherford RB. Management of peripheral arterial disease (PAD): TransAtlantic Inter-Society Consensus. J Vasc Surg 2000;31(Pt 2):S1–288.

57. Hunt SM, McEwen J, McKenna SP, eds. Measuring health status. Dover, NH:Croom Helm; 1986.

58. EuroQol Group. EuroQol – a new facility for the measurement of health-related quality of life. Health Policy 1990;16:199–208.

59. Bergner M, Bobbitt RA, Carter WB, et al. The Sickness Impact Profile: development and final revision of a health status measure. Med Care 1981;19:787–805.

60. Ware JE, Sherbourne CD. The MOS 36-item short-form health survey (SF-36). I. Conceptual framework and item selection. Med Care 1992;30:473–83.

61. Kaplan RM, Bush JW. Health-related quality of life measurement for evaluation and research and policy analysis. Health Psychol 1982;1:61–71.

62. Fowler FJ. Using patients' reports to evaluate medical outcomes. In: Tools for evaluating health technologies. Washington:US Government Printing Office; 1995:14–6.

63. Bosch JL, Hunink MGM. The relationship between descriptive and valuational quality-of-life measures in patients with intermittent claudication. Med Decis Making 1996;16:217–25.

64. Johnson BF, Evans L, Drury R, et al. Surgery for limb-threatening ischaemia: a reappraisal of the costs and benefits. Eur J Vasc Endovasc Surg 1995;9:181–8.

65. Duggan MM, Woodson J, Scott TE, et al. Functional outcomes in limb salvage vascular surgery. Am J Surg 1994;168:188–91.

66. Cook TA, Galland RB. Quality of life changes after angioplasty for claudication: medium-term results affected by co-morbid conditions. Cardiovasc Surg 1997;5:424–6.

67. Dardik A, Minor J, Watson C, Hands LJ. Improved quality of life among patients with symptomatic carotid artery disease undergoing carotid endarterectomy. J Vasc Surg 2001;33:329–33.

68. Rose GA. The diagnosis of ischemic heart pain and intermittent claudication in field surveys. Bull World Health Organ 1962;27:645–58.

69. Regensteiner JG, Steiner JF, Panzer RJ, Hiatt WR. Evaluation of walking impairment by questionnaire in patients with peripheral arterial disease. J Vasc Med Biol 1990;2:142–56.

70. Morgan MB, Crayford T, Murrin B, Fraser SC. Developing the Vascular Quality of Life Questionnaire: a new disease-specific quality of life measure for use in lower limb ischemia. J Vasc Surg 2001;33:679–87.

71. Chong PF, Garratt AM, Golledge J, et al. The intermittent claudication questonnaire: a patient-assessed condition-specific health outcome measure. J Vasc Surg 2002;36:764–71.

72. Marquis P, Comte S, Lehert P. International validation of the CLAU-S quality-of-life questionnaire for use in patients with intermittent claudication. Pharmacoeconomics 2001;19:667–77.

73. Perkins JM, Magee TR, Hands LJ, et al. Prospective evaluation of quality of life after conventional abdominal aortic aneurysm repair. Eur J Vasc Surg 1998;16:203–7.

74. Lloyd AJ, Boyle J, Bell PR, Thompson MM. Comparison of cognitive function and quality of life after endovascular or conventional aortic aneurysm repair. Br J Surg 2000;87:443–7.

75. Aquino RV, Jones MA, Zullo TG, et al. Quality of life assessment in patients undergoing endovascular or conventional AAA repair. J Endovasc Ther 2001;8:521–8.

76. Malina M, Nilsson M, Brunkwall J, et al. Quality of life before and after endovascular and open repair of asymptomatic AAAs: a prospective study. J Endovasc Ther 2000;7:372–9.

77. Inzitari D. Leukoaraiosis: an independent risk factor for stroke? Stroke 2003;34:2067–71.

CHAPTER
6

Vascular Laboratory Evaluation of Lower Extremity Arterial Occlusive Disease

Mary E Giswold, Andrew T Gentile, and Gregory L Moneta

KEY POINTS

- The non-invasive vascular laboratory is useful to confirm the presence and quantify the hemodynamic significance of lower extremity peripheral arterial disease (PAD).

- Plethysmography and applications of Doppler ultrasound are the two most commonly used techniques to evaluate PAD.

- Plethysmography is primarily used to evaluate digital arterial waveforms and pressures; these measurements are especially applicable to diabetic patients with medial calcinosis and suprasystolic ankle pressures.

- The ankle–brachial index is simple, reproducible, and allows categorization of PAD into severity subgroups that are of prognostic and clinical importance.

- Exercise testing is useful to quantify the hemodynamics of patients with intermittent claudication caused by PAD, but is especially useful in differentiating vasculogenic from neurogenic claudication.

- Arterial duplex scanning allows one to localize the anatomic site of a stenosis and quantify its hemodynamic significance based on systolic velocity ratios. It also can differentiate stenosis from occlusion and can be used to plan potential intervention (angioplasty or surgical reconstruction).

- Non-invasive testing provides essential, quantitative, objective physiologic data that serve as the scientific basis for modern therapeutic approaches to PAD patients.

INTRODUCTION

Because the differential diagnosis of chronic leg pain is quite broad, the ability to confirm the presence of arterial obstruction and quantify the hemodynamic and physiologic significance of detected lesions is of paramount importance. The non-invasive vascular laboratory has a critical role as an adjunct to the history and physical examination in providing an objective, quantitative diagnosis of lower extremity arterial occlusive disease and the functional abnormalities resulting from a decrease in limb blood flow.

HISTORY AND PHYSICAL EXAMINATION

The clinical history provides valuable information regarding the evaluation of patients with chronic lower extremity pain. In most patients, the clinical history, including questioning for coexistent atherosclerotic risk factors, coupled with the physical examination, is all that is necessary to firmly establish the diagnosis of exercise-induced muscular ischemia, intermittent claudication (IC), or ischemic extremity pain at rest.

Patients with exercise-induced leg or buttock pain should be specifically asked the location of the pain, its relationship to walking, the duration and severity of the symptoms, and symptomatic progression over time. Only exercise-induced muscular pain of the calf, thigh, or buttock, relieved within a few minutes of rest and reliably reproduced by further walking, can confidently be improved by lower extremity revascularization. Almost all patients with IC have diminished or absent lower extremity pulses. Occasionally, however, a patient may give a classic history of vasculogenic claudication yet have palpable pedal pulses at rest. Under these circumstances, exercise testing with post-exercise Doppler-measured ankle–brachial systolic blood pressure ratios is crucial to confirm the diagnosis of IC (see below).

Ischemic rest pain should be suspected when a patient complains of pain and/or numbness in the forefoot, toes, or instep. Ischemic rest pain is typically aggravated by elevating the leg and improved by placing the leg in a dependent position. It usually is worsened by exercise. Nocturnal leg cramps, which are frequently associated with lower extremity arterial occlusive disease, are themselves not manifestations of ischemic rest pain. However, true ischemic rest pain is frequently worse at night. Afflicted patients will often describe the need to sleep in a chair in order to keep the involved foot dependent; a position that provides some relief from ischemic pain because of the gravitational-induced increase in arterial blood flow. Because of the need to maintain the foot in a dependent position, many patients with chronic ischemic pain develop significant edema of the symptomatic extremity. It is important to note that edema is not a classic feature of arterial insufficiency but rather reflects prolonged dependency of the ischemic extremity rather than ischemia itself.

In addition to an absence of pedal pulses, patients with rest pain will frequently have thin, atrophic skin of the foot and lower leg, often with dependent rubor and pallor in elevation, and, ultimately, areas of cutaneous gangrene and ulceration. If the findings on physical examination are not consistent with vasculogenic ischemic pain, the physician should carefully inquire about a history of diabetes, thyroid disorders, vitamin deficiencies, or alcoholism, all of which can produce neuropathy with nocturnal foot dysesthetic discomfort similar to ischemic rest pain.

While the history and physical examination are clearly important in establishing the diagnosis of lower extremity arterial occlusive disease, the information obtained is by nature subjective and dependent on the skill of the observer. The location and hemodynamic significance of various athero-sclerotic lesions can only be grossly approximated by history and physical examination alone. This is clearly inadequate for monitoring individual lesions, and for predicting the magnitude and complexity of any revascularization procedure. For these reasons, together with an increasing appreciation of the importance of arterial hemodynamics in determining and following the outcome of reconstructive procedures, the non-invasive vascular laboratory has assumed a pivotal role in the modern practice of peripheral arterial surgery.

PERIPHERAL VASCULAR LABORATORY

The objectives of the modern non-invasive testing of patients with lower extremity arterial occlusive disease are to confirm the presence of arterial ischemia, to provide quantitative and reproducible physiologic data concerning its severity, and to document the location and hemodynamic significance of individual arterial lesions. Two broad categories of non-invasive techniques are used to evaluate lower extremity arterial occlusive disease: plethysmography and various applications of Doppler ultrasound. Each technique has advantages and disadvantages. Understanding what the tests can and cannot do is required for the optimal and cost-effective use of the vascular laboratory.

PLETHYSMOGRAPHY

Plethysmography preceded ultrasound in the evaluation of lower extremity ischemia. Plethysmography is based on the detection of volume changes in the limb in response to arterial inflow. In addition to volume flow, the basic technology can be modified to produce pulse waveforms and determine digital pressures. Mercury strain gauge plethysmography, air plethysmography (pulse volume recordings), and photoplethysmography all have been used clinically.

Volume flow

Calf or foot blood flow can be conveniently recorded with a mercury-in-silastic strain gauge. Measurements are based on detection of minute changes in the electrical resistance of the mercury column which depend on its length. Unfortunately, neither calf nor foot blood flow at rest differ between normal subjects and patients with even rather severe degrees of arterial insufficiency.[1] Hyperemic flow may be decreased in patients with arterial ischemia when compared with normal subjects, but these changes in volume flow are not routinely used to quantify precise differences in severity of arterial occlusive lesions.[2] For these reasons, measurements of volume flow have not proved useful in the evaluation of chronic lower extremity ischemia.

Pulse volume recordings

Air plethysmography can be used clinically to demonstrate pulse volume waveforms.[3] These pulsed volume recordings are obtained with partially inflated segmental blood pressure cuffs that detect volume changes sequentially down a limb. Volume changes beneath the cuffs resulting from systole and diastole cause small pressure changes within the cuffs, which, with the use of appropriate transducers, can be displayed as arterial wave-

forms. A normal pulse volume waveform is characterized by a sharp systolic upstroke and peak, and a prominent dicrotic notch on the downward portion of the curve. Such a waveform reflects normal arterial inflow to the portion of the extremity under the cuff. With increasing proximal arterial occlusion, the dicrotic notch is lost and the pulse peak wave becomes rounded, with loss of amplitude, and there are nearly equal upstroke and downstroke times. With very severe proximal occlusive disease, the pulse wave may be completely absent.[4] Pulse volume wave-forms are generally evaluated in a qualitative fashion based on the shape of the curve, with flat, dampened curves considered severely abnormal. Although quantitative interpretive criteria have been proposed, these criteria, which are based on amplitude and contour changes of the pulse volume curves, are not in widespread clinical use.[5] The lack of reliable, reproducible, quantitative data in pulse volume recordings, limits the utility of air plethysmography in the modern practice of vascular surgery.

Digital measurements

Perhaps the greatest current role for plethysmography is in the evaluation of digital pressures and waveforms. Air plethysmo-graphy, strain gauge plethysmography, and photoplethsymography can all be adapted for this purpose. Strictly speaking, photo-plethysmography is not a method to record volume change; rather, a photoelectrode is used to detect changes in cutaneous blood flow. This allows the technique to be readily used in combination with pneumatic cuffs to detect digital systolic pressures. These techniques are particularly useful in patients with pedal artery occlusive disease or highly calcified vessels, in whom Doppler-derived ankle blood pressures may not accurately reflect true intraluminal arterial pressure because of the relative incompressibility of the arterial walls. The presence of normal digital waveforms in patients with calcified proximal vessels indicates minimal restriction to blood flow despite the calcific arterial disease. Conversely, an obstructive digital wave-form in the presence of normal ankle pulses frequently indicates pedal artery occlusive disease, a situation frequently encountered in patients with diabetes or with distal atheroembolism (**Fig. 6.1**).

DOPPLER ULTRASOUND TECHNIQUES

Ultrasound has proved to be the single most important modality in the non-invasive evaluation of lower extremity ischemia. Ultrasound techniques are based on the principle that sound waves emitted from a transducer are reflected at the interface of two surfaces. By coupling the transducer with a receiver, and knowing the transmitting frequency and the acoustical charac-teristics of the transmitting medium, the reflected ultrasound waves can be analyzed for energy loss and frequency shift by the receiver. With appropriate technology, these reflected waves can then be processed to produce a picture (B-mode image) or a velocity waveform. The generation of velocity waveforms is based on the observation that an ultrasound wave undergoes a frequency shift proportional to the velocity of any moving object (e.g. red blood cells) encountered, the Doppler principle. The reflected waves can be processed into audible signals (continuous-wave Doppler) or displayed as an analog waveform similar to the plethysmographically derived waveforms. If the angle between the transmitting ultrasound beam and the flowing

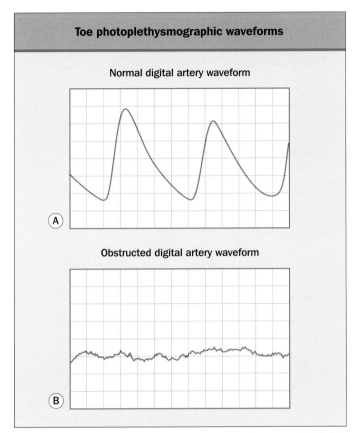

Figure 6.1 Toe photoplethysmographic waveforms. (A) Normal digital artery waveform. (B) Obstructed digital artery waveform.

Correlation between ankle–brachial index and severity of arterial ischemia.	
ABI	*Clinical status*
1.1 ± 0.1	Normal
0.6 ± 0.2	Intermittent claudication
0.3 ± 0.1	Ischemic rest pain
0.1 ± 0.1	Impending tissue necrosis

Table 6.1 Correlation between ankle–brachial index (ABI) and severity of arterial ischemia.

blood is known, quantitative measurements of systolic and diastolic blood flow velocities can be derived from the analog waveforms by using the Doppler equation.

Ankle–brachial systolic blood pressure index

The ankle-to-brachial systolic pressure ratio is the simplest application of Doppler ultrasound to the non-invasive vascular laboratory and is perhaps also the most useful. With a patient supine, a pneumatic pressure cuff placed just above the ankle is inflated to suprasystolic levels. As the cuff is deflated, a hand-held Doppler probe positioned over the posterior tibial or dorsalis pedis artery distal to the cuff is used to determine the systolic pressure – the cuff pressure at which distal blood flow, using the Doppler probe, is first heard as the cuff is deflated. The higher ipsilateral dorsal pedal or posterior tibial pressure is then divided by the higher Doppler-determined brachial artery systolic pressure, yielding an ankle–brachial index (ABI) for that lower extremity. Changes in systolic pressure are used because they are more sensitive to the presence of arterial occlusive disease than are changes in diastolic or mean pressure and because only systolic pressure can be accurately determined with the hand-held Doppler probe. By comparing ankle systolic pressure with brachial artery systolic pressure, the test is independent of day-to-day variations in arterial blood pressure, permitting quantitative comparison by serial examinations.

The ABI serves as an excellent indicator of the overall arterial supply of each lower extremity. A normal ABI is 1.0 to 1.1, with progressively lower values corresponding to worsening arterial disease (**Table 6.1**). This test, however, has several distinct limi-

tations. Significant bilateral subclavian or axillary artery occlusive disease may result in a falsely elevated ABI. In addition, patients with longstanding renal failure or diabetes may have medial calcinosis of the popliteal and tibial arteries. Such calcific arteries may be inadequately compressed by the ankle pressure cuff, resulting in a falsely elevated (suprasystolic) ankle pressure/ABI. Under these circumstances, qualitative analysis of Doppler-derived analog or plethysmographic waveforms or measurement of digital systolic pressures is more appropriate. Finally, in the presence of severe arterial occlusive disease, no arterial Doppler signal may be audible at the ankle. Under such circumstances, venous signals may be confused with arterial signals.

Segmental limb pressures

Multiple pneumatic cuffs may be used on the leg to determine the arterial blood pressure in different segments of the limb. These segmental leg pressures are compared with each other and with the higher brachial artery systolic pressure. Most laboratories prefer a four-cuff technique. Cuffs are placed: (1) as far proximal on the thigh as possible; (2) immediately above the knee; (3) just below the knee; and (4) just proximal to the malleolus. Theoretically, each cuff width should be 20% greater than the diameter of the limb at the point of application.[6] This would in most cases necessitate a single, wide, thigh cuff. Use of two cuffs above the knee, however, may permit a determination of iliac artery inflow, as well as superficial femoral artery disease. Narrower cuffs may be associated with the measurement of artifactually high pressures and do not permit more accurate disease localization. An awareness of this problem will help avoid confusion in the interpretation of segmental limb pressures.

The examination is performed by using the hand-held Doppler probe to detect the most prominent Doppler signal at the ankle. The high-thigh cuff is inflated first, until the Doppler signal at the ankle is no longer audible. The cuff is then deflated and the cuff pressure at which there is return of the Doppler signal at the ankle is the high-thigh pressure. The above-knee, below-knee and ankle pressures are similarly determined. If no Doppler signal is audible at the ankle, the popliteal artery is examined with the Doppler probe. Under such circumstances, only high-thigh and above-knee pressures can be determined. By comparing the pressures at various levels in the leg, one can predict with reasonable accuracy the location of the arterial occlusive lesions (**Fig. 6.2, Table 6.2**).

There are a number of potential problems and significant limitations in the interpretation of segmental limb pressures. In

Abnormal segmental limb pressures

	RIGHT		LEFT	
	Pressure	Leg/arm ratio	Pressure	Leg/arm ratio
Arm	152		150	
Upper thigh	156	1.02	122	0.80
Above knee	144	0.94	120	0.79
Below knee	124	0.81	90	0.59
Ankle D.P.	136	0.89	96	0.63
P.T.	144	0.94	96	0.63
Toe	88	0.57	66	0.43

Figure 6.2 Abnormal segmental limb pressures. The left limb has an iliac or common femoral artery lesion as well as a popliteal lesion. The right limb has a popliteal lesion.

Gradient location and corresponding anatomic location.

Gradient location	Corresponding anatomic location	Normal vertical gradient
Brachial–high thigh	Aorta, iliac artery, common femoral and superficial femoral arteries	+35–46mmHg
High thigh–above knee	Superficial femoral artery	–5–13mmHg
Above knee–high calf	Distal superficial femoral artery, popliteal artery	–12mmHg
High calf–ankle	Trifurcation vessels	–10–11mmHg
Ankle–toes	Pedal or digital arteries	–10mmHg

Table 6.2 Gradient location and corresponding anatomic location.

addition to cuff-induced artifacts, the high-thigh pressure is subject to particular difficulties in interpretation. Ideally, the high-thigh pressure should reflect iliac artery inflow to the groin. A diminished high-thigh pressure should indicate a pressure-reducing stenosis in the ipsilateral common or external iliac artery. A diminished high-thigh pressure, however, may also reflect a significant common femoral stenosis or tandem pressure-reducing lesions in both the profunda femoris and the proximal superficial femoral artery. As noted, calcified arteries may also result in artificially elevated pressures. In patients with multilevel disease, diminished proximal pressures may mask gradients that exist further down the leg. Finally, segmental pressure gradients give no information as to the nature of the pressure-reducing lesion. No differentiation is possible between short and long segment occlusions, or between occluded versus patent but highly stenotic arteries.

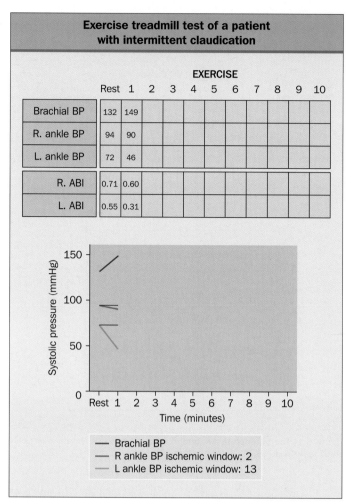

Exercise treadmill test of a patient with intermittent claudication

	Rest	EXERCISE									
		1	2	3	4	5	6	7	8	9	10
Brachial BP	132	149									
R. ankle BP	94	90									
L. ankle BP	72	46									
R. ABI	0.71	0.60									
L. ABI	0.55	0.31									

— Brachial BP
— R ankle BP ischemic window: 2
— L ankle BP ischemic window: 13

Figure 6.3 Exercise treadmill test of a patient with intermittent claudication. The ankle–brachial index drops significantly after 1min of exercise.

Exercise testing

Measurement of Doppler-determined pressures can be combined with treadmill exercise testing, assuming the patient does not have a significant medical contraindication to exercise. After determination of supine resting ankle pressures and the ABI, the patient is asked to walk continuously on a treadmill with a 10% incline at a predetermined rate, usually 1.5 miles per hour. The test lasts for 5min or until the patient is forced to stop because of claudication symptoms. The time to onset of symptoms, as well as the location of the symptoms, are recorded. At completion of the test, the patient is immediately placed supine and the ABIs are determined. If the ABI has dropped from the resting measurement, ABIs are determined every 30s until they return to normal. The greater the drop in the ABI with exercise, and the longer the time required to return to baseline, the more severe the patient's arterial occlusive disease (**Fig. 6.3**).

Whereas many laboratories perform exercise testing in all patients with suspected lower limb arterial insufficiency, the examination in most patients serves only to confirm the diagnosis suspected by history and physical examination. A patient with classic symptoms of claudication and absent peripheral pulses, combined with a diminished ABI in the appropriate lower extremity, does not require routine exercise testing for the determination of ABI decrease and recovery. However, exercise testing is indicated in preoperative patients, as the post-exercise recovery of ankle pressure provides an objective assessment of the potential postoperative benefit.

Exercise testing is particularly useful in the occasional patient with symptoms of claudication but palpable pedal pulses at rest, with a normal or near-normal ABI. Patients with claudication secondary to arterial insufficiency will show a significant decrease in the post-exercise ABI. In our vascular laboratory, the criteria for a positive exercise treadmill test include a decrease in the absolute ankle pressure of 20mmHg or 20%, or a decrease in the ABI of 0.2 in the symptomatic extremity after exercise testing.

With the exception of the rare patient with buttock claudication secondary to isolated internal iliac disease, failure of the ABI to decrease 20% with exercise, in association with a normal resting ABI, substantially rules out arterial insufficiency as the cause of the patient's exercise-induced leg pain. The frequently encountered condition of spinal stenosis and neurogenic claudication may be confused with arterial ischemia. These patients also typically present with symptoms of exercise-induced leg or calf pain, but careful questioning reveals atypical characteristics including occurrence of the pain with standing, occasional pain relief by leaning forward, worsening with coughing, and prolonged time requirement for pain abatement after exercise. In these patients, exercise testing reveals normal ankle pressures that do not decrease with exercise despite the onset of symptoms. Failure of the ankle pressures to decrease with exercise may also be a clue to the presence of other uncommon conditions, such as venous claudication and chronic exercise-induced compartment syndromes.

Doppler analog waveform analysis

Doppler analog waveforms may be obtained using a continuous-wave Doppler probe and analyzed in a qualitative fashion analogous to plethysmographic waveforms. Normal lower-extremity Doppler waveforms are triphasic with a reverse flow component in early diastole and low end-diastolic forward flow. The reverse flow component and low overall diastolic velocities reflect a relatively high end-organ resistance to blood flow in the resting extremity. With increasing proximal stenosis, the shape of the waveform changes. Initially, the reverse flow component is lost. With more severe degrees of stenosis, the rate of rise of the systolic upstroke is decreased, the amplitude of the waveform is diminished, and diastolic flow increases relative to systolic flow.

The primary clinical application of qualitative Doppler waveform analysis has been in assessing the adequacy of iliac artery inflow to the common femoral artery. An attenuated waveform recorded from the common femoral artery indicates proximal disease. Unfortunately, the technique cannot quantify stenosis or distinguish between iliac stenosis and occlusion. In addition, attenuated waveforms may be caused by superficial femoral artery disease or a combination of superficial femoral and aorto-iliac disease.

Peripheral arterial duplex scanning

Arterial duplex scanning provides detailed anatomic and hemodynamic information that cannot be determined by the indirect non-invasive tests (pulse volume recording, segmental pressures, ABI). Duplex scanning utilizes both B-mode ultra-

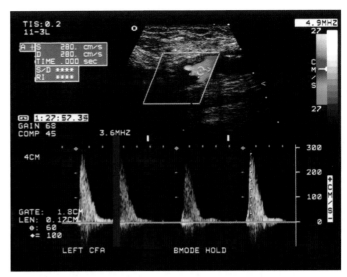

Figure 6.4 Arterial duplex of a left common femoral artery stenosis. The velocity is elevated and there is loss of the triphasic waveform.

sound and pulsed Doppler ultrasound. The combination of color Doppler and B-mode ultrasound allows assessment of anatomic and hemodynamic abnormalities from the infrarenal aorta to the distal tibial vessels. B-mode imaging alone cannot reliably distinguish hemodynamically significant soft plaque and thrombus from blood. However, Doppler ultrasound is able to detect the flow disturbances created by these lesions. B-mode ultrasound visualizes calcified plaque and localizes the artery of interest. This permits the precise placement of the Doppler sample volume at a known angle to the artery being examined. Knowledge of the angle of insonation allows quantitative determination of frequency shifts. Blood flow velocities can be calculated from the frequency shift to determine the degree of stenosis of an arterial lesion. Arterial duplex scanning has been prospectively compared with angiography to establish standard criteria for normal and diseased arteries.[7] In this study, the sensitivity of the duplex examination for detecting the presence of a hemodynamically significant lesion (>50%) ranged from 89% at the iliac artery to 68% at the popliteal artery. Overall sensitivities for predicting interruption of patency were 90% for the anterior tibial, 90% for the posterior tibial, and 82% for the peroneal artery. The sensitivity of arterial duplex mapping is not heavily influenced by the severity of atherosclerotic disease (**Fig. 6.4**).

Examination, equipment, and personnel

Although not absolutely necessary, color-flow imaging facilitates the duplex examination by aiding in rapid identification of the arteries, therefore decreasing the overall time for the examination. Color-flow is particularly useful for evaluating the iliac arteries, the popliteal trifurcation, and the tibial vessels. Also, color-flow can identify the presence and length of an arterial occlusion, as well as the distal site of reconstitution. Color-flow changes are not used to determine specific percent degrees of stenosis other than occlusion. The degree of stenosis of a sub-occlusive lesion is determined with velocity waveform analysis.

Lower extremity arterial duplex examination requires a variety of transducers. A 2MHz or 3MHz transducer is required for evaluating the iliac vessels. Infrainguinal vessels can be examined with a 5MHz transducer. Examining the superficial femoral artery in patients with large legs occasionally requires a lower-frequency transducer. Conversely, the tibial vessels are best examined with a higher-frequency transducer.

Using angle-corrected velocity recordings is of practical necessity when examining peripheral arteries. Varying body habitus and depth of vessels makes it impossible to insonate all portions of the peripheral arteries using a constant angle with the currently available technology. Although 60 degrees is considered the ideal angle of insonation, angles between 30 and 70 degrees are sufficiently accurate for the peripheral arterial examination.[8]

The complete lower extremity arterial duplex examination includes evaluation of the infrarenal aorta, the common and external iliac arteries, the profunda origin, the proximal, middle, and distal superficial femoral arteries, the popliteal artery, and the tibial vessels. The tibial arteries should be evaluated from the popliteal trifurcation to the level of the ankle. Examining patients after a fast of 8–12hours reduces abdominal gas and facilitates examination of the intra-abdominal vessels. The entire examination is performed with the patient in the supine position, except for the popliteal artery, which is best examined in the prone or lateral position.

Velocities should be routinely recorded from several sites along a vessel and from any site where a disturbance is identified. Areas both of high velocity, suggestive of a hemodynamically significant stenosis, and of low velocity, indicating a more proximal stenosis or occlusion, should be noted. **Table 6.3** demonstrates the normal duplex ultrasound velocities of normal arterial segments.

The lower extremity arterial duplex study is most efficient when it follows a physical examination, determination of segmental pressures, and exercise testing. If these tests are normal, arterial duplex is not indicated. Abnormalities in the physical examination and/or the segmental pressures can guide the technologist to examine certain areas with more detail. A complete arterial duplex study in a patient with complicated arterial anatomy usually requires 1–1.5 hours. (**Fig. 6.5**).

Velocity patterns and classifications of stenosis

Duplex-derived velocity waveforms of normal resting peripheral arteries are triphasic with a short reverse flow component at the end of systole. End-diastolic flow is near zero because of the high end-organ resistance associated with the peripheral circulation. The triphasic waveform is maintained throughout the leg

but the peak systolic velocities (PSV) decrease steadily from the iliac to the tibial vessels.

The hemodynamic significance of a given lesion is determined by analysis of duplex velocity waveforms. Important features that signify disease include the absence of the reverse flow component and an elevated peak systolic velocity. Traditionally, a 50% reduction in arterial diameter (equivalent to a cross-sectional surface area reduction of 75%) is considered to be associated with a significant drop in blood pressure across the lesion.

The original classification criteria derived for the non-invasive quantification of peripheral arterial stenosis were developed at the University of Washington (**Table 6.4**). This classification system uses spectral broadening to discriminate between lesions of 1–19% stenosis and those of 20–49% stenosis.[9] The assessment of spectral broadening, however, requires a constant Doppler angle, which is frequently not possible in peripheral duplex scanning. Therefore, analysis of varying degrees of spectral broadening has practical limitations in the evaluation of peripheral arterial disease.

The peak systolic velocity (PSV) ratio is also a widely accepted tool for grading the degree of stenosis. This ratio is based on the principle that the total flow at a lesion must be the same as the immediate pre- and post-stenotic area, and therefore a change in velocity is directly proportional to a change in cross-sectional area. The main advantage of the PSV ratio is that it is independent of changes in blood pressure, cardiac output, and vascular compliance. Typically, the velocity within a stenosis is compared with the velocity just proximal to the stenosis. Grading stenoses using the PSV ratio has been found to be highly reproducible.[10,11] A 50% stenosis in the lower extremity has been considered by different investigators to correlate with a PSV ratio from 1.4 to 3.0,[7,12–15] although a velocity ratio of 2.0 is used by most vascular laboratories as indicative of a 50% lesion.

Clinical applications

For the past decade, research efforts have focused on the ability of lower extremity duplex to replace contrast arteriography in the preoperative assessment of candidates for arterial intervention. Arterial duplex is clearly less invasive, less expensive, and safer than arteriography; however, this technology is highly operator-dependent. Also, the technical success rate of imaging the infrapopliteal arteries is reported to be 82–90%.[7] Nevertheless, successful lower extremity revascularization can be completed using only preoperative arterial duplex in up to 90% of cases.[16–18] Overall, the limiting factor with preoperative arterial duplex is the ability to accurately identify the best site for the distal anastomosis of a bypass graft, especially when the distal anastomotic site is below the knee.[19]

The role of duplex ultrasound scanning in the surveillance of lower extremity vein grafts has been well documented (**Figs 6.6 & 6.7**). Detection and repair of graft-threatening stenoses improves graft patency.[20–23] Twenty to thirty percent of vein grafts will develop a stenosis, which will require revision.[24] These lesions are readily identified and monitored for progression by duplex ultrasound. The recommended regimen for vein graft duplex surveillance is every 3 months for the first year and every 6 months thereafter. Approximately 80% of vein graft stenoses develop in the first postoperative year, but, because lesions can develop at any time, surveillance should be continued for the life of the graft. The examination involves

Duplex ultrasound blood flow velocities of normal lower extremity arterial segments.	
Artery	*Peak systolic velocity (cm/s)*
External iliac	119 ± 21
Common femoral	114 ± 25
Superficial femoral	91 ± 14
Popliteal	69 ± 14

Table 6.3 Duplex ultrasound blood flow velocities (mean ± standard deviation) of normal lower extremity arterial segments.

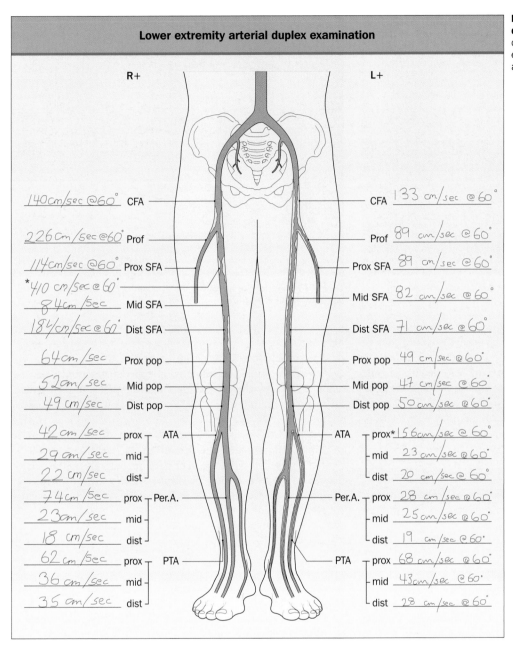

Figure 6.5 Lower extremity arterial duplex examination. This patient has diffuse arteriosclerosis of the left lower extremity and a right superficial femoral artery stenosis.

Degree of stenosis (%)	Criteria
0	Normal waveform velocities
1–19	Normal waveform velocities with spectral broadening
20–49	Marked spectral broadening, 30% increase in peak systolic velocity
50–99	Marked spectral broadening, 100% increase in peak systolic velocity, loss of reverse diastolic flow component of waveform
Occluded	No detectable flow signal in well-visualized artery

University of Washington duplex criteria for determination of peripheral arterial stenosis.

Table 6.4 University of Washington duplex criteria for determination of peripheral arterial stenosis.

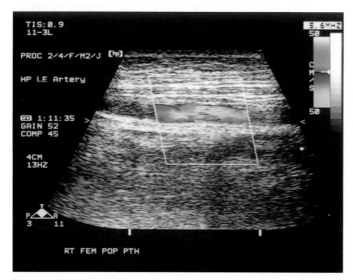

Figure 6.6 Arterial duplex of a right femoral popliteal reverse vein graft.

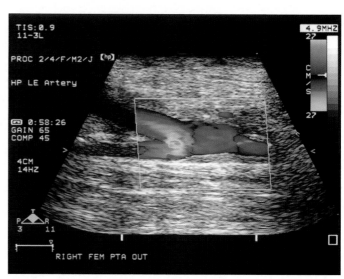

Figure 6.7 Arterial duplex of the distal anastomosis of a right femoral posterior tibial vein graft.

insonation of the proximal inflow artery, proximal anastomosis, mid-graft, distal anastomosis, and the distal outflow artery. A PSV ratio of 4, or a PSV above 300cm/s, indicates a critical graft stenosis, and arteriography and repair of the lesion should be considered.[25] If the PSV ratio is between 2 and 4, the patient should be re-evaluted in 3 months with a duplex examination.

SUMMARY

The non-invasive vascular laboratory provides critically important, objective information to supplement a careful history and physical examination in the evaluation of patients with chronic lower extremity ischemia. Optimal utilization of vascular testing will always depend on a sophisticated knowledge of vascular disease and detailed knowledge of the individual patient. A keen awareness of the limitations of each form of testing and potential sources of error is mandatory. Non-invasive vascular testing allows quantitative, physiologic assessment of lower extremity ischemia and provides the scientific basis for modern therapeutic approaches to the care of patients with arterial occlusive disease. Clearly, the vascular laboratory provides the objective diagnostic foundation on which the modern practice of vascular surgery is built.

REFERENCES

1. Yao JST, Nedham TN, Gourmos C. A comparative study of strain gauge plethysmography and Doppler ultrasound in the assessment of occlusive arterial disease of the lower extremities. Surgery 1972;71:4–9.
2. Yao JST, Flinn WR. Plethsymography. In: Kempczinski RF, Yao JST, eds. Practical noninvasive vascular diagnosis. Chicago:Yearbook Medical Publishers; 1987:80–94.
3. Darling RC, Raines JK, Brener BF. Quantitative segmental pulse volume recorder: a clinical tool. Surgery 1972;72:873–87.
4. Strandness DE. Peripheral arterial disease: a physiologic approach. Boston: Little, Brown; 1969:112–30.
5. Kempczinski RF. Segmental volume plethysmography: the pulse volume recorder. In: Kempczinski RF, Yao JST, eds. Practical noninvasive vascular diagnosis. Chicago:Yearbook Medical Publishers; 1987:140–53.
6. Krikendall WM, Burton AC, Epstein FH, et al. Recommendations for human blood pressure determination by sphygmomanometers: report of a subcommittee of the postgraduate education committee, American Heart Association. Circulation 1967;36:980–8.
7. Moneta GL, Yeager RA, Antonovic R, et al. Accuracy of lower extremity arterial duplex mapping. J Vasc Surg 1992;15:275–84.
8. Rizzo RJ, Sandager G, Astleford P, et al. Mesenteric flow velocity variations as a function of angle of insonation. J Vasc Surg 1990;11:688–94.
9. Jager KA, Ricketts HJ, Strandness DE. Duplex scanning for evaluation of lower limb arterial disease. In: Bernstein EF, ed. Noninvasive diagnostic techniques in vascular disease. St Louis:Mosby; 1985:619–31.
10. Whyman MR, Hoskins PR, Leng GC, et al. Accuracy and reproducibility of duplex ultrasound imaging in a phantom model of femoral artery stenosis. J Vasc Surg 1993;17:524–30.
11. Leng GC, Whyman MR, Donnan PT, et al. Accuracy and reproducibility of duplex ultrasonography in grading femoropopliteal stenoses. J Vasc Surg 1993;17:510–7.
12. Sacks D, Robinson ML, Marinelli DL, Perlmutter GS. Peripheral arterial Doppler ultrasonography: diagnostic criteria. J Ultrasound Med 1992;11:95–103.
13. Jager KA, Phillips DJ, Martin RL, et al. Noninvasive mapping of lower limb arterial lesions. Ultrasound Med Biol 1985;11:515–21.
14. Sensier Y, Hartshorne T, Thrush A, Nydahl S, Bolia A, London NJ. A prospective comparison of lower limb colour-coded duplex scanning with arteriography. Eur J Vasc Endovasc Surg 1996;11:170–5.
15. de Smet AA, Ermers EJ, Kitslaar PJ. Duplex velocity characteristics of aortoiliac stenoses. J Vasc Surg 1996;23:628–36.
16. Elsman BH, Legemate DA, van der Heijden FH, de Vos HJ, Mali WP, Eikelboom BC. Impact of ultrasonographic duplex scanning on therapeutic decision making in lower-limb arterial disease. Br J Surg 1995;82:630–3.
17. Ascher E, Mazzariol F, Hingorani A, Salles-Cunha S, Gade P. The use of duplex ultrasound arterial mapping as an alternative to conventional arteriography for primary and secondary infrapopliteal bypasses. Am J Surg 1999;178:162–5.
18. Mazzariol F, Ascher E, Salles-Cunha SX, Gade P, Hingorani A. Values and limitations of duplex ultrasonography as the sole imaging method of preoperative evaluation for popliteal and infrapopliteal bypasses. Ann Vasc Surg 1999;13:1–10.
19. Larch E, Minar E, Ahmadi R, et al. Value of color duplex sonography for evaluation of tibioperoneal arteries in patients with femoropopliteal

obstruction: a prospective comparison with anterograde intraarterial digital subtraction angiography. J Vasc Surg 1997;25:629–36.

20. Landry GJ, Moneta GL, Taylor LM, Jr, Edwards JM, Yeager RA, Porter JM. Patency and characteristics of lower extremity vein grafts requiring multiple revisions. J Vasc Surg 2000;32:23–31.

21. Johnson BL, Bandyk DF, Back MR, Avino AJ, Roth SM. Intraoperative duplex monitoring of infrainguinal vein bypass procedures. J Vasc Surg 2000;31:678–90.

22. Idu MM, Blankenstein JD, de Gier P, Truyen E, Buth J. Impact of a color-flow duplex surveillance program on infrainguinal vein graft patency: a five-year experience. J Vasc Surg 1993;17:42–52; discussion 52–3.

23. Lundell A, Lindblad B, Bergqvist D, Hansen F. Femoropopliteal-crural graft patency is improved by an intensive surveillance program: a prospective randomized study. J Vasc Surg 1995;21:26–33; discussion 33–4.

24. Passman MA, Moneta GL, Nehler MR, et al. Do normal early color-flow duplex surveillance examination results of infrainguinal vein grafts preclude the need for late graft revision? J Vasc Surg 1995;22:476–81; discussion 482–4.

25. Mills JL Sr, Wixon CL, James DC, Devine J, Westerband A, Hughes JD. The natural history of intermediate and critical vein graft stenosis: recommendations for continued surveillance or repair. J Vasc Surg 2001;33:273–8; discussion 278–80.

CHAPTER
7

The Medical Management of Claudication

Frank C T Smith

KEY POINTS

- Intermittent claudication is a manifestation of peripheral arterial disease, reflecting systemic atherosclerosis in which the coronary and cerebrovascular systems may also be involved.

- Treatment of claudication should now encompass secondary prevention for coronary and cerebrovascular events.

- Best medical treatment involves control of risk factors, including smoking cessation, supervised exercise, and control of hyperlipidemia, hypertension, diabetes, and hyperhomocysteinemia.

- Aspirin, clopidogrel, and the statins have established benefits in the prevention of secondary events.

- Naftidrofuryl and oxypentifylline have limited efficacy in improving walking capacity, but cilostazol has recently been shown to improve both pain-free walking distance and maximal walking distance, and appears to have a beneficial effect on quality of life.

INTRODUCTION

Peripheral arterial disease (PAD) involves the atherosclerotic occlusion of the arterial circulation to the lower limbs (**Fig. 7.1**). The condition is a common cause of morbidity in western countries and its increasing incidence reflects the growing proportion of elderly in the population.

PAD is part of a systemic disorder in which the coronary and cerebrovascular circulations may also be involved. Patients with PAD have an increased risk of ischemic heart disease and stroke, and the risk of death from cardiovascular causes in patients with PAD is equivalent to that in patients with a history of coronary or cerebrovascular disease.

The condition is characterized by intermittent claudication – muscular pain in one or both legs on walking, primarily affecting the calves, but which may also affect thigh and buttock muscles. The pain does not resolve on continued walking but is relieved by rest.

Sixty percent of patients with claudication die from coronary heart disease and 10% die from stroke.[1] The goals of managing claudication have recently broadened, therefore, to encompass prevention of coronary and cerebrovascular events.[2]

PREVALENCE AND INCIDENCE OF INTERMITTENT CLAUDICATION

Most epidemiologic studies have employed a standard World Health Organisation (WHO) questionnaire to diagnose claudication.[3] This diagnostic tool has acknowledged limitations in terms of being only moderately sensitive for the condition despite achieving high specificity, a deficit which has led to the development of more sensitive screening tools such as the Edinburgh Claudication Questionnaire.[4]

There is considerable variation in the prevalence of intermittent claudication in epidemiologic studies from different countries, ranging from 0.3% to 9%. In two UK studies, prevalences were 4.6% for Edinburgh men aged 55–74 years[5] and 7% in elderly men in Southampton.[6] The annual incidence is age related and ranges from 2–6 new cases per thousand population at age 50, to 5–10 new cases per thousand at age 70.[7,8] The variability in reported studies partially reflects differences in age structures of the examined populations.

NATURAL HISTORY OF CLAUDICATION

Morbidity

In patients with claudication, atherosclerotic disease progression tends to occur slowly and the condition has a relatively benign prognosis. Half of all patients may expect some improvement of symptoms, presumably owing to the development of collaterals or to adaption (either psychologic or because of changes in lifestyle). Improvement is more likely to occur in those patients who stop smoking. Symptoms deteriorate in approximately 25% of patients. Less than 5–10% of patients develop critical ischemia

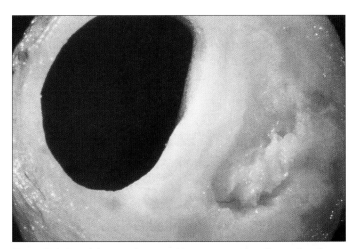

Figure 7.1 Arterial stenosis caused by an eccentric atherosclerotic plaque. There is liquefaction within the lipid core of the plaque, but the fibrous plaque cap remains intact. Stenosis or occlusion of the lower limb arteries is responsible for the symptom of intermittent claudication.

65

(rest pain, ischemic ulceration, or gangrene), and only 2% of patients eventually require an amputation.[9]

Mortality

Relative risk of death from all causes in claudicants, compared with the age-matched healthy population, is sex-dependent, ranging from approximately 1.6%[10] to 3.8%,[11] men being slightly more at risk than women. Cumulative 5-year mortality in men ranges from approximately 5% to 17%. Risk of death from cardiovascular causes is increased, the majority of excess mortality accounted for by fatal myocardial infarctions and strokes. In patients with known coronary artery disease, the presence of PAD is an independent risk factor for mortality, increasing the risk by 25% even after adjustment for other factors. Smoking, diabetes, hypertension, and elevated serum cholesterol also appear to confer increased risk.[12]

TREATMENT FOR INTERMITTENT CLAUDICATION

The traditional goals of treatment for intermittent claudication are to relieve the patient's symptoms of pain on walking, to increase walking capacity, and to improve quality of life. However, recognition of the inter-relationship of intermittent claudication with other manifestations of cardiovascular disease means that intervention should now be directed not only to improving focal symptoms but also to reducing the risk of coronary and cerebrovascular events. A recent consensus document has reviewed approaches to the diagnosis and treatment of PAD, providing a detailed discussion which places the use of appropriate medical and surgical therapeutic strategies in context.[9]

Control of risk factors for both claudication and the other sequelae of cardiovascular disease is central to the medical management of claudication. There is sufficient evidence to argue for risk factor modification in all patients with PAD regardless of the severity of symptoms.[13] Beyond this, the decision to intervene for claudication is dependent on the individual patient's quality of life and on the extent to which the symptoms interfere with the patient's occupation and daily activities.

Objective evaluation of the impact of claudication on an individual patient is potentially fraught with difficulties. The patient's assessment of his or her own walking distance, obtained when taking a medical history, is often unreliable. Patient and doctor may lack insight into the wide-ranging effects of the patient's symptoms on quality of life. Intermittent claudication has been shown to impact on sleep, emotional behavior, and social interactions, in addition to mobility.[14]

Quality-of-life questionnaires such as the non-disease-specific Medical Outcomes Short Form 36 Questionnaire (SF-36) or the disease-specific Walking Impairment Questionnaire (WIQ) may help define functional, physical, and mental limitations but need to be interpreted cautiously, particularly with respect to the effect of concomitant medical conditions.

Assessment

Routine investigations include measurement of fasting blood glucose or hemoglobin A1c (HbA1c) and lipid concentrations, a full blood cell count (to exclude anemia, polycythemia, leukemia, and thrombocythemia), urea, creatinine and electrolytes (for baseline assessment of renal function), and liver function tests

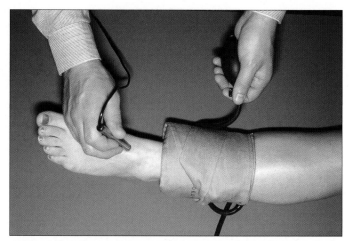

Figure 7.2 Continuous-wave Doppler measurement of ankle pressures. Continuous-wave Doppler measurement of ankle pressures is the primary investigation in assessment for intermittent claudication. Measurement of post-exercise pressures may increase the diagnostic sensitivity of the test.

(prior to and during statin therapy). Hypercoagulability screens and measurement of homocysteine levels should be performed selectively. An electrocardiogram (ECG) should be obtained. Many patients with claudication have a history of smoking, and a chest X-ray is mandatory to exclude an occult bronchial carcinoma.

Ankle–brachial pressure indices (ABPIs) of <0.9 at rest are useful in confirming the diagnosis of peripheral vascular disease and in helping to distinguish this from non-vascular causes of leg pain such as spinal stenosis (**Fig. 7.2**). Patients with leg pain on walking who have ABPIs of 0.91–1.30 should undergo an exercise test. Treadmill testing is helpful to define maximal walking distance (MWD) and pain-free walking distance (PFWD) but may not adequately simulate the patient's normal walking pace. In a patient with an ABPI of >0.9, a decrease by >20% post exercise is indicative of arterial disease.

Patients with ABPIs of >1.0 but with symptoms of claudication may have incompressible arteries. This clinical picture frequently occurs in diabetic patients due to calf vessel calcification. Other useful investigative modalities in this situation include Doppler assessment of toe pressures, the 'pole test'[15] (Doppler measurement of ankle pressures on leg elevation), and duplex ultrasound assessment of iliac, superficial femoral, and calf vessels (**Fig. 7.3**).

Magnetic resonance angiography is a valuable non-invasive adjunctive investigation for localizing stenotic or occlusive peripheral vascular disease, but, at present, digital subtraction angiography remains the investigation of choice when intervention by angioplasty or surgery is to be considered (**Fig. 7.4**).

MODIFICATION OF RISK FACTORS

Hyperlipidemia

Alterations in lipid metabolism are a major risk factor for all forms of atherosclerosis. There is evidence from several large epidemiologic studies demonstrating that elevated serum total cholesterol and low-density lipoprotein (LDL) cholesterol levels and decreased high-density lipoprotein (HDL) cholesterol levels are significantly associated with cardiovascular mortality.[16,17]

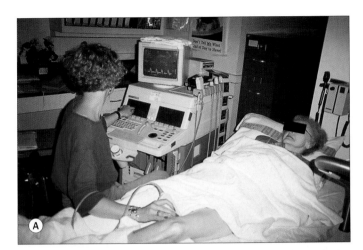

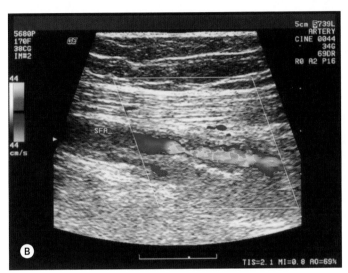

Figure 7.3 Duplex ultrasound. (A) Non-invasive duplex Doppler assessment of the lower limb arteries provides anatomic, morphologic, and hemodynamic information about the nature of vessel disease. (B) B-mode color-flow duplex ultrasound, showing a tight stenosis in the superficial femoral artery (SFA) of a claudicant. Turbulent blood flow in the vicinity of the stenosis is indicated by the change of color from blue to orange. Spectral analysis demonstrated a sixfold increase in blood flow velocity through the stenotic region.

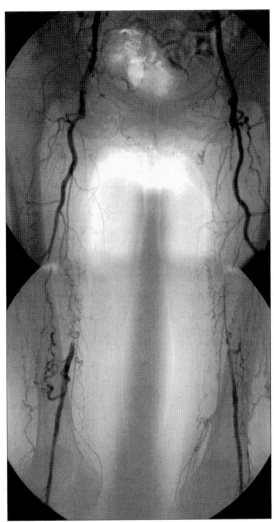

Figure 7.4 Digital subtraction angiography demonstrating bilateral superficial femoral artery occlusions, with development of extensive collateral circulations, in a patient with calf claudication in both legs.

The role of elevated triglyceride levels has been debated and it has been suggested that a strong association between triglyceride and cholesterol levels may account for the apparent effects of triglycerides. However, recent studies have shown conclusively that elevated triglyceride levels are also a strong and independent predictor of both ischemic heart disease and PAD.

Specific lipid fractions appear to be important in determining the extent and progression of atherosclerosis. Elevated total cholesterol, LDL cholesterol, triglycerides, and lipoprotein(a) are independent risk factors for PAD.[18,19] Increases in HDL cholesterol and apolipoprotein A-I confer protection.[19] For every increase of 10mg/dl in total cholesterol, the risk of PAD rises by approximately 10%. Increases in lipoprotein(a) appear to increase the risk of coronary disease by twofold and similar results have been noted in patients with PAD. Critical levels are 30mg/dL or greater. Apolipoprotein B, a large protein contained within LDL particles, has also been associated with development of PAD. In studies, higher levels of apolipoprotein B have been found in patients with peripheral vascular disease than in controls and there also appear to be differences in the apolipoprotein B gene locus between these groups.[20]

A meta-analysis of seven randomized controlled trials of lipid-lowering therapy in patients with PAD found inconsistencies in outcome with respect to changes in ABPIs and walking distances.[21] In these trials, 698 patients were treated with a variety of lipid-lowering therapies including diet, probucol, cholestyramine, and nicotinic acid, for periods of 4 months up to 3 years. The difference in mortality of 0.7% in treated patients versus 2.9% in controls did not achieve statistical significance. However, lipid-lowering therapy was effective in reducing disease progression as assessed by angiography and the severity of claudication.

Attempts to reduce lipid levels by diet alone achieved reductions of only 5–10% and a number of the drugs employed in the above studies have considerable side effects. In the Cholesterol Lowering Atherosclerosis Study, 188 men with both coronary disease and PAD were randomized to colestipol plus niacin or to placebo after initial diet control.[22] In the treated group, there was regression or stabilization of femoral atherosclerosis compared with the control group. In the St Thomas' Trial, a small number of patients ($n=25$) were treated with diet plus cholestyramine, nicotinic acid, or clofibrate for a mean period of 19 months, with an apparent beneficial effect on femoral atherosclerosis.[23]

Probucol is a drug that reduces LDL and HDL cholesterol concentrations. The Probucol Qualitative Regression Swedish Trial studied 303 patients with PAD who were treated by diet and cholestyramine and then by either probucol or placebo for 3 years.[24] No significant beneficial effect of probucol treatment was demonstrated on either femoral atherosclerosis or ABPIs. In the Program on the Surgical Control of the Hyperlipidemias (POSCH), ileal bypass was used to lower lipid concentrations and patients were followed up for 10 years.[25] This trial evaluated specific lower limb clinical endpoints. At 5 years, the relative risk of abnormal ABPIs in the treated group was 0.6 (95% confidence interval [CI], 0.4–0.9; absolute risk reduction, 15 percentage points; $p<0.01$), and that of claudication or limb-threatening ischemia, 0.7 (95% CI, 0.2–0.9; absolute risk reduction, 7 percentage points; $p<0.01$), compared with the control group.

The statins

The statins are a newer class of antilipidemic agent. These drugs are HMG-CoA reductase inhibitors and effectively reduce serum cholesterol (**Fig. 7.5**). However, they also have valuable ancillary effects on endothelial function, including plaque stabilization and antithrombogenic properties, and reduce plasma fibrinogen levels (**Table 7.1**).

The statins differ with respect to cytochrome P450 metabolism and drug interactions, but all may cause rhabdomyolysis. At present, only pravastatin and simvastatin are licensed for secondary prevention. Cerivastatin, which is metabolized by both cytochrome P450 3A4 and cytochrome P450 2C8, has recently been withdrawn because of potentially significantly higher rates of rhabdomyolysis when administered in combination with another drug, gemfibrozil. Statins should be used cautiously in patients with liver disease. Liver functions tests should be performed at baseline, and then repeated within 1 to 3 months of starting treatment and thereafter 6-monthly for 1 year.

To date, five major randomized controlled trials have shown a reduction in total mortality and major coronary events by lowering levels of serum cholesterol with statin therapy in patients with or without a history of cardiac disease.

A meta-analysis of these studies found that statin drug treatment was associated with mean reductions of total and LDL cholesterol of 20% and 28%, respectively, a 13% reduction in triglycerides, and a 5% increase in HDL cholesterol.[26] In the Long-term Intervention with Pravastatin in Ischemic Disease (LIPID) Study, a subgroup analysis of 905 out of 9014 patients with coronary heart disease and claudication showed a significant reduction in myocardial and cerebrovascular events in patients treated with pravastatin.[27] In the Heart Protection Study (HPS), statins were shown to reduce the risk of heart attack, stroke, and revascularization by at least a third in patients with PAD.[28] Average reductions in blood total and LDL cholesterol of 2mmol/L and 1.5mmol/L, respectively, were achieved. This study concluded that 5 years of statin therapy would prevent major vascular events in 70 of every 1000 patients with PAD.

The main reason for using these drugs to date, therefore, has been to reduce cardiovascular events. However, specifically with respect to PAD, the Scandinavian Simvastatin Survival Study (4S) found that the incidence of new-onset or worsening intermittent claudication was reduced by 38% in patients on statin therapy versus placebo, after 3 years (relative risk, 0.62; 95% CI, 0.44–0.88; absolute risk reduction, 1.3 percentage points).[29]

In further study, the effect of reducing serum lipoprotein(a) concentrations by plasma apheresis was investigated in 42 patients with primary hypercholesterolemia and extensive coronary atherosclerosis, who were randomized to receive simvastatin alone or simvastatin plus apheresis.[30] Follow-up was continued for 2 years. The peripheral arterial endpoints included assessment of femoral and tibial artery atherosclerotic disease by duplex ultrasonography. In the simvastatin-only group, the number of patients with

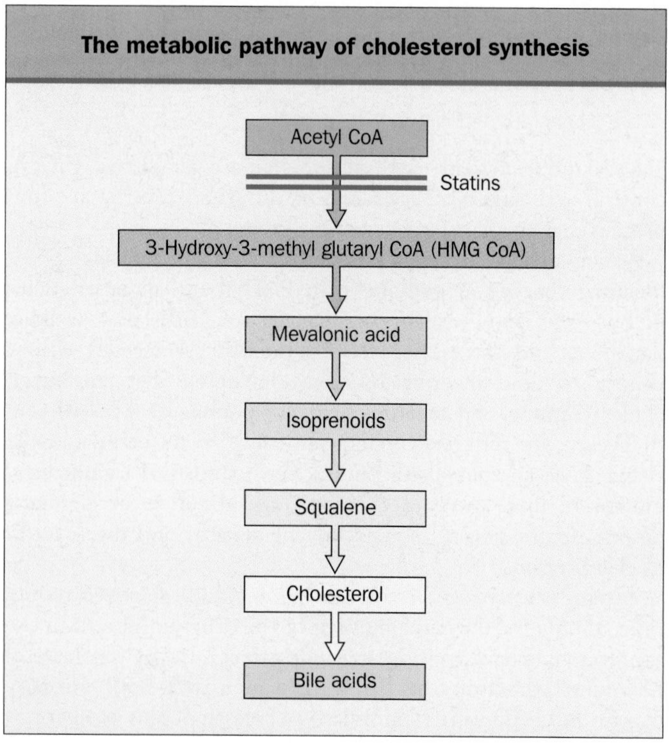

The metabolic pathway of cholesterol synthesis

Acetyl CoA

⟶ Statins

3-Hydroxy-3-methyl glutaryl CoA (HMG CoA)

Mevalonic acid

Isoprenoids

Squalene

Cholesterol

Bile acids

Figure 7.5 The metabolic pathway of cholesterol synthesis.
Blockade by statins (HMG-CoA reductase inhibitors) occurs at the first, rate-limiting step.

Non-lipid-lowering effects of statins.
Inhibition of vascular smooth muscle cell proliferation and migration
Improved endothelial function and vasomotion
Reduced oxygen-free radical production by activated macrophages
Reduced LDL oxidation
Reduced platelet aggregability
Increased fibrinolysis
Reduced fasting insulin concentrations

Table 7.1 Non-lipid-lowering effects of statins. LDL, low-density lipoprotein.

hemodynamically significant stenoses increased; in contrast, in those patients who were also treated by apheresis, the number decreased (p=0.002). Although apheresis has little practical scope as a routine therapy, these results achieved statistical significance and provide further evidence implicating lipoprotein(a) in peripheral atherogenesis.

In summary, lipid-lowering therapy benefits patients with PAD, who often have concomitant coronary and cerebrovascular disease. There is now a move toward the use of statins for secondary prevention, irrespective of the levels of cholesterol. Treatment benefits with statins appear similar in men and women and are independent of age, up to 75 years; however, there are insufficient data on treatment of patients above this age. The current aims of treatment of patients with PAD should be to lower total cholesterol concentrations to below 5mmol/L or by 20–25%, to lower LDL cholesterol levels to below 3mmol/L or by 30%, and to achieve a triglyceride concentration of less than 1.7mmol/L, with statins and dietary advice. Patients with very high cholesterol concentrations (>8mmol/L) may be suffering from a familial hyperlipidemia and should be referred to a specialist lipid clinic for advice, since these patients may benefit from combination therapies.

Hyperhomocysteinemia
High serum homocysteine levels are an independent risk factor for development of PAD.[31] Hyperhomocysteinemia may be related to an autosomal recessive inborn error of metabolism or be due to nutritional, physiologic, or pathologic factors, including dietary folate deficiencies and alterations in vitamin B_{12} metabolism. Patients with hyperhomocysteinemia and symptomatic PAD have a fourfold risk of vascular mortality and morbidity relative to patients with normal homocysteine levels.[32] Approximately one-third of patients with PAD have elevated serum homocysteine levels,[33] and for every 5μmol/L

rise in fasting homocysteine levels, there is an increase in relative risk of atherosclerotic disease of about 35% for men and 42% for women.

The mechanism of action of homocysteine is not fully elucidated, but is thought to involve facilitation of oxidation of LDL cholesterol. Homocysteine is implicated in the generation of oxygen-free radicals, which give rise to endothelial dysfunction with impaired nitric oxide (NO) generation and proliferation of smooth muscle cells, leading to acceleration of the process of atherosclerosis. It may also be implicated in blood hypercoagulability.

Homocysteine synthesis and metabolism is outlined in **Figure 7.6**. High serum homocysteine levels can be lowered by dietary supplementation with vitamins B_6 and B_{12}, and folate. However, at present, there exist no randomized clinical trials showing that lowering serum homocysteine concentrations confers a clinical benefit regarding claudication. These areas are currently being explored.

Diabetes mellitus
Lower limb arterial disease is a well-recognized complication of diabetes mellitus and may result from both macrovascular and microvascular disease. The incidence of claudication and low ABPIs is two- to sixfold higher in diabetic patients than in the age-matched population. Intensive control of blood glucose is well established in the treatment of microvascular complications of diabetes but the role of scrupulous diabetic control in prevention of macrovascular sequelae is less well defined.

In the UK Prospective Diabetes Study (UKPDS), 3867 patients with type 2 diabetes were randomized to receive either intensive care or 'usual care'.[34] Intensive care comprised treatment with either sulfonylureas or insulin; conventional care was achieved with diet therapy. Intensive care resulted in a significant reduction in the incidence of diabetes-related endpoints, including

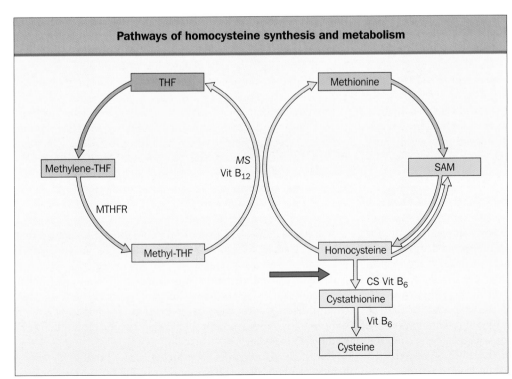

Pathways of homocysteine synthesis and metabolism

THF

Methylene-THF

MTHFR

Methyl-THF

MS Vit B_{12}

Methionine

SAM

Homocysteine

CS Vit B_6

Cystathionine

Vit B_6

Cysteine

Figure 7.6 Pathways of homocysteine synthesis and metabolism, and the involvement of vitamins B_6, B_{12}, and folate. The block arrow indicates the site of deficiency of the enzyme cystathionine synthase, which occurs in homocysteinuria, as a result of an autosomal recessive inborn error of metabolism. CS, cystathionine synthase; MS, methionine synthase; MTHFR, methylene tetrahydrofolate reductase; SAM, S-adenosyl methionine; THF, tetrahydrofolate.

myocardial infarction. The major part of this reduction was directly attributable to a reduction in microvascular-related complications. Risk of amputation, however, was not altered by intensive diabetic control.

In another important study, the Diabetes Control and Complications Trial (DCTT), 1441 patients with type 1 diabetes were treated by intensive or conventional insulin therapy.[35] There was a lower incidence of cardiovascular events in the intensively treated patients, which did not quite achieve statistical significance (p=0.08). However, there was a negligible difference in outcome with respect to peripheral vascular disease.

These results suggest that good blood glucose control in patients with type 1 or type 2 diabetes may not be sufficient to improve the outcome of associated peripheral vascular disease. The cornerstone of management here, therefore, is to attempt good diabetic control but in conjunction with aggressive management of other risk factors by, for example, diet, provision of adequate exercise, and control of smoking and blood pressure.

Hypertension

Hypertension has a strong association with the presence of PAD, the risk of claudication being increased up to threefold in hypertensive patients.[36] Treatment of hypertension may reduce cardiovascular deaths by 14% and the stroke rate by 38%, with a reduction in peripheral vascular events of 26%. However, there is little evidence to suggest that treatment alters either the progress of peripheral atherosclerosis or the symptoms of intermittent claudication.

Early studies suggested that treatment of hypertensive patients with beta-adrenergic antagonists aggravated the symptoms of claudication. These reports have been superseded by a meta-analysis of 11 randomized controlled trials, in which no detrimental effect of the drugs on walking distance or symptoms of claudication in patients with PAD was demonstrated.[37] The current view is that beta-blockers are safe to administer to patients with mild-to-moderate PAD but that if symptoms deteriorate after initial administration of these drugs, other appropriate antihypertensive medication – for instance, calcium antagonists, such as nifedipine – should be prescribed.

Angiotensin-converting enzyme (ACE) inhibitors may have a valuable cardioprotective role in patients with PAD. In large studies, ACE inhibitors such as ramipril have been shown to reduce death from vascular causes, non-fatal myocardial infarcts, and cerebrovascular accidents in hypertensive patients. However, the outcomes do not differ significantly between those patients with, and those without, PAD.

Smoking

Epidemiologic studies have shown that a lifetime of cigarette smoking approximately doubles the risk of morbidity and mortality from ischemic heart disease, compared with not smoking.[38] The risk is related to the amount and duration of smoking. Smoking cessation rapidly reduces this risk, although it may be up to 20 years – if ever – before the risk is completely reversed. Heavy smokers are three times more likely to develop intermittent claudication than are non-smokers, and the risks of developing critical limb ischemia or requiring amputation are three- to fivefold higher among patients with PAD who continue to smoke. Patients with PAD should therefore be encouraged and helped to stop smoking and to refrain from restarting.

The value and application of effective anti-smoking strategies have largely been neglected in everyday clinical practice. Unfortunately, long-term quit rates for behavioral interventions alone are poor, with only 15–30% of patients remaining abstinent after 1 year of treatment. However, there is good evidence that nicotine replacement therapy (NRT)[39] and oral bupropion[40] may improve smoking quit rates in motivated patients by two- to threefold at 1 year.

Cigarette smoking has two deleterious components: nicotine, which is addictive but plays no significant role in atherogenesis; and tar and other chemicals such as oxidizing agents, which exert powerful damaging atherogenic and carcinogenic effects, and impair lung function (**Fig. 7.7**). In using NRT, the strategy is to encourage patients to stop smoking abruptly. This precipitates nicotine withdrawal symptoms, which are alleviated by nicotine replacement via transdermal or sublingual routes or by nasal inhalation. (The oral bioavailability of nicotine is low). Transdermal and sublingual administration of NRT may be combined to achieve the plasma levels required to relieve symptoms of nicotine withdrawal, including agitation, sleep disturbance, and sympathetic nervous effects. NRT is then gradually reduced over 2–3 months.

Bupropion is an antidepressant that is licensed for use as part of a smoking-cessation program. In recent clinical trials, it has been demonstrated to be at least as effective as NRT in promoting smoking cessation.

Although the rationale for smoking cessation is still poorly understood and randomly applied by physicians, the cost-effectiveness of this intervention in patients with PAD compares favorably with that of other medical treatments such as statins and ACE inhibitors.

Exercise

Patients with intermittent claudication have diminished exercise performance and impaired overall functional and physical capacities. Peak oxygen consumption measured during treadmill testing is approximately half that of normal subjects and equivalent to that reported for patients with significant heart failure. Impairment in walking capacity is detrimental to other normal everyday functions and quality of life. Improvement of mobility per se, therefore, is an important goal for the patient with claudication.

Providing patients with advice to walk more has been shown to be largely ineffective, but formal supervised exercise training programs seem to have a beneficial effect. A recent Cochrane Review of 10 randomized trials of exercise therapy estimated an overall improvement in walking distance of approximately 150%.[41] Exercise was supervised in all but one of these trials, and, in the latter, evidence of unsupervised exercise was obtained from exercise log books and by providing patients with pedometers.

A meta-analysis of 21 exercise training programs showed that by training for at least 6 months, by walking to near-maximum pain tolerance, a significant improvement in pain-free and maximum walking distances was achieved.[42] However, similar dramatic improvements have also been reported in trials that have utilized shorter periods of exercise (1–3 months), with symptomatic improvement persisting beyond the period of supervised exercise.

The value of exercise in reducing cardiac risk is an added benefit of supervised exercise programs. Physical inactivity is an

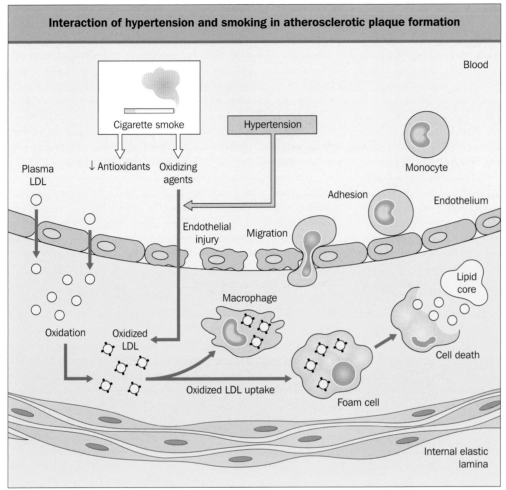

Interaction of hypertension and smoking in atherosclerotic plaque formation

Figure 7.7 Interaction of hypertension and smoking in atherosclerotic plaque formation. Monocytes adhere to the vascular endothelium and migrate to the intima. Low-density lipoprotein (LDL) also enters the intima, where it becomes oxidized and is taken up by monocytes to become foam cells. Foam-cell death, caused by apoptosis or due to necrosis induced by lipid peroxides, releases lipid, which is incorporated into the lipid core. Cigarette smoke contains oxidizing species whose passage across the endothelium is facilitated in the presence of hypertension. These oxidizing agents and the decreased levels of antioxidants found in smokers promote oxidation of LDL, speeding up the process of atherogenesis.

independent risk factor for atherosclerosis, and exercise has been shown to reduce blood pressure and to favorably influence the lipid profile and glucose metabolism in healthy persons. Furthermore, exercise rehabilitation reduces the risk of cardiovascular death after myocardial infarction by about 25%.

Exercise intensity – the rate at which work is performed – must be taken into consideration when designing an exercise program for an individual patient. It is important that the exercise intensity for aerobic work falls within the specific physiologic capabilities of each individual patient, and is sufficiently strenuous to produce a training response.

Various mechanisms have been implicated in the beneficial effects achieved by exercise training. Exercise training is not associated with a substantial increase in resting blood flow to the legs, and the changes that do occur fail to predict clinical responses. Improved cardiovascular fitness is a non-specific benefit of exercise, and upper limb training has also been shown to be effective in claudication. Some of the benefits are probably due to improved oxygen extraction by leg muscles. Alterations in muscle metabolism may also be implicated. Furthermore, training results in improvements in gait and walking efficiency.

Continued participation is an essential component of exercise therapy; thus, both initial and subsequent intensities of the training programs must be acceptable to the patient, who needs to remain motivated. The time of day at which a patient exer-

cises may affect compliance. Individuals who exercise regularly at the same time of day experience psychologic benefits at that time of day and are more likely to continue to comply with an exercise program.

In two trials comparing exercise therapy with angioplasty for claudication, conflicting data were obtained.[43,44] In the study from Oxford, exercise was found to be more effective than angioplasty at 1-year follow-up, but this advantage was lost at 70 months, when only one-third of patients still undertook exercise.[43] In the other trial, from Edinburgh, there was a benefit from angioplasty at 6 months, which was lost after 2 years.[44] Both trials, however, had relatively small numbers of patients, and data from large multicenter randomized trials of supervised exercise therapy versus angioplasty in patients with claudication are awaited.

Despite the demonstrated efficacy of exercise therapy, it has various limitations. Supervised exercise therapy is not readily available and unsupervised exercise therapy remains the mainstay of conservative treatment. Currently, in the UK, supervised exercise programs are available to only 27% of vascular surgeons.[45] Moreover, in the USA, exercise training programs are not covered by medical insurance, hindering their widespread use.

Exercise therapy appears to be cheaper and safer than surgery or angioplasty, but the optimal duration, intensity, and cost-effectiveness of exercise programs still have to be determined.

DRUG THERAPY

There is now unequivocal evidence for the value of antiplatelet agents in providing secondary protection against cardiovascular events in patients with PAD. No drug, however, has yet proved sufficiently effective in achieving a reduction or elimination of the symptoms of claudication to gain widespread acceptance or universal usage for improved walking, although a variety of drugs have been advocated for this purpose. These drugs have been reviewed in the recent TransAtlantic Inter-Society Consensus (TASC) document on the management of PAD.[9] The contents and recommendations of this document present a consensus view, devised and endorsed by 15 international societies, with representations from vascular surgery, radiology, angiology, and cardiology. The following drugs were classified as having some proven but small benefits in improving claudication distance: naftidrofuryl, oxypentifylline, cilostazol, and buflomedil. Use of the antiplatelet agents, the drugs listed above, and some of the other pharmacologic agents investigated for the treatment of claudication are discussed below.

Antiplatelet therapy
Aspirin

In patients with systemic cardiovascular disease, including those with PAD, current evidence suggests that antiplatelet drugs confer significant benefit, principally in terms of secondary prevention of vascular events.

In a recent meta-analysis of updated data from the Antithrombotic Trialists' Collaboration, results showed that among 9214 patients with PAD treated in 42 trials, allocation to antiplatelet therapy was associated with a proportional reduction of 23% (standard error, 8%) in serious vascular events

($p=0.004$) (**Fig. 7.8**).[46] Similar benefits were observed among patients with intermittent claudication, and those undergoing peripheral bypass surgery or peripheral angioplasty.

Aspirin is the most comprehensively investigated antiplatelet drug. Within a few days of beginning 75mg of aspirin daily, platelet cyclo-oxygenase-mediated production of thromboxane A_2 is virtually completely inhibited, producing an antithrombotic effect. In the Physicians' Health Study, a primary prevention trial, aspirin was found to reduce the subsequent need for arterial surgery.[47] Aspirin has also been shown to reduce vascular graft occlusion rates in patients with PAD who have previously undergone arterial bypass surgery.[48]

High doses of aspirin (500–1500mg/day), which carry greater potential risk of gastrointestinal (GI) side effects, seem to be no more effective than low doses (75–150mg). The addition of dipyridamole to aspirin does not appear to be associated with further significant reduction in serious vascular events.[46]

Ticlopidine and clopidogrel

Ticlopidine and clopidogrel are both thienopyridine drugs that inhibit platelet ADP-induced aggregation and activation. The effects of these agents could therefore be complementary to aspirin, which inhibits thromboxane-dependent activation. In patients with PAD, ticlopidine has been shown to reduce the risks of fatal and non-fatal myocardial infarction and stroke. However, the beneficial effects of ticlopidine have been partially negated by the substantial risk of thrombocytopenia, neutropenia, and thrombotic thrombocytopenic purpura. These significant side effects occur in 1 in 2000–4000 patients, and treatment therefore necessitates scrupulous hematological monitoring.

Clopidogrel is a second-generation thienopyridine with fewer side effects than ticlopidine. (The platelet inhibitory effects of

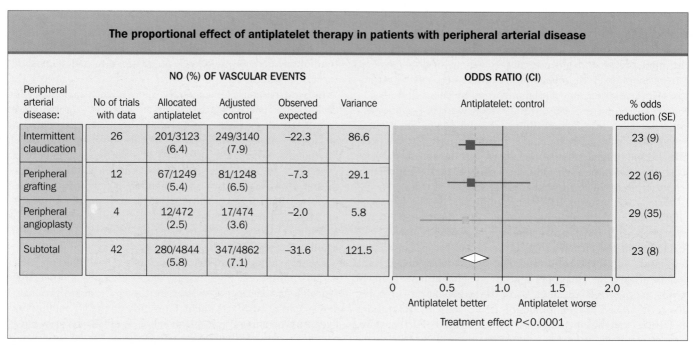

Figure 7.8 The proportional effect of antiplatelet therapy in 42 trials involving 9214 patients with peripheral arterial disease (PAD). The stratified ratio of odds of an event in treatment groups compared with that in control groups is plotted for each group of trials (square) together with its 99% confidence interval (horizontal line). Meta-analysis of the results for all categories of PAD is represented by the open diamond. Adjusted control totals were calculated after converting any unevenly randomized trials to even ones by counting control groups more than once. Other statistical calculations were based on actual numbers from individual trials. (Data from Antithrombotic Trialists' Collaboration.[46])

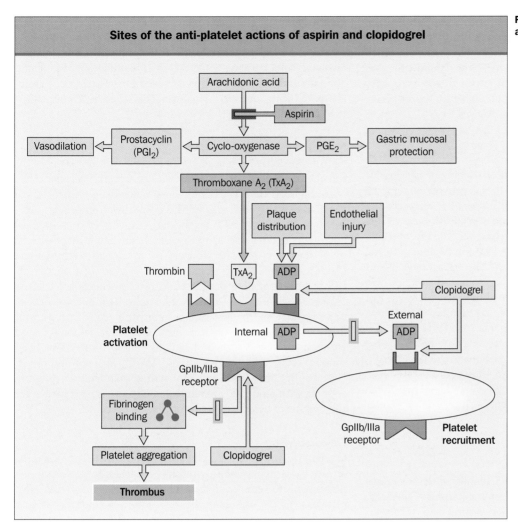

Sites of the anti-platelet actions of aspirin and clopidogrel

clopidogrel and aspirin are illustrated in **Figure 7.9**.) Evidence for the benefit of clopidogrel has principally been derived from the Clopidogrel versus Aspirin in Patients at Risk of Ischaemic Events (CAPRIE) trial.[49] This was a large randomized controlled trial conducted in 16 countries, comparing the benefits of clopidogrel, 75mg/day, with those of aspirin, 375mg/day. Over 19 000 patients participated in the trial. Primary outcome measures in this study had a composite endpoint including myocardial infarction, fatal or non-fatal ischemic stroke, or other vascular death. There was an overall risk reduction of 8.7% (p<0.05) in favor of clopidogrel compared with aspirin.

In this study, 6452 patients had either a history of claudication, with previous peripheral bypass surgery, or claudication with ABPIs of 0.85 or less. Subgroup analysis of these patients with moderate PAD showed an overall 23.8% risk reduction on treatment with clopidogrel (average event rate per year for aspirin, 4.86%, versus clopidogrel, 3.7%; p= 0.0028) (**Fig. 7.10**). Patients taking clopidogrel had a higher incidence of rash, diarrhea, and pruritis than those taking aspirin, but a lower incidence of GI disturbances and GI bleeds. An overlap in confidence intervals from negligible benefit to a 20% further reduction in vascular events in favor of clopidogrel in this trial means that the true size of any difference between aspirin and clopidogrel could not be reliably estimated.

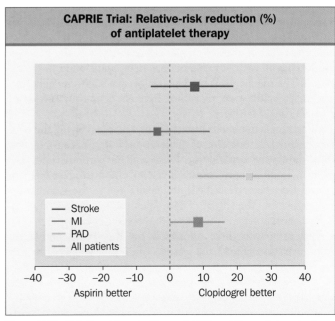

Figure 7.10 Relative-risk reduction and 95% confidence intervals, by disease subgroups, in patients with vascular disease who were treated with aspirin or clopidogrel in the CAPRIE Trial. MI, myocardial infarction; PAD, peripheral arterial disease. (From CAPRIE Steering Committee.[49])

Interest in combination therapy has been stimulated by the results of another large trial – the CURE (Clopidogrel in Unstable angina to prevent Recurrent Events) study[50] – which recently suggested improved outcome when clopidogrel was used in combination with aspirin in patients with acute coronary syndromes. However, the benefits of combination therapy have not yet been investigated in patients with PAD.

Glycoprotein IIb/IIIa inhibitors

Other recent trials involving combination therapy of aspirin plus glycoprotein IIb/IIIa antagonists in high-risk patients undergoing percutaneous coronary angioplasty have also suggested a significant benefit in terms of reduction of major vascular events over treatment with aspirin alone.[46] However, the glycoprotein IIb/IIIa antagonists were administered by intravenous infusion and benefits were offset by an increase in extracranial bleeds (not necessarily fatal), although no significant difference was observed in the incidence of intracranial bleeds, which was low (0.2% versus 0.1%). Again, combination therapy with these drugs has not yet been studied in patients with PAD.

Current evidence suggests that aspirin, at a dose of 75–150mg daily, is likely to be an appropriate antiplatelet regimen in PAD, unless patients have a definite contraindication to aspirin (e.g. allergy or appreciable gastric symptoms). Clopidogrel may be an appropriate alternative in such patients. The value of combination therapy has yet to be determined.

Cilostazol

Cilostazol is a phosphodiesterase type III inhibitor that increases cellular levels of cyclic adenosine monophosphate (cAMP). Cilostazol acts to inhibit platelet aggregation and thrombus formation, but also reduces vascular smooth muscle cell proliferation and has a direct effect as a vasodilator. Vasodilator-type drugs generally reduce systemic blood pressure, leading to a reduction in perfusion pressure of the lower limbs. They may also result in a 'steal' of blood from ischemic regions in which blood vessels are already maximally dilated; thus, the rationale for treatment with vasodilators has been questioned in claudication. The mechanisms by which cilostazol exerts its beneficial effects in claudication, therefore, have not been fully elucidated at this time.

Cilostazol is metabolized by hepatic routes involving the 3A4, 2C19, and 1A2 isoforms of cytochrome P450. Because of this, drugs inhibiting cytochrome P450, and in particular the 3A4 isoform, may increase serum levels of cilostazol. Various side effects have been described, principally due to the vasodilatory properties of the drug. These include headaches and GI disturbances.

The drug was first approved by the Food and Drug Administration (FDA) for use in claudicants in 1999. In four randomized placebo-controlled trials, cilostazol, at a dose of 50–100mg twice daily, has been shown to increase both PFWD and MWD.[51–54] Importantly, cilostazol also improved physical function and quality of life, as assessed by the SF-36 questionnaire.[52–54] Other beneficial endpoints have been increases in ABPI and raised serum HDL cholesterol concentrations. This drug, therefore, has some promise for the treatment of claudication.

Picotamide

Picotamide is an antiplatelet drug that inhibits thromboxane A_2 synthase, blocking thromboxane A_2 receptors. In a major trial involving 2304 patients with PAD, a 19% reduction of fatal and non-fatal ischemic events was achieved in the treatment group compared with controls.[55] However, this failed to achieve statistical significance.

Naftidrofuryl

Naftidrofuryl has been available in Europe, but not in the USA, for the treatment of claudication for several decades. The recommended dose is 200mg three times daily. It has a local anesthetic action and acts at the tissue level, improving oxygenation, increasing ATP levels, and reducing lactic acid, thus potentially attenuating symptoms of claudication. Mechanisms of action may include antagonism of 5-hydroxytryptamine (5-HT; serotonin).

In a review of nine double-blind placebo-controlled trials, a placebo response was seen in all studies, producing a mean improvement in PFWD of approximately 25%.[56] A further improvement of approximately 30% was seen in patients treated with naftidrofuryl, after 3–6 months. These results have been supported by two meta-analyses. MWD was not improved. Naftidrofuryl may lead to a slight symptomatic improvement in patients with moderate claudication but there is no evidence for any long-term benefit in terms of disease outcome.

Oxypentifylline

Oxypentifylline is a methylxanthine derivative that exerts its effects by reducing blood viscosity. It increases red blood cell deformability, reduces plasma fibrinogen levels, and has anti-platelet effects. The recommended dose is 400mg three times daily. Studies investigating the use of oxypentifylline as a treatment for claudication have provided conflicting evidence and have been bedevilled by variable methodology. Early controlled trials suggested a benefit over placebo in increasing initial claudication distance and absolute claudication distance. However, meta-analyses of randomized double-blind controlled trials have subsequently concluded that the limited amount and quality of reported data preclude reliable estimates of oxypentifylline efficacy and that there is insufficient evidence to support its widespread use.[57,58]

Buflomedil

Buflomedil is an agent with alpha-1 and alpha-2 adrenolytic effects. It decreases vasoconstriction and also has some anti-platelet effects, increases red cell deformability, and has a weak calcium antagonist effect. It has been available for the treatment of claudication in some countries for over 12 years. Two small studies have shown some benefit on absolute walking distance in claudicants, for treatment with buflomedil compared with placebo.

Antioxidants and chelation therapy

Oxidative injury is implicated in the pathogenesis of PAD and patients have diminished antioxidant capacity. Antioxidant vitamins C and E have been employed to reduce or attenuate this oxidative damage. However, there is little evidence of efficacy in this role in PAD.

Chelation therapy involves the use of repeated ethylene-diaminetetraacetic acid (EDTA) injections and concurrent treatment with vitamins, trace elements, and iron supplements. It has been suggested that this technique reduces the calcium content of atherosclerotic plaques, lowering LDL oxidation and facilitating activity of hydroxyl radical scavengers. Platelet adhesion is also diminished and chelation therapy appears to attenuate reperfusion injury. However, observed benefits of chelation therapy in randomized controlled trials, to date, are likely to have been due to powerful placebo responses.

Inositol nicotinate
This drug is licensed in the UK for the treatment of claudication (3–4g daily). Its mechanism of action is thought to involve vasodilation of skin blood vessels, fibrinolysis, and lipid lowering. It may also have a role in inhibition of oxidative metabolism in anoxic tissues. In randomized controlled trials, no significant benefits have been demonstrated for patients with PAD.

Cinnarizine
Cinnarizine is an antagonist to the endogenous vasoconstrictor substances 5-HT, angiotensin, and norepinephrine. It may also exert a beneficial effect on blood rheology. Current studies evaluating cinnarizine have not employed standardized methods of assessment and it is not possible to conclude that this drug is beneficial in PAD at this time.

Levocarnitine and propionyl levocarnitine
Various metabolic derangements occur in the skeletal muscle of patients with PAD. These anomalies include impairment of mitochondrial activity with accumulation of acyl carnitines, which are intermediates of oxidative metabolism. Diminished exercise performance is proportional to the accumulation of these metabolites. Both levocarnitine and propionyl levocarnitine (2g/day) have been used to treat these deleterious effects, the latter having a greater benefit. In a limited number of randomized trials, propionyl levocarnitine has been found to improve MWD and PFWD compared with placebo, with resultant beneficial effects on quality of life. However, data from larger, phase III trials are still awaited.

Prostaglandins
Prostacyclin (PGI$_2$) derivatives have been used extensively in the treatment of rest pain in critical ischemia and in patients with Raynaud's syndrome. However, few trials have critically investigated efficacy of these compounds in claudicants. One disadvantage has been that they are rapidly metabolized and, until recently, have required parenteral administration. Side effects are associated with their vasodilatory properties and include headaches, nausea, and facial flushing. In recent trials with oral analogs such as beraprost, positive – but statistically insignificant – effects on MWD and quality of life have been demonstrated. These were associated with a reduction in cardiovascular events. However, the results of larger-scale trials demonstrating a conclusive benefit are still awaited.

Immune modulation
Recently, a small double-blind prospective randomized trial has suggested that claudicants may derive some benefit, with improvement in MWD, when treated with autologous blood subjected to thermal, ultraviolet, and oxidative stresses.[59] This pilot study was carried out to investigate evidence gathered from anecdotal reports, and larger-scale trials are awaited.

SUMMARY

PAD is just one component of systemic atherosclerosis. Intermittent claudication, one of the most common symptoms of PAD, results in impaired functional capacity and diminished quality of life. To date, clinical trials in PAD have not received the emphasis accorded to ischemic heart disease and cerebrovascular disease. Despite this shortcoming, evidence is accumulating that patients with PAD should be considered for secondary prevention strategies in the same way as patients with coronary disease.

Antiplatelet agents reduce the risk of both fatal and non-fatal cardiovascular events. Aspirin should be considered for all patients with PAD, with clopidogrel as an effective alternative therapy where appropriate. Control of hyperlipidemia with statins also confers secondary protective effects. Smoking cessation and participation in a supervised exercise program are conservative measures that improve functional capacity and have other cardiovascular benefits. Various drugs including naftidrofuryl and oxypentifylline have been shown to have limited efficacy in improving walking capacity; more recently, cilostazol, too, has shown promise, not only improving PFWD and MWD but also resulting in enhanced quality of life. Other therapeutic avenues are still under investigation.

REFERENCES

1. Smith GD, Shipley MJ, Rose G. Intermittent claudication, heart disease risk factors and mortality: the Whitehall study. Circulation 1990; 82:1925–31.
2. Davies AH. The practical management of claudication. BMJ 2000; 321:911–2
3. Rose GA. The diagnosis of ischaemic heart pain and intermittent claudication in field surveys. Bull WHO 1962;27:645–58.
4. Leng GC, Fowkes FGR. The Edinburgh Claudication Questionnaire: an improved version of the WHO/Rose questionnaire for use in epidemiological surveys. J Clin Epidemiol 1992;45:1101–9.
5. Fowkes FGR, Houseley E, Cawood EHH, Macintyre CC, Ruckley CV, Prescott RJ. Edinburgh Artery Study: prevalence of asymptomatic and symptomatic peripheral vascular disease in the general population. Int J Epidemiol 1991;20:384–92.
6. Dewhurst G, Wood DA, Walker F, et al. A population survey of cardiovascular disease in elderly people: design, methods and prevalence results. Age Ageing 1991;20:353–60.
7. Kannel WB, McGee DL. Update on some epidemiological features of intermittent claudication: the Framingham Study. J Am Geriatr Soc 1985;33:13–8.
8. Leng GC, Lee AJ, Fowkes FGR, et al. Incidence, natural history and cardiovascular events in symptomatic and asymptomatic peripheral arterial disease in the general population. Int J Epidemiol 1996; 25:1172–81.
9. Dormandy JA, Rutherford RB. Management of peripheral arterial disease (PAD). TransAtlantic Inter-Society Consensus. J Vasc Surg 2000; 31:S1–296.
10. Leng GC, Fowkes FGR, Lee AJ, Dunbar J, Housley E, Ruckley CV. Use

of ankle brachial pressure index to predict cardiovascular events and death: a cohort study. BMJ 1996;313:1440–4.

11. Bainton D, Sweetnam P, Baker I, Elwood P. Peripheral vascular disease: consequence for survival and association with risk factors in the Speedwell prospective heart disease study. Br Heart J 1994;72:128–32.

12. Leng GC, Fowkes FGR. Epidemiology and risk factors for peripheral arterial disease. In: Beard JD, Gaines PA, eds. Vascular and endovascular surgery. Philadelphia:WB Saunders; 2001:1–26.

13. Hiatt WR. Medical treatment of peripheral arterial disease and claudication. N Engl J Med 2001;344:1608–21.

14. Khaira HS, Hanger R, Shearman CP. Quality of life in patients with intermittent claudication. Eur J Vasc Endovasc Surg 1996;12:65–9.

15. Smith FCT, Shearman CP, Simms MH, Gwynn BR. Falsely elevated ankle pressures in severe leg ischaemia: the pole test – an alternative approach. Eur J Vasc Surg 1994;8:408–12.

16. Martin MJ, Hulley SB, Browner WS, Kuller LH, Wentworth D. Serum cholesterol, blood pressure, and mortality: implications from a cohort of 361,662 men. Lancet 1986;2:933–6.

17. Gordon DJ, Probsfield JL, Garrison RJ et al. High-density lipoprotein cholesterol and cardiovascular disease. Four prospective American studies. Circulation 1989;79:8–15.

18. Murabito JM, D'Agostino RB, Silbershatz H, Wilson WF. Intermittent claudication. A risk profile from the Framingham Heart Study. Circulation 1997;96:44–9.

19. Johansson J, Egberg N, Hohnsson H, Carlson LA. Serum lipoproteins and hemostatic function in intermittent claudication. Arterioscler Thromb 1993;13:1441–8.

20. Monsalve MV, Young R, Jobsis J, et al. DNA polymorphism of the gene for apolipoprotein B in patients with peripheral arterial disease. Atherosclerosis 1988;70:123–9.

21. Leng GC, Price JF, Jepson RG. Lipid-lowering for lower limb atherosclerosis. Cochrane Database Syst Rev 2000;(2):CD000123.

22. Blankenhorn DH, Azen SP, Crawford DW, et al. Effects of colestipol-niacin therapy on human femoral atherosclerosis. Circulation 1991; 83:438–47.

23. Lewis B. Randomised controlled trial of the treatment of hyperlipidaemia on progression of atherosclerosis. Acta Med Scand Suppl 1985;701:53–7.

24. Walldius G, Erikson U, Olsson AG, et al. The effect of probucol on femoral atherosclerosis: the Probucol Quantitative Regression Swedish Trial (PQRST). Am J Cardiol 1994;74:875–83.

25. Buchwald H, Bourdages HR, Campos CT, Nguyen P, Williams SE, Boen JR. Impact of cholesterol reduction on peripheral arterial disease in the Program on the Surgical Control of the Hyperlipidemias (POSCH). Surgery 1996;120:672–9.

26. LaRosa JC, He J, Vupputuri S. Effect of statins on risk of coronary disease. A meta-analysis of randomized controlled trials. JAMA 1999; 282:2340–6.

27. Long-term Intervention with Pravastatin in Ischemic Disease (LIPID) Study Group. Prevention of cardiovascular events and death with pravastatin in patients with coronary heart disease and a broad range of initial cholesterol levels. N Engl J Med 1998;339:1349–57.

28. MRC/BHF Heart Protection Study of cholesterol-lowering therapy and of antioxidant vitamin supplementation in a wide range of patients at increased risk of coronary heart disease death: early safety and efficacy experience. Eur Heart J 1999;20:725–41.

29. Pedersen TR, Olsson AG, Faergeman O, et al. Effect of simvastatin on ischemic signs and symptoms in the Scandanavian Simvastatin Survival Study (4S). Am J Cardiol 1998;81:333–5.

30. Kroon AA, van Asten WN, Stalenhoef AF. Effect of apheresis of low-density lipoprotein on peripheral vascular disease in hypercholesterolemic patients with coronary artery disease. Ann Intern Med 1996;125:945–54.

31. Aronow WS, Ahn C. Association between plasma homocysteine and peripheral vascular disease in older persons. Coron Artery Dis 1998; 9:49–50.

32. Cheng SW, Ting AC, Wong J. Fasting total plasma homocysteine and atherosclerotic peripheral vascular disease. Ann Vasc Surg 1997; 11:217–23.

33. van der Berg M, Boers GH. Homocysteinuria: what about mild hyper-homocysteinaemia? Postgrad Med J 1996;72:513–8.

34. UK Prospective Diabetes Study (UKPDS) Group. Intensive blood-glucose control with sulphonylureas or insulin compared with conventional treatment and risk of complications in patients with type 2 diabetes (UKPDS 33). Lancet 1998;352:837–53. [Erratum, Lancet 1999;354:602]

35. Effect of intensive diabetes management on macrovascular events and risk factors in the Diabetes Control and Complications Trial. Am J Cardiol 1995;75:894–903.

36. Kannel WB, McGhee DL. Update on some epidemiologic features of intermittent claudication: the Framingham Study. J Am Geriatr Soc 1985;33:13–8.

37. Radack K, Deck C. Beta-adrenergic blocker therapy does not worsen intermittent claudication in subjects with peripheral arterial disease. A meta-analysis of randomized controlled trials. Arch Intern Med 1991;151:1769–76.

38. Doll R, Peto R, Wheatley K, Gray R, Sutherland I. Mortality in relation to smoking: 40 years' observations on male British doctors. BMJ 1994; 309:901–11.

39. Joseph AM, Norman SM, Ferry LH, et al. The safety of transdermal nicotine as an aid to smoking cessation in patients with cardiac disease. N Engl J Med 1996;335:1793–8.

40. Jorenby DE, Leischow SJ, Nides MA, et al. A controlled trial of sustained-release buproprion, a nicotine patch, or both for smoking cessation. N Engl J Med 1999;340:685–91.

41. Leng GC, Fowler B, Ernst E. Exercise for intermittent claudication. Cochrane Database Syst Rev 2000;(2):CD000990.

42. Garner AW, Poehlman ET. Exercise rehabilitation programs for the treatment of claudication pain. JAMA 1995;274:975–80.

43. Perkins JMT, Collin JC, Morris PJM. Angioplasty versus exercise for stable claudication: long-term results of a prospective randomised trial. Br J Surg 1995;82:557–8.

44. Whyman MR, Fowkes FGR, Kerracher E, Gillespie I, Lee M, Housley E. A randomised controlled trial of percutaneous balloon angioplasty (PTA) versus observation for intermittent claudication. Eur J Vasc Endovasc Surg 1996;12:167–72.

45. Stewart AHR, Lamont PM. Exercise for intermittent claudication. BMJ 2001;323:703–4.

46. Antithrombotic Trialists' Collaboration. Collaborative meta-analysis of randomised trials of anti-platelet therapy for prevention of death, myocardial infarction, and stroke in high risk patients. BMJ 2002; 324:71–86.

47. Goldhaber SZ, Manson JE, Stampfer MJ, et al. Low-dose aspirin and subsequent peripheral arterial surgery in the Physicians' Health Study. Lancet 1992;340:143–5.

48. Collaborative overview of randomised trials of anti-platelet therapy. II. Maintenance of vascular graft patency by anti-platelet therapy. BMJ 1994;308:159–68.

49. CAPRIE Steering Committee. A randomised, blinded trial of clopidogrel versus aspirin in patients at risk of ischaemic events (CAPRIE). Lancet 1996;348:1329–39.

50. CURE Study Investigators. Effects of clopidogrel in addition to aspirin in patients with non-ST segment elevation acute coronary syndromes. N Engl J Med 2001;345:494–502.

51. Dawson DL, Cutler BS, Hiatt WR, et al. A comparison of cilostazol and pentoxifylline for treating intermittent claudication. Am J Med 2000; 109:523–30.

52. Dawson DL, Cutler BS, Meissner MH, Strandness DEJ. Cilostazol has beneficial effects in treatment of intermittent claudication: results from a multicenter, randomized, prospective, double-blind trial. Circulation 1998;98:678–86.

53. Money SR, Herd JA, Isaacsohn JL, et al. Effect of cilostazol on walking distances in patients with intermittent claudication caused by peripheral vascular disease. J Vasc Surg 1998;27:267–74.

54. Beebe HG, Dawson DL, Cutler BS, et al. A new pharmacological treatment for intermittent claudication: results of a randomized multicenter trial. Arch Intern Med 1999;159:2041–50.

55. Balsano F, Violi F. Effect of picotamide on the clinical progression of peripheral vascular disease: a double-blind placebo-controlled study. Circulation 1993;87:1563–9.

56. Scottish Intercollegiate Guidelines Network. Drug therapy for peripheral vascular disease. Edinburgh:Scottish Intercollegiate Guidelines Network; 1998:27.

57. Hood SC, Moher D, Barber GG. Management of intermittent claudication with pentoxifylline: meta-analysis of randomized controlled trials. CMAJ 1996;155:1053–9.

58. Girolami B, Bernardi E, Prins MH, et al. Treatment of intermittent claudication with physical training, smoking cessation, pentoxifylline, or nafronyl: a meta-analysis. Arch Intern Med 1999;159:337–45.

59. McGrath C, Robb R, Lucas A, et al. A randomised, double-blind, placebo-controlled study to determine the efficacy of immune modulation therapy in the treatment of patents suffering from peripheral arterial occlusive disease with intermittent claudication. Eur J Vasc Endovasc Surg 2002;23:381–7.

CHAPTER

8

Interventional Treatment for Claudication

Dierk Vorwerk

KEY POINTS

- The Fontaine and Rutherford classifications offer clinically useful categorizations of patients with intermittent claudication (IC).

- IC may cause significant disability in the activities of daily living (lifestyle limitation) in some individuals but is unlikely to result in critical limb ischemia.

- Aortoiliac occlusive disease is generally more amenable to percutaneous intervention than is femoropopliteal occlusive disease.

- Lesion length, composition (calcification, thrombus), and morphology (concentric, eccentric) influence outcome of percutaneous intervention. TransAtlantic Inter-Society Consensus (TASC) classification should be used to guide determination of the appropriateness of percutaneous intervention.

- Balloon angioplasty with/without stenting is the best initial therapy for most TASC-A and TASC-B iliac lesions. Kissing balloon or stenting techniques are extremely useful for aortoiliac bifurcation lesions.

- Femoropopliteal lesions respond less favorably to percutaneous transluminal angioplasty (PTA) than do iliac lesions. For appropriate TASC lesions in this segment, PTA alone should be used, with stents reserved for complications and suboptimal PTA results. Femoropopliteal stents should not be routinely used.

INTRODUCTION

The title of this chapter might initially appear confusing since claudication is obviously a clinical symptom which is not strongly related to morphologic changes within the vasculature or to any specific type of treatment. It is well known that claudication is a relatively benign condition and lacks an aggressive tendency to deteriorate into a limb-threatening situation; nevertheless, affected patients may suffer significant limitations which are disabling and diminish quality of life.

Claudicants typically have limited disease of the aortoiliac, femoral, and popliteal arteries, with no major additional lesions in the subpopliteal arteries. Therefore, the techniques described in this chapter will mainly focus on these vascular provinces.

In contrast, patients with limb-threatening ischemia may show also iliac or femoral lesions in combination with lesions involving the lower leg arteries and small arteries of the foot. In such instances, however, treatment of the iliac and femoral arteries

does not differ technically from treatment of claudicants. The interventional treatment of patients with critical limb ischemia is subsequently addressed in Chapter 11.

OVERVIEW AND CLINICAL INDICATIONS FOR TREATMENT

It has generally been suggested that a surgical approach to peripheral vascular disease requires major clinical symptoms such as rest pain, non-healing ulceration, or, at least, severe claudication. Using the European classification of Fontaine, an advanced IIb or III stage is therefore accepted as requisite for invasive surgical management.

Endovascular treatment, however, is associated with low morbidity, an even lower mortality, as well as with satisfactory patient outcomes. Thus, it is fair to reconsider why an endovascular approach should be reserved only for those with severe clinical symptoms. Furthermore, occlusive arterial disease tends to occur earlier in life, owing to changed smoking and dietary habits among the population, and may affect individuals still in the active phases of a professional life.

On the other hand, intermittent claudication is not likely to worsen over time and only about 5% of claudicants ever develop critical limb ischemia if no important co-morbid factors such as diabetes are present. In light of this benign natural history, any proposed intervention should be associated with minimal risk and provide acceptable durability.

Problems of classification

Classification of intermittent claudication is difficult without the application of standardized methods. Patients are unreliable in defining their true walking distance, which may also be limited by their general physical abilities, coexisting angina pectoris, and their individual circumstances of living. Precise definition of walking distance requires a standardized treadmill test.

In the Fontaine classification, stage IIa defines a walking distance of more than 200m and IIb one of less than 200m. The Rutherford system distinguishes between category 1 (mild claudication), 2 (moderate), and 3 (severe). Comparing both systems, Fontaine stage IIa is equivalent to Rutherford category 1, while Fontaine stage IIb includes both Rutherford categories 2 and 3.[1] Nevertheless, while both systems offer an objective framework to provide guidelines for treatment and are very useful tools for scientific reporting, they may not totally reflect the degree of disability in an individual patient.

Lifestyle-limiting claudication

Intermittent claudication may affect a patient's life in various degrees and result in different levels of activity limitation. It is obvious that a patient with coexisting major angina pectoris or severe emphysema may not experience major disability even from severe peripheral arterial disease (PAD) since the coexisting diseases will limit that patient's walking capacity. An 85-year-old patient with significantly limited physical abilities may therefore be less affected from PAD than a young and active patient of 45 years. However, in an amputee, even mild claudication in the remaining leg may cause major restrictions of lifestyle since the patient is fully dependent on the remaining limb. People living in a flat area may not have major problems compared with those living in a mountainous region or on the seventh floor of an inner-city apartment block with no access to a lift. A younger individual previously used to an active sports life will hardly accept mild claudication since it is preventing that person from pursuing activities that are important to his or her lifestyle.

Therefore, in each patient, the individual circumstances of living should be taken into account before determining whether invasive therapy is indicated. Lifestyle-limiting claudication is an appropriate term and lifestyle alteration should be considered when evaluating a patient for potential interventional therapy.

Comparison of endovascular and surgical treatment

Endovascular therapy is perceived to be a less invasive form of therapy associated with good technical success and fair overall patency. For percutaneous transluminal angioplasty (PTA) of iliac lesions (data derived from five publications totaling 1264 procedures), an average complication rate of 3.6%, an initial success rate of 95%, and a 5-year patency rate of 61% have been reported.[1] The results of iliac stenting for stenoses (analysis of nine publications including 1365 patients) are somewhat better, with 99% technical success and 72% 5-year patency. The weighted average complication rate was 6.3%.[1] In femoropopliteal endovascular interventions (taken from eight publications reporting on 1469 procedures), the weighted average technical success was 90%, the complication rate was 4.3%, and the 3-year patency rate was 51%. Stents do not improve patency in the femoropopliteal segment, with a reported 3-year patency of 58%.

Surgery offers a limb-based 5-year patency of 91% for aortobifemoral bypasses; weighted average mortality was 3.3%. For femoropopliteal reconstruction, an average 5-year patency of 80% for vein bypasses and 65–75% for expanded polytetrafluoroethylene (ePTFE) bypasses has been reported. Combined mortality and amputation risk was calculated to be about 2.2% for aortobifemoral reconstructions and 1.4% for femoropopliteal reconstructions.[1]

One must consider that life expectancy of patients with intermittent claudication is limited compared with a non-claudicant control group. Mortality rates after 5, 10, and 15 years are approximately 30%, 50%, and 70%, respectively, although most patients will not die from peripheral vascular causes but rather from cardiac, cerebral, or non-vascular causes.[1]

Despite better clinical outcome for surgery, therefore, recommendation 37 of the TransAtlantic Inter-Society Consensus (TASC) proposes that surgery should be used as a treatment for intermittent claudication only in cases where other forms of medical therapy have been recommended but have either failed or been rejected for good reasons.[1] Furthermore there should be a high benefit-to-risk ratio for the proposed operation.[1] This is difficult to achieve in patients with mild-to-moderate claudication. Thus, endovascular therapy appears to be the method of

choice, if interventional therapy is required, in this subgroup of patients with mild–moderate intermittent claudication.

Lesion location

Claudication is mainly related to lesions in the aortoiliac or the femoropopliteal segments. It is less likely the result of infrapopliteal lesions and there is general agreement that treatment below the knee should be strictly limited to patients with critical limb ischemia, i.e. stage III and IV (Fontaine) or category 4 to 6 (Rutherford).

In the aortoiliac segment, a major proportion of lesions are amenable to percutaneous treatment with an acceptable outcome. In the femoropopliteal segment, overall success and long-term efficacy of percutaneous treatment is less and the lesion type becomes a more important determinant of success.

Thus, the location of a lesion and its type must be taken into consideration before treatment is recommended. While most aortoiliac lesions will be approachable with endovascular therapy, this is not generally true for femoropopliteal lesions. In addition, the risk of treatment is related to the lesion type and location, and requires careful consideration before embarking upon an endovascular approach.

Lesion morphology

Lesion morphology influences the technical success rate, long-term results, and also the risk of treatment. The TASC document therefore introduced a classification system to categorize lesions with regard to their appropriateness for either percutaneous treatment or surgery:

- focal type A lesions, which are ideal for percutaneous approach;
- type B lesions, in which the percutaneous approach is still the preferred technique;
- type C lesions, where the surgical approach should be preferred; and
- type D lesions, where surgery is the option of choice.

The TASC classification supersedes older classifications since it takes into account all available and published techniques including stent technology which offer a much wider variety of treatment and also an effective tool to deal with current acute complications of PTA such as occluding dissection or vascular rupture.

If we consider percutaneous therapy as the preferred method to deal with those patients presenting with mild or moderate claudication, treatment might be offered to those presenting with type A or B lesions, but should be discussed in depth with patients with type C lesions, since the risk and the potential benefit of treatment will be adversely affected by the underlying morphology (**Fig. 8.1**).

For iliac lesions, single stenoses up to 3cm in length both in the common iliac artery (CIA) and in the external iliac artery (EIA) are classified as type A lesions, while single stenoses of 3–10cm (not involving the common femoral artery [CFA]), tandem stenoses not longer than 5cm each, and unilateral occlusions of the CIA are classified as type B lesions. Bilateral long stenoses (5–10cm in length), unilateral EIA occlusions not extending into the CFA, and unilateral EIA stenoses extending into the CFA are classified as type C. More advanced lesions are classified as type D.

Based on this system of classification, many iliac lesions will meet the criteria for types A and B, opening a potentially growing

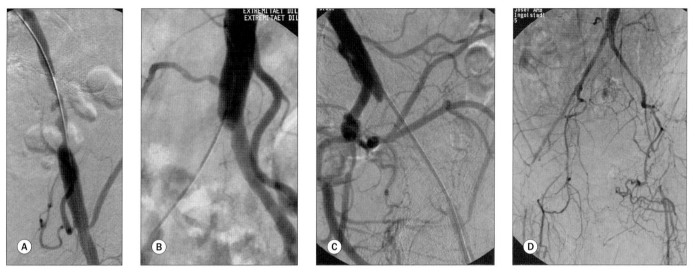

Figure 8.1 TASC classification of iliac lesions A to D, showing representative cases.

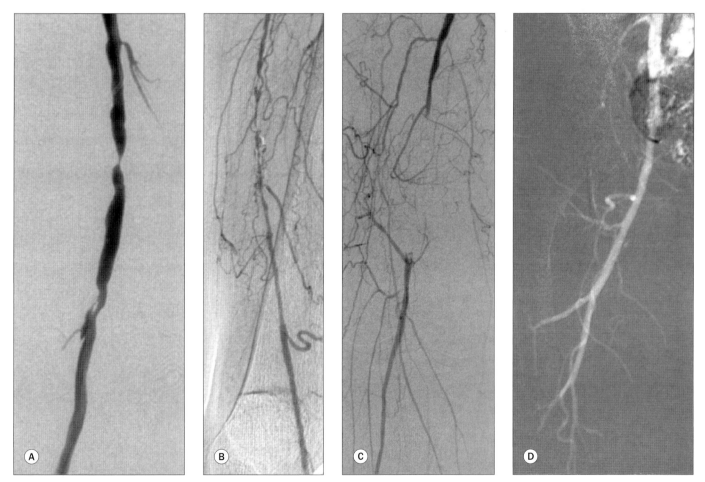

Figure 8.2 TASC classification of femoropopliteal lesions A to D, showing representative cases.

field for endovascular procedures if applied to mild and moderate claudicants. Our own experience suggests that percutaneous treatment may be appropriate in selected type C lesions, particularly for EIA occlusions not extending into the CFA. However, published data are lacking to support widespread adoption of this approach.

In the femoropopliteal segment (**Fig. 8.2**), type A lesions are single stenoses up to 3cm in length not involving the very proximal superficial femoral and the distal popliteal artery. Type B lesions are stenoses 3–5cm in length, heavily calcified stenoses, multiple lesions (each up to 3cm), and lesions with no sufficient tibial runoff (the latter are unlikely to meet the criteria of mild or moderate claudication). Type C lesions comprise stenoses or occlusions longer than 5cm and multiple mid-length lesions (3–5cm). Total common femoral, superficial femoral, and popliteal occlusions are classified as type D lesions. There was some dissension concerning the definition of type B lesions. Interventional radiologists represented by CIRSE wished to express their opinion that even longer lesions, up to 10cm, should be justifiably classified as type B instead of type C, claiming that the results reported are mainly due to underdeveloped techniques and instruments which have subsequently improved and no evidence exists comparing efficacy of PTA versus bypass surgery for lesions between 4 and 10cm.

In contrast to the iliac segment, fewer femoral artery lesions meet type A or B criteria, especially if limited to 5cm in length. Thus, fewer patients with mild and moderate claudication caused by femoropopliteal lesions will become ideal candidates for percutaneous treatment. Moreover, without limiting the importance of the TASC document, which certainly represents a step forward in a joint approach to peripheral vascular disease, the morphologic classification does not take into account some technical considerations that depend on the age and composition of a lesion. Particularly with respect to femoral occlusions, the degree of organization of the occluding thrombus, the composition of the lesion, and the relative location of the pre-existing stenosis are factors that are not readily predictable prior to initiation of intervention but which may influence the technical outcome of the intervention and its complication rate. Other than in the iliac arteries, liberal use of stents and stent-grafts may help to overcome a failed balloon angioplasty and to solve technical problems but does not result in an improved long-term efficacy. These associated potential drawbacks have to be carefully balanced against the potential benefits and need to be discussed in depth with the patient before treatment is performed, especially in association with only mild or moderate claudication. These considerations mainly restrict use of endovascular treatment in femoropopliteal lesions to stage IIb and IIa patients presenting with type A and less pronounced type B lesions.

Multilevel disease
Even mild symptoms may result from multilevel disease, i.e. an iliac stenosis and a concomitant, well-collateralized femoropopliteal lesion. There is some chance that intervention solely for the iliac stenosis may be sufficient to improve the clinical situation. Multilevel disease does not necessarily preclude endovascular treatment in such patients.

Adjuvant forms of treatment
It is widely accepted that smoking cessation and a well-conducted physical exercise program should precede any type of interventional treatment of intermittent claudication. The reality, however, is that in many institutions, it is most difficult to develop an infrastructure that provides state-of-the-art physical exercise in claudicants, and as far as smoking is concerned, there is a major difference between willing and doing.

Moreover, even with state-of-the-art exercise, a young patient may not recover completely from claudication in all his or her activities including sports. The process will be longer and may compromise the patient's abilities in professional life. Therefore, it might be worth considering, especially for the subgroup of young and active patients, whether they should be vigorously

treated with the axiom of physical exercise first or whether invasive treatment might be offered earlier in their course.

Conclusion
The decision regarding invasive treatment should be based on the individual circumstances in each patient presenting with claudication. Age, social life, physical abilities, and professional situation require consideration, and simple administration of rigid classification systems should be avoided. Under some circumstances, patients with mild-to-moderate claudication might become candidates for invasive treatment. Owing to its low morbidity and mortality, endovascular therapy should be considered as the method of choice unless precluded by morphologic or other factors. The type of percutaneous treatment, however, depends on the morphologic features of each particular lesion.

TECHNICAL OPTIONS OF TREATMENT

Percutaneous transluminal angioplasty
The basic endoluminal technique remains PTA. Over the years, balloon catheter technology has improved markedly. There is a variety available, ranging from non-compliant balloons holding the determined diameter, to semi-compliant balloons that allow pressure-guided adaptation of the definitive balloon diameter to the actual vessel diameter, and high-pressure balloons withstanding pressure up to 20atm as rated burst pressure, which might be exceeded by up to 50% (i.e. 30atm). The introduction diameter has been reduced to 6F introducer systems, or with smaller guidewires, down to 4F introducer sheath compatibility. Inflation and deflation time has become shorter and a smooth profile is maintained even after deflation. These improvements certainly contribute to the safety and ease of performance of the procedure; their influence on outcome, however, is difficult to determine.

Technical success of PTA is usually determined by the angiographic appearance of the lesion after PTA, improved flow and pulse, and by hemodynamic parameters such as pressure gradients across the lesion, particularly in iliac artery lesions.

Endovascular stents
The introduction of stent technology into the peripheral arterial arena has led to an enormous improvement in treatment, particularly with respect to iliac artery lesions. Since the late 1980s, stent implantation has rapidly increased.

In principle, two types of stents are available:

- balloon-expandable stents; and
- self-expanding stents.

Balloon-expandable stents are mounted on a balloon catheter and are passively enlarged to a desired diameter at the site of implantation by dilation of the balloon. Newer balloon-expandable stents are pre-crimped onto the balloon, permitting easy deployment. Older, hand-crimped stents are more difficult to employ in curved vessels and pose a risk of dislodgment from the balloon. Hand-crimping, however, allows use of a single type of stent for several vessel diameters, which is advantageous from an inventory standpoint. Balloon-expandable stents are usually short and made from stainless steel and are preferred for well-circumscribed lesions. They are advantageous if precise placement is required.

Self-expanding stents open actively after being released from a dedicated delivery system. The self-expanding character depends either on the braiding structure (Wallstent – BSIC, Watertown, USA – made from stainless steel) or on the type of alloy (nitinol). Most modern types of stents are made from nitinol, with different geometries of the stent structure. The Wallstent may be withdrawn even after partial deployment, which provides an additional safety feature in delicate situations, such as lesions near the iliac artery orifice. Although they are self-expanding, nitinol stents should not be moved after opening. Nitinol stents are less radiopaque compared with stainless steel, and visibility is enhanced by markers on the stent or the delivery system. Wallstents shorten considerably while nitinol stents do not. Self-expanding stents come in a variety of lengths up to 80mm and are of particular advantage in curved vessels, long lesions, and arterial occlusions. A recent innovation is the development of self-expanding stents that are deliverable through 6F introducer sheaths.

Especially in femoral arteries, neointimal overgrowth leading to significant restenosis is an unsolved problem. Therefore, drug-eluting stents that might help to reduce neointimal growth are being evaluated. Sirolimus (rapamycin) and taxol are the agents currently under investigation and will soon be released in North America for use in the coronary circulation. There has been some experimental work on radiating stents, but logistical problems and long-term sequelae with pronounced stenosis at the stent ends have prevented broad clinical application.

Stent-grafts

Stent-grafts currently play a limited role in the treatment of peripheral obstructive disease. Stent-grafts are stent bodies carrying a full jacket coating around their surface. While in bare stents, only a small percentage of the vessel surface is covered by foreign material, in stent-grafts there is a total coverage. There are two different clinically available coatings: Dacron and ePTFE. Animal experiments have shown that Dacron tends to stimulate a more pronounced neointimal growth compared with bare stents,[2] while ePTFE seems not to lead to a stimulated neointimal growth.[3] Again, the carrying stent might be balloon-expandable (Jomed stent graft, Jomed Inc.) or self-expanding (Wallgraft, BSIC, and Hemobahn, Gore Inc, Flagstaff, AZ, USA). Stent-grafts, especially in diameters larger than 8mm, require larger 9–11F introducer systems.

In the iliac segment, stent-grafts are predominantly used to treat aneurysmal disease or rare cases of rupture, perforation, or fistulae. In the femoral position, ePTFE stent-grafts have been used to treat long-segment stenoses and occlusions, and initial clinical results have been encouraging. Long-term results, however, are unavailable.

Atherectomy

Atherectomy catheters were introduced for the treatment of peripheral disease in the early 1990s. The most widely used device was a peripheral directed catheter – the Simpson atherectomy catheter (Guidant Inc, Brussels, Belgium). This device consists of a collecting chamber with a lateral opening and a rotating blade. An eccentric balloon presses the open chamber against the plaque while the rotating blade is advanced. The plaque material is cut and stored within the chamber. Then the balloon is deflated and the catheter is removed. The device was especially helpful to remove markedly eccentric and calcified plaques. Another indication was removal of neointimal tissue from self-expanding stents. In a general population of patients however, results after atherectomy did not show an improvement in patency compared with PTA alone. Unfortunately, the manufacturer withdrew the peripheral device from the market while the coronary device remains.

Mechanical recanalization instruments

There have been a number of other mechanical recanalization instruments described and used. Many of them have already disappeared from the market. Most of those available focus on the mechanical removal of fresh clots, which is a topic to be discussed in Chapter 11. Under particular circumstances, however, these devices might be of use in claudicants harboring stenotic lesions associated with subacute thrombosis. In such cases, aspiration thrombectomy is the most helpful, simple, and cost-effective technique available.

Subacute femoral artery thrombosis is another situation technically difficult to treat by endovascular means since there is a tendency toward poor response to PTA alone as well as a danger of distal embolization. A motor-driven rotational cutting and simultaneously aspirating system (Rotarex, Straub Medical, Switzerland) is promising to allow recanalization of this type of lesion. There is some anecdotal experience with ultrasonic clot maceration in subacute thrombosis but no large clinical trials have been published.

TREATMENT OPTIONS RELATIVE TO LESION LOCATION AND MORPHOLOGY

Aortoiliac arteries

The aorta and the iliac arteries have long been a primary field for percutaneous intervention. Ease of access to the lesion, the relatively large diameter of the target vessels, and the comparably benign outcome even of major complications contribute to the wide acceptance of percutaneous intervention for lesions in the aortoiliac system. Over the years, indications have broadened and now include treatment not only of focal stenoses but also of occlusive and aneurysmal disease. Introduction of vascular stents was particularly helpful to overcome technical problems and as a tool to treat major technical complications that otherwise would have required open surgical repair.

Aorta

While the suprarenal abdominal aorta is very rarely a target for percutaneous treatment, disease in the infrarenal segment may lend itself to PTA or related treatment. In more than 90% of cases, the cause of infrarenal aortic obstruction is atherosclerosis.[4] Clinically, solitary infrarenal aortic stenosis proximal to the aortic bifurcation is infrequent, but a stenosis of both the very distal aortic segment and the common iliac arteries is much more common. This may be complicated by an acute or sub-acute thrombosis of the aortic bifurcation. Small distal aortic caliber, especially in female patients, may be a predisposing factor. Atherosclerotic stenosis above the orifice of the inferior mesenteric artery is rare.[4]

Embolic occlusion of the distal aorta (saddle embolus) is much less frequent, but may occur in patients with mitral valve disease. Other rare causes of aortic obstruction are fibromuscular dysplasia, Takayasu's arteritis, and retroperitoneal fibrosis.

The typical age of patients with aortic obstruction ranges from 40 to 70 years. With respect to aortic occlusions, 55% are located at the level of the aortic bifurcation, 8% involve the entire infrarenal segment, and 37% involve aortic segments alone.[4] Collateral pathways are manifold via lumbar, epigastric, and mesenteric arteries.

Clinical symptoms of chronic aortic obstruction are bilateral claudication, predominantly with upper thigh symptoms, buttock pain, and erectile dysfunction in males. Symptoms must be differentiated from those of spinal stenosis. In occlusions, acute bilateral ischemia is present if no pre-existing stenotic process has promoted earlier development of collateral pathways. Aortic aneurysmal disease is increasingly becoming a field of interest for endovascular therapy, and such may be applied to selected patients with associated atherosclerotic occlusive disease. Endovascular treatment of aneurysms, however, is beyond the scope of this chapter.

Indications for percutaneous treatment

Indications for percutaneous versus surgical treatment largely depend on the location, extent, chronology (acute versus chronic), and morphology of the responsible lesion.

Accepted indications for PTA alone (**Fig. 8.3**) are:

• concentric segmental stenosis; and
• short-segment aortic bifurcation stenosis.

Balloon angioplasty may be followed by stent insertion in cases of either insufficient luminal gain or occurrence of significant dissection after PTA.

PTA is contraindicated if a complete calcified ring is present at the site of obstruction, as aortic rupture has been occasionally reported under such circumstances.[5] Owing to the Law of Laplace, the aorta is theoretically more easily prone to rupture than smaller-diameter vessels such as the iliac artery. In such instances, primary placement of a stent-graft might be considered.

Long-segment diffuse disease of both the aorta and iliac arteries is considered a contraindication to endovascular therapy; surgical aortobifemoral bypass grafts are generally a better choice.

Focal bifurcational aortic stenosis is treatable by PTA using a simultaneous 'kissing balloon' technique in order to dilate both the distal aortic segment and both iliac orifices. Stent implantation has been increasingly used to achieve a stable post-angioplasty widening by use of kissing stents in the distal aorta and both iliac arteries. In the case of distal aortic occlusion, few reports exist on remodeling the distal aortic segment or the aortic bifurcation by use of metallic stents.[6,7] In such difficult situations, use of advanced interventional techniques is certainly an advantage over simple balloon angioplasty.

Technical aspects

There are no major differences between the aortic and the iliac segment concerning techniques of lesion passage or traversal of occluded segments, whether they are located purely in the aorta or also involve the iliac segment. This is also true for balloon

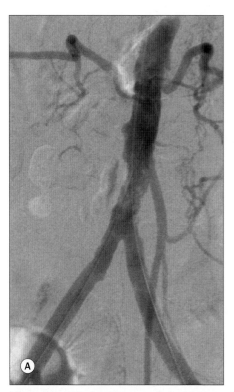
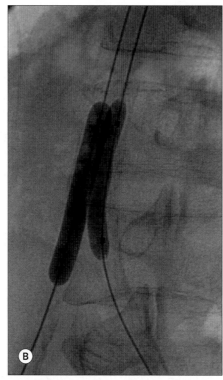
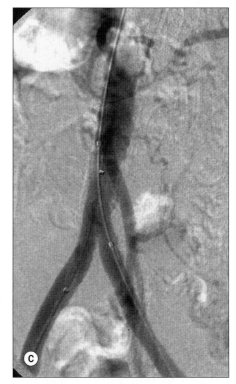

Figure 8.3 PTA of aortic stenosis in a 46-year-old male patient presenting with bilateral upper thigh claudication with symmetrical onset of symptoms after a walking distance of 250m. (A) Irregular calcific stenosis of infrarenal aorta; angiographically of moderate severity. (B) Bilateral 7mm kissing balloons in place. (C) After PTA, improved diameter of the aortic lumen. Patient became asymptomatic.

dilation, which does not differ significantly from angioplasty elsewhere. The relatively large diameter of the aortic lumen, however, presents certain technical issues.

Kissing or double balloon technique

Until recently, a major difficulty was the lack of suitable balloons of sufficient (16–20mm) diameter. Thus, a double or triple balloon technique was recommended to open the aortic stenosis to a sufficiently large diameter. With two or three kissing balloons that are inserted by a bifemoral and by an additional transbrachial approach, respectively, and are inflated simultaneously, the aortic lumen can be widened to its original diameter. The kissing technique is still recommended for dilatation of bilateral stenosis of the aortoiliac bifurcation and allows remodeling of the aortic bifurcation.

Single balloon technique

Recently, large-diameter balloons from 16 to 25mm have become available (Boston Scientific, Cordis), permitting the use of a single balloon technique by a unifemoral approach. With these balloons, it is strictly necessary to locate the balloon entirely within the aortic lumen, not overriding the bifurcation, in order to avoid overdilatation and rupture of the proximal iliac segment.

Stent insertion into the infrarenal aortic segment follows the same rules as elsewhere. Use of a stent of appropriate size, at least 14–16mm, is necessary to avoid undersizing. The largest stent diameter can be achieved by use of the balloon-expandable Palmaz XXL stent (Johnson and Johnson) that can be mounted on a large balloon and inflated up to 25mm in diameter.

Single stent technique

In lesions without involvement of the aortic bifurcation, a single stent can be implanted with no specific technical requirements. The stent type depends on the experience and preference of the interventionalist. Depending on the length of the stent and the location of the lesion, stent placement across the orifice of the inferior mesenteric artery may be unavoidable.

However, if the lesion ends very close to the bifurcation, placement of a single stent, especially of the balloon-expandable variety, may become difficult without overdilation of an iliac orifice. Under those circumstances, use of a self-expanding stent may be advantageous, while the aortic bifurcation is protected by a crossover catheter inserted from a contralateral approach. An alternative technique for very distal aortic lesions or bifurcational lesions is use of the kissing stents.

Kissing stent technique

Analogous to the kissing balloon method, stents of preferably an identical diameter and length are placed in kissing fashion within the distal aorta with their distal ends extending into the common iliac arteries. Very frequently, the stents tend to meet the opposite aortic wall. Thus – instead of being shaped in a kissing fashion – they cross each other, forming a mirror-sided artificial iliac orifice.

There are not very many reports of this technique and some questions remain open. Especially in stenotic lesions, it is not yet known whether there are potential sequelae from using two open stents that will remain partly non-endothelialized in their aortic portion, possibly causing embolic disease or an increased tendency for thrombosis. It is unclear whether covered stents would be advantageous in such cases.

If a kissing stent technique is applied, it is mandatory that the proximal ends of both stents parallel meticulously side by side to avoid a situation in which one stent compromises inflow into the other. Consequently, use of non-compressible, balloon-expandable stents such as the Palmaz stent (Johnson and Johnson) may be helpful.

Results

Aortic PTA has an excellent reported outcome compared with PTA at other sites. A primary success rate of 95% and a cumulative patency of 98% after 1 year and 80% after 5 years have been compiled from different series.[8]

There are only anecdotal reports of stent placement for aortic stenosis. Long et al.[9] reported two cases with successful stenting in Leriche syndrome. Dietrich[10] reported on six cases with chronic aortic occlusion that underwent thrombolysis and stenting by use of Palmaz stents. Long-term results are not available.

Complications

Complications that may occur after aortic dilation do not differ from those in other vascular provinces; however, they can be of greater potential clinical impact. While severe dissection, recollapse, or residual stenoses are simply treatable by additional stent implantation, aortic rupture, although reported rarely, is potentially life-threatening and therefore may require immediate surgery. To limit the extent of exsanguination, a large occlusion latex balloon (Boston Scientific) should be positioned just below the renal arteries or covering the site of rupture and left inflated until the patient is prepared for surgical repair. To avoid this complication, computerized tomography (CT) is recommended prior to the intervention, to exclude complete or near-complete circular calcification of the aortic wall, which is said to be a risk factor for rupture. A covered stent-graft may be placed across the site of rupture percutaneously; however, this method, to date, has only been reported for iliac arterial rupture and may risk occlusion of major collaterals and the inferior mesenteric artery.

Distal embolization develops in less than 1% of cases.[8] Subacute complications include thrombosis. This has not been reported for pure aortic dilation or stenting but is a risk in remodeling techniques of the aortic bifurcation. Thrombosis may be predisposed by adjacent aortic disease with plaques hanging over the stent orifice, thus causing inflow obstruction, or by adjacent outflow problems. If a technical reason has caused stent or post-PTA thrombosis, surgery is a reasonable option; if not, thrombolysis may be tried. Because of their large diameter, reobstruction of aortic stents occurs rarely but they may undergo repeat balloon dilatation similar to iliac stents. In kissing stents, obstruction may be caused by neointimal hyperplasia; such lesions are treatable by reballooning, atherectomy, or placement of a second stent.

TREATMENT OF ILIAC OCCLUSIVE DISEASE

Iliac occlusive disease accounts for approximately one-third of symptomatic lower extremity occlusive arterial lesions, while two-thirds are located infrainguinally. PTA lends itself to the

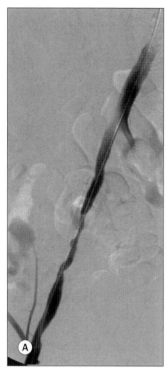 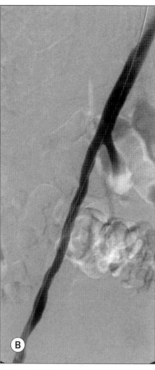

Figure 8.4 Iliac PTA without stent. (A) Eccentric long-segment stenosis of right external iliac artery. Usually, these lesions tend to show dissections after PTA. (B) After PTA with a 6mm balloon of 40mm length, smooth appearance of the treated lesion without dissection.

treatment of many iliac artery lesions, and technical as well as clinical results are satisfying (**Fig. 8.4**).

Clinically, intermittent claudication starting in the upper thigh together with lower limb claudication is the leading symptom of iliac arterial disease. Erectile dysfunction may also be present. In isolated iliac lesions, critical ischemia is rare if not associated with additional infrainguinal disease. Rarely, blue-toe syndrome

might be present if cholesterol embolization has occurred from an ulcerated plaque in the iliac axis.

Weakened femoral pulses and reduced ankle–arm index are simple clinical signs that can indicate iliac obstruction, which can be verified by direct or post-stenotic color-coded or duplex studies. For planning of a percutaneous intervention, magnetic resonance or conventional angiography is still most helpful.

Stent placement for stenotic iliac lesions should be performed if the angioplasty result is suboptimal (**Fig. 8.5**) as defined angiographically or by direct measurement of major pressure gradients. Since follow-up data are now available showing that iliac stent placement is relatively safe, a liberal approach is justified, although primary stenting of stenoses is not generally recommended owing to socioeconomic constraints and potential follow-up problems. Furthermore, primary stenting is not superior to successful PTA alone.[10] Thus, stenting is only performed for PTA failure or when technical requirements compromise success of simple PTA, such as for iliac occlusions. As previously outlined (see also **Fig. 8.1**) endovascular treatment is most appropriate for TASC A and B lesions.

Iliac artery stenoses

Although PTA has proved to be an effective procedure in the treatment of iliac stenoses, the indication for stent placement should be restricted to lesions which are not primarily amenable to PTA alone. An inadequate post-angioplasty result has been suggested as a general indication for stent placement, although the term remains ill defined. Residual pressure gradients are certainly a useful way to assess the angioplasty result,[11] but it is still unclear what the borderline gradient ultimately requiring additional intervention is, and, moreover, the decision should not be made without reference to both morphologic criteria and visibly reduced flow.

Long-segment stenoses with an irregular surface, aneurysmal formation, or markedly ulcerated plaques may be included in the group of complex lesions (**Fig. 8.1**). Eccentric stenoses and ostial lesions with extension to the aortic bifurcation are known

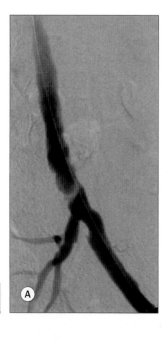 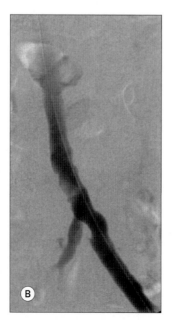 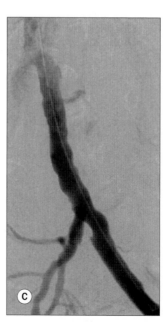

Figure 8.5 Very short eccentric stenosis of distal common iliac artery (left) undergoing secondary stenting. (A) Lesion before PTA. (B) After PTA, no major improvement has been achieved. (C) After implantation of a self-expanding nitinol stent, the lumen is widely patent.

not to respond well to balloon angioplasty alone. A stenotic lesion may respond well to initial balloon inflation but may collapse after balloon deflation, a process termed elastic recoil.

Such complications of PTA are well treatable by stent placement (**Fig. 8.5**). This includes not only intramural hematoma but also flow-obstructing dissection complicating PTA, which may be an acute indication for stent placement in order to maintain the vascular lumen, obviating emergency surgery.

Iliac restenosis after previous PTA does not generally require stent placement as there is no proof that stenting prevents restenosis under those circumstances. However, stenting may be considered from a technical point of view in cases in which the result of balloon angioplasty remains compromised.

Iliac artery occlusions

Percutaneous treatment of selected iliac occlusions is technically feasible. In cases of acute thrombosis, thrombolysis is an alternative to surgical thrombectomy and might precede PTA of an underlying lesion. Mechanical thrombectomy via a percutaneous access is still in its infancy and cannot be recommended as a routine approach since potential risks such as downward or crossover embolization are possible and no data are yet available to determine the overall complications of such a method.

In chronic occlusions with an occlusion time exceeding 3 months, balloon angioplasty alone, thrombolysis with subsequent balloon angioplasty and elective stenting, or mechanical passage of the occlusion followed by primary stent implantation have been described as alternative techniques (**Fig. 8.6**).

Metallic stents – and self-expandable endoprostheses in particular – offer a new concept of percutaneous revascularization in chronic iliac occlusion, which we believe is a primary indication.[12] Self-expandable stents are used to cover the occluding thrombotic material, thereby preventing peripheral dislodgment, a well-known complication of percutaneous recanalization of occlusions.

The indication for use of a metallic stent is almost always a technical one. Type and morphology of the lesion, the technical outcome of PTA, and complicated situations are important criteria for use of stenting.

Technical considerations in the iliac arteries
Percutaneous transluminal angioplasty

Iliac artery PTA is relatively simple to perform. A retrograde transfemoral approach affords the easiest access to such stenotic lesions. Crossover dilation may be performed in special indications such as double-sided stenoses in case both lesions should be dilated in one session or in case an external iliac stenosis extends far down into the CFA. After careful traversal of the diseased segment, a suitable balloon is placed across the lesion and dilation is performed either manually or by using a pressure-monitoring gauge (**Fig. 8.4**). Balloon size may be selected either by film-measuring or in digital subtraction angiography (DSA) images by use of graduated catheters that allow fairly exact measurement of the vessel size.

By leaving the wire in place across the lesion and using backflush angiography through a previously inserted sheath or by reinsertion of an angiographic catheter and downhill angiography, the post-dilatation result can be imaged. Backflush angiography was previously thought to be associated with a risk of retrograde dissection. However, in our experience with use of DSA this is an extremely rare event and sequelae are limited as long as the guidewire is left in place.

There is wide agreement that both the hemodynamic relevance of a lesion as well as post-PTA success can be accurately monitored by measuring the pressure gradient across the lesion. However, there is some dispute concerning criteria for success. A systolic pressure gradient of 10mmHg and less after peripheral drug-induced vasodilation is accepted by most authors to indicate successful PTA even if the morphologic result is not perfect. Some authors use a mean pressure gradient of 10mmHg.

There are no data to support anticoagulation following PTA of simple iliac lesions. We regularly keep our patients on full heparinization (500–1000IU/hour) for 12–24 hours and

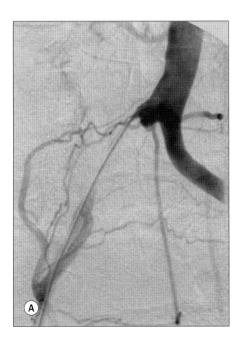
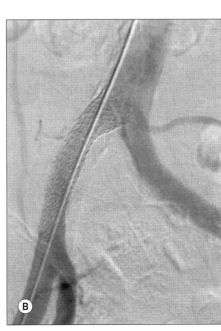

Figure 8.6 Chronic iliac artery occlusion.
(A) After guidewire traversal of the occluded segment, primary stenting is performed.
(B) After placement of a self-expanding nitinol stent and subsequent PTA, the segment is recanalized.

recommend lifetime acetylsalicylic acid (ASA, aspirin) medication (100mg/day).

Stent implantation

If balloon angioplasty fails by either morphologic or hemodynamic criteria, stent implantation can be considered. Technique depends on the type of stent employed. Most clinical series show similar results with various stents. Length and location of the lesion, experience of the investigator, and availability of appropriate size are important factors that may lead to preference of one or another type.

Precise placement is mandatory to avoid major complications, especially in cases where the stent must be placed close to the aortic bifurcation. While self-expanding Wallstents can be corrected during placement to a limited extent, balloon-expandable stents and self-expanding nitinol stents cannot undergo correction of their localization once inflation of the balloon has been started (**Fig. 8.5**).

Chronic iliac artery occlusions are primary indications for stent placement. We avoid pre-dilatation and place the stent directly into the occluded segment (**Fig. 8.6**). After stenting, careful balloon dilatation is performed to avoid dislodgment of occluding material.

Atherectomy

Directional atherectomy does not play a major role in the treatment of iliac arterial disease. This is because the ratio of introduction and working diameter in most atherectomy systems is relatively low, which requires a considerably large puncture to achieve atherectomy of larger iliac diameters from 8 to 12mm. The Simpson atherectomy catheter, the most widely used atherectomy system, requires an 11F sheath to sufficiently treat iliac lesions. Atherectomy may play an important role in the recanalization of stent reobstruction to debulk stents from reobstructing neointimal tissue.

Stent reobstruction

Directional atherectomy or repeat PTA are both applicable to cases of in-stent restenosis. If PTA is used, a balloon size in accordance with the outer diameter of the placed stent is recommended in order to maximally compress the neointima, especially if occurring within a self-expanding stent that does not allow overexpansion. If a balloon-expandable stent has been used, slight overdilatation of the stent is recommended in order to gain a larger diameter despite the presence of neointimal tissue. Some authors prefer atherectomy to debulk the stent. This is nicely achievable in smaller stents such as in the femorals, but may require very large instruments of 11F in iliac stents.

The treatment of stent occlusion is more difficult. Early acute occlusions are mainly due to technical problems and it is mandatory to address these problems to maintain long-term success. Recent thrombosis should be treated by thrombolysis followed by PTA and/or additional stent placement as required.

Late occlusion is mainly due to obstructing neointima within or adjacent to the stent. There is little published experience regarding treatment of complete stent occlusion at a chronic stage. Thrombolysis, atherectomy, and mechanical aspiration followed by balloon angioplasty are possible techniques. A relatively easy method is the use of the stent-in-stent technique. Following traversal of the occluded stent, a stent is placed within

the occluded segment, bridging it at both ends. The new stent is then carefully dilated, with a tendency to use an underdilation of 1–2mm in order to avoid distal embolization.

Results

Percutaneous transluminal angioplasty

For aortoiliac PTA, Becker and co-workers compiled data showing an average technical success of 92%, a 2-year patency of 81% (range 65–93%), and a 5-year-patency of 72% (range 50–87%) from available references in the literature including 2679 procedures.[13] Gardiner and colleagues described a total complication rate of 4.5% and a major complication rate requiring surgery of 2.7% in 224 iliac procedures.[14] More recently, Tegtmeyer et al. reported on a single-center series of 200 patients, with a technical success of PTA of 88%, a total complication rate of 10.5%, and a major complication rate of 6.5%.[15] Follow-up results reported a 2-year patency of 90% and a 5-year patency of 85% among patients whose initial treatment was successful. Secondary patency was 99% and 92% after 2 and 5 years, respectively.

Improvement of these results seems difficult to achieve. The type of the lesions that are treated, however, influences the technical results. The inclusion of eccentric lesions, calcified or ulcerated plaques, dissections, or iliac occlusions has a major impact on the technical outcome, and presumably on the long-term outcome, of iliac PTA. Stenting may be beneficial in such difficult cases and to treat complications of simple PTA.[13,16]

Stent implantation

We reported follow-up results of Wallstent placement in 118 patients with aortoiliac stenoses.[16] Mean length of the stenosed segment was 3±2cm; in 103 patients the lesion was <5cm, in 15 patients it was >5cm. Morphologically, 85 lesions were eccentric, 73 lesions showed major calcifications, and in 52 lesions, irregular margins were found.

A total of 142 stents were placed, with a mean of 1.2±0.5 stents per patient. Mean stented segment length was 4±2cm. Clinical stage improved in 112 patients; 89 patients improved by two or more stages (Fontaine classification). Mean ankle–arm index significantly improved to 0.92±0.17. The primary cumulative patency was 97% after 6 months, 95% after 1 year, and 88% after 2 years; 4-year-patency was 82%. Secondary or assisted patency was 97% after 6 months, 96% after 1 year, 93% after 2 years, and 91% at 4 years.

Chronic iliac occlusions

We also reported our experience with the treatment of 103 chronic iliac occlusions.[17] Mean length of the occluded segment was 5.1±3.1cm; in 44 patients the occlusion was <5cm (SCVIR class III), in 59 patients it was >5cm (SCVIR class IV).[10] The lesion included the orifice of the CIA in 48 patients and the orifice of the EIA in 41 patients. The lesion extended into the CFA in two patients. Mean ankle–arm index at rest was 0.48±0.2 prior to treatment. The mean angiographic follow-up period was 26±18 months and the mean clinical follow-up interval was 29±17 months.

A total of 154 stents were placed, with a mean of 1.6±0.7 stents per patient. Mean stented segment length was 6.1±3.3cm. Arterial flow was successfully re-established in 101 patients. In two patients, the stent entered the aorta subintimally, thus leading to a compression of the stent entrance. In both patients, further intervention was abandoned to avoid arterial rupture, and, despite heparinization, the new channel thrombosed within 24 hours. Thus, technical success of remodeling the vascular lumen was 98% (101 of 103 patients). Clinical stage improved in 99 patients. Mean ankle–arm index improved to 0.89±0.19. Primary patency was 92% after 6 months, 87% after 1 year, 83% after 2 years, and 78% at 3 years. Secondary or assisted patency was 95% after 6 months, 94% after 1 year, and 90% after 2 years. Three- and 4-year patencies were each 88%.

Palmaz and Strecker stents

For iliac stent placement, larger series with follow-up data are now available for three specific types of vascular endoprostheses: the Strecker stent, the Palmaz stent, and the Wallstent.[6,18] Device types differ with respect to stent design, radial expansile force, and surface geometry, all of which may theoretically influence respective long-term results.[19]

A multicenter study of the Palmaz stent including 486 patients revealed a technical success rate of 99% and a complication rate of 10%, with major complications reported in 4.7%. Clinical follow-up patency was 90% at 1 year and 84% at 2 years.[18]

Strecker and co-workers reported a technical success of 100% in 116 patients with iliac lesions who underwent implantation of a Strecker tantalum stent, with patencies of 95% at 1 and 2 years.[6] Long et al. reported on iliac implantation of Strecker stents in 64 patients. The technical success rate was 98%; the complication rate was 12%, but the rate of major complications was only 3.1%. Restenosis occurred in ten cases, and reocclusion in eight.[20]

Our results with the Wallstent compare quite favorably to those results reported for other types of stents. These results are equal to or even better than the data reported for other types of devices. However, it remains difficult to compare data from different series since numerous intrinsic and individual factors – including the lesion morphology, extent of disease, and outflow conditions – may also be of importance. In our series, only stenotic lesions were treated, and, compared with results in iliac occlusions, patency for treatment of stenoses was somewhat better.[16,17]

With respect to published data on the use of various types of metallic stents in the iliac arterial system, there is no obvious difference between such regarding technical success and mid-term patency.

Other stents

At present, minimal clinical results are available for other stents such as the Cragg non-covered nitinol stent and the low-profile Memotherm nitinol stent. Hausegger et al. reported the first clinical results with the Cragg stent, which showed a high technical success.[21] Starck et al. presented follow-up data on 203 patients with the Memotherm stent and reported a technical success of 98%. They used the stent in the iliac (44%) and femoropopliteal region (52%) and claimed to have achieved a better outcome than with the Strecker stent.[22] These preliminary data, however, are uncontrolled and non-randomized.

Atherectomy

Data are scarce for iliac atherectomy using the Simpson directional atherectomy catheter. A technical success rate of 85% and a 3-year patency ranging from 57% to 84% have been reported.[8] Maynar et al. preferentially used the system to treat the EIA, which is more accessible to atherectomy owing to its smaller diameter; 18-month patency was 87%.[23]

Reobstruction in stents

In cases of reobstruction, percutaneous reintervention is often feasible. We analyzed our results of such in 26 instances.[24] Percutaneous reintervention was effective in all ten cases of stent stenosis. For stent occlusion, the technical success rate was 88% (14 of 16 cases). Embolization was the major complication of reintervention, occurring in two of 26 cases. Patency after treatment of stent stenosis was 87% after 1 year, compared with a stent occlusion patency of 57%. Recurrent stent obstruction occurred in eight of 24 (33%) initially successful reinterventions.

Some authors prefer atherectomy as the method of choice for treatment of in-stent stenosis and occlusion. Available data are insufficient to compare different techniques of reintervention.

Complications

Iliac artery PTA is relatively safe. The overall complication rate after iliac PTA has been reported to be 8.1%, with major complications in 2.7% and major complications requiring surgery in 1.2%. The most frequent complications are related to access problems such as hematoma (2.9%) and pseudoaneurysm (0.5%), acute occlusion (1.9%), embolization (1.6%), and arterial rupture (0.2%). Mortality is very low, with a mean of 0.2%.[8]

Stenting is useful not only to improve the technical results of iliac PTA but also to deal with specific complications such as acute occlusion. Use of stents, however, has expanded the application of percutaneous techniques to cases that otherwise would have required open surgery.

Post stenting, the rate of complications in iliac arteries is relatively small. Using the Wallstent to treat iliac stenoses, there is a reported complication rate of 6.8%, with major complications – including subacute stent thrombosis – occurring in 3.4%.[16] For iliac occlusions, complications occurred in 11.7%. An additional surgical or percutaneous reintervention became necessary in six patients; thus, the major complication rate was 5.8%. The latter included arterial emboli, which was the most frequent type of complication in chronic arterial occlusions.[17]

In our series, stent reobstruction occurred in 7.6% of stenoses and 17.5% of occlusions. Stent reobstruction was due to stenosis in 44% and occlusions in 56%.

TREATMENT OF FEMOROPOPLITEAL OCCLUSIVE DISEASE

Treatment of femoropopliteal lesions in claudicants is more problematic than treatment of lesions in the iliac region, primarily because of lower technical success rates, higher complication rates, and poorer long-term success. Lesions in the femoropopliteal arterial segments are less likely to meet criteria that make them suitable for endovascular treatment. On the other hand, the versatility of endoluminal techniques extends treatment options in many patients. Depending on the type of lesion, a simple and limited intervention can often provide a considerable improvement for the patient.

The TASC classification for femoropopliteal lesions was previously outlined and is summarized in **Figure 8.2**. As with

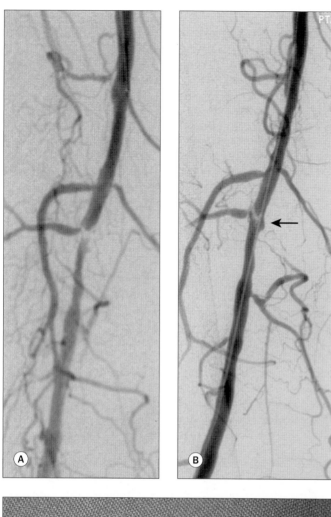

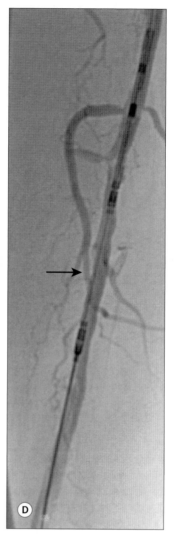

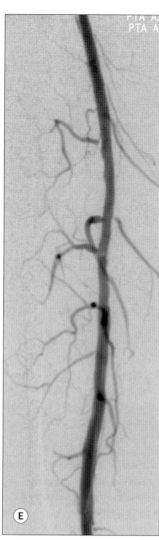

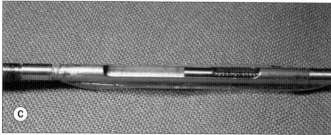

Figure 8.7 Femoral atherectomy by use of the Simpson atherectomy catheter. (A) Short eccentric femoral artery stenosis. (B) After PTA, insufficient result with residual stenosis and some dissection. (C) The Simpson atherectomy catheter with the collecting chamber and the round cutter. The eccentric balloon is not inflated. (D) The atherectomy catheter located across the lesion. (E) After atherectomy, full patency has been restored.

iliac lesions, TASC A and B femoropopliteal lesions are most suitable for endovascular approaches.

Additional morphologic factors (not included in the TASC classification)

Endovascular treatment of femoropopliteal occlusions, particularly those of recent onset, may be difficult. Simple PTA may result in distal embolization of thrombotic debris, which may aggravate the symptoms or create a limb-threatening situation. Even in short occlusions, PTA may be insufficient to adequately reopen the vessel, necessitating additional treatment such as stent placement. Reobstruction of stents, however, is more difficult to treat compared with simple restenosis. Eccentric calcified stenosis is difficult to treat reliably with PTA alone. Since stenting is a technical but not necessarily a long-term solution in treating such lesions, alternative techniques such as atherectomy (**Fig. 8.7**)

may be considered if available. Unfortunately, many of these 'niche' devices, such as the Simpson atherectomy catheter, are no longer on the market.

Techniques
Percutaneous transluminal angioplasty

Balloon angioplasty remains the endovascular workhorse for treating femoropopliteal lesions. Modern angiographic units permit precise and accurate measurement of the true arterial diameter, and, in conjunction with the use of semi-compliant balloons, adaptation to the arterial diameter is readily allowed. We prefer not to grossly overdilate the artery, in order to avoid dissection. Dilation times of 1–3min, using pressure gauges (**Fig. 8.8**), are preferred. Balloon lengths of 2 to 4cm are most commonly employed. In cases of major dissection, an initial attempt to improve the result should be repeat angioplasty with prolonged

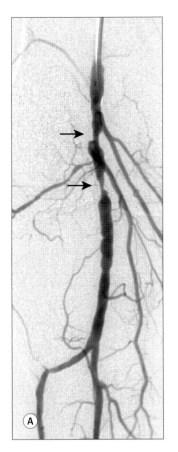
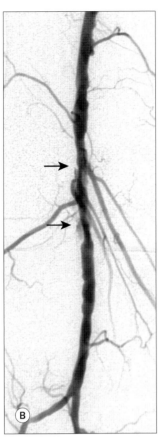
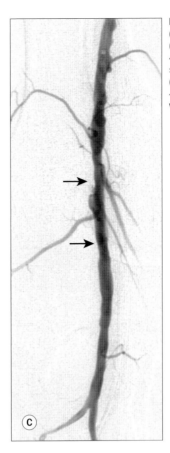

Figure 8.8 Prolonged dilatation.
(A) Tandem stenosis of popliteal artery (arrows). (B) After PTA for 45s with a 40mm-long balloon, major dissection is seen with residual stenosis (arrows). (C) After prolonged balloon inflation for 4min, dissections were gone and a wide lumen becomes visible (arrows).

balloon dilatation over 4–5min. In many cases, the result will be improved by this cost-effective and simple approach without the requirement for more complex techniques.

Stent placement

Use of stents for femoropopliteal lesions should be limited to those cases in which PTA in all its variations did not achieve a sufficient result. This is particularly true for occluding dissections (**Fig. 8.9**). Except in the iliac system, liberal deployment of stents cannot be recommended. If needed, the stent employed should be as short as possible. Balloon-expandable stents are preferable for longer lesions; if arterial angulation is an issue, a self-expanding stent may be useful.

The overall results of femoral stenting are disappointing. There are new developments with drug-eluting stents on the horizon, including those using sirolimus (rapamycin) and taxol. Initial results with sirolimus-eluting stents in the coronary circulation are very promising, but no data yet exist on their use in the femoral position. Radiation of stents at the time of primary insertion did not result in improved patency but was followed by an increased risk of thrombosis.

Stent-grafts

Stent-grafts still play a limited role in the treatment of femoropopliteal lesions. Expanded-PTFE-covered self-expanding stent grafts like the Hemobahn device (Gore Inc, Flagstaff, AZ, USA) yielded promising preliminary results in a multicenter trial, even in the femoropopliteal field, and stimulated the hope of a percutaneous alternative for those patients presenting with long femoro-

popliteal occlusions. Intermediate and long-term results, however, are not available.

Below the inguinal ligament, ePTFE covering should be used exclusively, since in animal experiments, it has shown much less tendency to induce neointimal growth compared with Dacron covering.[2,3]

A considerable disadvantage of stent-grafts, however, is that frequently, important collaterals are necessarily covered by the full body of the stent-graft. In case of reocclusion, these collaterals will no longer be available. This is particularly true for the popliteal artery, where development of compensating collaterals is limited. Therefore, we favor limiting the use of stent-grafts to the proximal two-thirds of the superficial femoral artery, especially in claudicants.

Results

Percutaneous transluminal angioplasty

In femoropopliteal endovascular interventions (taken from eight publications reporting on 1469 procedures), weighted average technical success was 90%, complication rate was 4.3%, and 3-year patency rate was 51%.[1]

Long-term patency is positively influenced by a good outflow tract (two or three infrageniculate arteries), absence of diabetes, and absence of residual stenosis. Residual stenosis could be addressed with stents, but there is no proof that stenting improves overall patency.

Hunink et al. performed a subgroup analysis of patients undergoing femoral PTA based on whether the treated lesion was an

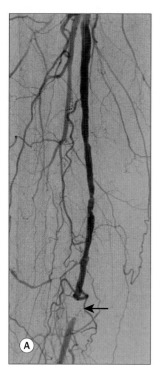

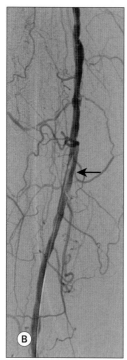

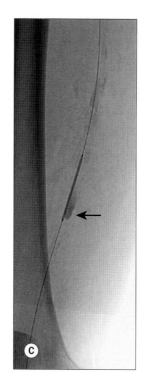

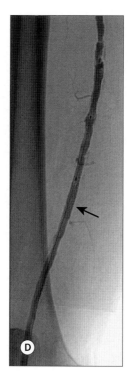

Figure 8.9 Femoral stenting. (A) Short occlusion of distal femoral artery (arrow). (B) After mechanical passage and PTA, a deep dissection (arrow) occurred, being refractory to prolonged balloon dilatation. (C) Since the antegrade dissection was growing [note the intramural deposit of contrast (arrow)], stent placement was performed (non-inflated stent before delivery). (D) After inflation of the balloon-dilated stent (arrow), patency is restored.

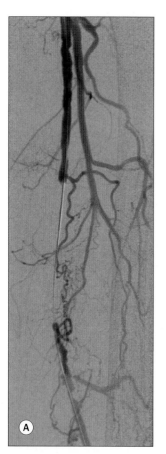

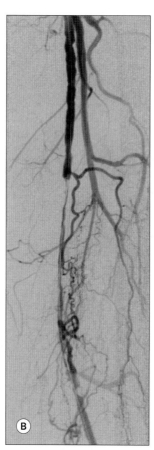

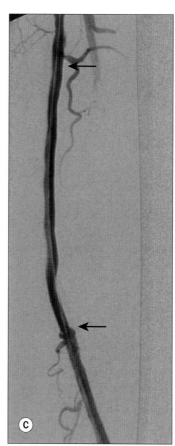

Figure 8.10 Femoral stent-graft. (A) Chronic occlusion of the middle segment of the left superficial femoral artery in a 43-year-old male patient in stage IIb (Fontaine). (B) After PTA by use of a 5mm balloon, no improvement of the possibly subintimal recanalization channel. (C) After placing a 6mm-wide Hemobahn endoprosthesis (arrows) and a non-covered balloon-expandable stent more distally on an eccentric plaque, patency is restored.

occlusion or a stenosis, as well as whether the runoff was good or poor, and found that each of these factors affected subsequent patency following intervention. Their reported five-year patencies for patients with good runoff were 62% for stenoses versus 48% for occlusions; corresponding patencies for those with poor runoff were 43% for stenoses and 27% for occlusions.[25]

Stents

Stent implantation into the femoropopliteal segments has not demonstrated increased patency compared with balloon angioplasty alone. In a meta-analysis, Muradin et al. reported a 3-year patency rate of 63–66% for stents compared with a rate of 61% for PTA of stenoses. They also found, however, that in patients with more severe disease and more complex lesions, stenting may confer a benefit to PTA alone.[26] Cejna and co-workers were unable to detect a significant difference between PTA alone and stenting in a randomized trial.[27]

Endoluminal radiation therapy with afterloading or beta-irradiation as well as drug-eluting stents may improve the overall results in the future. At present, stenting in the femoral arteries should be used as a bailout therapy in cases of PTA failure. Failure, however, needs to be defined strictly as severe dissection refractory to prolonged balloon dilatation, antegrade dissection with increasing obstruction, or severe residual obstruction. Minor irregularities of the wall are not sufficient to justify stenting.

Stent-grafts

Data are lacking on the utility of stent-grafts in the femoropopliteal arteries (**Fig. 8.10**). In a multicenter trial using the Hemobahn endoprosthesis, Lammer and co-workers achieved a primary patency rate of 90% after 6 months and 79% after 12 months, in 80 treated limbs. Secondary patency was 93% at 12 months.[28]

These encouraging results are contrasted by many single-center experiences in which endografts showed a high rate of thrombosis, frequently due to development of stenoses adjacent to the stent-graft itself.

Complications

The nature and variety of complications in femoropopliteal arteries do not differ principally from those in the aortoiliac area. They include dissection, perforation, and embolization of debris. With stents, risk of early thrombosis was a problem in the very beginning but may have been reduced by the administration of modern antiplatelet drugs.

When treating occlusions, distal embolization is potentially the most dramatic complication. Aspiration embolectomy in combination with selective thrombolysis is the treatment option of choice. Especially in claudicants, this significant risk needs to be well balanced against any potential benefit.

Adjunctive drug regimen

In iliac and femoral PTA in claudicants, heparinization during the intervention and for 24 hours thereafter, using either low-molecular-weight heparin or conventional heparin, is mostly sufficient. A dosage of 100mg of ASA daily is usually prescribed. After femoral stent placement or in cases with marked irregularities after PTA, heparinization may be prolonged up to 72 hours and an additional platelet inhibitor such as clopidogrel administered for a period of 4 to 6 weeks.

REFERENCES

1. The TASC Working Group. Management of peripheral arterial disease (PAD). TransAtlantic Inter-Society Consensus (TASC). J Vasc Surg 2000; 31:S1–296.
2. Schurmann K, Vorwerk D, Uppenkamp R, Klosterhalfen B, Bucker A, Gunther RW. Iliac arteries: plain and heparin-coated Dacron-covered stent-grafts compared with noncovered metal stents – an experimental study. Radiology 1997;203:55–63.
3. Cejna M, Virmani R, Jones R, et al. Biocompatibility and performance of the Wallstent and several covered stents in a sheep iliac artery model. J Vasc Interv Radiol 2001;12:351–8.
4. Vollmar J. Rekonstruktive Chirurgie der Arterien. Stuttgart:Thieme; 1996:207–14.
5. Berger T, Sörensen R, Konrad J. Aortic rupture. A complication of transluminal angioplasty. Am J Roentgenol 1986;146:373–4.
6. Strecker E, Hogan B, Liermann D, et al. Iliac and femoropopliteal vascular occlusive disease treated with flexible tantalum stents. Cardiovasc Intervent Radiol 1993;16:158–64.
7. Dietrich EB, Santiago O, Gustafson G. Preliminary observation on the use of the Palmaz stent in the distal portion of the abdominal aorta. Am Heart J 1993;125:490–500.
8. Rholl, K, Van Breda A. Percutaneous intervention for aortoiliac disease. In: Strandness E, Van Breda A, eds. Vascular diseases. New York: Churchill Livingstone; 1994:433–66.
9. Long A, Gaux J, Raynaud AC, et al. Infrarenal aortic stents: initial clinical experience and angiographic follow-up. Cardiovasc Intervent Radiol 1994;16:203–8.
10. Dietrich EB. Endovascular techniques for abdominal aortic occlusions. Int Angiol 1993;12:270–80.
11. Tetteroo E, Haaring C, van den Graaf Y, et al. Intraarterial pressure gradients after randomized angioplasty or stenting of iliac arterial lesions. Cardiovasc Intervent Radiol 1996;19:411–7.
12. Vorwerk D, Guenther RW. Mechanical revascularization of occluded iliac arteries with use of self-expandable endoprostheses. Radiology 1990; 175:411–5.
13. Becker G, Katzen B, Dake M. Noncoronary angioplasty. Radiology 1989; 170:921–40.
14. Gardiner G, Meyerovitz M, Stokes K, Clouse M, Harrington D, Bettmann M. Complications of transluminal angioplasty. Radiology 1986; 159:201–8.
15. Tegtmeyer C, Hardwell G, Selby B, Robertson R, Kron I, Tribble C. Results and complications of angioplasty in aortoiliac disease. Circulation 1991;83:I-53–I-60.
16. Vorwerk D, Günther RW, Schürmann K, Wendt G. Aortic and iliac stenoses: follow-up results of stent placement after insufficient balloon angioplasty in 118 cases. Radiology 1996;198:45–8.
17. Vorwerk D, Guenther R, Schürmann K, Wendt G, Peters I. Primary stent placement for chronic iliac artery occlusions: follow-up results in 103 patients. Radiology 1995;194:745–9.
18. Palmaz JC, Labored J, Rivera F, Encarnacion C, Lutz J, Moss J. Stenting of the iliac arteries with the Palmaz stent. Experience from a multi-center trial. Cardiovasc Intervent Radiol 1992;15:291–7.
19. Schatz R. A view of vascular stents. Circulation 1989;79:445–7.
20. Long A, Sapoval M, Beyssen B, et al. Strecker stent implantation in iliac arteries: patencies and predictive factors for long-term success. Radiology 1995;194:739–44.
21. Hausegger KA, Lafer M, Lammer J, et al. Iliac artery stenting – clinical experience with a nitinol prototype stent (Cragg stent). Cardiovasc Intervent Radiol 1993;16(Suppl):S25 (Abstr.).

22. Starck E, Dukiet C, Heinz C, Vierhauser S. Clinical experience with a new self-expanding nitinol stent. Cardiovasc Intervent Radiol 1995; 18(Suppl):S72 (Abstr.).

23. Maynar M, Reyes R, Cabrera P. Percutaneous atherectomy of iliac arteries. Semin Intervent Radiol 1988;5:253–5.

24. Vorwerk D, Günther RW, Schürmann K, Wendt G. Percutaneous treatment of late obstruction in iliac arterial stents. Radiology 1995; 197:479–84.

25. Hunink M, Wong J, Donaldson M, Meyerovitz M, de Vries J, Harrington D. Revascularization for femoropopliteal disease. A decision and cost-effectiveness analysis. JAMA 1995;274:165–71.

26. Muradin G, Bosch J, Stijnen T, Huninck M. Balloon dilation and stent implantation for treatment of femoropopliteal arterial disease: meta-analysis. Radiology 2001;221:137–45.

27. Cejna M, Schoder M, Lammer J. [PTA vs. stent in femoro-popliteal obstruction]. Radiologe 1999;39:144–50.

28. Lammer J, Dake M, Bleyn J, et al. Peripheral arterial obstruction: prospective study of treatment with a transluminally placed self-expanding stent-graft. International trial study group. Radiology 2000;217:95–104.

CHAPTER
9

Surgical Intervention

Amy B Reed and Magruder C Donaldson

KEY POINTS

- Surgical therapy for intermittent claudication (IC) is required in only approximately 5% of patients.

- In appropriately selected patients with IC, TransAtlantic Inter-Society Consensus (TASC) C and D lesions are best treated by surgical revascularization.

- Long-term patency of aortobifemoral bypass (ABF) is 85–90% at 5 years and 70–75% at 10 years. ABF is the most durable therapy for long-segment aortoiliac occlusive disease (AIOD).

- Extra-anatomic axillobifemoral grafting is useful in selected high-risk patients requiring operation for bilateral diffuse AIOD due to medical co-morbidities or anatomic considerations ('hostile abdomen', sepsis, etc.).

- Iliac endarterectomy, iliofemoral bypass, and femorofemoral bypass are useful approaches to patients with predominantly unilateral iliac occlusive disease not amenable to angioplasty.

- Femoropopliteal bypass for patients with IC should be preferentially performed with autologous vein. Prosthetic grafts are inferior not only below the knee but also above the knee.

- Femoropopliteal vein grafts should be routinely monitored by postoperative duplex surveillance.

- Profundaplasty is a critically important adjunctive procedure for patients undergoing operative intervention for IC. It is generally more useful when combined with an inflow or outflow reconstruction than when performed as an isolated procedure.

INTRODUCTION

Lower extremity intermittent claudication (IC) is defined clinically as muscular pain induced by exercise and relieved by rest. Claudication results from a lesion in the arterial system proximal to the affected muscle group, which limits the normal exercise-induced increase in limb blood flow and results in transient muscle ischemia. Subjective complaints of claudication vary in degree and significance, confounding efforts to determine its prevalence in the general population.[1] Studies have documented that more than half of patients with IC had never complained of this symptom to their physician, assuming the pain and difficulty with ambulation was a natural consequence of aging.[2,3] Using an objective definition of lower extremity peripheral arterial disease (PAD) as a resting ankle–brachial index (ABI) of less than 0.95, a 6.9% prevalence was encountered

in patients 45–74 years of age, only 22% of whom complained of IC.[4]

Although the presence of PAD may have less clinical significance with respect to the lower extremities, it is a strong marker for future cardiovascular events such as myocardial infarction (**Fig. 9.1**).[5] Results from several studies have shown 5- and 10-year mortality rates of 30% and 50%, respectively, among patients with PAD, the majority of deaths being due to cardiovascular complications.[6] A classic study from the Cleveland Clinic evaluated 1000 patients (381 with lower extremity ischemia) with coronary arteriography before elective vascular surgery and found normal coronary arteries in only 10%.[7] Twenty-eight percent of these patients had severe triple-vessel coronary disease or worse. Given these results and the high risk for future ischemic events, risk factor modification,[8–12] exercise,[13] and pharmacotherapy[14–16] should be recommended in all patients with lower extremity atherosclerosis, particularly before embarking on surgical intervention. Furthermore, the risk of progression of PAD to critical ischemia and limb threat is small over time. A summary of reports on the natural history of IC found overall 5-year rates of mortality of 29%, need for intervention of 25%, and risk of amputation of only 4%.[17] Over 55% of patients surviving had stable or improved claudication over the initial 5 years of history, with worsening of symptoms in only 16%. Intervention should therefore be limited to those patients who are truly disabled or develop signs or symptoms of resting ischemia and who are an acceptable risk for intervention.

EVALUATION

The symptoms associated with the peripheral vascular occlusive process vary with the location and extent of the disease (**Fig. 9.2**). Highly localized aortoiliac disease with occlusive lesions confined to the distal abdominal aorta and common iliac vessels occurs in only a small number of patients, and in the absence of more distal disease, rarely produces limb-threatening symptoms.[18] Women constitute a significant number of patients with localized aortoiliac disease, a pattern particularly prevalent among relatively younger female smokers. These patients typically present with claudication involving the proximal musculature of the thigh, hip, or buttocks. A number of male patients with aortoiliac disease complain of impotence.

While isolated superficial femoral artery occlusive disease occurs, many patients with IC have more diffuse disease. Twenty-five percent of claudicants have disease confined to the aortoiliac segment, while 65% have disease above and below the inguinal ligament, including disease limited to the superficial femoral artery. These patients are typically older, male, and more likely to have diabetes, hypertension, and associated

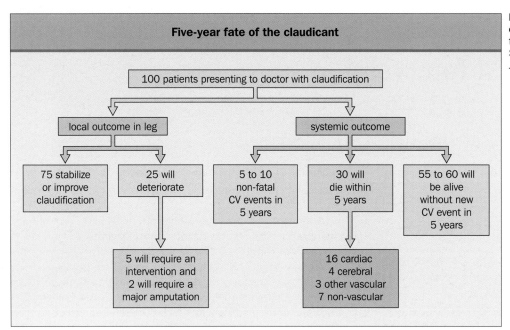

Figure 9.1 Five-year fate of the claudicant. (Adapted with permission from Report of the TransAtlantic Inter-Society Consensus (TASC) Group. J Vasc Surg (Suppl) 2000;31:S21.)

cerebrovascular and coronary atherosclerosis. Progression of the occlusive process is also more likely in such patients than in patients with more localized aortoiliac disease,[19–21] resulting in the development of critical ischemia in the form of rest pain or tissue necrosis.

The history and physical examination are usually sufficient to establish the diagnosis of vascular claudication, the likely anatomic location of arterial occlusive lesions, and the physiologic severity of the condition. For example, the characteristic triad of Leriche syndrome – defined as claudication in both legs, male impotence, and diminished or absent femoral pulses – corresponds to disease in the aortoiliac segments. Claudication limited to the calf muscle with a normal femoral pulse but reduced or absent popliteal and pedal pulses is characteristic of disease in the femoropopliteal segment. Measurement of the ABI in the clinic is a simple way of objectively establishing the presence of PAD and its severity.

Non-invasive laboratory study using segmental limb pressures and pulse volume recordings is a helpful adjunct to clinical assessment, particularly when physical findings are obscured by obesity or scarring from previous surgery, or the history is confusing. The laboratory is especially valuable in clarifying the functional importance of vascular disease in patients with claudication symptoms and in teasing out the vascular component of dysfunction when other potential problems such as arthritis and neurogenic conditions are present. For example, vascular claudication can be difficult to distinguish from neurogenic or musculoskeletal pain syndromes despite the fact that in most instances vascular claudication is relieved by standing after walking while pain caused by other etiologies is relieved only with sitting or lying down. Selective functional assessment of such complex patients using physiologic treadmill exercise study is a valuable adjunct to more routine studies performed at rest. Vascular laboratory measurements serve not only as objective confirmation of the severity of disease but also as baseline documentation by which to follow the course of disease.

Additional study by direct vascular imaging in patients with IC is generally indicated only when symptoms are severe enough to warrant intervention. Duplex ultrasound is used increasingly to image the arteries of the abdomen and lower extremities, sometimes with intervention based solely on ultrasound findings.[22–24] More commonly, magnetic resonance angiography (MRA) or abdominal aortography with bilateral lower extremity runoff is used to provide hard-copy images for interventional planning. Gadolinium-enhanced MRA is available in most centers and is increasingly supplanting contrast angiography for diagnostic and planning purposes, thus completely avoiding the small risk of allergic reaction and renal dysfunction associated with iodinated contrast agents. Computed tomographic angiography is an additional modality that may be applied in circumstances when MRA or angiography via arterial puncture is not feasible or advisable.

TREATMENT

Endovascular and surgical therapy for IC should be reserved for the minority of patients who have failed maximal non-operative measures including smoking cessation, weight reduction, exercise, and pharmacologic risk-factor modification. Patients must be fully aware of the potential risks of the initial procedure and potential complications associated with future failure of the revascularization effort, which might precipitate reintervention, and worsening of ischemia. In order to stratify the potential benefits of a particular procedure according to anticipated success, the TransAtlantic Inter-Society Consensus (TASC) Working Group divided lower extremity occlusive disease into aortoiliac and infrainguinal locations, categorizing the lesions according to preferred treatment options (**Fig. 9.2**).[6] Patients with short-segment iliac artery lesions (TASC-A) are generally treated with endovascular techniques. Longer stenotic segments of the iliac arteries (TASC-B) are frequently treated with endovascular therapy, but evidence for its superiority for these lesions is currently insufficient. Surgical treatment is usually undertaken for TASC-C lesions, though conclusive comparative evidence is lacking. Long-segment aortoiliac and multisegment occlusive

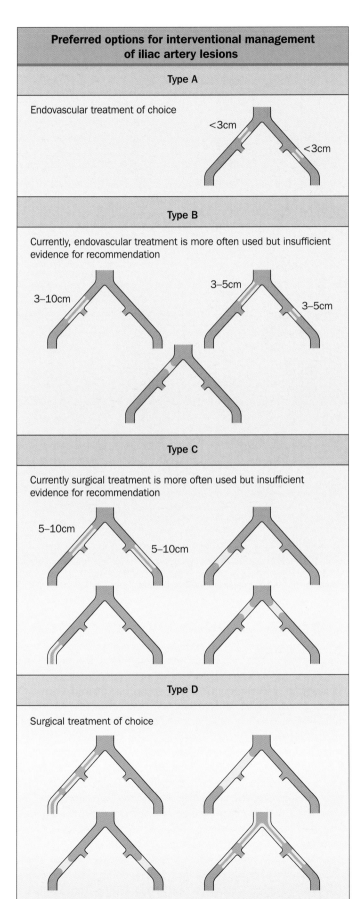

Preferred options for interventional management of iliac artery lesions

Type A

Endovascular treatment of choice

<3cm
<3cm

Type B

Currently, endovascular treatment is more often used but insufficient evidence for recommendation

3–10cm
3–5cm
3–5cm

Type C

Currently surgical treatment is more often used but insufficient evidence for recommendation

5–10cm
5–10cm

Type D

Surgical treatment of choice

Figure 9.2 Preferred options for interventional management of iliac artery lesions. (Adapted with permission from Report of the TransAtlantic Inter-Society Consensus (TASC) Group. J Vasc Surg (Suppl) 2000;31:S99.)

disease in TASC-D lesions is best treated by surgical revascularization. The TASC group also summarized the preferred treatment options for femoropopliteal lesions above the knee joint. Focal stenoses <3cm in length are preferentially treated by endovascular techniques. Results for serial stenoses <3cm long or a single occlusion <5cm are less favorable after endovascular therapy, but catheter-based treatment is still appropriate in some instances. Longer stenotic and obstructive lesions are best managed with surgical revascularization.

SURGICAL TREATMENT FOR AORTOILIAC OCCLUSIVE DISEASE

Direct pharmacologic management of vulnerable myocardium and preliminary cardiac intervention for appropriate individuals have improved surgical morbidity and mortality rates for revascularization of the aortoiliac arteries. For example, the 30-day operative mortality rate for bypass or endarterectomy using an abdominal approach has been reduced to less than 2% in many centers.[25–29] With acceptably low morbidity and excellent long-term patency rates, use of direct vascular reconstruction is reasonable in appropriately selected patients for IC, a condition which does not threaten life or limb.

Aortobifemoral bypass graft
Aortoiliac bypass is occasionally appropriate, using the common iliac bifurcation or external iliac arteries for the distal anastomosis. This procedure would be reasonable for a patient with proximal aortoiliac disease and normal external iliac arteries, and would be preferable to aortobifemoral bypass in such patients if the groins were inhospitable for one reason or another. In most patients, disease involves the external iliac arteries to some extent, and placement of the graft proximal to the groin leaves the patient exposed to progression of disease in the external iliac, with a relatively arduous revision necessary in the event of graft failure. Since it has become clear that tunneling a prosthetic graft across the hip joint to the groin does not cause graft failure due to kinking, aortobifemoral bypass has become the preferred procedure for most patients with diffuse infrarenal aortoiliac disease.

Aortobifemoral bypass surgery is started with bilateral groin incisions to expose both common femoral arteries, taking care to control lymphatic tissue to minimize the possibility of postoperative lymph leak with associated wound complications and infection. The posterior aspect of the inguinal ligament is divided over most of the distal external iliac artery to facilitate tunneling of the graft, taking care to avoid injury to the deep circumflex iliac vein (the 'vein of woe') crossing the external iliac artery just beneath the ligament. Dissection is carried distally to the common femoral artery bifurcation. If preoperative arteriography or intraoperative palpation reveals superficial femoral artery occlusion, the profunda femoris artery should be mobilized past any proximal disease, to the level of the medial and lateral femoral circumflex branches, to expose a more normal distal segment of the artery for possible profundaplasty at the time of construction of the distal anastomosis.

While the infrarenal abdominal aorta may be exposed by a variety of approaches, most surgeons prefer a transperitoneal midline incision from xiphoid to pubis. The retroperitoneum over the aorta is incised and the proximal abdominal aorta is

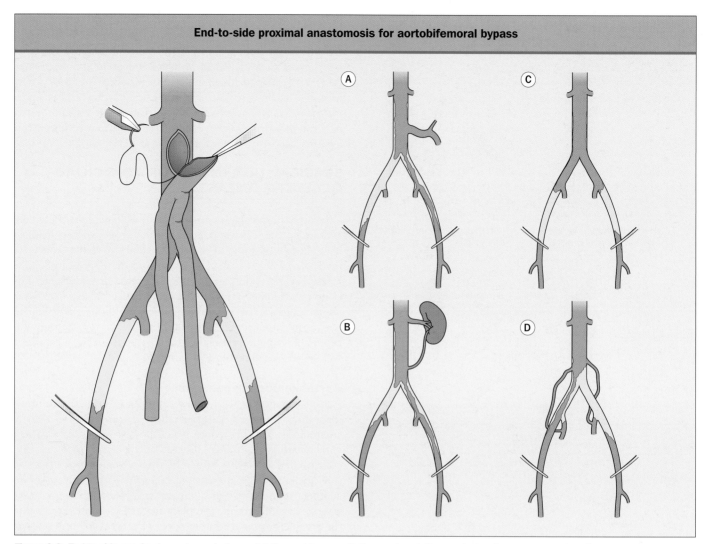

End-to-side proximal anastomosis for aortobifemoral bypass

Figure 9.3 End-to-side proximal anastomosis for aortobifemoral bypass. Patterns of aortoiliac occlusive disease appropriate for end-to-side proximal anastomosis of aortobifemoral bypass graft in order to preserve antegrade flow into important vascular beds. (Adapted from Brewster DC. Direct reconstruction for aortoiliac occlusive disease. In: Rutherford RB, ed. Vascular surgery, 5th edn. Philadelphia:WB Saunders; 2000:952.)

mobilized just below the renal arteries at the level of the left renal vein. Dissection proceeds distally, keeping to the right side of the anterior surface of the aorta to protect the inferior mesenteric artery to allow for possible reimplantation in the event of inadequate collateral flow to the left colon at the conclusion of surgery. The distal aorta is sufficiently mobilized for clamping at a level appropriate for the graft configuration chosen. A gentle atraumatic technique is necessary to avoid atheroembolization during dissection.

After completion of the femoral and aortic exposures, retroperitoneal tunnels are created from the aortic bifurcation to the groin to allow passage of the graft limbs. Gentle blunt dissection is carried out with both index fingers simultaneously, taking care to remain directly anterior to the common and external iliac arteries, posterior to the ureters and anterior to the deep circumflex iliac vein. Passage of the graft posterior to the ureters is an important detail that minimizes the potential of ureteral compression and hydronephrosis.

Once the dissection and tunneling are complete, the patient is systemically heparinized and the aorta cross-clamped infrarenally. The proximal anastomosis is constructed in an end-

to-end or end-to-side configuration. A good deal of controversy remains as to the proper configuration of the aortobifemoral bypass graft.[17,30-33] Some authors believe that the end-to-end technique reduces the incidence of late aortoduodenal fistula because the graft does not project as anteriorly as does the end-to-side anastomosis,[17,34,35] while others have not demonstrated any difference in complication or late patency rates between end-to-end and end-to-side grafts.[30-33] The end-to-end technique is best suited for patients who will not suffer any further hemodynamic compromise to the bowel and pelvic arterial beds from interruption of forward flow in the aorta, such as those with complete aortic occlusion below the renal arteries and those with patent external iliac arteries capable of retrograde flow from the groin into the internal iliacs. End-to-end anastomosis is mandatory in patients with aneurysmal disease of the infrarenal aorta. The end-to-side technique is reserved for those patients who have a patent and enlarged inferior mesenteric artery, a low-lying accessory renal artery arising from the distal aorta or proximal iliac artery, diffuse occlusive disease confined mainly to the external iliac arteries with an intact distal aorta and common iliac system, or those individuals with reconstituted

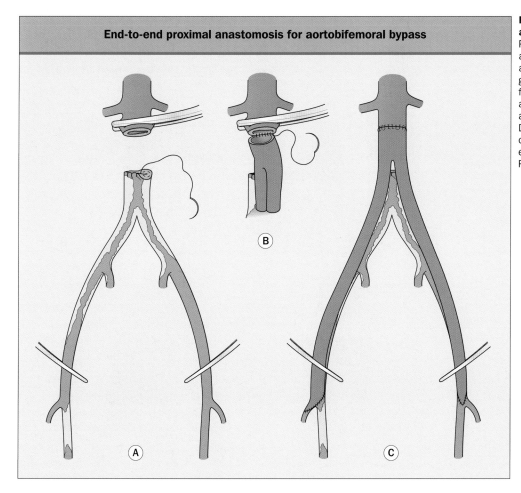

End-to-end proximal anastomosis for aortobifemoral bypass

Figure 9.4 End-to-end proximal anastomosis for aortobifemoral bypass. Pattern of aortoiliac occlusive disease appropriate for end-to-end proximal anastomosis of aortobifemoral bypass graft in which retrograde flow from femoral arteries will supply internal iliac arterial beds after occlusion of distal aorta. (Adapted from Brewster DC. Direct reconstruction for aortoiliac occlusive disease. In: Rutherford RB, ed. Vascular surgery, 5th edn. Philadelphia:WB Saunders; 2000:951.)

pelvic circulation via collateral arteries that might otherwise be lost in an end-to-end anastomosis (**Figs 9.3 & 9.4**).

The end-to-end proximal anastomotic technique requires transection of the aorta between two clamps below the renal arteries, allowing for localized thromboendarterectomy of the proximal aortic stump under direct visualization if necessary. A segment of aorta is usually resected and the distal aorta either oversewn or stapled (**Fig. 9.5**). Construction of an end-to-side anastomosis involves placement of a longitudinal aortotomy as proximal as possible below the renals after clamping in a relatively less diseased section of aorta. Although a partially occluding Satinsky clamp may be used when there is minimal disease, in most instances two clamps are best in order to facilitate exposure and selective flushing from each end of the aorta (**Fig. 9.6**). Care must be taken to remove all loose thrombus and debris from the excluded aortic segment between the occluding clamps.

The femoral anastomotic configuration is dependent on the amount of femoropopliteal occlusive disease present. If the superficial femoral artery is occluded, the profunda femoris will be the predominant runoff for the graft limb. If there is obvious disease at the profunda orifice, the common femoral arteriotomy should be extended down onto the first portion of the profunda femoris, where the toe of the graft limb will serve as a patch profundaplasty (**Fig. 9.7**). If the status of the profunda orifice is unclear from preoperative imaging and palpation, the initial common femoral arteriotomy may be kept short and extended onto the profunda only if a 3.5 or 4.0 dilator cannot be easily passed into the profunda. Orificial or proximal profunda disease

may be treated by endarterectomy, but care must be taken to avoid leaving a distal flap. Usually, endarterectomy is unnecessary and it is sufficient to simply open the profunda by patching with the hood of the bypass graft.

There is no evidence conclusively establishing superiority of one prosthetic graft material over another, and the choice can be made on the basis of handling characteristics and surgeon's preference. Dacron prostheses, optionally with either collagen or albumen coating to obviate the need for preclotting, are preferred by many because of absence of bleeding at suture holes, and flexibility and ease of manipulation. Others prefer expanded polytetrafluoroethylene (PTFE) for many of the same reasons. Regardless of which prosthetic graft is used, it is important to select the appropriate size based on the corresponding diameter of the patient's common femoral arteries. A 16 × 8mm bifurcated prosthesis is appropriate for most patients, with smaller grafts commonly used in females and larger ones in patients with an element of arteriomegaly or ectasia.

Early complications specific to aortobifemoral bypass grafting include:

- renal dysfunction caused by hemodynamic instability, atheroembolism, renal artery occlusion, or ureteral injury;
- colon ischemia due to interruption of inflow or collateral to the bed of the inferior mesenteric artery;
- lower extremity ischemia due to inflow occlusion or to embolism of thrombus or atheromatous debris; and
- impotence due to injury of the nervi erigentes or pelvic circulation.

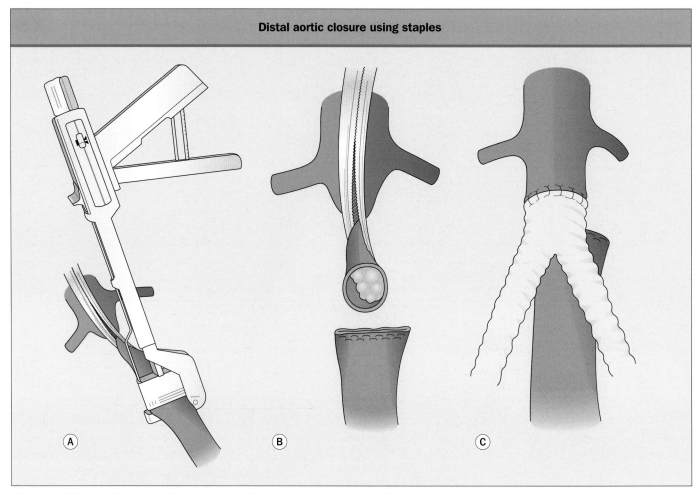

Distal aortic closure using staples

(A) (B) (C)

Figure 9.5 Distal aortic closure using staples. The distal aorta may be conveniently closed using staples in aortas relatively free of calcium in patients undergoing aortobifemoral bypass with end-to-end proximal anastomosis. (Adapted from Belkin M, Whittemore AD, Donaldson MC, Mannick JA. Aortoiliac occlusive disease. In: Moore WS, ed. Vascular surgery: a comprehensive review, 6th edn. Philadelphia:WB Saunders; 2002:512.)

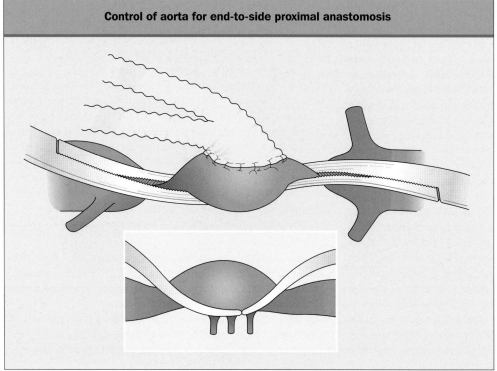

Control of aorta for end-to-side proximal anastomosis

Figure 9.6 Control of aorta for end-to-side proximal anastomosis. Method of clamping proximal aorta to allow occlusion and selective flushing of proximal and distal aorta, occlusion of lumbar arteries, and adequate exposure for local aortic thromboendarterectomy. (Adapted from Belkin MB et al. Aortoiliac occlusive disease. In: Moore WS, ed. Vascular surgery: a comprehensive review, 6th edn. Philadelphia:WB Saunders; 2002:513.)

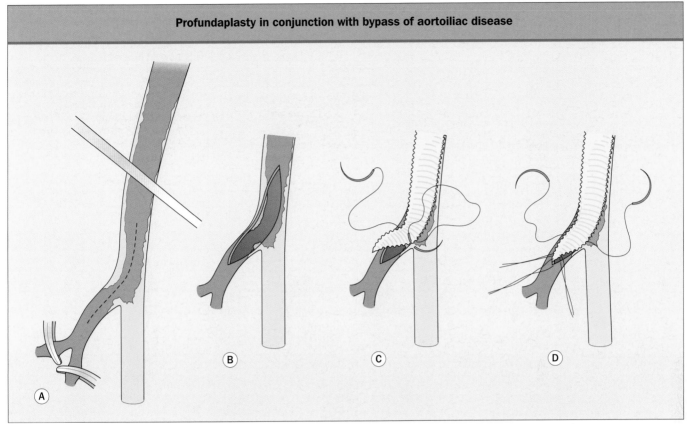

Profundaplasty in conjunction with bypass of aortoiliac disease

Figure 9.7 Profundaplasty in conjunction with bypass of aortoiliac disease. The distal anastomosis of a prosthetic inflow graft should include angioplasty over significant proximal disease in the profunda femoris artery when present. (Adapted from Brewster DC. Direct reconstruction for aortoiliac occlusive disease. In: Rutherford RB, ed. Vascular surgery, 5th edn. Philadelphia:WB Saunders; 2000:953.)

Long-term graft efficacy after aortobifemoral bypass is excellent, with cumulative patency rates of 85–90% at 5 years and 70–75% at 10 years. Younger patients with premature atherosclerosis and patients with small aortas, who are frequently female, have been shown to have inferior patency rates compared with the overall group of patients.[29]

Aortoiliac endarterectomy

First performed in the early 1950s,[36] aortoiliac endarterectomy is still an appropriate choice of treatment for candidates selected from the 5–10% of patients with IC who have disease limited to the distal aorta and common iliac arteries. Since diffuse disease is so much more common, many surgeons lack experience with endarterectomy and may prefer not to use the method for this reason. Patients most likely to be candidates include early-middle-aged females with occlusive disease of the middle and distal abdominal aorta, with limited extension into the proximal common iliac arteries. Patients who present with atheroembolization from disrupted focal aortoiliac plaque may be best treated by endarterectomy in order to avoid risk of further embolization from catheter manipulation during catheter-based therapy. The principal benefit of aortoiliac endarterectomy is avoidance of prosthetic grafts and attendant possible complications of infection. The procedure may be less appealing for males, owing to concern over interference with the nervi erigentes coursing over the aortic bifurcation and proximal common iliac arteries. The main contraindication to endarterectomy is the existence of a degenerated or aneurysmal arterial wall.

A midline abdominal incision allows good exposure of the aorta as described for aortobifemoral bypass. When the iliac arteries are involved, the retroperitoneal incision is extended down both common iliacs, leaving the tissue at and between the iliac origins undissected if possible in order to preserve the periaortic nervi erigentes which course lateral to the aorta and cross over the aortic bifurcation. The proximal external and internal iliac arteries are dissected out for clamping. Clamps are applied to the aorta at the level of the renal arteries and at the proximal internal and external iliac arteries, with bulldog clamps for lumbars and the inferior mesenteric artery. A longitudinal incision is made in the aorta at or above the target plaque and carried down to the aortic bifurcation. The endarterectomy plane is begun in the deep media, pushing the aortic wall away from the plaque. The plaque is transected below the level of the proximal aortic clamp. The distal endpoint is exposed by transverse or longitudinal counterincisions in the common iliac arteries, just proximal to the iliac bifurcation (**Fig. 9.8**). If the plaque does not taper to a satisfactory endpoint, it is sharply divided and mattress stitches are placed to tack it down. After irrigation with heparinized saline, backbleeding and forward flushing, the aortotomy is closed with a continuous monofilament suture. The iliac incisions are closed primarily or using a patch, depending upon arterial diameter and surgeon's preference.

Early complications specific to aortoiliac endarterectomy include limb ischemia related to embolization or dissection at the distal endpoint and hemorrhage from excessive thinning of an endarterectomized artery, most common when there is heavy

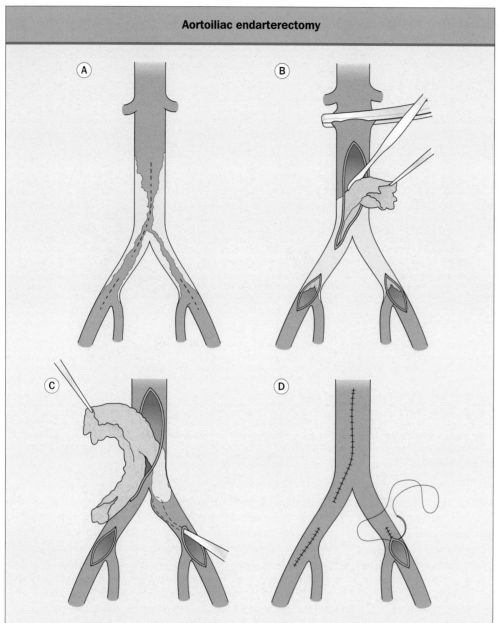

Aortoiliac endarterectomy

A B C D

Figure 9.8 Aortoiliac endarterectomy.
Method of aortoiliac endarterectomy using longitudinal aortotomy and distal common iliac arterotomies to gain access to disease localized to the distal aorta and proximal common iliac arteries, with primary closure. (Adapted from Brewster DC. Direct reconstruction for aortoiliac occlusive disease. In: Rutherford RB, ed. Vascular surgery, 4th edn. Philadelphia:WB Saunders; 1995:773.)

calcification of the plaque. Over time, aneurysmal dilatation of the endarterectomized segment and progressive atherosclerotic disease may necessitate reoperation. In carefully selected patients, the 5-year patency rate after aortoiliac endarterectomy is 80–90%.[37,38]

Axillofemoral bypass graft

Extra-anatomic bypass with axillofemoral grafting is used in patients with symptomatic aortoiliac disease who are deemed high risk for a major abdominal surgical procedure or who have a hostile abdomen due to prior irradiation, surgery, sepsis, or gastrointestinal stomas. Since few patients who meet these criteria are likely to complain solely of IC, axillofemoral reconstructions are most commonly utilized for patients with critical ischemia. Unilateral axillofemoral (axillounifemoral) bypass is infrequently used electively, but is appropriate as a temporizing measure

for aortic graft sepsis when the contralateral groin is infected or for temporary retrograde perfusion of the aorta during repair of a thoracoabdominal aneurysm. Because patency rates for axillofemoral grafts with distal anastomoses to both femoral arteries (axillobifemoral bypass) appear significantly superior to the axillounifemoral configuration, in part due to increased flow through the common axillary graft limb, the axillobifemoral option is preferred for most situations when feasible.[39,40]

Construction of the axillobifemoral bypass begins by assessment of the blood pressure in each arm, to select the optimal site for the proximal anastomosis. If pressures are equivalent, the right axillary artery is generally preferred as the donor because it has a lower risk of having or developing proximal occlusive disease than the left.[41] Routine preoperative arteriography has been recommended prior to axillofemoral bypass, because of evidence of significant inflow disease in 25% of patients, undetected by non-invasive testing in 75%.[42]

Tunneling for axillofemoral bypass graft

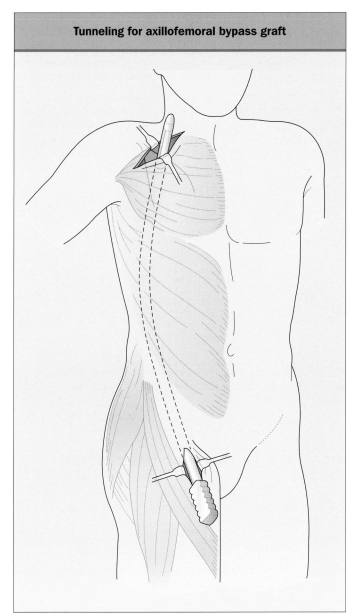

Figure 9.9 Tunneling for axillofemoral bypass graft. A long tunneling instrument is used to create space for the graft in a subcutaneous plane, anterior to the iliac spine, in the midaxillary line and under the pectoralis muscles on the chest wall, towards the proximal axillary artery. (Adapted from Taylor LM, Landry GJ, Moneta GL, Porter JM. Axillobifemoral bypass. In: Nyhus LM, Baker RJ, Fischer JE, eds. Mastery of surgery, 3rd edn. Boston:Little, Brown & Company; 1997:2040.)

The patient is positioned supine with the donor arm supported on a narrow arm board with slight flexion at the elbow in a 'hand-in-pants pocket' configuration. This posture relaxes the pectoralis muscles to facilitate tunneling and axillary artery exposure beneath the clavicle. Exposure of the first portion of the axillary artery is gained through a transverse infraclavicular incision, splitting the fibers of the pectoralis major muscle. The pectoralis minor may be divided, if necessary, to improve operative exposure. The axillary artery lies deep and superior to the axillary vein and inferior to the brachial plexus. The artery is isolated by dissection toward a palpable pulse or by following a branch of the thoracoacromial trunk, reflecting the vein either inferiorly or superiorly. The common femoral arteries are exposed

Proximal anastomotic region of axillofemoral bypass graft

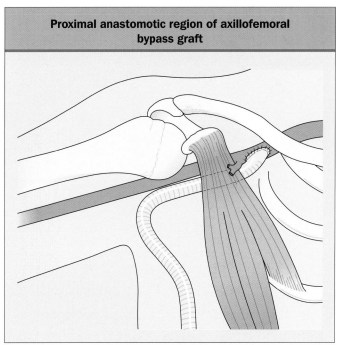

Figure 9.10 Proximal anastomotic region of axillofemoral bypass graft. The graft is connected to the anterior-inferior surface of the proximal axillary artery adjacent to the chest wall, with oblique course along the artery under the pectoralis muscles and some laxity (exaggerated in figure for emphasis) to avoid undue tension at the anastomosis when the arm is elevated. (Adapted from Taylor LM, Landry GJ, Moneta GL, Porter JM. Axillobifemoral bypass. In: Nyhus LM, Baker RJ, Fischer JE, eds. Mastery of surgery, 3rd edn. Boston:Little, Brown & Company; 1997:2040.)

through longitudinal groin incisions. A long tunneler is then passed from the ipsilateral groin incision in a subcutaneous plane in the midaxillary line and then beneath both pectoralis muscles along the chest wall (**Fig. 9.9**). Care is taken to direct the tunneler medial to the anterior iliac spine and to remain superficial to the costal margin. Grafts tunneled too far anterior to the midaxillary line are prone to kinking.[43] By using a long tunneler, a counterincision along the course of the graft can be avoided, thus eliminating a potential source of wound complications. A femorofemoral tunnel is then created in a gentle inverted C shape in the subcutaneous plane on the fascia of the external oblique and anterior rectus sheath.

Dacron and PTFE grafts have been used with equally good results, usually in an 8mm diameter with external supporting rings to minimize the risk of compression of the graft. The graft may be passed through the long tunnel before or after the proximal anastomosis is constructed. Once the patient is systemically heparinized, clamps are applied as proximally as possible on the axillary artery. The anastomosis is created proximal to the pectoralis minor muscle. An arteriotomy is made on the anterior-inferior aspect of the artery to allow gentle angulation of the anastomosis into the subcutaneous plane. Traumatic disruption of the axillary anastomosis has been reported with excessive arm abduction after having pulled the graft down to the groin too tightly[44] or when angling the anastomosis too acutely (<75°) with respect to the axillary artery (**Fig. 9.10**). The graft is flushed and clamped at its origin to allow reperfusion of the arm while the ipsilateral femoral anastomosis is constructed. The

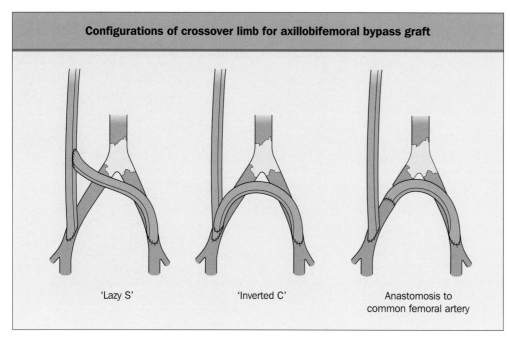

Configurations of crossover limb for axillobifemoral bypass graft

'Lazy S'   'Inverted C'   Anastomosis to common femoral artery

Figure 9.11 Configurations of crossover limb for axillobifemoral bypass graft. Configurations that minimize low flow in the ipsilateral short femoral limb may be preferable when there is compromised runoff from the short limb. (Adapted from Rutherford RB. Extra-anatomic bypass. In: Rutherford RB, ed. Vascular surgery, 5th edn. Philadelphia:WB Saunders; 2000:989.)

graft is copiously flushed once again just prior to final closure of the distal suture line and establishment of flow into the leg.

Several configurations have been advocated for the femoro-femoral portion of the bypass, though there is no conclusive evidence favoring one over another. Grafts are available with a pre-attached femoral sidearm, in which case the graft must be carefully positioned in the tunnels prior to creation of the axillary anastomosis, to assure optimal alignment of the sidearm. Most surgeons prefer constructing the sidearm by excising a window on the medial aspect of the axillofemoral limb, using one of several alternative configurations, including: (1) a 'lazy S' shape, involving an anastomosis just below the anterior iliac spine; (2) an 'inverted C' shape, with the anastomosis in the groin, just above or into the hood of the distal axillofemoral anastomosis; or even (3) dividing the distal external iliac artery and performing an end-to-end anastomosis between the femorofemoral prosthetic and the divided external iliac artery (**Fig. 9.11**). Configurations that eliminate the short arm of the graft system connected to the ipsilateral femoral artery may be preferred in situations when the runoff below the ipsilateral femoral artery is severely compromised, creating reduced flow in the short limb.

Early complications specific to axillofemoral bypass include injury to the axillary artery, axillary vein, and brachial plexus, in addition to inadvertent entry into the peritoneal or pleural cavity with the tunneler. Axillary anastomotic disruption and perigraft seroma are also occasionally associated with axillo-femoral grafting.

Patency rates for axillofemoral bypass are strongly influenced by the indications for the surgery and by the configuration and status of the runoff vessels at the groin. When the procedure is performed for aortic sepsis following aortic aneurysm resection, in the bifemoral configuration with patent superficial femoral artery runoff at the groins, 5-year primary patency rates may approach 90%. On the other hand, when performed for occlusive disease in the unilateral configuration with an occluded superficial femoral artery in the recipient groin, the long-term primary

patency rate may be expected to be much lower. Circumstances between these relative extremes can be expected to yield intermediate patency results. Secondary patency is substantially higher than primary patency, rewarding efforts to disobliterate and revise grafts when necessary.[45,46]

SURGICAL TREATMENT FOR ILIAC OCCLUSIVE DISEASE

Isolated iliac disease is relatively uncommon, as disease tends to affect both the aorta and the iliac arteries. Standard aorto-bifemoral bypass is the most definitive approach in good-risk younger patients, thus obviating any possible progression of disease in the less involved arteries over time. When the infrarenal aorta does not have significant disease and at least one common iliac artery is uninvolved, iliac disease may be successfully addressed independent of the aorta.[28,47] Since it can be assumed that atherosclerosis will eventually compromise the source of iliac inflow, this approach is most appealing among patients with minimal inflow disease at the outset and in whom longevity may be limited by age or concurrent illness.[48,49]

In addition to axillofemoral bypass, iliofemoral endarterectomy and iliofemoral or iliobifemoral bypass are options applicable to patients with suitable anatomy and excessive co-morbidity for major abdominal surgery. Femorofemoral bypass is an excellent option with good long-term success for patients with hemo-dynamically intact contralateral iliofemoral inflow to the groin. If necessary, mild-to-moderate iliac inflow disease may be corrected using catheter-based therapy in order to allow sub-sequent surgical bypass based on the improved inflow to the groin. This strategy has been used successfully for femoro-femoral and femorodistal grafting.[50,51]

Iliac endarterectomy
The role of iliac endarterectomy has diminished with increasing use of percutaneous transluminal angioplasty and stenting. Nonetheless, selected patients with suitable short-segment

involvement of either common or external iliac vessels have durable results after endarterectomy, particularly if the arteries are relatively large in caliber. This approach should not be used if there is aneurysmal change. Using the semi-closed technique without patching, endarterectomy obviates the need for prosthetic material and is thus an option when infection is a consideration. For patients with localized unilateral common iliac or external iliac occlusive disease, a retroperitoneal approach to the iliac fossa provides good access.[36,52,53] The common, internal, and external iliac artery are exposed through a 'kidney transplant' incision. Once proximal and distal control is achieved, techniques similar to those described above for aortoiliac endarterectomy disease may be utilized. A semi-closed approach may be employed via transverse arteriotomies with a ring endarterectomy loop to remove the core of disease, followed by transverse closure without the need for patch angioplasty. In smaller arteries, or when the disease ends adjacent to the iliac bifurcation, longitudinal arteriotomies may be used to facilitate exposure of the distal endpoint, in which case closure is performed with a patch angioplasty of vein or prosthetic material. Less commonly, a single arteriotomy may afford adequate exposure to handle very focal plaque. Concomitant common femoral endarterectomy, profundaplasty, or ipsilateral distal bypass may be combined with iliac endarterectomy in patients with unilateral multilevel disease.[52,54]

Iliofemoral bypass

When the disease has caused occlusion of the external iliac artery but has largely spared the distal aorta and ipsilateral common iliac artery, the common iliac may serve well as the site of inflow for bypass to the ipsilateral femoral artery, with adjunctive cross limb to the contralateral femoral artery if necessary.[51] Though axillofemoral bypass and femorofemoral bypass may be equally applicable in similar situations, iliofemoral grafts may be preferable because of generally more favorable long-term success. The iliobifemoral option may be chosen for patients with favorable ipsilateral anatomy and severe contralateral iliac disease who are felt to be high risk for aortobifemoral bypass. Alternatively, the unilateral iliofemoral bypass is a good choice for relatively healthy and active individuals with unilateral disease in whom a durable, strictly ipsilateral solution is desired. Occasionally, the unilateral graft is helpful if there is good reason to avoid the contralateral groin, such as sepsis or previous surgery. Presence of heavy calcification in the donor iliac artery on preoperative imaging makes this method less attractive because of potential difficulties in clamping and sewing the artery.

Exposure of the common iliac artery is obtained with a retroperitoneal incision extending obliquely from the anterior axillary line near the tip of the eleventh rib to 2–3cm below the umbilicus. The external and internal oblique muscles are divided. The medial extent of the incision may be terminated at the lateral edge of the rectus or with partial rectus incision in patients with wide costal margins. The transversus abdominus muscle is split in the line of its fibers and a pre-peritoneal plane developed and retracted medially. Use of a mechanical retractor system is of great help in gaining and maintaining adequate exposure of the deeper structures, particularly in relatively obese patients. The ureter is carefully mobilized away from the common iliac artery. The external and internal iliac artery origins are mobilized

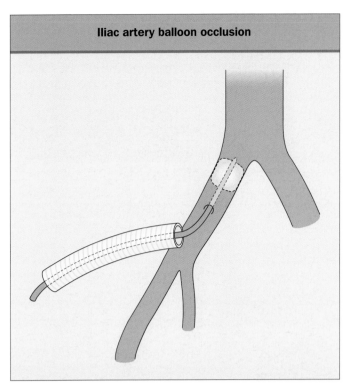

Figure 9.12 Iliac artery balloon occlusion. Method for balloon occlusion of a calcified common iliac artery during iliofemoral bypass grafting. The prosthetic graft is loaded on the balloon prior to insertion and inflation for control of inflow, then tailored to be sewn end-to-side into the arterotomy created by enlarging the iliac puncture using Potts scissors. Proximal iliac or distal aortic exposure should be adequate to control inflow as backup in the event of balloon failure.

sufficiently for later control with loops or clamps. The common iliac artery should be mobilized to its origin and the exposure extended to include the proximal contralateral iliac artery and distal aorta if there is heavy calcification and no favorable place for clamping. After exposing the common femoral artery through a longitudinal groin incision, a tunnel is created under the inguinal ligament anterior to the external iliac artery and under the ureter if it has been mobilized distal to the common iliac artery.

Proximal control of the common iliac artery is easily obtained with a clamp if the vessel is soft and generally free of disease. If there is circumferential or partially circumferential calcification, however, clamping may be difficult or may create a dissection or injury sufficient to compromise the anastomosis. Under these circumstances, it may be preferable to make use of a 5 or 6mm occluding balloon, passed through the graft and into the artery via a stab wound, to provide atraumatic inflow occlusion (**Fig. 9.12**). Most commonly, an 8mm prosthesis is an appropriate graft choice, constructing the proximal anastomosis using a continuous 'parachute' technique without tying down the heel and toe of the graft, in order to provide better visualization deep in the wound. If an additional graft limb is planned to the contralateral side, a cross limb may be attached to the graft in the retroperitoneum and passed across pre-peritoneally and under the contralateral inguinal ligament to the femoral artery. Alternatively, a femorofemoral bypass is constructed from the region of the ipsilateral femoral anastomosis across to the other femoral artery via the subcutaneous plane (**Fig. 9.13**).

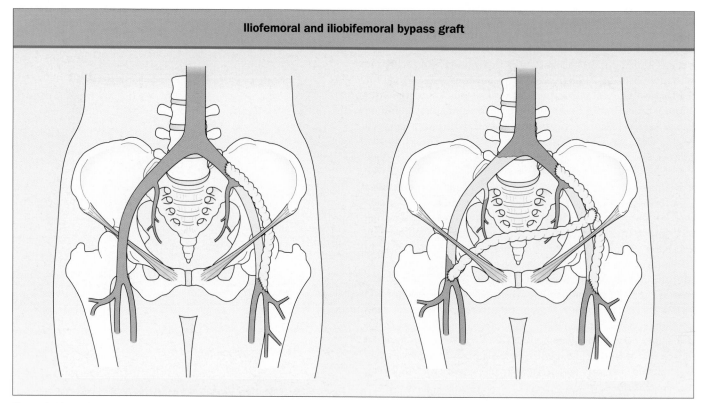

Figure 9.13 Iliofemoral and iliobifemoral bypass graft. Configurations of retroperitoneal iliofemoral bypass for unilateral external iliac occlusion (left) and iliobifemoral bypass for bilateral iliac occlusions with common iliac artery sparing (right). (Adapted from Belkin M, Whittemore AD, Donaldson MC, Mannick JA. Aortoiliac occlusive disease. In: Moore WS, ed. Vascular surgery: a comprehensive review, 6th edn. Philadelphia: WB Saunders; 2002:516.)

Although iliofemoral bypass was originally most commonly performed among patients judged unfit for transabdominal surgery, long-term patency rates have proven sufficient to allow indications to be extended to all patients with anatomically appropriate disease patterns.[51,55–57] Cumulative 5-year patency rates in the range of 80% are typical.[56] When applied for unilateral external iliac occlusion, patency rates for iliofemoral and femorofemoral bypass are equivalent in some reports,[58,59] but others demonstrate a small patency advantage for iliofemoral bypass, perhaps related to its antegrade configuration.[51,55–57,60] Other important advantages include avoidance of morbidity related to a second groin incision, and placement of the graft deep within the pelvis, where it is less susceptible to external compression or kinking.

Ilioiliac bypass

Under unusual circumstances, it may be advantageous to construct a bypass between a donor iliac and the contralateral iliac artery. This option is particularly appealing in patients who have had previous femoral artery procedures on either the donor or recipient side or in whom there is another compelling reason, such as sepsis, for avoiding one or the other groin. Another reason to avoid groin incisions might be a preference to preserve the groin for later distal bypass work. As for femorofemoral bypass, the donor iliac must be free of significant disease. The recipient-side anatomy consists of the relatively unusual pattern of common iliac occlusion with a virtually normal external iliac artery (**Fig. 9.14**). The external iliac arteries are exposed through an extraperitoneal plane via curvilinear oblique incisions parallel to and above the inguinal ligament. The prosthetic graft is tunneled through the pre-peritoneal plane via the space of Retzius, thus allowing deeper placement and better protection of the graft than is possible with femorofemoral bypass. The graft must be carefully routed past the bladder to avoid injury.

In a small series of patients undergoing ilioiliac bypass,[61] the cumulative patency rate was 96% at 4 years, demonstrating this technique to be an excellent option for selected patients with unilateral occlusive disease limited to the common iliac artery.

Femorofemoral bypass

Patients whose occlusive disease is confined to one iliac artery, with the aorta and contralateral iliac system free of hemodynamically significant disease, may be candidates for femorofemoral bypass. Typical candidates include patients in whom unilateral iliac lesions are not amenable to percutaneous therapy and in whom direct aortobifemoral bypass is judged unduly arduous or unnecessary. It is critical that the donor iliac artery is assessed before performing femorofemoral bypass. Presence of a normal femoral pulse on physical examination is a reassuring sign which should be followed by imaging using duplex ultrasound, MRA, or contrast angiography to be certain there is no anatomic lesion creating >50% diameter stenosis. If there is a lesion of questionable significance, hemodynamic assessment at preoperative angiography or early during surgery will establish its importance. Resting femoral artery pressure sampled through a needle or catheter should be no more than 10mmHg less than the

Ilioilial bypass graft

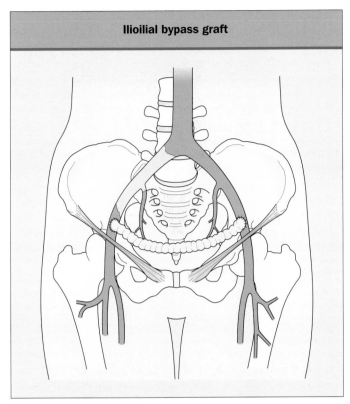

Figure 9.14 Ilioilial bypass graft. Configuration for graft crossing in pre-peritoneal plane from normal donor iliac artery to contralateral external iliac artery. (Adapted from Belkin M, Whittemore AD, Donaldson MC, Mannick JA. Aortoiliac occlusive disease. In: Moore WS, ed. Vascular surgery: a comprehensive review, 6th edn. Philadelphia:WB Saunders; 2002:516.)

Femorofemoral bypass graft

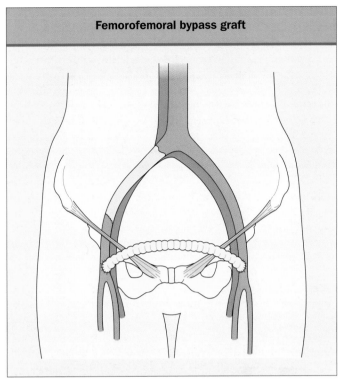

Figure 9.15 Femorofemoral bypass graft. Configuration of femorofemoral bypass with graft in deep subcutaneous plane above pubic rim in simple inverted 'U' pattern. To minimize kinking, the ends of the graft should approach the groins more parallel to the common femoral arteries than shown in figure. (Adapted from Belkin M, Whittemore AD, Donaldson MC, Mannick JA. Aortoiliac occlusive disease. In: Moore WS, ed. Vascular surgery: a comprehensive review, 6th edn. Philadelphia:WB Saunders; 2002:516.)

simultaneous pressure measured via a catheter in the radial artery or via a brachial cuff. The most precise assessment is obtained by advancing a catheter retrograde into the abdominal aorta and measuring pressure continuously as the catheter is pulled back through the lesion in question. Any pressure gradient is abnormal under these circumstances, and equivocal findings can be clarified by use of reactive hyperemia after thigh cuff occlusion or more readily by intra-arterial injection of a vasodilator such as papaverine. A 15% or greater drop in the femoral pressure with these maneuvers is consistent with the presence of signifi-cant inflow disease.[62] If a hemodynamically significant focal lesion is identified, it can be corrected by balloon angioplasty or stent. Inflow thus corrected has been found to be reliable when used for femorofemoral and femorodistal grafts.[50,51]

Femorofemoral bypass is particularly applicable to high-risk patients as it can be performed under local or regional anesthesia. The lower abdomen and upper thighs should be included in the sterile field to allow access to the external iliac arteries as well as the superficial and deep femoral arteries. Both common femoral arteries are exposed through longitudinal groin incisions. The incisions are connected via a subcutaneous suprapubic tunnel created by blunt dissection just anterior to the deep fascia. A gentle inverted U configuration is constructed well above the pubic rim to avoid compression (**Fig. 9.15**). The ends of the graft should approach the anastomotic regions parallel to the femoral arteries, with the arterotomies usually angled

obliquely toward the profunda femoral artery, in order to avoid kinking of the graft and to facilitate profundaplasty if necessary. Dacron and PTFE are equally suitable graft materials, usually in the 8mm diameter. Care must be taken to close the wounds without residual dead space, but to accommodate the graft as it transits from the deep tissue under the femoral sheath into the subcutaneous plane.

Reported primary patency rates of femorofemoral bypass are highly variable and range from 50% to 90% at 5 years, perhaps reflecting differences in patient selection criteria.[63] For example, under ideal circumstances with virtually normal iliofemoral artery inflow and patent superficial femoral artery outflow, primary patency may exceed 90%, compared with 50% when the superficial femoral artery is occluded. With close surveillance, reported secondary patency rates may exceed 90% at 4 years.[64] In patients with IC who have a patent superficial femoral artery, femorofemoral bypass patency rates can be expected to be similar to those for aortobifemoral bypass.[47] Hemodynamically, addition of the contralateral lower extremity to the runoff below the donor iliac artery results in increased volume and velocity of blood flow through the donor iliac system. Frequently, this results in significant dilatation of the donor iliac artery over time.[65] If the donor iliac artery is hemodynamically normal, it is capable of providing adequate flow to both limbs without creating a 'steal' phenomenon, which becomes a clinically important issue only if the donor iliac is stenotic.[66]

SURGICAL TREATMENT FOR FEMOROPOPLITEAL OCCLUSIVE DISEASE

Infrainguinal revascularization for IC typically addresses disease in the superficial femoral and popliteal arteries, with minimal involvement of the infrapopliteal runoff vessels. A distinct minority of patients with claudication have no satisfactory distal bypass target in the popliteal artery. Generally, their symptoms are severe and there may be reduction in the ABI to values of less than 0.4 and physical findings such as dependent rubor. Under such circumstances, bypass to tibial arteries is appropriate, and reported results are comparable to those obtained with more proximal infrainguinal targets.[67,68] Surgical intervention for IC is justified in appropriate low-risk individuals with limiting symptoms in light of low surgical operative mortality, excellent long-term palliation of symptoms, and low risk of late limb loss.

Femoropopliteal bypass

Femoropopliteal bypass is the most common surgical procedure performed for patients with IC caused by infrainguinal occlusive disease. Though controversy exists on whether to use autogenous saphenous vein or prosthetic material at the initial operation, most data support adherence to the basic principle that the procedure with the best expected long-term patency should be performed first. Above all, surgery to enhance function among patients with IC must strive to provide the least morbid and most durable procedure. Thus, prosthetic conduits with inferior durability compared with autogenous saphenous vein should be used infrequently. The most convenient distal target is the above-knee popliteal artery, but the below-knee popliteal should be used if there is any disease at all in the mid-popliteal artery, since progression of such disease will likely shorten durability of the graft. If autogenous vein is present but insufficient to reach the distal popliteal artery in cases with mild mid-popliteal artery plaque, a proximal popliteal anastomosis using vein is usually preferable to a distal anastomosis using prosthetic material.

Exposure of the common femoral artery and its branches is obtained through a standard longitudinal groin incision. The above-knee popliteal artery is exposed through a distal medial thigh incision with posterior retraction of the sartorius muscle. If the ipsilateral saphenous vein is being used as a conduit, the incision is placed to accommodate exposure of both vein and artery without creating large tissue flaps. Care is taken to avoid injury to the saphenous nerve, which exits the adductor canal into the subcutaneous plane adjacent to the saphenous vein just above the femoral condyle. The deep tissues are incised distal to the insertion of the adductor tendon for exposure of the popliteal space. The popliteal artery is identified exiting the adductor canal posterior to the femur, where it is dissected free from its surrounding veins at a location suitable for clamping and anastomosis.

The below-knee popliteal is exposed through a medial calf incision 1–2cm posterior and parallel to the edge of the tibia, extending proximally to the lower edge of the medial femoral condyle. If the greater saphenous vein is being used, the incision should be made directly over the vein in order to facilitate safe mobilization. The deep fascia is incised with care to avoid the overlying saphenous nerve, and the plane between the soleus muscle and the medial head of the gastrocnemius is developed bluntly, retracting the gastrocnemius posteriorly. With the popliteal space thus exposed, the artery is easily dissected free from the two adjacent veins.

Appropriate tunnels are created between the groin and distal incisions prior to systemic heparinization. Autogenous reversed or non-reversed grafts may be placed in the saphenous harvest bed without tunneling, as would be the case for veins left *in situ*. A sub-sartorial tunnel is also commonly used for vein grafts, and is preferable for prosthetic grafts in order to reduce the risk of graft infection. When grafts are extended to the below-knee popliteal artery, it is usually best to tunnel through the anatomic popliteal space between the two heads of the gastrocnemius muscle to avoid graft kinking or compression. This precaution is particularly useful for in-situ veins which would be unduly vulnerable to angulation as they were directed into the distal popliteal space if they were not mobilized to the distal thigh level to allow for anatomic tunneling.

Utilization of reversed greater saphenous vein, first reported by Kunlin in 1949,[69] solves the valve problem and eliminates the need for intraluminal manipulation, thus potentially minimizing overall trauma to the vein during preparation. To realize this advantage, exposure to warm ischemia time must be minimized during obligatory transfer of the vein from its bed, gentle flushing and dilation using culture medium, heparin/papavarine solution or heparinized blood, and reimplantation into the arterial system. The vein can be harvested through short longitudinal skin incisions with preservation of intervening cutaneous bridges, leaving it in its bed after ligation and division of side branches until full arterial dissection is complete. Veins with diameter smaller than 3.5mm after gentle inflation may not be sufficiently large to provide durable relief of claudication. Proximal and distal anastomoses are constructed with 5-0 or 6-0 monofilament suture. It is generally easier to perform the distal anastomosis first in order to facilitate exposure during the deeper portion of the procedure, passing the graft through the tunnel to the groin with care to avoid twisting and kinking. Size mismatch between the smaller distal end of the vein and a diseased and thickened common femoral artery may result in stenosis at the proximal graft anastomosis. This problem can be easily overcome by first creating a patch angioplasty of the femoral artery and sewing the vein graft into the patch (**Fig. 9.16**).

Utilization of in-situ saphenous vein grafting, first described by Hall[70] and perfected by Leather and colleagues,[71,72] offers the theoretical advantage of better size match between artery and vein both proximally and distally and potential for minimizing trauma to the vein related to the harvest process necessary for reversed and non-reversed vein methods. In exchange, there is potential for injury of the vein or retention of valve leaflets during valvulotomy, a technical requirement with a short but significant learning curve. When the vein is exposed over its entire length to allow ligation of branches and to guide valvulotomy using the modified Mills valvulotome, there may be a significant incidence of wound complications, reported as high as 44–77%.[73,74] Newer techniques with endoscopically guided valvulotomy and branch coil occlusion, or with valvulotomes which can be used 'blind' without direct visualization, have resulted in a reduction in wound complications.[75–78] The bypass is constructed by transecting the vein at the saphenofemoral junction and transposing the vein to the femoral artery in an end-to-side proximal anastomosis (**Fig. 9.17**). Arterial flow is

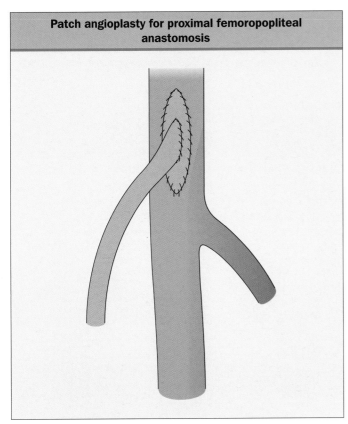

Patch angioplasty for proximal femoropopliteal anastomosis

Figure 9.16 Patch angioplasty for proximal femoropopliteal anastomosis. Patch angioplasty may be helpful in avoiding stenosis when constructing an anastomosis between a small-caliber graft and a heavily diseased artery with a thick anterior wall.

Once the femoropopliteal bypass is complete, intraoperative technical assessment is highly recommended. Completion arteriography is easily performed via hand injection of 20–25mL of iodinated contrast solution into the proximal graft, with or without inflow occlusion. A single injection is usually adequate to visualize the above-knee and below-knee popliteal anastomotic regions. If full runoff images are desired, a second injection may be performed with the film positioned lower on the leg. Arteriography may be facilitated by fluoroscopic imaging using digital C-arm, with injection of 5–10mL boluses of contrast solution during fluoroscopy and timed capture of the optimal image to store, review, magnify, and print. Angioscopy has been used to good advantage to better define endoluminal pathology when the vein is suspect. Operative duplex ultrasound to scrutinize the entire length of the graft has proved a valuable addition for detection of graft abnormalities and technical imperfections at the anastomoses. Immediate correction of defects that have a peak systolic flow velocity >180cm/s or a peak systolic flow velocity ratio >2.4, comparing velocity within the lesion with that in the normal proximal vein graft, has been proposed to reduce early graft failure and need for subsequent revision.[83]

Graft thrombosis occurs within 30 days of surgery in 2–7% of procedures, most often due to technical causes.[84] Wound complications occur because of flap necrosis related to vein harvesting; fat necrosis caused by desiccation or tight subcutaneous closure; lymphocele and lymph fistula due to lymphatic disruption; drainage from edema related to early reperfusion and lymphatic insufficiency;[85] and overt infection. Leg elevation and moderate elastic compression help alleviate the swelling, which typically subsides significantly over several weeks. A program of postoperative graft surveillance including use of duplex ultrasound and the ABI is an important strategy for prolonging graft durability.[86] Up to 25% of autogenous grafts develop areas of significant stenosis related to fibrous intimal hyperplasia during the first 2 years of follow-up. If detected, correction of these lesions with minor surgical revision or percutaneous methods before graft thrombosis significantly enhances late patency. Since most lesions occur early, routine surveillance at 3-month intervals has been suggested for the first postoperative year, with 6-monthly reviews thereafter. Frequent surveillance has not been shown to be efficacious in improving patency of prosthetic grafts, which are more susceptible to sudden thrombosis without anatomic precursor lesions.

Virtually all studies to date have documented the superiority of autogenous vein over prosthetic conduit for infrainguinal revascularization. When applied to patients with IC, primary patency rates for reversed greater saphenous vein have been reported to be between 47% and 88% at 5 years.[87–89] Results from one center revealed a higher 5-year primary patency rate of 81% for the in-situ technique[90] compared with 71% for veins used in the non-reversed configuration[79] among claudicators. The 5-year primary patency rate for above-knee femoropopliteal PTFE bypass is 60–75%, and for below-knee grafts, 40–65%, among claudicators.[91–94] Dacron has performed as well as PTFE in the above-knee position for claudication in prospective randomized trials comparing the two prosthetics.[95–97] Several comparative studies in the literature have found HUV to be superior to PTFE in terms of patency.[98,99]

In spite of inferior long-term efficacy, a strategy of preferential above-knee femoropopliteal bypass using prosthetic grafts has

established to the first competent venous valve. If the modified Mills valvulotome is being used, the instrument is introduced through transected side branches and the distal end of the vein to allow precise lysis of the valve leaflets. The distal vein is flushed to assure adequacy of inflow, then passed through the popliteal tunnel as appropriate, and the distal anastomosis is constructed with 5-0 or 6-0 monofilament suture.

The in-situ advantage of better size matching can be maintained by using ipsilateral or contralateral vein in non-reversed fashion after lysis of valves.[79] The vein is harvested and infused with heparinized saline solution introduced into the proximal end of the vein in order to deploy the valve leaflets in sequence. While infusing gently, the modified Mills valvulotome is introduced through a side branch or the distal end of the vein for valve lysis. Alternatively, valve lysis can be performed in a similar fashion after instituting graft inflow following completion of the proximal anastomosis.

Prosthetic materials including Dacron, human umbilical vein (HUV), and PTFE are available off the shelf and may be preferred because of ease and rapidity of insertion in the proximal femoropopliteal position. Given the increased technical demand in handling HUV, as well as a propensity for late dilatation and aneurysm formation,[80–82] PTFE and Dacron are currently more commonly chosen by most surgeons when suitable vein is unavailable. The procedure is simplified by the absence of vein harvest and preparation, with tunneling usually in the sub-sartorial or anatomic plane to avoid potential graft infection in the event of wound complications.

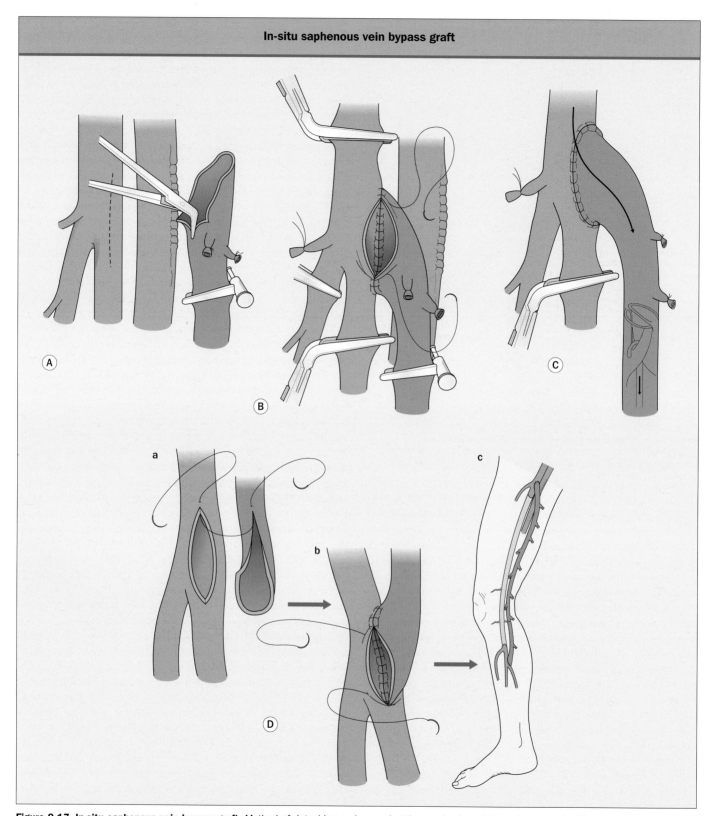

In-situ saphenous vein bypass graft

Figure 9.17 In-situ saphenous vein bypass graft. Method of detaching and preparing the proximal greater saphenous vein (A) and transposing it end-to-side from the common femoral vein to the femoral artery (B), followed by lysis of valve leaflets using a retrograde Mills valvulotome (C) and then completion of the distal anastomosis to the target artery after large branches are ligated (D). (Adapted from Whittemore AD, Belkin MB. Infrainguinal bypass. In: Rutherford RB, ed. Vascular surgery, 5th edn. Philadelphia:WB Saunders; 2000:1005.)

been favored by some surgeons for suitable patients with IC, in order to preserve the vein for future cardiac or tibial revascularization. In fact, less than 10% of patients who have undergone infrainguinal bypass require the vein for cardiac use within 5 years[100,101] and this number will undoubtedly remain small in the era of percutaneous transluminal coronary angioplasty and increased use of internal mammary and radial arteries as conduits. In the event of prosthetic occlusion, disobliteration is usually relatively easy, in distinction to vein occlusion, in which case a new bypass is often required. On the other hand, it has long been observed that occlusion of prosthetic grafts appears to result in more severe ischemia than occlusion of vein grafts. Consequently, prosthetic occlusion in patients initially operated upon for claudication may precipitate limb-threatening ischemia. In a recent report,[102] a 28% incidence of emergent revascularization occurred in patients within 4 years of PTFE femoropopliteal bypass compared with 3% in patients after bypass with autogenous greater saphenous vein. A significantly higher amputation rate of 44% was noted in the PTFE group compared with 19% in those with saphenous vein. Though new prosthetics may have improved long-term efficacy,[103] use of autogenous vein is still most appropriate for bypass among patients with IC.

Superficial femoral endarterectomy

Endarterectomy of the femoropopliteal segment was first described by Dos Santos in 1947,[104] just 2 years before Kunlin reported his experience with reversed greater saphenous vein for femoropopliteal bypass. The ensuing debate over which modality was optimal was resolved over subsequent years when it became clear that bypass was both safer and more effective than endarterectomy in most situations. Nonetheless, isolated common femoral or superficial femoral artery disease can be managed by endarterectomy with durable results in selected patients not amenable to percutaneous therapy.

Occlusive disease localized to the region of the adductor tendon at the distal end of Hunter's canal is common among patients with claudication. It is approached through a distal thigh incision as described for above-knee bypass, but with exposure of the superficial femoral artery above the tendon insertion, taking the tendon down if the disease is directly under it. If the lesion is less than 3cm in length, it can be managed by an open technique using a longitudinal arteriotomy through the disease to expose normal artery proximally and distally. Atheromatous media and intima are separated from the adventitia, and the lesion gently dissected to more normal artery. The specimen is transected sharply at both ends, and a mattress suture generally used to tack the distal intima to prevent distal dissection. The arteriotomy is then closed with a patch angioplasty, preferably using autogenous vein.

For lesions longer than 3cm, the semi-closed technique is appropriate, using either transverse or longitudinal arterotomies at the proximal and distal ends of the lesion to avoid the need for closure by long patch angioplasty. The distal end of the plaque is divided and the plaque is dissected in the endarterectomy plane in a retrograde fashion through the unopened vessel, using an endarterectomy spatula, hand-held loop dissector,[105] or air-powered oscillating loop.[106] If the lesion is particularly long, one or two counterincisions in the artery may be necessary. The dissection continues to the proximal arteriotomy, where the plaque is divided and extracted. The distal end of the plaque

may require tacking sutures. The arteriotomies are closed primarily if transverse, and with short patch angioplasty if longitudinal (**Fig. 9.18**).

Remote endarterectomy of long occlusive lesions in the superficial femoral artery associated with reconstitution of a normal proximal popliteal vessel can be performed with minimal surgery using a ring cutter designed by Moll, under fluoroscopic guidance.[107,108] After operative exposure of the arteries in the groin, the proximal superficial femoral artery is opened and the ring cutter advanced distally in the endarterectomy plane. When the device has reached the end of the lesion, the cutter divides the plaque and the specimen is removed. A guidewire is then threaded into the distal artery beyond the incised plaque, and a short stent deployed to tack the endpoint down.

Complications of all endarterectomy techniques include acute occlusion and early restenosis due to residual plaque, flaps, and reactive fibrosis. These complications are least likely after treatment of short lesions and more likely after long-segment endarterectomy. Long-term results are best for short lesions and therefore use of this technique for long-segment lesions among claudicators is not recommended under most circumstances. As for infrainguinal bypass, regular postoperative surveillance using duplex ultrasound is a critical strategy for detection of recurrent lesions which may be amenable to correction by minimal repeat surgery or percutaneous methods. A surveillance strategy is particularly important following long-segment endarterectomy of the superficial femoral artery. For example, using the remote ring-cutter technique,[107] a primary patency rate of 60% at 13 months was improved to assisted-primary patency of 83% after reintervention for stenosis in 25% of patients, using transluminal angioplasty.[108] Others[109] experienced less favorable results with a similar surveillance protocol after ring cutter use, however, with a 1-year primary patency rate of only 26%. Patency rates following long-segment endarterectomy, regardless of techniques, are generally inferior to reported results with autologous vein bypass.

Profundaplasty

Profundaplasty is most commonly used as an adjunct to an inflow procedure such as an aortobifemoral, axillofemoral, or femorofemoral bypass. Leeds and Gilfillan[110] and Morris and colleagues[111] were among the first to note that an increase in blood flow through the profunda femoris artery could significantly improve distal perfusion in the presence of an occluded superficial femoral artery, prompting interest in primary profundaplasty as a treatment option in selected patients.[112] Appropriate candidates include patients with disabling claudication and critical ischemia who have an occluded superficial femoral artery, profunda origin stenosis, and good arteriographic evidence of collaterals to the popliteal or tibial arteries.[113] Because few patients with IC meet these anatomic criteria and cannot undergo bypass or percutaneous therapy, use of isolated profundaplasty for claudication is increasingly rare.

The profunda femoris artery is exposed by dissecting out the common femoral artery and following it to the femoral bifurcation. The proximal superficial femoral artery is elevated on a tape, facilitating dissection along the anterior surface of the profunda until normal vessel is encountered, generally at the first major branch point 2–3 cm distal to the origin. A branch of the lateral circumflex femoral vein may require ligation to afford

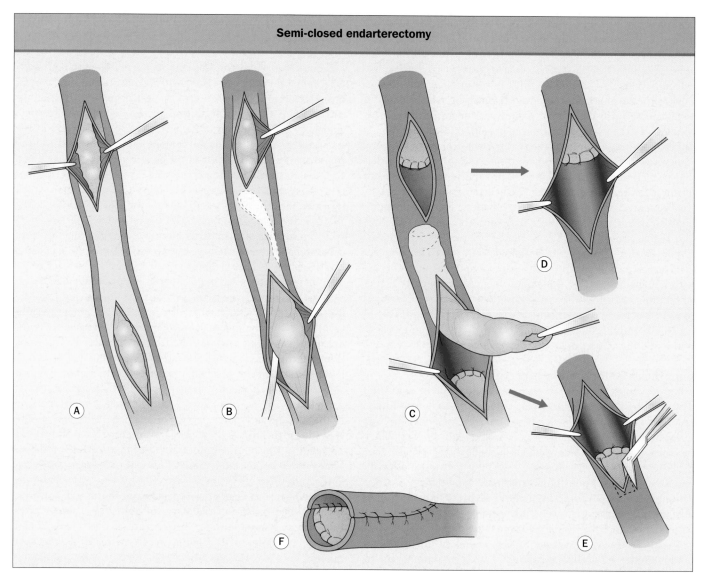

Semi-closed endarterectomy

Figure 9.18 Semi-closed endarterectomy. Method of performing semi-closed endarterectomy for lesions >3 cm in length using a spatula introduced through longitudinal arterotomies (A,B). Transverse arterotomy may be used in large vessels if visualization is adequate for precise control of the distal end of the plaque. Plaque is removed (C) and edges tacked down if necessary (D,E), with closure by patch in most cases (F). (Adapted from Haimovici H. Vascular surgery: principles and techniques. New York:McGraw-Hill; 1976:294.)

full exposure and all arterial branches are looped. Fibers of the femoral nerve must be protected as they cross the more distal profunda obliquely. After systemic heparinization, the common femoral artery and previously looped branches are occluded. The arteriotomy is begun on the common femoral artery and carried into the profunda until normal vessel is reached. If an endarterectomy is deemed appropriate, it is ended distally by sharply dividing the plaque, adding a tacking stitch if necessary. Saphenous vein, endarterectomized occluded superficial femoral artery, or prosthetic material can then be used to patch the artery closed (**Fig. 9.19**).[112,114,115]

Early complications specific to profundaplasty include dissection of the distal endpoint with thrombosis, lymphatic leak, and saphenous nerve injury. Because of the more extensive groin dissection usually required, lymphocele and lymph fistula are more common than for other femoral arterial exposures. Lymphatic complications can be reduced by avoiding transection

of lymph nodes during dissection, systematic ligation of lymph-bearing tissues in the medial part of the wound, and meticulous multilayer groin closure. Saphenous neuropathy is manifest by neuralgic pain over the medial thigh, and is best avoided by minimizing use of traction, electrocautery, and dissection applied adjacent to the oblique deep fascial edge crossing the plane of exposure of the more distal profunda. Reported cumulative primary patency rates after isolated profundaplasty are 83% at 30 days, 67% at 1 year, and 49% at 3 years, with results best among patients having good tibial outflow.[113]

ADJUNCTIVE THERAPY

A comprehensive medical regimen directed at controlling atherosclerosis is an important component of effective management of patients with IC. Exercise, tobacco abstinence, and pharmacologic reduction in cholesterol and control of hypertension

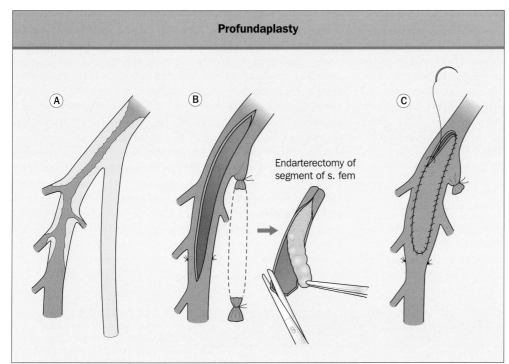

Profundaplasty

Ⓐ Ⓑ

Endarterectomy of
segment of s. fem

Ⓒ

Figure 9.19 Profundaplasty. Method of
patch angioplasty applicable to proximal
disease in profunda femoris in patients
with superficial femoral occlusion and
good collateral to distal arteries from
the profunda. Figure illustrates use of
endarterectomized superficial femoral
artery as patch; saphenous vein or
prosthetic are also applicable.
(Adapted from Towne JB, Bernhard VM.
Profundaplasty. In: Rutherford RB, ed.
Vascular surgery, 5th edn.
Philadelphia:WB Saunders;
2000:1023.)

are basic considerations. Use of adjunctive antithrombotic agents
after surgical or percutaneous interventions has emerged as an
important part of this strategy, though with due caution given
potential morbidity from hemorrhage.

Aspirin is routinely utilized prior to percutaneous therapy and
infrainguinal bypass and after aortoiliac surgery, to help diminish
platelet deposition at the site of intervention. A meta-analysis
published by the Antiplatelet Trialists' Collaboration in Britain
in 1994 analyzed over 100 000 patients in 174 randomized
trials of aspirin, as well as a small number of studies using
dipyridamole.[116] A 25% relative risk reduction in primary
myocardial infarction, stroke, and vascular occlusion was noted
among all patients, and a 21% risk reduction in those patients
with peripheral vascular disease, who were treated with
antiplatelet therapy as compared with placebo. Furthermore, a
30% reduction in the rate of occlusion was noted in coronary
artery bypass, coronary angioplasty, peripheral arterial procedures,
and hemodialysis access, at a mean of 19 months after intervention (p<0.00001). These results provide compelling support
for generalized use of aspirin, despite evidence from some
studies showing aspirin to have no significant effect on patency
of autogenous vein grafts.[117,118] Other agents found to be
effective compared with placebo include ticlopidine[119] and
clopidogrel. The Clopidogrel versus Aspirin in Patients at Risk of
Ischaemic Events (CAPRIE) trial noted an overall 8.7% relative
risk reduction of overall vascular morbidity when comparing
clopidogrel with aspirin.[16] Though more expensive than aspirin,
clopidogrel may be warranted in patients with evidence of
diffuse atherosclerosis who undergo intervention for IC.

Use of coumadin to prolong bypass graft patency has been
studied prospectively.[120] Some studies have reported improved
patency rates,[121,122] while others have shown no benefit.[123] A large
prospective randomized trial compared aspirin and high-dose

coumadin (international normalized ratio [INR] 3.0–4.5) and
found no overall graft patency advantage for either treatment.[124]
Given these data and the risk of hemorrhagic complications, oral
anticoagulation is best reserved for those few patients who
undergo surgery for IC in whom repeated failure of infrainguinal
bypass has occurred.

FUNCTIONAL OUTCOME AND COST-EFFECTIVENESS

Although surgery can successfully correct significant disease in
the aortoiliac and femoropopliteal segments of patients with IC,
the ultimate goal of therapy remains improvement of functional
impairment. Data support the value of surgery in this regard,
with reported improvement in resting ankle–brachial indices,
treadmill walking time, and self-reported walking ability 6 weeks
postoperatively.[125] Further data suggest that optimal functional
results occur when revascularization is restricted to patients less
than 70 years of age in whom there is no diabetes and in whom
restoration of a normal postoperative ABI could be anticipated.[126]

An important study used morbidity, mortality, graft patency,
and cost data collected from the literature to outline decision
and cost-effectiveness algorithms for choice of management
options for femoropopliteal disease.[127] Data on 4800 percutaneous
angioplasty patients and 4511 bypass patients were reviewed.
An analytical decision model was developed to examine the
choice between bypass surgery and angioplasty for lesions that
were amenable to either procedure. For example, results revealed
that for a typical 65-year-old man with disabling claudication
and a focal femoropopliteal stenosis or occlusion, a strategy
using initial angioplasty increased quality-adjusted life years
(QALY) and resulted in decreased lifetime expenditures
compared with strategies using initial bypass surgery. In fact,

under any circumstance when it could be predicted that the 5-year patency rate after angioplasty would likely exceed 30%, angioplasty emerged as the preferred initial intervention. Another recent study evaluated the cost-effectiveness of revascularization versus exercise therapy by meta-analysis of reports in the literature.[128] The analysis found that the expected gain in effectiveness achieved with bypass surgery for IC was small compared with the costs. Furthermore angioplasty, when feasible, was more effective than exercise alone and fell within the generally accepted range of cost-effectiveness.

SUMMARY

Although most patients with IC do not require revascularization, endovascular and surgical reconstruction can usually be completed successfully with low morbidity and mortality. Surgery should be offered to treat severe symptoms only after other forms of

management have failed or been rejected for appropriate reasons. If surgery is undertaken, it should have a high benefit-to-risk ratio with realistic expectations regarding functional outcome goals. One must take into account the natural history data regarding expected patient survival and limb amputation rates among claudicants managed without surgery.[129] Procedural morbidity and mortality must be carefully considered for each patient within the context of the surgeon's own institution, despite excellent statistics in the literature such as those from the Swedish Vascular Registry reporting a combined mortality and amputation rate of 2.2% for aortofemoral reconstruction and 1.4% for femoropopliteal reconstruction.[130] Once intervention has been chosen, surgery should be used in conjunction with catheter-based techniques, to achieve the best possible result for least possible cost and morbidity. With patency rates generally 20% or higher compared with percutaneous treatment for most lesions, surgical intervention remains an important and durable option for selected patients suffering from IC (**Figs 9.20 & 9.21**).

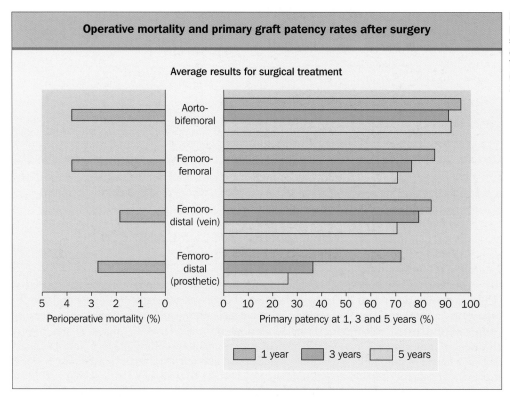

Figure 9.20 Operative mortality and primary graft patency rates after surgery. (Derived with permission from data assembled and reported by the TransAtlantic Inter-Society Consensus (TASC) Group. J Vasc Surg (Suppl) 2000;31:S234.)

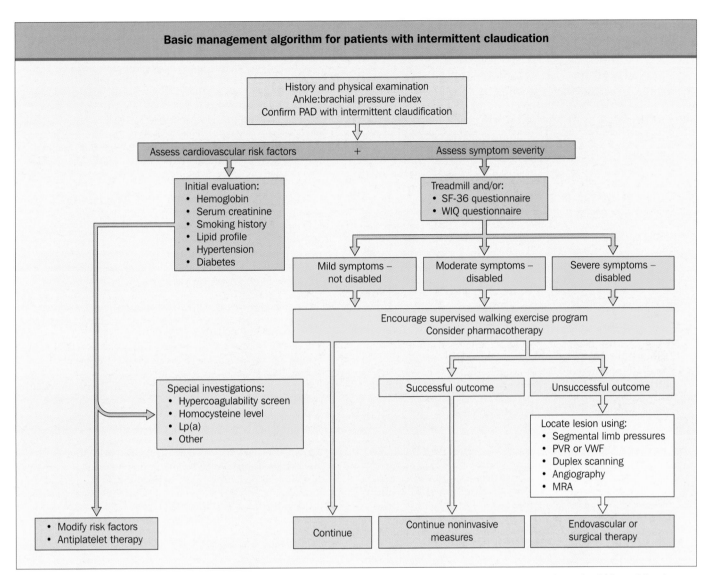

Figure 9.21 Basic management algorithm for patients with intermittent claudication. MRA, magnetic resonance angiography; PAD, peripheral arterial disease; PVR, pulse volume recording; SF-36, Medical Outcomes Short Form 36 Questionnaire; VWF, velocity waveform analysis; WIQ, Walking Impairment Questionnaire. (Adapted with permission from Report of the TransAtlantic Inter-Society Consensus (TASC) Group. J Vasc Surg (Suppl) 2000;31:S121.)

REFERENCES

1. Hiatt WR, Hoag S, Hamman RF. Effect of diagnostic criteria on the prevalence of peripheral arterial disease. The San Luis Valley Diabetes Study. Circulation 1995;91:1472–9.
2. Hughson WG, Mann JI, Garrod A. Intermittent claudication: prevalence and risk factors. BMJ 1978;1:1379–81.
3. Reid DD, Brett GZ, Hamilton PJ, et al. Cardiorespiratory disease and diabetes among middle-aged male Civil Servants. A study of screening and intervention. Lancet 1974;1:469–73.
4. Stoffers HE, Rinkens PE, Kester AD, et al. The prevalence of asymptomatic and unrecognized peripheral arterial occlusive disease. Int J Epidemiol 1996;25:282–90.
5. Criqui MH, Langer RD, Fronek A, et al. Mortality over a period of 10 years in patients with peripheral arterial disease. N Engl J Med 1992; 326:381–6.
6. Management of peripheral arterial disease (PAD). TransAtlantic Inter-Society Consensus (TASC). Eur J Vasc Endovasc Surg 2000;19(Suppl A):Si–xxviii, S1–250.
7. Hertzer NR, Beven EG, Young JR, et al. Coronary artery disease in peripheral vascular patients. A classification of 1000 coronary angiograms

and results of surgical management. Ann Surg 1984;199:223–33.
8. Smith I, Franks PJ, Greenhalgh RM, et al. The influence of smoking cessation and hypertriglyceridaemia on the progression of peripheral arterial disease and the onset of critical ischaemia. Eur J Vasc Endovasc Surg 1996;11:402–8.
9. Birkenstock WE, Louw JH, Terblanche J, et al. Smoking and other factors affecting the conservative management of peripheral vascular disease. S Afr Med J 1975;49:1129–32.
10. Hirsch AT, Treat-Jacobson D, Lando HA, et al. The role of tobacco cessation, antiplatelet and lipid-lowering therapies in the treatment of peripheral arterial disease. Vasc Med 1997;2:243–51.
11. Quick CR, Cotton LT. The measured effect of stopping smoking on intermittent claudication. Br J Surg 1982;69(Suppl):S24–6.
12. Reichard P, Nilsson BY, Rosenqvist U. The effect of long-term intensified insulin treatment on the development of microvascular complications of diabetes mellitus. N Engl J Med 1993;329:304–9.
13. Gardner AW, Poehlman ET. Exercise rehabilitation programs for the treatment of claudication pain. A meta-analysis. JAMA 1995;274: 975–80.

14. Dawson DL, Cutler BS, Hiatt WR, et al. A comparison of cilostazol and pentoxifylline for treating intermittent claudication. Am J Med 2000;109:523–30.

15. Money SR, Herd JA, Isaacsohl JL, et al. Effect of cilostazol on walking distances in patients with intermittent claudication caused by peripheral vascular disease. J Vasc Surg 1998;27:267–74; discussion 274–5.

16. CAPRIE Steering Committee. A randomised, blinded, trial of clopidogrel versus aspirin in patients at risk of ischaemic events (CAPRIE). Lancet 1996;348:1329–39.

17. McDaniel MD, Cronenwett JL. Basic data related to the natural history of intermittent claudication. Ann Vasc Surg 1989;3:273–7.

18. Brewster DC, Darling RC. Optimal methods of aortoiliac reconstruction. Surgery 1978;84:739–48.

19. Staple T. The solitary aortoiliac lesion. Surgery 1968;64:569.

20. Moore W, Cafferata HT, Hall AD, Blaisdell FW. In defense of grafts across the inguinal ligament. Ann Surg 1968;168:207.

21. Mozersky DJ, Sumner DS, Strandness DE. Long-term results of reconstructive aortoiliac surgery. Am J Surg 1972;123:503–9.

22. Ascher E, Mazzariol F, Hingorani A, et al. The use of duplex ultrasound arterial mapping as an alternative to conventional arteriography for primary and secondary infrapopliteal bypasses. Am J Surg 1999;178: 162–5.

23. Proia RR, Walsh DB, Nelson PR, et al. Early results of infragenicular revascularization based solely on duplex arteriography. J Vasc Surg 2001;33:1165–70.

24. Walsh DB, LaBombard E. Lower extremity bypass using only duplex ultrasonography: is the time now? Semin Vasc Surg 1999;12:247–51.

25. Whittemore A, Donaldson MC, Mannick JA, et al. Aortoiliac occlusive disease. Philadelphia, PA:WB Saunders; 1998:483–94.

26. Valentine RJ, Hansen ME, Myers SI, Cherva A, Clagett GP. The influence of sex and aortic size on late patency after aortofemoral revascularization in young adults. J Vasc Surg 1995;21:296–305; discussion 305–6.

27. Crawford ES, Bomberger RA, Glaeser DH, Saleh SA, Russell WL. Aortoiliac occlusive disease: factors influencing survival and function following reconstructive operation over a twenty-five-year period. Surgery 1981;90:1055–67.

28. Brewster DC. Current controversies in the management of aortoiliac occlusive disease. J Vasc Surg 1997;25:365–79.

29. Reed AB, Belkin M, Conte MS, Donaldson MC, Mannick JA, Whittemore AD. Aortobifemoral bypass in young adults: is it the gold standard? J Vasc Surg 2003 (in press).

30. Mikati A, Marache P, Watel A, et al. End-to-side aortoprosthetic anastomoses: long-term computed tomography assessment. Ann Vasc Surg 1990;4:584–91.

31. Rutherford RB, Jones DN, Martin MS, et al. Serial hemodynamic assessment of aortobifemoral bypass. J Vasc Surg 1986;4:428–35.

32. Ameli FM, Stein M, Aro L, et al. End-to-end versus end-to-side proximal anastomosis in aortobifemoral bypass surgery: does it matter? Can J Surg 1991;34:243–6.

33. Melliere D, Labastie J, Becquemin JP, et al. Proximal anastomosis in aortobifemoral bypass: end-to-end or end-to-side? J Cardiovasc Surg (Torino) 1990;31:77–80.

34. Robbs JV, Wylie EJ. Factors contributing to recurrent lower limb ischemia following bypass surgery for aortoiliac occlusive disease, and their management. Ann Surg 1981;193:346–52.

35. Sanders RJ, Kempczinski RF, Hammond W, DiClementi D. The significance of graft diameter. Surgery 1980;88:856–66.

36. Wylie E. Thromboendarterectomy for arteriosclerotic thrombus of major arteries. Surgery 1952;32:275–292.

37. Inahara T. Evaluation of endarterectomy for aortoiliac and aortoiliofemoral occlusive disease. Arch Surg 1975;110:1458–64.

38. van den Akker PJ, van Schilfgaarde R, Brand R, et al. Long-term results of prosthetic and non-prosthetic reconstruction for obstructive aorto-iliac disease. Eur J Vasc Surg 1992;6:53–61.

39. van den Dungen JJ, Boontje AH, Kropveld A. Unilateral iliofemoral occlusive disease: long-term results of the semi-closed endarterectomy with the ring-stripper. J Vasc Surg 1991;14:673–7.

40. Ascer E, Veith FJ, Gupta SK, et al. Comparison of axillounifemoral and axillobifemoral bypass operations. Surgery 1985;97:169–75.

41. Rutherford RB. Extra-anatomic bypass. In: Rutherford RB, ed. Vascular surgery, 5th edn. Philadelphia:WB Saunders; 2000:983.

42. Calligaro KD, Veith FJ, Gupta SK, et al. Unsuspected inflow disease in candidates for axillofemoral bypass operations: a prospective study. J Vasc Surg 1990;11:832–7.

43. Mannick JA, Williams LE, Nabseth DC. The late results of axillofemoral grafts. Surgery 1970;68:1038–43.

44. Taylor LM Jr, Park TC, Edwards JM, et al. Acute disruption of polytetrafluoroethylene grafts adjacent to axillary anastomoses: a complication of axillofemoral grafting. J Vasc Surg 1994;20:520–6; discussion 526–8.

45. Rutherford RB, Patt A, Pearce WH. Extra-anatomic bypass: a closer view. J Vasc Surg 1987;6:437–46.

46. el-Massry S, Saad E, Sauvage LR, et al. Axillofemoral bypass with externally supported, knitted Dacron grafts: a follow-up through twelve years. J Vasc Surg 1993;17:107–14; discussion 114–5.

47. Piotrowski JJ, Pearce WH, Jones DN, et al. Aortobifemoral bypass: the operation of choice for unilateral iliac occlusion? J Vasc Surg 1988;8:211–8.

48. Brener BJ, Brief DK, Alpert J. Femorofemoral bypass: a twenty-five year experience. In: Long-term results in vascular surgery. Norwalk, CT: Appleton & Lange; 1993:385–393.

49. Kalman PG. Unilateral retroperitoneal iliofemoral bypass. In: Ernst CB, Stanley JC, eds. Current therapy in vascular surgery, 4th edn. St Louis: Mosby; 2001:405–6.

50. Brewster DC, Cambria RP, Darling RC, et al. Long-term results of combined iliac balloon angioplasty and distal surgical revascularization. Ann Surg 1989;210:324–30; discussion 331.

51. Kalman PG, Hosang M, Johnston KW, Walker PM. Unilateral iliac disease: the role of iliofemoral bypass. J Vasc Surg 1987;6:139–43.

52. Taylor LM Jr, Freimanis IE, Edwards JM, Porter JM. Extraperitoneal iliac endarterectomy in the treatment of multilevel lower extremity arterial occlusive disease. Am J Surg 1986;152:34–9.

53. Vitale GF, Inahara T. Extraperitoneal endarterectomy for iliofemoral occlusive disease. J Vasc Surg 1990;12:409–13; discussion 414–5.

54. Brewster DC, Veith FJ. Combined aortoiliac and femoropopliteal occlusive disease. In: Veith FJ, Hobson RW 2nd, Williams RA, eds. Vascular surgery: principles and practice, 2nd edn. New York:McGraw-Hill; 1994:459–72.

55. Cham C, Myers KA, Scott DF, et al. Extraperitoneal unilateral iliac artery bypass for chronic lower limb ischaemia. Aust NZ J Surg 1988; 58:859–63.

56. Darling RC 3rd, Leather RP, Chang BB, et al. Is the iliac artery a suitable inflow conduit for iliofemoral occlusive disease: an analysis of 514 aortoiliac reconstructions. J Vasc Surg 1993;17:15–9; discussion 19–22.

57. Kalman PG, Hosang M, Johnston KW, Walker PM. The current role for femorofemoral bypass. J Vasc Surg 1987;6:71–6.

58. Lorenzi G, Domanin M, Costanini A, et al. Role of bypass, endarterectomy, extra-anatomic bypass and endovascular surgery in unilateral iliac occlusive disease: a review of 1257 cases. Cardiovasc Surg 1994;2:370–3.

59. Hanafy M, McLoughlin GA. Comparison of iliofemoral and femorofemoral crossover bypass in the treatment of unilateral iliac arterial occlusive disease. Br J Surg 1991;78:1001–2.

60. Sidawy AN, Menzoian JO, Cantelmo NL, LoGerfo FW. Retroperitoneal inflow procedures for iliac occlusive vascular disease. Arch Surg 1985; 120:794–6.

61. Couch NP, Clowes AW, Whittemore AD, et al. The iliac-origin arterial graft: a useful alternative for iliac occlusive disease. Surgery 1985;97:83–7.

62. Flanigan DP, Ryan TJ, Williams LR, et al. Aortofemoral or femoropopliteal revascularization? A prospective evaluation of the papaverine test. J Vasc Surg 1984;1:215–23.

63. Criado E, Farber MA. Femorofemoral bypass: appropriate application based on factors affecting outcome. Semin Vasc Surg 1997;10:34–41.

64. Ricco JB. Unilateral iliac artery occlusive disease: a randomized multicenter trial examining direct revascularization versus crossover bypass.

Association Universitaire de Recherche en Chirurgie. Ann Vasc Surg 1992;6:209–19.

65. da Gama AD. The fate of the donor artery in extraanatomic revascularization. J Vasc Surg 1988;8:106–11.

66. Donor limb vascular events following femoro-femoral bypass surgery. A Veterans Affairs Cooperative Study. Arch Surg 1991;126:681–5; discussion 685–6.

67. Conte MS, Belkin M, Donaldson MC, et al. Femorotibial bypass for claudication: do results justify an aggressive approach? J Vasc Surg 1995;21:873–80; discussion 880–1.

68. Byrne J, Darling RC 3rd, Chang BB, et al. Infrainguinal arterial reconstruction for claudication: is it worth the risk? An analysis of 409 procedures. J Vasc Surg 1999;29:259–67; discussion 267–9.

69. Kunlin J. Le traitement de l'arterite obliterante par le greffe veineuse. Arch Mal Coeur Vaiss 1949;42:371.

70. Hall KV. The great saphenous vein used "in situ" as an arterial shunt after extirpation of vein valves. Surgery 1962;51:492.

71. Leather RP, Powers SR, Karmody AM. A reappraisal of the in situ saphenous vein arterial bypass: its use in limb salvage. Surgery 1979; 86:453–61.

72. Leather RP, Shah DM, Chang BB, Kaufman JL. Resurrection of the in situ saphenous vein bypass. 1000 cases later. Ann Surg 1988;208: 435–42.

73. Reifsnyder T, Bandyk D, Seabrook G, et al. Wound complications of the in situ saphenous vein bypass technique. J Vasc Surg 1992;15: 843–8; discussion 848–50.

74. Dijk LCV, van Urk H, du Bois NA, et al. A new "closed" in situ vein bypass technique results in a reduced wound complication rate. Eur J Endovasc Surg 1995;10:162–7.

75. Rosenthal D, Matsuura JH, Clark MD. Current developments in endovascular in situ bypass grafting. Ann Vasc Surg 1999;13:637–40.

76. Rosenthal D, Herring MB, O'Donovan TG, et al. Endovascular infrainguinal in situ saphenous vein bypass: a multicenter preliminary report. J Vasc Surg 1992;16:453–8.

77. Rosenthal D, Dickson C, Rodriguez FJ, et al. Infrainguinal endovascular in situ saphenous vein bypass: ongoing results. J Vasc Surg 1994;20:389–94; discussion 394–5.

78. Gangadharan SP, Reed AB, Chew DK, et al. Initial experience with minimally invasive in situ bypass procedure with blind valvulotomy. J Vasc Surg 2002;35:1100–6.

79. Belkin M, Knox J, Donaldson MC, et al. Infrainguinal arterial reconstruction with nonreversed greater saphenous vein. J Vasc Surg 1996;24:957–62.

80. Dardik H. The use of glutaraldehyde-stabilized umbilical vein for lower extremity reconstruction. In: Greehalgh RM, ed. Vascular and endovascular surgical techniques: an atlas, 3rd edn. London:WB Saunders; 1994:373–87.

81. Dardik H, Miller N, Dardik A, et al. A decade of experience with the glutaraldehyde-tanned human umbilical cord vein graft for revascularization of the lower limb. J Vasc Surg 1988;7:336–46.

82. Hasson JE, Newton WD, Waltman AC, et al. Mural degeneration in the glutaraldehyde-tanned umbilical vein graft: incidence and implications. J Vasc Surg 1986;4:243–50.

83. Bandyk DF, Johnson BL, Gupta AK, Esses GE. Nature and management of duplex abnormalities encountered during infrainguinal vein bypass grafting. J Vasc Surg 1996;24:430–6; discussion 437–8.

84. Donaldson MC, Mannick JA, Whittemore AD. Causes of primary graft failure after in situ saphenous vein bypass grafting. J Vasc Surg 1992;15:113–8; discussion 118–20.

85. AbuRahma AF, Woodruff BA, Lucente FC. Edema after femoropopliteal bypass surgery: lymphatic and venous theories of causation. J Vasc Surg 1990;11:461–7.

86. Bandyk DF, Schmitt DD, Seabrook GR, et al. Monitoring functional patency of in situ saphenous vein bypasses: the impact of a surveillance protocol and elective revision. J Vasc Surg 1989;9:286–96.

87. Taylor LM Jr, Edwards JM, Porter JM. Present status of reversed vein bypass grafting: five-year results of a modern series. J Vasc Surg 1990;11:193–205; discussion 205–6.

88. Berkowitz HD, Greenstein SM. Improved patency in reversed femoral-

infrapopliteal autogenous vein grafts by early detection and treatment of the failing graft. J Vasc Surg 1987;5:755–61.

89. Donaldson MC, Mannick JA. Femoropopliteal bypass grafting for intermittent claudication: is pessimism warranted? Arch Surg 1980; 115:724–7.

90. Donaldson MC, Mannick JA, Whittemore AD. Femoral-distal bypass with in situ greater saphenous vein. Long-term results using the Mills valvulotome. Ann Surg 1991;213:457–64; discussion 464–5.

91. Veith FJ, Gupta SK, Ascer E, et al. Six-year prospective multicenter randomized comparison of autologous saphenous vein and expanded polytetrafluoroethylene grafts in infrainguinal arterial reconstructions. J Vasc Surg 1986;3:104–14.

92. Whittemore AD, Kent KC, Donaldson MC, et al. What is the proper role of polytetrafluoroethylene grafts in infrainguinal reconstruction? J Vasc Surg 1989;10:299–305.

93. Hunink MG, Wong JB, Donaldson MC, et al. Patency results of percutaneous and surgical revascularization for femoropopliteal arterial disease. Med Decis Making 1994;14:71–81.

94. Kent KC, Donaldson MC, Attinger CE, Couch NP, Mannick JA, Whittemore AD. Femoropopliteal reconstruction for claudication. The risk to life and limb. Arch Surg 1988;123:1196–8.

95. Post S, Kraus T, Muller-Reinartz U, et al. Dacron vs. polytetrafluoroethylene grafts for femoropopliteal bypass: a prospective randomised multicentre trial. Eur J Vasc Endovasc Surg 2001;22: 226–31.

96. Robinson BI, Fletcher JP, Tomlinson P, et al. A prospective randomized multicentre comparison of expanded polytetrafluoroethylene and gelatin-sealed knitted Dacron grafts for femoropopliteal bypass. Cardiovasc Surg 1999;7:214–8.

97. Abbott WM, Green RM, Matsumoto T, et al. Prosthetic above-knee femoropopliteal bypass grafting: results of a multicenter randomized prospective trial. Above-Knee Femoropopliteal Study Group. J Vasc Surg 1997;25:19–28.

98. Eickhoff JH, Broome A, Ericsson BF, et al. Four years' results of a prospective, randomized clinical trial comparing polytetrafluoroethylene and modified human umbilical vein for below-knee femoropopliteal bypass. J Vasc Surg 1987;6:506–11.

99. Aalders GJ, van Vroonhoven TJ. Polytetrafluoroethylene versus human umbilical vein in above-knee femoropopliteal bypass: six-year results of a randomized clinical trial. J Vasc Surg 1992;16:816–23; discussion 823–4.

100. Michaels JA. Choice of material for above-knee femoropopliteal bypass graft. Br J Surg 1989;76:7–14.

101. Houser SL, Hashmi FH, Jaeger VJ, et al. Should the greater saphenous vein be preserved in patients requiring arterial outflow reconstruction in the lower extremity? Surgery 1984;95:467–72.

102. Jackson MR, Belott TP, Dickason T, et al. The consequences of a failed femoropopliteal bypass grafting: comparison of saphenous vein and PTFE grafts. J Vasc Surg 2000;32:498–504; 504–5.

103. Devine C, Hons B, McCollum C. Heparin-bonded Dacron or polytetrafluoroethylene for femoropopliteal bypass grafting: a multicenter trial. J Vasc Surg 2001;33:533–9.

104. Santos JCD. Sur la desobstruction des thromboses arterieles anciennes. Mem Acad Chir 1947;73:409.

105. Cannon JA, Barker WF. Successful management of obstructive femoral atherosclerosis by endarterectomy. Surgery 1955;38:48.

106. Lerwick ER. Oscillating loop endarterectomy for peripheral vascular reconstruction. Surgery 1985;97:574–84.

107. Ho GH, Moll FL, Joosten PP, et al. The Mollring Cutter remote endarterectomy: preliminary experience with a new endovascular technique for treatment of occlusive superficial femoral artery disease. J Endovasc Surg 1995;2:278–87.

108. Rosenthal D, Schubart PJ, Kinney ER, et al. Remote superficial femoral artery endarterectomy: multicenter medium-term results. J Vasc Surg 2001;34:428–32; discussion 432–3.

109. Nelson PR, Powell RJ, Proia RR, et al. Results of endovascular superficial femoral endarterectomy. J Vasc Surg 2001;34:526–31.

110. Leeds F, Gilfillan R. Revascularization of the ischemic limb. Surgery 1961;82:25.

111. Morris G, Edwards W, Cooley D. Surgical importance of profunda femoris artery. Arch Surg 1961;82:52.

112. Martin P, Frawley JE, Barabas AP, Rosengarten DS. On the surgery of atherosclerosis of the profunda femoris artery. Surgery 1972;71:182–9.

113. Kalman PG, Johnston KW, Walker PM. The current role of isolated profundaplasty. J Cardiovasc Surg (Torino) 1990;31:107–11.

114. Rollins DL, Towne JB, Bernhard VM, Baum PL. Endarterectomized superficial femoral artery as an arterial patch. Arch Surg 1985;120:367–9.

115. Malone JM, Goldstone J, Moore WS. Autogenous profundaplasty: the key to long-term patency in secondary repair of aortofemoral graft occlusion. Ann Surg 1978;188:817–23.

116. Antiplatelet Trialists' Collaboration. Collaborative overview of randomised trials of antiplatelet therapy. II: Maintenance of vascular graft or arterial patency by antiplatelet therapy. BMJ 1994;308:159–68.

117. McCollum C, Alexander C, Kenchington G, et al. Antiplatelet drugs in femoropopliteal vein bypasses: a multicenter trial. J Vasc Surg 1991;13:150–61; discussion 161–2.

118. Jackson MR, Clagett GP. Antithrombotic therapy in peripheral arterial occlusive disease. Chest 2001;119(Suppl):283S–299S.

119. Becquemin JP. Effect of ticlopidine on the long-term patency of saphenous-vein bypass grafts in the legs. Etude de la Ticlopidine apres Pontage Femoro-Poplite and the Association Universitaire de Recherche en Chirurgie. N Engl J Med 1997;337:1726–31.

120. Flinn WR, Rohrer MJ, Yao JS, McCarthy WJ 3rd, Fahey VA, Bergan JJ. Improved long-term patency of infragenicular polytetrafluoroethylene grafts. J Vasc Surg 1988;7:685–90.

121. Kretschmer G, Wenzl E, Piza F, et al. The influence of anticoagulant treatment on the probability of function in femoropopliteal vein bypass surgery: analysis of a clinical series (1970 to 1985) and interim evaluation of a controlled clinical trial. Surgery 1987;102:453–9.

122. Kretschmer G, Herbst F, Prager M, et al. A decade of oral anticoagulant treatment to maintain autologous vein grafts for femoropopliteal atherosclerosis. Arch Surg 1992;127:1112–5.

123. Arfvidsson B, Lundgren F, Drott C, et al. Influence of coumarin treatment on patency and limb salvage after peripheral arterial reconstructive surgery. Am J Surg 1990;159:556–60.

124. Dutch Bypass Oral Anticoagulants or Aspirin (BOA) Study Group. Efficacy of oral anticoagulants compared with aspirin after infrainguinal bypass surgery (The Dutch Bypass Oral Anticoagulants or Aspirin Study): a randomised trial. Lancet 2000;355:346–51.

125. Regensteiner JG, Hargarten ME, Rutherford RB, Hiatt WR. Functional benefits of peripheral vascular bypass surgery for patients with intermittent claudication. Angiology 1993;44:1–10.

126. Zannetti S, L'Italien GJ, Cambria RP. Functional outcome after surgical treatment for intermittent claudication. J Vasc Surg 1996;24:65–73.

127. Hunink MG, et al. Revascularization for femoropopliteal disease. A decision and cost-effectiveness analysis. JAMA 1995;274:165–71.

128. de Vries SO, Visser K, de Vries JA, et al. Intermittent claudication: cost-effectiveness of revascularization versus exercise therapy. Radiology 2002;222:25–36.

129. Reunanen A, Takkunen H, Aromaa A. Prevalence of intermittent claudication and its effect on mortality. Acta Med Scand 1982;211:249–56.

130. Bergqvist D, Troeng T, Elfstrom J, et al. Auditing surgical outcome: ten years with the Swedish Vascular Registry – Swedvasc. The Steering Committee of Swedvasc. Eur J Surg Suppl 1998;581:3–8.

CHAPTER
10

Etiology and Natural History: Medical Management

Constantinos Kyriakides and John H N Wolfe

KEY POINTS

- Chronic lower extremity ischemia is associated with an increased risk of limb loss and vascular death.

- The incidence of critical limb ischemia (CLI) is between 500 and 1000 per million population per year.

- Up to 50% of patients with CLI will ultimately undergo major amputation.

- The 5-year mortality in patients with CLI is 70%. Of these, 35% will be cardiovascular deaths, with only 9% non-vascular deaths.

- The medical management of patients with CLI includes dealing with early treatment measures, such as control of pain and infection in the presence of tissue loss, as well as risk factor management including lifestyle modification.

INTRODUCTION

Chronic lower extremity ischemia is a common cause of morbidity and mortality in the western world and will likely increase in frequency and magnitude due to the growing elderly population. Patients are not only faced with disability in their legs and the risk of amputation, but they are also at an increased risk of angina, myocardial infarction, and stroke. The aim therefore should be to develop primary and secondary prevention strategies both to modify the progression of chronic lower extremity ischemia as well as to reduce the incidence of other adverse vascular events. In the first place, this requires accurate diagnostic criteria for chronic lower extremity ischemia, and secondly, differentiation between intermittent claudication (IC) and chronic critical limb ischemia (CLI).

Intermittent claudication, defined as pain in the leg musculature following activity, is the earliest and most frequent presentation of chronic lower extremity ischemia. Claudication pain is localized in the calf, thigh, or buttock musculature, depending on the distribution of the arterial compromise. As the disease progresses in severity, patients develop pain at rest, particularly when the legs are elevated in bed at night, which is relieved by dependency. In contrast to IC, ischemic 'rest pain' typically affects the foot. Further progression of the disease will then lead to severe tissue hypoperfusion, resultant ischemic ulceration and gangrene, with major amputation being the end result in over a third of these patients.[1] Significantly, CLI, which includes rest pain and tissue loss, is associated with an annual mortality of 20%.[1]

The development of primary and secondary prevention strategies for chronic lower extremity ischemia is based on a multidisciplinary approach, which aims to improve the outcome of the disease. This may include risk factor identification and modification such as lifestyle changes, pharmacotherapy, other forms of non-interventional treatment, as well as percutaneous intervention and surgery.

ETIOLOGY

Atherosclerotic arterial disease is responsible for almost all of lower limb arterial occlusive disease and consequently CLI. However, there are some rare conditions that tend to affect younger patients and it is imperative that they are diagnosed early. Too frequently, young fit people are brushed off with a diagnosis of 'muscle cramps'.

Persistent sciatic artery
This is a congenital anomaly whereby the embryonic axial limb artery (sciatic) fails to obliterate, and is commonly associated with failure of proper development of the iliofemoral segment. The persistent sciatic artery is prone to aneurysmal degeneration, which may cause thrombosis or distal embolization.[2]

Buerger's disease
Buerger's disease (also known as thromboangiitis obliterans) describes a clinical syndrome characterized by segmental thrombotic occlusions of the small and medium-sized arteries, usually of the distal lower limb. It tends to affect young men of Middle and Far Eastern origin who are heavy smokers. Associated vasospastic symptoms commonly occur and patients tend to present with rest pain and tissue loss.[2]

Cystic adventitial disease
Cystic adventitial disease is caused by a cystic abnormality of the adventitial layer of the arterial wall. Typically it is a condition that affects the popliteal artery, the contents of which resemble that of a ganglion, and occasionally the cysts may be in communication with the synovium of the knee joint. This process can also occur in arteries such as the femoral, which are at a distance from a synovial joint.[2]

Fibromuscular dysplasia
Although fibromuscular dysplasia primarily tends to affect the renal and carotid arteries, it can also involve the iliac and other arterial segments in young people. Thus, in young patients in whom atherosclerotic risk factors are lacking, this diagnosis should be considered and the common sites of involvement investigated.[2]

Popliteal artery entrapment

This condition most commonly occurs when the artery courses around the medial head of the gastrocnemius – though there are some variants – rather than between its two heads. The artery gets compressed during flexion. This tends to affect athletes. Eventually, aneurysmal degeneration, distal embolization, and thrombosis of the popliteal artery can occur.[2]

DIAGNOSTIC CRITERIA

Critical limb ischemia corresponds to stages III and IV of the Fontaine classification. This coincides with the Rutherford categories 4–6 of the Society for Vascular Surgery–International Society for Cardiovascular Surgery (SVS-ISCVS) Recommendations of Reporting Standards.[3] It has also been defined by the European Consensus Conference as persistently recurring rest pain requiring regular analgesia for more than 2 weeks, or ulceration, or gangrene at the foot, with an ankle systolic pressure less than 50mmHg or absent peripheral pulses in diabetics.[4] The various diagnostic criteria used to define CLI are summarized in **Table 10.1**.

Despite the multiplicity of definitions, the prevalence of CLI has been difficult to determine in population surveys. Thus, most of the epidemiologic data relate to the whole group of patients with chronic lower extremity ischemia. This is partly because the symptoms are uncharacteristic and easily confused with other causes of leg pain such as arthritis or venous disease, making them difficult to identify by questionnaire. In addition, it has not been possible to study accurately the natural history of CLI, as the significant majority of these patients will require surgical intervention. Nevertheless, detailed data can be obtained from hospital records as the majority of patients with CLI are referred to hospital for treatment.

Studies performed in the 1940s and late 1950s suggested that approximately 50% of patients with CLI, none of whom had undergone reconstructive surgery, would ultimately undergo major amputation.[5,6] In a more recent prospective study – published in 1986 – 25% of 428 patients with CLI needed a major amputation during the first year, although over 90% had undergone some form of intervention.[7] In 1995, the Vascular Surgical Society of Great Britain and Ireland (VSSGBI) published the results of a nationwide prospective survey of patients with CLI and reported an overall amputation rate of 21.5%, although just under 70% of the patients underwent some form of revascularization.[8] Major amputation was also associated with prolonged hospital stay compared with revascularization, and a greater requirement for institutional support. In contrast to these data, a Swedish study demonstrated that units with high revascularization rates did not necessarily have low amputation rates.[9] This unexpected finding may be explained by a difference in patient populations with different rates of disease severity.

The terms 'subcritical' and 'critical' ischemia have been suggested to better define the CLI population (**Table 10.2**).[10] We all recognize the critical foot, but to define it has proved elusive and every definition is flawed. However, by distinguishing between 'subcritical' and 'critical' when studying patients with leg ischemia, one may be able to more accurately predict the outcome of conservative management and surgery. A retrospective analysis of 20 recent publications consisting of 6118 patients with critical ischemia indicated that the lower risk ('subcritical')

Definitions of critical lower limb ischemia.
Fontaine classification[48]
• Stage III   Rest pain caused by arterial disease
• Stage IV   Ulceration and/or gangrene caused by arterial disease
International Vascular Symposium Working Party Definition[49]
• Severe rest pain requiring opiate analgesia for at least 4 weeks, *and either*
• Ankle pressure <40mmHg, *or*
• Ankle pressure <60mmHg in the presence of tissue necrosis or digital gangrene
Modified International Vascular Symposium Working Party Definition[50]
• Severe rest pain requiring opiate analgesia for at least 4 weeks, *and either*
• Ankle pressure <40mmHg, *or*
• Tissue necrosis or digital gangrene
First European Working Group Definition[51]
• Severe rest pain requiring opiate analgesia for at least 2 weeks, *or*
• Ulceration or gangrene, *and*
• Ankle pressure <50mmHg
Second European Consensus Document[40]
• Persistently recurring ischemic pain requiring analgesia for >2 weeks, *and* ankle systolic pressure <50mmHg, *and/or* toe systolic pressure <30mmHg, *or*
• Ulceration or gangrene of the foot or toes, *and* ankle systolic pressure <50mmHg, *or* toe systolic pressure <30mmHg

Table 10.1 **Definitions of critical lower limb ischemia.**

Critical ischemia groups with respect to outcome.	
Group	*Inclusion criteria*
Lower risk (subcritical ischemia)	Rest pain *and* ankle pressure >40mmHg
High risk (critical ischemia)	Rest pain *and* tissue loss *and/or* ankle pressure <40mmHg

Table 10.2 **Critical ischemia groups with respect to outcome.**

group achieved 27% limb survival without surgical intervention, compared with only 5% in the higher risk ('critical') group of patients, at 1 year.[10] For surviving patients in the 'subcritical' group, 100% cumulative graft patency was equivalent to only 64% resolution of symptoms at 1 year, indicating that 36% of surviving patients benefitted from conservative treatment. However, the limb salvage outcome following intervention was different in the 'critical' group. Here, 100% cumulative patency was equivalent to 93% limb salvage at 1 year, thus 93% of survivors benefitted from surgery. For this group, intervention was usually essential for limb viability to be maintained. There was no evidence that the use of pharmacotherapy, sympathectomy, or spinal cord stimulation could improve limb salvage for these patients.[10] There is, therefore, a group of patients with CLI (tissue loss ± an ankle pressure of <40mmHg) in whom radiologic or surgical intervention appears to be virtually imperative to save the limb. However, there is a less severely affected group of patients with CLI (tissues intact and an ankle pressure of >40mmHg) in whom limb loss does not appear to be inevitable and medical management may be effective.

PREVALENCE AND INCIDENCE

There is little direct information on the incidence of CLI. The European Working Group, on the basis of the number of major amputations, has estimated the incidence of CLI to range from 500 to 1000 per million population per year.[11] This takes into account the considerable number of deaths prior to amputation, plus the benefit obtained from reconstructive surgery in the majority of patients. Catalano documented the incidence of CLI in Northern Italy from three different perspectives in 1993.[12] Firstly, he prospectively observed the development of CLI in 200 patients with IC and a similar number of controls over a 7-year period. Secondly, he prospectively studied the number of hospitalizations for CLI in a sample of hospitals in Lombardy over a 3-month period. Finally, he documented the number of major amputations performed in various hospitals in the regions of Lombardy (6-month period) and Emilia Romagna (2-year period). He found the results from these three different approaches to be very similar, with the incidence of CLI varying from 450 to 652 patients per million per year, and the incidence of major amputation varying from 112 to 172 per million per year. Based on a national survey carried out in Britain and Ireland, the VSSGBI concluded that there were 20 000 patients with CLI in the population – an anuual incidence of 400 per million – 30% of whom were diabetic.[8] In addition, there are approximately 50 000 hospital admissions each year in England and Wales with a diagnosis of peripheral arterial disease (PAD), of which 15 000 have major reconstructive surgery or amputation.[13]

The TransAtlantic Inter-Society Consensus (TASC) on PAD has used prevalence studies on IC to extrapolate the incidence of CLI.[14] Assuming that the overall prevalence of IC is 3% and that 5% of patients with claudication will go on to develop CLI over the next 5 years, this gives an estimated incidence of CLI of 300 per million per year. In addition, TASC has calculated the incidence of CLI based on the number of major amputations performed, as reported in a number of well-designed studies. If one assumes that 90% of major amputations are performed for CLI and that only 25% of patients with CLI require a major amputation, the incidence of CLI is calculated at approximately 500 to 1000 per million per year. Based on all these incidences calculated by different methodologies, one would expect that for every 100 patients with IC in the population, one new patient per year will develop CLI.[14]

RISK FACTORS

There are a number of risk factors that have been shown to be associated with the development and progression of CLI. There

Risk factors in critical limb ischemia.

Risk factor	Evidence
Age	Direct
Family history	Indirect
Smoking	Direct
Diabetes	Direct
Hyperlipidemia	Indirect
Hypertension	Indirect

Table 10.3 Risk factors in critical limb ischemia.

are also specific risk factors that have been shown to be associated with IC, a condition more widely studied than CLI. In general, risk factors for the development of PAD can be divided into those that cannot be modified, such as age and family history, and those modifiable, such as cigarette smoking, diabetes, hyperlipidemia, and hypertension. Although the role of these risk factors has been individually assessed in various case-control studies and cross-sectional surveys, there is little evidence from long-term population studies (**Table 10.3**).

Age
The prevalence of IC and CLI increases with age, as do the rates of major limb amputation. In a Swedish 3-year prospective study of major lower limb amputation, approximately half the amputees were 80 years of age or more.[15] Similarly, in 1980, a Danish national discharge survey found the incidence of major lower limb amputation to rise from 3 per million per year for those younger than 40 years to 2260 per million per year for those older than 80 years.[16]

Family history
With regard to coronary artery disease, there is good evidence to suggest an association between family history of ischemic heart disease, particularly if it relates to death of a parent at a young age, and myocardial infarction.[17] However, not all of this risk can be explained by conventional risk factors such as smoking, hypertension, and hyperlipidemia. It is therefore likely that another familial risk factor must be present to account for the excess risk. However, to date, there are no published studies examining the association between family history and CLI.

Smoking
There appears to be an overall fourfold increase in the development of PAD in smokers compared with non-smokers in the general population.[18] Furthermore, the risks associated with smoking apply to all age groups and increase with the number of cigarettes smoked. In multivariate analyses, smoking has been shown to be the most important independent risk factor and to be more strongly linked to the development of PAD than coronary artery disease. Major amputation is commoner among persons with PAD who are heavy smokers and who continue to smoke.

Diabetes

Diabetes mellitus affects 2–5% of persons in the western world, yet up to 45% of all amputees are diabetic. Therefore, patients with diabetic peripheral arteriopathy are ten times more likely to need an amputation than are non-diabetic patients with PAD.

Hyperlipidemia

Although there are no studies linking hyperlipidemia with CLI, work has been published that shows an association with IC. Hospital-based studies and cross-sectional general-population surveys have indicated that the odds of having PAD associated with raised cholesterol levels range from 0.9 to 2.2.[18] However, although the odds are often raised, they do not always reach statistical significance, and are generally lower than the odds associated with smoking. Most studies that have used multivariate analysis have shown serum cholesterol to be an independent risk factor for the development of PAD.[19–21]

High-density lipoprotein (HDL), which transfers cholesterol from peripheral tissues and arterial walls back to the liver, tends to be at a lower serum level in claudicants than in normal controls, and there is an inverse relationship between serum levels of HDL and severity of PAD. Low serum HDL levels may also be related to cigarette smoking and reduced physical activity, although in the Edinburgh Artery Study the strong inverse relationship between HDL cholesterol and PAD was independent of smoking, other lipids, obesity, diabetes, and alcohol consumption.[22]

The chances of having PAD in patients with raised serum triglyceride levels are slightly higher than for raised cholesterol levels. However, unlike cholesterol, triglycerides do not show an independent relationship with IC when other risk factors such as smoking, cholesterol, and blood pressure are taken into account in multivariate analyses.

Hypertension

Hospital patients with IC generally have higher mean blood pressures than normal controls. In community-based studies, the odds of PAD are raised in those with high blood pressure, although frequently this association does not reach statistical significance. Considering that high blood pressure may be a consequence of arterial disease, the association with IC can be assessed only in follow-up population studies. To this effect, the Framingham Study found that hypertension (primarily systolic blood pressure) was associated with a threefold increase in risk of development of IC after a 26-year follow-up.[23]

PROGNOSIS

Some 60% to 90% of patients with CLI undergo some form of revascularization procedure, the rest undergoing a primary major amputation. It is therefore no longer possible to describe the natural history of the critically ischemic limb. The mortality rates of patients who present with CLI have been reported in a number of large single-center surgical series and tend to vary from 40% to 70% over a 3- to 5-year follow-up.[24–27] A UK study, published in 1986, reported a 1-year mortality rate of 18% in 400 unselected patients with CLI,[7] while a study from Switzerland, published in 1982, found a similar mortality rate over a 6-month period.[28] The ICAI group from Italy reported

that the mortality rate among approximately 500 patients with CLI to be in the region of 32% over a 2-year follow-up.[29] In addition, they found the overall incidence of vascular deaths (35%) to be much higher than that of non-vascular deaths (9%). Cardiovascular deaths tended to occur early (i.e. within the first year, rather than the second year, of follow-up).

Finally, one can get a good general idea on the prognosis of patients with CLI from multicenter trials that randomize between pharmacotherapy and placebo. Information about the spontaneous course of CLI can therefore be gathered from those patients who receive placebo treatment. However, these data have to be treated with some caution as they represent findings from only a subgroup of patients who have unreconstructable disease or in whom attempts at revascularization have failed. A number of such studies have published their results for this subgroup of patients and have found that, on average, 40% will undergo a major amputation within 6 months, whereas up to 20% will die. In most of these studies, less than 50% of the patients were alive and without major limb loss at 6 months.[30,31] De Weese and Rob found that 95% of their patients who presented with gangrene and 80% of those presenting with rest pain were dead within 10 years.[32]

MEDICAL MANAGEMENT

The management of patients with CLI is not dissimilar to that for claudicants, although the emphasis and urgency for rapid treatment is more pressing in the former group. For example, early treatment measures such as control of pain and infection in the presence of tissue loss are more relevant to patients with CLI. On the other hand, although risk factor management and

Medical treatments in critical limb ischemia.	
Treatment/Condition	Comment
Pharmacotherapy for pain control	Non-steroidal anti-inflammatory drugs and opiates, regular rather than 'on demand'
Epidural spinal cord stimulation	Not recommended at present
Ulcer care	Becaplermin (rhPDGF-BB) gel
Broad-spectrum antibiotics via intravenous access, for infected ulcers	
Prostacyclin analogs	Recommended for 4 weeks
Antiplatelet therapy	Recommended, although no direct evidence for CLI
Gene therapy	Not established, trials will have to be carried out
Co-morbidity	Particular emphasis on coronary artery disease
Risk factor profile	Should be aggressively targeted

Table 10.4 Medical treatments in critical limb ischemia (CLI).

lifestyle modifications are extremely important in the long-term outcome of patients with IC, they are less of a priority in patients with CLI. Within the context of this chapter, we will limit our discussion to the medical management of patients with CLI, as endovascular treatment and surgical intervention will be addressed in the following two chapters. The medical management of patients with CLI is summarized in **Table 10.4**.

Pain control

It is now appreciated that there can be rapid deterioration in a leg (presumably where a further artery occludes) leading to CLI. If there is tissue loss, CLI is unlikely to resolve without improving the blood supply in the leg. If, however, the skin is intact, judicious medical management can, in appropriate patients, maintain care through the acute event, following which, slow improvement may take place.

The clinician can use pain severity scores – such as a simple scale of 0 to 10, with '0' indicating no pain and '10' representing the most severe pain – to tailor analgesia. Regular use of the pain severity score for reassessment allows for more accurate provision of adequate analgesia. Initial attempts at pain relief should include the use of non-steroidal anti-inflammatory drugs (NSAIDs), but only after ensuring that renal function is normal. The use of opiate analgesia should be reserved as second-line treatment; this may need to be combined with laxatives, as some patients experience troublesome constipation. Regular use of analgesia rather than 'on demand' achieves better control of pain. Placing the affected limb in the dependent position can relieve some of the rest pain; thus, tilting the bed or the use of a reclining chair may be a helpful adjunct to pharmacotherapy.

Epidural spinal cord stimulation (SCS) has been in use since the 1960s for intractable rest pain – as an alternative to major amputation – in a number of European centers. The technique involves implantation of an electrode to the level of L3–L4 and a subcutaneous pulse generator. In addition to providing analgesia, SCS improves the arterial supply to the affected limb. In an uncontrolled study, 94% of the 38 patients treated with SCS experienced pain relief, and in half of the patients there was associated healing of ischemic ulcers.[33] In another uncontrolled study, 18 of 20 patients with CLI experienced immediate pain relief after SCS. Of these, 12 patients had continued pain relief, with healing of ischemic ulcers, and improved microcirculatory flow, as suggested by capillaroscopy.[34] Two controlled studies have been published on the efficacy of SCS in patients with end-stage CLI.[35,36] In the first study,[35] 51 patients were randomized either to SCS or to analgesia treatment only, with 18 months follow-up. Long-term pain relief was observed only in the SCS group. Tissue loss was significantly less in the SCS group, but the limb-salvage rate was not significantly different between the two groups. However, subgroup analysis (arguably inappropriate) indicated that in patients without arterial hypertension, SCS therapy resulted in a decreased amputation rate. In the second study,[36] 120 patients were randomized to receive either SCS in addition to best medical therapy or best medical therapy alone, and were followed up for a mean of 605 days. Although the amputation rate was lower in the SCS group, this failed to reach statistical significance. In addition, mortality rates were similar in both groups. On the basis of the available data, TASC do not recommend SCS as standard therapy for patients with inoperable CLI.[37]

Foot care

Patients with chronic CLI, particularly if complicated by diabetes, should be seen by a podiatrist and evaluated for proper foot care. In addition, the patient should be advised about heel care, avoiding any form of trauma, and extremes of heat or cold, to their feet. Even minimal physical trauma can convert a patient from having intact skin to an ischemic ulcer. Thus, local measures are extremely important in the overall management of these patients.

Ulcer and tissue loss management

Medical therapy for ulcers and tissue loss can be topical and systemic. Topical treatment is, by and large, empirical and based on experience with management of other ulcers. This includes topical antibiotics, growth factors, and debriding agents, although there is very little evidence for their use in terms of controlled randomized trials. Furthermore, there is a risk in using such agents, as some patients develop troublesome dermatitis, particularly with the use of topical antibiotics. Although the use of hydrophilic and seaweed dressings have been proposed and applied in this group of patients, there are no data to support their use. Alternatively, wet dressings soaked in saline can be applied a few times a day to clear the ulcers and reduce pain. Once the ulcer has dried, non-adherent dry dressings can be used. A number of studies have found the application of becaplermin (rhPDGF-BB) gel improves ulcer healing.[38] With the exception of neuropathic ulcers, topical therapy is unlikely to be successful as the sole mode of treatment. Ultimately, these patients require a revascularization procedure.

The use of systemic antibiotics is indicated in patients presenting with cellulitis. This is commonly seen in diabetics with ischemic wounds. Bacteriology tends to be polymicrobial; thus, intravenous broad-spectrum antibiotics should be administered to achieve adequate systemic levels.

Pharmacotherapy

The role of pharmacotherapy is to attempt to modify the effects of the low perfusion pressure on the distal microcirculation in order to alleviate rest pain and avoid amputation. Prostacyclin (PGI$_2$) is thought to have a major role in optimizing microvasculature autoregulation and preventing reciprocal potentiation of vascular endothelial, neutrophil, and platelet activation. Based on this knowledge, over the last few years, prostanoid pharmacotherapy has been widely tested in patients with CLI. Initially, PGE$_1$ was evaluated by intra-arterial administration, as it undergoes rapid pulmonary inactivation to 13,14-dihydro-PGE$_1$, although still displaying active biological activity on platelets comparable to its parent compound. In 1979, Szczeklik reported on the beneficial role of PGI$_2$ in five patients with unreconstructable CLI.[39] Since that first report, a number of 3- to 4-day trials have assessed the effects of intra-arterial or intravenous PGE$_1$ and PGI$_2$ in patients with end-stage PAD, with inconclusive results. Data are also available from long-term randomized trials on the systemic use of PGE$_1$, as well as the prostacyclin analogs ciprostene and iloprost, versus placebo in patients with Fontaine stages III and IV. The duration of treatment varied from 2 to 4 weeks, and the clinical end-points included relief of rest pain, analgesic consumption, and promotion of ulcer healing. Most of the studies showed a beneficial effect in at least one of the end-points, with greatest response in patients treated for 4 weeks. In addition, patients who were treated with iloprost were significantly less likely to undergo major amputation than were the placebo groups, during the treatment period and the 3–6-month follow-up. Furthermore, there was a significant reduction in mortality associated with limb salvage in the iloprost group over that follow-up period.[40] However, there are a number of limitations associated with these studies. Total ulcer healing was not used, as it was too uncommon an event after a few weeks of treatment. In addition, there was inter-observational variability, as well as poor-quality photographs where these were used. Furthermore, pain relief scoring relied on subjective assessment, and where patients developed side effects to prostanoid therapy, the potential for bias could have been introduced. With the currently available data, the recommendation from TASC is that use of prostanoids in end-stage CLI may be of use. Other vasoactive agents such as L-arginine and pentoxifylline have been used in patients with CLI but with inconclusive results.

There is a strong case for all patients with PAD to be treated with long-term antiplatelet therapy such as aspirin, ticlodipine, or, more recently, clopidogrel. Meta-analysis of the Final Report of the Second Cycle of the Antiplatelet Trialist Collaboration shows clear evidence that these antiplatelet agents reduce adverse vascular events (stroke, myocardial death, vascular death) by 25%, and also improve patency of peripheral arteries and grafts.[41] However, neither these trials nor the more recent Clopidogrel versus Aspirin in Patients at Risk of Ischaemic Events (CAPRIE) study[42] were conducted in patients with rest pain or tissue loss.

No clinical trials have been published on the use of unfractionated heparin for CLI, nor on oral anticoagulation. There is clearly a need to determine whether long-term oral anticoagulant therapy is useful in maintaining limb survival by conducting randomized trials.

Hyperbaric oxygen has been used in patients with non-healing ulcers who are not candidates for revascularization. However, it is very costly, and results so far have been inconclusive.

The benefit of hemodilution has not been fully evaluated in patients with chronic CLI. However, if a patient's hematocrit remains 50% despite cessation of smoking and rehydration, hemodilution may be considered. This treatment can cause significant side effects in some patients and should always be used cautiously.[43]

Gene therapy

Therapeutic angiogenesis was initially performed in patients with CLI by arterial gene transfer of vascular endothelial growth factor (VEGF) plasmid DNA ($phVEGF_{165}$).[44] Using a dose-escalating design, treatment was initiated with $100\mu g$ $phVEGF_{165}$. Three patients presenting with rest pain and treated with $1000\mu g$ were subsequently shown at 1-year follow-up to have improved blood flow to the ischemic limb and remain free of rest pain. With the increase in dose of $phVEGF_{165}$ to $2000\mu g$, angiographic and histologic evidence of new blood vessel formation became apparent. More recently, the use of intramuscular gene transfer (employed initially as a means of treating patients in whom vascular disease in the ischemic limb was too extensive to permit an intra-arterial approach) resulted in marked improvement in collateral vessel development in patients with CLI.[45] There was significant increase in the ankle–brachial pressure index, with associated ulcer healing and successful limb salvage. In addition, newly visible collaterals on either contrast or magnetic resonance angiography were observed. Lower extremity

edema from enhanced vascular permeability seemed to be the only untoward effect of VEGF administration. These findings indicate that intramuscular injection of naked DNA achieves constitutive expression of VEGF leading to therapeutic angiogenesis in patients with CLI, raising the need for proper randomized controlled trials. However, despite the apparent success of gene therapy, it should be interpreted with caution, as there is the theoretical risk for malignant development of cells concurrent with therapeutic angiogenesis.[1]

Treatment of co-morbidity

Patients with CLI are at the highest risk for subsequent myocardial infarction, stroke, and vascular death. In a study from the Cleveland Clinic, some degree of coronary atherosclerosis was present in 90% of patients undergoing routine coronary angiography before elective peripheral vascular reconstruction, with 28% of these patients having severe, three-vessel coronary disease.[46] Therefore, it is important to minimize the systemic risk of mortality for these patients, particularly if extensive revascularization surgery is planned. Patients with CLI are also likely to have impaired renal function. A multidisciplinary approach – with the involvement of cardiologists, renal physicians, and other specialists – is imperative in the ongoing management of patients with CLI. Furthermore, improvement of coexisting cardiac failure will certainly improve peripheral tissue perfusion, which will inevitably lead to improvement in the CLI of the patient.

Modification of risk factor profile

Patients with CLI have the same cardiovascular risk factor profile as claudicants, although their risk of cardiovascular events and mortality is much higher. Therefore, aggressive risk factor modification is warranted.

Cigarette smoking is associated with the various stages of progression of PAD through to CLI. In patients with severe disease, graft patencies for both vein and prosthetic conduits are improved by stopping smoking. Furthermore, amputation rates are higher in persistent smokers.[47] Five-year survival rates are also correlated with smoking. Thus, in patients with end-stage CLI, smoking cessation is still highly beneficial.

Hypertension is a risk factor for all forms of cardiovascular disease, including peripheral vascular disease. However, maintaining an adequate blood pressure is essential for limb perfusion. Aggressive treatment of hypertension in patients with CLI may compromise limb perfusion, resulting in worsening ischemic rest pain or delayed healing of ischemic ulcers. Consequently, use of beta-blocking antihypertensive agents should be carefully considered in CLI and patients should be closely monitored.

Diabetes is an important risk factor for all forms of PAD and also greatly contributes to CLI. In addition to being at increased risk of atherosclerotic arterial occlusive disease, patients with diabetes mellitus are prone to developing neuropathy and associated ulceration. Thus, a comprehensive approach to treating patients with diabetes would include proper footwear, with attention to trauma from poorly fitting shoes. Patients with non-healing ulcers often need to be treated in hospital with intravenous antibiotics. Finally, long-term blood sugar control is important in limiting diabetes-related complications.

Hyperlipidemia is another risk factor that is associated with all forms of cardiovascular disease. Thus, in patients with CLI, the goals of cholesterol-lowering therapy are to reduce the risk of myocardial infarction and stroke, as well as to delay the progression of peripheral atherosclerosis.

Pharmacotherapy and nephrotoxicity

Many of these patients have impaired renal function, and commonly used nephrotoxic drugs must be used with caution or avoided altogether. These include NSAIDs, statins, biguanides, cephalosporins, angiotensin-converting enzyme (ACE) inhibitors, beta-blockers, thiazide diuretics, and many others.

SUMMARY

Chronic lower extremity ischemia is becoming an increasingly common cause of morbidity and mortality in the western world, in part due to the growth of the elderly population. Ill health is secondary both to the risk of limb loss and to an increased risk of angina, myocardial infarction, and stroke. Thus, CLI is associated with an annual mortality of 20%.

Atherosclerotic arterial disease is by far the commonest cause of chronic lower extremity ischemia, although other rare causes should be considered, particularly in the younger age groups. These include persistent sciatic artery, Buerger's disease, cystic adventitial disease, fibromuscular dysplasia, and popliteal artery entrapment.

Although CLI has been defined by a number of authorities, its prevalence has been difficult to determine in population surveys. Thus, most of the epidemiologic data relates to the whole group of patients with chronic lower extremity ischemia. It is estimated that the incidence of CLI ranges between 500 and 1000 per million population per year. In addition, up to 50% of patients with CLI will ultimately undergo major amputation, half of these within the first year of presentation.

The mortality rates of patients who present with CLI have been reported as high as 70% over a 3- to 5-year follow-up. Of these, 35% will be cardiovascular deaths with only 9% non-vascular deaths. In addition, cardiovascular deaths tend to occur within the first year of follow-up. Similarly, up to 95% of patients who present with gangrene and 80% of those presenting with rest pain will die within 10 years.

The medical management of patients with CLI includes dealing with early treatment measures, such as control of pain and infection in the presence of tissue loss, as well as risk factor management, including modification of lifestyle. The clinician can use pain severity scores to tailor analgesia; regular reassessment with such allows for more accurate provision of adequate analgesia. Pain relief should be administered regularly, and should include the use of NSAIDs, with opiate analgesia reserved as second-line treatment. SCS may be of use in some patients, as uncontrolled studies have shown benefits of such with regard to both pain control and ulcer healing; however, it cannot be

recommended as standard therapy, as randomized studies have failed to show any significant benefit or improved mortality.

Patients with chronic CLI, particularly if it is complicated by diabetes, should be seen by a podiatrist and evaluated for proper foot care. In addition, advice should be given about heel care.

Medical therapy for ulcers and tissue loss can be topical or systemic. A number of studies have found the application of rhPDGF-BB gel to improve ulcer healing. However, with the exception of neuropathic ulcers, topical therapy is unlikely to be successful as the sole mode of treatment. Ultimately, these patients require revascularization. The use of intravenous broad-spectrum antibiotics is indicated in patients presenting with cellulitis, commonly seen in diabetics with ischemic wounds.

Over the last few years, prostanoid pharmacotherapy has been widely tested in patients with CLI. Data are available from long-term randomized trials on the systemic use of PGE_1, ciprostene, and iloprost. The duration of treatment varied from 2 to 4 weeks and the clinical endpoints included relief of rest pain, analgesic consumption, and promotion of ulcer healing. Most of the studies showed a beneficial effect in at least one of the endpoints, with greatest response in patients treated for 4 weeks. In addition, patients were significantly less likely to undergo major amputation and there was a significant reduction in mortality associated with limb salvage in the iloprost group over that follow-up period. Although there are a number of limitations associated with these studies, prostanoid pharmacotherapy in end-stage CLI may be of use.

Patients with PAD should be treated with long-term anti-platelet therapy such as aspirin, ticlodipine, and clopidogrel, as these agents reduce adverse vascular events, including stroke, myocardial death, and vascular death, by 25%, and also improve patency of peripheral arteries and grafts. However, there are no data available in patients with rest pain or tissue loss. Other forms of therapy include heparin, hyperbaric oxygen, hemodilution, and gene therapy with recombinant VEGF, but none of these constitute standard treatment at the present time.

Patients with CLI are at a higher risk for subsequent myocardial infarction, stroke, and vascular death, and are also more likely to have impaired renal function. It is therefore important to minimize the systemic risk of mortality for these patients, particularly if extensive revascularization surgery is planned. A multidisciplinary approach with the involvement of cardiologists, renal physicians, and other appropriate specialists, is imperative in the further management of these patients.

Cigarette smoking is associated with the various stages of progression of PAD through to CLI, and amputation rates are also higher in persistent smokers. Five-year survival rates, too, correlate with smoking; thus, in patients with end-stage CLI, smoking cessation is still highly beneficial. In addition, hypertension, diabetes mellitus, and hyperlipidemia are independently associated with chronic lower extremity ischemia, and appropriate therapy should be instigated in all affected patients.

REFERENCES

1. Ouriel K. Peripheral arterial disease. Lancet 2001;358:1257–64.
2. Beard JD, Gaines PA. Treatment of chronic lower limb ischaemia. In: Beard JD, Gaines PA, eds. Vascular and endovascular surgery. London: Harcourt; 2001:55–9.
3. Ad Hoc Committee on Reporting Standards. Suggested standards for reports dealing with lower extremity ischaemia. J Vasc Surg 1986;4:80–94.
4. European Working Group on Critical Limb Ischaemia. Second European Consensus Document on Chronic Critical Leg Ischaemia. Eur J Vasc Surg 1992;6(Suppl A):1–32.

5. Hines EA, Barker NW. Arteriosclerosis obliterans. Am J Med Sci 1940;200:717–30.

6. Cranley JJ, Krause RJ, Strasser ES. Limb survival with and without definitive surgical treatment in obliterative arterial disease. Surgery 1959;45:32–9.

7. Wolfe J. Defining the outcome of critical limb ischaemia: a one year prospective study. Br J Surg 1986;73:321.

8. Vascular Society of Great Britain and Ireland (VSSGBI). Critical limb ischaemia: management and outcome. Report of a national survey. Eur J Vasc Endovasc Surg 1995;10:108–13.

9. The Westcoast Vascular Surgeons (WVS) Study Group. Variation of rates of vascular surgical procedures for chronic critical limb ischaemia and lower limb amputation rates in western Swedish countries. Eur J Vasc Endovasc Surg 1997;14:310–4.

10. Wolfe JH, Wyatt MG. Critical and subcritical ischaemia. Eur J Vasc Endovasc Surg 1997;13:578–82.

11. European Working Group on Critical Limb Ischaemia. Second European Consensus Document on Chronic Critical Limb Ischaemia. Circulation 1991;84(Suppl):1–26.

12. Catalano M. Epidemiology of critical limb ischaemia: north Italian data. Eur J Med 1993;2:11–4.

13. Department of Health and Social Security UK. Hospital inpatient enquiry. London:Office of Population Censuses and Surveys; 1986.

14. Dormandy JA, Rutherford RB. Management of peripheral arterial disease (PAD). TASC Working Group. TransAtlantic Inter-Society Concensus (TASC). J Vasc Surg 2000;31(1 Pt 2):S22.

15. Liedberg E, Persson BM. Increased incidence of lower limb amputation for arterial occlusive disease. Acta Orthop Scand 1983;54:230–4.

16. Eickhoff JH, Hansen HJ, Lorentzen JE. The effect of arterial reconstruction on lower limb amputation rate. An epidemiological survey based on reports from Danish hospitals. Acta Chir Scand Supp, 1980;502:181–7.

17. Phillips AN, Shaper AG, Pocock SJ, Walker M. Parental death from heart disease and the risk of heart attack. Eur Heart J 1988;9:243–51.

18. Leng,CL, Fowkes FGR. Epidemiology and risk factors for peripheral arterial disease. In: Beard JD, Gaines PA, eds. Vascular and endovascular surgery. London:Harcourt; 2001:9–10.

19. Schroll M, Munck O. Estimation of peripheral arteriosclerotic disease by ankle blood pressure measurements in a population study of 60-year-old men and women. J Chronic Dis 1981;34:261–9.

20. Fowkes FG, Housley E, Cawood EH, et al. Edinburgh Artery Study: prevalence of asymptomatic and symptomatic peripheral arterial disease in the general population. Int J Epidemiol 1991;20:384–92.

21. Hale WE, Marks RG, May FE, et al. Epidemiology of intermittent claudication: evaluation of risk factors. Age Ageing 1988;17:57–60.

22. Fowkes FG, Housley E, Riemersma RA, et al. Smoking, lipids, glucose intolerance, and blood pressure as risk factors for peripheral atherosclerosis compared with ischemic heart disease in the Edinburgh Artery Study. Am J Epidemiol 1992;135:331–40.

23. Kannel WB, McGee DL. Update on some epidemiologic features of intermittent claudication: the Framingham Study. J Am Geriatr Soc 1985;33:13–8.

24. Ouriel K, Fiore WM, Geary JE. Limb-threatening ischemia in the medically compromised patient: amputation or revascularization? Surgery 1988;104:667–72.

25. Griffith CD, Callum KG. Limb salvage surgery in a district general hospital: factors affecting outcome. Ann R Coll Surg Engl 1988;70:95–8.

26. Veith FJ, Gupta SK, Samson RH, et al. Progress in limb salvage by reconstructive arterial surgery combined with new or improved adjunctive procedures. Ann Surg 1981;194:386–401.

27. Hickey NC, Thomson IA, Shearman CP, Simms MH. Aggressive arterial reconstruction for critical lower limb ischaemia. Br J Surg 1991;78:1476–8.

28. Schneider E, Gruntzig A, Bollinger A. [Percutaneous transluminal angioplasty (PTA) in stages III and IV of peripheral arterial occlusive disease]. Vasa 1982;11:336–9 (in German).

29. Long-term mortality and its predictors in patients with critical leg ischaemia. The I.C.A.I. Group (Gruppo di Studio dell'Ischemia Cronica Critica degli Arti Inferiori). The Study Group of Critical Chronic Ischemia of the Lower Exremities. Eur J Vasc Endovasc Surg 1997; 14:91–5.

30. Belch JJ, McKay A, McArdle B, et al. Epoprostenol (prostacyclin) and severe arterial disease. A double-blind trial. Lancet 1983;1:315–7.

31. Treatment of limb threatening ischaemia with intravenous iloprost: a randomised double-blind placebo controlled study. U.K. Severe Limb Ischaemia Study Group. Eur J Vasc Surg 1991;5:511–6.

32. De Weese JA, Rob CG. Autogenous vein grafts ten years later. Surgery 1966:6:775–84.

33. Augustinsson LE, Carlsson CA, Holm J, Jivegard L. Epidural electrical stimulation in severe limb ischemia. Pain relief, increased blood flow, and a possible limb-saving effect. Ann Surg 1985;202:104–10.

34. Jacobs MJ, Jorning PJ, Beckers RC, et al. Foot salvage and improvement of microvascular blood flow as a result of epidural spinal cord electrical stimulation. J Vasc Surg 1990;12:354–60.

35. Jivegard LE, Augustinsson LE, Holm J, Risberg B, Ortenwall P. Effects of spinal cord stimulation (SCS) in patients with inoperable severe lower limb ischaemia: a prospective randomised controlled study. Eur J Vasc Endovasc Surg 1995;9:421–5.

36. Klomp HM, Spincemaille GH, Steyerberg EW, Habbema JD, van Urk H. Spinal-cord stimulation in critical limb ischaemia: a randomised trial. ESES Study Group. Lancet 1999;353:1040–4.

37. Dormandy JA, Rutherford RB. Management of peripheral arterial disease (PAD). TASC Working Group. TransAtlantic Inter-Society Consensus (TASC). J Vasc Surg 2000;31(1 Pt 2):S264–5.

38. Wieman TJ. Clinical efficacy of becaplermin (rhPDGF-BB) gel. Becaplermin Gel Studies Group. Am J Surg 1998;176(2A Suppl): 74S–79S.

39. Szczeklik A, Nizankowski R, Skawinski S, Szczeklil J, Gluszko P, Gryglewski RJ. Successful therapy of advanced arteriosclerosis obliterans with prostacyclin. Lancet 1979;1:1111–4.

40. Second European Consensus Document on chronic critical leg ischemia. Circulation 1991;84(4 Suppl):IV1–26.

41. Antiplatelet Trialists' Collaboration. Collaborative overview of randomised trials of antiplatelet therapy. II: Maintenance of vascular graft or arterial patency by antiplatelet therapy. BMJ 1994;308:159–68.

42. CAPRIE Steering Committee. A randomised, blinded, trial of clopidogrel versus aspirin in patients at risk of ischaemic events (CAPRIE). Lancet 1996;348:1329–39.

43. Wolfe JH, Waller DG, Chapman MB, et al. The effect of hemodilution upon patients with intermittent claudication. Surg Gynecol Obstet 1985;160:347–51.

44. Isner JM, Walsh K, Symes J, et al. Arterial gene therapy for therapeutic angiogenesis in patients with peripheral artery disease. Circulation 1995;91:2687–92.

45. Baumgartner I, Pieczek A, Manor O, et al. Constitutive expression of phVEGF165 after intramuscular gene transfer promotes collateral vessel development in patients with critical limb ischemia. Circulation 1998;97:1114–23.

46. Hertzer NR, Beven EG, Young JR, et al. Coronary artery disease in peripheral vascular patients. A classification of 1000 coronary angiograms and results of surgical management. Ann Surg 1984;199:223–33.

47. McGrath MA, Graham AR, Hill DA, et al. The natural history of chronic leg ischemia. World J Surg 1983;7:314–8.

48. Fontain R, Kim M, Kieny R. Die Chirurgische Behandlung der peripheren Durch-Blutungsstorungen. Helv Chir Acta 1954;21:499.

49. Bell PRF, Charlesworth D, De Palma RG. The definition of critical ischemia of the limb. Working party of the International Vascular Symposium (Editorial). Br J Surg 1982; 69;S2.

50. Tyrrell MR, Wolfe JH. Critical leg ischaemia: an appraisal of clinical definitions. Joint Vascular Research Group. Br J Surg 1993;80:177–80.

51. European consensus on critical limb ischaemia. Lancet 1989;1:737–8.

CHAPTER

11

Endovascular Treatment

Bruce H Gray

KEY POINTS

- Patients with critical limb ischemia have multilevel, systemic atherosclerosis and a reduced life expectancy.

- Aortoiliac disease can frequently be treated with endovascular angioplasty and stenting.

- Superficial femoral artery occlusive disease is amenable to endovascular treatment; however, recurrence is high.

- Stenting of superficial femoral artery disease should be reserved for failed angioplasty.

- Balloon-expandable stents perform well in common iliac arteries; self-expanding stents are used for all other lower extremity lesions.

- Thrombus-dominant occlusions can be treated with laser-assisted angioplasty.

- Tibial angioplasty is technically feasible and reserved for poor candidates for surgical reconstruction.

- Use of anticoagulant and antiplatelet medications are important to the success of the endovascular procedure.

- After revascularization, frequent follow-up with non-invasive functional studies is necessary to optimize outcome.

INTRODUCTION

Balloon angioplasty – percutaneous transluminal angioplasty (PTA) – has remained the cornerstone of percutaneous revascularization since the pioneering work of Gruntzig, Dotter and Judkins over 30 years ago.[1,2] Although balloon angioplasty for peripheral arterial disease (PAD) was initially limited to claudicants with simple, focal, short lesions in the aortoiliac distribution, the application of PTA with stents, stent-grafts, laser-light, and advanced pharmacotherapies has enabled endovascular treatment regardless of disease distribution or degree of ischemia. Further refinement of guidewires, sheaths, and adjunctive medications has allowed traversal of even the longest lesions, enabling technical success. However, restenosis remains the Achilles heel of PTA. Recent advances including drug-coated stents, brachytherapy, and other pharmacotherapies have shown promise to address this inherent weakness.

Endovascular percutaneous therapy is complementary to traditional open surgery (bypass, endarterectomy). Two small randomized trials have compared surgical bypass with balloon angioplasty for the treatment of aortoiliac and femoropopliteal disease.[3,4] These studies concluded that the two procedures lead to similar patency and amputation rates. However, surgery has remained the principal treatment for patients with critical limb ischemia (CLI). The issues include training bias of physicians, technical expertise, and perceived maximal benefit of surgery in CLI patients.

In light of these recent endovascular advances, how does a physician assess the benefit and risk of multiple treatment options? Important factors to consider include:

- the anatomic level of disease (TransAtlantic Inter-Society Consensus [TASC] classification);
- degree of ischemia at presentation (i.e. claudication, rest pain, gangrene);
- functional status (i.e. ambulatory, homebound, bedridden);
- co-morbidities (i.e. obesity, heart disease, age), and;
- technical factors (bypass target, integrity of autologous vein).

This chapter will explore the use of endovascular therapies for CLI patients according to the distribution of disease in the aortoiliac, femoral-popliteal, and/or tibial level.

GENERAL CONCEPTS

Initial evaluation and anatomic assessment

It is important before formulating a revascularization plan to distinguish between hemodynamically significant and non-significant lesions. Non-invasive studies – pulse volume recordings (PVR), segmental pressures – provide functional information and allow quantification of the hemodynamic significance of critical lesions. They can further quantify the hemodynamic significance of collateralization, and establish a baseline for comparative purposes. Segmental pressures across the iliac, femoral, tibial, and toe should be measured (**Fig. 11.1**). Segmental pressure gradients *at rest* of 10mmHg are sometimes significant, a 20mmHg gradient is usually significant, and gradients more than 30mmHg are always significant.[5] For example, a patient with a resting ankle–brachial index (ABI) of 0.4 who has a 10mmHg pressure drop across the iliac segment, a 50mmHg drop across the superficial femoral artery (SFA)/popliteal artery, and a 20mmHg drop across the tibials, will require correction of at least the SFA component. In contrast, a drop of 60mmHg across the iliac segment, with a 20mmHg drop through the SFA and tibials implies that the iliac lesion is most significant and should be initially treated. Then if the clinical response were inadequate, correction of the infrainguinal lesion would be necessary. Resolving these gradients and improving the corresponding PVR waveform can predict successful revascularization. Failure to correct the 'functionally important' lesion will result in poor outcomes.[6]

Anatomic studies such as a digital subtraction arteriogram provide the road map for revascularization. Arteriography with

Lower extremity pulse volume recording

Pulses	Femoral	Popliteal	DP	Post tibial	Other
Right	4	0	0	0	
Left	4	4	4	4	

RESTING SEGMENTAL PULSE VOLUME AND SYSTOLIC PRESSURE DATA

RT Brachial: 100mmHg

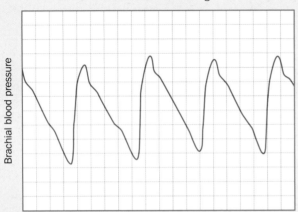

LT Brachial: 100mmHg

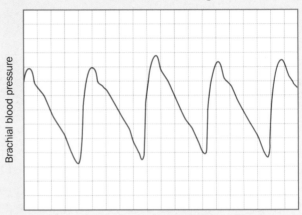

RT Thigh: 90mmHg

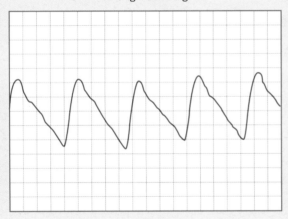

LT Thigh: 100mmHg

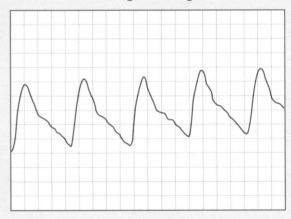

RT Calf: 60mmHg

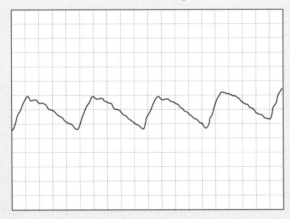

LT Calf: 100mmHg

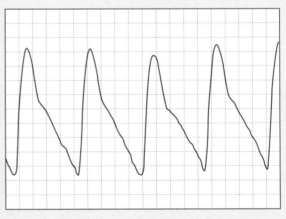

(A)

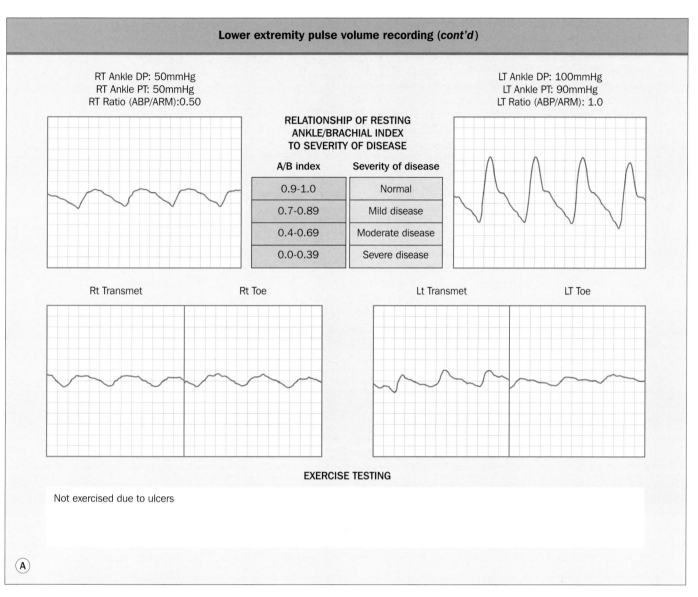

Lower extremity pulse volume recording (*cont'd*)

RT Ankle DP: 50mmHg
RT Ankle PT: 50mmHg
RT Ratio (ABP/ARM):0.50

LT Ankle DP: 100mmHg
LT Ankle PT: 90mmHg
LT Ratio (ABP/ARM): 1.0

RELATIONSHIP OF RESTING
ANKLE/BRACHIAL INDEX
TO SEVERITY OF DISEASE

A/B index	Severity of disease
0.9-1.0	Normal
0.7-0.89	Mild disease
0.4-0.69	Moderate disease
0.0-0.39	Severe disease

Rt Transmet   Rt Toe   Lt Transmet   LT Toe

EXERCISE TESTING

Not exercised due to ulcers

(A)

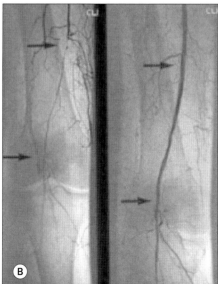

(B)

Figure 11.1 Measurement of segmental pressures. (A) Pulse volume recording demonstrating the functional significance of a right superficial femoral artery (SFA) occlusion. Note the 30mmHg drop across the right SFA and the 10mmHg drop across the tibials. (B) Arteriogram of a popliteal artery with diffuse stenotic disease treated with balloon angioplasty.

posterior-anterior, lateral, and oblique projections can identify most lesions. Contralateral oblique projections may be needed to unmask proximal external iliac artery lesions obscured by internal iliac artery overlap. Ipsilateral oblique projections of the femoral arteries uncover proximal SFA and profunda lesions. Lateral projections of the popliteal artery may be necessary in patients with orthopedic knee prostheses or in patients with non-atherosclerotic diseases. Lateral foot films identify the dorsalis pedis and plantar arch vessels best. Patients with extensive disease can be challenging to image with the aortic injections only. Selective catheter placement at each level can provide the most useful anatomic and hemodynamic information.

Intra-arterial pressure gradients are an essential component to procedural success and are complementary to the pre-procedural non-invasive studies. Intra-arterial gradients are usually much higher than gradients obtained non-invasively. Iliac lesions of significance will usually impart >20mmHg gradient, with complete resolution of the gradient as the interventional endpoint. Superficial femoral and popliteal lesions induce large gradients and are more difficult to resolve with endovascular techniques. An 80mmHg gradient across the SFA that can be reduced to 20mmHg may be perfectly acceptable. Measurement of pressure gradients across the tibials are compromised by the catheter itself and typically are not useful.

Magnetic resonance angiography (MRA) and duplex ultrasound have been used with increasing frequency to facilitate revascularization therapy. The use of non-nephrotoxic agents and avoidance of needles, catheters, and wires make MRA attractive. The quality and resolution of MRA has improved dramatically and MRA is gradually replacing diagnostic angiography. Duplex ultrasound provides excellent information in patients with single-level disease, but falters with multilevel disease.[7,8] Limitations in imaging obese patients, the external iliac artery, or the tibioperoneal trunk leave duplex as a screening test in many CLI patients.

Selection of procedure

One must understand the natural history of the disease in context of the history and physical examination before making therapeutic decisions. Not all patients with CLI could or should undergo revascularization. Patients with extensive necrosis, infectious gangrene, or those who are non-ambulatory may be best served with primary amputation. Ambulatory patients with long arterial occlusions, heavily calcified arteries (usually diabetic), and who have adequate autologous venous conduit are best served with bypass surgery. However, many patients are poor surgical candidates because of medical co-morbidities, compromised bypass target, or poor venous conduit, and, despite advanced vascular disease, would be best treated endovascularly. These treatments are not mutually exclusive and should be viewed as complementary. Safe, effective treatment requires the selective application of all the available tools.

Percutaneous access site

Potential percutaneous access sites include the radial, brachial, axillary, femoral, popliteal, and pedal arteries. The common femoral artery (CFA) is the most convenient, safest, and easiest access site for most diagnostic and therapeutic procedures (**Fig. 11.2**). It can be accessed in an antegrade and/or retrograde direction. The contralateral CFA is usually the best site for the

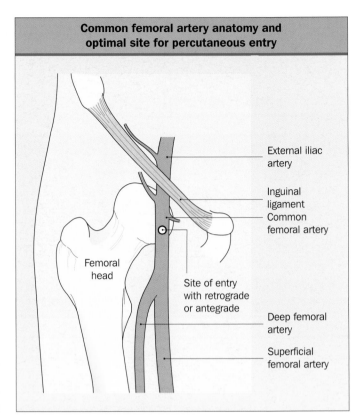

Common femoral artery anatomy and optimal site for percutaneous entry

External iliac artery

Inguinal ligament

Common femoral artery

Femoral head

Site of entry with retrograde or antegrade

Deep femoral artery

Superficial femoral artery

Figure 11.2 Depiction of common femoral artery anatomy and optimal site for percutaneous entry.

initial diagnostic study. From this site, therapeutic intervention on the contralateral distal common iliac, external iliac, common femoral, profunda femoral, and superficial femoral artery can be done. Ipsilateral, retrograde CFA access is best to treat proximal lesions of the common iliac artery. Ipsilateral, antegrade CFA access can be used for mid- to distal SFA, popliteal, and tibial intervention. These distal lesions can also be done from the contralateral side, but catheter manipulation is much simpler with the antegrade approach. Retrograde popliteal artery approach is excellent for proximal SFA occlusions with or without involvement of the CFA.[9] Retrograde pedal artery access enables traversal of proximal tibial occlusions when the antegrade approach is unsuccessful.[10] Axillary, brachial, or radial artery sites may be helpful in patients with aortic occlusions, but distance to the lower extremities limits the therapeutic application (**Fig. 11.2**).

Percutaneous needle entry into the artery should be a single stick, anterior wall puncture only. The Seldinger technique (anterior through posterior wall) should be avoided since arterial closure devices can only close a single, anterior wall arteriotomy. Arterial puncture high in the CFA may predispose to retro-peritoneal bleeding, whereas low punctures at the level of the SFA have a higher incidence of arteriovenous fistula, hematoma, and pseudoaneurysm formation. Occasionally, unplanned use of fibrinolytic therapy is necessary and a single wall puncture will reduce groin complications associated with fibrinolysis. Pulseless sticks can be challenging, but there are several helpful techniques (**Table 11.1**).

**Helpful tricks to obtain percutaneous
needle access to pulseless arteries.**

1.	Identify flow with a Doppler 'Smart' needle
2.	Directly puncture calcification in the artery wall under fluoroscopy
3.	Inject contrast from a remote site and puncture the contrast column on road map
4.	Direct needle to 1cm in from the inferior/medial border of the femoral head

Table 11.1 Helpful tricks to obtain percutaneous needle access to pulseless arteries.

Wires

There are many different wires (entry wire, support or exchange wires, small-vessel wires, glide wires) that are available for therapeutic interventions. Initial entry wires (0.035in) usually have a slight J-shape that reforms as the wire passes through the needle into the artery. This wire design rarely passes sub-intimally, avoiding iatrogenic dissection. Exchange wires are long and sturdy and are important for coaxial catheter exchanges to reduce the risk of losing wire access. Support wires improve the trackability and deliverability of balloon catheters and stents, but are poor in crossing lesions. Wires with slippery coatings (glide wires) facilitate traversal of occlusions and should not be used through entry needles since the coating can be sheared. After crossing a lesion with a glide wire, it should be exchanged for a support wire to avoid inadvertent loss of wire access. Small-caliber wires (0.014–0.018in) enable access into tibial vessels with small-vessel balloons, lasers, and stents.

Sheaths and catheters

Sheaths provide stable arterial access, minimize blood loss, and improve catheter manipulation. They are sized according to their inner diameter. The outer diameter varies from 1.6 to 2.7 French (F) sizes larger, depending on the brand. Most diagnostic and simple angioplasty procedures can be done through a 4F or 5F sheath. Balloon-expandable stents require at least a 6F sheath, while self-expanding stents usually need a 7F sheath. Long, flexible sheaths are needed for contralateral work. These radially supported sheaths minimize kinking when placed over the aortic bifurcation. Thin, smooth-walled sheaths produce a smaller arteriotomy and are preferred when access is from the upper extremity.

Pigtail catheters are the mainstay for diagnostic aortography and can be used to cross over the bifurcation. When they fail, pre-shaped selective catheters can be used. Some catheters have a slippery glide coating that improves trackability. Trackability enables a catheter to advance through tortuous anatomy without pulling the wire out of position. The combination of glide-coated wires and catheters enables traversal of almost any lesion. Catheters can also have markers for measuring, radiopaque tips for better visibility, and tapering ends for improved crossability.

Balloons

Balloons differ in diameter, length, material strength, compliance, shaft size, shoulders, profile, and coaxial versus mono-rail design. Balloon angioplasty causes a controlled injury to the

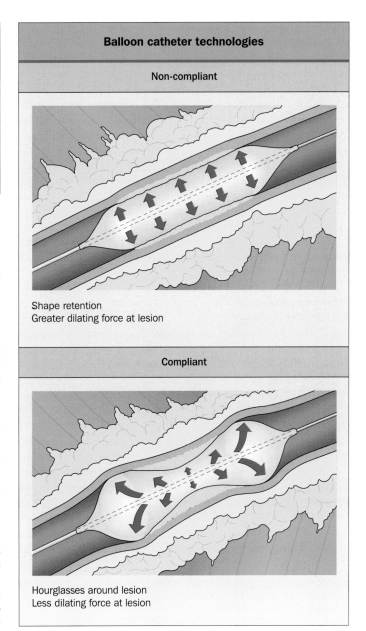

Balloon catheter technologies

Non-compliant

Shape retention
Greater dilating force at lesion

Compliant

Hourglasses around lesion
Less dilating force at lesion

Figure 11.3 Balloon catheter technologies.

vessel wall, producing localized dissection, plaque fracture, and medial/adventitial layer stretching. Dissections are usually non-flow limiting and are anticipated with concentric plaques. Eccentric plaque is more resistant, with expansion of the free wall accounting for improved luminal diameter. Stretching or disruption of the internal elastic lamina predisposes to intimal hyperplasia.[11]

Non-compliant balloons assume their intended diameter even at high pressures and are the mainstay for peripheral intervention. Non-compliant balloons inflate to pre-set diameters and pressures. Compliant balloons are prone to overstretching in areas of less plaque and do not exert equal forces without balloon distortion (**Fig. 11.3**). Some balloons are considered non-compliant at low pressures and then become compliant or enlarge further at higher pressures. This enables the operator to alter the final balloon size by adjusting the balloon pressure. Atherosclerotic lesions can typically be dilated at 8 atmospheres of pressure or less. Intimal hyperplasia requires higher pressure to compress and stretch. Most balloons are made of polypropylene, polyethylene, or nylon. Nylon is non-compliant, puncture resistant, and works well for stent delivery and postdilating. Compliant balloons should not be used for stent deployment. Smaller-profile balloons improve crossability. Upon deflation, most balloons do not rewrap to their predilation diameter, so distal lesions should be crossed and dilated first, followed by more proximal lesions. Monorail designs or 'rapid-exchange' technology has been extrapolated from coronary technology and applied in the periphery. These monorail systems allow the use of shorter wires, speeding up catheter exchange at the expense of pushability. Balloon inflation times vary according to operator preference. Maintaining the inflated balloon for 3–30min reduces the incidence of dissection and stent use, but does not improve the long-term patency of PTA compared with shorter inflation times.[12,13]

Pharmacotherapies
Antiplatelet agents
Adjunctive medications for endovascular procedures include antiplatelet therapy, anticoagulant therapy, and fibrinolytic therapy. All patients with PAD should receive long-term antiplatelet therapy and it should be started prior to the procedure. Antiplatelet agents including aspirin, ticlopidine, clopidogrel, dipyridamole, and picotamide have shown a statistically significant reduction in cardiovascular events.[14,15] These agents also improve patency after PTA and stenting. Aspirin has the most rapid onset of action (within minutes) and peak action (<30min), produces about 20% platelet inhibition, and its effects last 5–7 days. It is the most cost-effective antiplatelet agent and the most effective dosing regimen is 75–150mg/day.[14]

Ticlopidine and clopidogrel provide additive antiplatelet inhibition to aspirin up to 40%. This translates into a reduction of serious adverse events by 9% over aspirin alone.[16] Clopidogrel takes 5 days to reach peak activity with the daily dose of 75mg. Loading doses of 300–450mg reduce this to hours. The risk of significant neutropenia is higher with ticlopidine, so clopidogrel is preferred. Long-term use of clopidogrel in all PAD patients can be supported; however, cost may be the limiting factor.[15,17] Dipyridamole combined with aspirin produced no greater effect on vascular risk reduction than aspirin alone.[14] Picotamide, a thromboxane synthase inhibitor that is available only in Europe, is comparable to aspirin in reducing the risk of a cardiovascular event.[14]

Oral glycoprotein IIb/IIIa agents have not proved superior to aspirin alone in several clinical studies involving cardiovascular patients.[15] Intravenous glycoprotein (Gp) IIb/IIIa agents for peripheral intervention have been infrequently used. These agents at full dose suppress platelet activity by >80% and substantially reduce the risk of acute arterial closure at the time of intervention. These agents – abciximab (ReoPro; Centocor, Malvern, PA, USA), eptifibatide (Integrilin; Scering-Plough Corporation, San Francisco, CA, USA), and tirofiban hydrochloride (Aggrastat; Merck, Whitehouse Station, NJ, USA) – escalate bleeding risk at the catheter entry site over unfractionated heparin (UFH).[18] Abciximab, an antibody, binds non-competitively to the GpIIb/IIIa receptor site with high affinity. The drug therefore has a short plasma half-life but a prolonged receptor blockade. The drug dosing is unchanged by renal insufficiency and its

effects can be reversed with platelet infusion. Eptifibatide and tirofiban have low molecular weight, bind competitively to the GpIIb/IIIa receptor, and have a longer plasma half-life. They are excreted in the urine and dosing must be adjusted in patients with renal insufficiency. Their effects cannot be reversed with platelet infusions, but resolve with time. The cost:benefit ratio has not been studied in CLI interventions. Intravenous GpIIb/IIIa inhibitors should be considered for long SFA, popliteal, or tibial revascularizations that have a high risk of acute closure. The strategy to use full-dose GpIIb/IIIa inhibitor with reduced dose (one-half to one-quarter) fibrinolytic has shown promise for subacute thromboses.[19] Combination therapy has not reduced the lytic infusion time over monotherapy, so further safety data will be required to support widespread use.

Anticoagulant therapy
Anticoagulation should be used routinely for peripheral interventions. Standard bolus doses of UFH (60–80 units/kg) can elevate the activated clotting time (ACT) above 250s and are given after catheter insertion. This range minimizes the risk of peri-catheter/sheath thrombosis and allows for prolonged balloon inflation times. The heparin half-life of 60–90min coupled with its inexpense and low allergic risk make it the ideal anticoagulant. Newer agents such as low-molecular-weight heparin, bivalirudin (Angiomax), or recombinant hirudin (Refludin), can be helpful, particularly in patients sensitive to UFH. Bivalirudin, a direct thrombin inhibitor, has a shorter half-life and less platelet activation, but costs 10–20 times more than UFH. Refludin, another direct thrombin inhibitor, can be used in patients allergic to heparin. This drug provides better thrombus penetration than UFH and may complement fibrinolysis.

Fibrinolytic therapy
Fibrinolytic therapy – streptokinase, urokinase, tissue plasminogen activator (tPA), recombinant tPA (r-tPA), tenecteplase, staphylokinase – has been used clinically for patients with acute arterial occlusion and for the pretreatment of chronic lesions.[19–25] Chemical clearance of the main artery and small resistance vessels without further endothelial trauma can simplify treatment of the underlying lesion. Efficacy is limited by the age of the thrombus, drug delivery, and lack of flow through the occlusion. Systemic infusions are ineffective, requiring intra-thrombus catheter delivery. Other concerns of fibrinolytic therapy include a higher bleeding complication rate, drug expense, and prolonged ischemia time.[20,21] The feared complication of intracranial hemorrhage (ICH) occurs in up to 2.9% of intra-arterial catheter infusions and is associated with at least 78% mortality.[22] Specific risk factors for ICH include recent CVA or TIA (within 2–6 months), intracranial neoplasm, uncontrolled hypertension, and concomitant warfarin therapy. In such patients, fibrinolytic therapy should be avoided. The concomitant use of anticoagulation may contribute to bleeding risk; however, the safety margin produced with less than full dose (activated partial thromboplastin time 1.5–2 times control) heparin is unknown.[21]

Urokinase was used extensively in the USA until removal from the market in 1998. It was reintroduced in 2002. Typical doses range from 240 000 down to 60 000 units/hour and are infused from 4 to 36 hours.[19,20,22] The dose is usually tapered to the lower range, after 4 hours, after re-establishing flow with the higher doses. Urokinase directly activates plasminogen, is less antigenic, and poses a lower bleeding risk with greater efficacy, compared with streptokinase. Streptokinase is of historical interest only.

Tissue plasminogen activator has been used extensively for peripheral arterial thromboses in Europe.[23,24] The fibrin specificity of r-tPA does not spare the patient of a systemic fibrinolytic state with typical doses. Weight-based doses have varied from 0.025 to 0.1mg/kg/hour. Alternatively, non-weight-based doses of 0.25–10mg/hour have been used. When given at 2mg/hour, the fibrinogen level stays above 65% of baseline in 84% of patients, infrequently dropping below 50%.[23] The lytic response can be quite rapid (6 hours or less) when fixed doses above 5mg/hour are used.[24] The risk of ICH with this drug appears to be higher than with traditional urokinase infusions.[22] Total dose limitation to 0.9mg/kg or 100mg does not eliminate this risk even though the drug is infused in a slow continuous fashion. Current practice is to use 1 or 2mg/hour (fixed dose) limited to 24 hours.

Reteplase (Retavase), a direct plasminogen activator, appears to be safe and effective for arterial occlusions.[25] Empiric dosing with the drug has been 0.5 or 1.0U/hour. This drug has a longer half-life (18min) than r-tPA (4–5min). The bleeding risks associated with a slow continuous infusion of this drug are unknown. Some authors have used heparin quite sparingly with reteplase (100–500U/hour).[25] Reteplase activates platelets more intensely than Alteplase (r-tPA), so concomitant use with GpIIb/IIIa inhibitors may be helpful.

Exit strategies

Arteriotomy closure devices have influenced endovascular intervention. These devices promote prompt hemostasis, enabling early ambulation, and avoidance of anticoagulation interruption.[26] Because of closure devices there is less reservation to use large sheath sizes, and multiple or remote access sites. Some devices close the arteriotomy with suture (Perclose) or a collagen/disk sandwich (Angioseal). Others expedite the clotting process with extra-arterial collagen (Vasoseal) or thrombin (Duett). Routine use can be justified by early ambulation and prompt discharge while minimizing access site bleeding. The number of major groin complications is not lessened with closure devices. Major complications before closure devices of hematoma and pseudo-aneurysm have been replaced with infection, acute closure of the access site, and limb ischemia.[26] There is a learning curve to using each device and the development of tactile feel is required to produce consistently good results.

REVASCULARIZATION OPTIONS FOR AORTOILIAC DISEASE

The treatment of atherosclerotic aortoiliac disease has evolved from surgical endarterectomy to aortobifemoral bypass grafting to endovascular balloon angioplasty with stenting. Excellent results can be realized with each of these techniques in appropriately selected patients. Stenting has broadened the applicability of endovascular treatment to patients with iliac occlusions and those in need of concomitant infrainguinal bypass. Percutaneous endovascular therapy is typically advocated as the initial treatment option, reserving bypass surgery for treatment failures, patients with severe ischemia, and patients with extensive disease, particularly with lesions extending into the CFA.

Morphologic stratification of iliac lesions.
TASC-A iliac lesions
• Single stenosis of CIA or EIA (unilateral or bilateral) <3cm in length
TASC-B iliac lesions
• Single stenosis of iliac not involving CFA, 3–10cm in length
• Two stenoses of CIA or EIA not involving CFA, <5cm in length
• Unilateral CIA occlusion
TASC-C iliac lesions
• Bilateral stenoses of CIA and/or EIA not involving CFA, 5–10cm in length
• Unilateral EIA occlusion not involving CFA
• Unilateral EIA stenosis extending into CFA
• Bilateral CIA occlusion
TASC-D iliac lesions
• Extensive stenoses of entire CIA, EIA, and CFA, >10cm in length
• Unilateral occlusion of CIA and EIA
• Bilateral EIA occlusions
• Iliac stenosis adjacent to abdominal aortic or iliac aneurysm

Table 11.2 Morphologic stratification of iliac lesions.[5] CFA, common femoral artery; CIA, common iliac artery; EIA, external iliac artery.

Anatomic characteristics

The TASC document provides guidelines for the treatment of chronic arterial disease.[5] Atherosclerotic disease of the aortoiliac segment is categorized according to complexity. The morphologic stratification of iliac lesions is summarized in **Table 11.2**. As the complexity of the lesion increases, the preferred treatment shifts from percutaneous endovascular to open surgical techniques. For instance, focal short lesions of the aorta, common iliac artery, and proximal external iliac artery are considered the simplest and most amenable to endovascular revascularization (**Fig. 11.4**). Diffuse, extensive, complex, multilevel, occluded segments of the infrarenal abdominal aorta and iliac arteries are better suited to surgical treatment (**Fig. 11.5**). Many patients have disease that does not fall into either extreme. The treatment decision must take into account multiple factors, including life expectancy, age, co-morbid medical conditions, presumed procedural risk, previous procedures (bypass or PTA), and operator ability and experience.

When stenoses of the aorta, common iliac and external iliac are less than 3cm in length, the optimum procedure is PTA.[8] The aortoiliac segment should be treated initially in patients with multilevel disease.

TASC-A aortoiliac lesions
PTA

Early studies (pre-stent era prior to 1992) of aortoiliac PTA were typically performed for TASC-A lesions (**Fig. 11.4**).

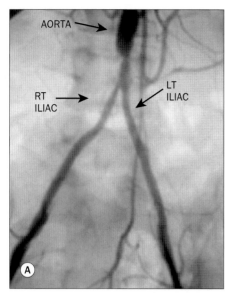

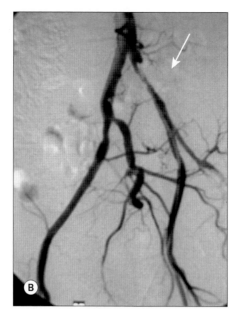

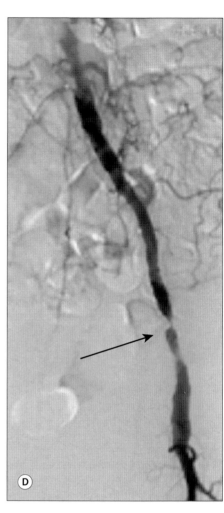

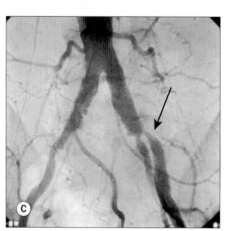

Figure 11.4 TASC-A lesions of the aortoiliac distribution: (A) aorta, (B) common iliac, (C) proximal external iliac, (D) distal external iliac artery without involvement of the common femoral artery.

Cumulative results of iliac PTA report primary patency rates varying from 67–92% at 1 year to 54–78% at 5 years of follow-up. The failure rate during the first year is thought to be 10%, with a late failure rate of 3% per year.[27] The patency rates associated with PTA of the common iliac artery are better than those associated with the external iliac artery by approximately 20%.[27,28] This trend is particularly evident in women, presumably due to their smaller-diameter vessels. Stand-alone PTA works well for focal lesions, except for lesions at the aortic bifurcation (which is really an extension of aortic plaque into the origin of the common iliac artery).[29] After PTA, this plaque is prone to elastic recoil.

In a non-randomized patient series, Laborde et al. noted that patients with diffuse disease (Type III = TASC C or D) had lower patency rates at 36 months (91.6% versus 60.1%, p<0.05) and higher complication rates (4% versus 11.5%, p<0.05) as compared with patients who had focal disease (Types I & II = TASC A or B).[30] When considering a non-specific series of aortoiliac patients treated with PTA only, occlusions seem to carry a higher initial technical failure rate (up to 27%).[5] Once successfully angioplastied, the 1-year primary patency rates were 60–94%. When initial failure rates are factored out of the patency rates, occlusions are similar to stenoses. The length of the lesion and patency of the ipsilateral SFA are thought to be the most significant predictors of primary patency.[31–37]

Complication rates are higher for occlusions (ranging from 3.1% to 10.6%) and are usually associated with access-site hemorrhage or pseudoaneurysm. Vessel rupture, symptomatic embolization, and/or flow-limiting dissections causing acute closure occur infrequently (<5%).[38,39] Distal embolization can occur from these lesions both before and after PTA. Using Doppler ultrasound, the occurrence of emboli is particularly frequent in the first 2 hours after PTA. The clinical significance of these embolic signals are unknown, since symptomatic distal emboli are infrequent.[40] The procedures can be performed on an outpatient basis with the use of arteriotomy closure devices.[41]

Iliac stents

The currently available stents are permanent and metal. Balloon-expandable stents are typically stainless-steel tubes. Self-expanding stents are made from stainless-steel mesh or nitinol. Nitinol, an alloy of nickel and titanium, has thermal

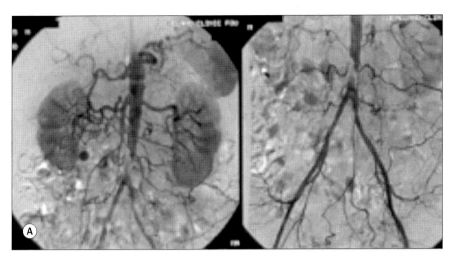

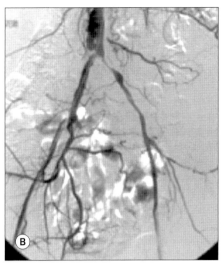

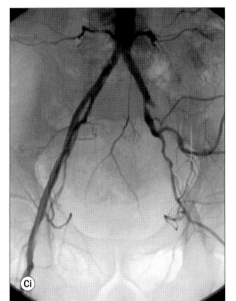

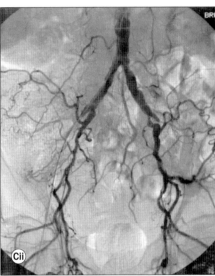

Figure 11.5 **TASC-C and TASC-D lesions of the aorta (A) and iliac arteries (B,C).**

memory and expands at normal body temperature. There is no ideal stent for aortoiliac intervention.[42] The self-expanding stents are usually longer and easy to deploy in contralateral lesions. Balloon-expanding stents foreshorten minimally and can be placed with a high degree of accuracy, and are particularly suited to aortic bifurcation lesions.[29] Restenosis rates are independent of the type of stent used.[8] Stents can limit recoil and maintain maximal luminal diameter.[29] Stents also reduce the pressure gradient at the lesion site, which is a strong determinant of favorable clinical outcome.[32] Stents have been reported to reduce the initial technical failure rate to 2–5%.[31] Controversy remains as to the appropriate threshold to warrant stent placement. Examining different reported thresholds (5 or 10mmHg difference in peak systolic pressure or mean pressure) shows that secondary stent placement would be indicated in 4% to 87% of cases.[33]

Maximizing stent deployment can be achieved with the use of intravascular ultrasound (IVUS). Incomplete deployment of balloon-expandable stents, which was not appreciated with conventional arteriography, can be seen in 27% of stents or 45%

of patients.[43] In a study by Buckley and colleagues,[44] the patency of iliac stenting was improved from 69% to 100% (p<0.001) at 6-month follow-up when using IVUS rather than an arteriographic endpoint. Secondary intervention was also drastically reduced from 23% (five of 22 patients) to 0% (p<0.05). IVUS better defined the diameter endpoint after stent deployment, by altering the post-dilation balloon size, since underdeployment was the most frequent IVUS finding.

The Dutch Iliac Stent Trial compared PTA with direct stent placement versus primary PTA with selective stent placement.[34] Selective stenting was necessary in 43% of patients due to a residual systolic pressure gradient of 10mmHg or more. There were 12 patients with short segment occlusions (TASC B), ten of which required stenting. These patients had intermittent claudication and not CLI. The primary technical and hemodynamic success rate was 97%. The clinical success rates were the same in each group (76% versus 78%) at 2-year follow-up. Hemodynamic success (as noted with ABIs) was 85% in both groups. Patency rates (as determined with color duplex) were 71% in the direct-stent group versus 70% in the selective-stent

135

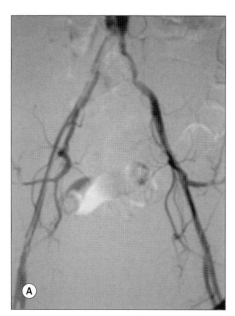 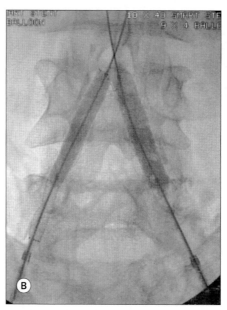 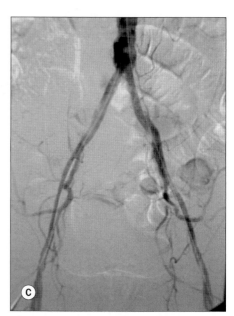

Figure 11.6 TASC-B aortoiliac lesions. Arteriogram of symmetrical common iliac artery stenoses (TASC B) (A). S/P percutaneous transluminal angioplasty with primary stenting using the kissing balloon technique (B,C).

group. The reintervention rates were 7% and 4%, respectively. Quality of life improved significantly after intervention (p<0.05). Complications (4% direct stent, 7% selective stent) were typically associated with the percutaneous access site. Surgical intervention was necessary in only two patients. Overall, this study provides supportive data for the safety and efficacy of endovascular treatment of focal lesions. Furthermore, selective stenting was equivalent to direct stenting for these lesions. Selective stenting for TASC-A lesions seems cost-effective as long as the reintervention rates are low. Exceptions to this may be the patient with extremely calcified marble-like atheroma that angioplasty and stents cannot displace.

TASC-B and TASC-C aortoiliac lesions
These stenotic lesions are between 3 and 10cm in length and may extend into the CFA (**Table 11.2, Figs 11.6 & 11.7**). Occlusions are shorter and do not involve the entire iliac segment (common or external iliac artery) as in TASC-D lesions (**Fig. 11.8**).

PTA/Stenting
A meta-analysis comparing the results of PTA with/without stenting for aortoiliac disease found that regardless of lesion type, direct stenting improved primary patency by 10%. Direct stenting also reduced the late failure rate by 39%.[5] In a clinical retrospective study in 288 patients, a patency rate of 84% at 24 months was seen with direct stenting.[31] Claudication was the indication in 72% of cases, with external iliac involvement in 30%. Multiple segments were treated in 56% of patients. The reintervention rate was only 5.6%, with subsequent surgical intervention in 3.8%. Factors associated with initial success included the need for multiple stents, a higher degree of stenosis, a lower severity of baseline ischemia, younger age, and the pre-procedural patency of the ipsilateral SFA. Late success was influenced favorably by SFA patency and a higher degree of initial stenosis. Although it was not statistically significant, external iliac artery intervention was less durable than common

iliac artery intervention.[31] Lee et al. have shown that the strategy of direct stenting improves primary patency and lowers reintervention rates for external iliac lesions.[45]

Powell and colleagues studied the effectiveness of endovascular treatment of multi-segment iliac occlusive disease.[46,47] They reviewed the treatment of 207 iliac artery segments in 87 patients. Stents were used selectively in 56% of the segments. The indications were claudication in 60% and CLI in 40%. All patients had at least two iliac segments treated, with initial hemodynamic success in 72%. Symptoms resolved in 88%, with a complication rate of 11%. Endovascular reintervention was performed in 29% and subsequent surgical intervention in 14%. The primary and primary-assisted patency rate at 12 months was 61% and 87%, and at 36 months was 43% and 72%, respectively. Durability was negatively affected by external iliac artery involvement, reducing the patency rates by half. External iliac artery lesions were three times more likely to require reintervention, since recurrent stenosis occurred at the previous treatment site most often (75%).[47] Direct rather than selective stenting of external iliac artery lesions may be a more appropriate strategy.

There are no randomized trials comparing surgical and endovascular procedures to determine the 'best' approach for patients with TASC-B and TASC-C lesions. If angioplasty with direct stenting is technically feasible, then it should be considered for the initial procedure for patients with CLI.

Stenting prior to infrainguinal bypass
Timaran et al. have shown that PTA with stenting of iliac inflow disease is effective at maintaining the patency of infrainguinal bypass grafts.[48] They compared the patency rates of infrainguinal bypass in patients who had previously undergone PTA alone, PTA with stenting, or aortobifemoral bypass. The 5-year patency rates were 46%, 68%, and 61%, respectively (p=0.02). The strategy of PTA with stenting, rather than aortobifemoral bypass, prior to infrainguinal bypass reduces the cumulative

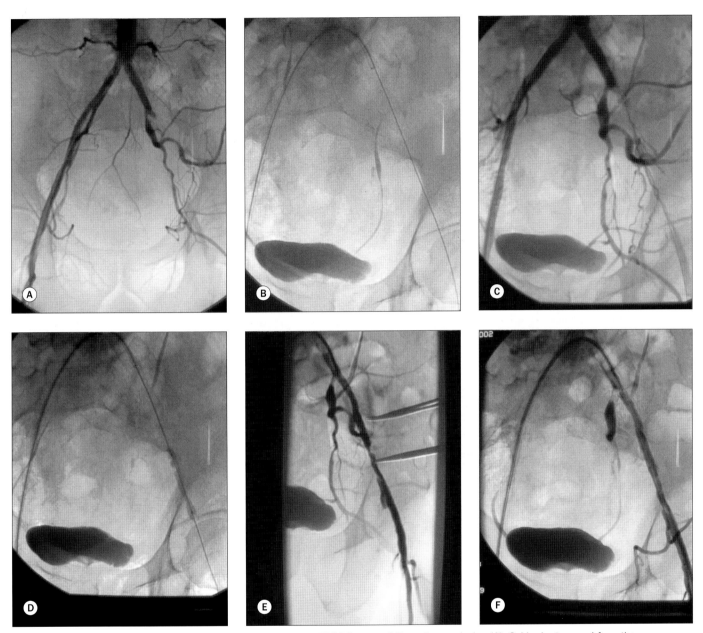

Figure 11.7 TASC-C aortoiliac lesions. Pelvic arteriogram showing TASC-C external iliac artery occlusion (A). Guidewire traversal from the contralateral approach (B) with contrast confirmation of luminal position (C). Distal external iliac artery (EIA) percutaneous transluminal angioplasty (PTA) (D) with residual stenosis in the EIA (E). S/P stent in EIA (F).

procedural morbidity and mortality in patients with multilevel disease. Direct stenting rather than selective stenting is supported by these data. Angioplasty and stenting of an ipsilateral iliac stenosis as inflow for a femoral-femoral graft is an acceptable option in poor-risk patients with a contralateral iliac occlusion.[49] SFA patency (~50% of patients) enhances the durability of crossover grafts.

TASC-D aortoiliac lesions

Extensive disease of the entire aortoiliac segment or lesions associated with aneurysmal disease fall into this category (**Table 11.2, Figs 11.8 & 11.9**). In good surgical candidates, aortobifemoral bypass is preferred. In poor surgical candidates, extra-anatomic bypass has been the treatment. Data regarding endovascular treatment of these lesions have been limited; most studies do

not include TASC-D lesions. Treatment with stand-alone PTA often leaves a residual pressure gradient, limiting hemodynamic success. Direct stenting typically requires multiple stents, escalating costs and increasing the likelihood of restenosis. Alternative strategies include pretreatment with thrombolytic therapy, laser-assisted angioplasty, or the use of covered stents.

Covered stents

Covered stents have the theoretical advantage of excluding the diseased segment. The covering can trap atheroma and thrombus, preventing further debris, while maintaining luminal diameter, although the data supporting their use are scant. They have been successfully employed to treat isolated iliac artery aneurysms, dissections, and traumatic iliac artery perforations.[50,51] Covered stents comprise either stainless-steel or nitinol

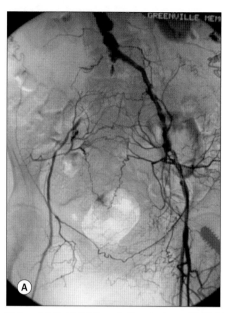
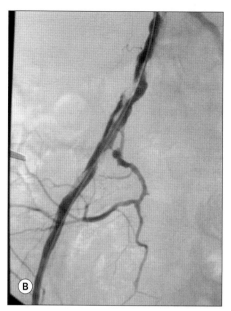
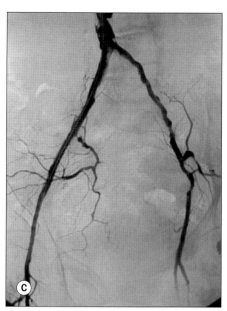

Figure 11.8 TASC-D aortoiliac lesions. (A) TASC-D lesion in a patient with diffuse aortoiliac disease and an occluded superficial femoral artery. (B) Percutaneous transluminal angioplasty induced dissection of the right common iliac artery. (C) Stenting of the common and external iliac artery. Note, the asymptomatic left iliac was not treated, to simplify the procedure.

stents covered with Dacron or polytetrafluoroethylene (PTFE) (**Table 11.3**). The Hemobahn (Viabahn in the USA; WL Gore & Associates, Flagstaff, AZ, USA) endoprosthesis is a flexible, self-expanding, endoluminal prosthesis made of an expanded PTFE (ePTFE) tube inside a nitinol, sinusoidally shaped, helically wrapped stent. The prosthesis does not shorten during expansion. Results of an international study using the Hemobahn for iliac occlusive disease were excellent.[52] Sixty-one limbs in 53 patients were treated, either in the common (n=32) or external iliac (n=29) artery. Only 7% of lesions were longer than 10cm, the rest being TASC C or less. The primary and secondary patency rates at 12 months were 91% and 95%, respectively. The overall complication rate was 17%; major complications were only 2.1%. Two embolic events and one occlusion occurred and were treated successfully with fibrino-

lytic therapy. One major and one minor infection occurred. Fever and local pain were not observed in this study; in contrast, these have been seen with the Cragg EndoPro System 1 (Minimally Invasive Technologies, La Ciotat, France) in 26% of patients.[53,54] The Cragg EndoPro System 1 is a polyester-covered stent-graft that is no longer available. The Wallgraft (Boston Scientific, Boston, MA, USA), a Dacron-covered wire-mesh stent, demonstrates early patency at least as high as non-covered stents, especially with large vessels. Preliminary results show 92% patency at 12 months,[55] but long-term data have not been published. Theoretically, in-stent restenosis should be reduced, but it remains to be seen how the long-term results will compare against those achieved with non-covered stents and with aortobifemoral bypass. The thrombosis rate of covered stents is high in the SFA, less so in the iliac artery. Stent-graft diameter (<7mm) and lesion length (>10cm) seem to be important variables for thrombosis.[52–54] Long-term anticoagulation is advocated for SFA use, but antiplatelet therapy is adequate for iliac use.

Thrombolysis, thrombectomy, or laser
Most occlusions of the aortoiliac segment are thrombus-dominant rather than plaque-dominant. Removal of chronic thrombus prior to PTA may lower the risk of embolization. This also simplifies the lesion, allowing direct treatment of the underlying stenosis with PTA with/without stenting.[56] Guidewire traversal provides some insight regarding the use of thrombolysis, thrombectomy, or laser for occlusions of uncertain duration.[57] Thrombus of recent organization is easy to cross and lyse, whereas more-aged thrombus is firm and adherent to the arterial wall, and more resistant to thrombolysis or thrombectomy (**Fig. 11.9**). Thrombolysis increases procedural time and bleeding risk.[58] Laser-light energy has been shown to ablate chronic thrombus.[59] The channel through the occlusion is larger than the catheter itself with thrombus removal. Recanalization

Covered stents for complex lesions.	
Stent-graft	*Description*
Wallgraft (Boston Scientific)	Wallstent with Dacron covering
Corvita (Boston Scientific)	Nitinol with PTFE
Hemobahn (now Viabahn) (WL Gore & Associates)	Nitinol with PTFE
AneuRx (Medtronic)	Nitinol with Dacron
Precedent (Boston Scientific)	Nitinol with PTFE
aSpire (VA)	Helical flat wire; nitinol with PTFE (Partly covered)
Jostent (Jomed)	Balloon-expandable steel with PTFE

Table 11.3 Covered stents for complex lesions.
PET, polyethyleneterephthalate; PTFE, polytetrafluoroethylene.

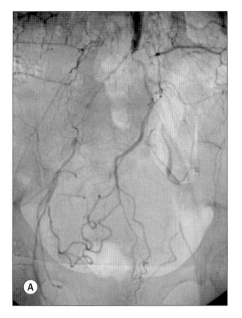

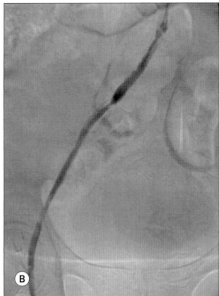

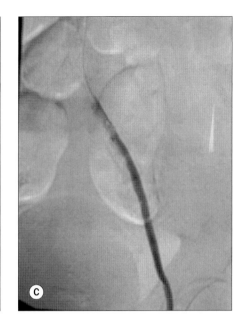

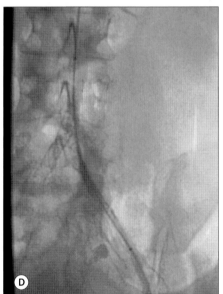

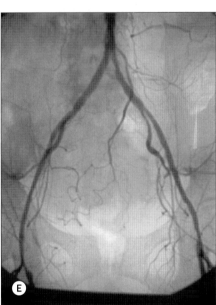

Figure 11.9 Aortic occlusion with thrombus in both common and external iliac arteries (A). POSSIS catheter thrombectomy of each iliac limb (B,C) followed by catheter-directed fibrinolysis in aorta and left iliac limb (D). Completion arteriogram (E) after overnight infusion of Retavase.

of plaque-dominant occlusions leaves a channel the size of the catheter. Subsequent PTA and stenting is required. Thermal injury to the vessel is avoided with the use of pulsed laser light (Excimer; Spectranetics, Colorado Springs, CO, USA). The safety and efficacy of this approach remains to be determined. Each of these modalities will be discussed more fully in the next section on femoropopliteal disease.

REVASCULARIZATION OPTIONS FOR FEMOROPOPLITEAL DISEASE

Femoropopliteal disease is more common than iliac disease and is the most common site of peripheral arterial involvement.[60,61] The atherosclerotic plaque can involve the entire 30cm artery or it can be focal and discrete, illustrating the heterogeneity of lesions (**Figs 11.10–11.14**). Stenoses of the SFA are typically short, with 79% less than 5cm, whereas occlusions are rarely less

than 5cm (9%).[62] In-situ thrombosis converts atherosclerotic stenoses into occlusions. Often, the anatomy of the contralateral limb may provide a comparative basis as to the extent of atherosclerotic plaque since disease is often symmetrical (**Fig. 11.12**). This distinction is pivotal for endovascular intervention since procedure can be modified to treat the thrombus and/or plaque specifically.

Endovascular techniques spare autologous saphenous vein, can be done with local anesthesia, and minimize inpatient hospitalization and the need for outpatient extra-care facilities. PTA carries a lower procedural risk than surgery, with less durability. Early failure of PTA merely leaves the patient with unresolved limb ischemia without precluding surgical options. It rarely increases the risk of limb loss above the heightened risk associated with the disease condition. Late failure does not necessarily result in a return of the patient's original symptoms since clinical benefit outpaces patency.[63]

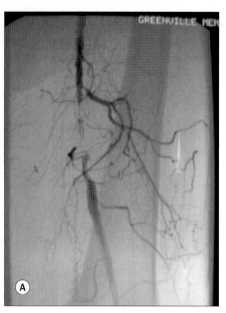
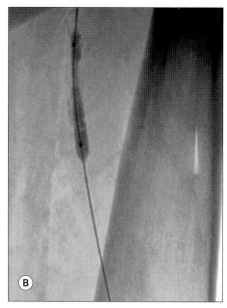
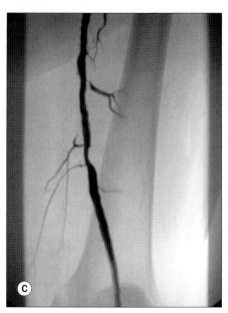

Figure 11.10 TASC-C lesion. TASC-C lesion of the left superficial femoral artery (A) treated with percutaneous tranluminal angioplasty (B), and completion arteriogram with mild residual stenosis not stented (C).The patient has venous insufficiency, weighs 350 pounds, and has a non-healing ulceration on the lower leg of mixed arteriovenous origin.

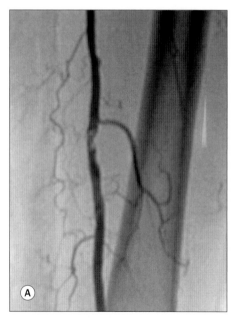
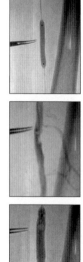
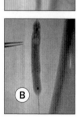
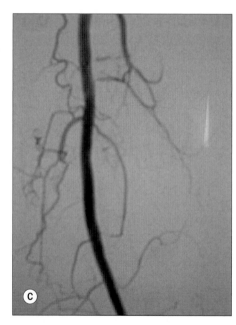

Figure 11.11 Ischemic toes due to thromboemboli from a left superficial femoral artery lesion (A). The resting ankle–brachial index (ABI) was 0.87, with palpable pulses. Treated with percutaneous transluminal angioplasty (B), eccentric residual stenosis prompted a short self-expanding stent (B,C).

In CLI patients, direct flow into the foot needs to be established, so tibial intervention may also be necessary (**Figs 11.15–11.17**). Concomitant treatment of tibial disease may also increase the durability of SFA angioplasty.[64] Early failure of PTA is predicated on the length of the lesion while runoff integrity predicts long-term success.

Anatomic considerations

There is no universal definition for 'short' or 'long' SFA lesions (**Table 11.4**). Long lesions have been arbitrarily defined as greater than 5, 7, or even 10cm in length. Conversely, lesions less than 5, 7, or 10cm have been designated as short. Long lesions (whether defined as greater than 5, 7, or 10cm) treated endovascularly have less durability with PTA.[48–51] Since there is

little procedural difference with lesions less than 5cm, the treatment of short lesions (TASC A–C) will be discussed collectively and long lesions (>5–10cm, TASC D) will be discussed separately (**Figs 11.14 & 11.15**).

TASC-A, TASC-B and TASC-C femoropopliteal lesions
Technique

Irrespective of stenosis or occlusion, high initial technical success rates can be achieved with current technology for short lesions. The use of 'glide' wires allows the traversal of virtually any occlusion. The wire shape and resistance as it traverses the lesion, coupled with the contour of the balloon on inflation, distinguishes an intimal from subintimal traversal. Intimal traversal uses the tip of the wire to steer through the occlusion.

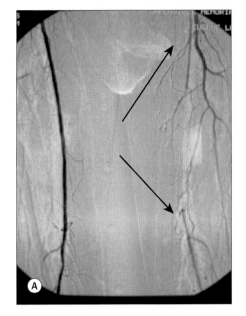

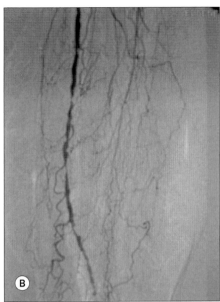

Figure 11.12 Atherosclerotic plaque.
(A) Thrombus-dominant left superficial femoral artery (SFA) occlusion using the right SFA as comparison. The size of the SFA proximal or distal to the occlusion is small due to lack of perfusion and improves with revascularization. (B) Plaque-dominant left SFA.

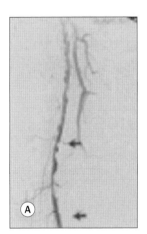

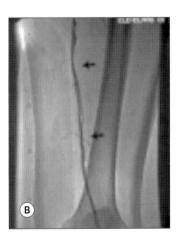

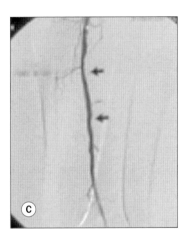

Figure 11.13 Diffuse atherosclerosis of the left superficial femoral artery (A) treated with balloon angioplasty (B). Dissection occurred in the area of greatest plaque burden and was treated with stent (C). The pressure gradients between the arrows were 40mmHg (A), 22mmHg (B), and 6mmHg (C).

The balloon will have a 'waist' at the site of atherosclerotic plaque. Subintimal traversal pushes a loop of the wire under the plaque proximally and re-enters the true lumen distal to the plaque. The balloon will be smooth in contour on inflation without the 'waist' of the plaque. Subintimal traversal, even unintentional, occurs commonly when crossing occlusions.

PTA

Most femoropopliteal studies are composed of patients with claudication rather than CLI. In general, PTA of lesions <5cm in length has a patency of 59–93% at 1 year.[64–71] In a population of CLI patients, SFA patency was 78% at 3 years after PTA in lesions <5cm when two or three tibial vessels were patent versus 25% when none or one tibial vessel was patent, emphasizing the importance of patent tibial vessels.[65] Occlusions had a lower patency rate than stenoses (31% versus 61%) at 5 years, when the initial technical success rate was included. Analysis after exclusion of these initial technical failures showed that the durability was unchanged by the presence of an occlusion.

Blair et al. conducted a retrospective study comparing PTA with bypass surgery in CLI patients.[66] Clinical improvement was seen in 72% (39/54) of PTA patients, with a limb salvage of 78%. Bypass surgery patency was 68% at 2 years, with a limb salvage of 90%. Hemodynamic benefit was better with bypass but limb salvage rates were not statistically different. Reintervention rates were higher with PTA as compared with bypass surgery. This study supports the contention that despite late restenosis of the PTA-treated patients, the clinical impact on limb salvage is not substantially different. Lofberg et al. evaluated the results of femoropopliteal PTA in 92 patients with CLI.[67] The technical success rate was 88%, with primary patency of 32% for lesions <5cm. Limb salvage was 86%, and survival only 51%, at 5 years. Jamsen et al. reported on 100 consecutive CLI patients treated with femoropopliteal PTA.[68] Lifelong follow-up of each patient revealed that 32 patients underwent repeat PTA, 11 surgical revascularization, and 51 (37 major) amputations. Limb salvage was 65%, 60%, and 60%, at 3, 5, and 8 years, while survival rates were 41%, 26%, and 16%, respectively. This high mortality rate, secondary to cardiovascular causes, makes endovascular therapy appealing for TASC A–C lesions even if secondary procedures are necessary.

Unsuccessful PTA occurs secondary to eccentric stenoses, extensive dissection, acute thrombosis, perforation, atheroemboli, or significant residual stenosis. Acute closure due to dissection

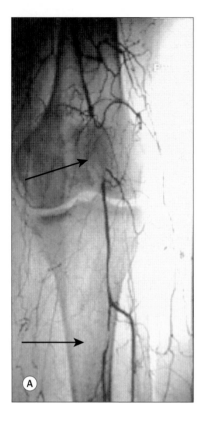

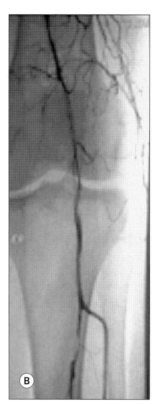

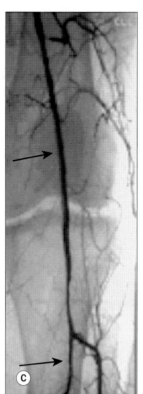

Figure 11.14 Femoropopliteal disease.
(A) Arteriogram of left popliteal artery and tibioperoneal trunk occlusions. (B) Excimer laser atherectomy of popliteal occlusion. (C) Completion arteriogram after percutaneous transluminal angioplasty of popliteal and tibioperoneal trunk.

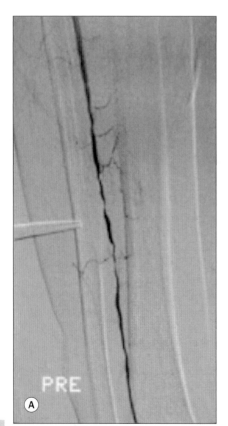

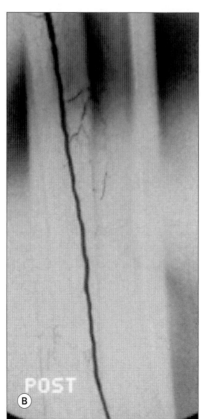

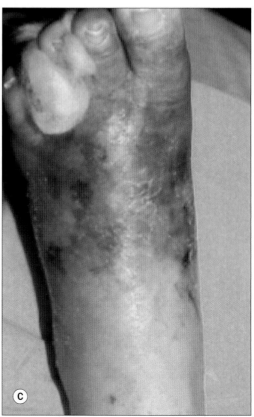

Figure 11.15 Tibial intervention. (A) Arteriogram of isolated anterior tibial artery with diffuse atherosclerosis. (B) Treated with rotational atherectomy. (C) Trash foot from emboli with atherectomy.

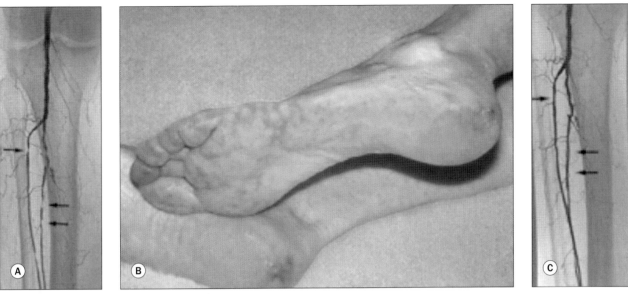

Figure 11.16 Isolated tibial artery disease in a diabetic with ischemic ulceration atheroemboli (A,B) treated with stand-alone Excimer laser (C).

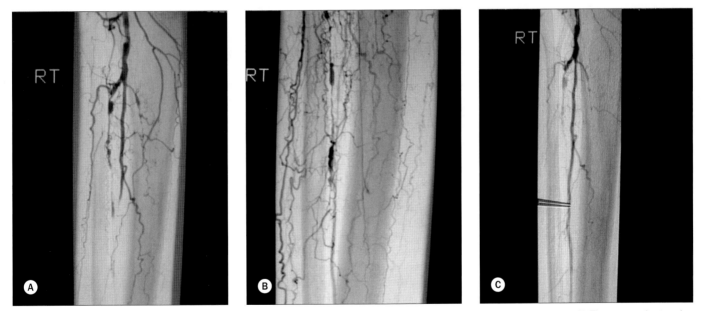

Figure 11.17 Tibial intervention. (A) Tibial occlusions in a patient with no autologous vein for femoperoneal artery bypass. (B) The peroneal artery is shown to be patent distally. (C) Final arteriogram after percutaneous transluminal angioplasty of the tibio-peroneal trunk and peroneal artery. Reestablishment of inline flow to the foot was achieved.

and/or thrombosis can occur in 4–7%.[69] An important endpoint after intervention is the re-establishment of brisk pedal pulses. This physical examination finding corresponds to improved ABIs and volume flow. The restenosis rate at 12 months is significantly lower (24% versus 64%) when the 24-hour post-interventional ABI is greater than 0.9.[70] Restenosis or recoil occurs within 3 months of the procedure and is not intimal hyperplasia. Restenosis within the first year is usually due to intimal hyperplasia and recoil. Restenosis occurs in 35–50% of non-iliac peripheral arterial angioplasties within the first year.[71]

Short-segment stents

Both balloon-expandable and self-expanding stents have been used in the SFA, mainly to treat claudication patients. Balloon-

expandable stents can be deformed by trauma or external compression, making self-expanding stents the prefered option.[72] Stents can be placed at the time of successful angioplasty (direct or primary stenting) or with failed angioplasty (secondary stenting) (**Fig. 11.11**). Three randomized trials in patients with short femoropopliteal lesions have shown no improvement in long-term success after primary stent placement as compared with PTA alone. Two of these trials were small and compared PTA with PTA and balloon-expandable stents. They showed a 1-year PTA patency of 63–85% compared with 62–63% with stenting.[73,74] The largest randomized trial of PTA versus PTA/stent, using the Vascucoil (Intratherapeutics, MN, USA), consisted of 267 patients with 368 lesions. The mean lesion length was 3.5cm. Acute angiographic success rates were 94%

Morphological stratification of superficial femoral and popliteal artery lesions.
TASC-A femoropopliteal lesions
• Single, focal stenosis <3cm in length
TASC-B femoropopliteal lesions
• Single SFA stenosis 3–10cm in length
• Heavily calcified or multiple stenoses <3cm in length
TASC-C femoropopliteal lesions
• Single stenosis or occlusion >5cm in length
• Multiple stenoses, each 3–5cm in length
TASC-D femoropopliteal lesions
• Occlusion of entire SFA or popliteal artery

Table 11.4 Morphological stratification of superficial femoral and popliteal artery lesions.[5] SFA, superficial femoral artery.

with PTA and 98% with PTA/stent. Restenosis rates at 9 months were 43% with PTA versus 46% with PTA/stent. The complication rates were higher in the PTA group (8.4%) as compared with the stent group (1.5%) (Rosenfield K, personal communication). Based upon these data, the Food and Drug Administration (FDA) approved the use of these stents for failed angioplasty (secondary stenting). There was no statistical difference to advocate the use of primary stenting for short-segment SFA lesions. Cost-effectiveness analysis also suggests that these favorable lesions should initially be treated with PTA.[75,76]

The shear force of blood flow through the SFA is different than that for the larger iliac arteries. This heightens the risk of acute thrombosis with SFA stents. Rousseau et al. reported an acute thrombosis rate of 25% and suggested that anticoagulation was necessary when self-expanding stents were used in the SFA.[77] Do-Dai-Do et al. confirmed this risk with three early thromboses in patients not treated with warfarin.[78] In contrast, White et al. treated short-segment SFA disease without warfarin and noted only two of 32 cases thrombosed within 30 days.[79] Therefore, for short lesions, antiplatelet agents (aspirin and clopidogrel) may suffice, whereas long lesions should receive anticoagulation as well.

Since the restenosis rate is substantial, routine non-invasive laboratory testing should be performed. This is particularly true during the first year. We suggest routine duplex ultrasound surveillance every 3 months for the first year and then twice-yearly thereafter. Not all patients with restenosis will require reintervention, since the clinical benefit not infrequently outlasts the anatomic patency.[63]

Atherectomy

Atherectomy catheters, either rotational or directional, are designed to remove plaque. This debulking strategy, used as a stand-alone procedure or concomitantly with PTA, has not improved upon the results of PTA alone.[80–83] Directional atherectomy (i.e. Simpson Atherocath, DVI, Redwood, CA, USA) consists of a circular cutting blade that excises plaque when pressed against the diseased side of the arterial wall with an inflated balloon on the back side of the catheter. The retained tissue samples are removed, debulking the lesion, and can be evaluated histologically. The depth of cutting with this device is difficult to control, often debulking to the media, which increases the risk of intimal hyperplasia. Restenosis rates at 6 months range from 15% to 65%.[80,81] This technique is more time-consuming than PTA, requires a larger sheath, cannot remove heavily calcified plaque, and must be done ipsilateral to the lesion. These disadvantages have limited the use of atherectomy to removal of eccentric short focal lesions or retained valve cusps.

The Transluminal Extraction Catheter (TEC; Interventional Technologies, San Diego, CA, USA) and Rotablator (Heart Technologies, Redmond, WA, USA) are examples of rotational atherectomy devices. A sharp cutting blade (TEC) or diamond-studded metal tip (Rotablator) spins rapidly, shaving atheroma from the vessel wall as it passes over a guidewire. The TEC device aspirates the debris, while the Rotablator sends it distally. The new channel is only as large as the catheter itself, requiring ancillary PTA. Thirty to forty percent of initially successful procedures fail within the first 6 months, limiting the enthusiasm for debulking.[82] TEC is most effective in removing soft or thrombus-containing occlusions. Currently, there is no niche role for rotational atherectomy in treating SFA disease. Three other atherectomy devices are under study: the Pullback atherectomy catheter, the Redha-Cut catheter, and the Xtrak device. The clinical utility of these has yet to be shown.[83]

TASC-D femoropopliteal lesions
Long-segment SFA PTA

Patients with CLI are frequently found to have long-segment occlusions of the SFA. Many are unsuitable for open bypass surgery because of medical co-morbidities. Stand-alone PTA for long SFA lesions has a high incidence of restenosis. Primary patency rates from 23% at 6 months to 69% at 18 months in lesions <10cm have been reported.[84,85] Matsi et al. reported rates of 56% in lesions <15cm and 23% in lesions >15cm at 1 year.[86] Strategies to improve these results have included intentional subintimal angioplasty, laser-assisted angioplasty, fibrinolytic therapy, stents, drug-eluting stents, stent-grafts, and adjunctive brachytherapy.

Bolia and Bell advocate intentional subintimal angioplasty for these lesions. They reported an initial technical success of 80% in 200 patients (mean lesion length 11.5cm, range 2–37cm).[87] Life table analysis excluding technical failures revealed primary patency rates of 71% and 58% at 1 and 3 years, respectively. There were two major (1%) and 13 minor (6.5%) complications, with a 30-day mortality rate of 1.5%. These results are impressive. However, this technique may not be unique to this study. Unintentional subintimal traversals of SFA occlusions are common and probably make up a significant portion of occlusive lesions treated with endovascular methods.

Laser-assisted angioplasty has had a resurgence since technical improvements of pulsed (rather than continuous) light; use in a saline medium, and slow, gradual progression through the lesion. The use of pulsed light allows the heat to dissipate, minimizing thermal injury seen with earlier-generation lasers. Performing the laser procedure with continuous saline infusion limits dissections caused by acoustic trauma induced in contrast or blood. Excimer-laser (308nm) light resolves chronic thrombus and some plaque without producing thermal injury. PTA after laser therapy can produce an excellent channel without a stent (**Fig. 11.14**). Laser-assisted angioplasty was performed in 411 patients with SFA occlusions averaging 19.5cm in length.[88] The initial technical success rate was 83% from the contralateral approach, but improved to 93% when a second access site (ipsilateral or popliteal) was used. The primary, primary-assisted, and secondary patency rates were 33%, 65%, and 75%, respectively. Stents were used in only 7.3% of patients. Restenosis usually occurred in a focal area, predictably at the site of greatest plaque burden. Repeat PTA or PTA with spot stenting was used for secondary intervention, producing high secondary patency rates. Acute reocclusion, perforation, distal thrombosis or embolization occurred in only 7.1%. This study highlights the benefit of laser assistance to simplify long occlusions by removing coexistent thrombus prior to PTA. Secondary procedures are common but lead to reasonable results in these long lesions.

Fibrinolytic therapy can also simplify occlusions by conversion into stenoses. The Surgery versus Thrombolysis for Ischemia of the Lower Extremity (STILE) trial compared r-tPA, urokinase, and primary surgical treatment for patients with lower limb ischemia of less than 6 months duration.[56] The study was terminated early, after 393 of a planned 1000 patients had been randomized. There was a significant incidence of ongoing/recurrent ischemia in the thrombolysis patients (45% versus 24%, p<0.001). These chronic occlusions were more difficult to traverse, leading to initial technical failure in 28%. This occurred more frequently in bypass grafts (41%) as compared with native arteries (22%). Recombinant tPA achieved arterial patency more rapidly than urokinase (8 hours versus 24 hours, p<0.05); however, the regimens were equally efficacious. Heparin was infused concomitantly (~500–1000U/hour). Hospital stay was shorter for lysis patients (10 days versus 14 days, p=0.04). Lysis reduced the magnitude of the subsequent surgical procedure in 56% of patients. Patients with more chronic ischemia (>14 days) required fewer amputations with surgery (10% versus 18%, p=0.08). Survival was not different in the overall treatment categories except in diabetics treated with lysis (94% versus 68%, p=0.014). Consequently, fibrinolytic therapy for chronic SFA disease has been limited to treating embolic complications after PTA.

Bare stents
Self-expandable stents that have been used in the SFA include the Wallstent, Symphony, Memotherm, SMART (shape memory alloy recoverable technology), Vascucoil, and Protégé. The Wallstent (Meditech, Boston Scientific, Boston, MA, USA) is a flexible, multistrand metal mesh that is self-expandable when unconstrained. It has to foreshorten to fully expand, making precise deployment and wall apposition difficult. Nitinol (nickel–titanium alloy) stents expand at body temperature and exert more radial force than the Wallstent. They do not foreshorten significantly and more consistently appose the arterial wall. They are the preferred stent when angioplasty fails. These stents cross the lesion easily even with a contralateral approach. Most should be sized 1mm larger than the dilating balloon: exceptions include the Vascucoil, which should not be over-

sized, particularly in a heavily diseased artery. Slow deployment allows more complete expansion. Post-dilating with a short-length balloon (not one that covers the entire length of the stent) improves wall apposition and also helps to avoid unnecessary angioplasty outside the stent.

Stenting of these long lesions improves initial technical success but fails to improve the long-term durability (**Figs 11.11 & 11.12**).[89–93] In two studies with stents covering lesions greater than 10cm, the restenosis rate at 12 months was 39–43%.[63,90] Occlusions have a higher restenosis rate than stenoses (38% versus 10%) at 12 months.[94] Restenosis occurs in flexible or rigid stent types and is more likely to occur with multiple stents. Henry et al. reported a restenosis rate of 33% when more than four Palmaz stents were placed in the SFA as compared with 4% with a single stent.[95] They also noted restenosis to be more prominent in the distal SFA as compared with the proximal two-thirds (4% versus 18%). This variable is difficult to assess independently since longer lesions are treated with more stents and lesion length is a strong negative predictor. Patency is consistently better in patients with claudication compared with those with CLI.

Drug-eluting stents
Drug-eluting stents have the potential to revolutionize the treatment of long-SFA disease if the early reports from the SIRROCO trial hold up. In this small, randomized European study of 36 patients, the mean lesion length was over 8cm, making this a high-risk group for restenosis. Randomization was between a bare SMART stent (Cordis, Johnson & Johnson, Miami, FL, USA) and a SMART stent coated with sirolimus (rapamycin). There was no restenosis at 6 months in the sirolimus-eluting stent group, compared with 23% in the bare-stent group.[96] The stent minimizes elastic recoil and negative remodeling while the drug coating inhibits the development of intimal hyperplasia. Many other coated stents will be forthcoming.

Covered stents
Stent-grafts have been used in the femoropopliteal distribution. The different types were outlined in the iliac section (**Table 11.3**). The Dacron-covered nitinol stent (Cragg EndoPro System 1) has performed poorly.[53,97] Early thrombosis was seen in 17%, post-implantation pain and fever in 40%, and late failure in 83%.[97] The Hemobahn (Viabahn) PTFE/nitinol stent-graft has less thrombotic events, less post-implantation symptoms, and better patency rates.[52,98] The 1-year primary patency was 73–79% and secondary patency was 83–93%. The PTFE endograft seems to inhibit intimal hyperplasia and has less thrombogenicity than Dacron. The stent prevents negative remodeling and may offer a distinct advantage over bare stenting for long SFA lesions.

Brachytherapy
Endovascular brachytherapy may be a promising treatment after PTA, to prevent restenosis. The Peripheral Artery Radiation Investigational Study (PARIS) used an iridium-192 gamma-radiation source with a prescribed dose of 14Gy in 40 patients with SFA lesions averaging almost 10cm in length.[99] The angiographic restenosis rate at 6 months was 17% and the clinical restenosis rate at 12 months was 13%. This study supports the use of brachytherapy after PTA. Brachytherapy has also been

used after stenting in a small study of 33 patients with an average lesion length of 12cm and stent length of 17cm.[100] At 6 months, 70% (23 of 33 arteries) were considered patent. Seven of the ten early failures had sudden thrombotic occlusion and were treated with fibrinolysis. Only four of the 33 arteries (12%) had in-stent restenosis due to intimal hyperplasia.

Patients who potentially would benefit most from these less invasive procedures have the worst procedural prognosis. In summary, multiple endovascular modalities are necessary if meaningful patency rates are to be achieved for long SFA lesions. The treatment needs to minimize coexistent thrombus, simplifying the PTA, employ stent or stent-graft selectively, and use ancillary treatment to reduce the risk of intimal hyperplasia and acute thrombosis. Frequent follow-up is necessary.

TIBIAL ARTERY INTERVENTION

Typically, patients with multilevel disease and CLI have been treated with femorotibial bypass. Isolated tibial artery disease is unusual except in diabetics and immunosuppressed patients. The application of coronary artery techniques (small balloon and wires) improves accessibility and initial technical success rates, particularly in non-calcified arteries. Unfortunately, these vessels are frequently calcified, not allowing PTA to stretch the vessel wall easily. **Table 11.5** summarizes the TASC classification of tibial artery lesions. Complex lesions would consist of any lesion >4cm in length and carry the worst prognosis with PTA. Techniques utilizing cutting balloons, small self-expanding stents, or laser-light energy can offer an endovascular alternative. The new low-profile balloon-expandable stents are deliverable, but may be prone to external compression in this location, limiting utility. Treatment should be restricted to patients who lack surgical alternatives and have limb-threatening ischemia.

In a study conducted in our institution, tibial artery revascularization was performed on 213 limbs (290 arteries) in 204 patients.[101] The average number of arteries per limb revascularized was 1.36. The degree of ischemia pre-procedure was Rutherford 3 in 30.1% (64 limbs), Rutherford 4 in 24.4% (52 limbs), and Rutherford 5 in 45.5% (97 limbs). The tibial arteries were stenotic in 64.8% (188 arteries) and occluded in 35.2% (102 arteries), with a technical success rate of 93.8%. Hemodynamic improvement was shown by an increase in the ABI from 0.43+/–0.11 to 0.75+/–0.11 at 18.3 months of follow-up. Technical failure occurred only in occluded arteries (18) and correlated to the length of the occlusion. The failure rate was 3.0% with occlusions <4cm, compared with 34.4% with occlusions >4cm. Major amputations occurred in 26/213 limbs (12.2%) and minor amputations in 22/213 limbs (10.3%), supporting the use of PTA in these patients.

PTA can be performed with a cutting balloon (CB) or intentional subintimal angioplasty. The CB consists of surgical microtomes mounted on the balloon. The CB can dilate recalcitrant lesions such as calcified stenoses, ostial lesions, and in-stent restenosis.[102] These lesions are commonly seen in diabetics with tibial artery calcification. No clinical data on tibial intervention are available using the CB, but it is conceptually attractive. Midterm results are available for subintimal PTA of tibial occlusions in CLI patients (n=40).[103] Technical success was 78%, clinical success 68%, and complications occurred in 12.5%. Limb salvage and survival were 81% and 78%, respectively, at 1 year.

Rotational atherectomy is not a viable alternative in most CLI patients.[82] The debris sent distally may further compromise the runoff (**Fig.11.15**). Debulking with stand-alone laser light offers an alternative since the size of the catheter matches the vessel. This avoids balloon trauma and flow-limiting dissections in these small vessels. The LACI trial studied 25 limbs in 23 patients with Rutherford category 5 or 6 ischemia. This study combined

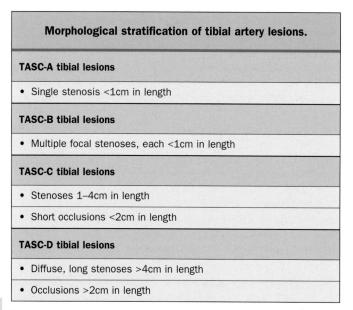

Morphological stratification of tibial artery lesions.
TASC-A tibial lesions
• Single stenosis <1cm in length
TASC-B tibial lesions
• Multiple focal stenoses, each <1cm in length
TASC-C tibial lesions
• Stenoses 1–4cm in length
• Short occlusions <2cm in length
TASC-D tibial lesions
• Diffuse, long stenoses >4cm in length
• Occlusions >2cm in length

Table 11.5 Morphological stratification of tibial artery lesions.[5]

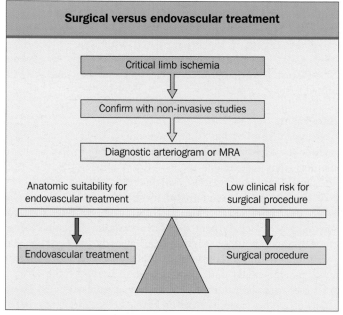

Figure 11.18 Surgical versus endovascular treatment. MRA, magnetic resonance angiography.

laser-assisted angioplasty of the femoral and tibial arteries (mean 3.1 lesions per limb) with bailout stents (41%) and prospectively followed the patients (**Figs 11.17 & 11.18**). Wound healing was 89% and bypass-free limb salvage was 70% at 6 months. There were three technical failures (12%).[101] Runoff targets were identified in four patients after endovascular therapy, who then underwent successful bypass. Endovascular therapy and bypass surgery are not mutually exclusive; nor are interventionalists and surgeons in the care of CLI patients.

Simple tibial lesions can be treated with PTA. Cutting balloons may improve success in recalcitrant lesions. Stents improve flow dynamics after suboptimal angioplasty. Excimer-laser light may debulk plaque without thermal injury or need for subsequent PTA. The options are more extensive than the data from which qualified efficacy statements can be based.

SUMMARY

There is increasing evidence as to the effectiveness of endovascular therapy for patients with CLI. Patients who are at high risk for loss of life or limb have the most to gain with low-risk revascularization procedures. These procedures are not exclusive of traditional surgical treatment and should be viewed as complementary to such. Technological advances in balloons, laser light, stents (bare, covered, coated), and pharmacotherapies, allow application to a wider variety of clinical and anatomic problems. **Figures 11.18–11.21** summarize our approach to endovascular therapy of CLI. The aortoiliac component of multilevel disease should be treated initially. Aortoiliac PTA with stenting provides excellent results irrespective of concomitant infrainguinal treatment. Patients with tissue loss require re-establishment of direct flow to the foot, which usually involves SFA and tibial revascularization. Endovascular strategies for SFA occlusions should start by removing the coexistent thrombus before treating the underlying atherosclerotic plaque. Covered or coated stents may prove to be useful, providing long-term benefit. After successful revascularization, close surveillance is required while maintaining a low threshold for reintervention.

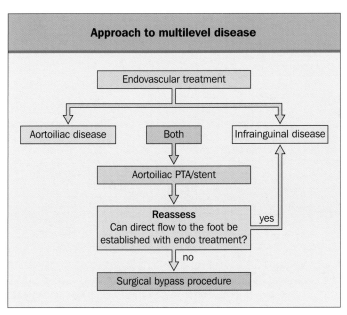

Figure 11.19 Approach to multilevel disease. PTA, percutaneous transluminal angioplasty.

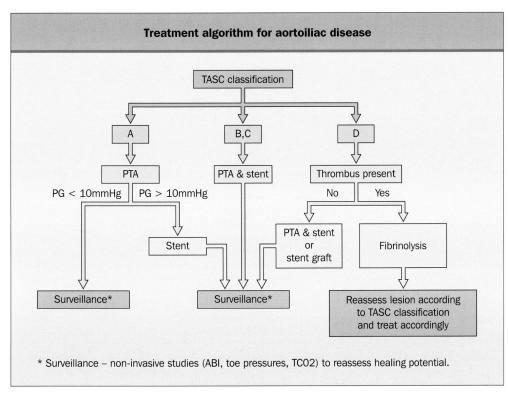

Figure 11.20 Treatment algorithm for aortoiliac disease. ABI, ankle–brachial index; PG, pressure gradient; PTA, percutaneous transluminal angioplasty; TASC, TransAtlantic Inter-Society Consensus.

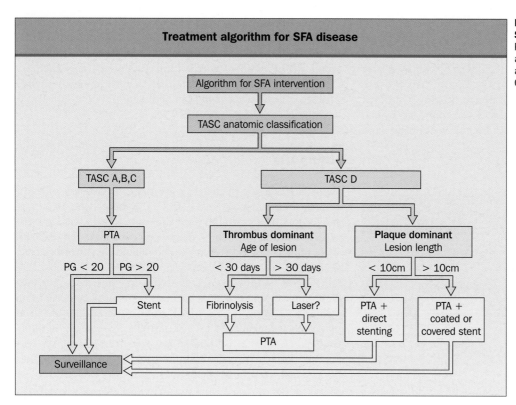

Figure 11.21 Treatment algorithm for SFA disease. PG, pressure gradient; PTA, percutaneous transluminal angioplasty; SFA, superficial femoral artery; TASC, TransAtlantic Inter-Society Consensus.

REFERENCES

1. Dotter CT, Judkins MP. Transluminal treatment of atherosclerotic obstruction: description of a new technique and a preliminary report of its application. Circulation 1964;30:654.

2. Gruntzig A, Kumpe DA. Technique of percutaneous angioplasty with Gruntzig balloon catheter. Am J Radiol 1979;132:547.

3. Wolf GL, Wilson SE, Cross AP, et al. Surgery or balloon angioplasty for peripheral vascular disease: a randomized clinical trial. J Vasc Interv Radiol 1993;4:639–48.

4. Holm J, Arfvidsson B, Jivegard L, et al. Chronic lower limb ischaemia: a prospective randomized controlled study comparing the 1-year results of vascular surgery and percutaneous transluminal angioplasty. J Vasc Endovasc Surg 1991;5:517–22.

5. Management of peripheral arterial disease (PAD). TASC Working Group. Transatlantic Inter-Society Consensus (TASC). J Vasc Surg 2000;31(1 Pt 2):S1–S296.

6. Krajewski LP, Olin JW. Atherosclerosis of the aorta and lower-extremity arteries. In: Young JR, Bartholomew JR, Olin JW, eds. Peripheral vascular diseases, 2nd edn. St Louis:Mosby; 1996:215–6.

7. Allard L, Cloutier G, Durand LG, Roederer GO, Langlois YE. Limitations of ultrasonic duplex scanning for diagnosing lower limb stenosis in the presence of adjacent segment disease. J Vasc Surg 1994;19:650–7.

8. Polak JF, Karmel MI, Mannick JA, O'Leary DH, Donaldson MC, Whittemore AD. Determination of the extent of lower-extremity peripheral arterial disease with color-assisted duplex sonography: comparison with angiography. Am J Radiol 1990;155:1085–9.

9. Saha S, Gibson M, Magee TR, et al. Early results of retrograde transpopliteal angioplasty of iliofemoral lesions. Cardiovasc Intervent Radiol 2001;24:378–82.

10. Ansel GM, George BS, Botti CF Jr, et al. Infrapopliteal endovascular techniques: indications, techniques, and results. Curr Interv Cardiol Rep 2001;3:100–8.

11. Barth KH, Virmani R, Froelich J, et al. Paired comparison of vascular wall reactions to Palmaz stents, Strecker tantalum stents, and Wallstents in canine iliac and femoral arteries. Circulation 1996; 93:2161–9.

12. Zorger N, Manke C, Lenhart M, et al. Peripheral arterial balloon angioplasty: effect of short versus long balloon inflation times on the morphologic results. J Vasc Interv Radiol 2002;13:355–60.

13. Soder H, Manninen HI, Rasanen HT, et al. Failure of prolonged dilation to improve long-term patency of femoropopliteal artery angioplasty: results of a prospective trial. J Vasc Interv Radiol 2002; 13:361–70.

14. Antithrombotic Trialists' Collaboration. Collaborative meta-analysis of randomized trials of antiplatelet therapy for prevention of death, myocardial infarction, and stroke in high risk patients. BMJ 2002;324:71–86.

15. Agnelli G. Rationale for the use of platelet aggregation inhibitors in PAD patients. Vasc Med 2001;6(Suppl 1):13–5.

16. CAPRIE Steering Committee. A randomized, blinded, trial of clopidogrel versus aspirin in patients at risk of ischaemic events (CAPRIE). Lancet 1996;348:1329–39.

17. Gaspoz JM, Coxson PG, Goldman PA, et al. Cost effectiveness of aspirin, clopidogrel, or both for secondary prevention of coronary heart disease. N Engl J Med 2002;346:1800–6.

18. Shlansky-Goldberg R. Combination therapy in peripheral vascular disease: the rationale of using both thrombolytic and antiplatelet drugs. J Am Coll Surg 2002;194(Suppl 1):S103–13.

19. Duda SH, Banz K, Ouriel K, et al. Cost-effectiveness analysis of treatment of subacute peripheral artery occlusions with thrombolysis with and without adjunctive abciximab. J Vasc Interv Radiol 2001;21:S70.

20. Ouriel K, Vieth F, Sasahara AA. A comparison of recombinant urokinase with vascular surgery as initial treatment for acute arterial occlusion of the legs: Thrombolysis of Peripheral Arterial Surgery (TOPAS) Investigators. N Engl J Med 1998;338:1105–11.

21. Weaver F, Toms C. The practical implications of recent trials comparing thrombolytic therapy with surgery for lower extremity ischemia. Semin Vasc Surg 1997;10:49–54.

22. Ouriel K, Gray BH, Clair DG, et al. Complications associated with the use of urokinase and recombinant tissue plasminogen activator for catheter-directed peripheral arterial and venous thrombolysis. J Vasc Interv Radiol 2000;11:295–8.

23. Earnshaw JJ, Comerota A. Towards international consensus in peripheral arterial thrombolysis. Br J Surg 1997;84:1332–3.

24. Braithwaite BD, Birch PA, Poskitt KR. Accelerated thrombolysis with high dose bolus t-PA extends the role of peripheral thrombolysis but may increase the risks. Clin Radiol 1995;50:747–50.

25. Martin U, Kaufmann B, Neugebauer G. Current clinical use of reteplase for thrombolysis. A pharmacokinetic-pharmacodynamic perspective. Clin Pharmacokinetic 1999;36:265–76.

26. Silber S. Rapid hemostasis of arterial puncture sites with collagen in patients undergoing diagnostic and interventional cardiac catheterization. Clin Cardiol 1997;20:981–92.

27. Johnston KW. Iliac arteries: reanalysis of results of balloon angioplasty. Radiology 1993;186:207–12.

28. Bosch JL, van der Graaf Y, Hunink MGM, for the Dutch Iliac Stent Trial Study Group. Health-related quality of life after angioplasty and stent placement in patients with iliac artery occlusive disease. Circulation 1999;99:3155–60.

29. Schneinert D, Schroder M, Balzer JO, et al. Stent-supported reconstruction of the aortoiliac bifurcation with the kissing balloon technique. Circulation 1999;100:II-295.

30. Laborde JC, Palmaz JC, Rivera FJ, et al. Influence of anatomic distribution of atherosclerosis on the outcome of revascularization with iliac stent placement. J Vasc Interv Radiol 1995;6:513–21.

31. Sullivan TM, Childs MB, Bacharach MJ, et al. Percutaneous transluminal angioplasty and primary stenting of the iliac arteries in 288 patients. J Vasc Surg 1997;25:829–39.

32. Nawaz S, Cleveland T, Gaines P, et al. Aortoiliac stenting: determinants of clinical outcome. Eur J Vasc Endovasc Surg 1999;17:351–9.

33. Kamphuis AGA, van Engelen AD, Tetteroo E, et al, for the Dutch Iliac Stent Trial Study Group. Impact of different hemodynamic criteria for stent placement after suboptimal iliac angioplasty. J Vasc Interv Radiol 2000;10:741–56.

34. Tetteroo E, van der Graaf Y, Bosch JL, et al, for the Dutch Iliac Stent Trial Study Group. Randomised comparison of primary stent placement versus primary angioplasty followed by selective stent placement in patients with iliac-artery occlusive disease. Lancet 1998; 351:1153–9.

35. Jorgensen B, Skovgaard N, Norgard J, et al. Percutaneous transluminal angioplasty in 226 iliac artery stenoses: role of the superficial femoral artery for clinical success. Vasa 1992;21:382–6.

36. Laborde JC, Palmaz JC, Rivera FJ, et al. Influence of anatomic distribution of atherosclerosis on the outcome of revascularization with iliac stent placement. J Vasc Interv Radiol 1995;6:513–21.

37. Uher P, Nyman U, Forssell C, et al. Percutaneous placement of stents in chronic iliac and aortic occlusive disease. Eur J Vasc Endovasc Surg 1999;18:114–21.

38. Tegtmeyer CJ, Hartwell GD, Selby JB, et al. Results and complications of angioplasty in aortoiliac disease. Circulation 1991;83(Suppl I): I-53–I-60.

39. Jeans WD, Armstrong S, Cole SEA, et al. Fate of patients undergoing transluminal angioplasty for lower-limb ischemia. Radiology 1990; 177:559–64.

40. Al-Hamali S, Baskerville P, Fraser S, et al. Detection of distal emboli in patients with peripheral arterial stenosis before and after iliac angioplasty: a prospective study. J Vasc Surg 1999;29:345–51.

41. Chamberlin JR, Lardi AB, McKeever LS, et al. Use of vascular sealing devices (Vasoseal and Perclose) versus assisted manual compression (Femostop) in transcatheter coronary interventions requiring abciximab (Reopro). Catheter Cardiovasc Interv 1999;47:143–7.

42. Duda SH, Wiskirchen J, Tepe G, et al. Physical properties of endovascular stents: an experimental comparison. J Vasc Interv Radiol 2000;11:645–9.

43. Navarro F, Sullivan TM, Bacharach JM. Intravascular ultrasound assessment of iliac stent procedures. J Endovasc Ther 2000;7:315–9.

44. Buckley CJ, Arko FR, Mettauer M, et al. Intravascular ultrasound scanning improves long-term patency of iliac lesions treated with balloon angioplasty and primary stenting. J Vasc Surg 2002;35:316–23.

45. Lee ES, Steenson CC, Trimble KE, et al. Comparing patency rates between external iliac and common iliac artery stents. J Vasc Surg 2000;31:889–94.

46. Powell RJ, Fillinger M, Bettmann M, et al. The durability of endovascular treatment of multisegment iliac occlusive disease. J Vasc Surg 2000;31:1178–84.

47. Powell RJ, Fillinger M, Walsh DB, et al. Predicting outcome of angioplasty and selective stenting of multisegment iliac artery occlusive disease. J Vasc Surg 2000;32:564–9.

48. Timaran CH, Stevens SL, Freeman MB, et al. Infrainguinal arterial reconstructions in patients with aortoiliac occlusive disease: the influence of iliac stenting. J Vasc Surg 2001;34:971–8.

49. Schneider JR, Besso SR, Walsh DB, et al. Femorofemoral versus aortobifemoral bypass: outcome and hemodynamic results. J Vasc Surg 1994;19:43–57.

50. Sanchez LA, Patel AV, Ohki T, et al. Midterm experience with the endovascular treatment of isolated iliac aneurysms. J Vasc Surg 1999;30:907–14.

51. Scheinert D, Ludwig J, Steinkamp HJ, et al. Treatment of catheter-induced iliac artery injuries with self-expanding endografts. J Endovasc Ther 2000;7:213–20.

52. Lammer J, Dake MD, Bleyn J, et al. Peripheral arterial obstruction: prospective study of treatment with a transluminally placed self-expanding stent-graft. Radiology 2000;217:95–104.

53. Henry M, Amor M, Cragg A, et al. Occlusive and aneurysmal peripheral arterial disease: assessment of a stent-graft system. Radiology 1996; 201:717–24.

54. Link J, Mueller-Huelsbeck S, Brossmann J, et al. Perivascular inflammatory reaction after percutaneous placement of covered stents. Cardiovasc Intervent Radiol 1996;19:345–7.

55. Kumins NH, Owens EL, Oglevie SB, et al. Early experience using the Wallgraft in the management of distal microembolism from common iliac artery pathology. Ann Vasc Surg 2002,16:181–6.

56. The STILE Investigators. Results of a prospective randomized trial evaluating surgery versus thrombolysis for ischemia of the lower extremity: the STILE Trial. Ann Surg 1994;220:251–68.

57. Motarjeme A, Gordon GI, Bodenhagen K. Thrombolysis and angioplasty of chronic iliac artery occlusions. J Vasc Interv Radiol 1995;6:66S–72S.

58. Bucek RA, Schnurer G, Haumer M, et al. Long-term results of systemic thrombolysis therapy in aorto-iliac occlusive disease. Vasa 2001; 30:212–8.

59. Visona A, Perissinotto C, Lusiani L, et al. Percutaneous Excimer laser angioplasty of lower limb vessels: results of a prospective 24-month follow-up. Angiology 1998;49:91–8.

60. Hertzer NR. The natural history of peripheral vascular disease: implications for its management. Circulation 1991;83(Suppl 1):I-12–I-19.

61. McDaniel MD, Cronenwett JL. Basic data related to the natural history of intermittent claudication. Ann Vasc Surg 1989;3:273–7.

62. Juergens JL, Barker NW, Hines EA Jr. Arteriosclerosis obliterans: review of 520 cases with special reference to pathogenic and prognostic factors. Circulation 1960;21:188–95.

63. Gray BH, Sullivan TM, Childs MB, et al. High incidence of restenosis/ reocclusion of stents in the percutaneous treatment of long-segment superficial femoral artery disease after suboptimal angioplasty. J Vasc Surg 1997;25:74–83.

64. Horvath W, Oertl M, Haidinger D. Percutaneous transluminal angioplasty of crual arteries. Radiology 1990;177:565–9.

65. Jeans WD, Armstrong S, Cole SEA, et al. Fate of patients undergoing transluminal angioplasty for lower-limb ischemia. Radiology 1990; 177:559–64.

66. Blair JM, Gewertz BL, Moosa H, et al. Percutaneous transluminal angioplasty versus surgery for limb-threatening ischemia. J Vasc Surg 1989;9:698–703.

67. Lofberg AM, Karacagil S, Ljungman C, et al. Percutaneous transluminal angioplasty of the femoropopliteal arteries in limbs with chronic critical lower limb ischemia. J Vasc Surg 2001;34:114–21.

68. Jamsen T, Manninen H, Tulla H, et al. The final outcome of primary infrainguinal percutaneous transluminal angioplasty in 100 consecutive patients with chronic critical limb ischemia. J Vasc Interv Radiol 2002;13:455–63.

69. Gardiner GA Jr, Meyerovitz MF, Harrington DP, et al. Dissection complicating angioplasty. Am J Radiol 1985;145:627–31.

70. Krepel VM, van Andel GJ, van Erp WF, et al. Percutaneous transluminal angioplasty of the femoropopliteal artery: initial and long term results. Radiology 1985;156:325–8.

71. Johnston KW, Rae M, Hogg-Johnston SA, et al. Five-year results of a prospective study of percutaneous transluminal angioplasty. Ann Surg 1987;206:403–13.

72. Rosenfield K, Schainfeld R, Pieczek A, et al. Restenosis of endovascular stents from stent compression. J Am Coll Cardiol 1997;29:328–38.

73. Cejna M, Thurnher S, Illiasch H, et al. PTA versus Palmaz stent placement in femoropopliteal artery obstructions: a multicenter prospective randomized study. J Vasc Interv Radiol 2001;12:23–31.

74. Vroegingeweij D, Vos LD, Tielbeek AV, et al. Ballooon angioplasty combined with primary stenting versus balloon angioplasty alone in femoropopliteal obstructions: a comparative randomized study. Cardiovasc Intervent Radiol 1997;20:420–5.

75. Muradin GS, Myriam Hunink MG. Cost and patency rate targets for the development of endovascular devices to treat femoropopliteal arterial disease. Radiology 2001;218:464–9.

76. Hunink MGM, Wong JB, Donaldson MC, et al. Revascularization for femoropopliteal disease: a decision and cost-effectiveness analysis. JAMA 1995;274:165–71.

77. Rousseau HP, Raillat CR, Joffre FG, et al. Treatment of femoropopliteal stenosis by means of self-expandable endoprostheses: midterm results. Radiology 1989;172:961–4.

78. Do-Dai-Do, Triller J, Walpoth BH, et al. A comparison study of self-expandable stents versus balloon angioplasty alone in femoropopliteal artery occlusions. Cardiovasc Intervent Radiol 1992;15:306–12.

79. White GH, Liew SCC, Waugh SC, et al. Early outcome and intermediate follow-up of vascular stents in the femoral and popliteal arteries without long-term anticoagulation. J Vasc Surg 1995;21:270–81.

80. Graor RA, Whitlow PL. Transluminal atherectomy for occlusive peripheral vascular disease. J Am Coll Cardiol 1990;15:1151–8.

81. Simpson JB, Selmon MR, Robertson GC, et al. Transluminal atherectomy for occlusive peripheral vascular disease. Am J Cardiol 1988;61:96G–101G.

82. Ahn SS, Auth DC, Marcus DR, et al. Removal of focal atheromatous lesions by angioscopically guided high-speed rotary atherectomy: preliminary experimental observations. J Vasc Surg 1988;7:292–300.

83. Yoffe B, Yavnel L, Altshuler A, et al. Preliminary experience with the Xtrak debulking device in the treatment of peripheral occlusion. J Endovasc Ther 2002;9:234–40.

84. Murray RR Jr, Hewes RC, White RI, et al. Long-segment femoropopliteal stenoses: is angioplasty a boon or a bust? Radiology 1987;162:473–6.

85. Murray JG, Apthorp LA, Wilkins RA. Long-segment (>10 cm) femoropopliteal angioplasty: improved technical success and long-term patency. Radiology 1995;195:158–62.

86. Matsi PJ, Manninen HI, Vanninen RL, et al. Femoropopliteal angioplasty in patients with claudication: primary and secondary patency in 140 limbs with 1–3 year follow-up. Radiology 1994;191:727–37.

87. Bolia A, Bell PRF. Femoropopliteal and crural artery recanalization using subintimal angioplasty. Semin Vasc Surg 1995;8:253–64.

88. Scheinert D, Laird JR Jr, Schroder M, et al. Excimer laser-assisted recanalization of long, chronic superficial femoral artery occlusions. J Endovasc Ther 2001;8:156–66.

89. Capek P, McLean GK, Berkowitz HD. Femoropopliteal angioplasty: factors influencing long-term success. Circulation 1991;83(Suppl 1): I-70–I-80.

90. Zollikofer CL, Antonucci F, Pfyffer M, et al. Arterial stent placement with use of the Wallstent: midterm results of clinical experience. Radiology 1991;179:449–56.

91. Saproval MR, Long AL, Raynaud AC, et al. Femoropopliteal stent placement: long-term results. Radiology 1992;184:833–9.

92. Martin EC, Katzen BT, Benanti JF, et al. Multicenter trial of the Wallstent in the iliac and femoral arteries. J Vasc Interv Radiol 1995; 6:843–9.

93. Gray BH, Olin JW. Limitations of percutaneous transluminal angioplasty with stenting for femoropopliteal arterial occlusive disease. Semin Vasc Surg 1997;10:8–16.

94. Do-Dai-Do, Triller J, Walpoth BH, et al. A comparison study of self-expandable stents vs balloon angioplasty alone in femoropopliteal artery occlusions. Cardiovasc Intervent Radiol 1992;15:306–12.

95. Henry M, Amor M, Ethevenot G, et al. Palmaz stent placement in iliac and femoropopliteal arteries: primary and secondary patency in 310 patients with 2–4 year follow-up. Radiology 1995;197:167–74.

96. Duda SH, Pusich B, Richter G, et al. Sirolimus-eluting stents for the treatment of obstructive superficial femoral artery disease: six-month results. Circulation 2002;106:1505–9.

97. Ahmadi R, Schillinger M, Maca T, et al. Femoropopliteal arteries: immediate and long-term results with a dacron-covered stent-graft. Radiology 2002;223:345–50.

98. Bauermeister G. Endovascular stent-grafting in the treatment of superficial femoral artery occlusive disease. J Endovasc Ther 2001;8:315–20.

99. Waksman R, Laird JR, Jurkovitz CT, et al. Intravascular radiation therapy after balloon angioplasty of narrowed femoropopliteal arteries to prevent restenosis: results of the PARIS feasibility clinical trial. J Vasc Interv Radiol 2001;12:915–21.

100. Wolfram RM, Pokrajac B, Ahmadi R, et al. Endovascular brachytherapy for prophylaxis against restenosis after long-segment femoropopliteal placement of stents: initial results. Radiology 2001;220:724–9.

101. Gray BH, Laird JR, Ansel GM, Shuck JW. Complex endovascular treatment for critical limb ischemia in poor surgical candidates. J Endovasc Ther 2002;9:599–604.

102. Engelke C, Morgan RA, Belli AM. Cutting balloon percutaneous transluminal angioplasty for salvage of lower limb arterial bypass grafts: feasibility. Radiology 2002;223:106–14.

103. Vraux H, Hammer F, Verhelst R, et al. Subintimal angioplasty of tibial vessel occlusions in the treatment of critical limb ischaemia: mid-term results. Eur J Vasc Endovasc Surg 2000;5:441–6.

CHAPTER
12
Surgical Intervention

Nicholas J M London

KEY POINTS

- The optimal management of a patient with critical limb ischemia (CLI) often requires a combination of endovascular and open surgical techniques.

- Preoperative independent mobility best predicts postoperative status after infrainguinal bypass for CLI.

- Patients with CLI have a profoundly reduced quality of life that is immediately improved by successful treatment of CLI.

- Primary amputation is more expensive than bypass for CLI.

- Autologous vein is the conduit of choice for infrainguinal bypass.

- Poor runoff status and poor-quality vein conduit are significant risk factors for graft occlusion.

- No patient should be denied an attempted reconstruction based on results of preoperative arteriography alone.

- The results of infrainguinal *in situ* and reverse vein bypass are similar.

- Between 15% and 25% of infrainguinal vein bypass grafts are technically flawed, and some form of post-reconstruction quality control is essential.

- There is a strong body of evidence in favor of duplex surveillance of vein grafts whereas there is no evidence for duplex surveillance of prosthetic grafts.

- All patients with CLI should be prescribed an antiplatelet agent. The addition of warfarin to an antiplatelet agent carries a considerable risk of major hemorrhage and should only be used therefore in patients with 'high-risk' vein or prosthetic grafts.

INTRODUCTION

Chronic lower extremity ischemia progressing to critical limb ischemia (CLI) is nearly always the result of arterial obstruction due to atherosclerosis. Although there are other rare causes of arterial obstruction, such as distal embolization in the 'blue toe syndrome', these conditions will not be discussed here. Similarly, this chapter will not discuss the relative role of endovascular techniques and surgery because this will depend on local facilities and expertise. CLI usually results from multilevel disease and it is often possible to treat one level of disease by percutaneous transluminal angioplasty (PTA) while another component is best

managed surgically. This combined approach lessens the magnitude of therapy and can either take the form of PTA in the angiography suite prior to surgery or an 'on-table' angioplasty can be performed at the same time as the surgical procedure.

Although at one time lumbar sympathectomy was used for the treatment of CLI, in modern vascular surgical practice, operative lumbar sympathectomy has little part to play. However, for the occasional patient in whom it is not possible to treat CLI by either endovascular or surgical methods, a chemical lumbar sympathectomy may provide useful analgesia. For these reasons, the techniques of lumbar sympathectomy will not be discussed, nor will the recently described, and as yet unproven, technique of distal venous arterialization.[1]

PATIENT SELECTION

A detailed social history is essential for the optimal management of the patient with CLI. In particular it is vital that the clinician assesses the functional status of the threatened limb. Thus, the bed-bound patient using an ischemic leg to transfer to and from a wheelchair or from wheelchair to toilet poses a different management issue than the bed-bound patient who never uses the leg. The clinician should also clarify whether a dying leg reflects a dying patient, or whether it is an isolated event in an otherwise reasonably fit patient. There may be occasions when the general condition of the patient is so poor and the chances of survival limited by co-morbidity, that it is appropriate simply to make the patient comfortable. There may be occasions when a reasonably fit patient has lost so much tissue in the foot that any attempt to save it is futile. Similarly, patients who have developed fixed flexion contractions of the knee and the hip are usually best managed by primary amputation. These decisions are best made in consultation with the patient, relatives, and the rehabilitation team looking after the patient.

It has been shown that preoperative independence and mobility best predict postoperative status after infrainguinal bypass for CLI.[2] Thus, only 4% of survivors who are not living independently before surgery achieve independent living 6 months post-operatively. It would seem, therefore, that there is little point in undertaking extensive revascularization in the hope of achieving independence for a patient already requiring care in a nursing home. Conversely, 99% of survivors who live independently before developing the need for limb salvage surgery remain independent 6 months after surgery. Certainly, age itself should not be considered a contraindication to surgery and there are a number of studies reporting benefit in patients over the age of 80 years.[3–5]

IMPACT OF SURGERY ON QUALITY OF LIFE IN PATIENTS WITH CLI

It has been shown using the Nottingham Health Profile that compared with a normal control population, patients with CLI have a profoundly reduced quality of life.[6] Studies evaluating the impact of successful surgical revascularization on quality of life have uniformly shown that a patent graft following infrainguinal arterial reconstruction for CLI results in an immediate and lasting improvement in health-related quality of life. Conversely, symptomatic graft occlusion leads to a reduction in quality of life. Amputation results in a striking deterioration in physical function, particularly after failed secondary revascularization. A successful patent graft particularly improves the domains of physical functioning, social functioning, and pain.[7–10]

ECONOMICS AND COST-EFFECTIVENESS

The precise costs of procedures will vary between countries and between institutions within countries. Also, the cost of health care is continually increasing and it is therefore not possible to compare costs quoted by studies performed in different eras. For these reasons, this section will focus on the comparative cost of various approaches. A number of studies both from Europe and North America[11–14] have shown that the overall costs 1 year after intervention are between 1.5 and two times greater for primary amputation than for femorodistal grafting. These studies have included in the costs of femoro-distal grafting the costs of graft failure and secondary amputation. The main reason that primary amputation costs more is the community costs in the first year after amputation. In general, two to three times as many patients who undergo successful primary reconstruction are able to return home compared with those who undergo amputation. A study from Finland by Luther[13] has shown that among patients undergoing amputation the total costs for those already in an institution is one-sixth of that required by patients who return home after amputation. This substantial difference results from the longer hospital stay, longer survival, and home care of the group who were not institutionalized prior to amputation. Interestingly, a study from Sheffield by Singh et al.[15] has shown that over 1 year there was no significant difference in the cost of managing a patient with CLI by angioplasty or surgical reconstruction. This is because the major costs in both groups were related to the length of inpatient stay, which was similar in the two groups. Presumably, this reflects the fact that the length of hospital stay is related more to the state of the foot and social factors than the specific intervention received.

FACTORS AFFECTING OUTCOME

A number of studies have investigated the factors influencing graft patency, limb salvage, and mortality rate after lower limb bypass procedures for CLI. Although most surgeons would attempt a bypass procedure in the presence of one or two adverse risk factors, the presence of numerous adverse risk factors may influence the decision whether to attempt a bypass. In addition, knowledge of the risk factors discussed below is important with respect to informed consent and counseling the patient about the risks and likely outcome of bypass surgery.

Gender

The literature concerning the effect of gender on outcome after infrainguinal bypass is contradictory and the issue not resolved. Thus, some authors identify female gender as an adverse risk factor with respect to long-term survival[16] and graft patency,[16–18] whereas others do not.[19–22] However, there does seem to be a consensus that the combination of female gender and diabetes significantly reduces 3-year postoperative survival, graft patency, and limb salvage.[16,19]

Age

With increasing age, a number of important risk factors become more prevalent. These include diabetes, female gender combined with diabetes, and cardiac risk factors. A multivariate analysis, which took account of these confounding factors, found no independent effect of age on operative mortality, graft patency, leg salvage, or survival.[19] Thus, age itself should not be a contraindication to infrainguinal bypass surgery.

Diabetes

There is disagreement concerning the influence of diabetes on the patency of infrainguinal bypass grafts. Some authors conclude that diabetes has no effect[21,23–26] or even improves outcome,[27,28] while others conclude that diabetes adversely affects outcome.[17,19,29–31] One of the reasons for these differences may be the nature of the analyses performed. Thus, some authors who have found diabetes to be a risk factor for graft occlusion in univariate analysis have found that this disappears on multivariate analysis.[16,19,29] This suggests that although diabetic patients are more likely to have risk factors for graft occlusion than non-diabetics, diabetes itself is not a significant risk factor. Contrary to previous studies,[16,19] a recent paper from Hamdan et al.[32] has reported that diabetes is not associated with an increased postoperative mortality after vascular surgery. Diabetic patients do however have a markedly reduced long-term survival compared with non-diabetics.[16,19,32]

Renal failure

There seems little doubt that patients with chronic renal failure who require lower limb revascularization have a high perioperative mortality[33,34] and poor long-term survival.[35] However, there is also evidence that providing autologous vein is used, acceptable graft patencies can be achieved.[35,36] Certainly, it would seem that for hemodialysis-dependent patients, the use of prosthetic material is of questionable benefit.[35]

Smoking

Although Rutherford et al.[27] reported that smoking significantly reduces late graft patency, others, somewhat surprisingly, have not found this association.[17,23,25,26,29] This is probably because smoking history is not a true reflection of smoking activity.[29] However, in view of the overall health benefits of smoking cessation, all patients who smoke should be encouraged to desist.

Graft material
Vein versus prosthetic
Although prosthetic materials can achieve acceptable results for below-knee bypass grafts,[37] there is no doubt that the best results below the knee are obtained with autologous vein.[18,23,25,27,29,37] Until recently, the situation above the knee had been less clear.[38–40]

However, a recently published prospective randomized study from Boston[40] convincingly showed that the 5-year patency of above-knee saphenous vein grafts is significantly superior to that of polytetrafluoroethylene (PTFE) or human umbilical vein grafts. This study randomized 752 patients and had a follow-up of 5 years. In patients with critical ischemia, the 5-year patency of saphenous vein was 68% compared with 52% and 37% for human umbilical vein and PTFE, respectively.

It has recently been reported that for both above- and below-knee grafts, the proportion of graft occlusions that result in limb-threatening ischemia is significantly greater for PTFE than for vein grafts.[41] Thus, prosthetic grafts not only have lower patency rates than vein grafts but in addition the consequences of graft failure are more severe in prosthetic grafts than in vein grafts. With respect to composite vein–prosthetic grafts, it has been shown that below-knee composite grafts have poor patency rates[42] and offer no advantage over prosthetic grafts alone.[43,44] Thus, for grafts both above and below the knee, autologous vein is undoubtedly the conduit of choice.

Source of vein

Although there are descriptions of the use of cryopreserved saphenous vein allografts, the patencies are poor[45,46] and their only use may be as an interim or temporary conduit through infected fields.[47] The options for autogenous vein are the ipsilateral long and/or short saphenous, the ipsilateral superficial femoral-popliteal vein, the contralateral saphenous veins, or arm veins. Any of these veins can be joined or spliced together to produce a vein of adequate total length. There is no doubt that the first choice is ipsilateral long saphenous vein. However, this vein is available in only approximately 45% of cases.[48,49] The ipsilateral short saphenous vein is a good alternative that can frequently be used without the need to join it to other vein.[50]

The use of the superficial femoral-popliteal vein as an infrainguinal bypass conduit was introduced by Schulman et al. in 1981[51] and has subsequently been used by others.[52,53] While there seems no doubt that the superficial femoral-popliteal vein provides excellent patency rates,[51,52] harvesting the vein is more difficult than for saphenous vein and 20–30% of patients are troubled by postoperative limb swelling.[54]

Although some surgeons routinely use long saphenous vein from the contralateral leg,[55] others are reluctant to do so because of the chance that the patient may require contralateral lower limb bypass at a future date. It has been reported that at 2 years after surgery for CLI, 20% of patients will have developed critical ischemia in the contralateral limb,[56] and that by 5 years, 30% of patients will have required intervention for contralateral CLI.[57] Multivariate analysis has shown that diabetes, coronary artery disease, an ankle–brachial pressure index (ABPI) below 0.7, and age less than 70 years are all significant independent predictors of the need for contralateral intervention.[57] Although based on these data it would seem unwise to use the contralateral long saphenous vein in patients less than 70 years of age or in diabetics, Chew et al.[55] have routinely used the contralateral long saphenous vein when required, without compromising the contralateral leg, even in diabetics.

Kakkar[58] suggested the use of arm vein for lower limb bypass grafting in 1969, and since then, a number of authors have described its use.[59–62] The incidence of diseased veins in the arm is as high as 63%,[61] considerably higher than the value of 12%

for the long saphenous vein.[63,64] Many of these abnormalities are thought to result from previous phlebotomy and/or intravenous cannulation and this explains why the incidence of disease in the more accessible forearm cephalic vein is 49%, while in the less accessible basilic vein is only 12%.[61] It has been reported that the patency of composite arm vein is significantly less than that of single-length arm vein (29% versus 52% at 5 years).[59] However, Marcaccio et al.[61] found that if angioscopy was used to detect and 'upgrade' diseased arm veins, the patency of composite grafts was no different from that of single-length grafts. This would seem to imply that providing the surgeon is technically proficient, composite arm vein grafts are acceptable if the conjoined vein segments are disease-free. Certainly, composite vein grafts are preferable to prosthetic grafts[60,65] and are preferable to single-length long saphenous vein that contains narrowed, diseased areas.[66]

Vein quality and diameter
Diameter

Most vascular surgeons believe that the size and quality of the venous conduit are among the most important determinants of long-term patency of infrainguinal bypass grafts. There is disagreement concerning the minimum useable vein diameter. Thus, Bergamini et al.[23] consider 2.0mm to be the minimum diameter whereas Shah et al.[21] consider 4.0mm to be the minimum. Wengerter et al.[67] demonstrated increasing graft patency with graft diameters ranging from 3.0 to 4.0mm, and Sumner[68] has shown, based on theoretical considerations, that long vein grafts with diameters less than 3.0mm produce unacceptably high pressure gradients. Varty et al.[66] concluded that vein grafts with a diameter less than 3.0mm are at increased risk of developing stenoses, whereas Idu et al.[25] concluded that grafts less than 3.5mm in diameter are at increased risk of such. Based on the data available, it would appear preferable to use vein with a diameter greater than 3.0mm.

It should be noted that in patients with poor limb perfusion, the saphenous vein may be underfilled and the resting diameter may not reflect the ability of the vein to dilate under arterial pressure. It has been suggested that measurements of the long saphenous vein diameter with venous occlusion cuffs can predict subsequent diameter 12 months after surgery.[69] Davies et al.[69] found that if the minimum resting diameter of the vein regarded as being suitable for bypass is 3.0mm, this venous occlusion technique can increase the vein utilization rate by 22% by identifying veins less than 3.0mm that dilate up beyond 3.0mm with venous occlusion.

Vein quality

Vein quality can be assessed either macroscopically or microscopically. Although the latter may be of importance with respect to the development of vein graft stenosis, it is primarily of research interest.[70,71] The macroscopic vein appearance is crucially important to the practicing vascular surgeon because it profoundly influences both early and late graft patency.[64,72] Thus, Panetta et al.[64] found that 63 (12%) of 513 infrainguinal vein bypasses contained abnormalities such as thick walls, postphlebitic occlusions, postphlebitic stenoses, calcification, or varicosities. Preoperative duplex was able to identify 62% of these macroscopically abnormal veins. The remaining abnormalities were detected intraoperatively (see below).

153

Site of distal anastomosis, runoff, and plantar arch status

Although it has been shown that the patency of above-knee bypass grafts is better than that of below-knee grafts,[29] it has also been shown that the patencies of below-knee vein grafts that are anastomosed to tibial vessels are as good as for those placed onto the below-knee popliteal artery itself.[23,73] Many studies conclude that poor runoff is an independent risk factor for graft failure[18,29–31,74,75] and it has also been suggested that lack of continuity of the calf vessels with the plantar arch is a significant risk factor for graft occlusion.[74,76–80] It has been suggested that grafts to the peroneal artery do not do as well as grafts to the anterior or posterior tibial arteries.[81] However, there is a substantial body of literature that contradicts this view,[21,82–84] and the single most important factor is that the artery chosen for the distal anastomosis is disease-free distally and is in continuity with the pedal arch.

GENERAL CONSIDERATIONS PRIOR TO SURGERY

There is now a substantial body of evidence that patients with peripheral vascular disease should be prescribed an antiplatelet agent such as aspirin or clopidogrel and that this agent should be continued in the perioperative period.[85,86] Similarly, there is compelling evidence that perioperative β-blocker use reduces mortality and improves event-free survival for up to 2 years after major non-cardiac surgery.[86,87] The need for vigilance with respect to the medical management of patients with CLI has been highlighted by a recent Danish study showing that only a minority of patients with CLI are receiving adequate risk factor management.[88] All patients who smoke should be encouraged to stop.

Although intraoperative anticoagulation with intravenous heparin has been widely believed to provide adequate protection against thromboembolic phenomena, it has been shown that 18% of patients undergoing lower limb vascular reconstruction without specific deep vein thrombosis (DVT) prophylaxis develop postoperative DVT.[89] A randomized controlled trial comparing low-molecular-weight heparin with unfractionated heparin for the prevention of postoperative DVT in patients undergoing femorodistal bypass reported that the postoperative DVT rate was 3.4%, with no significant difference between the two heparin types.[90] These studies, taken in conjunction with the general literature on the subject, suggest that patients undergoing lower limb revascularization should receive DVT prophylaxis. However, a recent study from North Carolina[91] found the rate of DVT in patients undergoing infrainguinal reconstruction without routine DVT prophylaxis to be 2.8% and concluded that routine prophylaxis is not indicated. However, it is noteworthy that 25% of all patients in this study were anticoagulated for other reasons.

With respect to antibiotic prophylaxis, it is recommended that this should be used in the context of clean operations whenever intravascular prosthetic material is inserted or if deep infection would pose a catastrophic risk. Thus, although vascular procedures are usually clean, they frequently qualify for prophylaxis. The agent used for prophylaxis should be active against staphylococci. Although there is no evidence to support a prolonged course of antibiotic prophylaxis in vascular patients,

most surgeons continue prophylaxis for at least 24 hours, and for longer in patients with indwelling central venous or arterial lines.[92]

PREOPERATIVE IMAGING

Imaging of the arterial tree has already been covered in Chapter 6. This section will therefore address specific issues that are pertinent to lower limb bypass grafting. Two of the most important aspects of preoperative imaging are defining the arterial runoff vessels and determining the availability and suitability of vein that can be used as a bypass conduit.

Imaging of the arterial system

It is advantageous to initially image the arterial tree by non-invasive techniques. This allows the surgeon to assess the potential role of endovascular techniques, and if PTA is chosen, a non-invasive arterial map facilitates an endovascular approach. In addition, it is much easier to have an informed discussion with the patient about the available treatment options if the surgeon has a non-invasive arterial map to hand.[93] The two most commonly used non-invasive techniques for imaging the arterial tree are color duplex scanning and magnetic resonance angiography (MRA).[94–96] The choice will depend on local facilities and expertise. Duplex scanning has the advantages that it can be performed as part of a single-visit assessment and provides both an anatomic and a hemodynamic map (**Fig. 12.1**). It is also cheaper than MRA. The major disadvantages of color duplex scanning are that it is operator-dependent and time-consuming. Both duplex scanning and MRA may demonstrate distal vessels not seen on digital subtraction angiography (DSA).[94,95,97,98] A number of studies have shown that it is safe to proceed to lower limb arterial reconstruction based solely on the results of duplex scanning.[95,99,100]

One of the major disadvantages of intra-arterial DSA is that in the face of severe proximal arterial obstruction, it may fail to show patent distal vessels revealed by intra-operative arteriography.[101] Additional approaches that have proved useful are pulse-generated runoff (PGR)[77,102] and dependent Doppler.[103,104] The principle of PGR is that blood flow is generated in patent calf arteries by application of a pulsatile pressure (250mmHg at a rate of 50 per min) to a sphygmomanometer cuff placed around the upper calf. Patent arteries can then be detected at the ankle by insonation with a 10 MHz Doppler ultrasound probe. An alternative and simpler approach is that of dependent Doppler examination (**Fig. 12.2**). This technique allows the accurate detection of calf vessels that have continuity with the pedal arch. The leg is placed in a dependent position and a Doppler signal obtained in the first web space over the area of the deep plantar artery. Individual calf vessels are then compressed in turn at the ankle joint. If only one calf vessel communicates with the pedal arch, then the Doppler signals are obliterated. If more than one tibial vessel is in continuity with the arch, compression results in attenuation of the pedal arch signal. The vessel that gives the greatest attenuation is defined as the major inflowing vessel to the arch.

A number of authors have developed 'runoff scores' based on preoperative angiography, PGR, or Doppler, or a combination of these modalities.[76–78,105] Most of these scoring systems have a low positive predictive value and high negative predictive value for amputation (e.g. 50% and 97%, respectively).[78] This means

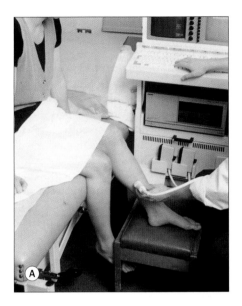

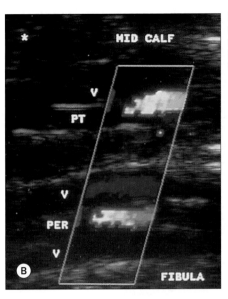

Figure 12.1 Duplex scanning. (A) The tibial vessels are best scanned with the leg dependent. (B) This scan shows the peroneal (PER) and posterior tibial (PT) arteries and associated veins (V) at mid-calf level.

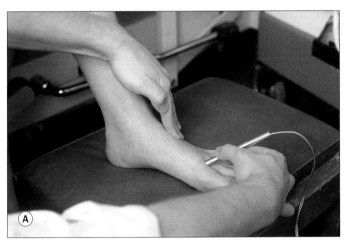

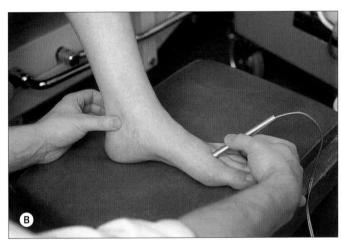

Figure 12.2 Dependent Doppler. The leg is placed in a dependent position and a Doppler signal obtained in the first web space over the area of the deep plantar artery. Individual calf vessels are then compressed in turn at the ankle joint (A, the dorsalis pedis; B, the posterior tibial artery). If only one calf vessel communicates with the pedal arch, the Doppler signal is obliterated. If more than one tibial vessel is in continuity with the arch, compression results in attenuation of the pedal arch signal. The vessel that gives the greatest attenuation is defined as the major inflow vessel to the arch.

that these systems are better at predicting patency rather than occlusion and most surgeons would therefore not deny a patient the chance of vessel exploration with intraoperative pre-reconstruction arteriography on the basis of an unfavorable score.

Imaging of the venous system

It has been shown by a number of authors that preoperative duplex scanning of the superficial veins of the legs and arms can identify veins that are not visible clinically and in addition can size veins (**Fig. 12.3**) and detect veins with macroscopic disease caused by postphlebitic sclerosis (**Fig. 12.4**), calcification, or varicosities.[64,106,107] If a vascular technologist marks the site of the chosen vein with a skin marker, this greatly aids exposure of the vein and reduces the likelihood of undermining skin flaps that may then become necrotic. In addition, the technologist can use a venous occlusion technique (see above) to identify veins less than 3.0mm diameter that might be suitable as a bypass conduit.

ANESTHETIC CONSIDERATIONS

Lower limb bypass surgery can be performed under general anesthesia, epidural anesthesia, or local infiltration anesthesia.[103,108] The choice will often be determined by the precise nature of the planned surgery and the cardiorespiratory status of the patient. Although there is a growing consensus that those patients undergoing major vascular surgery who receive combined general and epidural anesthesia with postoperative epidural anesthesia have significantly lower cardiac morbidity than those receiving general anesthesia alone,[109] not all studies support this viewpoint.[110–112] It has been reported that epidural anesthesia after lower limb vascular reconstruction reduces platelet hyperaggregability as compared with general anesthesia[113] and that there is relatively less inhibition of fibrinolysis after epidural anesthesia.[114] It has also been shown that epidural anesthesia significantly decreases peripheral resistance and increases graft blood flow in femorodistal grafts.[115] However, in patients undergoing lower limb vascular

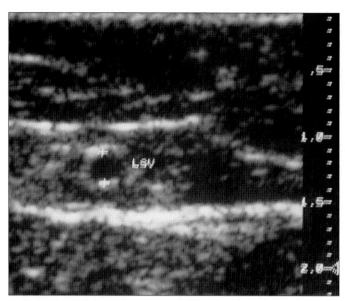

Figure 12.3 Small saphenous vein. Even with venous occlusion, this long saphenous vein (LSV) will not dilate beyond 2mm and is not therefore suitable for use as a bypass conduit.

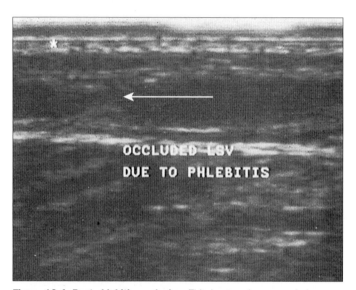

Figure 12.4 Post-phlebitic occlusion. This long saphenous vein has been occluded (arrow) by previous phlebitis.

reconstruction, it has not been convincingly shown that there is a significant difference in graft thrombosis rate between those who receive epidural anesthesia and those who receive general anesthesia.[112,115] Currently, therefore, the choice between general anesthesia and epidural anesthesia should be based on traditional anesthetic considerations.

Among the potential risks of epidural anesthesia is epidural hematoma, particularly in patients who receive large doses of anti-coagulants or fibrinolytic agents. Effective epidural anesthesia may provide such adequate pain relief that graft thrombosis is not immediately recognized and temperature differences between the limbs may be incorrectly ascribed to epidural anesthesia. An additional anesthetic consideration is that if the patient is to undergo arterial reconstruction using arm vein, it is important to ensure that the anesthetist does not cannulate the arm vein chosen as a bypass conduit!

SURGICAL STRATEGY

Precise surgical strategy will depend on the distribution of obstructive arterial disease, the cardiorespiratory status of the patient, the nature and extent of any previous abdominal or lower limb procedures, and the availability and location of autogenous vein. One of the intellectual challenges facing the surgeon is to 'tailor the procedure' to the patient. Thus, the operative strategy needs to take into account the length of available autogenous vein and the potential inflow and outflow sites. While it is not sensible to compromise the principles of unimpaired inflow and outflow sites, for the patient with limited autogenous vein it may be possible to move the inflow site more distally by PTA of proximal disease prior to or during surgery[116] or to move the outflow site more proximally by using on-table PTA of distal disease.[117]

Broadly speaking, surgical treatments can be divided into suprainguinal bypass, profundaplasty/endarterectomy, and infrainguinal bypass. Sometimes a combination of approaches is required. Techniques for suprainguinal bypass have already been discussed in Chapter 9, hence this chapter will discuss only the aspects that are particularly relevant to patients with CLI. However, this chapter will discuss profundaplasty/ endarterectomy, infrainguinal bypass, and related issues in detail.

Suprainguinal bypass

There is no doubt that in patients without significant cardio-respiratory or renal impairment, an aortobifemoral bypass graft gives excellent results. In those patients with aortic occlusions or bilateral iliac artery disease, the alternative is axillobifemoral bypass. The choice of axillary artery should be determined by measuring both brachial artery pressures and using the axillary artery with the higher pressure as the donor side. If both pressures are the same, then traditionally the axillary artery on the same side as the affected leg is used. Although axillobifemoral bypass has poorer patency than aortobifemoral bypass, it has been shown that the patency of an axillobifemoral bypass is superior to that of axillounifemoral bypass.[118] Graft material is usually 10 or 8mm externally supported PFTE or Dacron and the graft is tunneled down under pectoralis major and minor and then subcutaneously to the groin. Use of a long tunneler precludes the need for counter-incision. It has been shown in a randomized trial that the use of an axillobifemoral graft with a symmetrical flow-splitter at the bifurcation reduces the risk of the crossover limb occluding.[119] The patency rate of the prosthesis with a flow-splitter was 85% at 2 years as compared with 38% for a prosthesis with a 90°-angled bifurcation. Interestingly, in this series, patency was not influenced by anticoagulant therapy or by the nature of the outflow tract. The graft infection rate was 6%.

In patients with unilateral iliac disease, the options are femorofemoral or iliofemoral bypass. Femorofemoral bypass is performed from one common femoral artery to the other via vertical groin incisions. The graft is usually 10 or 8mm externally supported Dacron or PTFE tunneled subcutaneously, and the 5-year patency rate can be as high as 82%.[120] The alternative procedure, iliofemoral bypass, has the advantage of avoiding bilateral groin incisions and the associated risks of infection. Another advantage of an iliofemoral graft is that it can be tunneled behind the rectus sheath, and the groin preserved for radiologic access if angioplasty of the donor iliac artery is subsequently required. A recent study from Belgium reported primary and secondary 3-year patency rates for iliofemoral cross-over grafting of 94% and 100%, respectively, and limb salvage of 87% at 3 years.[121]

Profundaplasty/endarterectomy
Profundaplasty
Although profundaplasty is most commonly performed as part of an inflow procedure such as aortobifemoral bypass,[122] it may have a role as an isolated procedure in selected patients with CLI.[123,124] The indication for profundaplasty is in patients with a superficial femoral artery occlusion with a significant stenosis (>50%) or occlusion of the origin of the profunda femoris artery and who lack autogenous vein for a bypass. Criteria for successful outcome after isolated profundaplasty include the presence of well-developed distal profunda femoris artery collaterals and patent tibial vessels. Cumulative 3-year limb salvage rates of 83%[123] and 76%[124] have been reported. Kalman et al.[124] noted that the best results were obtained in those with two or three patent tibial arteries.

Endarterectomy
Although not commonly performed nowadays, it should not be forgotten that iliofemoral endarterectomy is a technique that may still have a role in the patient with critical ischemia. A recent series from France reported 5- and 10-year actuarial limb salvages of 98% and 90%, respectively.[125] An alternative to open endarterectomy is endarterectomy through a single arteriotomy using a ring cutter.[126] Although described and used predominantly in the superficial femoral artery segment, the technique has also been used with success in the iliac arteries.[126]

Infrainguinal bypass
Before discussing detailed operative techniques, it is necessary to consider general operative strategies and planning for infrainguinal bypass procedures.

General considerations
There is no doubt that femorodistal reconstruction can be very demanding of a surgeon's time, technical skills, and patience. There is also no doubt that a successful outcome requires meticulous attention to detail, gentle tissue handling, and an unwillingness to accept technical imperfection. With this in mind, these procedures should be performed in an environment that is not time-constrained, and it is invaluable to have at least two experienced surgeons, particularly if vein needs to be harvested from a number of different sites. Many surgeons find loupe magnification greatly facilitates these procedures, in particular the distal anastomosis. Intraoperative assessment and quality control is facilitated by an operating theater that is equipped with either mobile or static DSA equipment. Finally, it is well established that surgeon-determined judgmental or technical error accounts for the majority of graft failures in the first month after surgery,[127] and it cannot be stressed enough that it is highly preferable to spend time and effort getting these procedures right first time. Early graft thrombosis not only poses a difficult challenge for the surgeon but also markedly decreases secondary graft patency[23,31,128,129] and increases the morbidity and mortality of these procedures.

Choice and use of bypass material
As discussed above, there is no doubt that the preferred bypass conduit is autogenous vein. The importance of using good-quality vein cannot be overstressed and it is preferable to use composite vein grafts composed of good-quality vein than to use a single length of vein that contains diseased segments. Composite vein–prosthetic grafts offer no advantage over prosthetic grafts alone, and the alternative to autogenous vein, therefore, is a prosthetic graft.

Reversed vein versus in-situ vein
Since its first description by Kunlin in 1949,[130] reversed saphenous vein has been the most commonly used method for autogenous vein bypass. The in-situ technique was first described in 1965[131] and became increasingly popular in the early 1970s with the development of a valve stripper that can be inserted through the open end of the greater saphenous vein.[132] The major proposed theoretical advantage of the in-situ technique is that it keeps the vasa vasorum intact and thereby preserves the endothelial lining. However, it has been shown that the valve stripper causes extensive endothelial and smooth muscle damage, which is more severe in the case of in-situ vein than reversed vein.[133,134] A number of prospective randomized studies[135–139] and a large retrospective comparative review[140] have concluded that the incidence of vein graft stenosis and long-term patency of reversed and in-situ grafts are remarkably similar. Thus, the decision concerning in-situ or reversed vein should be made on an individual patient basis and not in the belief that either technique provides superior long-term patency.

One of the major disadvantages of the in-situ technique is that the use of an ipsilateral long saphenous vein is mandatory and this is not available in 30–40% of limbs.[21,138] It has been suggested that one potential advantage of the in-situ technique is that it allows the use of smaller-caliber vein because it allows a better match to the recipient distal artery.[141] However, small veins have been shown to perform badly for both the in-situ and the reversed technique[135–139] and, as discussed above, it would not seem sensible to use vein less than 3mm in diameter. One of the advantages of the in-situ technique is that in the event of graft thrombosis it is relatively easy to unblock the graft because the valves have been lysed. Unblocking a reversed vein graft with intact valves can be more difficult.

Angioscopy of bypass vein
Angioscopy has been used both to detect unsuspected venous disease[142] and for the minimally invasive construction of in-situ vein grafts.[143] Sales et al.[142] used angioscopy to examine 32 long saphenous veins prior to their use as bypass conduits and found a significantly better 1-year patency in an angioscopically normal compared with an abnormal group (70% versus 14%). More recently, Thorne et al.[144] used angioscopy to inspect roughly one-third of in-situ vein bypasses prior to the formation of the distal anastomosis. Interestingly, angioscopy detected partially occluding thrombus in 16% of veins but itself damaged the vein in 9% of cases. Although the 1-year primary patency was significantly better in those bypasses that had undergone angioscopy, the secondary patencies were not different. It is also interesting to note that this study was hampered by angioscope breakage and there is no doubt that one of the problems with angioscopy

is the delicate nature of the equipment and the costs of repair or replacement.

Angioscopically assisted in-situ vein bypass became very popular in the early 1990s with the angioscope being used to assist valve lysis and aid vein branch identification and occlusion. It was hoped that angioscopy would reduce operative morbidity, shorten hospital stay, and improve graft patency. A prospective study by Clair et al.[143] in 1994 randomized 59 patients and concluded that angioscopically assisted in-situ bypass conferred no benefit in terms of operative morbidity, hospital stay, or graft patency. A more recent multicenter study[145] randomized 273 patients undergoing in-situ vein bypass to an angioscopically assisted or a conventional procedure. The angioscopic group underwent angioscopically guided valvulotomy and side-branch occlusion using an angioscopic Side Branch Occlusion system. The 3-year primary patency, secondary patency, and limb salvage rates were similar. However, small veins (<3.0mm diameter) in the angioscope group fared badly, with a 1-year graft thrombosis rate of 15%. Wound complications, length of hospital stay, and overall costs were less in the angioscope group. Therefore, it would appear that angioscopically assisted in-situ bypass does have advantages providing the vein is >3.0mm in diameter. For smaller veins, instrumentation damage to the vein and subsequent graft thrombosis would appear to outweigh the benefits.

Prosthetic grafts

If it is not possible to use autologous vein, prosthetic grafts are an alternative. There is controversy regarding the role of prosthetic infrainguinal grafts to a single calf vessel and many surgeons would not use a prosthetic graft in this context. Careful patient selection is crucial and it should be borne in mind that the most important determinants of short- and long-term patency are the state of the runoff, the completeness of the plantar arch, and the degree of continuity between the two.[74,146] The choice of graft material lies between PTFE and Dacron. Although most surgeons prefer PTFE, there is little clinical evidence that it is better than Dacron. A recent randomized trial comparing PTFE with gelatin-sealed Dacron for femoropopliteal bypass found no difference in 3-year primary patency (52% versus 47%, respectively),[146] and a randomized trial comparing PTFE with heparin-bonded Dacron found that the latter had a significantly superior 3-year patency (55% versus 42%).[147] It should be noted that in both studies, the majority of bypasses were to the above-knee popliteal artery.

It has been shown in a prospective randomized study that the patency of below-knee PTFE grafts is improved by the addition of a vein cuff at the distal anastomosis.[148] This study did not include patients with bypass grafts to single calf vessels. However, it would seem reasonable to extrapolate the results and to use a vein cuff in this situation. It has been demonstrated in a prospective randomized study that the addition of a distal arteriovenous fistula to a vein cuff does not improve the patency of PTFE grafts to infrapopliteal vessels.[149]

Selection of inflow site

The inflow for infrainguinal bypass grafts has traditionally been based on the common femoral artery. However, there is no reason that more distal arteries cannot serve as inflow sites providing that there is no significant arterial obstruction proximally. Thus, a number of authors have described the use of the superficial femoral, profunda femoris, and popliteal arteries as inflow sites.[28,150–152] The potential advantages of these distal origin grafts include the increased likelihood of using autogenous vein and reduced surgical morbidity and recovery time. Mills et al.[151] reported secondary patency rates of 89%, 87%, and 87% for reversed vein bypasses originating from the common femoral, superficial femoral, and popliteal arteries, respectively. Distal origin grafts may be particularly useful in diabetic patients. Indeed, Reed et al.[28] have recently reported that the 5-year graft patency and limb salvage of distal origin grafts is higher in diabetic than non-diabetic patients (73% versus 45% and 84% versus 69%, respectively). A possible explanation for this finding is the typical diabetic pattern of disease, with relative sparing of inflow vessels above the knee.

If there is doubt about the suitability of a possible inflow site at the time of surgery, intra-arterial pressure measurements at rest and after papaverine can be helpful.[153] The principle is to compare the intra-arterial pressure at the proposed inflow site with brachial or radial arterial pressure. The inflow artery is punctured by a needle connected to a pressure transducer; the brachial or radial artery is also punctured, and the pressures compared. A resting systolic pressure difference of greater than 10mmHg is significant. After recording the inflow artery/brachial pressure ratio, papaverine (30mg) is injected into the inflow artery and the percentage fall in the ratio measured. A fall of 15% after papaverine is considered significant.[154]

Isolated popliteal segment

The most commonly used definition of an isolated popliteal segment is a distally occluded popliteal artery without direct runoff or with runoff into a single infrapopliteal artery that is patent for a distance of less than 5cm.[155,156] Although it would seem unlikely that a graft to an isolated popliteal segment will remain patent for long, the published results are surprisingly good. In a prospective randomized study of patients with an isolated popliteal artery segment, Darke et al.[157] found that the 1-year patency of bypasses to the isolated segment was not significantly different to that of bypasses to a reconstituted distal vessel lower in the calf (79% versus 70%, respectively). The conduit used in the majority of the patients in this study was in-situ vein.

Kram et al.[155] reported a 10-year experience of 217 femoro-popliteal bypasses to isolated popliteal artery segments. The majority (98%) of these procedures were for critical ischemia and the majority (85%) of bypass conduits were PTFE. Although the 5-year secondary patency for the saphenous vein group was significantly higher than for the PTFE group (74% versus 56%), the 5-year limb salvage rates were the same (78%). Other authors have also reported reasonable limb salvage results using PTFE grafts to an isolated popliteal segment.[156,158,159] It would appear, therefore, that in patients with an isolated popliteal artery segment who only have a short length of autogenous vein, a bypass to the isolated segment is a good option. If there is no autogenous vein available, then a PTFE bypass to an isolated popliteal artery segment is a reasonable option.

Pre-reconstruction intraoperative arteriography

The principles behind pre-reconstruction intraoperative angiography are to identify distal vessels that may not have been revealed by preoperative investigations[98,101] and to be absolutely certain that the site chosen for the distal anastomosis is appropriate. Some surgeons[103] do not perform preoperative angiography in the presence of a normal femoral pulse and instead always perform pre-reconstruction intraoperative angiography. Most surgeons use pre-reconstruction intraoperative arteriography selectively, depending on the results of preoperative imaging. The technique most commonly used is to study the preoperative investigations and then expose the most proximal site that will provide visualization of the predicted distal bypass target artery. The vessel is then cannulated with a small-gauge butterfly needle and 10–20mL of an ionic contrast medium is manually injected under X-ray screening.

Post-reconstruction quality control

Although a large number of techniques have been used to provide quality control for femorodistal bypass grafting, the three most commonly used are angioscopy,[160,161] post-reconstruction arteriography,[160,161] and duplex scanning.[162] Comparisons of angioscopy with arteriography have shown that angioscopy is better at detecting abnormalities within the conduit[160,161] but that angioscopy can miss abnormalities beyond the distal anastomosis. Miller et al.[161] prospectively randomized 293 patients undergoing infrainguinal bypass grafts to angioscopy or completion arteriography. Although more abnormalities were detected by angioscopy than by arteriography, this did not result in improved 1-month patency rates in the angioscopy group.

Gilbertson et al.[163] compared duplex with arteriography and angioscopy in a small series of 20 in-situ vein grafts. The results of this study suggest that angioscopy may be of particular value for in-situ vein grafts because it is particularly good at detecting residual competent valves or unligated tributaries. A recent report from Johnson et al.[162] has described the use of papaverine-augmented intraoperative completion duplex scans to provide quality control for infrainguinal bypass procedures. There was a 15% intraoperative revision rate, and a normal intraoperative duplex scan on initial imaging or after revision was associated with a 30-day graft thrombosis rate of only 0.2%.

It is pertinent to note that regardless of the quality-control technique used, the overall intraoperative graft revision rate is high (15–25%) in most studies. Thus, until the best technique or combination of techniques for quality control is defined, the important point is that some form of quality control is essential and the technique used will depend on local facilities and expertise.

Use of a tourniquet

The use of tourniquets in infrainguinal bypass surgery was first described by Bernhard et al.[164] in 1980 and since then a number of other authors have described their use. Distal vascular control during femorodistal reconstruction can be awkward. Vascular clamps, silastic slings, intraluminal flow arresters, and intraluminal balloons are commonly used methods of obtaining vascular control. These techniques may not work well in the presence of calcified vessels, may cause intimal flaps, and can clutter the operative field and reduce visibility and access. Proponents of the tourniquet technique argue that many of these technical problems are reduced and suggest that the reduced intimal trauma produced by tourniquets may improve both short and long-term patency rates.[165] The latter point, however, has not been proven. The technique most commonly used is to obtain

proximal vessel control in the normal way with clamps or slings, expose (but not mobilize) the distal vessels, if necessary tunnel the graft, heparinize the patient, exsanguinate the leg, apply the tourniquet at mid-thigh level, and then perform the distal anastomosis.[166]

OPERATIVE TECHNIQUES

The operative techniques for suprainguinal bypass have been discussed in Chapter 9 and this section will therefore discuss profundaplasty and infrainguinal bypass techniques. The latter will be described in detail.

Profundaplasty

A vertical groin incision is made over the common femoral artery and is carried approximately 5cm proximal to the inguinal crease. The length of profunda femoris artery requiring exposure will determine the distal extent of the incision. The common femoral artery and its branches are then exposed, as is the superficial femoral artery for 4–5cm from its origin. This allows the superficial femoral artery to be mobilized, which then facilitates dissection of the profunda femoris artery. The origin of the profunda femoris artery from the posterior aspect of the common femoral artery is identified and the dissection then continues down its anterior surface. At this point, the surgeon has to be aware that a number of large veins cross anterior to the profunda femoris artery, including the lateral circumflex femoral vein. These veins need to be carefully ligated and divided (**Fig. 12.5**). The length of dissection down the profunda femoris artery depends on the distal extent of disease within the artery. This is best ascertained by palpation. The dissection down the profunda femoris artery should continue to the first set of branches beyond the disease so that distal control can be obtained.

In patients who have had previous groin surgery and vascular repair, an alternative approach is to expose the mid-portion of the profunda femoris artery through an anterior thigh incision. The sartorius muscle is retracted laterally to expose the superficial femoral vessels, which are then retracted medially (**Fig. 12.6**). The fascia deep to the superficial artery is incised to expose the profunda femoris vessels between the first and second perforator branches. An approach lateral to the sartorius may also be employed to expose the profunda femoris artery.

Once the dissection has been completed, 5000 units of heparin is given intravenously and the vessels controlled by whatever means the surgeon prefers. A vertical incision is made in the anterior aspect of the common femoral artery, which then continues down the anterior wall of the profunda femoris for 1cm or more beyond the transition between abnormal and normal artery. Thromboendarterectomy is carried out as far as the transition zone, at which point it may be necessary to place tacking sutures (**Figs 12.7A & B**). The arteriotomy is then closed with a patch (**Fig. 12.7C**) that can either be formed from a segment of adjacent occluded endarterectomized superficial femoral artery or from saphenous vein (preferably a major branch of the long saphenous vein rather than the long saphenous vein itself), or by a prosthetic patch. The latter should only be used if no vein is available. The patch is tailored and sutured in such a way that it produces a gradually tapering lumen.

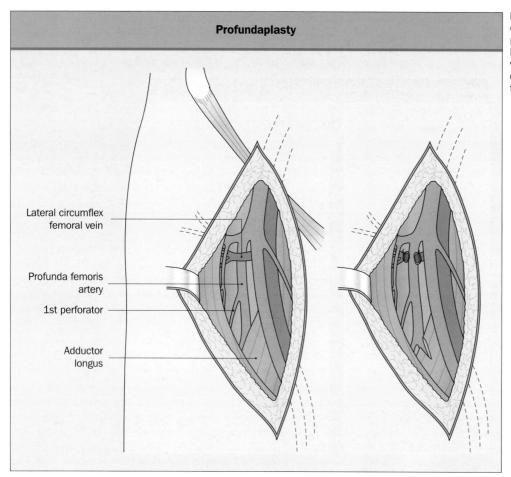

Profundaplasty

Lateral circumflex femoral vein

Profunda femoris artery

1st perforator

Adductor longus

Figure 12.5 Profundaplasty. A number of large veins cross anterior to the profunda femoris artery, including the lateral circumflex femoral vein. These veins need to be carefully ligated and divided in order to expose the profunda femoris artery.

Infrainguinal bypass
General
The patient should be prepared for surgery as previously described (see above). This should usually include subcutaneous heparin DVT prophylaxis, prophylactic antibiotics, and pre-operative duplex marking of the vein intended for use. In the case of arm vein, it is important to ensure that the anesthetist does not use the intended vein for intravenous access. If arm vein is to be used, the arms should be abducted and placed on arm boards. The patient usually lies supine unless it is intended to use a posterior approach, in which case the patient is placed prone. Exposure of many of the lower limb vessels is facilitated if the knee is flexed, and it is useful to have a heavy sandbag that can be placed under the sole of the foot to hold the leg in a flexed position.

Vessel exposure
Common femoral/profunda femoris /superficial femoral artery
If just the common femoral artery or the origin of the profunda femoris or superficial femoral artery needs exposure, then the preferred incision is an oblique incision placed above and parallel to the groin crease (**Fig. 12.8**). This is because oblique incisions for vascular access at the groin are associated with a decreased incidence of wound infection compared with conventional vertical incisions.[167] If, however, it is necessary to dissect some distance down the profunda femoris or superficial femoral artery, then a vertical incision is preferred. The

common femoral artery is exposed from the level of the inguinal ligament to its bifurcation, and the proximal superficial femoral artery and profunda femoris artery are mobilized and control is obtained. If it is necessary to expose the distal profunda, the technique described above for profundaplasty is followed. It is straightforward to follow the superficial femoral artery down the thigh by extending the vertical incision and dissecting the superficial femoral artery out of the loose areolar tissue surrounding it.

Above-knee popliteal artery
The above-knee popliteal artery is exposed through a medial thigh incision (**Fig. 12.8**) to expose the sartorius muscle, which is then retracted posterolaterally. The underlying deep fascia distal to the adductor magnus tendon is incised over the abductor canal, and the popliteal artery is dissected free of accompanying structures as it lies posterior to the femur. The artery is then mobilized as far as necessary distally. This is best determined by palpation. Flexion of the knee facilitates distal dissection.

Below-knee popliteal artery
The below-knee popliteal artery is exposed through a medial calf incision posterior to the medial femoral condyle (**Fig. 12.8**), extending distally medial to the tibial crest. Care should be taken not to damage the underlying saphenous vein, which should be carefully mobilized. The deep muscular fascia is incised and the medial head of gastrocnemius is reflected posteriorly to

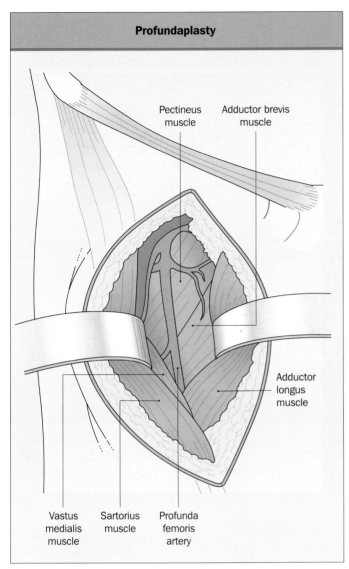

Profundaplasty

Pectineus muscle

Adductor brevis muscle

Adductor longus muscle

Vastus medialis muscle

Sartorius muscle

Profunda femoris artery

Figure 12.6 Profundaplasty. The mid portion of the profunda femoris artery is exposed by lateral retraction of the sartorius muscle and medial retraction of the superficial femoral vessels.

expose the popliteal artery. The distal popliteal artery is mobilized from the popliteal vein, which usually lies medially. Great care should be taken not to damage surrounding veins. By following the dissection distally, the tibioperoneal trunk can be exposed, as can the origin of the anterior tibial artery.

Anterior tibial artery

The anterior tibial artery can be exposed at its origin as it leaves the below-knee popliteal artery, as described above. More commonly, however, the anterior tibial artery is approached through a longitudinal incision over the anterior compartment of the leg (**Figs 12.8 & 12.9**) and is exposed by reflection of the anterior tibial muscle anteromedially and the digital extensor muscles laterally. The vessels are found lying on the interosseous membrane close to the tibia.

Posterior tibial artery

The proximal posterior tibial artery is best isolated by continued dissection down the tibioperoneal trunk as described above. The

mid-posterior tibial artery is exposed through a medial calf incision (**Figs 12.8 & 12.9**). The distal posterior tibial artery is exposed through an incision just posterior to the medial malleolus (**Fig. 12.8**), and its medial and lateral plantar branches are exposed by extension of the incision on to the medial surface of the foot.

Peroneal artery

The proximal peroneal artery can be exposed by continuation of dissection down the tibioperoneal trunk as described above. There are a number of techniques for exposure of the distal peroneal artery. One technique using a lateral approach involves placing a longitudinal incision over the distal fibula (**Figs 12.8 & 12.10**), mobilizing the long peroneal muscle from the fibula and reflecting it posteriorly along with the flexor hallucis longus. A 10cm length of fibula is then resected and the peroneal artery and its accompanying veins are located just deep to a thin layer of fascia lying on the surface of the posterior tibial muscle. This lateral approach can be followed by postoperative pain and distal lower extremity edema, and an alternative is a posterior approach to the peroneal artery (**Fig. 12.11**). This approach is particularly useful when the inflow source is the popliteal artery and the conduit to be used is to lesser saphenous vein. The patient is placed prone on the operating table and a longitudinal incision is made in the midline at the level of the proposed anastomosis to the peroneal artery. The mid-peroneal artery is exposed by splitting the fibers of the gastrocnemius and soleus muscles. This can be facilitated with the use of a hand-held intraoperative pencil Doppler probe. The distal peroneal artery is readily isolated by medial displacement of the lateral body of the gastrocnemius and soleus muscles, followed by incision of the deep investing fascia in lateral to tendo calcaneus. The flexor hallucis longus muscle is retracted laterally and the fibula is palpated as a landmark running immediately lateral to the artery.[168] Up to 15cm of the vessel can be exposed before it bifurcates into anterolateral and posteromedial collateral branches running to the anterior and posterior tibial arteries, respectively.

Dorsalis pedis artery

This vessel is easily exposed through a longitudinal incision on the dorsum of the foot just lateral to the extensor hallucis longus tendon (**Fig. 12.9**). It is important that a wide skin bridge is provided between the arterial incision and that required for exposure and subsequent mobilization of the distal saphenous vein.

In-situ bypass

In-situ bypass can be performed either by exposing the entire length of the long saphenous vein, or, if an angioscope is used to identify vein tributaries, by means of multiple small discontinuous incisions. As described above, a further extension of the use of the angioscope is occlusion of patent tributaries with small metal coils. Although there is little doubt that these angioscopic approaches are appealing, there is a significant learning curve and operative times can be significantly prolonged. The in-situ method requires that the proximal anastomosis be initially constructed after transection of the saphenofemoral junction and closure of the common femoral venotomy. The proximal anastomosis is usually located in the distal common femoral

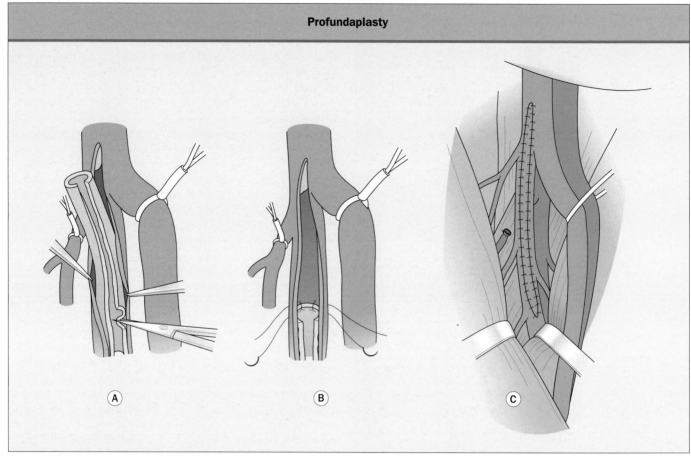

Profundaplasty

Figure 12.7 Profundaplasty. (A) Endarterectomy of profunda femoris artery. (B) After completion of the endarterectomy, the distal intimal flap is tacked down and the arteriotomy is closed with a patch (C).

artery but the precise site is dictated by the level of the saphenofemoral junction. It is usual to mobilize a segment of proximal saphenous vein and to excise the cusps of the first venous valve under direct vision. Once control of the relevant inflow arteries has been obtained, an arteriotomy is made in the distal common femoral artery, and, if necessary, a preliminary endarterectomy can be performed. The anastomosis is then constructed using conventional techniques, and, after completion of such, arterial flow is established through the vein to the level of the first competent valve. Valve lysis is then achieved using a valvulotome such as those developed by Hall or Mills. The efficacy of valve lysis can be assessed by observing the flow out of the open end of the graft. An arteriotomy is made in the distal target vessel and the anastomosis performed using a fine monofilament suture. Some surgeons like to perform the distal anastomosis with a fine catheter in the distal artery to reduce the chance of technical error.

Non-reversed saphenous vein

If the ipsilateral long saphenous vein is not available and it is felt that the practical advantages of the in-situ technique, such as a better size match between the artery and vein at the proximal and distal anastomoses, are desirable, then an alternative approach, as described by Beard et al.,[169] may be used. In this approach, the vein is harvested from its bed and the proximal valve is then excised under direct vision. The proximal anastomosis is completed and the valves are lysed as described for the in-situ bypass operation. The graft may then be tunneled if necessary and the distal anastomosis performed.

Reversed long saphenous vein

Vein may be harvested either through one long incision or through numerous short longitudinal skin incisions with intervening cutaneous bridges. The tributaries of the vein are divided and ligated. After excision, the reverse vein is gently flushed with heparinized saline and then stored in the flush solution until use. Either the proximal or distal anastomosis may be performed first. The advantage of performing the proximal anastomosis first is that it is easier to detect kinking of the vein. The vein is then tunneled using an appropriate tunneling device down to the relevant distal target artery. It is important after tunneling to ensure that the vein is not kinked and that there is an adequate length of vein with the leg in the extended position. The chances of kinking can also be minimized by marking the anterior surface of the vein with methylene blue prior to tunnelling and ensuring that the marks remain on the anterior surface of the vein after tunneling. Although it is usual to tunnel the vein down the medial side of the leg, it is entirely acceptable, if necessary, to tunnel the vein along the anterior lateral thigh and calf to the anterior tibial artery.

Arterial exposure

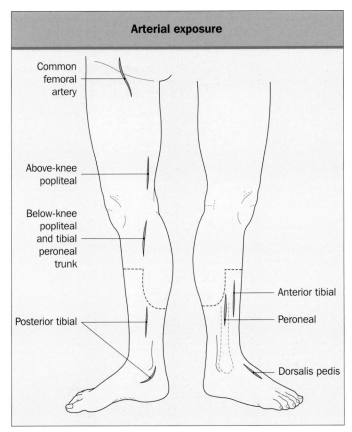

Figure 12.8 Arterial exposure. Sites of incisions for exposure of major lower limb arteries.

Approaches to tibial arteries

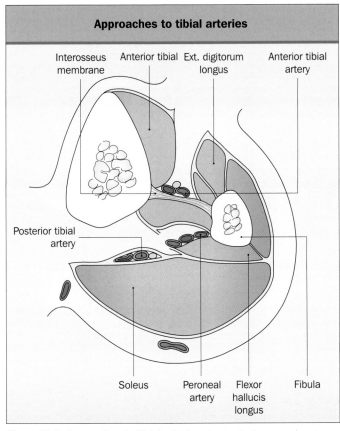

Figure 12.9 Approaches to tibial arteries. Anatomical approaches to the anterior tibial, peroneal, and posterior tibial arteries in the mid calf.

Lateral approach to peroneal artery

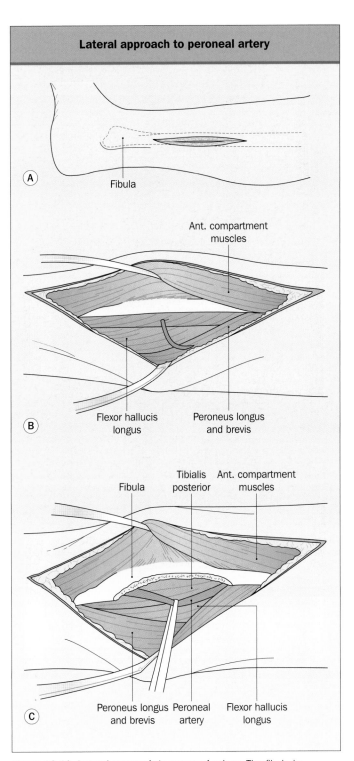

Figure 12.10 Lateral approach to peroneal artery. The fibula is exposed and a 10cm length resected to reveal the peroneal artery and vein lying beneath it.

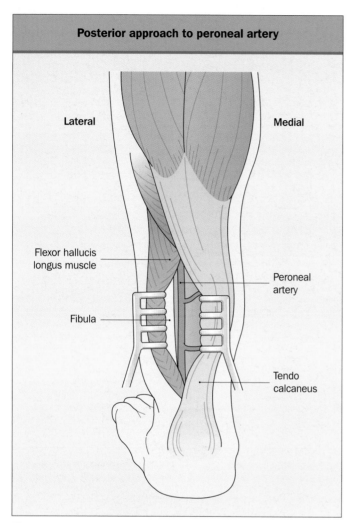

Figure 12.11 Posterior approach to peroneal artery. The tendo calcaneus is retracted medially and flexor hallucis longus is retracted laterally to expose the peroneal artery.

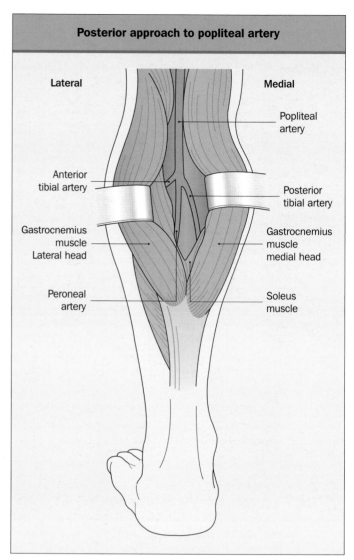

Figure 12.12 Posterior approach to popliteal artery. The two heads of the gastrocnemius muscle are separated and the proximal soleus muscle is divided to reveal the proximal tibial vessels.

Pedal bypass

A number of authors have shown that with careful patient selection, excellent results can be achieved with bypass to the foot.[170,171] This approach may be of particular value in patients with diabetes.[28,172] Ouriel[171] has described a posterior approach to popliteal-crural bypass. The patient is placed in a prone position and the short saphenous vein is used as the bypass conduit.[173] The popliteal artery is exposed through a posterior midline short saphenous vein harvest incision that is placed between the two heads of the gastrocnemius muscle (**Fig. 12.12**). The proximal 10cm of the soleus muscle can then be divided to expose the proximal portion of the crural vessels. Only the first 2cm of the anterior tibial artery can be exposed, but this can be extended by dividing the interosseous membrane. The exposures of the peroneal and posterior tibial arteries are shown in **Figures 12.11 and 12.13** respectively. The anterior tibial artery is exposed through the standard anterior lateral incision by externally rotating the leg to bring the cleft between the anterior tibial and extensor hallucis longus muscles into an accessible view. If the anterior tibial artery is the target vessel,

the vein can be tunneled from the posterior fossa to the anterior tibial artery through the interosseous membrane.

Optimizing the use of autogenous vein

There are a number of techniques that can be used to optimize the use of autogenous vein and these are shown diagrammatically in **Figures 12.14–12.16**.

Prosthetic bypass

As discussed above, if a prosthetic bypass is to be used with a distal anastomosis to the below-knee popliteal artery or more distal, a vein cuff should be utilized. The three types of vein cuff commonly used are illustrated in **Figure 12.17**.

PHARMACOTHERAPY

Intraoperative

Although a number of small studies have examined the effect of intraoperative iloprost on graft patency, the largest study is from the Iloprost Bypass International Study Group.[174] This

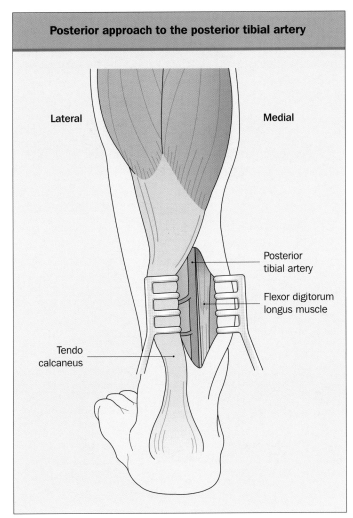

Posterior approach to the posterior tibial artery

Lateral

Medial

Posterior
tibial artery

Flexor digitorum
longus muscle

Tendo
calcaneus

Figure 12.13 Posterior approach to the posterior tibial artery. The tendo calcaneus is retracted laterally and the flexor digitorum longus muscle is retracted medially to reveal the posterior tibial artery.

prospective, multicenter, placebo-controlled study randomized 516 patients undergoing femorodistal bypass surgery (424 vein, 92 prosthetic) to receive either intravenous iloprost or placebo intraoperatively, followed by daily 6-hour infusions for the first three postoperative days. All patients had critical ischemia and in 97.5% of cases the distal anastomosis was distal to the below-knee popliteal artery. Iloprost had no effect on 1-year primary patency or limb salvage in either the prosthetic or the vein group.

Postoperative
Antiplatelet agents
There have been a large number of relatively small trials that have suggested that aspirin improves the patency of infrainguinal bypass grafts, in particular prosthetic grafts.[175] Although this finding is of interest, its relevance to clinical practice has been diminished by the fact that all patients with peripheral vascular disease should be on an antiplatelet agent anyway, because of the cardio- and cerebroprotective effects of such.[176] It has also been shown that these agents should be continued in the perioperative period.[85] If patients are intolerant of aspirin, clopidogrel is an excellent, although more expensive, alternative.[177]

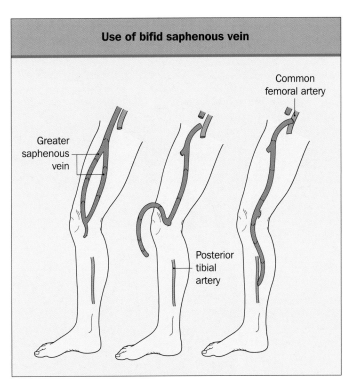

Use of bifid saphenous vein

Common
femoral artery

Greater
saphenous
vein

Posterior
tibial
artery

Figure 12.14 Use of bifid saphenous vein. One proximal end of the bifid vein is divided and rotated to become the distal end of the graft. The proximal half of the graft is kept *in situ* and the valves lysed with a valvulotome. The distal rotated segment is reversed and valve lysis is not therefore necessary.

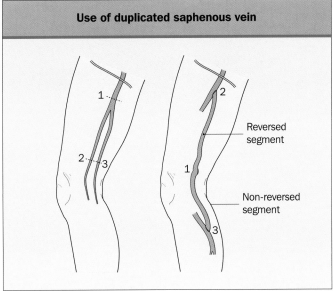

Use of duplicated saphenous vein

Reversed
segment

Non-reversed
segment

Figure 12.15 Use of duplicated saphenous vein. Both branches of the saphenous vein are mobilized and the trunk with the largest diameter reversed and used for the proximal part of the graft. The smaller branch is used as a distal non-reversed segment and its valves lysed. The excised bifurcation zone is sutured.

Anticoagulants
There has been only one long-term placebo-controlled study assessing the effect of anticoagulation on long-term infrainguinal bypass patency.[178] This study randomized 130 patients undergoing infrainguinal vein bypass to phenprocoumon or placebo and

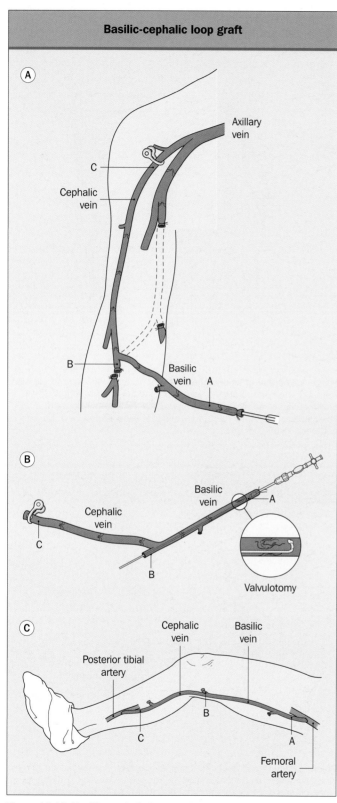

Basilic-cephalic loop graft

Figure 12.16 Basilic–cephalic loop graft. The basilic and cephalic veins are mobilized (A) and the valves of the distended basilic vein lysed (B). The proximal basilic vein is then placed in 'non-reversed ' orientation (C), while the distal cephalic segment is used in the reversed orientation. (Modified from LoGerfo FW, Paniszyn CW, Menzoian J. A new arm vein graft for distal bypass. J Vasc Surg 1987;5:889–91.)

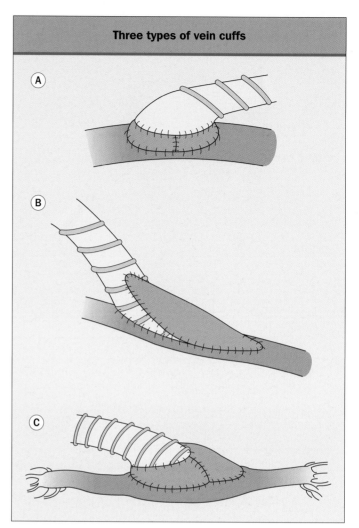

Three types of vein cuffs

Figure 12.17 Three types of vein cuffs. (A) Miller collar; (B) Taylor patch; (C) St Mary's boot.

reported a significant improvement in graft patency, limb salvage, and patient survival in the phenprocoumon group. The Dutch Bypass or Oral anticoagulants or Aspirin (BOA) study randomized 2690 patients undergoing infrainguinal bypass to aspirin or oral anticoagulants.[179] Analysis of the data revealed no overall difference between the two groups. However, subgroup analysis revealed that oral anticoagulation significantly improved the patency of vein grafts compared with aspirin, with a relative risk of graft occlusion of 0.69 (confidence interval [CI] 0.64–0.88), whereas aspirin significantly increased the chances of a prosthetic graft remaining patent by 1.26 (CI 1.03–1.55). It is important to note that patients randomized to oral anticoagulation in this study had a relative risk of a major bleeding episode of 1.96 (CI 1.42–2.71).

Sarac et al.[180] randomized 56 patients with high-risk infrainguinal vein grafts to receive aspirin alone or a combination of aspirin plus warfarin. Patients randomized to warfarin were anticoagulated immediately after surgery with intravenous heparin. High-risk grafts were defined as those with a suboptimal venous conduit, poor arterial runoff, or redo infrainguinal bypass grafting. The 3-year primary patency was significantly higher in the warfarin-plus-aspirin group (74% versus 51%), as was the 3-year limb salvage (81% versus 31%). However, this improved outcome was gained at the expense of significantly more postoperative wound hematomas in the warfarin-plus-aspirin group (32% versus 3.7%). One-quarter of the wound hematomas in the warfarin-plus-aspirin group required operative evacuation.

More recently, Johnson et al.[181] have reported the results of a Veterans Affairs Cooperative study that included 665 patients with infrainguinal bypasses who were randomized to aspirin alone or aspirin plus warfarin. The addition of warfarin to aspirin had no effect on vein bypass patency but did reduce the risk of prosthetic bypass occlusion by a factor of 0.62 (CI 0.42–0.92). There were twice as many major hemorrhagic events in those taking warfarin and the risk of death was increased by a factor of 1.41 (CI 1.09–1.84).

There seems no doubt from the above studies in patients with peripheral vascular disease that combining an anticoagulant with aspirin carries significant risks. The same risks have been noted in other patient groups. Thus, a meta-analysis[182] of the effects of combining aspirin with warfarin in patients with angina has shown an excess of major bleeding in those taking warfarin plus aspirin compared with those taking aspirin alone (odds ratio 1.95; CI 1.27–2.98).

The fact that all patients with peripheral vascular disease should be on an antiplatelet agent for cardio- and cerebro-protection means that the decision to be made in the case of the patient with an infrainguinal bypass graft is whether to add an anticoagulant to the antiplatelet agent. Current evidence suggests that for prosthetic grafts and 'high-risk' vein grafts there may be some benefit in terms of graft patency. However, this improved patency is gained at the expense of roughly doubling the risk of a major hemorrhage compared with taking aspirin alone. A reasonable approach, therefore, is to use anticoagulants selectively and only anticoagulate patients with 'high-risk' vein or prosthetic grafts providing the patient does not have a raised baseline risk of a hemorrhagic event.

GRAFT SURVEILLANCE

The principle behind a graft surveillance program is to detect failing grafts before they occlude. Graft occlusion during the first postoperative month most commonly results from technical error or poor runoff. After 1 month, the commonest cause of graft occlusion is intimal hyperplasia causing a localized graft stenosis (**Figs 12.18 & 12.19**). Up to 30% of vein grafts will develop a patency-threatening stenosis in the first two postoperative years. It has been shown that only one-third of hemodynamically significant graft stenoses cause symptoms or diminished pulses[183] and that serial ABPI measurements are insensitive.[184] Color duplex scanning can detect stenoses (**Fig. 12.20**) and the criterion most commonly used is the peak systolic velocity ratio (PSVR) across the stenosis. Repair has been recommended for stenoses with a PSVR above 3.0 or 4.0.[185,186] The treatment options are interposition vein graft, surgical vein patch angioplasty, or PTA (**Fig. 12.21**).

Although there is no doubt that color duplex scanning can detect graft stenoses, there is controversy regarding the effectiveness of graft surveillance programs. Lundell et al.[187] randomized patients with infrainguinal vein grafts to intensive duplex surveillance or not, and found that intensive surveillance significantly improved secondary patency at 3 years (82% versus 56%). In contrast, a randomized controlled study by Ihlberg et al.[188] failed to show any benefit from duplex

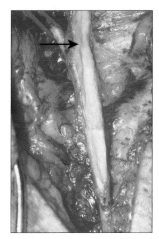

Figure 12.18 Vein graft stenosis. Operative photograph of a vein graft stenosis (arrowed).

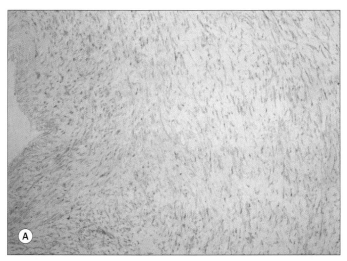

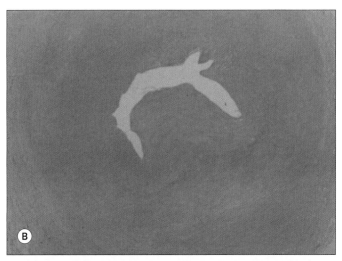

Figure 12.19 Histology of vein graft stenosis. Photomicrograph of a vein graft stenosis stained with anti-smooth-muscle actin and Alcian blue/PAS. The former stains smooth muscle cells red and the latter stains matrix mucopolysaccharides blue. It can be seen that the intimal hyperplastic lesion contains large numbers of smooth muscle cells that are producing copious extracellular matrix.

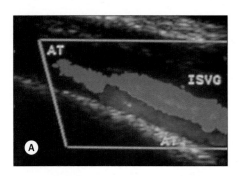
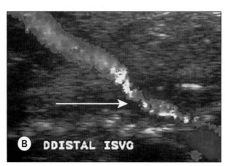

Figure 12.20 Duplex scanning. (A) A normal in-situ vein graft (ISVG) is seen joining the anterior tibial artery (AT). (B) In the distal portion of this in-situ vein graft there is a flow disturbance (arrow) that was causing a peak systolic velocity ratio of 4.5 across the stenosis.

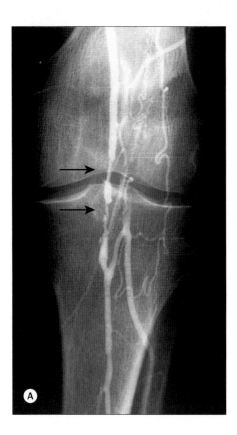
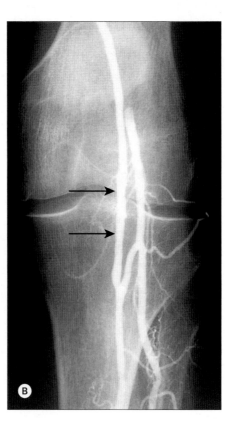

Figure 12.21 Percutaneous transluminal angioplasty of vein graft stenoses. Two stenoses (arrows) in vein graft to below-knee popliteal artery before (A) and after (B) angioplasty.

surveillance. However, only 60% of patients randomized to duplex surveillance actually received a duplex scan and 8% of patients in the non-surveillance group underwent duplex surveillance at the request of their surgeon. The graft revision rate was also quite low in this report. The results of this study are therefore difficult to interpret. Visser et al.[189] in Europe and Wixon et al.[190] in North America have examined the cost-effectiveness of vein graft duplex surveillance and have concluded that in patients with CLI it is highly effective and leads to a reduction in major amputation and, consequently, in costs. Overall, there is a strong body of evidence in favor of duplex surveillance of vein grafts. Conversely, there is agreement that surveillance of prosthetic grafts is not worthwhile.[187,191,192]

MANAGEMENT OF GRAFT THROMBOSIS

Early graft thrombosis, within 30 days of surgery, can result from technical error, poor-quality conduit, poor inflow, poor outflow, or hypotension in the immediate postoperative period.

In addition, there are a small number of grafts, particularly prosthetic grafts, that occlude in the immediate postoperative period for no identifiable reason. Graft failure between 1 month and 2 years usually results from intimal hyperplasia; after 2 years, progression of atherosclerosis in either inflow or outflow arteries becomes increasingly important. Early graft thrombosis will often result in acute critical ischemia requiring immediate re-operation, whereas late graft thrombosis will more frequently result in the return of preoperative symptoms. Although in the latter situation there is no need for immediate surgery to save the leg, there is no doubt that the longer a graft remains thrombosed, particularly a vein graft, the more difficult it is to unblock. An underlying principle behind the management of all thrombosed grafts is the need to ascertain and correct the cause or causes of the graft failure. It is particularly helpful in this respect if the surgeon performing the original procedure records in the operation note any areas of concern or likely causes of graft failure. Most surgeons would consider revised thrombosed grafts as 'high risk' and, in the absence of contraindications, would anticoagulate the patient.

Early graft thrombosis

Early graft thrombosis frequently results in severe acute ischemia and requires an immediate re-operation. The return to theater should not be delayed by arteriography because this can be performed on table. It is, however, invaluable to request a vascular technologist to search for and mark any useable vein in the contralateral leg or arms. This should not, however, significantly delay the return to theater. If for any reason the return to theater is unavoidably delayed, the surgeon may have to consider performing a fasciotomy. Finally, these re-operative procedures are particularly demanding and are greatly aided by the assistance of a 'fresh' experienced vascular surgeon.

Vein grafts

The distal incision is reopened, and, after anticoagulation with intravenous heparin, a linear venotomy is made in the hood of the graft. Any visible clot is removed with fine forceps and a balloon catheter is passed distally. An on-table arteriogram is then performed to examine the state of the runoff vessels. If there is fresh clot in the vessels, this can be removed by direct infusion of tissue plasminogen activator (5–10mg in 50mL saline infused over 20min) into the vessels. If there is long-standing runoff disease, this can be dealt with either by extension of the bypass or by on-table PTA. The choice of approach will depend on factors such as the availability of additional autogenous vein and the nature of the distal disease. Although thrombus in the body of the graft can sometimes be removed using a balloon catheter passed up from the distal venotomy, it is frequently necessary to expose the proximal anastomosis and remove thrombus through a proximal venotomy. Reversed vein grafts can be particularly troublesome because of intact valves obstructing the passage of balloon catheters. The technique described by Pit and Lawson[193] is particularly useful in this respect (**Fig. 12.22**).

If a cause for the graft thrombosis can be identified and corrected using the original vein graft, then a completion arteriogram including the full length of the graft should be performed to ensure that there are indeed no remaining problems. If the vein graft itself cannot be unblocked or is an inadequate conduit, then every effort should be made to replace it with alternative autogenous vein, including, if necessary, composite vein. If no additional autogenous vein can be found, the decision regarding the use of a prosthetic graft is based on the state of the runoff, the completeness of the plantar arch, and the degree of continuity between the two.[74,146] If a prosthetic graft is used, it has to be accepted that the risk of infection is increased in the circumstance of an often-prolonged revision procedure occurring soon after the primary operation.

If the techniques described above do not demonstrate a cause for graft failure, a final investigation once graft flow has been established is to measure the pressure (see above) in the inflow artery. If pressure measurements reveal an inflow problem, this is best dealt with by on-table PTA. Sometimes no cause for the early failure of a vein graft can be found, and in this circumstance, simple thrombectomy can result in long-term patency.

Prosthetic grafts

The surgical principles underlying the management of the early thrombosis of a prosthetic graft are the same as those for a vein graft. However, the graft itself is usually easier to unblock and

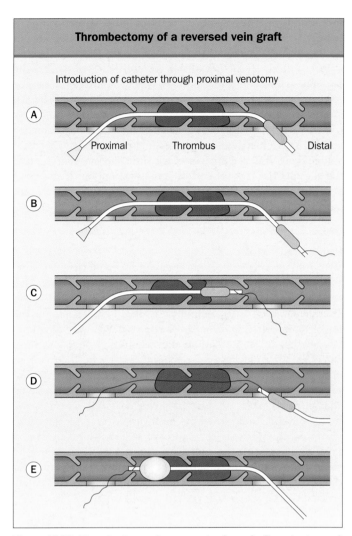

Thrombectomy of a reversed vein graft

Introduction of catheter through proximal venotomy

(A) Proximal   Thrombus   Distal

(B)

(C)

(D)

(E)

Figure 12.22 Thrombectomy of a reversed vein graft. Thrombectomy of a reversed vein graft using a Fogarty balloon catheter is impeded by the presence of valves. The graft is opened with small proximal and distal incisions and a Fogarty catheter introduced through the proximal incision (A). A thread is attached to the catheter tip (B) that is then pulled through the graft and out of the proximal incision (C). The distal thread is now attached to the catheter tip, which is then pulled up through the valves against their flow direction (D). The catheter balloon is then inflated and thrombectomy proceeds (E). Steps (D) and (E) can be repeated as required. (Adapted from Pit & Lawson.[193])

it is more common to not find an identifiable cause of graft failure. If a below-knee prosthetic graft has not had a vein cuff placed at the distal anastomosis, then one should be inserted. If no cause for graft failure can be found, one approach, in theory, is to replace the prosthetic with autologous vein. However, in practice, most surgeons would only use a prosthetic graft for the primary procedure if vein was not available, and it is unlikely, therefore, that vein would be available at this point.

Late graft thrombosis

Late graft thrombosis does not usually lead to acute ischemia and in some cases may not lead to a recurrence of the patient's preoperative symptoms. The first course of action, therefore, may be a risk/benefit discussion with the patient concerning the need for and potential benefits of reintervention. If reintervention is required, then the arterial system of the affected limb should be investigated by duplex scanning. If this reveals disease that is amenable to PTA, then this is an excellent solution to the problem. However, this option is rarely available, since the original bypass procedure was performed because the original arterial disease was not suitable for PTA. If further surgery is required, the patient should have all of his or her remaining leg and arm veins mapped so that the surgeon can assess the available options. If vein mapping reveals sufficient length to replace the thrombosed graft, then this is the best option. If sufficient vein is not available, the options depend on the type of graft that has thrombosed.

Vein grafts

Vein grafts that have been thrombosed for more than 48 hours are usually impossible to unblock using surgical techniques. One approach to the problem which can be used for up to 14 days after graft thrombosis is thrombolysis. Initial enthusiasm for the use of thrombolysis in thrombosed vein grafts has been tempered by the risks of hemorrhagic complications and poor long-term patencies.[194,195] Thus, although the success rate for thrombolysis of thrombosed vein grafts can be as high as 100%,[194] up to 25% of patients suffer a serious hemorrhage and up to 75% require an adjunctive radiologic or surgical procedure.[195] It would seem, therefore, that thrombolysis is best viewed as a technique to open up a thrombosed vein graft prior to a radiologic or surgical procedure to correct the underlying cause of the graft failure. In view of the risks of thrombolysis, it is probably best reserved for those occasions when there is insufficient autogenous vein to replace a thrombosed vein graft.

Prosthetic grafts

Unlike with vein grafts, it is usually possible to unblock prosthetic grafts using conventional surgical techniques, and, conversely, the results of thrombolysis of occluded prosthetic grafts are poor. If autogenous vein is not available, then one approach is surgical graft thrombectomy combined with on-table thrombolysis in an attempt to rid the distal runoff vessels of thrombus. The nature of any corrective procedure will be determined by the findings of on-table arteriography. Chronic runoff vessel disease can be dealt with either by on-table PTA or by a distal extension of the prosthetic bypass. Distal or proximal anastomotic intimal hyperplasia is best managed by patch angioplasty using vein.

A PERSONAL VIEW

The preceding sections have summarized the evidence for a number of approaches to the management of CLI. In this section, I will summarize my own approach to such, not in the belief that my method is necessarily the best, but it does at least provide the reader one approach to the problem. My initial investigation of the patient with CLI is always a color duplex scan of the lower limb arterial tree. Based on this scan, I then decide whether a PTA is possible. If a PTA is technically feasible, I will discuss the pros and cons of such an approach with the patient, including the complication rate. If a PTA looks unlikely to be technically possible or successful, I will then request a scan of the patient's lower limb veins and, if necessary, the arm vein as well. If no autogenous vein is available, this would make me more likely to request an attempted angioplasty in a borderline case; if autogenous is available, I would proceed to surgery. I routinely perform a dependent Doppler examination to confirm that the proposed target distal vessel is in continuity with the pedal arch. I would never proceed to a primary amputation in a patient in whom I was intending to salvage the leg without intraoperative pre-reconstruction arteriography.

I routinely use subcutaneous low-molecular-weight heparin thromboprophylaxis and at least three doses of antibiotic prophylaxis. I try to tailor the operative plan to the individual patient. In particular, it is often possible to use autogenous vein by being creative about inflow and outflow sites, including if required, pre- and intraoperative PTA. I would use contralateral long saphenous vein or arm vein or composite autologous vein rather than a prosthetic graft. I always request preoperative duplex marking of the intended venous conduit: this is to detect diseased segments and to minimize undermining skin flaps. I routinely use loupe magnification. Although I only rarely request preoperative arteriography, as discussed above I routinely perform pre-reconstruction arteriography, the site of which is dictated by a preoperative duplex scan. I favor a reversed vein technique because I find that valve lysis in small veins can be difficult and also because I like to tunnel the vein deep to thigh or calf wounds that if they become infected may threaten an underlying in-situ vein graft. I routinely perform completion arteriography in the expectation that approximately 20% of grafts will harbor a technical error that requires correction. I would only use a prosthetic graft if the patient had excellent runoff that was in continuity with the plantar arch. If I use a prosthetic graft, I always use a vein cuff if the outflow is below the knee. I always enter vein grafts into a surveillance program, but never do so with prosthetic grafts. A remarkably similar approach is utilized by many experienced North American surgeons.[196,197]

REFERENCES

1. Taylor RS, Belli AM, Jacob S. Distal venous arterialisation for salvage of critically ischaemic inoperable limbs. Lancet 1999;354:1962–5.
2. Abou-Zamzam AM, Lee RW, Moneta GL, Taylor LM, Porter JM. Functional outcome after infrainguinal bypass for limb salvage. J Vasc Surg 1997;25:287–95.
3. O'Brien TS, Lamont PM, Crow A, et al. Lower limb ischaemia in the octogenerian: is limb salvage surgery worthwhile? Ann R Coll Surg Engl 2002;75:445–7.
4. Nehler MR, Moneta GL, Edwards JM, et al. Surgery for chronic lower extremity ischemia in patients eighty or more years of age: operative results and assessment of postoperative independence. J Vasc Surg 1993;18:618–24.
5. Scher LA, Veith FJ, Ascer E, et al. Limb salvage in octogenarians and nonagenarians. Surgery 1986;99:160–5.
6. Klevsgard R, Hallberg IR, Risberg B, Thomsen MB. Quality of life associated with varying degrees of chronic lower limb ischaemia: comparison with a healthy sample. Eur J Vasc Endovasc Surg 1999; 17:319–25.

7. Chetter IC, Spark JI, Scott DJ, et al. Prospective analysis of quality of life in patients following infrainguinal reconstruction for chronic critical ischaemia. Br J Surg 1998;85:951–5.
8. Tangelder MJD, McDonnell J, Van Busschbach JJ, et al. Quality of life after infrainguinal bypass grafting surgery. J Vasc Surg 2002; 29:913–9.
9. Albers M, Fratezi AC, De Luccia N. Assessment of quality of life of patients with severe ischemia as a result of infrainguinal arterial occlusive disease. J Vasc Surg 1992;16:54–9.
10. Holtzman J, Caldwell M, Walvatne C, Kane R. Long-term functional status and quality of life after lower extremity revascularization. J Vasc Surg 1999;29:395–402.
11. Humphreys WV, Evans F, Watkin G, Williams T. Critical limb ischaemia in patients over 80 years of age: options in a district general hospital. Br J Surg 1995;82:1361–3.
12. Johnson BF, Evans L, Drury R, et al. Surgery for limb threatening ischaemia: a reappraisal of the costs and benefits. Eur J Vasc Endovasc Surg 1995;9:181–8.
13. Luther M. Surgical treatment for chronic critical leg ischaemia: a 5 year follow-up of socioeconomic outcome. Eur J Vasc Endovasc Surg 1997; 13:452–9.
14. Cheshire NJ, Wolfe JH, Noone MA, Davies L, Drummond M. The economics of femorocrural reconstruction for critical leg ischemia with and without autologous vein. J Vasc Surg 1992;15:167–74.
15. Singh S, Evans L, Datta D, Gaines P, Beard JD. The costs of managing lower limb-threatening ischaemia. Eur J Vasc Endovasc Surg 1996; 12:359–62.
16. Magnant JG, Cronenwett JL, Walsh DB, et al. Surgical treatment of infrainguinal arterial occlusive disease in women. J Vasc Surg 1993; 17:67–76.
17. Enzler MA, Ruoss M, Seifert B, Berger M. The influence of gender on the outcome of arterial procedures in the lower extremity. Eur J Vasc Endovasc Surg 1996;11:446–52.
18. Tangelder MJ, Algra A, Lawson JA, Eikelboom BC. Risk factors for occlusion of infrainguinal bypass grafts. Eur J Vasc Endovasc Surg 2000;20:118–24.
19. Luther M, Lepantalo M. Femorotibial reconstructions for chronic critical leg ischaemia: influence on outcome by diabetes, gender and age. Eur J Vasc Endovasc Surg 1997;13:569–77.
20. Harris EJ, Taylor LM, Moneta GL, Porter JM. Outcome of infrainguinal arterial reconstruction in women. J Vasc Surg 1993;18:627–34.
21. Shah DM, Darling RC 3rd, Chang BB, et al. Long-term results of in situ saphenous vein bypass. Analysis of 2058 cases. Ann Surg 1995; 222:438–46.
22. Eugster T, Gurke L, Obeid T, Stierli P. Infrainguinal arterial reconstruction: female gender as risk factor for outcome. Eur J Vasc Endovasc Surg 2002;24:245–8.
23. Bergamini TM, Towne JB, Bandyk DF, Seabrook GR, Schmitt DD. Experience with in situ saphenous vein bypasses during 1981 to 1989: determinant factors of long-term patency. J Vasc Surg 1991; 13:137–47.
24. Tordoir JH, van der Plas JP, Jacobs MJ, Kitslaar PJ. Factors determining the outcome of crural and pedal revascularisation for critical limb ischaemia. Eur J Vasc Surg 1993;7:82–6.
25. Idu MM, Buth J, Hop WC, et al. Factors influencing the development of vein-graft stenosis and their significance for clinical management. Eur J Vasc Endovasc Surg 1999;17:15–21.
26. Burger DH, Kappetein AP, van Bockel JH, Breslau PJ. A prospective randomized trial comparing vein with polytetrafluoroethylene in above-knee femoropopliteal bypass grafting. J Vasc Surg 2000;32:278–83.
27. Rutherford RB, Jones DN, Bergentz SE, et al. Factors affecting the patency of infrainguinal bypass. J Vasc Surg 1988;8:236–46.
28. Reed AB, Conte MS, Belkin M, et al. Usefulness of autogenous bypass grafts originating distal to the groin. J Vasc Surg 1954;35:48–54.
29. Budd JS, Brennan J, Beard JD, et al. Infrainguinal bypass surgery: factors determining late graft patency. Br J Surg 1990;77:1382–7.
30. Seeger JM, Pretus HA, Carlton LC, et al. Potential predictors of outcome in patients with tissue loss who undergo infrainguinal vein bypass grafting. J Vasc Surg 1999;30:427–35.
31. Olojugba DH, McCarthy MJ, Reid A, et al. Infrainguinal revascularisation in the era of vein-graft surveillance – do clinical factors influence long-term outcome? Eur J Vasc Endovasc Surg 1999;17:121–8.
32. Hamdan AD, Saltzberg SS, Sheahan M, et al. Lack of association of diabetes with increased postoperative mortality and cardiac morbidity. Arch Surg 2002;137:417–21.
33. Gerrard DJ, Ray SA, Barrio EA, et al. Effect of chronic renal failure on mortality rate following arterial reconstruction. Br J Surg 2002; 89:70–3.
34. Peltonen S, Biancari F, Lindgren L, et al. Outcome of infrainguinal bypass surgery for critical leg ischaemia in patients with chronic renal failure. Eur J Vasc Endovasc Surg 1998;15:122–7.
35. Meyerson SL, Skelly CL, Curi MA, et al. Long-term results justify autogenous infrainguinal bypass grafting in patients with end-stage renal failure. J Vasc Surg 2001;34:27–33.
36. Chang BB, Paty PS, Shah DM, Kaufman JL, Leather RP. Results of infrainguinal bypass for limb salvage in patients with end-stage renal disease. Surgery 1990;108:742–6.
37. Sayers RD, Raptis S, Berce M, Miller JH. Long-term results of femorotibial bypass with vein or polytetrafluoroethylene. Br J Surg 1998;85:934–8.
38. Mamode N, Scott RN. Graft type for femoro-popliteal bypass surgery Cochrane Database Syst Rev 2000;(2):CD001487.
39. Kumar K, Crinnion JN, Ashley S, Case WG, Gough MJ. Conduit of choice for above-knee femoropopliteal bypass. Br J Surg 1995;82:556.
40. Johnson WC, Lee KK. A comparative evaluation of polytetra-fluoroethylene, umbilical vein, and saphenous vein bypass grafts for femoral-popliteal above-knee revascularization: a prospective randomized Department of Veterans Affairs cooperative study. J Vasc Surg 2000;32:268–77.
41. Jackson MR, Belott TP, Dickason T, et al. The consequences of a failed femoropopliteal bypass grafting: comparison of saphenous vein and PTFE grafts. J Vasc Surg 2000;32:498–504.
42. McCarthy WJ, Pearce WH, Flinn WR, et al. Long-term evaluation of composite sequential bypass for limb-threatening ischemia. J Vasc Surg 1992;15:761–9.
43. Londrey GL, Ramsey DE, Hodgson KJ, Barkmeier LD, Sumner DS. Infrapopliteal bypass for severe ischemia: comparison of autogenous vein, composite, and prosthetic grafts. J Vasc Surg 1991;13:631–6.
44. Fichelle JM, Marzelle J, Colacchio G, et al. Infrapopliteal polytetra-fluoroethylene and composite bypass: factors influencing patency. Ann Vasc Surg 1995;9:187–96.
45. Harris RW, Schneider PA, Andros G, et al. Allograft vein bypass: is it an acceptable alternative for infrapopliteal revascularization? J Vasc Surg 1993;18:553–9.
46. Walker PJ, Mitchell RS, McFadden PM, James DR, Mehigan JT. Early experience with cryopreserved saphenous vein allografts as a conduit for complex limb-salvage procedures. J Vasc Surg 1993;18:561–8.
47. Fujitani RM, Bassiouny HS, Gewertz BL, Glagov S, Zarins CK. Cryopreserved saphenous vein allogenic homografts: an alternative conduit in lower extremity arterial reconstruction in infected fields. J Vasc Surg 1992;15:519–26.
48. Taylor LM Jr, Edwards JM, Porter JM. Present status of reversed vein bypass grafting: five-year results of a modern series. J Vasc Surg 1990; 11:193–205.
49. Donaldson MC, Whittemore AD, Mannick JA. Further experience with an all-autogenous tissue policy for infrainguinal reconstruction. J Vasc Surg 1993;18:41–8.
50. Chang BB, Paty PS, Shah DM, Leather RP. The lesser saphenous vein: an underappreciated source of autogenous vein. J Vasc Surg 1992;15:152–6.
51. Schulman ML, Badhey MR, Yatco R. Superficial femoral-popliteal veins and reversed saphenous veins as primary femoropopliteal bypass grafts: a randomized comparative study. J Vasc Surg 1987;6:1–10.
52. Sladen JG, Reid JD, Maxwell TM, Downs AR. Superficial femoral vein: a useful autogenous harvest site. J Vasc Surg 1994;20:947–52.
53. Wells JK, Hagino RT, Bargmann KM, et al. Venous morbidity after superficial femoral-popliteal vein harvest. J Vasc Surg 1999; 29:282–9.

54. Taylor SM, Fujitani RM, Myers JC, Mills JL. Combined coronary artery bypass and abdominal aortic aneurysmectomy: appropriate management in selected cases. South Med J 1993;86:974–6.

55. Chew DK, Owens CD, Belkin M, et al. Bypass in the absence of ipsilateral greater saphenous vein: safety and superiority of the contralateral greater saphenous vein. J Vasc Surg 2002;35:1085–92.

56. de Vries SO, Donaldson MC, Hunink MG. Contralateral symptoms after unilateral intervention for peripheral occlusive disease. J Vasc Surg 1998;27:414–21.

57. Tarry WC, Walsh DB, Birkmeyer NJ, et al. Fate of the contralateral leg after infrainguinal bypass. J Vasc Surg 1998;27:1039–47.

58. Kakkar VV. The cephalic vein as a peripheral vascular graft. Surg Gynecol Obstet 1969;128:551–6.

59. Londrey GL, Bosher LP, Brown PW, et al. Infrainguinal reconstruction with arm vein, lesser saphenous vein, and remnants of greater saphenous vein: a report of 257 cases. J Vasc Surg 1994;20:451–6.

60. Calligaro KD, Syrek JR, Dougherty MJ, et al. Use of arm and lesser saphenous vein compared with prosthetic grafts for infrapopliteal arterial bypass: are they worth the effort? J Vasc Surg 1997;26:919–24.

61. Marcaccio EJ, Miller A, Tannenbaum GA, et al. Angioscopically directed interventions improve arm vein bypass grafts. J Vasc Surg 1993;17:994–1002.

62. Tisi PV, Crow AJ, Shearman CP. Arm vein reconstruction for limb salvage: long-term outcome. Ann R Coll Surg Engl 1996;78:497–500.

63. Miller A, Stonebridge PA, Jepsen SJ, et al. Continued experience with intraoperative angioscopy for monitoring infrainguinal bypass grafting. Surgery 1991;109:286–93.

64. Panetta TF, Marin ML, Veith FJ, et al. Unsuspected preexisting saphenous vein disease: an unrecognized cause of vein bypass failure. J Vasc Surg 1992;15:102–10.

65. Kreienberg PB, Darling RC 3rd, Chang BB, et al. Early results of a prospective randomized trial of spliced vein versus polytetrafluoroethylene graft with a distal vein cuff for limb-threatening ischemia. J Vasc Surg 2002;35:299–306.

66. Varty K, London NJ, Brennan JA, Ratliff DA, Bell PR. Infragenicular in situ vein bypass graft occlusion: a multivariate risk factor analysis. Eur J Vasc Surg 1993;7:567–71.

67. Wengerter KR, Veith FJ, Gupta SK, Ascer E, Rivers SP. Influence of vein size (diameter) on infrapopliteal reversed vein graft patency. J Vasc Surg 1990;11:525–31.

68. Sumner DS. Haemodynamics and rheology of vascular disease: applications to diagnosis and treatment. In: Haimovici H, ed. Haimovici's vascular surgery. Cambridge:Blackwell Science; 1996:104–23.

69. Davies AH, Magee TR, Hayward JK, Baird RN, Horrocks M. Prediction of long saphenous vein graft adaptation. Eur J Vasc Surg 1994;8:478–81.

70. Davies AH, Magee TR, Baird RN, Sheffield E, Horrocks M. Pre-bypass morphological changes in vein grafts. Eur J Vasc Surg 1993;7:642–7.

71. James DC, Durrani T, Wixon CL, et al. Preimplant vein intimal thickness is not a predictor of bypass graft stenosis. J Surg Res 2001;96:1–5.

72. Stansby G. Vein quality in vascular surgery. Lancet 1998;351:1001–2.

73. Shah DM, Paty PS, Leather RP, et al. Optimal outcome after tibial arterial bypass. Surg Gynecol Obstet 1993;177:283–7.

74. Schweiger H, Klein P, Lang W. Tibial bypass grafting for limb salvage with ringed polytetrafluoroethylene prostheses: results of primary and secondary procedures. J Vasc Surg 1993;18:867–74.

75. Copeland GP, Edwards P, Wilcox A, Wake PN, Harris PL. GORA: a scoring system for the quantification of risk of graft occlusion. Ann R Coll Surg Engl 1994;76:132–5.

76. Panayiotopoulos YP, Edmondson RA, Reidy JF, Taylor PR. A scoring system to predict the outcome of long femorodistal arterial bypass grafts to single calf or pedal vessels. Eur J Vasc Endovasc Surg 1998;15:380–6.

77. Scott DJ, Horrocks EH, Kinsella D, Horrocks M. Preoperative assessment of the pedal arch using pulse generated runoff and subsequent femorodistal outcome. Eur J Vasc Surg 1994;8:20–5.

78. Alback A, Biancari F, Saarinen O, Lepantalo M. Prediction of the immediate outcome of femoropopliteal saphenous vein bypass by angiographic runoff score. Eur J Vasc Endovasc Surg 1998;15:220–4.

79. Biancari F, Alback A, Ihlberg L, et al. Angiographic runoff score as a predictor of outcome following femorocrural bypass surgery. Eur J Vasc Endovasc Surg 1999;17:480–5.

80. Toursarkissian B, D'Ayala M, Stefanidis D, et al. Angiographic scoring of vascular occlusive disease in the diabetic foot: relevance to bypass graft patency and limb salvage. J Vasc Surg 2002;35:494–500.

81. Elliott BM, Robison JG, Brothers TE, Cross MA. Limitations of peroneal artery bypass grafting for limb salvage. J Vasc Surg 1993;18:881–8.

82. Plecha EJ, Seabrook GR, Bandyk DF, Towne JB. Determinants of successful peroneal artery bypass. J Vasc Surg 1993;17:97–105.

83. Raftery KB, Belkin M, Mackey WC, O'Donnell TF. Are peroneal artery bypass grafts hemodynamically inferior to other tibial artery bypass grafts? J Vasc Surg 1994;19:964–8.

84. Bergamini TM, George SM Jr, Massey HT, et al. Pedal or peroneal bypass: which is better when both are patent? J Vasc Surg 1994; 20:347–55.

85. Neilipovitz DT, Bryson GL, Nichol G. The effect of perioperative aspirin therapy in peripheral vascular surgery: a decision analysis. Anesth Analg 2001;93:573–80.

86. Sonksen J, Gray R, Hickman PJ. Safer non-cardiac surgery for patients with coronary artery disease. BMJ 1998;317:1400–1.

87. Poldermans D, Boersma E, Bax JJ, et al. The effect of bisoprolol on perioperative mortality and myocardial infarction in high-risk patients undergoing vascular surgery. Dutch Echocardiographic Cardiac Risk Evaluation Applying Stress Echocardiography Study Group. N Engl J Med 1999;341:1789–94.

88. Bismuth J, Klitfod L, Sillesen H. The lack of cardiovascular risk factor management in patients with critical limb ischaemia. Eur J Vasc Endovasc Surg 2001;21:143–6.

89. Hollyoak M, Woodruff P, Muller M, Daunt N, Weir P. Deep venous thrombosis in postoperative vascular surgical patients: a frequent finding without prophylaxis. J Vasc Surg 2001;34:656–60.

90. Farkas JC, Chapuis C, Coombe S, et al. A randomised controlled trial of a low-molecular-weight heparin (Enoxaparin) to prevent deep-vein thrombosis in patients undergoing vascular surgery. Eur J Vasc Surg 1993;7:554–60.

91. Passman MA, Farber MA, Marston WA, et al. Prospective screening for postoperative deep venous thrombosis in patients undergoing infrainguinal revascularization. J Vasc Surg 2000;32:669–75.

92. Mangram AJ, Horan TC, Pearson ML, Silver LC, Jarvis WR. Guideline for Prevention of Surgical Site Infection, 1999. Centers for Disease Control and Prevention (CDC) Hospital Infection Control Practices Advisory Committee. Am J Infect Control 1999;27:97–132.

93. Ligush J Jr, Reavis SW, Preisser JS, Hansen KJ. Duplex ultrasound scanning defines operative strategies for patients with limb-threatening ischemia. J Vasc Surg 1998;28:482–90.

94. Eiberg JP, Lundorf E, Thomsen C, Schroeder TV. Peripheral vascular surgery and magnetic resonance arteriography – a review. Eur J Vasc Endovasc Surg 2001;22:396–402.

95. Pemberton M, Nydahl S, Hartshorne T, et al. Can lower limb vascular reconstruction be based on colour duplex imaging alone? Eur J Vasc Endovasc Surg 1996;12:452–4.

96. Roditi G. Contrast-enhanced magnetic resonance angiography. Br J Surg 2002;89:817–20.

97. Dorweiler B, Neufang A, Kreitner K-F, Schmiedt W, Oelert H. Magnetic resonance angiography unmasks reliable target vessels for pedal bypass grafting in patients with diabetes mellitus. J Vasc Surg 2002; 35:766–72.

98. Lujan S, Criado E, Puras E, Izquierdo LM. Duplex scanning or arteriography for preoperative planning of lower limb revascularisation. Eur J Vasc Endovasc Surg 2002;24:31–6.

99. Mazzariol F, Ascher E, Hingorani A, et al. Lower-extremity revascularisation without preoperative contrast arteriography in 185 cases: lessons learned with duplex ultrasound arterial mapping. Eur J Vasc Endovasc Surg 2000;19:509–15.

100. Avenarius JK, Breek JC, Lohle PNM, van Berge Henegouwen DP, Hamming JF. The additional value of angiography after colour-coded duplex on decision making in patients with critical limb ischaemia. A prospective study. Eur J Vasc Endovasc Surg 2002;23:393–7.

101. Sayers RD, Naylor AR, London NJ, et al. The additional value of intraoperative angiography in infragenicular reconstruction. Eur J Vasc Endovasc Surg 1995;9:211–7.

102. Harris RA, Kumar P, Collin J, et al. Preoperative prediction of graft patency for infrapopliteal arterial bypass using pulse-generated runoff. Eur J Vasc Endovasc Surg 1999;17:429–33.

103. Hickey NC, Thomson IA, Shearman CP, Simms MH. Aggressive arterial reconstruction for critical lower limb ischaemia. Br J Surg 1991;78:1476–8.

104. McCarthy MJ, Nydahl S, Hartshorne T, et al. Colour-coded duplex imaging and dependent Doppler ultrasonography in the assessment of cruropedal vessels. Br J Surg 1999;86:33–7.

105. Scott DJ, Hunt G, Beard JD, Hartnell GG, Horrocks M. Arteriogram scoring systems and pulse generated run-off in the assessment of patients with critical ischaemia for femorodistal bypass. Br J Surg 1989;76:1202–6.

106. Leopold PW, Shandall A, Kupinkski AM, et al. Role of B-mode venous mapping in infrainguinal in situ vein-arterial bypasses. Br J Surg 1989; 76:305–7.

107. Bagi P, Schroeder T, Sillesen H, Lorentzen JE. Real time B-mode mapping of the greater saphenous vein. Eur J Vasc Surg 1989; 3:103–5.

108. Barkmeier LD, Hood DB, Sumner DS, et al. Local anesthesia for infrainguinal arterial reconstruction. Am J Surg 1997;174:202–4.

109. Buggy DJ, Smith GS. Epidural anaesthesia and analgesia: better outcome after major surgery? BMJ 1999;319:530–1.

110. Rivers SP, Scher LA, Sheehan E, Veith FJ. Epidural versus general anesthesia for infrainguinal arterial reconstruction. J Vasc Surg 1991; 14:764–8.

111. Christopherson R, Beattie C, Frank SM, et al. Perioperative morbidity in patients randomized to epidural or general anesthesia for lower extremity vascular surgery. Perioperative Ischemia Randomized Anesthesia Trial Study Group. Anesthesiology 1993;79:422–34.

112. Pierce ET, Pomposelli FB Jr, Stanley GD, et al. Anesthesia type does not influence early graft patency or limb salvage rates of lower extremity arterial bypass. J Vasc Surg 1997;25:226–32.

113. Naesh O, Haljamae H, Hindberg I, et al. Epidural anaesthesia prolonged into the postoperative period prevents stress response and platelet hyper-aggregability after peripheral vascular surgery. Eur J Vasc Surg 1994; 8:395–400.

114. Rosenfeld BA, Beattie C, Christopherson R, et al. The effects of different anesthetic regimens on fibrinolysis and the development of postoperative arterial thrombosis. Perioperative Ischemia Randomized Anesthesia Trial Study Group. Anesthesiology 1993;79:435–43.

115. Hickey NC, Wilkes MP, Howes D, Watt J, Shearman CP. The effect of epidural anaesthesia on peripheral resistance and graft flow following femorodistal reconstruction. Eur J Vasc Endovasc Surg 1995;9:93–6.

116. Brewster DC, Cambria RP, Darling RC, et al. Long-term results of combined iliac balloon angioplasty and distal surgical revascularization. Ann Surg 1989;210:324–31.

117. Gross GM, Johnson RC, Roberts RM, Fisher DF, AbuRahma A. Results of peripheral endovascular procedures in the operating room. J Vasc Surg 1996;24:353–62.

118. LoGerfo FW, Johnson WC, Corson JD, et al. A comparison of the late patency of axillobifemoral and axillounilateral femoral grafts. Surgery 1977;81:33–40.

119. Wittens CH, van Houtte HJ, van Urk H. European Prospective Randomised Multi-centre Axillo-bifemoral Trial. Eur J Vasc Surg 1992; 6:115–23.

120. Farber MA, Hollier LH, Eubanks R, Ochsner JL, Bowen JC. Femorofemoral bypass: a profile of graft failure. South Med J 1990; 83:1437–43.

121. Defraigne JO, Vazquez C, Limet R. Crossover iliofemoral bypass grafting for treatment of unilateral iliac atherosclerotic disease. J Vasc Surg 1999;30:693–700.

122. Edwards WH, Jenkins JM, Mulherin JL Jr, Martin RS 3rd, Edwards WH Jr. Extended profundaplasty to minimize pelvic and distal tissue loss. Ann Surg 1990;211:694–702.

123. Hansen AK, Bille S, Nielsen PH, Egeblad K. Profundaplasty as the only reconstructive procedure in patients with severe ischemia of the lower extremity. Surg Gynecol Obstet 1990;171:47–50.

124. Kalman PG, Johnston KW, Walker PM. The current role of isolated profundaplasty. J Cardiovasc Surg (Torino) 1990;31:107–11.

125. Radoux JM, Maiza D, Coffin O. Long-term outcome of 121 iliofemoral endarterectomy procedures. Ann Vasc Surg 2001;15:163–70.

126. Ho GH, Moll FL, Hedeman Joosten PP, et al. Endovascular remote endarterectomy in femoropopliteal occlusive disease: one-year clinical experience with the ring strip cutter device. Eur J Vasc Endovasc Surg 1996;12:105–12.

127. Donaldson MC, Mannick JA, Whittemore AD. Causes of primary graft failure after in situ saphenous vein bypass grafting. J Vasc Surg 1992;15:113–8.

128. Whittemore AD, Clowes AW, Couch NP, Mannick JA. Secondary femoropopliteal reconstruction. Ann Surg 1981;193:35–42.

129. Belkin M, Donaldson MC, Whittemore AD, et al. Observations on the use of thrombolytic agents for thrombotic occlusion of infrainguinal vein grafts. J Vasc Surg 1990;11:289–94.

130. Kunlin J. Le traitement de l'arterite obliterante par la greffe veineuse. Arch Mal Coeur Vaiss 1949;42:371–2.

131. May AG, DeWeese JA, Rob CG. Arterialized in situ saphenous vein. Arch Surg 1965;91:743–50.

132. Skagseth E, Hall KV. In situ vein bypass. Experiences with new vein valve strippers. Scand J Thorac Cardiovasc Surg 1973;7:53–8.

133. Sayers RD, Watt PA, Muller S, Bell PR, Thurston H. Endothelial cell injury secondary to surgical preparation of reversed and in situ saphenous vein bypass grafts. Eur J Vasc Surg 1992;6:354–61.

134. Sayers RD, Watt PA, Muller S, Bell PR, Thurston H. Structural and functional smooth muscle injury after surgical preparation of reversed and non-reversed (in situ) saphenous vein bypass grafts. Br J Surg 1991;78:1256–8.

135. Harris PL, How TV, Jones DR. Prospectively randomized clinical trial to compare in situ and reversed saphenous vein grafts for femoropopliteal bypass. Br J Surg 1987;74:252–5.

136. Harris PL, Veith FJ, Shanik GD, et al. Prospective randomized comparison of in situ and reversed infrapopliteal vein grafts. Br J Surg 1993; 80:173–6.

137. Moody AP, Edwards PR, Harris PL. In situ versus reversed femoropopliteal vein grafts: long-term follow-up of a prospective, randomized trial. Br J Surg 1992;79:750–2.

138. Wengerter KR, Veith FJ, Gupta SK, et al. Prospective randomized multicenter comparison of in situ and reversed vein infrapopliteal bypasses. J Vasc Surg 1991;13:189–97.

139. Watelet J, Soury P, Menard JF, et al. Femoropopliteal bypass: in situ or reversed vein grafts? Ten-year results of a randomized prospective study. Ann Vasc Surg 1997;11:510–9.

140. Lawson JA, Tangelder MJ, Algra A, Eikelboom BC. The myth of the in situ graft: superiority in infrainguinal bypass surgery? Eur J Vasc Endovasc Surg 1999;18:149–57.

141. Leather RP, Shah DM, Chang BB, Kaufman JL. Resurrection of the in situ saphenous vein bypass. 1000 cases later. Ann Surg 1988; 208:435–42.

142. Sales CM, Goldsmith J, Veith FJ. Prospective study of the value of prebypass saphenous vein angioscopy. Am J Surg 1995;170:106–8.

143. Clair DG, Golden MA, Mannick JA, Whittemore AD, Donaldson MC. Randomized prospective study of angioscopically assisted in situ saphenous vein grafting. J Vasc Surg 1994;19:992–9.

144. Thorne J, Danielsson G, Danielsson P, et al. Intraoperative angioscopy may improve the outcome of in situ saphenous vein bypass grafting: a prospective study. J Vasc Surg 2002;35:759–65.

145. Rosenthal D, Arous EJ, Friedman SG, et al. Endovascular-assisted versus conventional in situ saphenous vein bypass grafting: cumulative patency, limb salvage, and cost results in a 39-month multicenter study. J Vasc Surg 2000;31:60–8.

146. Robinson BI, Fletcher JP, Tomlinson P, et al. A prospective randomized multicentre comparison of expanded polytetrafluoroethylene and gelatin-sealed knitted Dacron grafts for femoropopliteal bypass. Cardiovasc Surg 1999;7:214–8.

147. Devine C, Hons B, McCollum C. Heparin-bonded Dacron or polytetrafluoroethylene for femoropopliteal bypass grafting: a multicenter trial. J Vasc Surg 2001;33:533–9.

148. Stonebridge PA, Prescott RJ, Ruckley CV. Randomized trial comparing infrainguinal polytetrafluoroethylene bypass grafting with and without vein interposition cuff at the distal anastomosis. J Vasc Surg 1997; 26:543–50.

149. Hamsho A, Nott D, Harris PL. Prospective randomised trial of distal arteriovenous fistula as an adjunct to femoro-infrapopliteal PTFE bypass. Eur J Vasc Endovasc Surg 1999;17:197–201.

150. Veith FJ, Gupta SK, Samson RH, et al. Superficial femoral and popliteal arteries as inflow sites for distal bypasses. Surgery 1981; 90:980–90.

151. Mills JL, Taylor SM, Fujitani RM. The role of the deep femoral artery as an inflow site for infrainguinal revascularization. J Vasc Surg 1993; 18:416–23.

152. Logason K, Barlin T, Jonsson M-L, Bostrom A, Hardemark HG, Karacagil S. The importance of Doppler angle of insonation on differentiation between 50–69% and 70–99% carotid artery stenosis. Eur J Vasc Endovasc Surg 2001;21:311–3.

153. Tweedie JH, Ballantyne KC, Callum KG. Direct arterial pressure measurements during operation to assess adequacy of arterial reconstruction in lower limb ischaemia. Br J Surg 1986;73:879–81.

154. Flanigan DP, Williams LR, Schwartz JA, Schuler JJ, Gray B. Hemodynamic evaluation of the aortoiliac system based on pharmacologic vasodilatation. Surgery 1983;93:709–14.

155. Kram HB, Gupta SK, Veith FJ, et al. Late results of two hundred seventeen femoropopliteal bypasses to isolated popliteal artery segments. J Vasc Surg 1991;14:386–90.

156. Karacagil S, Almgren B, Bowald S, Eriksson I. Bypass grafting to the popliteal artery in limbs with occluded crural arteries. Am J Surg 1991; 162:19–23.

157. Darke S, Lamont P, Chant A, et al. Femoro-popliteal versus femorodistal bypass grafting for limb salvage in patients with an "isolated" popliteal segment. Eur J Vasc Surg 1989;3:203–7.

158. Loh A, Chester JF, Taylor RS. PTFE bypass grafting to isolated popliteal segments in critical limb ischaemia. Eur J Vasc Surg 1993;7:26–30.

159. Samson RH, Showalter DP, Yunis JP. Isolated femoropopliteal bypass graft for limb salvage after failed tibial reconstruction: a viable alternative to amputation. J Vasc Surg 1999;29:409–12.

160. Woelfle KD, Kugelmann U, Bruijnen H, Storm G, Loeprecht H. Intraoperative imaging techniques in infrainguinal arterial bypass grafting: completion angiography versus vascular endoscopy. Eur J Vasc Surg 1994;8:556–61.

161. Miller A, Marcaccio EJ, Tannenbaum GA, et al. Comparison of angioscopy and angiography for monitoring infrainguinal bypass vein grafts: results of a prospective randomized trial. J Vasc Surg 1993; 17:382–96.

162. Johnson BL, Bandyk DF, Back MR, Avino AJ, Roth SM. Intraoperative duplex monitoring of infrainguinal vein bypass procedures. J Vasc Surg 2000;31:678–90.

163. Gilbertson JJ, Walsh DB, Zwolak RM, et al. A blinded comparison of angiography, angioscopy, and duplex scanning in the intraoperative evaluation of in situ saphenous vein bypass grafts. J Vasc Surg 1992;15:121–7.

164. Bernhard VM, Boren CH, Towne JB. Pneumatic tourniquet as a substitute for vascular clamps in distal bypass surgery. Surgery 1980;87:709–13.

165. Ciervo A, Dardik H, Qin F, et al. The tourniquet revisited as an adjunct to lower limb revascularization. J Vasc Surg 2000;31:436–42.

166. Eyers P, Ashley S, Scott DJ. Tourniquets in arterial bypass surgery. Eur J Vasc Endovasc Surg 2000;20:113–7.

167. Chester JF, Butler CM, Taylor RS. Vascular reconstruction at the groin: oblique or vertical incisions? Ann R Coll Surg Engl 1992;74:112–4.

168. Mukherjee D. Posterior approach to the peroneal artery. J Vasc Surg 1994;19:174–8.

169. Beard JD, Wyatt M, Scott DJ, Baird RN, Horrocks M. The non-reversed vein femoro-distal bypass graft: a modification of the standard in situ technique. Eur J Vasc Surg 1989;3:55–60.

170. Shah DM, Darling RC 3rd, Chang BB, et al. Is long vein bypass from groin to ankle a durable procedure? An analysis of a ten-year experience. J Vasc Surg 1992;15:402–7.

171. Ouriel K. The posterior approach to popliteal-crural bypass. J Vasc Surg 1994;19:74–9.

172. Dorweiler B, Neufang A, Schmitt DD, Oelert H. Pedal bypass for limb salvage in patients with diabetes mellitus. Eur J Vasc Endovasc Surg 2002;24:309–13.

173. Goyal A, Shah PM, Babu SC, Mateo RB. Popliteal-crural bypass through the posterior approach with lesser saphenous vein for limb salvage. J Vasc Surg 2002;36:708–12.

174. Effects of perioperative iloprost on patency of femorodistal bypass grafts. The Iloprost Bypass International Study Group. Eur J Vasc Endovasc Surg 1996;12:363–71.

175. Watson HR, Belcher G, Horrocks M. Adjuvant medical therapy in peripheral bypass surgery. Br J Surg 1999;86:981–91.

176. Collaborative overview of randomised trials of antiplatelet therapy. I: Prevention of death, myocardial infarction, and stroke by prolonged antiplatelet therapy in various categories of patients. Antiplatelet Trialists' Collaboration. BMJ 1994;308:81–106.

177. A randomised, blinded, trial of clopidogrel versus aspirin in patients at risk of ischaemic events (CAPRIE). CAPRIE Steering Committee. Lancet 1996;348:1329–39.

178. Kretschmer G, Herbst F, Prager M, et al. A decade of oral anticoagulant treatment to maintain autologous vein grafts for femoropopliteal atherosclerosis. Arch Surg 1992;127:1112–5.

179. Efficacy of oral anticoagulants compared with aspirin after infrainguinal bypass surgery (The Dutch Bypass Oral Anticoagulants or Aspirin Study): a randomised trial. Lancet 2000;355:346–51.

180. Sarac TP, Huber TS, Back MR, et al. Warfarin improves the outcome of infrainguinal vein bypass grafting at high risk for failure. J Vasc Surg 1998;28:446–57.

181. Johnson WC, Williford WO. Department of Veterans Affairs Cooperative Study. Benefits, morbidity, and mortality associated with long-term administration of oral anticoagulant therapy to patients with peripheral arterial bypass procedures: a prospective randomized study. J Vasc Surg 2002;35:413–21.

182. Secondary prevention of ischaemic cardiac events. Clinical Evidence 2002; 7 June: www.clinicalevidence.org.

183. Moody P, Gould DA, Harris PL. Vein graft surveillance improves patency in femoro-popliteal bypass. Eur J Vasc Surg 1990;4:117–21.

184. Green RM, McNamara J, Ouriel K, DeWeese JA. Comparison of infrainguinal graft surveillance techniques. J Vasc Surg 1990;11:207–14.

185. Olojugba DH, McCarthy MJ, Naylor AR, Bell PR, London NJ. At what peak velocity ratio value should duplex-detected infrainguinal vein graft stenoses be revised? Eur J Vasc Endovasc Surg 1998;15:258–60.

186. Mills JL Sr, Wixon CL, James DC, et al. The natural history of intermediate and critical vein graft stenosis: recommendations for continued surveillance or repair. J Vasc Surg 2001;33:273–8.

187. Lundell A, Lindblad B, Bergqvist D, Hansen F. Femoropopliteal-crural graft patency is improved by an intensive surveillance program: a prospective randomized study. J Vasc Surg 1995;21:26–33.

188. Ihlberg L, Luther M, Tierala E, Lepantalo M. The utility of duplex scanning in infrainguinal vein graft surveillance: results from a randomised controlled study. Eur J Vasc Endovasc Surg 1998;16:19–27.

189. Visser K, Idu MM, Buth J, Engel GL, Hunink MG. Duplex scan surveillance during the first year after infrainguinal autologous vein bypass grafting surgery: costs and clinical outcomes compared with other surveillance programs. J Vasc Surg 2001;33:123–30.

190. Wixon CL, Mills JL, Westerband A, Hughes JD, Ihnat DM. An economic appraisal of lower extremity bypass graft maintenance. J Vasc Surg 2000;32:1–12.

191. Dunlop P, Sayers RD, Naylor AR, Bell PR, London NJ. The effect of a surveillance programme on the patency of synthetic infrainguinal bypass grafts. Eur J Vasc Endovasc Surg 1996;11:441–5.

192. Lalak NJ, Hanel KC, Hunt J, Morgan A. Duplex scan surveillance of infrainguinal prosthetic bypass grafts. J Vasc Surg 1994;20:637–41.

193. Pit MJ, Lawson JA. A simple technique for thombectomy of a reversed saphenous vein arterial bypass graft. J Vasc Surg 1993;7:452–3.

194. Seabrook GR, Mewissen MW, Schmitt DD, et al. Percutaneous intraarterial thrombolysis in the treatment of thrombosis of lower extremity arterial reconstructions. J Vasc Surg 1991;13:646–51.
195. Berridge DC, Al Kutoubi A, Mansfield AO, Nicolaides AN, Wolfe JH. Thrombolysis in arterial graft thrombosis. Eur J Vasc Endovasc Surg 1995;9:129–32.
196. Mills JL. Reverse vein bypass. In: Mills JL, ed. Management of chronic lower limb ischemia. London:Arnold; 2000.
197. Mills JL. Complex reconstruction. In: Mills JL, ed. Management of chronic lower limb ischemia. London:Arnold; 2000.

CHAPTER

13

Diabetic Foot Problems

Frank B Pomposelli Jr and Christoph Domenig

KEY POINTS

- In patients with diabetes mellitus, the presence of neuropathy and ischemia promotes the development of foot ulcers, pressure necrosis, non-healing wounds, and secondary infection.

- Soft tissue infection is usually multimicrobial, often involves tendon or bone, and can cause extensive tissue destruction.

- Treatment of complications of infection and/or neuropathy often requires surgery; if inadequate circulation is present, it must be corrected or measures to treat infection and/or neuropathy will ultimately fail.

- The concept of 'small vessel disease' is erroneous and has no place in the diagnosis or management of foot ischemia, which is due to atherosclerosis.

- Atherosclerosis in the ischemic diabetic foot usually involves the tibial or peroneal arteries (tibial artery disease) but almost always spares the foot arteries.

- In the treatment of foot ischemia, a carefully planned approach, including the prompt control of infection when present, and an extreme distal arterial reconstruction to maximize foot perfusion, often to the foot arteries, should lead to rates of limb salvage in patients with diabetes which equal or exceed those achieved in the non-diabetic patient population.

- There is an increasing role for percutaneous treatment of chronic ischemia and ulcers.

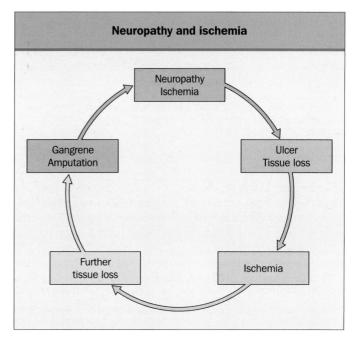

Figure 13.1 Neuropathy and ischemia. The presence of neuropathy and ischemia sets the stage for the development of ulcers (neuro-ischemic ulcers) and tissue loss. If ischemia is not corrected with appropriate arterial reconstruction, tissue loss will occur and will ultimately lead to gangrene and amputation.

For the physician involved in the care of these patients, understanding how neuropathy, ischemia, and infection are impacting on the individual patient with a foot complication is essential if the foot is to be salvaged. In the following discussion, neuropathy, infection, and ischemia will be discussed in detail separately, but it is important to understand that they seldom work in isolation and must be treated simultaneously in a successful treatment plan.

NEUROPATHY

Neuropathy is a common complication of diabetes mellitus and is included in the triad of pathologic conditions characteristic for this disease – namely, retinopathy, nephropathy, and neuropathy.

Pathophysiology

Diabetic neuropathy is a polyneuropathy affecting the autonomic and the somatic nervous systems, leading to a complex and polymorphous group of disorders.

The pathogenesis of diabetic neuropathy is not fully understood. Possible explanations for the development of these

INTRODUCTION

Problems related to the foot remain the most common cause for hospitalization for patients with diabetes mellitus.[1,2] Up to 20% of the 12 to 15 million people in the US with diabetes mellitus will be hospitalized for a foot problem at least once during their lifetime. The annual healthcare cost for this problem alone exceeds one billion dollars.[3] The pathologic combination of neuropathy and ischemia sets the stage for foot ulcers, pressure necrosis, and non-healing wounds. The resultant loss of continuity of the 'skin envelope' often leads to destructive multimicrobial infection and further tissue loss. A vicious cycle is created, which will ultimately lead to gangrene and amputation (Fig. 13.1). This scenario explains the high risk of limb amputation that all patients with diabetes face. In the US, patients with diabetes account for more than two-thirds of people undergoing non-traumatic limb amputations annually, even though they comprise only 12% of the population.

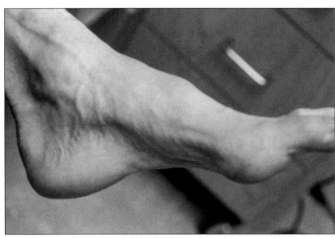

Figure 13.2 The 'claw' position. Motor neuropathy causes loss of normal balance between flexor and extensor muscles through decreased neural stimulation, causing atrophy of the intrinsic muscles of the foot. The plantar arch is exaggerated and the toes are fixed in a 'claw' position.

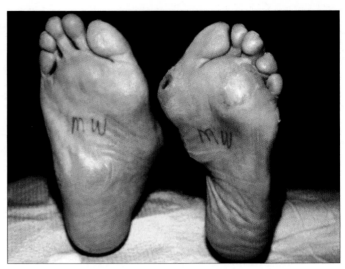

Figure 13.3 Neuropathic arthropathy (Charcot foot). Severe foot deformity and collapse of the normal architecture of the foot leads to abnormal bony prominences ('rocker bottom deformity'). These prominences are frequent causes of ulceration.

disorders are based on theories of changes in nerve supplying blood vessels (vasa nervorum) or abnormalities in metabolism. The vascular theory is based on observations of thickening of the nutrient vessels, which may occlude with progression, resulting in ischemic injury to the nerve. A more popular theory for the pathogenesis of neuropathy is the increased activity of the polyol (sorbitol) pathway.[4] Accumulation of sorbitol has been demonstrated in aortic intima and media. Excess sorbitol may be toxic, resulting in demyelination and impaired velocity of peripheral nerve conduction. These pathologic findings have been reported in human diabetic neuropathy.[5] Several studies have suggested that a decrease in neurotrophic factors may be important for the development of diabetic neuropathy.[6,7] As with microangiopathic complications of retinopathy and nephropathy, the severity of neuropathy tends to be related to the duration of diabetes.

Neuropathy involving the autonomic system may result in the shunting away of blood through arteriovenous connections in the microcirculation.[8] This leads to decreased tissue perfusion, even in the presence of normal arterial supply. The second interaction between neuropathy and perfusion involves the nocioceptive reflex. When a (peripheral) sensory fiber is stimulated, the signal travels to the central nerve cell body and the spinal cord and then to other axon branches (axon reflex). This reflex releases substance P from the nerve, which triggers mast cells to release histamine, resulting in a 'wheal and flare'. This response to a noxious stimulus is greatly attenuated in diabetic patients, and may precede clinically apparent neuropathy.[9] The absence of this reflex may contribute to the diminished inflammatory response to infection of the foot and the common clinical error of underestimating the severity of the infection.

Motor neuropathy decreases the neural stimulation of the intrinsic muscles of the foot and leads to atrophy and wasting of these muscles which are important in maintaining digital stability at the metatarsophalangeal joint level, and increased tonus of the long flexors. With intrinsic muscle wasting, the metatarsal bones are fixed, and the toes are drawn up in a 'claw' position (**Fig. 13.2**). The resultant foot deformity creates abnormal pressure points beneath the metatarsal heads and over the dorsum and the tip of the toes, which may lead to ulcers.

The major predisposing factor for plantar ulceration is peripheral sensory neuropathy, because these patients are unable to detect painful stimuli or injury to the lower extremity. High-pressure penetrating injuries, low-pressure repetitive stress from walking or standing, especially in a foot deformed by neuropathy, and thermal injury may go unrecognized due to loss of pain sensation and can lead to ulcers, necrosis, and tissue loss.[10]

Joints can be affected by neuropathy as well. Neuropathic arthropathy (Charcot foot) may be described as a relatively painless, progressive, and degenerative arthropathy of single or multiple joints. In diabetic patients, the areas primarily affected are the joints of the foot and the ankle (**Fig. 13.3**). In the presence of severe sensory neuropathy, proprioception is lost and the joints of the foot are subjected to extreme ranges of motion without 'warning'. This leads to capsular and ligamentous stretching, joint laxity, distension and subluxation – without any discomfort for the patient. As weight bearing continues and instability increases, the dislocated articular surfaces grind on adjacent bone and may result in osteochondral fragmentation and joint fractures. During the period of joint destruction, a natural hyperemic response occurs which is often mistaken for infection. This promotes resorption of debris and softening of normal bony structures. These osteoporotic areas are more susceptible to trauma and a vicious circle of continued bony destruction is created, in which the end result is collapse of the normal architecture of the foot and severe foot deformity.

Clinical presentation

On inspection, the neuropathic foot often has a characteristic appearance. The toes may be clawed (see above). The skin is usually dry and may be cracked due to the loss of sweating and oil secretion (autonomic neuropathy). Heavy, thick callus, which may ulcerate over time, is often evident at points of increased pressure and weight bearing. Atrophy of small muscles of the foot may or may not be apparent, but if wasting of the small muscles of the hand is observed, it can be assumed that those in the foot are affected as well. Color and temperature changes can range from hyperemic and warm in a patient with an acute Charcot fracture, to pale and cool in a patient with ischemia as well as neuropathy. In addition, in the presence of arteriovenous shunting, an ischemic foot may appear pink and relatively warm even with significant loss of arterial perfusion.

In Charcot foot, collapse of the arch, a 'rocker bottom' deformity (**Fig. 13.3**), or other severe abnormalities may be seen. Crepitus on passive range of motion of involved joints and excessive subluxation is a common finding with acute fractures. The foot may or may not be painless.

The loss of pinprick sensation is the most discriminant physical finding with neuropathy. Loss of soft touch sensation tends to be preserved even in moderate to severe neuropathy, and ankle reflexes are almost always absent in older patients. Testing for vibration sense can be useful in detecting the younger patient at risk for developing clinically significant neuropathy later in life.

Diagnosis
The presence of neuropathy can usually be determined by taking a careful history and physical examination. Loss of pinprick and vibratory sensation can be determined by the use of Semms–Weinstein filaments (**Fig. 13.4**) and a tuning fork. Occasionally, nerve conduction or electromyelographic studies may be helpful, but are not essential. Plain-film radiographs are helpful in the diagnosis of Charcot disease, foreign bodies, and infection. Radiologically, the osteoarthropathy takes on the appearance of a severely destructive form of degenerative arthritis.

Computed tomography (CT) and magnetic resonance imaging (MRI) scans may be required, especially when planning foot reconstructive surgery. Computerized methods to demonstrate points of high pressure under the sole have been developed. With 'pedobarography', specially designed sensors can be embedded within the insoles of the patient's shoe and pressures under the soles of both feet can be recorded while the patient is standing still or during walking (**Fig. 13.5**). Increased forces exerted on different areas of the sole can be visualized and analyzed both before and after treatment.[11]

Management
The first step in the treatment of any type of neuropathic complication is restriction of weight bearing of the involved extremity. Patients who have ulcers complicated by limb-threatening infection (see below) and non-compliant patients will require hospitalization and bed rest. Treatment of infection and ischemia if present (see below) must be undertaken simultaneously at this time.

For uncomplicated neuropathic ulcers, topical therapy and non-weight bearing will often heal the ulcer. A trial of outpatient care is usually the first step. Patients should be instructed not to soak or bathe the foot. Weight bearing can be limited by the use of a walker, crutches, or a wheelchair. The ulcer should be protected from excessive pressure by an accommodating pad around the lesion, which will distribute the pressure around the ulcer to surrounding tissues. Topical dressing care with saline-impregnated gauze, topical antibiotic ointments, or other agents designed to maintain a moist environment should be used. Heavy callus around the edges of the lesion should be trimmed away.

Shoes are usually replaced with a stiff-soled 'healing sandal' (**Fig. 13.6**) until the ulcer has closed. Once healed, custom-

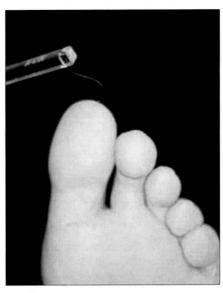

Figure 13.4 Assessment of loss of pin-prick sensation using Semms–Weinstein filaments. The monofilament should be applied firmly in order to create a bend.

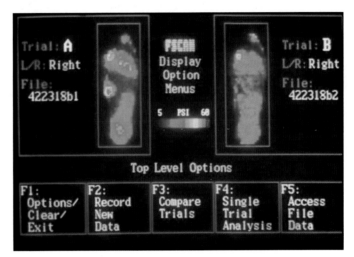

Figure 13.5 Pedobarography. Points of high pressure under the sole are recorded by sensors embedded within the insoles of the patient's shoes. Increased forces being exerted on the midfoot (left panel) and over the first metatarsal head can be visualized and analyzed before and after treatment.

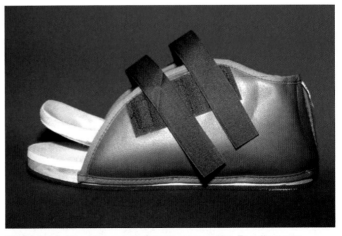

Figure 13.6 Management of diabetic neuropathy. To relieve any pressure from healing ulcers, shoes are replaced by a stiff-soled healing sandal until the ulcer has closed. A custom-molded orthotic protects the foot during weight bearing.

molded orthotics and extra-depth shoes, running shoes, or custom-molded shoes in the case of severe foot deformity are prescribed to prevent future recurrence. Patient education about the dangers of neuropathy along with proper footwear and regular podiatric care are essential preventive measures. When conservative measures fail, surgical therapy to correct underlying bony deformities or mechanical derangements may be indicated.

The combined presence of neuropathy and ischemia should not rule out treatment of ischemia. In the presence of neuropathy, arterial revascularization is even more important to bring maximal circulation to the foot to allow healing.

In the management of the Charcot foot, the goal is to protect the affected extremity, prevent further collapse and deformity, and to protect the opposite foot. The first step of treatment is an extended period of non-weight bearing (3–6 months) and cast or splint immobilization to promote eventual healing of the joint. In the initial phase of treatment, hospitalization may be required to provide proper treatment of potentially infected ulcers and reduce swelling of the affected foot. The duration of immobilization is determined by the anatomic location of the fracture and evidence of healing, acquired by clinical examination and foot X-rays. It is important to realize that the use of accommodative footwear is essential to long-term management. Surgery is rarely indicated. A stabilizing procedure is done most safely after a quiescent stage of the disease has been reached. Amputation is reserved for those rare patients with severe uncorrectable deformity, chronic ulcers that have caused extensive osteomyelitis making the foot unsalvageable, or after failed open reconstructions.

INFECTION

The infected foot is the most common cause of hospitalization for the diabetic patient, accounting for more in-hospital days than any other complication of diabetes.[1]

Pathophysiology

Sensory neuropathy results in sensory loss to pain and pressure, which leads to unrecognized trauma and ulcers. Autonomic neuropathy leads to loss of sweating and oil secretion, causing cracks and fissures. Both are causes of skin breakdown and open a portal of entry for bacteria. The signs of infection are often diminished due to the reduced neurogenic inflammatory response.

Metabolic state, arterial insufficiency

Hyperglycemia causes a relative immunocompromised state in which patients are more prone to infections of any kind.[12] Manifest proteinuria leads to loss of albumin, which affects tissue nutrition. Furthermore, infection causes increased metabolism and oxygen demand to combat infection. In the ischemic foot, inability to meet the increased oxygen requirement of infection may accelerate and exacerbate tissue necrosis. Increased blood flow is necessary, therefore, and inadequate circulation must be detected and treated when present or measures to treat infection will ultimately fail.

Classification/Microbiology

Non-limb-threatening infections are superficial ulcers, without bone or joint involvement, in which systemic signs of infection are limited or absent. There should be no evidence of severe limb ischemia. In microbiologic specimens, the most prevalent pathogens are an aerobic gram-positive cocci, usually *Staphylococcus aureus*, coagulase-negative staphylocci, or streptococci. Gram-negative bacilli and anaerobes are occasionally present but not common in these infections.

Limb-threatening infections are classified as deep ulcers involving tendon, bone, or joint, or any infection with associated tissue necrosis (wet gangrene) or those with evidence of concomitant severe ischemia (**Fig. 13.7**). Cellulitis is frequent and lymphangitis may be present. Systemic signs include fever, rigors,

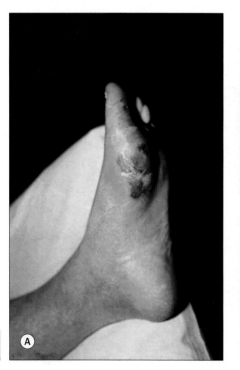
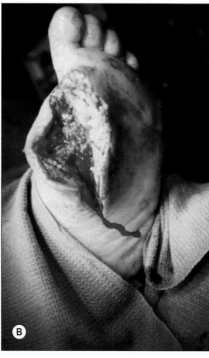

Figure 13.7 Deep space infection of the forefoot caused by ulceration of the plantar surface over the first metatarsal head. (A) Note the diffuse swelling, erythema, and subcuticular hemorrhage. The drainage from the ulcer had a foul odor and the patient was febrile and hyperglycemic. (B) Extensive necrosis of the underlying fascia and septic arthritis of the metatarsophalangeal joint was seen at surgery. An open first-ray amputation was performed.

Pathogens detected in microbiologic specimens from patients with moderate/severe (limb-threatening) diabetic foot infections.	
Pathogens	*Patients (%) with pathogens isolated*
Monomicrobial	16
Polymicrobial	80
Staphylococcus aureus	56
Coagulase-negative staphylococci	13
Streptococci	36
Enterococci	29
Klebsiella sp.	5
Proteus sp.	7
Other gram-negatives	6–44
Pseudomonas aeruginosa	7
Anaerobes	42
Fungi	3

Table 13.1 Pathogens detected in microbiologic specimens from patients with moderate/severe (limb-threatening) diabetic foot infections. (Modified from Grayson ML. Diabetic foot infections. Antimicrobial therapy. Infect Dis Clin North Am 1995;9:143–61.)

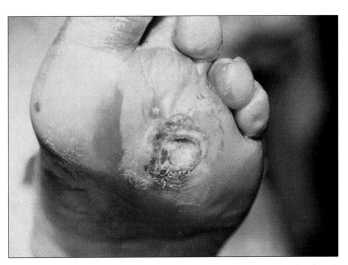

Figure 13.8 Penetrating ulcer located at a pressure point over the fourth metatarsal head, with resulting deep space abscess and osteomyelitis.

and stupor. Severe hyperglycemia is usually present. Bacteremia and septic shock can occur, making such infections life threatening. In microbiologic specimens, a polymicrobial flora consisting of gram-positive organisms (staphylococci, streptococci, enterococci), gram-negative organisms (*Escherichia coli*, proteus), and anaerobes (peptostreptococci, bacteroides, clostridia) is almost always present (**Table 13.1**). More chronic infections or those already partially treated with antibiotics may include additional 'opportunistic' species (*Enterobacter*, *Pseudomonas*, yeast).

The presence of anaerobes should always be suspected in any ulcer with foul-smelling drainage or a deep space abscess.

Osteomyelitis
Soft tissue ulceration and infection of the ischemic and neuropathic diabetic foot can lead to osteomyelitis and/or septic arthritis. Most cases of osteomyelitis in diabetic patients originate from penetrating ulcers at pressure points beneath the metatarsal heads (**Fig. 13.8**). Extension of osteomyelitis into the joint space can cause loss of the subchondral bone plate and joint space narrowing associated with septic arthritis. Spontaneous fracture, subluxation, and dislocation of the bones and joints may follow.

Clinical presentation/Diagnosis
Since many diabetic patients have a blunted neurogenic inflammatory response, typical inflammatory signs of infection may be absent or diminished.

Elevated blood glucose levels can sometimes be the first and only sign of sepsis; fever can be absent. Leukocytosis is often absent due to impaired leukocyte function.[12,13] Careful palpation of the foot for areas of tenderness or fluctuance is a very important means to detect undrained abcesses in deeper tissue planes. Undermining of infected foot ulcers is common, making it imperative that all ulcers be carefully probed and inspected, and superficial eschar unroofed, to look for potential deep space abscesses, which are not readily apparent from visual inspection of the foot. The use of a sterile metallic probe to probe the ulcer will not only determine the ulcer depth and extent, but will also allow the examiner to determine whether bony structures are involved or not. In a study by Grayson et al.[14], palpating bone on probing the pedal ulcer had a positive predictive value of 89% for osteomyelitis.

X-rays of the foot should be obtained in every patient with suspected foot infection. It is the first line to determine the presence of a foreign body, gas, osteolysis, or joint effusions. A bone scan may be positive 24 hours after the onset of osteomyelitis, and a three-phase bone scan can be useful in distinguishing osteomyelitis from cellulitis. Unfortunately, the specificity of radionuclide scans is poor in diabetic foot infections. Radiolabeled leukocyte scans are more specific, but may give false-negative results when antibiotic treatment has been initiated prior to study.[15] MRI has shown to be a highly sensitive diagnostic tool (up to 100%), but is only about 80% specific, since osteomyelitis and fracture may appear similar.[16]

Management
Antibiotic therapy
Patients with limb-threatening infections require hospitalization and intravenous antibiotics in the initial treatment period, to ensure adequate serum drug concentrations. Cultures from the depths of the ulcer should be taken immediately. Establishment of high serum drug concentrations is essential when local host factors such as reduced arterial supply, edema, devitalized tissue, and altered tissue pH might impede delivery or impair efficacy of the drug(s) at the site of infection. Until culture data are available, initial antibiotic therapy is empiric, based on probable species present. Empiric antibiotic regimens are dictated by institutional preferences, availability, and cost, but must cover gram-positive, gram-negative, and anaerobic organisms, since

most infections in diabetics are polymicrobial.[1,17] Our antibiotic protocol has undergone many changes over the last 15 years. Currently, a combination of levofloxacin and metronidazole is our empiric 'first-line' choice. In a prospective study, the fluoroquinolone levofloxacin proved superior to other antibiotics tested for the treatment of diabetic foot infections.[18] Major advantages of levofloxacin are its potent activity against both gram-positive and gram-negative organisms, the high tissue concentrations obtained with oral administration, and the ability to use it in penicillin-allergic patients. Metronidazole is added to cover anaerobic bacteria against which levofloxacin has no activity.[19] We have recently been evaluating the efficacy of the oral administration of the above regimen in severe infections requiring hospitalization. Once culture data are available, antibiotics must be adjusted appropriately. When possible, less-broad-spectrum agents should be used, to prevent development of resistance.

Incision and drainage

Diabetic patients do not tolerate undrained pus or devitalized infected tissue. In those patients with abscess formation, septic arthritis, necrotizing fasciitis, etc., prompt incision, drainage (**Fig. 13.9**), and debridement, including partial open toe, ray, or forefoot amputation, must be performed as indicated.[20]

The incision should be longitudinal and such that the skin is opened further than the subcutaneous tissue, which again is opened further than the underlying deep tissue plane, so that no undermined areas or pockets in which pus can accumulate remain. Tendon sheaths should be probed as proximal as possible and should be opened and the tendon excised if infected. Large drainage incisions do heal when infection is controlled and the circulation to the foot is adequate!

Wounds should be packed open with saline-impregnated gauze to promote continued drainage and changed two to three times a day. Wounds should be examined daily. Bedside or operative debridement should be repeated as needed.

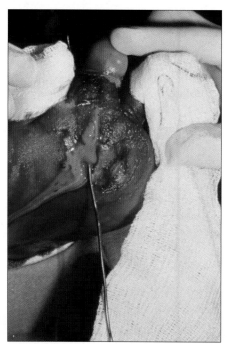

Figure 13.9 Incision and drainage of an infected ulcer. The probe tracks along the flexor tendon of the toe and exits in the web space. Such infections are usually polymicrobial and often contain anaerobic organisms.

Pedal osteomyelitis must be treated by an early aggressive approach, including appropriate antibiotic therapy, surgical debridement, and/or open amputation as needed. In our experience, long-term antibiotics without excision of infected bone is rarely successful in these patients.

ISCHEMIA

The management of ischemic complications of the diabetic foot has changed dramatically in the last two decades. The results of lower extremity arterial reconstruction have improved to the point where most patients can now be successfully treated. Unfortunately, inappropriate pessimism remains, leading to many needless and avoidable amputations. Our experience suggests that there should be no difference in the principles applied or outcomes expected for diabetic and non-diabetic patients with lower extremity ischemia.

Pathophysiology

The most important principle in treating foot ischemia in patients with diabetes is recognizing that the cause of their ischemia is macrovascular occlusion of the leg arteries due to atherosclerosis. Some years ago, many clinicians incorrectly assumed that gangrene, non-healing ulcers, and poor healing of minor amputations or other foot procedures were due to microvascular occlusion of arterioles – so-called small vessel disease. This flawed concept originated from a study by Goldenberg and co-workers, who performed soft tissue microscopic evaluation of amputated limb specimens from diabetic patients. They observed a periodic acid–Schiff (PAS)-positive material occluding the arterioles and named this process 'arteriolosclerosis'.[21] A subsequent prospective study[22] of amputation specimens from diabetic and non-diabetic patients, however, demonstrated no histologic evidence of an arteriolar occlusive lesion associated with diabetes. Probably the best argument against the existence of 'small vessel disease' may be the observation that the results of lower extremity bypass grafting in diabetic patients equal or exceed those achieved in non-diabetic patients.[23] In the minds of many clinicians and their patients, this concept of 'small vessel disease' has resulted in a very pessimistic attitude towards treatment of ischemia in diabetic patients that all too often leads to unnecessary limb amputation without attempted arterial reconstruction. This attitude and approach is antiquated, inappropriate, and must be discouraged. In our opinion, rejection of the small vessel theory alone could probably decrease the forty-fold increase of major limb amputation a person with diabetes faces during his or her lifetime compared with non-diabetic counterparts.

Histologically, atherosclerosis in the diabetic patient is similar to that in non-diabetic patients, but there are clinically relevant differences. Previous studies have demonstrated that diabetes is a strong independent risk factor for atherosclerotic coronary,[24,25] cerebrovascular, and peripheral vascular disease.[26] The likelihood of cardiovascular mortality is higher; generalized atherosclerosis is more prevalent and progresses more rapidly in diabetic patients. In those patients presenting with ischemic symptoms of the lower extremity, gangrene and tissue loss is more likely to be present than in non-diabetics. Diabetic patients with coronary atherosclerosis and significant polyneuropathy are more likely to develop 'silent ischemia' – the absence of typical anginal symptoms or symptoms of myocardial infarction.[27]

These findings suggest that arterial reconstruction in these patients would be associated with a higher risk of a perioperative myocardial infarction and/or death. Indeed, Eagle and colleagues,[28] and more recently Lee et al.,[29] identified diabetes mellitus as an independent risk factor for adverse cardiac events for patients undergoing major surgery. In our own experience, this has not been true. For diabetic patients undergoing lower extremity arterial reconstruction, the in-hospital mortality rate was 1%, and long-term graft patency, limb salvage, and patient survival rates were comparable or better than for non-diabetic patients treated over the same time period.[23] In a larger study, reviewing the outcomes of more than 6000 arterial reconstructive procedures of all types, perioperative mortality rates were no different for patients with or without diabetes.[30]

From the vascular surgeon's perspective, the most important difference in lower extremity atherosclerosis in the diabetic patient is the location and distribution of the atherosclerotic lesions in the artery supplying the foot.[31] In patients with diabetes, the most significant occlusive lesions are typically found in crural arteries, distal to the knee joint, but arteries of the foot are spared (**Fig. 13.10**).

Advanced ischemia may be present even when the aortoiliac segment and superficial femoral artery are patent, an uncommon finding in the non-diabetic patient with limb ischemia. This 'tibial artery disease' requires a different approach to arterial reconstruction and presents special challenges for the surgeon.

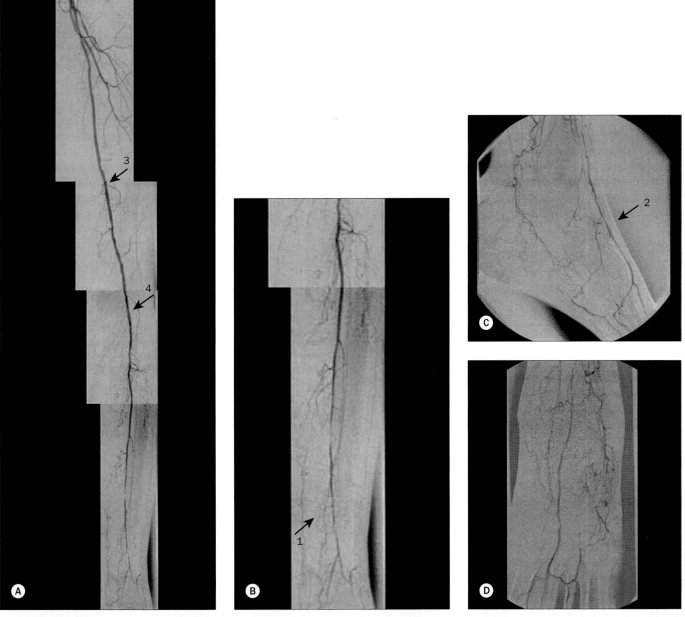

Figure 13.10 Location of the arteriosclerotic lesions in diabetic patients. The most significant lesions are found at the crural level distal to the knee joint. The foot arteries are usually spared, especially the dorsalis pedis artery. 1, peroneal artery; 2, dorsalis pedis artery; 3, superficial femoral artery; 4, popliteal artery.

Patient selection criteria

Some asymptomatic patients with diabetes will have evidence of peripheral vascular disease manifested by absence of palpable leg or foot pulses. In such patients, the disease is well compensated and no surgical treatment is indicated.

For patients presenting with typical symptoms that require surgery, several factors must be taken into consideration. Certain patients may not be appropriate candidates for arterial reconstruction based on their overall health status. Elderly patients with severe dementia and/or other organic brain syndromes who are non-ambulatory, bedridden, or have severe flexion contractures of the knee and/or hip have no prospect of rehabilitation and are inappropriate candidates for revascularization procedures. Age alone, however, is not a contraindication for arterial reconstruction. We recently evaluated our results with arterial reconstruction in those patients 80 years of age or older at the time of surgery. Graft patency, limb salvage, and perioperative mortality rates were similar to those of younger patients. Moreover, two important quality-of-life outcomes – the ability to ambulate and return to living at home – were analyzed. One year after surgery, more than 80% were still ambulatory and residing in their homes.[32]

Patients with terminal cancer with very short life expectancy or similar lethal co-morbidities do poorly and are probably better served by primary amputations. Some patients present with an unsalvageable foot due to extensive necrosis resulting from ischemia and/or infection and require primary amputation.

Patients with salvageable ischemic foot lesions complicated by active infection need to have the infection controlled prior to vascular surgical intervention (see Infection). These efforts may include open debridement and drainage, or partial foot amputation, in addition to antibiotics, and may delay vascular surgery for several days. Waiting longer than necessary in order to 'sterilize wounds' is inappropriate and may result in further necrosis and tissue loss, and loss of opportunity to save the foot. During this period, which rarely lasts longer than 5 days, contrast arteriography and other presurgical evaluations such as testing for coronary disease (when necessary) can be performed. Once cellulitis, lymphangitis, and edema have improved or resolved, especially in any areas of expected incisions for bypass, vascular surgery can be undertaken without further delay.

Patients with limb ischemia and signs and symptoms of coronary artery disease need to have stabilization of their cardiac disease prior to lower extremity arterial reconstruction. Rarely, coronary artery interventions may be required prior to arterial reconstruction. The value of routine screening tests for occult coronary ischemia remains unclear. Virtually all diabetic patients with lower extremity ischemia have occult coronary artery disease.[33] Attempting to quantify the degree of coronary artery disease with dipyridamole–thallium imaging testing has occasionally proved useful in stratifying patients at excessive risk for cardiac morbidity and mortality; however, most patients with severely abnormal scans usually have obvious clinical signs or symptoms as well.[34] As a result, we rely mostly upon the patient's clinical presentation and electrocardiogram in determining when further evaluation is needed and use imaging studies selectively in patients with unclear or atypical symptoms. We are convinced that frequent use of invasive perioperative cardiac monitoring, including pulmonary arterial catheters in selected patients, along with anesthesia management by personnel experienced in treating patients with ischemic heart disease, and managing these patients in a specialized, monitored unit with cardiac monitoring capabilities, in the early postoperative period, has significantly reduced the perioperative cardiac morbidity and mortality in our patients.

The presence of renal failure presents special challenges. When acute renal failure occurs, most commonly following contrast arteriography, surgery is delayed until renal function is stabilized or returns to baseline. Affected patients will demonstrate a transient elevation of serum creatinine levels without other symptoms. It is rare that such patients will become anuric or require hemodialysis. If there are severe concerns about renal function, magnetic resonance angiography (MRA) can usually provide adequate images to plan arterial reconstruction.[35]

Patients with dialysis-dependent end-stage renal disease can safely undergo arterial reconstruction, with reasonable initial graft patency rates. However, gangrene and tissue loss are frequently present and the healing response is poor, even with restoration of arterial blood flow. Studies have demonstrated that graft patency and limb salvage in these patients are lower than in patients without renal failure.[36,37] In some patients, despite patent arterial bypass grafts, amputation has been required. In our experience, long-term survival has been exceedingly poor for this group. Careful patient selection is therefore extremely important in this particular patient population. To determine which patients with chronic renal failure are most likely to have a favorable outcome from arterial reconstructive surgery and which patients are better served with primary amputation remains a difficult problem and requires further study.

Vascular evaluation and diagnostic studies

Patients requiring surgical intervention for lower extremity arterial insufficiency usually present with severely disabling intermittent claudication or signs and symptoms of limb-threatening ischemia. The location of discomfort can suggest the location of the lesion. Patients with tibial arterial occlusive disease will have calf claudication and may complain of foot discomfort or numbness with walking. Nocturnal muscle cramping is a common complaint of diabetic patients, but is not a typical symptom of vascular disease and should not be mistaken for intermittent claudication.

Studies on the natural history of intermittent claudication have demonstrated that progression to limb-threatening ischemia is uncommon.[38] Most patients with intermittent claudication do not require surgical intervention. Conservative treatment options include cessation of tobacco use, risk factor reduction for arteriosclerosis, weight reduction when necessary, and an extensive exercise program involving walking.[39] Administration of pentoxifylline and cilostazol has been shown to improve walking distance in patients with claudication due to atherosclerosis.[40,41] Both drugs need to be taken for several weeks before improvement in walking distance can be anticipated. In most cases, exercise and risk reduction will lead to improvement of symptoms. Our approach is to add a medication later if necessary. Surgical intervention for claudication is reserved for patients presenting with a very limited functional capacity who are unable to work due to their symptoms. However, very distal procedures to the pedal or tarsal vessels are reserved for foot or limb salvage.

Most diabetic patients requiring arterial reconstructive surgery have limb-threatening ischemia. The most common problem is

Presenting symptoms in our series of 1032 bypass grafts to the dorsalis pedis artery.		
Indication	*n*	*%*
Ulcer	547	53
Gangrene	384	37
Rest pain	55	5
Claudication	26	3
Failing graft	20	2
Total	1032	100

Table 13.2 Presenting symptoms in our series of 1032 bypass grafts to the dorsalis pedis artery. Most patients presented with a non-healing ulcer with or without associated gangrene or infection.

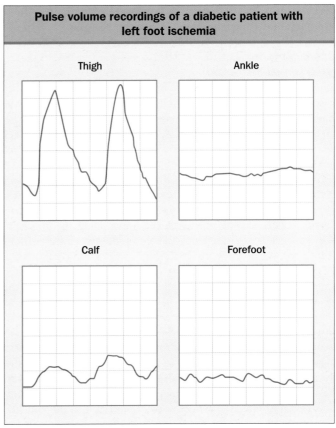

Figure 13.11 Pulse volume recordings of a diabetic patient with left foot ischemia. The severely abnormal calf waveform suggests popliteal artery occlusion and flat waveforms at the ankle and forefoot level are consistent with additional tibial arterial occlusive disease.

a non-healing ulcer with or without associated gangrene or infection (**Table 13.2**). Some patients are referred after a minor surgical procedure in the foot fails to heal because of ischemia. Patients with limb-threatening ischemia can also present with ischemic rest pain with or without associated tissue loss. Ischemic rest pain typically occurs in the distal foot, particularly the toes. It is exacerbated by recumbency and relieved by dependency. It is important, but sometimes difficult, to distinguish rest pain from painful diabetic neuropathy, which may also be subjectively worse at night. Neuropathic patients may present with no rest pain in spite of severe ischemia, due to complete loss of sensation. Non-invasive vascular laboratory studies are particularly useful in patients presenting with pain in the foot and absent pulses where the etiology is unclear and may be due to either ischemia or painful diabetic neuropathy. Patients with severe ischemia will usually have ankle–brachial indices of less than 0.4. In diabetic patients, however, care must be taken in interpreting ankle pressures since many patients will have artificially elevated ankle pressures due to calcification of the arterial wall.[42] Approximately 10% of patients will have incompressible vessels, making ankle pressures incalculable. Pulse volume recordings are useful since they are unaffected by calcification of vessels (**Fig. 13.11**). Some centers have found toe pressures[42] and transcutaneous oxygen measurements[43] to be useful in diabetic patients. Following surgery, non-invasive testing can be used to quantify the degree of improvement in distal circulation. Postoperative duplex ultrasonography of vein grafts has been useful in detecting areas of stenosis caused by intimal hyperplasia, which can be corrected before they cause graft thrombosis.[44]

Non-invasive testing, however, adds little information to the evaluation of the patient with obvious signs of foot ischemia and absent foot pulses. If the posterior tibial and dorsalis pedis artery pulses are non-palpable in patients in whom typical signs and symptoms of ischemia are present, no further non-invasive testing is necessary and contrast arteriography should be performed straight away.

Arteriography

The ultimate goal of arterial reconstructive surgery in diabetic patients is to restore maximal blood supply to the foot. Ultimately, the decision of when to perform a tibial bypass or a

pedal bypass is based on a carefully performed arteriogram. The outflow target artery should be relatively free of occlusive disease and demonstrate unimpeded arterial flow into the arteries of the foot. In general, the most proximal artery distal to the occlusion and meeting these two criteria is chosen. Because of the propensity for diabetic patients to have occlusive lesions in the tibial arteries, it is essential that arteriograms not be terminated at the mid-tibial level, but that they incorporate the complete infrapopliteal circulation, including the foot vessels. Iliac artery atherosclerosis accompanies lower extremity atherosclerosis in approximately 10–20% of patients with diabetes. When hemodynamically significant stenosis is present, angioplasty of iliac lesions with or without placement of a stent is almost always possible and will improve arterial inflow for the subsequent bypass procedure. Moreover, this can be performed at the same setting as for the diagnostic arteriogram. It is our preference to exclusively use intra-arterial digital subtraction angiography (DSA) to evaluate the lower extremity arterial circulation. For patients with moderate renal insufficiency (creatinine <2.5mg/dL), hydration with normal saline solution prior to angiography will usually prevent significant deterioration of renal function.

For patients with more marginal renal function, MRA can provide images of the distal circulation sufficient to plan the arterial reconstruction. Although some authors claim MRA is superior to DSA,[35] we have found that intra-arterial DSA continues to provide the best-quality images (**Fig. 13.10**) and reserve MRA for those patients in whom the administration of contrast is potentially harmful or contraindicated.

Management
Arterial reconstruction

One of the most important developments in vascular surgery has been the demonstration that autogenous saphenous vein gives the best short- and long-term results for distal bypass. In a large, multicenter, prospective randomized trial, 6-year graft patency of saphenous vein grafts was more than four times that of prosthetic grafts.[45]

For more than five decades, the standard conduit for lower extremity revascularization has been the reversed greater saphenous vein.[46] An inherent problem with reversing the vein – which is necessary to overcome the impediment of flow from valves – is a size discrepancy that results between the arteries and veins when they are connected. Vein grafts that have a diameter of less than 4mm at the distal end can thrombose when connected to the much larger common femoral artery in the groin, because of size discrepancy. For many years, some vascular surgeons would routinely discard saphenous veins that were smaller than 4mm at the distal end. Methods were developed to render the valves incompetent to allow the vascular surgeon to use the vein non-reversed or 'in situ'. However, no such valve lysis technique was widely accepted until the late 1970s, when Leather[47] described a new method, using a modified Mills valvulotome, which cut the valves atraumatically and quickly. The technique was quickly incorporated into the repertoire of most vascular surgeons. This led to the conclusion that the in-situ bypass was superior to the reversed saphenous vein graft; however, evidence to support this concept is lacking.[48] When in-situ bypasses are compared with reversed saphenous vein grafts, no apparent superiority is evident.[49] In our own experience, we have frequently used both procedures and have observed essentially identical results with both configurations.[50]

In the 1980s, the first series of bypass grafts with inflow taken from the popliteal artery was reported.[51] The results were equivalent to those achieved with arterial reconstructions taking inflow from the common femoral artery. These results have been confirmed by other groups, including our own,[52,53] and represent another important advance in arterial reconstruction in patients with diabetes. In diabetic patients, the superficial femoral artery is frequently spared from significant disease, allowing the popliteal artery to be used as a source of inflow for the distal vein graft. Doing so shortens the operative procedure and avoids potentially troublesome wound complications in the groin. Short vein grafts are also advantageous in patients with a limited length of adequate saphenous vein. Theoretically, shorter vein grafts should also have higher flow rates and possibly better long-term patency. Our experience with extreme distal bypasses has shown that popliteal inflow is possible in about 60% of diabetic patients undergoing lower extremity vascular reconstruction.[50]

When the greater saphenous vein is unavailable owing to previous harvesting or vein stripping, alternative sources of conduits must be used. Alternative vein grafts such as contralateral saphenous vein, arm vein, or lesser saphenous vein can be used. We have generally not harvested the greater saphenous vein from the opposite extremity in patients with diabetes. Our experience has demonstrated that in patients with missing

ipsilateral saphenous vein, the likelihood of requiring another vascular reconstruction in the contralateral extremity approaches 40% at 3 years following the first operation.[54] Moreover, in our tertiary care practice, many patients do not have adequate available contralateral saphenous vein owing to its use for other vascular procedures, including coronary artery bypass. When the greater saphenous vein is not available, our vein conduit of choice has been arm vein. Our results with arm vein grafts have been improving by performing angioscopy to identify and exclude vein segments with strictures or recanalization (webs) induced by previous venepuncture and thrombosis (**Fig. 13.12**). Using the angioscope to 'upgrade' the quality of arm vein grafts not only enhances results with these grafts but also further reduces the number of patients requiring the use of a prosthetic conduit.[55] Creation of composite grafts made of various segments of arm vein, including the cephalic-basilic vein loop graft,[56] can provide sufficient conduit length to reach from the groin to the mid-calf or foot vessels in many patients. Our results with arm vein grafts have recently been reported.[57] The results were inferior to those with de-novo reconstructions done with saphenous vein, but significantly better than those reported with prosthetic conduits.

The choice of outflow artery is made from the lower extremity arteriogram including the foot vessels. Our experience has demonstrated that in 10% of cases, a foot artery, usually the dorsalis pedis artery, is the only suitable outflow vessel, and in an additional 15% of patients, the dorsalis pedis artery will appear to be the best target vessel in comparison to other patent but diseased tibial vessels. As a result, we began performing bypasses to the dorsalis pedis artery in the early 1980s. Early results were encouraging, and we standardized our surgical technique and broadened our indications by giving the dorsalis pedis artery equal consideration as an outflow target.[58] Our published results with bypasses to the dorsalis pedis artery have demonstrated graft patency and limb salvage approaching 80% and 90% at 5 years, respectively.[59] Moreover, even in the presence of foot infection, pedal bypass can be performed safely as long as spreading sepsis is controlled prior to surgery.[60] Although pedal artery bypass represents the most 'extreme' type of distal arterial reconstruction, it is almost always possible,

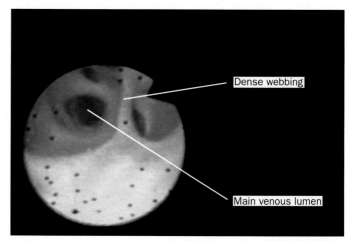

Figure 13.12 Angioscopy of the lumen of an arm vein, demonstrating dense 'webbing'. These lesions occur as a result of previous venipunctures. Segments of vein with these findings are not suitable for use as bypass conduits.

Outflow target arteries for lower extremity arterial bypasses performed by the Division of Vascular Surgery of the Beth Israel Deaconess Medical Center in the year 2000.		
Outflow target artery	n	%
Dorsalis pedis	68	27
Tibial	69	28
Peroneal	16	7
Above-knee popliteal	32	13
Below-knee popliteal	40	16
Other	21	9
Total	246	100

Table 13.3 Outflow target arteries for lower extremity arterial bypasses performed by the Division of Vascular Surgery of the Beth Israel Deaconess Medical Center in the year 2000. Bypasses to the dorsalis pedis artery constituted approximately 27% of all lower extremity arterial reconstructions (unpublished data).

particularly when the vascular surgeon is flexible in terms of how the vein graft is prepared and where the proximal anastomosis is placed.

Distal arterial reconstruction presents specific technical challenges to the vascular surgeon and requires meticulous attention to detail. The distal target arteries are usually small (1–2mm in diameter) and often calcified. Harvesting of an adequate venous conduit is essential but can be difficult.

Since the inception of dorsalis pedis artery bypass a significant decline in all amputations performed for ischemia has been observed.[61] Currently, bypasses to the dorsalis pedis artery constitute approximately one-quarter of all lower extremity arterial reconstructions in our patients with diabetes mellitus (Table 13.3).

It is important to recognize that pedal artery bypass is not the only procedure applicable to patients with diabetes. The goal of treatment is to restore maximal arterial flow to the foot. The preoperative arteriogram is the key piece of information needed in planning an appropriate surgical procedure. If a bypass to the popliteal or tibial artery will restore maximal arterial flow to the level of the foot, it should be done. Since the quality of the venous conduit is the most important determinant in long-term success, using the shortest length of high-quality venous conduit necessary to achieve this goal is the basic principle. Each operation must be individualized based on the patient's available venous conduit and arterial anatomy as demonstrated in the preoperative arteriogram.

SUMMARY

This chapter has reviewed the principles of evaluation, diagnosis, and treatment of arterial disease in patients with lower extremity ischemia in diabetes. Rejection of the small vessel disease hypothesis and understanding the location of atherosclerotic disease in the lower extremity of patients with diabetes are key to effecting proper treatment. Understanding the interplay of neuropathy, infection, and ischemia is essential to ultimate success. When treating foot ischemia, a carefully planned approach, including prompt control of infection when present, a high-quality digital subtraction arteriogram, and an extreme distal arterial reconstruction to maximize foot perfusion, should lead to rates of limb salvage in patients with diabetes which equal or exceed those achieved in non-diabetics.

REFERENCES

1. Gibbons GW, Eliopoulos GM. Infection of the diabetic foot. In: Kozak GP, Campbell DR, Frykberg RG, et al., eds. Management of diabetic foot problems, 2nd edn. Philadelphia:WB Saunders; 1984: 121–30.
2. Edmonds ME. The diabetic foot: pathophysiology and treatment. Clin Endocrinol Metab 1986;15:889–916.
3. Grunfeld C. Diabetic foot ulcers: etiology, treatment, and prevention. Adv Intern Med 1992;37:103–32.
4. Kozak GP, Giurini JM. Diabetic neuropathies: lower extremities. In: Kozak GP, Campbell D, Frykberg R, et al., eds. Management of diabetic foot problems, 2nd edn. Philadelphia:WB Saunders; 1995:43–52.
5. Gabbay KH. The sorbitol pathway and the complications of diabetes. N Engl J Med 1973;288:831–6.
6. Apfel SC. Introduction to diabetic neuropathy. Am J Med 1999; 107(2B):1S.
7. Ishii DN. Implication of insulin-like growth factors in the pathogenesis of diabetic neuropathy. Brain Res Brain Res Rev 1995;20:47–67.
8. Boulton AJ, Scarpello JH, Ward JD. Venous oxygenation in the diabetic neuropathic foot: evidence of arteriovenous shunting? Diabetologia 1982;22:6–8.
9. Walmsley D, Wiles PG. Early loss of neurogenic inflammation in the human diabetic foot. Clin Sci (Lond) 1991;80:605–10.
10. Kosiak M. Etiology and pathology of ischemic ulcers. Arch Phys Med Rehabil 1959;40:62–9.
11. Lobmann R, Kayser R, Kasten G, et al. Effects of preventative footwear on foot pressure as determined by pedobarography in diabetic patients: a prospective study. Diabet Med 2001;18:314–9.
12. Tan JS, Anderson JL, Watanakunakorn C, et al. Neutrophil dysfunction in diabetes mellitus. J Lab Clin Med 1975;85:26–33.
13. Bagdade JD, Root RK, Bulger RJ. Impaired leukocyte function in patients with poorly controlled diabetes. Diabetes 1974;23:9.
14. Grayson ML, Gibbons GW, Balogh K, et al. Probing to bone in infected pedal ulcers. A clinical sign of underlying osteomyelitis in diabetic patients. JAMA 1995;273:721–3.
15. Johnson JE, Kennedy EJ, Shereff MJ, et al. Prospective study of bone, indium-111-labeled white blood cell, and gallium-67 scanning for the evaluation of osteomyelitis in the diabetic foot. Foot Ankle Int 1996; 17:10–6.
16. Marcus CD, Ladam-Marcus VJ, Leone J, et al. MR imaging of osteomyelitis and neuropathic osteoarthropathy in the feet of diabetics. Radiographics 1996;16:1337–48.
17. Grayson ML, Gibbons GW, Habershaw GM, et al. Use of ampicillin/sulbactam versus imipenem/cilastatin in the treatment of limb-threatening foot infections in diabetic patients. Clin Infect Dis 1994;18:683–93.
18. Goldstein EJ, Citron DM, Nesbit CA. Diabetic foot infections. Bacteriology and activity of 10 oral antimicrobial agents against bacteria isolated from consecutive cases. Diabetes Care 1996;19:638–41.
19. Ellison MJ. Vancomycin, metronidazole, and tetracyclines. Clin Podiatr Med Surg 1992;9:425–42.
20. Gibbons GW. The diabetic foot: amputations and drainage of infection. J Vasc Surg 1987;5:791–3.
21. Goldenberg SG, Alex M, Joshi RA, et al. Nonatheromatous peripheral vascular disease of the lower extremity in diabetes mellitus. Diabetes 1959;8:261–73.

22. Strandness DE, Priest RE, Gibbons GW. Combined clinical and pathological study of diabetic and nondiabetic peripheral arterial disease. Diabetes 1964;13:366–72.

23. Akbari CM, Pomposelli FB Jr, Gibbons GW, et al. Lower extremity revascularization in diabetes: late observations. Arch Surg 2000;135:452–6.

24. Kannel WB, McGee DL. Diabetes and cardiovascular disease. The Framingham study. JAMA 1979;241:2035–8.

25. Smith JW, Marcus FI, Serokman R. Prognosis of patients with diabetes mellitus after acute myocardial infarction. Am J Cardiol 1984;54:718–21.

26. Petersen CM, Kaufman J, Jovanovic L. Influence of diabetes on vascular disease and its complications. In: Moore WS, ed. Vascular surgery: a comprehensive review, 5th edn. Philadelphia:WB Saunders; 1998:146–67.

27. Zarich S, Waxman S, Freeman RT, et al. Effect of autonomic nervous system dysfunction on the circadian pattern of myocardial ischemia in diabetes mellitus. J Am Coll Cardiol 1994;24:956–62.

28. Eagle KA, Coley CM, Newell JB, et al. Combining clinical and thallium data optimizes preoperative assessment of cardiac risk before major vascular surgery. Ann Intern Med 1989;110:859–66.

29. Lee TH, Marcantonio ER, Mangione CM, et al. Derivation and prospective validation of a simple index for prediction of cardiac risk of major noncardiac surgery. Circulation 1999;100:1043–9.

30. Hamdan AD, Saltzberg SS, Sheahan M, et al. Lack of association of diabetes with increased postoperative mortality and cardiac morbidity: results of 6565 major vascular operations. Arch Surg 2002;137:417–21.

31. LoGerfo FW, Coffman JD. Current concepts. Vascular and microvascular disease of the foot in diabetes. Implications for foot care. N Engl J Med 1984;311:1615–9.

32. Pomposelli FB Jr, Arora S, Gibbons GW, et al. Lower extremity arterial reconstruction in the very elderly: successful outcome preserves not only the limb but also residential status and ambulatory function. J Vasc Surg 1998;28:215–25.

33. Nesto RW. Screening for asymptomatic coronary artery disease in diabetes. Diabetes Care 1999;22:1393–5.

34. Zarich SW, Cohen MC, Lane SE, et al. Routine perioperative dipyridamole 201Tl imaging in diabetic patients undergoing vascular surgery. Diabetes Care 1996;19:355–60.

35. Carpenter JP, Baum RA, Holland GA, et al. Peripheral vascular surgery with magnetic resonance angiography as the sole preoperative imaging modality. J Vasc Surg 1994;20:861–9; discussion 869–71.

36. Korn P, Hoenig SJ, Skillman JJ, et al. Is lower extremity revascularization worthwhile in patients with end-stage renal disease? Surgery 2000;128:472–9.

37. Johnson BL, Glickman MH, Bandyk DF, et al. Failure of foot salvage in patients with end-stage renal disease after surgical revascularization. J Vasc Surg 1995;22:280–5; discussion 285–6.

38. Dormandy J, Heeck L, Vig S. The natural history of claudication: risk to life and limb. Semin Vasc Surg 1999;12:123–37.

39. Hertzer NR. The natural history of peripheral vascular disease. Implications for its management. Circulation 1991;83(2 Suppl):I12–9.

40. Dawson DL, Cutler BS, Hiatt WR, et al. A comparison of cilostazol and pentoxifylline for treating intermittent claudication. Am J Med 2000;109:523–30.

41. Gillings DB. Pentoxifylline and intermittent claudication: review of clinical trials and cost-effectiveness analyses. J Cardiovasc Pharmacol 1995;25(Suppl 2):S44–50.

42. Weitz JI, Byrne J, Clagett GP, et al. Diagnosis and treatment of chronic arterial insufficiency of the lower extremities: a critical review [published erratum appears in Circulation 2000;102:1074]. Circulation 1996;94:3026–49.

43. Hauser CJ, Klein SR, Mehringer CM, et al. Superiority of transcutaneous oximetry in noninvasive vascular diagnosis in patients with diabetes. Arch Surg 1984;119:690–4.

44. Bandyk DF, Seabrook GR, Moldenhauer P, et al. Hemodynamics of vein graft stenosis. J Vasc Surg 1988;8:688–95.

45. Veith FJ, Gupta SK, Ascer E, et al. Six-year prospective multicenter randomized comparison of autologous saphenous vein and expanded polytetrafluoroethylene grafts in infrainguinal arterial reconstructions. J Vasc Surg 1986;3:104–14.

46. Kunlin J. Le traitment de làrterite obliterante par la greffe veinuse. Arch Mal Coeur Vaiss 1949;42:371.

47. Leather RP, Powers SR, Karmody AM. A reappraisal of the in situ saphenous vein arterial bypass: its use in limb salvage. Surgery 1979;86:453–61.

48. Cambria RP, Megerman J, Brewster DC, et al. The evolution of morphologic and biomechanical changes in reversed and in-situ vein grafts. Ann Surg 1987;205:167–74.

49. Taylor LM Jr, Edwards JM, Porter JM. Present status of reversed vein bypass grafting: five-year results of a modern series. J Vasc Surg 1990;11:193–205; discussion 205–6.

50. Pomposelli FB Jr, Jepsen SJ, Gibbons GW, et al. A flexible approach to infrapopliteal vein grafts in patients with diabetes mellitus. Arch Surg 1991;126:724–7; discussion 727–9.

51. Ascer E, Veith FJ, Gupta SK, et al. Short vein grafts: a superior option for arterial reconstructions to poor or compromised outflow tracts? J Vasc Surg 1988;7:370–8.

52. Cantelmo NL, Snow JR, Menzoian JO, et al. Successful vein bypass in patients with an ischemic limb and a palpable popliteal pulse. Arch Surg 1986;121:217–20.

53. Stonebridge PA, Tsoukas AI, Pomposelli FB Jr, et al. Popliteal-to-distal bypass grafts for limb salvage in diabetics. Eur J Vasc Surg 1991;5:265–9.

54. Holzenbein TJ, Pomposelli FB Jr, Miller A, et al. Results of a policy with arm veins used as the first alternative to an unavailable ipsilateral greater saphenous vein for infrainguinal bypass. J Vasc Surg 1996;23:130–40.

55. Stonebridge PA, Miller A, Tsoukas A, et al. Angioscopy of arm vein infrainguinal bypass grafts. Ann Vasc Surg 1991;5:170–5.

56. Balshi JD, Cantelmo NL, Menzoian JO, et al. The use of arm veins for infrainguinal bypass in end-stage peripheral vascular disease. Arch Surg 1989;124:1078–81.

57. Faries PL, Arora S, Pomposelli FB Jr, et al. The use of arm vein in lower-extremity revascularization: results of 520 procedures performed in eight years. J Vasc Surg 2000;31(1 Pt 1):50–9.

58. Pomposelli FB Jr, Jepsen SJ, Gibbons GW, et al. Efficacy of the dorsal pedal bypass for limb salvage in diabetic patients: short-term observations. J Vasc Surg 1990;11:745–51; discussion 751–2.

59. Pomposelli FB Jr, Marcaccio EJ, Gibbons GW, et al. Dorsalis pedis arterial bypass: durable limb salvage for foot ischemia in patients with diabetes mellitus. J Vasc Surg 1995;21:375–84.

60. Tannenbaum GA, Pomposelli FB Jr, Marcaccio EJ, et al. Safety of vein bypass grafting to the dorsal pedal artery in diabetic patients with foot infections. J Vasc Surg 1992;15:982–8; discussion 989–90.

61. LoGerfo FW, Gibbons GW, Pomposelli FB Jr, et al. Trends in the care of the diabetic foot. Expanded role of arterial reconstruction. Arch Surg 1992;127:617–20; discussion 620–1.

CHAPTER
14

Amputation

Mark R Nehler

KEY POINTS

- Diabetes mellitus, cigarette smoking, and a reduced ankle–brachial index are major risk factors for lower limb amputation.

- Diabetes mellitus accounts for the majority of non-traumatic lower limb amputations.

- The majority of patients requiring amputation for critical limb ischemia (CLI) have had symptoms of <6 months duration. Patients with chronic intermittent claudication infrequently progress to CLI requiring amputation.

- Primary BKA healing rates are highly variable but consistently lower than AKA healing rates.

- Mortality for major limb amputation (6–13%) greatly exceeds that for nearly all other major vascular procedures, reflecting the comorbidities of this patient population rather than the magnitude of the operation.

INTRODUCTION

Major lower extremity amputation, like many procedures in modern vascular surgery, is performed by several surgical specialties. However, vascular surgeons frequently perform major lower extremity amputations, as these patient populations generally require other vascular care. The principles of major lower extremity amputation are similar to those of other surgical care designed to remove infected or non-viable tissue (resection for ischemic bowel, resection for diverticulitis, or resection for chronic lung infection). The goals of the operation are:

- complete removal of diseased or infected tissue;
- relief of pain;
- eventual incisional wound healing; and
- providing the most functional possible amputation stump

These goals take on variable priorities depending on the age of the patient and other co-morbidities, as well as the etiology of the process necessitating major lower extremity amputation. For example, a young trauma patient with great ambulatory potential and many years to take advantage of this may undergo several operations, including muscular free-flap grafting in order to preserve the knee joint with a transtibial amputation (below-the-knee amputation; BKA). Conversely, an elderly patient with severe chronic obstructive pulmonary disease may be best served with a transfemoral amputation (above-the-knee amputation; AKA), with efforts then being concentrated on providing home wheelchair access, as eventual prosthetic wear and limited

ambulation is not realistic due to cardiopulmonary limitations, and uncomplicated primary incisional wound healing is of greatest importance. The goal of this section is to familiarize the reader with the data regarding technical and functional success which support clinical decisions in the patient undergoing major lower extremity amputation.

EPIDEMIOLOGY

Three important risk factors for major lower extremity amputation are diabetes, tobacco use, and level of ankle–brachial index.[1–3] The incidence of major lower extremity amputation has declined slightly in the last two decades, probably due to improvements and more widespread performance of lower extremity arterial bypass. Although occasional young patients lose limbs due to trauma, the majority of major limb losses are due to the complications of diabetes, such as neuropathy, atherosclerosis, or both. One of the greatest risk factors for major lower extremity amputation is a previous amputation. This is true for the risk of a contralateral amputation in a patient with ipsilateral AKA or BKA[4,5] and also for an ipsilateral BKA/AKA in a patient with previous minor limb amputation (digit, ray, or transmetatarsal).[4,6,7] This is largely due to the multifactorial etiology of the prior amputation (patient weight, compliance, neuropathy, peripheral vascular disease), usually involving both lower extremities, as well as detrimental mechanical factors for the remaining lower extremity, including changes in weight distribution following either minor or major lower extremity amputation. From 20–70% of patients presenting with acute limb ischemia will require amputation, due to lack of collateral circulation and inadequate time for referral to vascular centers.[8,9] Critical limb ischemia (CLI) patients with necrosis/ulceration have a greater risk of eventual amputation than those with isolated rest pain.[4,10]

It has been assumed that patients with CLI who eventually undergo major lower extremity amputation have an antecedent history of steady symptomatic progression from claudication, to rest pain/necrosis. Available data would indicate that this is the exception rather than the rule. Dormandy reported that over half of 713 patients undergoing BKA in a randomized pharmaceutical trial had no ischemic symptoms 6 months prior to surgery.[11] The vast majority of multiple natural history studies examining patients with claudication have demonstrated that only a minority of patients go on to develop CLI in a 5–10 year period.[12] The author believes that the majority of patients undergoing major limb amputation have come from the asymptomatic state directly to rest pain or necrosis via one of two mechanisms. Patients either suffer 1) a major acute event (cardiac, stroke, orthopedic, etc.) leading to a significant reduction in cardiopulmonary or functional status and then develop limb threat due either to a reduction in cardiac output or pressure necrosis in an area with pre-existing marginal peripheral circulation; or 2) Minor trauma in a marginally perfused extremity or loss of an important arterial collateral. Patients in the first group have significant global issues that are in part responsible for CLI/amputation and are therefore more likely to have limited functional and/or survival post-amputation. Patients in the second group may benefit from early intervention with potential limb salvage, or at least knee salvage, and eventual prosthesis. Finally, a subgroup of patients undergoing interventions for claudication will suffer failures with deterioration in their antecedent vascular anatomy to the point of CLI. It is unknown what percentage of patients this subgroup comprises, but reported series of bypass for claudication report minimal limb loss over 4–5 years.[13–16] However, patients with premature atherosclerosis appear to fare poorly over time.[17–20]

The ratio of AKA to BKA is approximately one and has not changed appreciably in the last two decades.[21–25] Therefore, despite the potential functional benefits of saving the knee joint (this will be discussed in more detail later), due to age and multiple co-morbid conditions, there continues to be a substantial group of patients who will never gain ambulatory status with a prosthesis and are better served with a procedure that has a superior primary healing rate.[26] Several epidemiologic studies from Europe demonstrate that 85% of major limb amputations were performed for CLI.[27–29] Such data reinforce the role of the vascular surgeon in the care of the amputee.

OPERATIVE MORBIDITY/MORTALITY

Despite being a vascular procedure that gains less attention, both in training and in the literature, than endovascular surgery, open aortic repair, carotid endarterectomy, and limb salvage operations, the reported success with BKA is sobering. Primary BKA healing rates vary widely (**Table 14.1**). Up to 30% of patients who fail to heal will undergo a repeat amputation to save the knee joint and half of these will ultimately require an AKA. In contrast, the primary healing rate for an AKA is a more consistent 70%, with 90% ultimately healing after further revision procedures.[30,31] Wound healing failure can be attributed to secondary trauma from falls in the postoperative period and/or difficulties in obtaining primary wound healing in dysvascular tissue ± concomitant venous and lymphedema. Many vascular surgeons and rehabilitation services use early stump casting

Below-knee amputation healing rates.					
Authors	Year	n	Primary healing %	Secondary healing %	Reamputation %
Finch et al.[91]	1980	61	75	13	12
Kazmers et al.[92]	1986	84	75	–	25
Tripses & Pollak[93]	1981	64	67	13	20
Rush et al.[85]	1981	110	76	–	24
Creaney et al.[94]	1981	46	70	–	30
Burgess et al.[95]	1982	37	81	5	14
Yamanaka & Kwong[75]	1983	23	74	9	17
Ratcliff et al.[96]	1984	37	75	–	15
O'Dwyer & Edwards[97]	1985	203	56	19	25
Holstein[98]	1985	144	78	–	22
Kay et al.[99]	1987	33	76	15	9
Christensen & Klarke[49]	1986	28	68	21	11
Dowd[100]	1986	61	69	13	18
Gregg[22]	1986	92	84	–	16
Harrison et al.[23]	1987	109	75	–	9
Silverman et al.[101]	1987	32	–	91	9
Ruckley et al.[80]	1991	191	60	23	–
Inderbitzi et al.[102]	1992	66	67	35	–
Dormandy et al.[11]	1994	713	59	11	19
McWhinnie et al.[87]	1994	96	75	16	9
*For surviving patients.					

Table 14.1 Below-knee amputation healing rates.

for protection against trauma and control of edema. A single randomized trial (total of 51 patients) did not demonstrate any benefits in wound healing in postoperative casting following BKA compared to standard soft dressing (85 versus 83% healing).[32] A more recent randomized trial (total of 56 patients) examining the effect of casting on healing of chronic (≥ 3 months duration) postoperative BKA wounds did demonstrate a benefit for casting (healing time of 71 versus 97 days).[33] The prevailing belief that the majority of patients undergoing BKA will heal in 6 weeks without problems and be ready for prosthesis is clearly unduly optimistic and largely incorrect. Healing times in BKA are often measured in months, rather than weeks.[34,35] This observation is similar to that in limb salvage series, in healing of open foot wounds and distal leg incisions following successful revascularization.[36,37] Therefore, healing dysvascular tissue below the knee is a problem, irrespective of the approach.

In an effort to improve primary healing rates, a substantial amount of literature has accumulated regarding measures to assess the adequacy of the arterial circulation to support healing of a BKA. Not surprisingly, since the issue appears multifactorial and arterial circulation is merely one component of the problem, these efforts have not been conclusive. However, adequate arterial circulation is necessary for any chance of a BKA to be subject to the wide range of healing rates documented. Historically, the clinical examination of the leg by the operating surgeon involved consideration of skin integrity, warmth, absence of wounds, viable muscle on palpation, and capillary refill. The presence of a popliteal pulse indicates adequate vascularity, but its absence does not predict failure.[38] An absent femoral pulse, however, is an ominous sign and the circulation should be further investigated prior to BKA. The clinical judgment of the operating surgeon (tissue bleeding, viable muscle, and wounds without tension) has been demonstrated to be reasonably accurate (75–85%) in several large clinical series (combined, involving around 1000 patients).[30,39,40]

The utility of preoperative vascular laboratory studies in the prediction of amputation success is unclear. Quantification of skin temperature has not been useful.[41,42] Measurement of Doppler-derived arterial pressures has yielded conflicting results. Several decades ago, investigators suggested that a below-knee pressure of 70 torr appeared to correlate close to 100%, with eventual BKA healing in two series totaling close to 200 patients.[43,44] However, other studies have failed to reproduce these results.[42,45,46] Inaccuracy of Doppler pressure to predict BKA healing is likely due to the frequent arterial calcification in patients with CLI and the multifactorial etiology of BKA failure.

Transcutaneous oxygen (TCO$_2$) determination has also been evaluated as a predictor for BKA healing. These measurements can be difficult to perform in individual vascular laboratories as they are dependent on multiple examinations in areas of the skin in question and need a controlled environment. Multiple groups have shown that a TCO$_2$ ≥ 35 mmHg at the below-knee level predicts BKA healing in 95% of patients.[42,47–49] Skin perfusion measurements via photoplethysmography (20mmHg) and laser Doppler (30mmHg) have also been used to predict BKA amputation healing. In several small series consisting of fewer than 100 patients, healing of 80–90% of BKAs has occurred using those parameters.[38,50,51] A number of other methods to determine skin perfusion, including laser Doppler velocimetry,[52] isotopic measurement,[53,54] and fluorescein dye measurement[55] have been

studied to predict BKA healing. At present, these are collectively best considered as research tools without significant practical utility to the practicing vascular surgeon.

Major amputations are frequently performed in extremely ill, end-stage patients. This is demonstrated in a review from the Veteran Affairs (VA) National Surgical Quality Improvement Program (NSQIP).[56] From 1991 to 1995, 1909 BKAs and 2152 AKAs were performed in VA hospitals in the USA. Thirty-day mortality was 6.3% for BKA and 13.3% for AKA. This is in striking contrast to the 2.7% 30-day mortality for the more technically challenging abdominal aortic aneurysm repair in the recently reported VA small aneurysm trial,[57] clearly demonstrating the frailty of the amputation population, and in particular those patients who are felt to not benefit functionally from preservation of the knee joint. A large series from Keagy and colleagues reported similar findings.[30] In 1028 consecutive amputations over a 13-year period, operative mortality was 7%.

The most common reported cause of perioperative death following major amputation is cardiac.[30] Other significant morbidities beyond wound issues include thromboembolism, stroke, aspiration pneumonia, and renal failure. Deep venous thrombosis (DVT) is considered a significant perioperative problem in amputees. These patients are usually fairly sedentary preoperatively and occasionally harbor hypercoaguable conditions. In an early study, Barnes et al. failed to demonstrate any DVT in 35 of 87 amputees.[58] The non-consecutive nature of these data and lack of color flow Duplex makes this finding suspect. Yeager et al. prospectively evaluated 72 major amputation patients with perioperative Duplex ultrasound and found eight patients with popliteal venous thrombus (11%).[59] Others have reported similar findings.[60]

Most amputees have kinesthetic sensations (feelings of volume, length, etc.) in the immediate postoperative period, which persist over time. A study of 58 patients, via pain questionnaires, at 8 days and 6 months post-amputation demonstrated an 85% incidence of such kinesthetic symptoms.[61] Chronic postoperative amputation pain can be divided into two groups, residual limb (stump pain) and phantom limb pain, with a reported prevalence in the range of 50–80% of patients.[62] Both central and peripheral pain mechanisms appear to be involved, including ectopic activity originating from afferent fibers in a neuroma and cortical reorganization/spinal cord sensitization.[63] A recent community-based survey of phantom limb symptoms in 255 amputees is instructive.[64] Approximately 70% reported either residual or phantom limb pain. For most patients, the pain is episodic in nature and not particularly troublesome. In approximately one in four patients, however, the symptoms are very disabling. In addition, there are some data to suggest that the duration and intensity of pre-amputation limb pain plays a role in early post-amputation residual limb and phantom limb pain.[61]

Therapy for residual and phantom limb pain has been disappointing, in part due to the unclear mechanisms involved. Sodium channel blockers (lidocaine) and opioids have traditionally been the agents used. Preemptive epidural infusions, early regional nerve blocks with perineural infusions, and mechanical vibratory sensation have been advocated. Gabapentin, clonidine, and tricyclic antidepressants have also been used. Halbert et al.[65] summarized the data for efficacy as consisting of a few randomized trials (many with success in the treatment arm barely greater than controls)[66–71] and case reports/small series.[70,72–74] They concluded that there is currently a large gap between research and clinical practice in the management of residual and phantom limb pain in amputees.

TECHNICAL ISSUES

Despite the significant variability in technical success of BKA, there has not been a substantial amount of technical innovation or change in the operative approach in the last two decades. Isolated reports of unique flap design including side to side[75] and sagittal,[76] notwithstanding, the two techniques for BKA that have predominated are the long posterior and the skew flap technique. The creation of a long posterior musculocutaneous flap with the gastrocnemius muscle, or the 'Burgess' technique, has been the predominant method used, particularly in the USA.[77] This technique requires adequate quality skin in the posterior leg to create the flap, and has the advantage of being a relatively simple procedure. The anterior incision is made approximately one hand-breadth below the tibial tuberosity, with posterior extension distally for the flap. Once the fascia is divided, the anterior compartment is then divided. Next, the tibia is divided at or just proximal to the anterior skin incision. The lateral compartment is divided to expose the fibula, which is transected 1–2cm more proximal than the tibia. The posterior compartment is then divided in an oblique manner to remove most of the soleus and leave the gastrocnemius muscle for the flap. After vascular control, the fascia is approximated followed by the skin. A tourniquet can be used to minimize blood loss.

Despite the ease of this technique, several problems are common. For example, in patients with an obese or muscular calf, it can be difficult to close the neuromuscular flap without dog-ear deformities. These may delay prosthetic fitting, as the prosthetist uses massage and compression following stump healing to shape the stump. Another problem is that the incision line for the skin and fascia lies directly over the cut edge of the tibia. This is the area of maximal wound tension, and is therefore most likely to break down with any trauma. Due to the tenuous covering of the tibia, trauma may lead to exposed bone.

Based on these drawbacks, the skew flap amputation was designed in 1982 (**Figs 14.1 & 14.2**).[78] This technique has the advantage of displacing the skin incision lateral to the tibial stump. In addition, a single comparative study of TCO_2 levels in 10 skew flap amputees compared to 10 Burgess flap amputees demonstrated better global flap perfusion with the skew flap, possibly due to the limited distal extension.[79] Harrison reported improved healing rates in BKAs with skew flap compared to the Burgess technique in a retrospective review of approximately 200 BKAs using both techniques.[23] However, a more recent randomized, multicenter trial from Scotland showed identical findings in both groups (total of 191 patients). Primary healing without complication at 1 week was 60% and eventual need for revision was 16% versus 17%.[80]

Through-the-knee amputations have been advocated because of increased limb length, compared to an AKA with improved functionality for future prosthetic wear. This technique has the disadvantage of requiring long flap coverage, with potential healing complications. In a single series of 12 patients,[81] 60% primary healing was achieved and two of the ten surviving patients required AKA conversion for infection. Seven patients

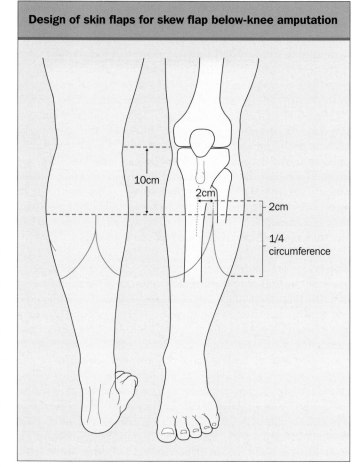

Figure 14.1 Design of skin flaps for skew flap below-knee amputation. (Redrawn from Ruckley et al[80] with permission).

were able to ambulate to some extent. Based on the patient population and later discussions regarding function, this procedure has limited application but may be useful in the rare patient who is a good ambulatory candidate with technical issues precluding BKA.

A final technical note worth discussing is cryoamputation in the critically ill patient requiring major lower extremity amputation, usually due to acute ischemia or overwhelming infection. Many of these patients present severely dehydrated, oliguric, and may have significant electrolyte abnormalities due to hyperglycemia and glycosuria. Cryoamputation offers a physiologic amputation of the limb to provide time for the patient to be resuscitated prior to definitive amputation. A review by Hunsaker et al. illustrates the technique.[82] Fifty-six procedures over a 12-year period were performed, with a mortality rate of 14%. Ninety-three percent of patients presented with systemic sepsis. All patients were operated on in an elective manner following stabilization. These authors used a Styrofoam cooler with a section hole placed in one end for the extremity. Dry ice is used to cool the extremity, and tape is used to seal the cooler. A heating pad is used to prevent transfer of cold proximally in the extremity. Analgesics are given for pain until the nerve fibers freeze. Others have also reported the successful use of cryoamputation, although its precise role in the practice of modern amputation surgery is uncertain.[83,84]

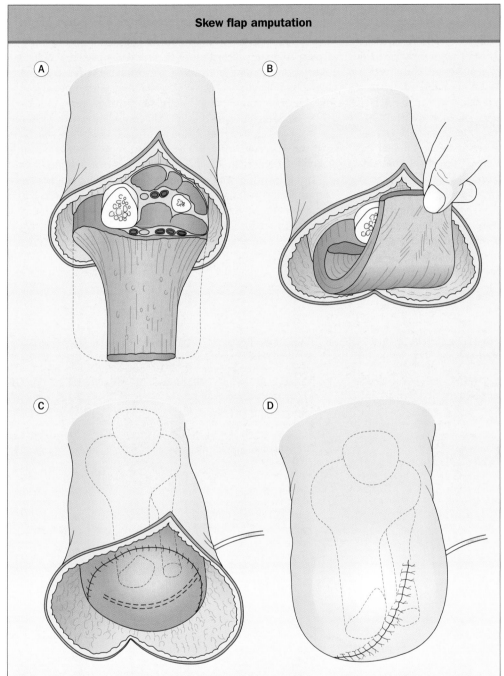

Skew flap amputation

(A) (B) (C) (D)

Figure 14.2 Skew flap amputation.
(A) Gastrocnemius muscle, with deep fascia attached, is narrowed. (B) The posterior flap is brought forward. (C) The anterior border of the tibia is covered by suturing the posterior flap to deep fascia and periosteum. (D) The flaps are closed over a vacuum drain. Note that the suture line does not lie directly in front of divided bone. (Redrawn from Ruckley et al[80] with permission).

FUNCTIONAL OUTCOME/SURVIVAL

Patient survival in the NSQIP amputation series for BKA and AKA was 57% and 39% at 3 years, respectively, again emphasizing the palliative nature of these procedures in most patients.[56] Other reports have found similar poor survival following major limb amputation.[5,70,85] In addition to mortality, significant ongoing morbidity occurs in both the remaining stump (BKA) and contralateral limb following major lower extremity amputation. At 2 years, 15% of patients with an initially successful BKA require conversion to an AKA, and an additional 15% will suffer a major contralateral amputation.[10]

A significant amount of functional outcomes data from clinical series of major limb amputation has been reported. Most of these data have focused on the percentage of surviving patients who wear a prosthesis and ambulate to any extent. Interestingly, the results vary widely from series to series.[22,25,31,34,35,86–90] From 15–96% of patients with successful BKA were able to walk with or without assist devices with prosthesis. Some of the reason for the variability is differing definitions of success (wearing the prosthesis any time during the day versus walking independent of the home), differing patient populations (younger diabetics versus older patients with CLI), and different settings (academic, private practice, Veterans Affairs, and European). The ambulatory success for eventual AKA patients was one-third to one-half that of BKA patients. The review by Houghton et al. summarizes the data for patients with CLI.[24] Four hundred and forty major amputations (BKA/AKA ratio roughly one) were performed in eight major London hospitals over a 2-year period. Seventy-five patients (17%) died prior to discharge. One hundred thirteen were not considered rehabilitation candidates, with 252 referred to prosthetics/rehabilitation. At 2 years, 54 more patients had died and 19 had become non-ambulatory for non-vascular reasons (stroke, heart failure, etc.). Of the 179 remaining patients, 52 could walk briefly inside their home and 21 could walk outside their home. Currently, functional outcomes in major amputation for CLI include moderate BKA and a few AKA patients wearing prostheses. Although many BKA patients can ambulate in their homes, few are able to be completely wheelchair free. The number of AKA patients walking is minimal and a negligible number are wheelchair free. The number of ambulatory patients declines over time for a variety of reasons.

SUMMARY

Major lower extremity amputation is a procedure common to all vascular surgeons, regardless of their practice patterns. Although a substantial amount of effort and research has focused on maintaining limb length and preserving the knee joint if possible, the amputee population calls some of these principles into serious question. Affected patients are usually elderly, with systemic disease, and approaching the end of life. Operative mortality is substantial, and wound healing and morbidity significantly higher for BKA than AKA. Prosthetic wear is the emphasized goal of both patient and rehabilitation programs preoperatively, but the reality is that many of these artificial limbs are of a cosmetic nature over time. Major limb amputation for CLI is a palliative procedure in a disadvantaged population, and efforts to maximize pain relief and wound healing should take precedence in many patients.

REFERENCES

1. Hirsch AT, Treat-Jacobson D, Lando HA, Hatsukami DK. The role of tobacco cessation, antiplatelet and lipid-lowering therapies in the treatment of peripheral arterial disease. Vasc Med 1997;2:243–51.
2. Beckman JA, Creager MA, Libby P. Diabetes and atherosclerosis: epidemiology, pathophysiology, and management. JAMA 2002;287:2570–81.
3. McDermott MM, Feinglass J, Slavensky R, Pearce WH. The ankle–brachial index as a predictor of survival in patients with peripheral vascular disease. J Gen Intern Med 1994;9:445–9.
4. Isakov E, Budoragin N, Shenhav S, Mendelevich I, Korzets A, Susak Z. Anatomic sites of foot lesions resulting in amputation among diabetics and non-diabetics. Am J Phys Med Rehabil 1995;74:130–3.
5. Whitehouse FW, Jurgenson C, Block MA. The later life of the diabetic amputee. Another look at fate of the second leg. Diabetes 1968;17:520–1.
6. Murdoch DP, Armstrong DG, Dacus JB, Laughlin TJ, Morgan CB, Lavery LA. The natural history of great toe amputations. J Foot Ankle Surg 1997;36:204–8.
7. Nehler MR, Whitehill TA, Bowers SP, et al. Intermediate-term outcome of primary digit amputations in patients with diabetes mellitus who have forefoot sepsis requiring hospitalization and presumed adequate circulatory status. J Vasc Surg 1999;30:509–17.
8. Allen DR, Smallwood J, Johnson CD. Intra-arterial thrombolysis should be the initial treatment of the acutely ischaemic lower limb. Ann R Coll Surg Engl 1992;74:106–10.
9. Marty B, Wicky S, Ris HB, et al. Success of thrombolysis as a predictor of outcome in acute thrombosis of popliteal aneurysms. J Vasc Surg 2002;35:487–93.
10. Dormandy J, Heeck L, Vig S. Major amputations: clinical patterns and predictors. Semin Vasc Surg 1999;12:154–61.
11. Dormandy J, Belcher G, Broos P, et al. Prospective study of 713 below-knee amputations for ischaemia and the effect of a prostacyclin analogue on healing. Hawaii Study Group. Br J Surg 1994;81:33–7.
12. McDaniel MD, Cronenwett JL. Basic data related to the natural history of intermittent claudication. Ann Vasc Surg 1989;3:273–7.
13. Byrne J, Darling RC III, Chang BB, et al. Infrainguinal arterial reconstruction for claudication: is it worth the risk? An analysis of 409 procedures. J Vasc Surg 1999;29:259–67.
14. Donaldson MC, Mannick JA. Femoropopliteal bypass grafting for intermittent claudication: is pessimism warranted? Arch Surg 1980;115:724–7.
15. Kent KC, Donaldson MC, Attinger CE, Couch NP, Mannick JA, Whittemore AD. Femoropopliteal reconstruction for claudication. The risk to life and limb. Arch Surg 1988;123:1196–8.
16. Conte MS, Belkin M, Donaldson MC, Baum P, Mannick JA, Whittemore AD. Femorotibial bypass for claudication: do results justify an aggressive approach? J Vasc Surg 1995;21:873–80.
17. Valentine RJ, Jackson MR, Modrall JG, McIntyre KE, Clagett GP. The progressive nature of peripheral arterial disease in young adults: a prospective analysis of white men referred to a vascular surgery service. J Vasc Surg 1999;30:436–44.
18. Valentine RJ, Myers SI, Inman MH, Roberts JR, Clagett GP. Late outcome of amputees with premature atherosclerosis. Surgery 1996;119:487–93.
19. Valentine RJ, Kaplan HS, Green R, Jacobsen DW, Myers SI, Clagett GP. Lipoprotein (a), homocysteine, and hypercoagulable states in young men with premature peripheral atherosclerosis: a prospective, controlled analysis. J Vasc Surg 1996;23:53–61, discussion.
20. McCready RA, Vincent AE, Schwartz RW, Hyde GL, Mattingly SS, Griffen WO Jr. Atherosclerosis in the young: a virulent disease. Surgery 1984;96:863–9.
21. Bunt TJ, Manship LL, Bynoe RP, Haynes JL. Lower extremity amputation for peripheral vascular disease. A low-risk operation. Am Surg 1984;50:581–4.
22. Gregg RO. Bypass or amputation? Concomitant review of bypass arterial grafting and major amputations. Am J Surg 1985;149:397–402.
23. Harrison JD, Southworth S, Callum KG. Experience with the 'skew flap' below-knee amputation. Br J Surg 1987;74:930–1.
24. Houghton AD, Taylor PR, Thurlow S, Rootes E, McColl I. Success rates for rehabilitation of vascular amputees: implications for preoperative assessment and amputation level. Br J Surg 1992;79:753–5.
25. Jamieson MG, Ruckley CV. Amputation for peripheral vascular disease in a General Surgical Unit. J R Coll Surg Edinb 1983;28:46–50.
26. Eskelinen E, Eskelinen A, Hyytinen T, Jaakkola A. Changing pattern of major lower limb amputations in Seinajoki Central Hospital 1997–2000. Ann Chir Gynaecol 2001;90:290–3.
27. Pernot HF, Winnubst GM, Cluitmans JJ, De Witte LP. Amputees in Limburg: incidence, morbidity and mortality, prosthetic supply, care utilisation and functional level after one year. Prosthet Orthot Int 2000;24:90–6.
28. Rommers GM, Vos LD, Groothoff JW, Schuiling CH, Eisma WH. Epidemiology of lower limb amputees in the north of The Netherlands: aetiology, discharge destination and prosthetic use. Prosthet Orthot Int 1997;21:92–9.
29. Pohjolainen T, Alaranta H. Ten-year survival of Finnish lower limb amputees. Prosthet Orthot Int 1998;22:10–6.
30. Keagy BA, Schwartz JA, Kotb M, Burnham SJ, Johnson G Jr. Lower extremity amputation: the control series. J Vasc Surg 1986;4:321–6.

31. Kihn RB, Warren R, Beebe GW. The 'geriatric' amputee. Ann Surg 1972;176:305–14.

32. Baker WH, Barnes RW, Shurr DG. The healing of below-knee amputations: a comparison of soft and plaster dressing. Am J Surg 1977;133:716–8.

33. Vigier S, Casillas JM, Dulieu V, Rouhier-Marcer I, D'Athis P, Didier JP. Healing of open stump wounds after vascular below-knee amputation: plaster cast socket with silicone sleeve versus elastic compression. Arch Phys Med Rehabil 1999;80:1327–30.

34. Stirnemann P, Walpoth B, Wursten HU, Graber P, Parli R, Althaus U. Influence of failed arterial reconstruction on the outcome of major limb amputation. Surgery 1992;111:363–8.

35. Pollock SB Jr, Ernst CB. Use of Doppler pressure measurements in predicting success in amputation of the leg. Am J Surg 1980; 139:303–6.

36. Abou-Zamzam AM Jr, Moneta GL, Lee RW, Nehler MR, Taylor LM Jr, Porter JM. Peroneal bypass is equivalent to inframalleolar bypass for ischemic pedal gangrene. Arch Surg 1996;131:894–8.

37. Nicoloff AD, Taylor LM Jr, McLafferty RB, Moneta GL, Porter JM. Patient recovery after infrainguinal bypass grafting for limb salvage. J Vasc Surg 1998;27:256–63.

38. Dwars BJ, van den Broek TA, Rauwerda JA, Bakker FC. Criteria for reliable selection of the lowest level of amputation in peripheral vascular disease. J Vasc Surg 1992;15:536–42.

39. Harris JP, Page S, Englund R, May J. Is the outlook for the vascular amputee improved by striving to preserve the knee? J Cardiovasc Surg (Torino) 1988;29:741–5.

40. Lim RC Jr, Blaisdell FW, Hall AD, Moore WS, Thomas AN. Below knee amputation for ischemic gangrene. Surg Obstet Gynecol 1967; 125:493–501.

41. Burnham SJ, Wagner WH, Keagy BA, Johnson G Jr. Objective measurement of limb perfusion by dermal fluorometry. A criterion for healing of below-knee amputation. Arch Surg 1990;125:104–6.

42. Wagner WH, Keagy BA, Kotb MM, Burnham SJ, Johnson G Jr. Non-invasive determination of healing of major lower extremity amputation: the continued role of clinical judgment. J Vasc Surg 1988;8:703–10.

43. Barnes RW, Shanik GD, Slaymaker EE. An index of healing in below-knee amputation: leg blood pressure by Doppler ultrasound. Surgery 1976;79:13–20.

44. Nicholas GG, Myers JL, DeMuth WE Jr. The role of vascular laboratory criteria in the selection of patients for lower extremity amputation. Ann Surg 1982;195:469–73.

45. Barnes RW, Thornhill B, Nix L, Rittgers SE, Turley G. Prediction of amputation wound healing. Roles of Doppler ultrasound and digit photoplethysmography. Arch Surg 1981;116:80–3.

46. Cederberg PA, Pritchard DJ, Joyce JW. Doppler-determined segmental pressures and wound-healing in amputations for vascular disease. J Bone Joint Surg Am 1983;65:363–5.

47. Bacharach JM, Rooke TW, Osmundson PJ, Gloviczki P. Predictive value of transcutaneous oxygen pressure and amputation success by use of supine and elevation measurements. J Vasc Surg 1992;15:558–63.

48. Katsamouris A, Brewster DC, Megerman J, Cina C, Darling RC, Abbott WM. Transcutaneous oxygen tension in selection of amputation level. Am J Surg 1984;147:510–7.

49. Christensen KS, Klarke M. Transcutaneous oxygen measurement in peripheral occlusive disease. An indicator of wound healing in leg amputation. J Bone Joint Surg Br 1986;68:423–6.

50. Adera HM, James K, Castronuovo JJ Jr, Byrne M, Deshmukh R, Lohr J. Prediction of amputation wound healing with skin perfusion pressure. J Vasc Surg 1995;21:823–8.

51. van den Broek TA, Dwars BJ, Rauwerda JA, Bakker FC. Photo-plethysmographic selection of amputation level in peripheral vascular disease. J Vasc Surg 1988;8:10–3.

52. Mars M, McKune A, Robbs JV. A comparison of laser Doppler fluxmetry and transcutaneous oxygen pressure measurement in the dysvascular patient requiring amputation. Eur J Vasc Endovasc Surg 1998;16:53–8.

53. Avci S, Musdal Y. Skin blood flow level and stump healing in ischemic amputations. Orthopedics 2000;23:33–6.

54. Harris JP, McLaughlin AF, Quinn RJ, Page S, May J. Skin blood flow measurement with xenon-133 to predict healing of lower extremity amputations. Aust N Z J Surg 1986;56:413–5.

55. Lund F, Jogestrand T. Video fluorescein imaging of the skin: description of an overviewing technique for functional evaluation of regional cutaneous blood perfusion in occlusive arterial disease of the limbs. Clin Physiol 1997;17:619–33.

56. Feinglass J, Pearce WH, Martin GJ, et al. Postoperative and late survival outcomes after major amputation: findings from the Department of Veterans Affairs National Surgical Quality Improvement Program. Surgery 2001;130:21–9.

57. Lederle FA, Wilson SE, Johnson GR, et al. Immediate repair compared with surveillance of small abdominal aortic aneurysms. N Engl J Med 2002;346:1437–44.

58. Barnes RW, Slaymaker EE. Postoperative deep vein thrombosis in the lower extremity amputee: A prospective study with Doppler ultrasound. Ann Surg 1976;183:429–32.

59. Yeager RA, Moneta GL, Edwards JM, Taylor LM Jr, McConnell DB, Porter JM. Deep vein thrombosis associated with lower extremity amputation. J Vasc Surg 1995;22:612–5.

60. Fletcher JP, Batiste P. Incidence of deep vein thrombosis following vascular surgery. Int Angiol 1997;16:65–8.

61. Jensen TS, Krebs B, Nielsen J, Rasmussen P. Phantom limb, phantom pain and stump pain in amputees during the first 6 months following limb amputation. Pain 1983;17:243–56.

62. Kooijman CM, Dijkstra PU, Geertzen JH, Elzinga A, van der Schans CP. Phantom pain and phantom sensations in upper limb amputees: an epidemiological study. Pain 2000;87:33–41.

63. Nikolajsen L, Staehelin JT. Phantom limb pain. Curr Rev Pain 2000; 4:166–70.

64. Ehde DM, Czerniecki JM, Smith DG, et al. Chronic phantom sensations, phantom pain, residual limb pain, and other regional pain after lower limb amputation. Arch Phys Med Rehabil 2000;81:1039–44.

65. Halbert J, Crotty M, Cameron ID. Evidence for the optimal management of acute and chronic phantom pain: a systematic review. Clin J Pain 2002;18:84–92.

66. Wu CL, Tella P, Staats PS, et al. Analgesic effects of intravenous lidocaine and morphine on postamputation pain: a randomized double-blind, active placebo-controlled, crossover trial. Anesthesiology 2002;96:841–8.

67. Dellemijn PL, Vanneste JA. Randomised double-blind active-placebo-controlled crossover trial of intravenous fentanyl in neuropathic pain. Lancet 1997;349:753–8.

68. Lambert A, Dashfield A, Cosgrove C, Wilkins D, Walker A, Ashley S. Randomized prospective study comparing preoperative epidural and intraoperative perineural analgesia for the prevention of postoperative stump and phantom limb pain following major amputation. Reg Anesth Pain Med 2001;26:316–21.

69. Nikolajsen L, Ilkjaer S, Christensen JH, Kroner K, Jensen TS. Randomised trial of epidural bupivacaine and morphine in prevention of stump and phantom pain in lower-limb amputation. Lancet 1997; 350:1353–7.

70. Jahangiri M, Jayatunga AP, Bradley JW, Dark CH. Prevention of phantom pain after major lower limb amputation by epidural infusion of diamorphine, clonidine and bupivacaine. Ann R Coll Surg Engl 1994;76:324–6.

71. Finsen V, Persen L, Lovlien M, et al. Transcutaneous electrical nerve stimulation after major amputation. J Bone Joint Surg Br 1988; 70:109–12.

72. Rusy LM, Troshynski TJ, Weisman SJ. Gabapentin in phantom limb pain management in children and young adults: report of seven cases. J Pain Symptom Manage 2001;21:78–82.

73. Vichitrananda C, Pausawasdi S. Midazolam for the treatment of phantom limb pain exacerbation: preliminary reports. J Med Assoc Thai 2001;84:299–302.

74. Carabelli RA, Kellerman WC. Phantom limb pain: relief by application of TENS to contralateral extremity. Arch Phys Med Rehabil 1985; 66:466–7.

75. Yamanaka M, Kwong PK. The side-to-side flap technique in below-the-knee amputation with long stump. Clin Orthop 1985;75–9.

76. Au KK. Sagittal flaps in below-knee amputations in Chinese patients. J Bone Joint Surg Br 1989;71:597–8.

77. Burgess EM, Romano RL, Zettl JH, Schrock RD Jr. Amputations of the leg for peripheral vascular insufficiency. J Bone Joint Surg Am 1971;53:874–90.

78. Robinson KP, Hoile R, Coddington T. Skew flap myoplastic below-knee amputation: a preliminary report. Br J Surg 1982;69:554–7.

79. Johnson WC, Watkins MT, Hamilton J, Baldwin D. Transcutaneous partial oxygen pressure changes following skew flap and Burgess-type below-knee amputations. Arch Surg 1997;132:261–3.

80. Ruckley CV, Stonebridge PA, Prescott RJ. Skewflap versus long posterior flap in below-knee amputations: multicenter trial. J Vasc Surg 1991;13:423–7.

81. Cull DL, Taylor SM, Hamontree SE, et al. A reappraisal of a modified through-knee amputation in patients with peripheral vascular disease. Am J Surg 2001;182:44–8.

82. Hunsaker RH, Schwartz JA, Keagy BA, Kotb M, Burnham SJ, Johnson G Jr. Dry ice cryoamputation: a twelve-year experience. J Vasc Surg 1985;2:812–6.

83. Bunt TJ. Physiologic amputation. Preliminary cryoamputation of the gangrenous extremity. AORN J 1991;54:1220–4.

84. Winburn GB, Wood MC, Hawkins ML, et al. Current role of cryoamputation. Am J Surg 1991;162:647–50.

85. Rush DS, Huston CC, Bivins BA, Hyde GL. Operative and late mortality rates of above-knee and below-knee amputations. Am Surg 1981;47:36–9.

86. Hagberg E, Berlin OK, Renstrom P. Function after through-knee compared with below-knee and above-knee amputation. Prosthet Orthot Int 1992;16:168–73.

87. McWhinnie DL, Gordon AC, Collin J, Gray DW, Morrison JD. Rehabilitation outcome 5 years after 100 lower-limb amputations. Br J Surg 1994;81:1596–9.

88. Robinson KP. Long posterior flap amputation in geriatric patients with ischaemic disease. Ann R Coll Surg Engl 1976;58:440–51.

89. Ecker ML, Jacobs BS. Lower extremity amputation in diabetic patients. Diabetes 1970;19:189–95.

90. Siriwardena GJ, Bertrand PV. Factors influencing rehabilitation of arteriosclerotic lower limb amputees. J Rehabil Res Dev 1991;28:35–44.

91. Finch DR, Macdougal M, Tibbs DJ, Morris PJ. Amputation for vascular disease: the experience of a peripheral vascular unit. Br J Surg 1980;67:233–7.

92. Kazmers M, Satiani B, Evans WE. Amputation level following unsuccessful distal limb salvage operations. Surgery 1980;87:683–7.

93. Tripses D, Pollak EW. Risk factors in healing of below-knee amputation. Appraisal of 64 amputations in patients with vascular disease. Am J Surg 1981;141:718–20.

94. Creaney MG, Chattopadhaya DK, Ward AS, Morris-Jones W. Doppler ultrasound in the assessment of amputation level. J R Coll Surg Edinb 1981;26:278–81.

95. Burgess EM, Matsen FA III, Wyss CR, Simmons CW. Segmental transcutaneous measurements of pO_2 in patients requiring below-the-knee amputation for peripheral vascular insufficiency. J Bone Joint Surg Am 1982;64:378–82.

96. Ratliff DA, Clyne CA, Chant AD, Webster JH. Prediction of amputation wound healing: the role of transcutaneous pO_2 assessment. Br J Surg 1984;71:219–22.

97. O'Dwyer KJ, Edwards MH. The association between lowest palpable pulse and wound healing in below knee amputations. Ann R Coll Surg Engl 1985;67:232–4.

98. Holstein PE. Skin perfusion pressure measured by radioisotope washout for predicting wound healing in lower limb amputation for arterial occlusive disease. Acta Orthop Scand Suppl 1985;213:1–47.

99. Kay SP, Moreland JR, Schmitter E. Nutritional status and wound healing in lower extremity amputations. Clin Orthop 1987;253–6.

100. Dowd GS. Predicting stump healing following amputation for peripheral vascular disease using the transcutaneous oxygen monitor. Ann R Coll Surg Engl 1987;69:31–5.

101. Silverman DG, Roberts A, Reilly CA, et al. Fluorometric quantification of low-dose fluorescein delivery to predict amputation site healing. Surgery 1987;101:335–41.

102. Inderbitzi R, Buttiker M, Pfluger D, Nachbur B. The fate of bilateral lower limb amputees in end-stage vascular disease. Eur J Vasc Surg 1992;6:321–6.

CHAPTER
15 Etiology and Natural History: Diagnosis and Evaluation

John Byrne

KEY POINTS

Acute leg ischemia:

- The incidence of acute leg ischemia is 14 per 100 000 population per year, accounting for 12% of operations in an average vascular unit.

- With the decline of rheumatic heart disease and an increased prevalence of atherosclerosis, acute arterial thrombosis accounts for most episodes of acute leg ischemia.

- Trauma remains an important source of acute ischemia in the young but in the elderly, vascular trauma is often iatrogenic due to endovascular procedures.

- Angiograms and duplex imaging are invaluable in planning intervention but assessment of limb viability and the urgency of revascularization remains clinical.

- Life expectancy for patients with acute leg ischemia is similar to many cancers; only 17–44% are still alive at 5 years, significantly fewer than age-matched controls.

- Patients with a thrombosis survive twice as long as those with emboli but are twice as likely to lose their limb.

- In the absence of intervention, two-thirds of patients come to amputation. Thrombosis (versus embolism), total ischemic time, advanced age, and omission of postoperative anticoagulation predict a greater chance of amputation.

Acute arm ischemia:

- Arm ischemia accounts for one-fifth of limb ischemia (2.4 cases/100 000 population/year), but has a better prognosis for both life and limb.

- Arm ischemia is due to embolism in 80% of patients, usually associated with atrial fibrillation. Conservative treatment is associated with a significant rate of limb dysfunction.

In general:

- Overall, vascular specialists have better limb salvage rates than general surgeons. In the 21st century, where expertise is available, all acute arm and leg ischemia should be managed by a vascular specialist.

INTRODUCTION

Acute limb ischemia can be the simplest vascular condition to diagnose and the most perplexing to manage. The need for urgent intervention is usually clear. However, clinical decisions can be more difficult in the anesthetized or ventilated patient, or at extremes of age.

In acute limb ischemia, the surgeon is faced with the conundrum of urgent restoration of blood flow, yet collecting sufficient information to avoid a cascade of inappropriate interventions. Initial symptoms improve in some patients with anticoagulation but gauging the urgency of revascularization requires careful judgment. Not all acutely ischemic limbs are salvageable, and primary amputation can be both appropriate and life-saving. Rarely, profound limb ischemia is a manifestation of terminal illness, and palliation, rather than aggressive attempts at salvage, may be the best approach.

Thromboembolic events still account for over 90% of cases of acute limb ischemia. The remainder are due to trauma and iatrogenic accidents. Acute limb ischemia is often taxing and surgeons may need to employ a full armamentarium, from simple embolectomy to extra-anatomic and tibial bypass.

Despite the nihilism and frustration that sometimes attends management of acute ischemia, attempts at limb salvage are worthwhile and satisfying. Initial diagnosis and clinical evaluation are crucial in achieving good outcomes.

ACUTE LEG ISCHEMIA

Diagnostic criteria
Clinical evaluation

Acute limb ischemia is defined by the TransAtlantic Inter-Society Consensus (TASC) Working Group[1] as 'any sudden decrease or worsening in limb perfusion causing a potential threat to extremity viability'. The emphasis is on threat to limb viability. It excludes sudden changes in limb perfusion that do not endanger the limb, such as acute onset claudication. At present, there are no reliable hematologic or radiologic markers of limb viability. Initial assessment of the 'threatened limb', therefore, remains clinical.

History
Pain

Pain is usually the first symptom. With embolus or trauma, the pain is acute. However, with in-situ arterial thrombosis, the onset is more insidious. Once established, however, the pain is usually severe. It requires opiates but can be resistant to narcotic analgesia. The patient complains of diffuse pain throughout the entire affected limb – a distinguishing point from the rest pain of chronic ischemia, which is limited to the forefoot. In the neonate with acute ischemia due to iatrogenic intervention, or the elderly, confused patient, no history may be forthcoming at all.

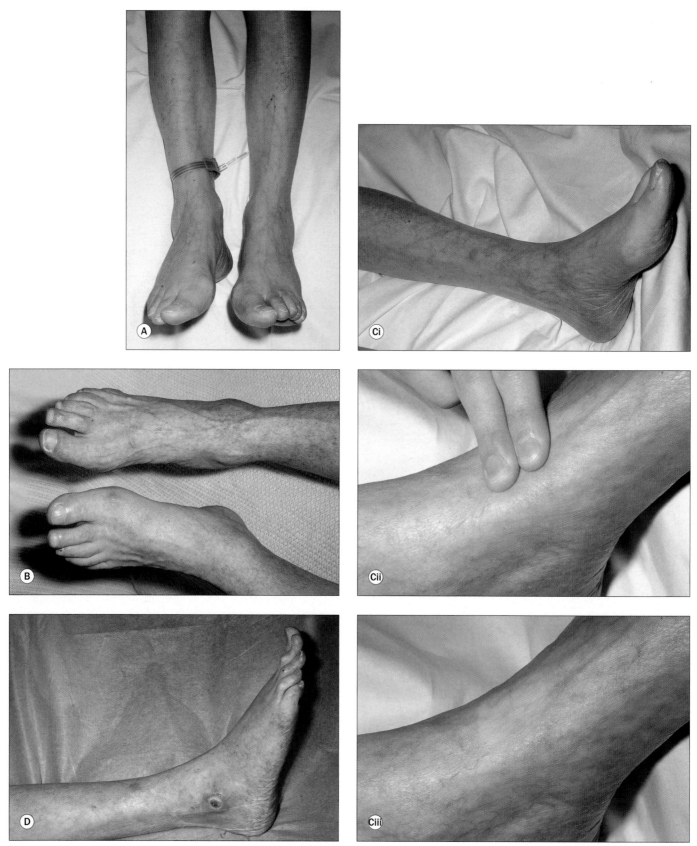

Figure 15.1 Acute leg ischemia. (A) Category 1 – time for investigations. (B) Category 2a. (C) Category 2b – acute arterial ischemia. Skin still blanches. (D) Category 3. Prior below-knee popliteal graft with a Miller cuff for critical ischemia. Patient presented with profound anesthesia of right foot and paralysis. Above-knee amputation was the outcome.

Pain accompanies acute leg ischemia, with one exception. In acute aortic thrombosis with profound leg ischemia, the first symptom may be paralysis and not pain. This has led to patients being referred inadvertently to a neurologist or physician. Indeed, Batz[2] reported that 84% of patients with acute aortic occlusion presented with paralysis and only 14% with pain; with 55% referred for a neurologic opinion.

Paresthesia

Paresthesia, when present, is a clear indication of deterioration of sensory neurologic function and a sign of progressive ischemia. Proprioception and light sensation are conveyed by small myelinated fibers and are lost early in acute ischemia. Larger sensory nerves convey temperature, pain, and pressure, and these are maintained unless ischemia is prolonged.

Paralysis

Paralysis is an ominous symptom. It ought to be termed, more properly, 'loss of motor function', as it reflects ischemic myopathy rather than nerve hypoperfusion. Loss of function of the intrinsic muscles of the foot occurs first. Absent foot dorsiflexion and plantar flexion indicate loss of function of the flexors and extensors of the lower leg. In patients with paralysis, there is no place for expectant management with anticoagulants. Paralysis indicates the need for urgent restoration of blood flow.

Clinical examination
Pallor

Pallor indicates obstruction of a major arterial trunk to the leg. In the absence of collateral circulation, this will produce a marble white, waxy leg with absent capillary refill and collapsed veins ('venous guttering'). In arterial thrombosis, initial pallor may be followed by gradual improvement, with return of skin perfusion and capillary refill over 6–12 hours due to opening of pre-formed collaterals (**Figs 15.1A & B**). Capillary refill on blanching of the skin indicates the limb is still retrievable, even if the skin is mottled and cyanosed (**Fig. 15.1C**). However, 'fixed staining' (cyanosed or purple areas of skin that fail to blanch on pressure) indicates that the capillaries have thrombosed and ruptured. Such limbs are unsalvageable (**Fig. 15.1D**).

Perishing cold

This is easy to elicit, especially when compared to the contralateral extremity. However, both legs will be equally cold in patients with aortic occlusion. It is difficult to correlate the extent of coolness with the level of arterial occlusion, but if the thigh and buttock are cool and cyanosed, an aorto-iliac occlusion is likely.

Pulselessness

Pulselessness is the absolute prerequisite of acute ischemia. In the presence of a full set of pulses, arterial ischemia can be excluded. The caveats are venous gangrene, where limb nutrition is severely impaired despite palpable pedal pulses, and 'blue toe syndrome' due to atheroemboli lodging in the digital arteries. An intact set of pulses in the contralateral leg suggests an embolic process; absent pulses in the healthy leg reflect diffuse peripheral arterial disease and point to in-situ thrombosis. The discovery of a popliteal artery aneurysm in either leg will also point to the diagnosis.

Embolus or thrombus?

There is good evidence that patients with arterial thrombosis, yet who are subjected to embolectomy, have a particularly poor outcome[3]. *Acute arterial thrombosis* is associated with a previous history of intermittent claudication. However, in very elderly and housebound patients, or those with angina or chronic obstructive pulmonary disease (COPD), there may be no such history due to their inability to reach their claudication distance in the course of their daily routine. A history of claudication may be obtainable in as few as 40% of patients with arterial thrombosis.[4] On angiography, mature collaterals are seen and the arteries appear diffusely diseased. *Acute arterial embolus* usually arises in patients with no history of claudication. Ischemia is often profound on presentation. Emboli typically lodge at an arterial bifurcation, most frequently the femoral artery (50%) or the 'trifurcation' of the tibial vessels. 'Saddle emboli' are now rare and most instances of aortic occlusion are due to 'in-situ' thrombosis. Angiographically, there is a diagnostic sharp cut-off ('meniscus sign') with normal proximal arteries (**Fig. 15.2**). Simultaneous asymptomatic emboli may be seen. Emboli usually occur in the setting of atrial fibrillation, recent cardioversion, or arterial manipulation (surgery or angiography). Cambria and Abbott[4] went as far as to state that a diagnosis of embolism should seldom be made in a patient who does not have atrial fibrillation. In fact, 80% of emboli are due to atrial fibrillation, 10% due to prior myocardial infarction and 10% due to aneurysms or other causes.

Assessing limb viability

Assessing viability can be difficult. A scoring system has been derived by the Society of Vascular Surgery/International Society for Cardiovascular Surgery(SVS/ISCVS) (see **Table 15.1**). It was initially devised in 1986[5] and modified in 1997,[6] and requires clinical assessment of motor and sensory function and use of a

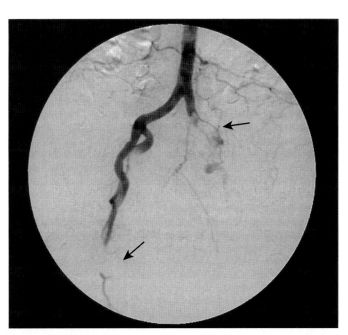

Figure 15.2 Bilateral lower arterial emboli affecting left common iliac and right common femoral arteries. Note normal vessels and classic 'meniscus signs' on both sides. Emboli are frequently multiple and can occasionally cause bilateral ischemia.

SVS/ISCVS criteria for limb viability.					
		Findings		**Doppler signals**	
Category	Description/Prognosis	Sensory loss	Muscle weakness	Arterial	Venous
I. Viable	Not immediately threatened	None	None	Audible	Audible

II. Threatened
     a. Marginally
     b. Immediately
	Salvageable if promptly treated
	Salvageable with immediate revascularization
		Minimal or none
		More than toes; often rest pain
			None
			Mild, moderate
				(Often) inaudible
				(Usually) inaudible
					Audible
					Audible

III. Irreversible	Major tissue loss or permanent nerve damage inevitable	Profound, anesthetic	Profound, paralysis (rigor)	Inaudible	Inaudible

Table 15.1 SVS/ISCVS criteria for limb viability. Clinical categories of acute limb ischemia (based on SVS/ISCVS classification).

hand-held Doppler probe. While not tested prospectively, it at least offers guidance. There will, inevitably, be a small number of patients who will not fit comfortably into any category.

I. *Viable*. This category usually comprises patients with acute-on-chronic arterial thrombosis (see **Fig. 15.1A**). The onset is sudden, but sensation is preserved and normal motor function is present. The leg is noticeably cooler. Doppler examination detects both arterial and venous signals. Patients in this group require no immediate intervention and can be anticoagulated while investigations are organized.

II. *Threatened* (a – marginally threatened; b – immediately threatened). All legs in this category need urgent intervention. However, there is still time for angiography in level IIa ischemia, as long as close surveillance of the leg is maintained. In level IIb ischemia, immediate revascularization is needed. Reduced skin sensation is found in both categories. In marginally threatened legs, the reduction in sensation will be minimal (**Fig. 15.1B**); in immediately threatened limbs, the reduction will be more profound (**Fig. 15.1C**). Loss of motor function indicates an immediately threatened limb. In general, arterial Doppler signals are inaudible in threatened legs, but venous signals are still present. Of course, these two subdivisions are slightly artificial. In practice, patients present as part of a continuous clinical spectrum.

III. *Irreversible*. A cold cyanosed limb with fixed staining and calf muscle rigor is clearly unsalvageable (see **Fig. 15.1D**). Sensory loss is profound and Doppler examination fails to elicit either arterial or venous signals. Such patients are usually systemically unwell and require expeditious amputation.

The pragmatic approach

In daily practice, a more practical approach is often employed. Jivegård et al.[7] suggested that muscle weakness with skin cyanosis or mottling mandated emergency revascularization. Patients without this combination were low risk and did not develop gangrene when managed conservatively, irrespective of etiology. In a 1998 survey,[8] Swedish surgeons ranked loss of motor function as the main indicator for immediate surgery. Doppler signals, as suggested by the SVS/ISCVS, were ranked very low. Using Jivegård's criteria,[7] emergency revascularization was employed in 30% of patients.

Investigations
Non-invasive investigations

1) *Duplex imaging* is usually confirmatory and is quick, non-invasive and non-nephrotoxic. Reconstructive surgery can be planned on the basis of duplex alone.[9] Alternatively, it can indicate options for catheter-directed thrombolytic therapy.

2) *Magnetic resonance angiography (gadolinium/contrast enhanced)* has the advantage of using non-nephrotoxic contrast agents. With improvements in software, this technique is becoming quicker to perform. While it can provide consistent anatomic detail of the aorto-iliac arterial segment, reliable images of the infra-inguinal vessels are more difficult to obtain. The technique has not, at present, been validated in the assessment of the acutely ischemic leg and it is uncertain how it correlates with contrast angiography in planning thrombolytic therapy.

3) *Computed tomographic angiography* may have a role in the future. The anatomic detail provided by this imaging modality is superb. However, its role has not been validated and it still requires intravenous iodinated contrast agents, which may affect renal function.

Invasive investigation

Arteriography remains the 'gold standard' investigation for acute leg ischemia. It accurately delineates the arterial tree of the affected leg and permits a coherent approach to reconstruction. It also allows for immediate catheter-directed thrombolysis or angioplasty. However, despite its advantages, it is time-consuming. In patients with severe ischemia, urgent restoration of blood flow is paramount, so surgical revascularization is the priority. If necessary, on-table angiography can be performed, although the quality of these images in the emergency setting can be inconsistent (**Fig. 15.3**).

Additional investigations

In the patient with acute leg ischemia, the need for ancillary investigations is often unclear and their benefits questionable.

i) *Thrombophilia screening* There is scant evidence to support routine thrombophilia screening in most patients with acute arterial thrombosis. Screening should be limited to situations where results will have a tangible impact on patient care.[10] The

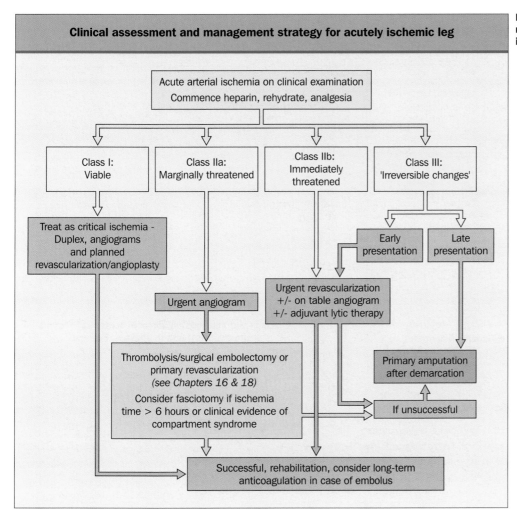

Clinical assessment and management strategy for acutely ischemic leg

Acute arterial ischemia on clinical examination
Commence heparin, rehydrate, analgesia

Class I:
Viable

Class IIa:
Marginally threatened

Class IIb:
Immediately threatened

Class III:
'Irreversible changes'

Treat as critical ischemia -
Duplex, angiograms
and planned
revascularization/angioplasty

Early presentation

Late presentation

Urgent angiogram

Urgent revascularization
+/- on table angiogram
+/- adjuvant lytic therapy

Thrombolysis/surgical embolectomy or
primary revascularization
(see Chapters 16 & 18)

Consider fasciotomy if ischemia
time > 6 hours or clinical evidence of
compartment syndrome

Primary amputation
after demarcation

If unsuccessful

Successful, rehabilitation, consider long-term
anticoagulation in case of embolus

Figure 15.3 Clinical assessment and management strategy for acutely ischemic leg.

TASC report committee[1] recommended that a thrombophilia screen and measurement of homocysteine levels be performed in all young patients with acute arterial thrombosis or those who have a strong family history of thrombotic events or no other obvious predisposing cause for thrombosis.

ii) *Echocardiography* This technique forms part of the routine work-up of most patients with an acute embolus by some surgeons. Most often, this is a transthoracic echocardiogram (TTE). However, this frequently fails to demonstrate any cardiac thrombus or valvular pathology. The left atrial appendage is the most common source of thrombus, but is poorly visualized by transthoracic echocardiography. Transesophageal echocardiography (TEE), on the other hand, is more invasive but readily demonstrates the left atrium and ascending aorta with greater resolution. It also detects very low flow pre-thrombotic areas ('spontaneous echocontrast'). In the setting of peripheral arterial embolism, TEE has been shown to be significantly better than transthoracic imaging in detecting cardiac lesions.[11] However, echocardiography rarely influences patient management. Many will be warfarinized empirically, regardless of echocardiogram findings. It is difficult, even in the presence of detectable cardiac defects, such as atrial septal aneurysms or patent foramen ovale, to prove conclusively that they are the source of emboli. TTE, in fact, alters management in fewer than 5% of patients with systemic emboli. TEE

causes discomfort to the patient, and, after a negative TTE, will alter management in fewer than 4% of patients (see **Table 15.2**).[11]

The decision for palliative care

During assessment of acute leg ischemia, it must be recognized that there are a small group of patients in whom intervention is inappropriate.[12] In these patients, acute leg ischemia is a manifestation of severe co-morbid disease, most often cardiac or stroke-related. Often they are elderly and most will not have been mobile prior to the acute event. The emphasis in these patients is adequate analgesia. The decision not to intervene ought to be made by a senior vascular specialist in consultation with the patient and their family.

Prevalence and incidence
National incidences of leg ischemia
The Nordic studies

Much of the early epidemiologic data came from Sweden. In 1984, Dryjski and Swedenborg[13] estimated the crude incidence of acute leg ischemia in Greater Stockholm (population 1.5 million) to be 9/100 000, with a peak incidence of 180/100 000 in patients over 90 years of age. Subsequently, Ljungman and colleagues[14] analyzed temporal trends in acute ischemia over a 19-year interval (1965–1983) in Uppsala (population 1.3 million).

Rational approach to echocardiography in acute leg ischemia.
TTE not indicated:
Known heart disease associated with thromboembolism, e.g. atrial fibrillation, prosthetic valve, mitral stenosis, acute myocardial infarction
Patient unfit for anticoagulation or cardiac surgery
TTE indicated:
Undiagnosed cardiac condition, e.g. murmur and fever, abnormal electrocardiogram, cardiomegaly
Young patients (<65 years) with acute embolus, to exclude major sources, e.g. atrial myxoma, mitral stenosis
TEE indicated:
Young patients (<65 years) with acute embolus and negative TTE
Undiagnosed cardiac condition, but negative TTE

Table 15.2 Rational approach to echocardiography in acute leg ischemia. TTE, transthoracic echocardiography; TEE, transesophageal echocardiography.

They demonstrated an annual increase of 2.7–3.9% over the study interval. Some of this might be expected in an aging population; however, even when age-adjusted, there was a 2.7% annual increase in men, but no increase in women. The Swedish Vascular Registry (Swedvasc) was established in 1987. In 1998, it reported an average national incidence of acute leg ischemia of 13/100 000 population.[15] The Finnish vascular registry (Finnvasc) covers a population of 5 million.[16] While no incidence figures are available, the committee identified 509 cases of acute ischemia over 23 months (see **Figs 15.4A & B**).

The British studies

In 1989, Clason and colleagues[17] suggested that the incidence of acute leg ischemia in south-east Scotland was 3.7/100 000 population. This report was based on a survey of patients referred to the regional specialist unit in Edinburgh. The Gloucestershire study[18] in 1997 proposed a definition of acute limb ischemia as 'sudden deterioration in the circulation of a previously symptom-free leg at rest'. This definition is remarkably close to that subsequently adopted by the TASC group in 2000. The incidence of acute leg ischemia was estimated for the county of Gloucestershire (population 540 000) for a single year (1994) using hospital charts, general practice records, and death certificates. The incidence was 14/100 000 population. When thrombosed vascular grafts were included, the incidence in Gloucestershire rose to 16/100 000.

Acute versus chronic ischemia

Acute leg ischemia is less common than chronic ischemia. From data supplied by national vascular registers,[19] acute leg ischemia accounts for 11.9% of operations undertaken by vascular surgeons. Chronic ischemia, by comparison, comprises 40.2% of vascular reconstructions. This would reflect the experience of many vascular surgeons.

National incidences of leg ischemia: the Nordic Studies

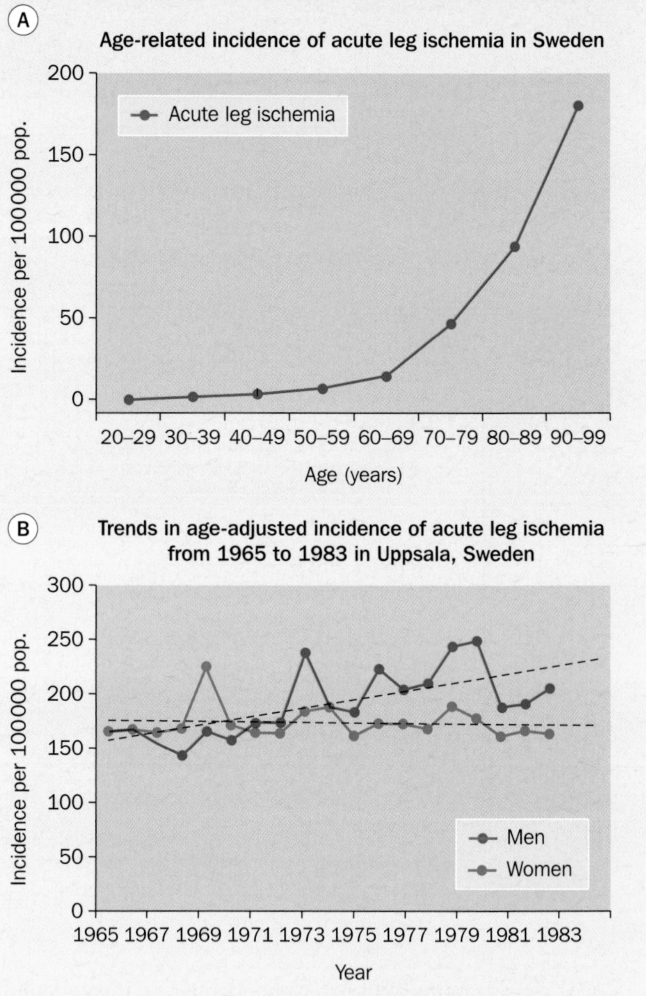

Figure 15.4 National incidences of leg ischemia: the Nordic Studies. (A) Age-related incidence of acute leg ischemia in Sweden.[13] (B) Trends in age-adjusted incidence of acute leg ischemia from 1965 to 1983 in Uppsala, Sweden.[14]

Changing patterns of embolic and thrombotic disease

The relative incidence of acute arterial thrombosis and embolism have altered over the past decades (see **Figs 15.5A & B**). However, in many series the diagnosis is based on clinical grounds and is often incorrect when compared to operative findings. In up to 19% of patients with a suspected cardiac embolus, the diagnosis will ultimately be acute thrombosis. Despite this, there is little doubt that the incidence of acute arterial embolism has declined substantially. This has mirrored the decline in rheumatic fever. Cardiac surgery has also had an impact on the prevalence of rheumatic lesions. At the same time, the 'at-risk' population for arterial thrombosis has increased with the aging of most Western populations. Data from single centers[20] suggest that embolic disease is now responsible for as few as 9% of episodes of acute leg ischemia. However, population data suggest that the change has been more gradual. Data from Sweden[15] covering 1987–1995 show that the incidence of embolism has

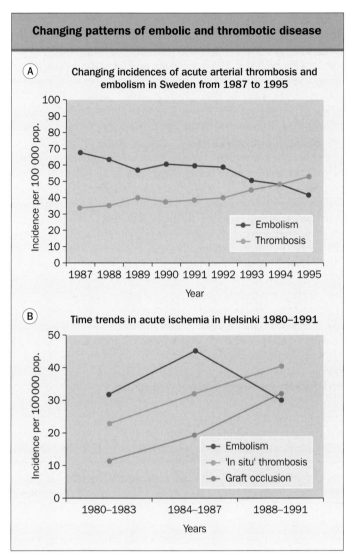

Figure 15.5 **Changing patterns of embolic and thrombotic disease.**
(A) Changing incidences of acute arterial thrombosis and embolism in
Sweden from 1987 to 1995.[15] (B) Time trends in acute ischemia in
Helsinki, 1980-1991.[22]

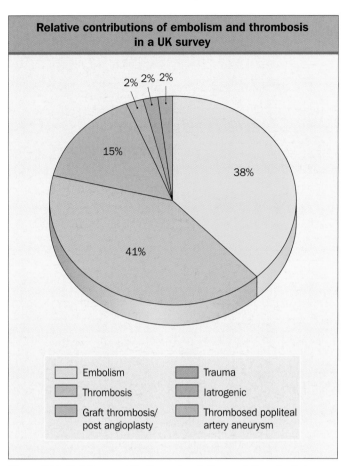

Figure 15.6 **Relative contributions of embolism and thrombosis in a
UK survey.**[21]

declined from 65% to 43% (**Fig. 15.5A**). Finnish data from
1980–1991 show that the number of patients presenting with
acute arterial embolus has actually remained constant, but the
number of patients with in-situ thrombosis and graft thrombosis
have both increased substantially[21] (**Fig. 15.5B**). A survey of
British vascular surgeons in 1998 also showed less dramatic
differences (in-situ thrombosis 41%; embolus 38%; graft occlusion
15%; trauma, iatrogenic injuries and popliteal aneurysms 6%)
(**Fig. 15.6**).[22]

Circadian and seasonal incidences
Evidence is accumulating for a circadian pattern to cardiovascular events.[23] Transient myocardial ischemia has a diurnal
peak, usually within 1–2 hours of awakening. Neural and hormonal
factors follow a diurnal variation too, as do vasoconstrictors such
as norepinephrine and renin. Fibrinogen and factor VIII also
have a morning peak, and plasma fibrinolytic activity has a
morning trough. Analysis of the circadian incidence of acute leg

ischemia has shown that it, too, has a morning peak, with a large
cluster of events around 9 am (**Fig. 15.7A**).[24] Interestingly,
paroxysmal atrial fibrillation also has a morning peak.

While a circadian variation in acute leg ischemia is plausible,
seasonal variations in the incidence of cardiovascular events are
more questionable. In 1983 it was reported that the incidence
of brachial and femoral emboli peaked in winter.[25] However,
a review of the monthly incidence of acute leg ischemia in
Edinburgh showed no significant monthly variation.[26] The
Finnvasc study group revisited the question in 2000 in a study
of 1550 patients.[27] They found that admissions for acute leg
ischemia peaked in winter, but that the difference was not
significant. They concluded that patients with acute limb ischemia
seek help in a non-uniform seasonal pattern (**Fig. 15.7B**).

Risk factors
Risk factors for embolism
In patients with acute leg ischemia, 75% of arterial emboli are
attributed to a cardiac source. Today, most emboli are due to
atrial fibrillation secondary to ischemic heart disease rather than
to rheumatic heart disease. A 25-year review of cardiac disease
in patients with acute arterial embolus in Queensland was
illustrative (**Fig. 15.8**).[28] From 1961–1985, the incidence of
rheumatic heart disease fell from 37.5% to 10.1%, while the
incidence of atherosclerotic heart disease rose from 37.5% to
68.1%.

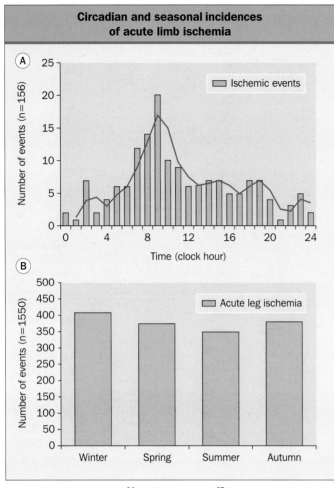

Figure 15.7 (A) Circadian[24] and (B) seasonal[27] incidences of acute limb ischemia.

Recent cardiac ischemia also is a risk factor. Myocardial infarction results in an area of dyskinesia that promotes the formation of 'mural thrombus'. Thrombus is found at post-mortem in up to 40% of patients with acute myocardial ischemia. Ventricular aneurysms may also develop and become a source for recurrent emboli. The destination of cardiac emboli also follows a distinct pattern: the leg is most often affected (50–60%), followed by the arm (15–20%), brain (15–20%), and mesenteric vessels (5%) (see **Fig. 15.9**).

Other, rarer causes of cardiac emboli are: mechanical heart valves, bacterial endocarditis, atrial myxoma, and paradoxical emboli.

The other 25% of emboli are thought to arise from aneurysms or atherosclerotic plaques ('atheroembolism'), where plaque ulceration showers cholesterol-rich emboli into the distal circulation. In one recent series,[29] aortic aneurysms accounted for 24% of atheroemboli and popliteal artery aneurysms for 10%. The rest were due to atherosclerotic plaques. However, even within this 'athero-embolic' group, the pattern has altered. With the increasing number of endovascular interventions, 'spontaneous' leg embolism now accounts for only 55% of episodes; the remainder are caused by endovascular procedures (38%) or intra-operative manipulation (7%).

Risk factors for acute arterial thrombosis

Peripheral arterial occlusive disease is the main marker for acute arterial thrombosis. However, within this group, certain patients are at higher risk.

Hypercoagulable states are particular risk factors for thrombosis (**Table 15.3**).[10] *Activated protein C resistance (APC-R)* is present in 12% of Caucasians. In 90% of cases, APC-R is attributable to a mutation in the factor V gene (factor V Leiden). It predicts early graft thrombosis and is found in 35% of patients under 51 years of age with leg ischemia. *Hyperhomocysteinemia* is an independent risk factor for atherosclerosis but elevated homocysteine levels (>13μmol/L) also significantly increase the risk of acute arterial thrombosis (odds ratio, 7.8).[30] Defects in the *endogenous fibrinolytic system* seem important. In

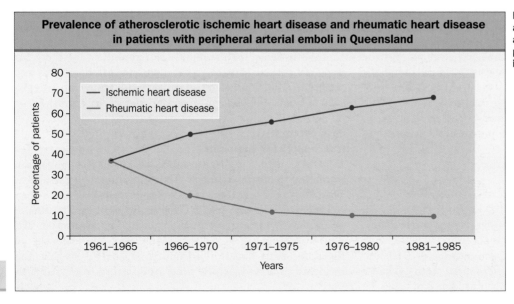

Figure 15.8 Prevalence of atherosclerotic ischemic heart disease and rheumatic heart disease in patients with peripheral arterial emboli in Queensland.[28]

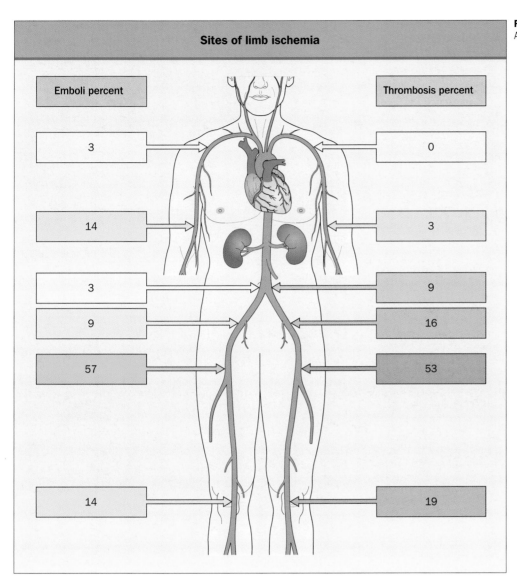

Sites of limb ischemia

Emboli percent		Thrombosis percent
3		0
14		3
3		9
9		16
57		53
14		19

Figure 15.9 Sites of limb ischemia.
Adapted from Dryjski.[42]

young patients with unexplained arterial thrombosis, deficient tissue-type plasminogen activator has been found in 45% and elevated plasminogen activator inhibitor 1 in 59%. *Antiphospholipid antibody syndrome (APS)* is characterized by the presence of *lupus anticoagulants* and *anticardiolipin antibodies*. Up to 30% of patients with APS will suffer arterial or venous thrombosis during their lives. Peripheral arterial reconstructions in patients with APS are 5.6 times more likely to fail. Other coagulation disorders that predispose to premature arterial thrombosis are: *hyperfibrinogenemia, elevated von Willebrand factor, 'sticky platelet syndrome'*, and *heparin-induced thrombocytopenia*.

The association between venous thrombosis and malignancy was recognized by Trousseau in 1865. Less common is the association between cancer and arterial thrombosis. Arterial thrombosis has been reported in association with lung, breast, and gastrointestinal cancers. When it occurs as the initial manifestation of malignancy, it is associated with a high risk of amputation and short survival.

The popliteal artery has been described as a sinister harbinger of pathology. Popliteal disease which results in acute arterial thrombosis can be particularly difficult to manage. In elderly

men, *thrombosed popliteal artery aneurysms* account for 10% of acute arterial occlusions. Up to 50% are bilateral, and amputation rates can be high. *Popliteal artery entrapment syndrome* is caused by compression of a healthy popliteal artery by an anomalous medial head of gastrocnemius. This ought to be considered in an otherwise fit and healthy man under 40 years of age with severe acute leg ischemia. Frequently, there will be a history of claudication, but occasionally, this syndrome presents with acute thrombosis. It is bilateral in 25% of cases. *Cystic adventitial disease of the popliteal artery* is much less common, but can cause popliteal artery compression; patients usually present with claudication, not acute ischemia.

Other conditions that predispose to thrombosis are aortic dissection and intra-arterial injection of narcotics by drug abusers. *Aortic dissection* ought to be considered in any patient who complains of severe chest pain before developing acute ischemia. Lower limb vessels are involved in 10% of patients, and rarely acute leg ischemia may be the first presentation of acute aortic dissection.[31] *Intra-arterial injection* of narcotics causes intense vasospasm of the entire artery. It is also a constant source of acute ischemia in young people in Western countries.

205

Hypercoagulable syndromes in acute leg ischemia.
Test for the following only in patients with acute arterial thrombosis at an early age, a strong family history of thrombosis, or with no other obvious predisposing cause:
1. Disorders of natural anticoagulants • Antithrombin III, protein C & protein S deficiency • Activated protein C resistance ('factor V Leiden'/point mutation on factor V gene)
2. Hyperhomocysteinemia (>13μmol)
3. Impaired endogenous fibrinolysis • Inadequate release of tissue-type plasminogen activator (t-PA) • High level of plasminogen activator inhibitor (PAI-1)
4. Lipoprotein (a) (>20mg/dL)
5. Antiphospholipid antibodies (more correctly family of antibodies) • Include: lupus anticoagulants (LA) and anticardiolipin antibodies (ACA) • LA + ACA + clinical syndrome = antiphospholipid antibody syndrome
6. Myeloproliferative disorders • Polycythemia rubra vera • Essential thrombocythemia (ET) – platelet count >1 000 000/μL
7. Heparin-induced thrombocytopenia (HIT) • HIT + clinical thrombosis = HIT-associated thrombosis (HITT)
8. Hematologic malignances • Multiple myeloma • Waldenström's macroglobulinemia
9. Others • Hyperfibrinogenemia • Elevated von Willebrand factor • Sticky platelet syndrome • Elevated factor VIII

Table 15.3 Hypercoagulable syndromes in acute leg ischemia.[10]

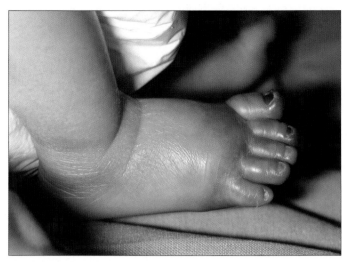

Figure 15.10 Neonate with acute ischemia due to iatrogenic intervention.

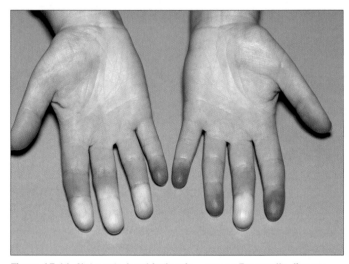

Figure 15.11 Not acute hand ischemia – severe Raynaud's disease.

Risk of iatrogenic trauma

As the number of percutaneous and endoluminal procedures increases, the risk of vascular injury also rises (**Fig. 15.10**). The risk of acute ischemia in diagnostic angiography is low at 0.1–0.15%. It rises to 1–2% in patients undergoing balloon angioplasty or stent insertion. Reports from endovascular series suggest a 4% incidence of acute leg ischaemia.[32] Acute leg ischemia is well recognized in patients undergoing cardiac surgery. In one large series covering 7620 procedures,[33] the overall incidence of acute leg ischemia was 0.85%, the majority (86%) due to injury during intra-aortic balloon pump insertion. Overall, 27% of aortic balloon pumps are associated with leg ischemia.

Military and civilian trauma

Motor vehicle accidents account for most blunt arterial injuries. The mechanism of injury is fracture or dislocation in three-quarters of cases. Less commonly, injury is due to traction or contusion. In approximately two-thirds of cases, there will be complete disruption of the artery; in one-third of cases, intimal or medial tears will be found. Motorcycle accidents and crush injuries appear to be associated with a disproportionately high incidence of arterial disruption. Increasingly, gunshot injuries are featuring in civilian trauma.

Lessons from the Korean and Vietnam wars heavily influenced the management of vascular injuries. Recent conflicts, such as Afghanistan, Lebanon and the Balkans, have also contributed to our understanding. Data from both Afghanistan and Croatia confirm that the superficial femoral artery is the most commonly injured major vessel in modern conflict, followed by the brachial artery. In up to 40% of cases, there will also be a major venous injury. Concomitant venous injury increases the risk of amputation. A quarter will also have a major bony injury. As with non-traumatic ischemia, total ischemia time correlates with risk of amputation – 22% if treated within 12 hours, 93% if the delay is greater than 12 hours.

Differential diagnosis

Vasospastic disorders are rarely a cause of acute ischemia, as the history is usually long-standing. The initial appearances of a patient with an exacerbation of Raynaud's disease or acrocyanosis may be deceptive (**Fig. 15.11**). A duplex scan will provide

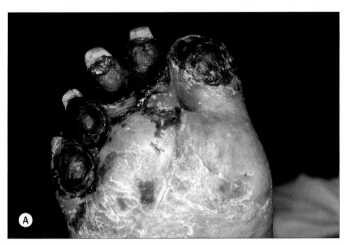

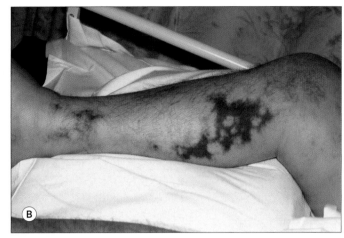

Figure 15.12 Venous gangrene in a 56-year-old man with an occult primary malignancy.

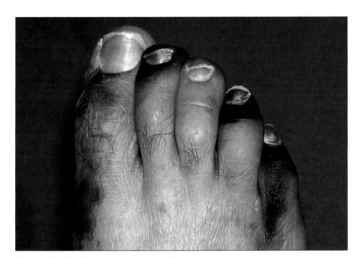

Figure 15.13 Meningococcal septicemia.

objective confirmation of the integrity of the vessels. Similarly, *arteritis* seldom causes acute ischemia. Takayasu's disease rarely affects the legs and Buerger's disease presents as chronic, not acute, ischemia. *Phlegmasia cerulea dolens* (**Fig. 15.12**) and the rarer entity, *phlegmasia alba dolens*, are extreme manifestations of extensive deep venous thrombosis. The affected foot may be cool and cyanosed and 'fixed staining' may be present. The leg may also be swollen, making pulse examination difficult. Awareness of the condition and duplex examination usually resolve any doubts. *Congestive cardiac failure* with a low cardiac index and decreased peripheral perfusion may confuse the unwary. Palpable pulses will confirm viability of the limb. Rarely, a vascular specialist may be asked to see patients with thrombotic complications of *meningococcal septicemia* (**Fig. 15.13**)

Prognosis
Natural history
Understandably, there are few contemporary studies on the natural history of acute leg ischemia. In 1948, Warren and Linton described 24 patients with acute arterial emboli seen at the Massachusetts General Hospital from 1937 to 1946.[34] The amputation rate was high: 17/24 (71%). They also described an additional 32 legs in which 'conservative therapy' was employed.

This consisted of lumbar sympathectomy, papaverine, and a special boot to apply intermittent compression. A small number of patients also received heparin. In this group, the amputation rate was 38%. A subsequent review of unoperated patients in the same institution from 1937–1953 with lower limb emboli showed an in-hospital mortality of 33–58%, with aorto-iliac occlusions associated with a particularly high mortality.[35] In 1950, Haimovici reported the outcome of 300 patients with acute leg ischemia.[36] There was a 13% mortality rate and 27% developed gangrene. Contemporary operative mortality rates are 8.5–15.7%, with limb salvage rates of 81.1–89.4%.[37,38]

Life expectancy with acute leg ischemia
Acute leg ischemia is associated with poor long-term survival. Data from Portland show a cumulative survival rate of 85% at 1 month and 51% at 36 months.[20] Swedish figures for 1965–1983 showed 4-year survival rates of 33–43%. Aune and Trippestad, in 1998, looked specifically at 5-year survival rates in Norwegian patients with acute ischemia and compared them with expected survival rates in the general population.[39] The 5-year survival rate for patients treated for an acute arterial embolus was 17%, significantly lower than the expected survival rate of 62% (**Fig. 15.14A**). More patients with acute arterial thrombosis lived to 5 years, but the 44% survival rate was still lower than the expected 74% (**Fig. 15.14B**). Explanations commonly advanced for the discrepancy between survival after embolism and thrombosis are the older age profile of patients with embolic disease and the greater incidence of cardiac disease.

However, other factors also affect survival after treatment of acute leg ischemia. Age at presentation and poor cardiac function appear to be associated consistently with higher mortality. Cardiac function accurately predicts survival. Patients in New York Heart Association (NYHA) class III–IV (angina or dyspnea with usual activity or at rest) had a six times higher mortality than those in NYHA class I–II (no symptoms or only on severe exertion).[40] Jivegard and colleagues looked at patients with acute leg ischemia due to presumed embolic disease.[41] They found a 60% mortality rate within 10 days in patients with a cardiac index <1.7L/min/m^2. Data from the Finnish national vascular database in 1994 also confirmed that cardiac and pulmonary disease adversely affected survival. Not unexpectedly, Dryjski and Swedenborg showed that patients over 80 years of age with

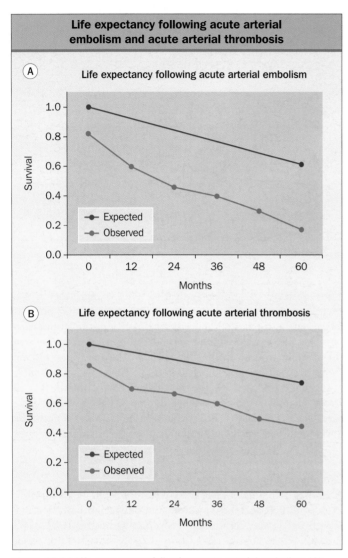

Figure 15.14 Life expectancy following acute arterial embolism (A) and acute arterial thrombosis (B).[39]

acute arterial thrombosis had a 50% mortality compared to a 5% mortality in patients younger than 60 years.[42] Population studies from Sweden in 1996 showed 5-year survival rates of 31% in patients with acute ischemia over 80 years of age.[43] In patients under 50 years of age, 5-year survival was 86%.

Predictors of limb salvage

In general, patients with acute arterial embolism are more likely to die; those with acute arterial thrombosis are more likely to require amputation. Cambria and Abbott reported the outcome of patients with acute leg ischemia.[4] Limb salvage rates were significantly lower in patients with acute arterial thrombosis than those with embolism (63% versus 81%). More contemporary reports support this. Data from the Finnvasc registry in 1994 also reported higher amputation rates after thrombosis when compared to embolus (26% versus 10%).[16] The Swedish vascular registry analyzed outcomes in 1189 patients and confirmed the risk of amputation in thrombosis to be twice that of embolic disease.[14]

There are other factors that predict a poorer chance of limb salvage. Patients who present with established leg ischemia fare

worse than those presenting early. The risk of amputation in patients with symptoms for over 25 hours is four times greater (odds ratio, 4.3) than in those with symptoms for less than 6 hours.[15]

Other prognostic indicators of limb loss may not be so obvious. The Thrombolysis or Peripheral Arterial Surgery (TOPAS) trial prospectively collected data on 544 patients with acute leg ischemia from 113 centers worldwide.[44] Univariate analysis of the data showed that eight factors predicted the likelihood of being alive with a viable limb at 1 year (amputation-free survival). Patients at higher risk were: non-white patients, aged less than 65 years, body weight less than 160 pounds (72kg), history of malignancy, neurological or cardiac disease, mottled skin at presentation, and rest pain. Most of these factors are predictable, as patients with severe systemic disease or more profound ischemia at presentation would be expected to fare worse. However, race, age, and body mass as prognostic indicators are more difficult to explain, especially as Dryjski and Swedenborg had previously shown significantly lower chance of limb salvage in octogenarians compared to patients under 60 years.[42]

Postoperative management may affect limb salvage (**Fig. 15.15**). Abbott and colleagues emphasized the importance of anticoagulation in improving survival and limb salvage rates. In 1998, the Swedish registry confirmed that postoperative anticoagulation significantly reduces amputation rates (odds ratio, 0.3).[45] In 2000, Campbell et al. reported the results at 2-year follow-up of 287 British patients with acute leg ischemia.[46] Patients who were warfarinized had significantly less chance of recurrent acute ischemia (7% versus 17%).

ACUTE ARM ISCHEMIA

Acute arm ischemia is uncommon but has a better prognosis than leg ischemia. It is usually not limb-threatening, due to the rich network of collateral vessels supplying the arm. However, the consequences of a poor outcome can be devastating. Conservative therapy will suffice in some patients, but can leave others with debilitating forearm claudication. Whether to operate or not in a patient with a viable arm at time of presentation remains contentious.

Diagnostic criteria
Acute arm ischemia can be divided into three categories: acute embolic events, iatrogenic trauma, and uncommon conditions.

Clinical evaluation – history & examination
In non-traumatic arm ischemia, the patient presents with a history of acute onset 'coldness' in their hand, often exacerbated by using the affected limb. Often they will also give a history of transient pain and paresthesia. Objectively, the hand will feel cooler than the healthy limb and appear noticeably paler (**Fig. 15.16**). Motor function is preserved, although initially the hand may be a little weaker than normal. Examination will confirm absent radial, ulnar, brachial, or axillary pulses, depending on the level of occlusion. Usually, within 24 hours of instigating heparin, the hand will be appreciably 'pinker' and movement restored. 'Mottling' of the arm or hand is rare in embolic disease. Using the SVS/ISCVS system, most cases are class I or IIa ischemia.[6]

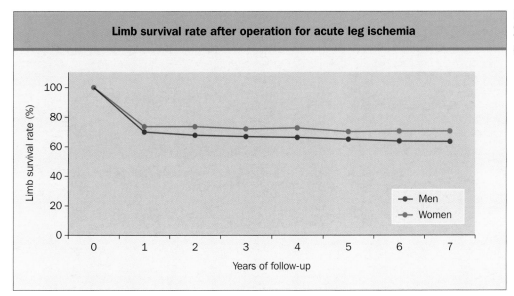

Figure 15.15 Limb survival rate after operation for acute leg ischemia. The amputation rate stabilizes after 6 months.[43]

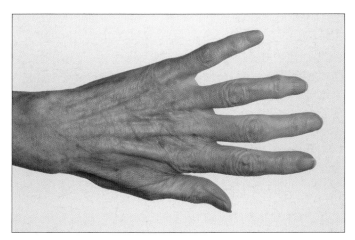

Figure 15.16 Acutely ischemic hand due to brachial artery embolism.

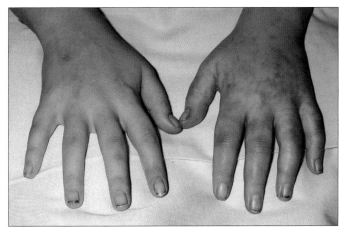

Figure 15.17 Acute ischemia of the left hand due to intra-arterial injection of narcotics.

In trauma, however, pain and paresthesia are often present from the outset, with marked pallor and loss of motor function. Pulses are absent distal to the injury. All these injuries are class IIb or III ischemia. Urgent surgical revascularization is needed.

Obviously, there are several conditions which may mimic acute arm ischemia (**Figs 15.11 & 15.17**). Often, a precise history will suggest the diagnosis.

Investigations – indications for imaging
Arterial imaging
In practice, many patients are successfully managed on clinical grounds alone. For example, in a patient with arm ischemia and atrial fibrillation, brachial embolectomy under local anesthesia is usually effective. Therefore, it is difficult to be dogmatic about the role of investigations. However, in a minority of patients in whom the clinical picture is less clear, clinical imaging is required. Patients with acute ischemia and previous axillary or subclavian artery surgery, e.g. axillofemoral or carotid-subclavian bypass, should undergo duplex imaging and angiography. A history compatible with thoracic outlet syndrome, clinical evidence of a subclavian artery aneurysm, or suspicion of 'in-situ' thrombosis

also mandate angiography. Persistent digital microemboli ('blue finger syndrome') or isolated digital ischemia are also clear indications for an angiogram.

Few authors have looked specifically at the place of diagnostic imaging. A review of 251 patients with acute arm ischemia from Munich in 2001 suggested that angiograms are needed in as few as 4% of patients.[47] Based on their experience, these authors stated that diagnostic angiograms are only indicated in the absence of a carotid pulse or in patients with generalized atherosclerosis and a long occlusion.

Ancillary investigations
The arguments for and against echocardiography are identical to those in acute leg ischemia. Most patients will be warfarinized empirically following successful brachial embolectomy. Therefore, using the criteria for leg ischemia, it is possible to rationalize the use of TTE and TEE.

Incidence
Acute arm ischemia accounts for one-fifth of all episodes of acute limb ischemia (see **Fig. 15.18**). There seems to be a female

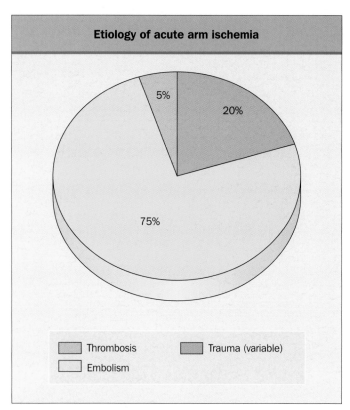

Figure 15.18 Etiology of acute arm ischemia.

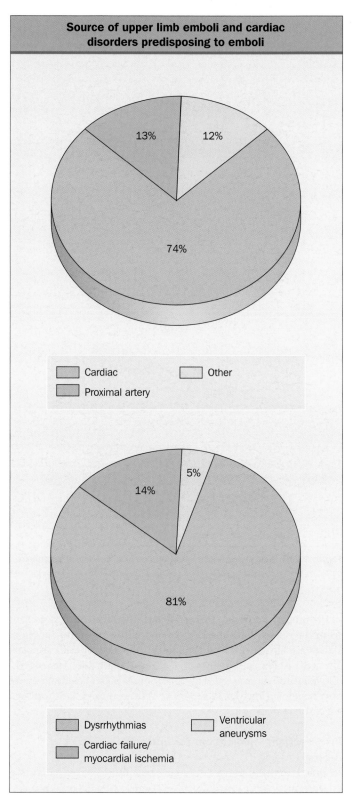

Figure 15.19 Source of upper limb emboli[48] **and cardiac disorders predisposing to emboli.**[47]

preponderance in all series, of approximately 2:1. Patients with acute arm ischemia are also slightly older than those with acute leg ischemia (67 years versus 62 years). Most of the published series include only those patients who have surgery. In reality, between 9–30% of patients seen by vascular specialists are managed conservatively as they are either unfit for surgery or have minimal symptoms. In Dryjski and Swedenborg's survey of acute limb ischemia in Stockholm, the incidence of acute arm ischemia was 1.13/100 000 population.[13] Most current estimates would suggest an incidence of 1.2–3.5/100 000 population.

Risk factors for acute non-traumatic arm ischemia
Embolus
Embolic occlusions account for three-quarters of acute arm ischemia. The majority of arm emboli are cardiac in origin (approximately 75%), the other 25% being extra-cardiac or of indeterminate origin. Cardiac emboli are usually due to dys-rhythmias (81%), chiefly atrial fibrillation. Recent myocardial infarction or heart failure (14%) are also important. A minority (5%) will be accounted for by ventricular aneurysms, atrial myxomas, and paradoxical emboli (**Fig. 15.19**).

With regard to extra-cardiac emboli, the aorta, brachiocephalic, and subclavian arteries account for approximately 13% of acute arm ischemia due to atherosclerotic plaque embolization ('atheroemboli') or extrinsic compression due to fibrous bands or cervical ribs. Subclavian artery aneurysms are rare but can be a source of embolic material. Even rarer causes are malignant emboli and fibromuscular dysplasia. In 12% of cases, no embolic source will be found.

Emboli usually lodge in the brachial artery (60%). The next most common site is the axillary artery (26%). There is a slightly greater frequency of emboli in the right arm, possibly due to the brachiocephalic artery being closer to the heart.

Thrombosis

'In-situ' thrombosis of the arm is rare. Approximately 5% of community episodes of acute arm ischemia are due to thrombosis. Eyers and Earnshaw suggest that the more proximal the occlusion, the more likely it is to be thrombosis.[48] As with acute leg ischemia, patients who are initially misdiagnosed and subjected to inappropriate embolectomy fare worse. The most common predisposing cause is atherosclerotic plaques, although thoracic outlet syndrome, aneurysms, and arteritis are also implicated. Less common causes include hypercoagulable conditions, malignancy (Trousseau's syndrome), and radiotherapy injury.

Prognosis
Natural history

Untreated patients with acute arm ischemia fare relatively well. All natural history series pre-date the development of the Fogarty embolectomy catheter in 1963. Warren and Linton reported the Massachusetts General Hospital experience in 1948 of 14 patients who received no treatment.[34] In all cases, the arm survived, and no information was provided about subsequent function. Abbott et al. analyzed all non-operated patients with arm ischemia presenting to a single center from 1937–1953.[45] These authors showed an in-hospital mortality rate of 17%. By 1980, mortality rates for acute arm ischemia had fallen to 6%.

Mortality rates and long-term survival

Postoperative survival rates in acute arm ischemia are good. However, acute non-traumatic arm ischemia is a marker of reduced long-term survival. Hernandez-Richter et al. quote a 5-year survival rate for patients of 56% following brachial embolectomy.[47] When specifically compared to outcomes for patients with leg ischemia, however, patients with arm ischemia fare better. Stonebridge et al. reported that patients with arm ischemia had a 5% in-hospital mortality rate versus 30% for leg ischemia.[49] While patients with arm ischemia were older and had a similar incidence of cardiac dysrhythmias, they had significantly fewer cardiopulmonary symptoms.

Arm function and recurrent embolization

The reported operative mortality rate after brachial embolectomy is 5.5–19.2%. Following successful brachial embolectomy, 95–98% of patients will be symptom-free, with as few as 2% reporting long-term claudication.

Conservatively managed patients are probably underrepresented in the literature. In the few reported series, assessment of symptoms and disability tends to be inconsistent. However, in a series of 95 patients reported in 1964, 32% were left with abnormal function of the arm. In 1977, Savelyev et al. reported that 75% of patients managed conservatively had a poor functional outcome.[50] More recently, Galbraith and colleagues confirmed that 50% of their conservatively managed patients had persistent forearm claudication.[51]

Recurrent embolization was reported in 11% of patients managed in Edinburgh, despite full anticoagulation. All had ongoing atrial fibrillation. Recurrent emboli are also more likely when the underlying cause was acute myocardial ischemia. In patients who are not anticoagulated, the outlook is worse, with up to 33% experiencing recurrent emboli. As might be expected, recurrent embolization is associated with a higher mortality rate.

Summary

Acute limb ischemia remains a major problem for the vascular specialist. Most patients with acute limb ischemia are elderly; many have significant co-morbidities. The incidence of acute limb ischemia is slowly increasing. This reflects the aging population and increased prevalence of peripheral vascular disease. Accordingly, the most common cause of leg ischemia is now acute arterial thrombosis. Embolic disease is still the main cause of non-traumatic arm ischemia.

Improvements in limb salvage rates have been dramatic since the 1950s. However, even with improved limb salvage techniques, only 70% of patients leave hospital with an intact limb. Of the remaining 30%, half will die and half will require major amputations. Only 10–15% of these amputees regain any degree of independent activity. Early, appropriate intervention can save life and limb. There is compelling evidence that outcomes are better when these patients are treated by vascular specialists.[22] Approximately 30% of those admitted with acute leg ischemia require immediate surgical revascularization, either bypass or embolectomy. Where the diagnosis of embolus can confidently be made, embolectomy is immediately effective. The other patients ought to have angiography, unless they are unfit for further intervention. The role of magnetic resonance angiography and computed tomographic angiography remain uncertain and with best intentions, ancillary investigations are probably overused. Ultimately, assessment remains clinical, and early treatment the best indicator of outcome.

REFERENCES

1. Management of peripheral arterial disease (PAD). TransAtlantic Inter-Society Consensus (TASC). Section C: acute limb ischaemia. Eur J Vasc Endovasc Surg 2000;19(Suppl A):S115–43.
2. Batz W, Bruckner R [Symptoms and therapy of aortic bifurcation embolism]. Chirurg 1985;56:166–9.
3. Jivegard L, Holm J, Schersten T. The outcome in arterial thrombosis misdiagnosed as arterial embolism. Acta Chir Scand 1986;152:251–6.
4. Cambria RP, Abbott WM. Acute arterial thrombosis of the lower extremity. Its natural history contrasted with arterial embolism. Arch Surg 1984;119:784–7.
5. Suggested standards for reports dealing with lower extremity ischemia. Prepared by the Ad Hoc Committee on Reporting Standards, Society for Vascular Surgery/North American Chapter, International Society for Cardiovascular Surgery. J Vasc Surg 1986;4:80–94.
6. Rutherford RB, Baker JD, Ernst C, et al. Recommended standards for reports dealing with lower extremity ischemia: revised version. J Vasc Surg 1997;26:517–38.
7. Jivegard L, Bergqvist D, Holm J. When is urgent revascularization unnecessary for acute lower limb ischaemia? Eur J Vasc Endovasc Surg 1995;9:448–53.
8. Jivegard L, Wingren U. Management of acute limb ischaemia over two decades: the Swedish experience. Eur J Vasc Endovasc Surg 1999; 18:93–5.
9. Bostrom A, Ljungman C, Hellberg A, et al. Duplex scanning as the sole preoperative imaging method for infrainguinal arterial surgery. Eur J Vasc Endovasc Surg 2001;23:140–5.

10. Deitcher SR, Carman TL, Sheikh MA, Gomes M. Hypercoagulable syndromes: evaluation and management strategies for acute limb ischemia. Semin Vasc Surg 2001;14:74–85.
11. Egeblad H, Andersen K, Hartiala J, et al. Role of echocardiography in systemic arterial embolism. A review with recommendations. Scand Cardiovasc J 1998;32:323–42.
12. Campbell WB, Verfaillie P, Ridler BM, Thompson JF. Non-operative treatment of advanced limb ischaemia: the decision for palliative care. Eur J Vasc Endovasc Surg 2000;19:246–9.
13. Dryjski M, Swedenborg J. Acute ischemia of the extremities in a metropolitan area during one year. J Cardiovasc Surg (Torino) 1984;25:518–22.
14. Ljungman C, Adami HO, Bergqvist D, Berglund A, Persson I. Time trends in incidence rates of acute, non-traumatic extremity ischaemia: a population-based study during a 19-year period. Br J Surg 1991; 78:857–60.
15. Bergqvist D, Tröeng T, Elfstrom J, et al. Eur J Surg 1998;164(Suppl 581):1–45.
16. Kuukasjarvi P, Salenius JP. Perioperative outcome of acute lower limb ischaemia on the basis of the national vascular registry. The Finnvasc Study Group. Eur J Vasc Surg 1994;8:578–83.
17. Clason AE, Stonebridge PA, Duncan AJ, Nolan B, Jenkins AM, Ruckley CV. Acute ischaemia of the lower limb: the effect of centralizing vascular surgical services on morbidity and mortality. Br J Surg 1989; 76:592–3.
18. Davies B, Braithwaite BD, Birch PA, Poskitt KR, Heather BP, Earnshaw JJ. Acute leg ischaemia in Gloucestershire. Br J Surg 1997;84:504–8.
19. Salenius JP, Lepantalo M, Ylonen K, Luther M. Treatment of peripheral vascular diseases – basic data from the nationwide vascular registry FINNVASC. Ann Chir Gynaecol 1993;82:235–40.
20. Yeager RA, Moneta GL, Taylor LM Jr, Hamre DW, McConnell DB, Porter JM. Surgical management of severe acute lower extremity ischemia. J Vasc Surg 1992;15:385–91.
21. Luther M, Alback A. Acute leg ischaemia – a case for the junior surgeon? Ann Chir Gynaecol 1995;84:373–8.
22. Campbell WB, Ridler BM, Szymanska TH. Current management of acute leg ischaemia: results of an audit by the Vascular Surgical Society of Great Britain and Ireland. Br J Surg 1998;85:1498–503.
23. Maemura K, Layne MD, Watanabe M, Perrell MA, Nagai R, Lee ME. Molecular mechanisms of morning onset of myocardial infarction. Ann NY Acad Sci 2001;947:398–402.
24. Manfredini R, Gallerani M, Portaluppi F, Salmi R, Zamboni P, Fersini C. Circadian variation in the onset of acute critical limb ischaemia. Thromb Res 1998;92:163–9.
25. Clark CV. Seasonal variation in incidence of brachial and femoral emboli. BMJ (Clin Res Ed) 1983;287:1109.
26. John TG, Stonebridge PA. Seasonal variation in operations for ruptured abdominal aortic aneurysm and acute lower limb ischaemia. J R Coll Surg Edinb 1993;38:161–2.
27. Kuukasjarvi P, Salenius JP, Lepantalo M, Luther M, Ylonen K. Weekly and seasonal variation of hospital admissions and outcome in patients with acute lower limb ischaemia treated by surgical and endovascular means. Int Angiol 2000;19:354–7.
28. Englund R, Magee HR. Peripheral arterial embolism: 1961–1985. Aust NZ J Surg 1987;57:27–31.
29. Sharma PV, Babu SC, Shah PM, Nassoura ZE. Changing patterns of atheroembolism. Cardiovasc Surg 1996;4:573–9.
30. Kottke-Marchant K, Green R, Jacobsen DW, et al. High plasma homocysteine: a risk factor for arterial and venous thrombosis in patients with normal coagulation profiles. Clin Appl Thromb Hemost 1997; 34:239–44.
31. Pacifico L, Spodick D. ILEAD – ischemia of the lower extremities due to aortic dissection: the isolated presentation. Clin Cardiol. 1999; 22:353–6.
32. Fairman RM, Velazquez O, Baum R, et al. Endovascular repair of aortic aneurysms: critical events and adjunctive procedures. J Vasc Surg 2001;33:1226–32.
33. Allen RC, Schneider J, Longenecker L, Kosinski AS, Smith RB III, Lumsden AB. Acute lower extremity ischemia after cardiac surgery. Am J Surg 1993;166:124–9.
34. Warren R, Linton RR. The treatment of arterial embolism. N Engl J Med 1948;238:421–9.
35. Warren R, Linton RR, Scannell JG. Arterial embolism. Recent progress. Ann Surg 1954;140: 311–7.
36. Haimovici H. Peripheral arterial embolism. A study of 330 unselected cases of embolism of the extremities. Angiology 1950;1:20–45.
37. The STILE Investigators. Results of a prospective randomized trial evaluating surgery versus thrombolysis for ischemia of the lower extremity. The STILE trial. Ann Surg 1994;220:251–66.
38. Ouriel K, Veith FJ, Sasahara AA. A comparison of recombinant urokinase with vascular surgery as initial treatment for acute arterial occlusion of the legs. Thrombolysis or Peripheral Arterial Surgery (TOPAS) Investigators. N Engl J Med 1998;338:1105–11.
39. Aune S, Trippestad A. Operative mortality and long-term survival of patients operated on for acute lower limb ischaemia. Eur J Vasc Endovasc Surg 1998;15:143–6.
40. Dregelid EB, Stangeland LB, Eide GE, Trippestad A. Patient survival and limb prognosis after arterial embolectomy. Eur J Vasc Surg 1987; 1:263–71.
41. Jivegard L, Arfvidsson B, Frid I, Haljamae H, Holm J. Cardiac output in patients with acute lower limb ischaemia of presumed embolic origin – a predictor of severity and outcome? Eur J Vasc Surg 1990;4:401–7.
42. Dryjski M, Swedenborg J. Acute nontraumatic extremity ischaemia in Sweden. A one-year survey. Acta Chir Scand 1985;151:333–9.
43. Ljungman C, Holmberg L, Bergqvist D, Bergstrom R, Adami HO. Amputation risk and survival after embolectomy for acute arterial ischaemia. Time trends in a defined Swedish population. Eur J Vasc Endovasc Surg 1996;11:176–82.
44. Ouriel K, Veith FJ. Acute lower limb ischemia: determinants of outcome. Surgery 1998;124:336–41.
45. Abbott WM, Maloney RD, McCabe CC, Lee CE, Wirthlin LS. Arterial embolism: a 44 year perspective. Am J Surg 1982;143:460–4.
46. Campbell WB, Ridler BM, Szymanska TH. Two-year follow-up after acute thromboembolic limb ischaemia: the importance of anticoagulation. Eur J Vasc Endovasc Surg 2000;19:169–73.
47. Hernandez-Richter T, Angele MK, Helmberger T, Jauch KW, Lauterjung L, Schildberg FW. Acute ischemia of the upper extremity: long-term results following thrombembolectomy with the Fogarty catheter. Langenbecks Arch Surg 2001;386:261–6.
48. Eyers P, Earnshaw JJ. Acute non-traumatic arm ischaemia. Br J Surg 1998;85:1340–6.
49. Stonebridge PA, Clason AE, Duncan AJ, Nolan B, Jenkins AM, Ruckley CV. Acute ischaemia of the upper limb compared with acute lower limb ischaemia: a 5-year review. Br J Surg 1989;76:515–6.
50. Savelyev VS, Zatevakhin II, Stepanov NV. Artery embolism of the upper limbs. Surgery 1977;81:367–75.
51. Galbraith K, Collin J, Morris PJ, Wood RF. Recent experience with arterial embolism of the limbs in a vascular unit. Ann R Coll Surg Engl 1985;67:30–3.

CHAPTER
16

Thrombolytic Therapy for Acute Peripheral Arterial Occlusion

Kenneth Ouriel

KEY POINTS

- Acute occlusion of a peripheral artery is a catastrophic event. Whether occurring as a result of in-situ thrombosis of a native artery or bypass graft, or from embolization, the acute ischemia threatens both the patient's leg and life.

- Traditionally, open surgical intervention has been the 'gold standard' treatment for these patients. However, the multiplicity and complexity of medical co-morbidities account for a high rate of perioperative morbidity and mortality. Thus, a non-surgical alternative is attractive.

- The non-surgical approach, however, must be associated with a similar rate of limb salvage, and other untoward events must not occur at increased frequency.

- Catheter-directed thrombolytic therapy has been studied in this regard, offering the potential to restore arterial perfusion without the need for open surgery in many cases. Thrombolysis has been criticized, however, on the basis of associated hemorrhagic complications, a slow rate of thrombus dissolution, and an unacceptable risk of rethrombosis.

- There exist several prospective, randomized trials that have evaluated these issues. An analysis of these studies sheds some light on the safety and efficacy of thrombolytic strategies as initial interventions in patients with acute leg ischemia.

Early (in-hospital or 30-day) rates of amputation and death in selected series of patients with recent peripheral arterial occlusion, treated with primary open surgical intervention.

Study	Year	Amputation rate	Mortality rate
Blaisdell et al[1]	1978	25%	30%
Jivegård et al[2]	1988	–	20%
Rochester[5]	1994	14%	18%
STILE[7]	1994	5%	6%
TOPAS[6]	1998	2%	5%

Table 16.1 Early (in-hospital or 30-day) rates of amputation and death in selected series of patients with recent peripheral arterial occlusion, treated with primary open surgical intervention.

Patients with acute occlusion of a peripheral artery or bypass graft present with sudden onset of pain, progressing to sensory loss and, later, paralysis. The rapidity of onset is correlated with the extent of the thrombotic process and the amount of pre-existing collateral pathways. Whether from in-situ thrombosis of a native artery or bypass graft or from embolization, the acute ischemia threatens both the patient's leg and life. Mortality is closely linked with the presence of medical co-morbidities such as coronary artery disease rather than being directly associated with the ischemic process itself; in-hospital mortality rates exceed 20% in this group of individuals.[1,2]

Treatment begins with early heparin anticoagulation to limit the propagation of thrombus and prevent clinical deterioration, although there are few objective data on which to base this practice.[1,3,4] Anticoagulation is followed by urgent surgical intervention, employing thrombectomy, bypass grafting, and other techniques to restore adequate arterial flow to the affected leg. Such an approach, however, is associated with a high rate of complications, including major amputation and death. A now classic study by Blaisdell, published in the late 1970s, documented amputation and mortality rates in excess of 25% each, following open surgical repair for acute leg ischemia.[1] Jivegård and colleagues observed a 20% mortality rate in patients treated operatively.[2]

Despite advances in surgical technique and perioperative care, the risk of morbidity and mortality following open surgical intervention remains unacceptably high (**Table 16.1**).[5–8] What factors explain this finding? Clearly, the baseline medical status of patients with acute peripheral arterial occlusion underlies the observation. Patients are frequently elderly, with a high rate of cardiac and other co-morbidities. They are ill equipped to tolerate the insult of ischemia of an extremity, let alone an invasive surgical intervention to relieve the obstruction. A multivariate analysis of the data from the Rochester series uncovered several variables that were predictive of poor outcome, irrespective of the type of treatment instituted.[9] A summary of available literature would appear to confirm that individuals with acute limb-threatening ischemia comprise one of the sickest subgroup of patients that the peripheral vascular surgeon is asked to treat.[10]

There is some evidence that a less invasive intervention is better tolerated in this very ill group of patients.[2] Today, many centers employ intra-arterial thrombolytic therapy as the initial intervention, infusing thrombolytic agents directly into the occluding thrombus. Agents such as urokinase,[11] alteplase,[12] and reteplase[13] provide a less invasive means of restoring adequate arterial perfusion, addressing the unmasked culprit lesion responsible for the occlusion with an endovascular or open surgical procedure performed electively after adequate patient preparation. Thus, although thrombolytic therapy does not always obviate the need for an endovascular or open surgical procedure to correct the underlying causative lesion, use of these agents as initial therapy may allow the more invasive modalities to be deterred until the patient can be better prepared for a major intervention.[14]

But percutaneous thrombolytic therapy has not been a panacea for patients with acute leg ischemia. In fact, thrombolytic therapy has been criticized, citing a high rate of re-occlusion, high cost and low rate of patency.[15,16] The conclusions of these studies, however, were based on improper expectations for therapy. The need for subsequent intervention to address unmasked lesions was often neglected, the endpoint of patency was the focus rather than survival, and long-term outcome was contrasted with primary surgical revascularization, rather than re-do operative procedures. Moreover, poor technique, inadequate devices, and inferior agents colored the initial experiences with catheter-directed thrombolytic therapy. For instance, the now well-accepted principle of ensuring infusion of the thrombolytic agent directly into the substance of the occluding thrombus was not always ardently adhered to. End-hole catheters were employed; it was not until the late 1980s that multisided-hole catheters were available. Finally, streptokinase (SK) was the most frequently used agent until the landmark article of McNamara and Fischer in 1985 documented improved results with locally administered high-dose urokinase.[11]

THE THROMBOLYTIC AGENTS

Pharmacology

All available thrombolytic agents in clinical use are plasminogen activators (**Table 16.2**). As such, they do not directly degrade fibrinogen. Rather, they are trypsin-like serine proteases that have high specific activity directed at the cleavage of a single peptide bond in the plasminogen zymogen, converting it to plasmin. Plasmin is the active molecule that cleaves fibrin polymer to cause the dissolution of thrombus. Milstone first recognized the

importance of plasminogen in 1941, when it was noted that clots formed with highly purified fibrinogen and thrombin were not lysed by streptococcal fibrinolysin unless a small amount of human serum (plasminogen) was added.[17] Recognizing this direct role of plasminogen, early investigators attempted to dissolve occluding thrombi with the administration of exogenous plasmin. Free plasmin, however, was ineffective as a thrombolytic agent. Plasmin is extremely unstable at physiologic pH, with auto-degradation, accounting for the failure of these attempts. Effective thrombolysis can only be achieved when fibrin-bound plasminogen is converted to its active form, plasmin, at the site of the thrombus.

The dependence of fibrinolysis on adequate circulating levels of plasminogen is best illustrated by studies of the fibrinolytic potential of blood drawn from patients receiving intravenous administration of thrombolytic agents for acute myocardial infarction.[18] Blood obtained soon after the start of thrombolytic administration displayed a great degree of in-vitro fibrinolytic potential. Aliquots of plasma drawn from the patients and then added to radiolabeled clots in test tubes produced rapid dissolution of the clots. By contrast, similar aliquots drawn from patients after 20min of thrombolytic administration had considerably less thrombolytic potential. The explanation for this observation relates to the amount of plasminogen present in the blood. Prolonged thrombolytic administration consumed all of the endogenous plasminogen and, despite continued administration of thrombolytic agent, no further clot lysis was possible.

History of thrombolytic therapy

In 1933, Tillett and Garner at the Johns Hopkins Medical School discovered that filtrates of broth cultures of certain strains of hemolytic streptococcal bacteria had fibrinolytic properties.[19] This streptococcal byproduct was originally termed streptococcal fibrinolysin. The purity of this agent, however, was poor. Clinical use, of necessity, awaited adequate purification. Tillett and Sherry

Properties of the components of the fibrinolytic scheme.			
Component	Molecular weight	Plasma $t_{1/2}$	Properties
Streptokinase	48 000	16 min/90 min	Complexes with plasmin(ogen) to gain activity
Urokinase	32 000/54 000	14 min	Direct plasminogen activator
r-Urokinase	32 000	7 min	Similar in most respects to natural urokinase
r-Prourokinase	49 000	7 min	Little intrinsic activity, converted to urokinase
rt-PA	68 000	3.5 min	Exhibits great degree of fibrin activity and specificity
TNK-tPA	65 000	15 min	A modified t-PA with a longer half-life
Reteplase	39 000	14 min	A truncated t-PA with a longer half-life
Plasminogen	88 000	2.2 days	Binds to fibrin, converted to active plasmin
Plasmin	88 000	0.1s	Serine protease that cleaves fibrin
Alpha$_2$-antiplasmin	70 000	3 days	Inactivates free plasmin
PAI-1	52 000	Unknown	Inactivates the plasminogen activators

Table 16.2 Properties of the components of the fibrinolytic scheme. PAI-1, plasminogen activator inhibitor-1; rt-PA, recombinant tissue plasminogen activator; TNK-tPA, tenecteplase; t-PA, tissue plasminogen activator.

administered streptokinase intrapleurally to dissolve loculated hemothoraces in the late 1940s,[20] but intravascular administration was not attempted until the following decade. Tillett first reported intravascular administration of a thrombolytic agent in an article published in 1955.[21] A concentrated and partially purified streptokinase (SK) (Varidase®, Lederle Laboratories) was injected into 11 patients. This investigation was performed with the intent to gain data on the safety of the agent in volunteers; in no case was the SK administered to dissolve pathologic thrombi. Fever and hypotension developed as the amount of SK approached therapeutic levels. Whereas fever was generally mild and controllable with antipyretics, hypotension was sometimes prominent. The mean fall in systolic pressure was 31mmHg and three of the patients manifested systolic pressures below 80mmHg. These untoward reactions were more likely to be the result of contaminants in the preparation, rather than the SK itself. Despite these reactions, systemic proteolysis was observed, with a decrease in fibrinogen and plasminogen, concurrent with a mild increase in the prothrombin time.

These early studies were followed by reports on the use of SK in patients with occluding vascular thrombi. In 1956, EE Cliffton, at the Cornell University Medical College in New York, was responsible for the first brief description of the clinical effectiveness of intravascular thrombolytic administration, and the following year, he published his results in 40 patients with occlusive thrombi treated with a SK-plasminogen combination.[22] The location of the thrombi was diverse, and included peripheral arterial thrombi, venous thrombi, pulmonary emboli, retinal occlusions, and, in two patients, occlusive carotid thrombi. Cliffton's clinical results were far from exemplary: recanalization was not uniform and bleeding complications were frequent. Nevertheless, he must be credited with the first use of thrombolytic agents for the treatment of pathologic thrombi, as well as with the first use of catheter-directed administration of a thrombolytic agent.

Classification of thrombolytic agents

Several schemes may be used to classify thrombolytic agents. The agents may be grouped by their mechanism of action: those that directly convert plasminogen to plasmin versus those that are inactive zymogens and require transformation to an active form before they can cleave plasminogen. Thrombolytic agents can also be grouped by their mode of production: those that are manufactured via recombinant techniques versus those that are of bacterial origin. Of interest, recombinant agents harvested from a bacterial expression system such as *Escherichia coli* do not contain carbohydrates, while products of mammalian hybridoma (e.g. recombinant prourokinase from mouse hybridoma SP2/0 cells) are fully glycosylated.

Thrombolytic agents can be classified by their pharmacologic actions: those that are 'fibrin-specific' (bind to fibrin but not fibrinogen) versus those that are non-specific, and those that have a great degree of 'fibrin-affinity' (bind avidly to fibrin) versus those that do not (**Table 16.3**). We have found it most useful to classify thrombolytic agents into groups based on the origin of the parent compound. It is most efficient to divide the agents into four groups: the streptokinase compounds, the urokinase compounds, the tissue plasminogen activators, and an additional, miscellaneous group consisting of novel agents distinct from those agents in the three other groups.

Properties of the thrombolytic agents.		
Agent	*Fibrin specificity*	*Fibrin affinity*
Streptokinase	Low	Low
APSAC	Low	Intermediate
Urokinase	Low	Low
Prourokinase	High	Low
t-PA	High	High
TNK-tPA	Very high	High
Reteplase	High	Low
Bat PA	Very high	Low

Table 16.3 Properties of the thrombolytic agents. APSAC, anisoylated plasminogen-streptokinase activator complex; TNK-tPA, tenecteplase; t-PA, tissue plasminogen activator.

Streptokinase compounds

Streptokinase, originating from the streptococcus bacteria, was the first thrombolytic agent to be described.[19] SK is a 50kDa molecule with a biphasic half-life comprising a rapid $t_{\frac{1}{2}}$ of 16min and a second, slower $t_{\frac{1}{2}}$ of 90min. Whereas the initial half-life is accounted for by the formation of a complex between the molecule and SK antibodies, the second half-life represents the actual biologic elimination of the protein. SK differs from other thrombolytic agents with respect to the stoichiometry of plasminogen binding. Whereas other agents directly convert plasminogen to plasmin, SK must form an equimolar stoichiometric complex with a plasmin or plasminogen molecule to gain activity. Only then can this SK-plasmin(ogen) complex activate a second plasminogen molecule to form active plasmin; thus, two plasminogen molecules are utilized in SK-mediated plasmin generation.

Streptokinase suffers from the limitation of antigenic potential. Preformed antibodies exist to a certain extent in all patients who have been infected with the streptococcus bacterium. Similarly, patients with exposure to SK may have high antibody titers on repeat exposure. These neutralizing antibodies inactivate exogenously administered SK. SK antibodies may be overwhelmed through the use of a large initial bolus of SK. Some investigators have recommended measurement of antibody titers prior to beginning SK therapy, gauging the loading dose on the basis of this titer.[23] While SK administration may be complicated by allergic reactions such as urticaria, pyrexia, periorbital edema, and bronchospasm, the major untoward effect associated with SK is hemorrhage. SK-associated hemorrhage may be no different from bleeding associated with any thrombolytic agent. The primary cause is likely to be the actions of the systemic agent on the thrombi sealing the sites of vascular disintegrity. The generation of free plasmin, however, can contribute to the problem, with degradation of fibrinogen and other serum clotting proteins, as well as the release of fibrin(ogen)-degradation products that are potent anticoagulants themselves and exacerbate the coagulopathy.

Recognizing potential limitations with SK, anisoylated plasminogen-streptokinase activator complex (APSAC) was

215

developed by pharmacologists at Beecham Laboratories.[24] APSAC has a longer half-life than SK, since acylation renders the complex less susceptible to degradation. Because of this property, it was anticipated that APSAC would be associated with a reduced risk of rethrombosis. Contrary to expectations, APSAC offered little clinical benefit over SK or recombinant tissue plasminogen activator (rt-PA) when studied in the setting of acute coronary occlusion,[25] and, at present, APSAC is not used to treat thrombi in the peripheral vasculature.

Urokinase compounds

The fibrinolytic potential of human urine was first described by Macfarlane in 1947.[26] The active molecule was extracted, isolated and named 'urokinase' in 1952.[27] This urokinase-type plasminogen activator is a serine protease composed of two polypeptide chains, occurring in a low-molecular weight (32kDa) and high-molecular weight (54kDa) form. The high-molecular weight form predominates in urokinase isolated from urine, while the low-molecular weight form is found in urokinase obtained from tissue culture of kidney cells. Unlike SK, urokinase directly activates plasminogen to form plasmin; prior binding to plasminogen or plasmin is not necessary for activity. Also in contrast to SK, preformed antibodies to urokinase are not observed. The agent is non-antigenic, and untoward reactions of fever or hypotension are rare.

Presently, the most commonly employed urokinase in the USA is of tissue-culture origin, manufactured from human neonatal kidney cells (Abbokinase®, Abbott Laboratories). Urokinase has been fully sequenced, and a recombinant form of urokinase (r-UK) was tested in a single trial of patients with acute myocardial infarction and in two multicenter trials of patients with peripheral arterial occlusion.[28] r-UK is fully glycosylated, since it is derived from a murine hybridoma cell line. r-UK differs from Abbokinase® in several respects. Firstly, r-UK has a higher molecular weight than Abbokinase. Secondly, r-UK has a shorter half-life than its low-molecular weight counterpart. Despite these differences, however, the clinical effects of the two agents have been similar.

A precursor of urokinase was discovered in urine in 1979.[29] Prourokinase was characterized and subsequently manufactured by recombinant technology using *E. coli* (non-glycosylated) or mammalian cells (fully glycosylated). This single-chain form is an inactive zymogen, inert in plasma, but can be activated by kallikrein or plasmin to form active two-chain urokinase. This property accounts for amplification of the fibrinolytic process – as plasmin is generated, more prourokinase is converted to active urokinase, and the process is repeated. Prourokinase is relatively fibrin specific, that is, its fibrin degrading (fibrinolytic) activity greatly outweighs its fibrinogen degrading (fibrinogenolytic) activity. This feature is explained by the preferential activation of fibrin-bound plasminogen found in a thrombus over free plasminogen found in flowing blood. Non-selective activators such as SK and urokinase activate free and bound plasminogen equally and induce systemic plasminemia with resultant fibrinogenolysis and degradation of clotting factors V and VII.

Given the potential advantages of prourokinase over urokinase, Abbott Laboratories produced a recombinant form of prourokinase (r-prourokinase) from a murine hybridoma cell line. This recombinant agent was named Prolyse® (Abbott Laboratories) and is converted to active two-chain urokinase by plasmin and kallikrein. Prolyse® has been studied in the settings of myocardial infarction, stroke, and peripheral arterial occlusion. To date, it appears that r-prourokinase offers the advantages associated with an agent that does not originate from a human cell source. Fibrin specificity, however, may be lost at the higher dose levels necessary to effect more rapid thrombolysis than Abbokinase®.[8]

Tissue plasminogen activators

Tissue plasminogen activator is a naturally occurring fibrinolytic agent produced by endothelial cells and intimately involved in the balance between intravascular thrombogenesis and thrombolysis.[30] Natural t-PA is a single-chain (527-amino acid) serine protease with a molecular weight of approximately 65kDa. Plasmin hydrolyzes the Arg275-Ile276 peptide bond, converting the single-chain molecule into a two-chain moiety. In contrast to most serine proteases (e.g. urokinase), the single-chain form of t-PA has significant activity. t-PA has potential benefits over other thrombolytic agents. The agent exhibits significant fibrin specificity. In plasma, the agent is associated with little plasminogen activation. At the site of the thrombus, however, the binding of t-PA and plasminogen to the fibrin surface induces a conformational change in both molecules, greatly facilitating the conversion of plasminogen to plasmin and dissolution of the clot. t-PA also manifests the property of fibrin affinity, that is, it binds strongly to fibrin. Other fibrinolytic agents such as prourokinase do not share this property of fibrin affinity.

Recombinant t-PA was produced in the 1980s after molecular cloning techniques were used to express human t-PA DNA. Activase® (Genentech), a predominantly single-chain form of rt-PA, was eventually approved in the USA for the indications of acute myocardial infarction and massive pulmonary embolism. rt-PA has been studied extensively in the setting of coronary occlusion. In the Global Use of Strategies To Open Occluded Coronary Arteries (GUSTO)-I study of approximately 41 000 patients with acute myocardial infarction, rt-PA was more effective than SK in achieving vascular patency.[31] Despite a slightly greater risk of intracranial hemorrhage with rt-PA, overall mortality was significantly reduced.

In an effort to lengthen the duration of bioavailability of t-PA, the molecule has been systematically bioengineered. Initial investigations identified regions in kringle 1 and the protease portion of t-PA that mediated hepatic clearance, fibrin specificity, and resistance to plasminogen activator inhibitor. Three sites were modified to create tenecteplase (TNK-tPA), a novel molecule with a greater half-life and fibrin specificity. The longer half-life of TNK-tPA allowed successful administration as a single bolus for acute myocardial infarction, in contrast to the requirement for an infusion with rt-PA. In addition, TNK-tPA manifests greater fibrin specificity than rt-PA, resulting in less fibrinogen depletion. In studies of acute coronary occlusion, TNK-tPA performed at least as well as rt-PA, concurrent with greater ease of administration.[32]

Similar to TNK-tPA, the novel recombinant plasminogen activator reteplase comprises the kringle 2 and protease domains of t-PA. Reteplase was developed with the goal of avoiding the necessity of a continuous intravenous infusion, thereby simplifying ease of administration. Reteplase (Retavase®, Centocor), produced in *E. coli* cells, is non-glycosylated, demonstrating a lower fibrin-binding activity and a diminished affinity for hepatocytes. This latter property accounts for a longer half-life than rt-PA, potentially enabling bolus injection versus prolonged infusion. The fibrin affinity of reteplase was only 30% of that exhibited with t-PA, similar to urokinase. The decrease in fibrin affinity was hypothesized to reduce the incidence of distant bleeding complications, in a manner similar to that of SK over rt-PA in the GUSTO trial.[31] In fact, several properties of reteplase may account for a decreased risk of hemorrhage, including poor lysis of platelet-rich, older clots.[33] To date, reteplase has demonstrated some benefit over rt-PA in the GUSTO III study for acute myocardial infarction.[34]

Miscellaneous agents

There exist a wide variety of novel thrombolytic agents, all of which have undergone extensive preclinical study but few of which have been evaluated in patients. Vampire bat plasminogen activator ('bat PA'), was cloned and expressed from the saliva of the vampire bat *Desmodus rotundus*.[35] This agent manifests extraordinary fibrin specificity, the plasminogenolytic activity being over 100 000 times greater in the presence of fibrin. The half-life of bat PA is five to nine times longer than that of rt-PA, offering some potential advantages with respect to ease of administration. To date, clinical trials have been limited to Phase I study with healthy volunteers.[36]

Fibrolase is a metalloproteinase, originating from venom of the southern copperhead snake.[37] It is a unique fibrinolytic agent which does not require plasminogen for its activity. Rather, the agent directly degrades fibrin without the requirement of any other blood components.[38] Since the agent is not dependent on plasminogen, older thrombi and those with low levels of plasminogen may be better treated with fibrolase than with the plasminogen activators. Fibrolase is inactivated by alpha-2 macroglobulin, potentially limiting the systemic effects of the agent when administered through a catheter-directed approach. There now exists a recombinant form of fibrolase, but to date no clinical trials have been completed.

Staphylokinase is a byproduct of *Staphylococcus aureus* bacterium, originally mentioned in the classic streptococcal fibrinolysin work of Tillett and Garner in 1933.[19] Staphylokinase has been produced by recombinant techniques and has been studied in the settings of myocardial infarction, peripheral arterial occlusion, and deep venous thrombosis.[39,40] Like SK, staphylokinase is inactive and must bind to plasminogen to activate other plasminogen molecules. Unlike SK, staphylokinase is relatively fibrin-specific and spares circulating plasminogen and fibrinogen. Unfortunately, staphylokinase is antigenic, although less so with certain recombinant mutants.

CLINICAL TRIALS OF THROMBOLYTIC THERAPY

There have been three well-controlled, randomized comparisons of thrombolytic therapy versus primary operation in patients with recent peripheral arterial occlusion. From the start, one must realize that thrombolytic therapy alone is seldom sufficient therapy. Successful pharmacologic dissolution of thrombus must be followed by definitive therapy to address the underlying lesion that caused the occlusion. In fact, when no such lesion can be found, the risk of early rethrombosis is unacceptably high.[41] As testimony to this caveat, Sullivan et al. observed post-

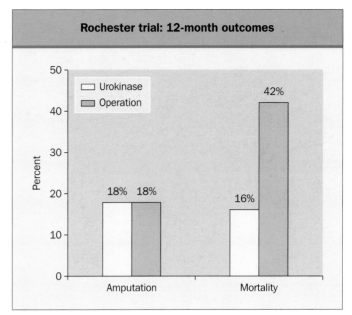

Figure 16.1 Rochester trial: 12-month outcomes. The rate of amputation was identical in the two treatment groups in the Rochester trial, but the mortality rate was significantly lower in patients assigned to thrombolytic therapy.

thrombolysis 2-year patency rates of 79% in bypass grafts with a flow-limiting lesion identified and corrected by angioplasty or surgery versus only 9.8% in patients without such lesions.

The first study of thrombolysis versus surgery, the Rochester series, compared urokinase to primary operation in 114 patients presenting with what has subsequently been called 'hyperacute ischemia'.[42] Enrolled patients in this trial all had severely threatened limbs (Rutherford Class IIb) with a mean symptom duration of approximately 2 days. This was a single-center trial that was funded by the Thrombolysis and Thrombosis Program Project NIH grant at the University of Rochester. After 12 months of follow-up, 84% of patients randomized to urokinase were alive, compared to only 58% of patients randomized to primary operation (**Fig. 16.1**). By contrast, the rate of limb salvage was identical at 80%. A closer inspection of the raw data revealed that the defining variable for mortality differences was the development of perioperative cardiopulmonary complications. The rate of long-term mortality was high when such complications occurred but was relatively low when they did not. It was only the fact that such complications occurred more commonly in patients taken directly to the operating theatre that explained the greater long-term mortality rate in the operative group.

The second prospective, randomized analysis of thrombolysis versus surgery was the Surgery or Thrombolysis for the Ischemic Lower Extremity (STILE) trial.[7] Genentech (South San Francisco, CA, USA), the manufacturer of the Activase brand of rt-PA, funded the study. At its termination, 393 patients were randomized to one of three treatment groups: rt-PA, urokinase, or primary operation. Subsequently, the two thrombolytic groups were combined for purposes of data analysis when the outcome was found to be similar. While the rate of the composite endpoint of untoward events was higher in the thrombolytic patients, the rate of the more relevant and objective endpoints

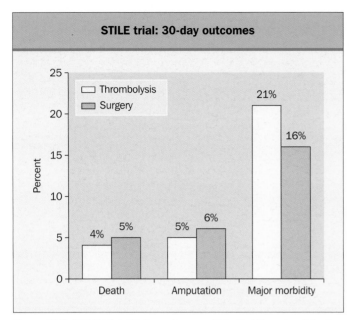

Figure 16.2 STILE trial: 30-day outcomes. Note that the rate of death and amputation are similar.

of amputation and death were equivalent (**Fig. 16.2**). Articles then appeared in the literature, comprising subgroup analyses of the STILE data, one relating to native artery occlusions[43] and one to bypass graft occlusions.[44] Thrombolysis appeared to be more effective in patients with graft occlusions. The rate of major amputation was higher in native arterial occlusions treated with thrombolysis (10% thrombolysis versus 0% surgery at 1 year; p=0.0024). By contrast, amputation was lower in patients with acute graft occlusions treated with thrombolysis

(p=0.026). These data suggest that thrombolysis may be of greatest benefit in patients with acute bypass graft occlusions of less than 14 days' duration.

The third and final randomized comparison of thrombolysis and surgery was the Thrombolysis Or Peripheral Arterial Surgery (TOPAS) trial, funded by Abbott Laboratories (Abbott Park, IL). Following completion of a preliminary dose-ranging trial in 213 patients,[45] 544 patients were randomized to a recombinant form of urokinase or primary operative intervention.[6] After a mean follow-up of 1 year, the rate of amputation-free survival was identical in the two treatment groups: 68.2% and 68.8% in the urokinase and surgical patients, respectively (**Table 16.4**). While this trial failed to document improvement in survival or limb salvage with thrombolysis, 31.5% of the thrombolytic patients were alive without amputation with nothing more than a percutaneous procedure after 6 months of follow-up (**Table 16.5**). After 1 year, this number had decreased only slightly, with 25.7% alive, without amputation and with only percutaneous interventions. Thus, the original goal of the TOPAS trial, to generate data on which regulatory approval of recombinant urokinase would be based, was not achieved. Nevertheless, the findings confirmed that acute leg ischemia could be managed with catheter-directed thrombolysis, achieving similar amputation and mortality rates but avoiding the need for an open surgical procedure in a significant percentage of patients.

Status of thrombolytic agents in the USA

Until a few years ago, in the USA, urokinase was the most commonly used agent for peripheral arterial indications. In late 1998, the United States Food and Drug Administration raised questions about the manufacturing of this agent. Abbott Laboratories, the manufacturer, voluntarily suspended shipment of urokinase. Manufacturing changes were made, and in late

Results of the TOPAS trial, demonstrating similar mortality rates and amputation-free survival rates after thrombolysis or surgery.

Intervention	Native artery occlusions (n=242)			Bypass graft occlusions (n=302)		
	Urokinase (n=122)	Surgery (n=120)	p value	Urokinase (n=150)	Surgery (n=152)	p value
Complete dissolution of clot on final angiogram – no./total no. of patients	67/112 (60%)	NA	–	100/134 (75%)	NA	–
Increase in ankle–brachial index*	0.44±0.04	0.52±0.04	0.15[†]	0.48±0.03	0.50±0.03	0.76[†]
Mortality (%):						
6 month	20.8	15.9	0.33[†]	12.1	9.4	0.45[†]
1 year	24.6	19.6	0.36[†]	16.2	15.0	0.77[†]
Amputation-free survival (%):						
6 month	67.6	76.1	0.15[†]	75.2	73.9	0.79[†]
1 year	61.2	71.4	0.10[†]	68.2	68.8	0.91[†]

*Mean ± standard error.
[†]The p value was based on one-way analysis of variance.
[†]The p value was based on Kaplan–Meier analysis.

Table 16.4 Results of the TOPAS trial, demonstrating similar mortality rates and amputation-free survival rates after thrombolysis or surgery. NA, not applicable. (Adapted from Ouriel et al.[6] Copyright © 2004 Massachusetts Medical Society. All rights reserved.)

The Thrombolysis Or Peripheral Arterial Surgery (TOPAS) trial.				
Intervention or outcome	*Urokinase group (n=272)*		*Surgery group (n=272)*	
	6 months	*1 year*	*6 months*	*1 year*
Operative intervention	*No. of interventions*			
Amputation	48	58	41	51
Above the knee	22	25	19	26
Below the knee	26	33	22	25
Open surgical procedures	315	351	551	590
Major	102	116	177	193
Moderate	89	98	136	145
Minor	124	137	238	252
Percutaneous procedures	128	135	55	70
Worst outcome[†]	*% of patients*			
Death	16.0	20.0	12.3	17.0
Amputation	12.2	15.0	12.9	13.1
Above the knee	5.6	6.5	6.1	7.5
Below the knee	6.6	8.5	6.8	5.6
Open surgical procedures	40.3	39.3	69.0	65.4
Major	23.6	24.3	39.3	39.3
Moderate	10.3	8.7	16.3	13.4
Minor	6.4	6.3	13.4	12.7
Endovascular procedures	16.9	15.4	2.1	1.7
Medical treatment alone	14.6	10.3	3.7	2.8

[†]Worst outcome is the most severe event that occurred over the specified time period.

Table 16.5 The Thrombolysis Or Peripheral Arterial Surgery (TOPAS) trial. The thrombolytic group in the TOPAS trial achieved similar rates of limb loss and mortality without the need for open surgical intervention in a significant number of patients. (Adapted from Ouriel et al.[6] Copyright © 2004 Massachusetts Medical Society. All rights reserved.)

2002, the agent was returned to the marketplace. At present, centers in the USA rely on urokinase, rt-PA, and reteplase when treating patients with peripheral arterial occlusions.

Comparison of thrombolytic agents

There have been few well-designed clinical comparisons of various thrombolytic agents in the peripheral vasculature. There exist a variety of in-vitro studies and retrospective clinical trials, most pointing to improved efficacy and safety of urokinase and rt-PA over SK.[46,47] In an analysis of data collected in a prospective, single institution registry at the Cleveland Clinic Foundation, urokinase demonstrated a diminished rate of bleeding complications when compared with rt-PA.[48] Efficacy was not evaluated in this trial.

There have been two prospective, randomized comparisons of urokinase and rt-PA, neither of which was blinded. Meyerovitz

and associates from the Brigham and Women's Hospital randomized 32 patients with peripheral arterial or bypass graft occlusions of less than 90 days' duration to rt-PA (10mg bolus, 5mg/hour to a maximum of 24 hours) or urokinase (60 000IU bolus, 4000IU/min for 2 hours, 2000IU/min for 2 hours, then 1000IU/min to a maximum of 24 hours' total administration).[49] There was significantly greater systemic fibrinogen degradation in the rt-PA group (p=0.01), indicating that the fibrin specificity of rt-PA was lost at this dose. rt-PA achieved more rapid initial thrombolysis, but efficacy was identical in the two groups by 24 hours. The trade-off to more rapid thrombolysis was a trend towards a higher rate of bleeding complications in the rt-PA treated patients (p=0.39)

The second randomized comparison of urokinase and rt-PA was the STILE trial, a three-armed multicenter comparison of urokinase (250 000IU bolus, 4000IU/min for 4 hours, then 2000IU/min for up to 36 hours), rt-PA (0.05 to 0.1mg/kg/hour for up to 12 hours) and primary operation.[7] There was one intracranial hemorrhage in the urokinase group (0.9%) and two in the rt-PA group (1.5%, no significant difference). Although actual rates of overall bleeding complications and efficacy were not reported for the two thrombolytic groups, the authors remarked that there were no significant differences detected in any of the outcome variables. In a subsequent 're-analysis' of the data, reported in 1999, the frequency of complete clot lysis was similar with urokinase and rt-PA at the time of the early arteriographic study.[50] This recent information suggests that the rate of thrombolysis may be similar, in contrast to the popularly held view that rt-PA is a much more rapidly acting agent.

A multicenter, blinded trial compared the results of thrombolysis with urokinase versus r-urokinase in 300 patients with peripheral arterial occlusion.[51] These data were never published. There were no significant differences noted between the two agents. A North American multicenter trial compared three different doses of r-prourokinase to urokinase in 241 patients with lower extremity arterial occlusions of fewer than 14 days' duration.[8] While the higher r-prourokinase dose was associated with a slightly greater percentage of patients with complete (>95%) clot lysis at 8 hours, there was a mild increase in the rate of bleeding complications compared with either the urokinase or the lower dose r-prourokinase groups. The fibrinogen levels fell in the higher r-prourokinase group, suggesting that fibrin specificity is lost at the higher doses of this compound.

SUMMARY

Knowledge of the properties of the thrombolytic agents and the clinical trials that compare the agents to one another and to surgical therapy is prerequisite to the appropriate care of patients with peripheral arterial occlusion. Thrombolytic agents offer a less invasive approach to thrombotic occlusions, with the opportunity to address the unmasked, causative lesions directly. Correction of these lesions can often be accomplished through an endovascular approach such as percutaneous angioplasty and stenting. Even when a new bypass graft must be placed, the procedure can frequently be performed in an elective setting after adequate patient preparation. Following clinical principles based on objective data should result in improved outcome for patients with peripheral arterial occlusion.

REFERENCES

1. Blaisdell FW, Steele M, Allen RE. Management of acute lower extremity arterial ischemia due to embolism and thrombosis. Surgery 1978; 84:822–34.

2. Jivegård L, Holm J, Scherstén T. Acute limb ischemia due to arterial embolism or thrombosis: influence of limb ischemia versus pre-existing cardiac disease on postoperative mortality rate. J Cardiovasc Surg 1988;29:32–6.

3. Holm J, Scherstén T. Anticoagulant treatment during and after embolectomy. Acta Chir Scand 1972;138:683–7.

4. Caruana JA, Gutierrez IZ, Andersen MN, et al. Factors that affect the outcome of peripheral arterial embolization. Arch Surg 1981;116:423–50.

5. Ouriel K, Shortell CK, DeWeese JA, et al. A comparison of thrombolytic therapy with operative revascularization in the initial treatment of acute peripheral arterial ischemia. J Vasc Surg 1994; 19:1021–30.

6. Ouriel K, Veith FJ, Sasahara AA. A comparison of recombinant urokinase with vascular surgery as initial treatment for acute arterial occlusion of the legs. N Engl J Med 1998;338:1105–11.

7. Anonymous. Results of a prospective randomized trial evaluating surgery versus thrombolysis for ischemia of the lower extremity. The STILE trial. Ann Surg 1994;220:251–66.

8. Ouriel K, Kandarpa K, Schuerr DM, Hultquist M, Hodkinson G, Wallin B. Prourokinase versus urokinase for recanalization of peripheral occlusions, safety and efficacy: the PURPOSE trial. J Vasc Interv Radiol 1999;10:1083–91.

9. Ouriel, K, Veith, FJ. Acute lower limb ischemia: determinants of outcome. Surgery 1998;124:336–42.

10. Dormandy J, Heeck L, Vig S. Acute limb ischemia. Semin Vasc Surg 1999;12:148–53.

11. McNamara TO, Fischer JR. Thrombolysis of peripheral arterial and graft occlusions: improved results using high-dose urokinase. AJR American Journal of Roentgenology 1985;144:769–75.

12. Semba CP, Murphy TP, Bakal CW, Calis KA, Matalon TA. Thrombolytic therapy with use of alteplase (rt-PA) in peripheral arterial occlusive disease: review of the clinical literature. The Advisory Panel. J Vasc Interv Radiol 2000;11:149–61.

13. Ouriel K, Katzen B, Mewissen MW, et al. Reteplase in the treatment of peripheral arterial and venous occlusions: a pilot study. J Vasc Interv Radiol 2000;11:849–54.

14. McNamara TO. Thombolysis as the initial treatment for acute lower limb ischemia. In: Comerota AJ, ed. Thrombolytic therapy for peripheral vascular disease. Philadelphia:JB Lippincott Company; 1995:253–68.

15. Faggioli GL, Peer RM, Pedrini L, et al. Failure of thrombolytic therapy to improve long-term vascular patency. J Vasc Surg 1994;19:289–96.

16. Korn P, Khilnani NM, Fellers JC, et al. Thrombolysis for native arterial occlusions of the lower extremities: clinical outcome and cost. J Vasc Surg 2001;33:1148–57.

17. Milstone H. A factor in normal human blood which participates in streptococcal fibrinolysis. J Immunol 1941;42:116.

18. Onundarson PT, Haraldsson HM, Bergmann L, Francis CW, Marder VJ. Plasminogen depletion during streptokinase treatment or two-chain urokinase incubation correlates with decreased clot lysability ex vivo and in vitro. Thromb Haemost 1993;70:998–1004.

19. Tillett WS, Garner RL The fibrinolytic activity of hemolytic streptococci. J Exp Med 1933;58:485–502.

20. Tillett WS, Sherry S. The effect in patients of streptococcal fibrinolysin (streptokinase) and streptococcal desoxyribonuclease on fibrinous, purulent, and sanguinous pleural exudations. J Clin Invest 1949;28:173.

21. Tillett WS, Johnson AJ, McCarty WR. The intravenous infusion of the streptococcal fibrinolytic principle (streptokinase) into patients. J Clin Invest 1955;34:169–85.

22. Cliffton EE. The use of plasmin in humans. Ann NY Acad Sci 1957; 68:209–29.

23. Jostring H, Barth U, Naidu R. Changes of antistreptokinase titer following long-term streptokinase therapy. In: Martin M, Schoop W, Hirsh J, eds. New concepts of streptokinase dosimetry. Vienna:Hans Huber; 1978:110.

24. Smith RAG, Dupe RJ, English PD, Green J. Fibrinolysis with acyl-enzymes: a new approach to thrombolytic therapy. Nature 1981;290:505.

25. ISIS-3 Collaborative Group. ISIS-3: a randomized comparison of strepto-kinase vs tissue plasminogen activator vs anistreplase and of aspirin plus heparin vs aspirin alone among 41,299 cases of suspected acute myocardial infarction. Lancet 1992;339:753.

26. Macfarlane RG, Pinot JJ. Fibrinolytic activity of normal urine. Nature 1947;159:779.

27. Sobel GW, Mohler SR, Jones NW, Dowdy ABC, Guest MM. Urokinase: an activator of plasma fibrinolysin extracted from urine. Am J Physiol 1952;171:768–9.

28. Credo RB, Burke SE, Barker WM, et al. Recombinant urokinase (r-UK): biochemistry, pharmacology, and clinical experience. In: Sasahara AA, Loscalzo J, eds. New therapeutic agents in thrombosis and thrombolysis. New York:Marcel Dekker, Inc; 1997:513–37.

29. Husain SS, Lipinski B, Gurewich V, inventors. Isolation of plasminogen activators useful as therapeutic and diagnostic agents (single-chair, high-fibrin affinity urokinase).1979 US Patent 4,381,346.

30. Hoylaerts M, Rijken DC, Lijnen HR, Collen D. Kinetics of the activation of plasminogen by human tissue plasminogen activator: role of fibrin. J Biol Chem 1982;257:2912.

31. The GUSTO Investigators. An international randomized trial comparing four thrombolytic therapies for acute myocardial infarction. N Engl J Med 1993;329:673–82.

32. Cannon CP, Gibson CM, McCabe CH, et al. TNK-tissue plasminogen activator compared with front-loaded alteplase in acute myocardial infarction: results of the TIMI 10B trial. Thrombolysis in Myocardial Infarction (TIMI) 10B Investigators. Circulation 1998;98:2805–14.

33. Meierhenrich R, Carlsson J, Seifried E, et al. Effect of reteplase on hemostasis variables: analysis of fibrin specificity, relation to bleeding complications and coronary patency. Int J Cardiol 1998;65:57–63.

34. Anonymous. A comparison of reteplase with alteplase for acute myocardial infarction. The Global Use of Strategies to Open Occluded Coronary Arteries (GUSTO III) Investigators. N Engl J Med 1997; 337:1118–23.

35. Gardell SL, Duong LT, Diehl RE. Isolation, characterization and cDNA cloning of a vampire bat salivary plasminogen activator. J Biol Chem 1989;264:17947–52.

36. Schleuning WD, Bhargava A, Donner P. Desmodus rotundus (Vampire Bat) plasminogen activator DSPAalpha$_1$: A superior thrombolytic created by evolution. In: Sasahara AA, Loscalzo J, eds. New therapeutic agents in thrombosis and thrombolysis. New York:Marcel Dekker, Inc; 1997:603–23.

37. Ahmed NK, Gaddis RR, Tennant KD, Lacz JP. Biological and thrombolytic properties of fibrolase – a new fibrinolytic protease from snake venom. Haemostasis 1990;20:334–40.

38. Ahmed NK, Tennant KD, Markland FS, Lacz JP. Biochemical characteristics of fibrolase, a fibrinolytic protease from snake venom. Haemostasis 1990;20:147–54.

39. Heymans S, Verhaeghe R, Stockx L, Collen D. Feasibility study of catheter-directed thrombolysis with recombinant staphylokinase in deep venous thrombosis. Thromb Haemost 1998;79:517–9.

40. Heymans S, Vanderschueren S, Verhaeghe R, et al. Outcome and one year follow-up of intra-arterial staphylokinase in 191 patients with peripheral arterial occlusion. Thromb Haemost 2000;83:666–71.

41. Sullivan KL, Gardiner GAJ, Kandarpa K, et al. Efficacy of thrombolysis in infrainguinal bypass grafts. Circulation 1991;83(2:Suppl): I99-105.

42. Ouriel K; Shortell CK; DeWeese JA, et al. A comparison of thrombolytic therapy with operative revascularization in the initial treatment of acute peripheral arterial ischemia. J Vasc Surg 1994;19:1021–30.

43. Weaver FA, Comerota AJ, Youngblood M, Froehlich J, Hosking JD, Papanicolaou G. Surgical revascularization versus thrombolysis for nonembolic lower extremity native artery occlusions: results of a prospective randomized trial. The STILE Investigators. Surgery versus Thrombolysis for Ischemia of the Lower Extremity. J Vasc Surg 1996;24:513–21.

44. Comerota AJ, Weaver FA, Hosking JD et al. Results of a prospective, randomized trial of surgery versus thrombolysis for occluded lower extremity bypass grafts. Am J Surg 1996;172:105–12.

45. Ouriel K, Veith FJ, Sasahara AA. Thrombolysis or peripheral arterial surgery: phase I results. TOPAS Investigators. J Vasc Surg 1996;23:64–73.

46. van Breda A, Robison JC, Feldman L, et al. Local thrombolysis in the treatment of arterial graft occlusions. J Vasc Surg 1984;1:103–12.

47. Ouriel K, Welch EL, Shortell CK, Geary K, Fiore WM, Cimino C. Comparison of streptokinase, urokinase, and recombinant tissue plasminogen activator in an in vitro model of venous thrombolysis. J Vasc Surg 1995;22:593–7.

48. Ouriel K, Gray BH, Clair DG, Olin JW. Complications associated with the use of urokinase and recombinant tissue plasminogen activator for catheter-directed peripheral arterial and venous thrombolysis. J Vasc Intervent Radiol 2000;11:295–8.

49. Meyerovitz M, Goldhaber SZ, Reagan K, et al. Recombinant tissue-type plasminogen activator versus urokinase in peripheral arterial and graft occlusions: a randomized trial. Radiology 1990;175:75–8.

50. Comerota AJ. A re-analysis of the STILE data. Presentation given at the Montefiore Symposium, New York, NY, USA; 1999.

51. Abbott Laboratories Venture Group. A comparison of urokinase and recombinant urokinase in the treatment of peripheral arterial occlusion. Data on file, Abbott Laboratories; 1994.

CHAPTER

17

Practical Techniques in Surgical and Endovascular Management of Acute Limb Ischemia

Jonathan D Beard and Jonothan J Earnshaw

KEY POINTS

- The practical management of acute leg ischemia remains a challenge, as it involves one of the most complex decision pathways in vascular surgery.

- A successful outcome depends upon an experienced team (vascular radiologist and surgeon) with access to, and the ability to use, the full range of available techniques.

- Treatment should be based on the severity of the ischemia rather than the underlying cause.

- An arteriogram should be obtained in all patients with a threatened limb, time and availability permitting.

- The arteriogram catheter must not be removed until a decision on the treatment pathway (percutaneous or surgical) has been agreed.

- The role of conventional balloon catheter embolectomy is diminishing due to the decreasing incidence of cardiac embolism and the proliferation of new endovascular techniques.

- Despite several large trials, the precise role of each treatment modality remains unclear.

INTRODUCTION

The question of whether thrombolysis is better than surgery for acute limb ischemia (ALI) has been addressed by large randomized studies such as the Surgery or Thrombolysis for the Ischemic Lower Extremity (STILE) and the Thrombolysis Or Peripheral Arterial Surgery (TOPAS) trials (see Chapter 16). Like all new therapies, thrombolysis was adopted with great enthusiasm, followed by increasing caution. The question remains as to what is the precise role of each of the treatments and their relationship to each other. Many patients with ALI require a combination of endovascular and conventional surgery; thrombolysis may reveal a chronic occlusion that requires surgical bypass. Although the incidence of ALI seems to be increasing, the role of conventional balloon catheter embolectomy is diminishing. The reasons for this include:

- availability of percutaneous techniques such as thrombolysis, aspiration thrombectomy, and mechanical thrombectomy;
- less frequent cardiac embolism due to rheumatic heart disease; and
- more frequent thrombosis due to the increasing incidence of peripheral arterial disease (PAD) and bypass grafting.

Patients with cardiac embolism may also suffer from PAD as atherosclerosis is frequently systemic. This increases the difficulty in establishing the cause of the ischemia (see Chapter 15).

The implication of all these changes is that 'blind' embolectomy by a trainee surgeon is no longer acceptable as a treatment for ALI. The management of ALI can involve one of the most complex decision pathways in vascular surgery. A successful outcome depends upon an experienced team (vascular radiologist and surgeon) with access to, and the ability to use, the full range of available techniques. Outcome seems best when decisions about treatment are made based on the severity of the ischemia, rather than the cause.

SELECTION OF TREATMENT

The severity of leg ischemia is often defined according to the Society of Vascular Surgery/International Society for Cardiovascular Surgery (SVS/ISCVS) criteria.[1] This classification is useful for reporting results but is of less use when planning treatment. The TransAtlantic Inter-Society Consensus (TASC) recommends three categories based on the severity of ischemia[2] as this, rather than the underlying cause, determines the care pathway; these categories are described below.

1) Viable leg

There is acute onset of a painful, cold leg but no neurologic deficit and an audible arterial Doppler signal at the ankle. The cause is often acute thrombosis of an atherosclerotic artery or previous bypass graft. Such patients can be treated with anticoagulation while awaiting urgent arteriography. Thromboembolectomy is unlikely to successfully treat thombosis of a stenosed artery or graft. The therapeutic alternatives in these patients are surgical reconstruction or percutaneous thrombolysis.

2) Threatened leg

There is usually loss of sensation, variable loss of motor function, and no audible arterial Doppler signal at the ankle. These patients require emergency intervention, especially if the calf muscles are tender. An acute white leg with no prior history of claudication, normal contralateral pulses, and atrial fibrillation makes embolism the likely cause but in many cases it is difficult to differentiate between embolism and thrombosis (Fig. 17.1). There is some debate about whether preoperative angiography provides beneficial information or wastes valuable time. When the femoral pulse is absent, imaging helps to exclude alternative diagnoses, such as dissection, and to plan inflow surgery or

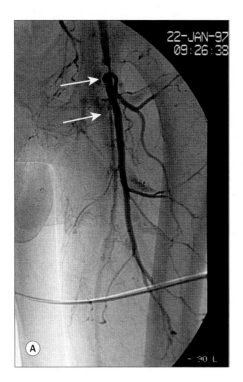

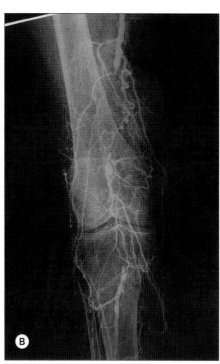

Figure 17.1 (A) Angiogram of a typical embolus lodged at the bifurcation of the common femoral artery (CFA) (arrows) with poor filling of the superficial femoral artery (SFA) below this. Contrast this appearance with a typical thrombosis of the popliteal artery (B). The extensive collaterals suggest a pre-existing stenosis.

stenting. Patients without motor loss can also be treated with accelerated thrombolysis if a suitable lesion is found, while percutaneous aspiration embolectomy and mechanical thrombectomy are now alternatives to conventional balloon catheter thromboembolectomy. Therefore, there are good reasons for all such patients to undergo arteriography, when time and availability permit. The arteriogram catheter should not be removed until a decision on the treatment pathway (percutaneous or surgical) has been agreed. Otherwise, the puncture site may bleed if thrombolysis is performed subsequently.

3) Dead leg
This is irreversible acute ischemia, with a complete neurologic deficit of the leg, tense muscles, and fixed skin staining. Such patients require resuscitation and amputation if they are to survive but the prognosis is often poor. Terminal care seems to be the kindest option for moribund patients with severe comorbidity.[3]

Thrombosed popliteal aneurysm
The presence of an easily palpable contralateral popliteal pulse or an ipsilateral popliteal mass raises the possibility of a thrombosed popliteal aneurysm (**Fig. 17.2**). Duplex ultrasound imaging will confirm the diagnosis. The bulk of thrombus within the aneurysm restricts the use of thrombolysis because of the high risk of massive distal embolization,[4] the slow clearance, and large amount of residual thrombus after recanalization. If thrombolysis does have a role to play, then it is to open runoff vessels for distal bypass grafting. This is achieved by placing a catheter through the popliteal artery into a tibial vessel and then lysing it until a distal vessel becomes patent for bypass. Alternatively, surgical exploration may be performed, with intraoperative angiography and thrombolysis to clear the runoff,[5] prior to exclusion bypass.

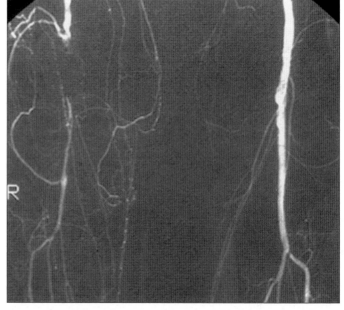

Figure 17.2 Angiogram showing occlusion of a right popliteal aneurysm. The ectatic left popliteal artery provides a clue to the diagnosis. A duplex scan confirmed thrombosis of a 3cm popliteal aneurysm.

Ischemic arm
Acute limb ischemia of the arm is usually embolic in origin, as PAD of the upper limb is rare. The same classification regarding the severity of ischemia can be used, but most patients with features sufficiently severe to warrant intervention can proceed to balloon catheter thromboembolectomy without an arteriogram. The exception are those with an absent subclavian pulse. Some surgeons advise initial conservative treatment with anticoagulation, and operation only if the arm does not improve. There is

a risk that a patient will be left with neurologic symptoms and forearm claudication if a threatened limb is left untreated.[6]

GENERAL MANAGEMENT

Patients presenting with ALI are often in poor general health, which is one reason why the condition has such a high mortality rate, often from associated cardiovascular disease. Blood should be taken for full blood count, coagulation profile, urea, electrolytes, and glucose. An electrocardiogram (EKG) and chest radiograph should be requested, a central venous cannula and urethral catheter inserted, and monitoring with an EKG and pulse oximetry commenced. Twenty-four per cent oxygen should be given by face mask, as there is some experimental evidence of its benefit.[7] Further oxygen therapy is determined by the results of blood gas analysis.

Dehydration is common and is treated with an intravenous infusion of 5% dextrose by central venous line, if indicated, together with appropriate treatment of cardiac failure and/or arrhythmia with diuretics and digoxin. An adequate diuresis will also reduce the risk of renal impairment due to contrast toxicity. Morphine is usually required for pain relief and is best given by an intravenous pump. Intramuscular analgesia should be avoided because of the risk of bleeding if thrombolysis is used. Intravenous unfractionated heparin (5000U) should be given immediately, followed by a heparin infusion to maintain an activated partial thromboplastin time ratio of >2. The aim is to restrict propagation of thrombus and reduce the risk of futher embolization (if this is the cause); there is some evidence that heparinization improves the prognosis.[8] Anticoagulation may, however, prevent the use of epidural anesthesia if surgery is required. Many patients are not fit for general anesthesia and an epidural also provides excellent postoperative analgesia. Heparin may be withheld temporarily if surgery under epidural is contemplated.[2]

SURGICAL MANAGEMENT

With the increasing age of the population, underlying atherosclerosis often complicates ischemia, even if the cause is primarily embolic. Consequently, complex secondary procedures may well be necessary if initial balloon catheter thromboembolectomy fails. Operation under local anesthesia may be preferred in a slim patient with a clear-cut embolus and high cardiac risk but although wound analgesia can be achieved, the embolectomy and arteriography remain painful. Pain during embolectomy and arteriography can be abolished by intra-arterial injection of plain 1% lidocaine (lignocaine).[9] An anesthetist should always be present during surgery (even when done under local anesthetic) to monitor the EKG and oxygen saturation, administer sedation or analgesia, and convert to general anesthesia, if required. Obesity, confusion, and the likelihood of additional procedures seem to be good reasons for general or epidural anesthesia.

Femoral artery exploration

Femoral embolectomy remains the standard surgical treatment for lower-limb threatening ALI. Both groin and entire leg should be prepared to permit surgical access and intraoperative arteriography. The foot is placed in a sterile transparent bag for easy inspection. The common femoral artery bifurcation is exposed via

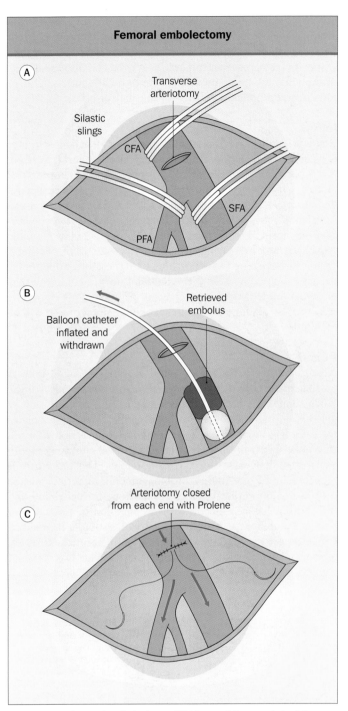

Femoral embolectomy

Figure 17.3 Femoral embolectomy. (A) Via an oblique groin incision, a transverse arteriotomy is made in a soft portion of the CFA, after control of the bifurcation with slings. (B) The thromboembolus is retrieved by gentle inflation and withdrawal of the balloon catheter. The arteriotomy is closed with 4/0 Prolene from each end, after flushing with heparinized saline (C). CFA, common femoral artery; SFA, superficial femoral artery.

an oblique groin incision, which reduces wound-healing problems, and the vessels controlled with silastic slings (**Fig. 17.3**). It is important to take care not to damage the long saphenous vein and its lateral tributary. The former may be required for a bypass graft and the latter can be used to patch the arteriotomy, if the femoral artery is severely diseased. Clamps should be avoided initially because they fragment thrombus that may otherwise be removed intact. A transverse arteriotomy is made in the common femoral artery proximal to the bifurcation, avoiding any obvious plaque. A transverse arteriotomy is easier to close without narrowing and it can be converted to a diamond shape for proximal anastomosis if a bypass is required. Any thrombus at the bifurcation can be removed by gentle suction or forceps and momentary release of the sling or clamp.

Inflow

If pulsatile inflow is not present then a 5F or 6F balloon catheter is passed proximally up the iliac artery into the aorta, inflated, and withdrawn. Pressure should be applied to the contralateral femoral artery during this procedure to prevent contralateral embolization. A saddle embolus of the aortic bifurcation can usually be retrieved by bilateral femoral embolectomy, withdrawing both balloons simultaneously to prevent the saddle embolus from ball-valving from side to side. If the catheter cannot be passed up the iliac artery, then the surgeon should try to shape the tip into a 'J'. If this does not work, a guidewire may be passed under fluoroscopic control. If good inflow cannot be achieved, then a femoro-femoral or axillofemoral bypass will be required.

Runoff

Next, a 3F or 4F balloon catheter is passed as far distally as possible down both the profunda and superficial femoral arteries. Force should not be used if resistance is met, as dissection or perforation may result. The balloon should be inflated only as the catheter is withdrawn, and the amount of inflation adjusted to avoid excessive intimal friction. Inflation of the balloon with air is safer than saline for the same reason. The procedure is repeated until no more thromboembolic material can be retrieved. Conventional embolectomy is performed blind and the surgeon has no control over the direction of the catheter past the popliteal trifurcation.[10] Use of an end-hole balloon catheter permits selective catheterization of the tibial arteries, over a guidewire, under fluoroscopic control (**Fig. 17.4**). Use of a guidewire also reduces the risk of an intimal dissection. It is

better to fill the artery with contrast and leave the balloon filled with air, which can then be seen as a negative image. Filling the balloon with contrast makes inflation and deflation difficult, due to the viscosity of the contrast.

Completion arteriography

A completion arteriogram should always be performed because persistent thrombus may be present even if the catheter passes to the foot.[11] Backbleeding is of no prognostic value as it may arise from established proximal collaterals. Most operating theaters now have excellent fluoroscopic facilities capable of high-quality arteriography. If a C-arm image intensifier is not available, the surgeon can use a film cassette wrapped in a towel under the leg, centred on the knee. Fifty milliliters of contrast medium infused rapidly down the superficial femoral artery (SFA) via a Tibbs cannula or umbilical catheter, with a silastic snugger to prevent backflow, will give good images of the distal vessels. If the SFA is chronically occluded, contrast can be infused down the profunda femoris artery. The contrast should be flushed out with 100mL of heparin saline and if no thrombus is present, the arteriotomy is closed with 5/0 Prolene. The surgeon should use a double needle suture cut in two, starting from each corner of the arteriotomy, remembering to pass the needles from in to out on the distal side of the arteriotomy to avoid an intimal flap. On removing the clamps the foot should become pink with palpable pulses.

Intraoperative thrombolysis

If the arteriogram shows persistent occlusion (usually at the popliteal trifurcation), an infusion of 100 000U of streptokinase or 10mg of recombinant tissue plasminogen activator (r-tPA) in 100mL heparin saline can be given via the Tibbs cannula or umbilical catheter in boluses over 30 minutes and the arteriogram repeated (**Fig. 17.5**). This results in complete lysis in about a third of cases and partial lysis facilitating further embolectomy

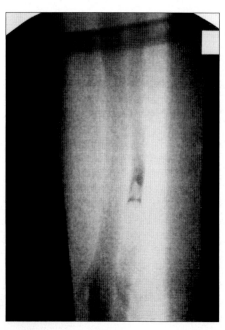

Figure 17.4 Balloon catheter embolectomy using the 'negative contrast' method. The artery is filled with contrast and the air-filled balloon withdrawn under fluoroscopic control. The embolus and balloon show up clearly against the contrast-filled artery.

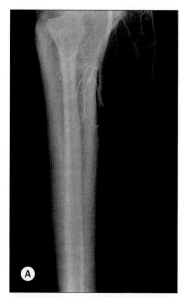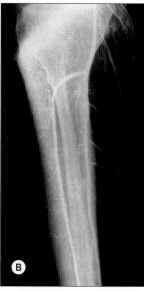

Figure 17.5 Intraoperative arteriogram after balloon catheter embolectomy, showing persistent occlusion of the popliteal trifurcation (A). A short infusion of 10mg rt-PA resulted in complete lysis of the residual thrombus (B).

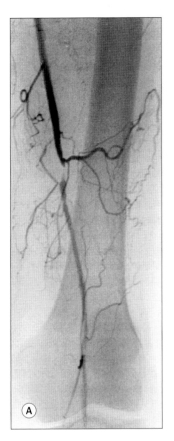

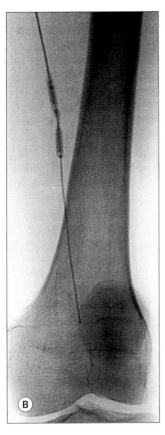

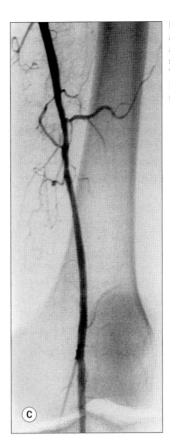

Figure 17.6 Intraoperative angiogram after balloon catheter embolectomy and lysis showing an underlying severe stenosis of the distal SFA (A). This was succesfully treated by intraoperative balloon angioplasty (B and C).

or bypass in another third.[12–14] The technique may also be used to lyse residual thrombus in the tibial arteries during popliteal exploration or repair of a popliteal aneurysm.[5] Intraoperative thrombolysis seems effective because the lack of blood flow ensures a high concentration of lytic agent despite the low dose, which reduces the problem of systemic bleeding complications. If an underlying stenosis of the superficial femoral artery is revealed, on-table balloon angioplasty may be attempted (**Fig. 17.6**). Thrombolysis may also be continued postoperatively in patients with no 'reflow' after thromboembolectomy. Law et al[15] used 58 000U/hour of urokinase and achieved limb salvage in seven of 12 patients. The angiographic appearance of blushing or tufting due to extravasation of contrast from the muscle capillaries is a bad prognostic sign.

Popliteal exploration

Persistent distal occlusion requires exploration of the below-knee popliteal artery. A skin incision is made on the medial side of the knee, extending down from the femoral condyle, making sure to preserve the long saphenous vein. The origins of the anterior tibial artery, tibioperoneal trunk, posterior tibial artery, and peroneal artery should be controlled with slings. Access often requires extensive dissection and division of the anterior tibial vein which crosses in front of the trifurcation (**Fig. 17.7**). If the popliteal artery is disease-free, a transverse arteriotomy may be used, but this is rarely the case. A longitudinal arteriotomy is usually the best option, as it can be extended into the tibioperoneal trunk, if required. Selective embolectomy of each tibial artery is performed with a 2F or 3F catheter. Thrombus lodged at the adductor hiatus may also be successfully retrieved retrogradely via a popliteal embolectomy if the femoral approach

fails. Persistent occlusion of the SFA and/or popliteal artery will require a femoropopliteal/tibial bypass graft. A longitudinal popliteal arteriotomy should be repaired with a vein patch. The fascial layer should not be closed and if there is any suggestion of muscle tension, the skin incision should also be left open.

Tibial embolectomy

Tibial embolectomy should be considered if embolectomy and/or intraoperative thrombolysis via the popliteal artery fail because of distal mature thrombus or atheroembolism (trash foot). The anterior and posterior tibial arteries are exposed at the ankle level via short vertical incisions. A 2F embolectomy catheter is passed up to the popliteal level and down into the foot via a small transverse arteriotomy.[16,17] It is important to take care not to split the arteriotomy when withdrawing the balloon. Simms performed tibial embolectomy in 22/233 surgical procedures for ALI. Overall limb salvage was only 50% at 6 months but six of seven trashed feet were salvaged (unpublished data). Wyfells et al. employed an adjuvant intraoperative infusion of urokinase during 16 tibial embolectomies in 12 legs and continued the infusion postoperatively in 14 arteries that did not lyse after the intraoperative bolus.[18] Four patients required concomitant bypass grafting and four required transfusion for bleeding.

Upper limb embolectomy

Upper limb embolectomy is usually performed via the brachial approach. This can normally be done under local anesthesia but the same requirements regarding monitoring and the presence of an anesthetist apply.[6] The entire arm, axilla, and supraclavicular fossa should be prepared and the arm placed on a board with the hand in a transparent bowel bag. Surgical exposure is via a lazy

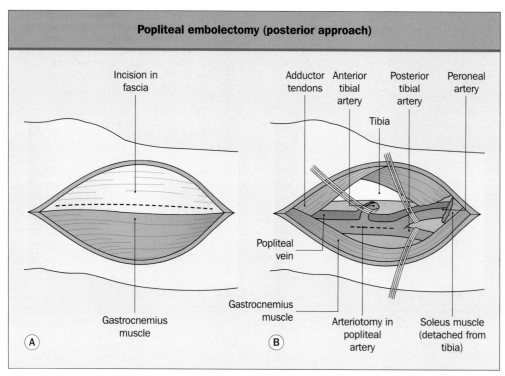

Popliteal embolectomy (posterior approach)

Incision in fascia

Gastrocnemius muscle

(A)

Adductor tendons Anterior tibial artery Posterior tibial artery Peroneal artery

Tibia

Popliteal vein

Gastrocnemius muscle

Arteriotomy in popliteal artery

Soleus muscle (detached from tibia)

(B)

Figure 17.7 Popliteal embolectomy. The medial incision extends down from the femoral condyle and is deepened by incising the fascia anterior to gastrocnemius (A). Division of the proximal attachment of the soleus to the back of the tibia and one of the tibial veins is required to completely expose the popliteal trifurcation (B). The arteriotomy must cross the origin of the anterior tibial artery and requires closure with a vein patch.

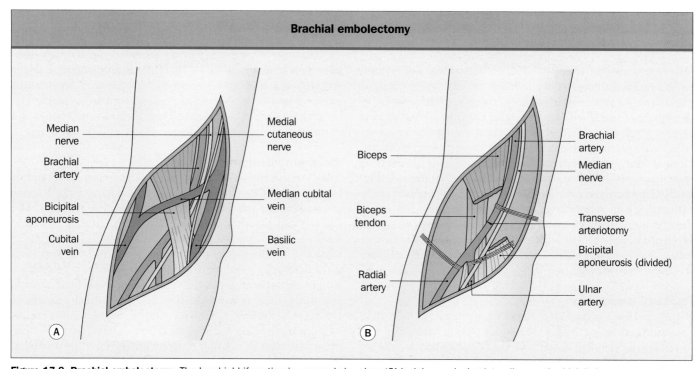

Brachial embolectomy

Median nerve

Brachial artery

Bicipital aponeurosis

Cubital vein

(A)

Medial cutaneous nerve

Median cubital vein

Basilic vein

Biceps

Biceps tendon

Radial artery

(B)

Brachial artery

Median nerve

Transverse arteriotomy

Bicipital aponeurosis (divided)

Ulnar artery

Figure 17.8 Brachial embolectomy. The brachial bifurcation is exposed via a lazy 'S' incision, swinging laterally over the bicipital aponeurosis to end in the midline (A). The bifurcation is controlled with slings after division of the bicipital aponeurosis, taking care to protect the median nerve. A 120 degree transverse arteriotomy should be made proximal to the bifurcation and then closed with 6/0 interrupted Prolene sutures (B).

'S' incision swinging laterally over the bicipital aponeurosis to end in the midline, over the bifurcation of the brachial artery (**Fig. 17.8**). The medial cutaneous nerve of the forearm and cubital veins should be preserved if possible. Damage to the nerve results in an irritating paresthesia and the vein is a useful conduit or patch. Additional local anesthetic may result in a temporary median nerve palsy, which should be anticipated.

The brachial artery and the origins of the radial and ulnar arteries are controlled with silastic slings, and clamps should be avoided if possible. A transverse arteriotomy is made proximal to the bifurcation and a 3F or 4F embolectomy catheter passed up the brachial artery if pulsatile inflow is not present. The runoff is then cleared with a 2F or 3F embolectomy guided selectively down the radial and ulnar arteries in turn. The arteriotomy is closed using interrupted 6/0 Prolene. Hematoma formation is common, so it is wise to apply a well-padded crepe bandage, after carefully checking that the radial pulse is present.

Failed brachial embolectomy is rare, as the runoff vessels are accessible, but occasionally distal embolectomy is required via the radial artery at the wrist. Failure to establish inflow should raise the possibility of a subclavian aneurysm or chronic proximal disease. This is the reason why the subclavian pulse should be palpated and a preoperative arteriogram or duplex scan requested if a proximal aneurysm or occlusion is suspected. Sometimes a larger embolus lodged in the axillary or subclavian artery cannot be retrieved via the smaller caliber brachial artery. This will require retrieval via an axillary or supraclavicular approach.

Fasciotomy

Revascularization of ischemic muscle can result in considerable swelling within the fascial compartments of the leg. This compartment syndrome will lead to further muscle and nerve damage if not relieved. All muscle compartments should be decompressed via full-length skin and fascial incisions from knee to ankle if any muscle tenseness is present, or when ischemia has been prolonged (see Chapter 18).[19]

FURTHER MANAGEMENT

The operating surgeon should document the pulse status of the limb at the end of the operation. The surgeon should also decide whether reintervention is worthwhile if it becomes clear that reperfusion is inadequate. The wounds, pulse status, color, and capillary refilling of the extremity should be documented hourly. Wound hematomas are common because of anticoagulation,[20] and are best drained unless small.

Revascularization of an ischemic limb results in a sudden venous return of blood with low pH and a high potassium concentration. The anesthetist must be prepared to correct these, as hypotension and arrhythmias may occur. Reperfusion of a large mass of ischemic tissue results in a systemic inflammatory reaction caused by neutrophil activation. This may cause multiple organ dysfunction including renal and pulmonary failure (see

Chapter 18). Initial reperfusion with a hypertonic perfusate containing anti-oxidants, combined with venous drainage, reduces this systemic injury.[21] Renal function may be further impaired by myoglobinuria and this can be avoided by maintaining a good diuresis but it is important to beware of pushing a patient with poor cardiac reserve into heart failure. Established renal failure will require hemofiltration and/or dialysis. Careful monitoring on a high-dependency unit is beneficial for all patients with significant co-morbidity. Inotropes may be required for cardiac or renal support.

Following embolectomy, anticoagulation with unfractionated heparin and then warfarin is continued as this reduces the risk of recurrent embolism, especially if atrial fibrillation (AF) is present.[20,22,23] A search for a proximal source should be undertaken in patients with clearcut embolism who do not have AF. This includes an abdominal ultrasound scan to exclude an aneurysm, a 24-hour EKG to exclude paroxysmal arrythmias, and an echocardiogram to exclude cardiac thrombus or valvular pathology. There is little evidence regarding the role of anticoagulation in patients without AF.[24] In many patients, an individual decision will need to be made, based on the risks of warfarinization and the state of the distal circulation.

INTRA-ARTERIAL THROMBOLYSIS

Standard low-dose thrombolysis

Every radiologist who undertakes intra-arterial thrombolysis will have their own personal method. Each will use a subtly different technique but the following schedule emphasizes the important components of an episode of intra-arterial thrombolysis (see **Fig. 17.9**).[25]

Preoperative diagnosis

The diagnosis of acute leg ischemia is normally a clinical one. It is necessary to confirm the diagnosis, usually by intra-arterial angiography. There are advantages in using non-invasive methods such as duplex imaging or magnetic resonance angiography. These techniques, however, are often not available in an emergency. The principle of investigation is to establish the length and site

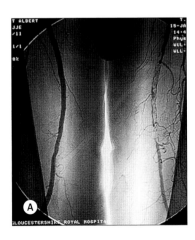

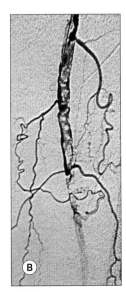

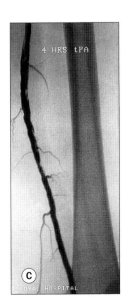

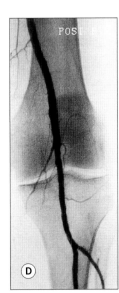

Figure 17.9 Low-dose intra-arterial thrombolysis.
(A) Superficial femoral artery thrombosis of 14 days' duration.
(B) Thrombogram after catheter insertion.
(C) After 4-hour lysis with t-PA 0.5mg/hour, the superficial femoral artery was patent but with a mid-point stenosis.
(D) Good result after angioplasty.

of obstruction and the presence of any runoff vessels. This can be difficult in patients with acute leg ischemia whose distal vessels do not opacify due to the lack of collaterals. If angiography is used, the radiologist should minimize the number of arterial punctures and use small arterial catheters without a sheath, to reduce the risk of subsequent bleeding.

Catheter insertion
Once the diagnosis is confirmed, an infusion catheter needs to be inserted within the arterial obstruction. The occlusion is usually approached from the contralateral groin if it is above the inguinal ligament or in the proximal superficial femoral artery, using the diagnostic catheter puncture site if possible. The approach is from the ipsilateral groin for distal femoropopliteal occlusions and will often require a second puncture. An introducer sheath facilitates catheter changes during progression of thrombolysis but does leave a larger puncture site for later hemostasis. The infusion catheter is inserted several centimeters into the thrombus. The catheter size used is usually 3F or 4F with a single end hole. Catheters with multiple side holes can be used, provided that all the side holes are situated within the thrombus. A mistake made by early radiologists was to leave the catheter proximal to the thrombus, with resulting poor outcomes. If a guidewire is used to place the infusion catheter, this can be used to probe the arterial occlusion. If the guidewire crosses the occlusion (guidewire traversal test), this is an excellent predictor that successful thrombolysis will ensue. If the thrombus is impenetrable, it is likely the arterial occlusion is chronic. Occasionally, infusion of the lytic agent just proximal to a chronic occlusion will soften it sufficiently for a catheter to be inserted.

Low-dose infusion
Conventionally, 0.5 to 1mg of tPA, or its equivalent, are infused per hour. A reasonable volume of fluid should be infused so that a steady concentration of lytic drug is maintained (5–10mL fluid per hour). Concomitant heparin is used by some radiologists to prevent pericatheter thrombosis. Other additional maneuvers that speed the duration of lysis include lacing and debulking. Radiologists sometimes lace the entire length of the thrombus with lytic drug, which can speed up the process. Debulking using aspiration embolectomy can also accelerate thrombolysis (see below). Once the infusion is running, sequential angiography is performed. Usually, an initial angiogram after 4 hours confirms the position of the catheter and commencement of lysis; after this, angiography should be performed at least every 12 hours until the occlusion is lysed. The infusion is stopped if there is no clot lysis between two 12-hour angiograms, or if complications ensue. If the occlusion is long, it will often be necessary to advance the infusion catheter as the occlusion is gradually lysed. Some radiologists feel it is better to lyse the occlusion from distal to proximal by sequentially withdrawing the catheter to try and prevent distal embolization. Often, successful thrombolysis uncovers a significant arterial stenosis. Angioplasty may be performed at any stage during the lytic process and some radiologists perform it as early as possible, as soon as a stenosis is identified. Angioplasty should certainly not be left until days after a successful procedure, as re-thrombosis is highly likely. The fundamental principle of intra-arterial thrombolysis is to establish forward flow as soon as possible.

Monitoring
Patients should be monitored in a suitable area. Ideally, a ward staffed by specialist vascular nurses or a high-dependency unit should be employed. Clinicians who feel that lysis should only be performed in a high-dependency unit run the risk that this procedure will not be able to be carried out if a bed is not available there. Vital signs and arterial puncture sites should be monitored carefully for signs of bleeding. The legs should also be observed and regular Doppler examination checked. Dehydration should be avoided: patients can receive oral fluids but it is best to avoid giving them food, just in case urgent surgery becomes necessary. Supplemental oxygen is beneficial.[7] Intra-arterial thrombolysis can be uncomfortable and analgesia is important. If oral analgesia is not adequate, intravenous opiate infusion is better than intramuscular injections, which run the risk of bruising. The most efficient way of caring for patients having intra-arterial thrombolysis is to use a care pathway that contains reminders of all of these items. Regular hematologic monitoring does not seem to improve outcome and therefore is not necessary.

After thrombolysis
Once successful thrombolysis has been achieved, the infusion catheter should be removed as soon as possible. Groin puncture sites will need firm pressure, often for 20–30 minutes. Pressure should not occlude the artery, as this can cause rethrombosis. Arterial closure devices can be useful in this situation. There is a rebound risk of hypercoagulability after thrombolysis, and patients should be anticoagulated with heparin for at least 48 hours. The activated partial thromboplastin time should be monitored carefully, as this can be prolonged by tPA therapy. The role of prolonged anticoagulation is as controversial here as after embolectomy. Some vascular surgeons anticoagulate patients with coumadin for long periods. Others feel that antiplatelet medication alone is satisfactory in those who have high flow through a vessel treated with angioplasty and good runoff. Duplex follow-up is advisable, particularly if the cause of occlusion has not been found.

Accelerated methods of thrombolysis
Conventional low-dose intra-arterial thrombolysis takes between 18 and 30 hours to clear most arterial occlusions. This may be too long for a patient with a threatened leg, who may have established muscle and skin damage at this stage. Several techniques speed the duration of lysis, either by using special catheters or by varying the lytic schedules (**Fig. 17.10**).

Pulse spray thrombolysis
For this procedure, an infusion catheter with multiple side holes shaped as slits is employed (**Fig. 17.11**). A special infusion pump is attached to the catheter, and this delivers small pulses of lytic agent throughout the thrombus as a fine spray. This technique partially macerates the occlusion as well as delivering drug throughout its whole length. The technique speeds thrombolysis, and good results have been published.[26,27] However, the equipment required is expensive.

High-dose bolus lysis
Various methods of altering lytic infusions have been tested. One that has been investigated in a randomized controlled trial

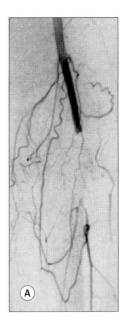
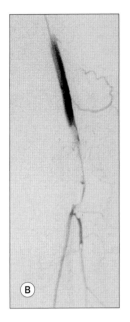
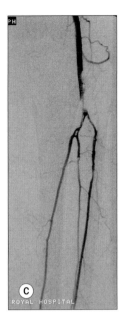
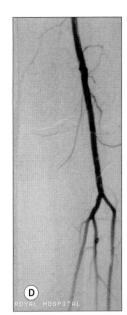

Figure 17.10 Accelerated thrombolysis. (A) Acute left popliteal artery embolus in a patient in atrial fibrillation. (B) Partial lysis after 30 minutes of high-dose t-PA. (C) Small amount of residual clot after 4 hours. (D) Continued lysis resulted in fully patent vessel after 12 hours.

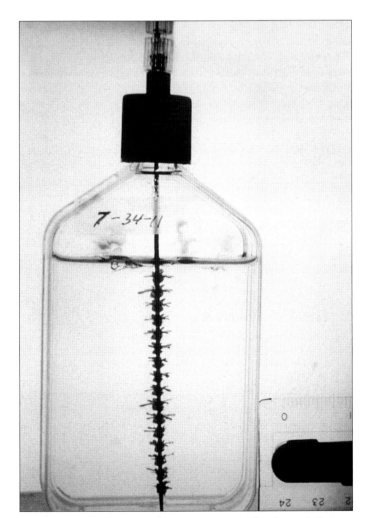

Figure 17.11 Illustration of pulse spray lysis catheter in a gelatin bottle. Note the multiple side holes.

is high-dose bolus lysis.[28] Three 5mg boluses of tPA are given over 30 minutes, laced into the full length of the occlusion. If after this time there is no improvement on the angiogram, lysis is abandoned and the patient is taken for surgery. This is termed the trial of lysis. If after 30 minutes there has been some dissolution of the thrombus, an infusion of 3.5mg of tPA per hour is continued for the next 4 hours. The majority of patients have complete or partial thrombolysis by the end of the 4 hours. If not, treatment can be continued, but the dose is usually reduced to 0.5 to 1mg an hour. The median duration of lysis using this technique is reduced from 24 to 7 hours (**Fig. 17.12**).

The use of accelerated thrombolysis means that patients with a threatened limb and a partial neurologic deficit can be treated by endovascular means. There is no specific clinical advantage and none of the trials has shown improved results with accelerated thrombolysis over conventional techniques in equivalent patients. In patients with a viable leg and no neurosensory deficit, radiologists are free to choose which technique they prefer, and an individual decision is acceptable.

Minimizing the risks of intra-arterial thrombolysis

Many vascular surgeons and radiologists believe that intra-arterial thrombolysis is a particularly dangerous undertaking. However, if managed carefully, the risks of intra-arterial thrombolysis need be no greater than those of major surgery. Bleeding is the most common complication and can be severe in up to 10% of patients. Minor puncture site bleeding is more common and can be seen in up to half of the procedures (**Fig. 17.13**). Usually, simple pressure over the groin, possibly with a sandbag can keep oozing under control. If a significant groin hematoma occurs, or there are signs of major blood loss or shock, thrombolysis will need to be stopped. Resuscitation and blood transfusion will then need to be given. Considerable retroperitoneal bleeding is possible, and occurs particularly after high antegrade arterial

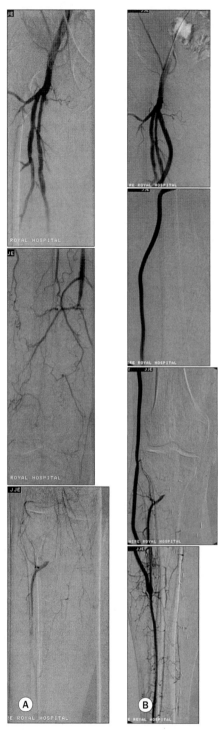

Figure 17.12 Occluded femoropopliteal polytetrafluoroethylene graft (A) treated successfully with high-dose bolus t-PA within 4 hours (B).

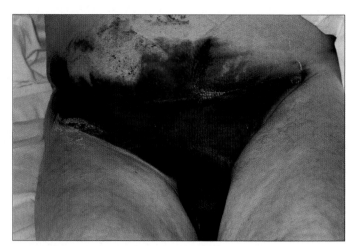

Figure 17.13 Extensive groin hematoma after successful intra-arterial thrombolysis.

Unfortunately, monitoring hematologic profiles does not seem to be clinically useful as it seldom affects the conduct of a thrombolytic episode. The only coagulation factor that predicts bleeding complications is a low plasma fibrinogen level.

Stroke is the most feared complication of intra-arterial thrombolysis, occurring in approximately 2% of procedures. In fact, only 50% of the strokes are hemorrhagic; the other 50% are thrombotic due to the nature of the high-risk patient group being treated. If a stroke occurs during thrombolysis, urgent brain computed tomography is required. If the stroke is hemorrhagic, clearly, thrombolysis should be stopped; the dilemma is whether or not to continue thrombolysis in a patient who has a thrombotic occlusion. The incidence of stroke during thrombolysis means that pre-treatment consent is a very important part of counselling.

Distal embolization occurs in up to 10% of patients, due to the break-up of thrombus during lysis. In most patients, continued infusion clears the small distal occlusions. If the foot does not improve after 4 hours of continued thrombolysis, surgical embolectomy is required to retrieve the distal thrombus. The highest risk of distal embolization is during the thrombolysis of an acutely thrombosed popliteal aneurysm.[4]

Re-thrombosis is rare after properly conducted thrombolysis. If it occurs, the reason is usually that the thrombolysis was inadequate or that an underlying stenosis has remained.

Optimizing the results of thrombolysis

The best results for thrombolysis are achieved when a team of experienced radiologists and surgeons work together to make the decisions about treatment and share the responsibility of carrying out the thrombolytic procedure. The fact that the randomized trials alluded to in the previous chapter have failed to show an advantage of thrombolysis over surgery, means that the optimal treatment of leg ischemia is performed by clinicians familiar with both techniques and who use them appropriately in individually selected patients. Thrombolysis driven by protocol and using care pathways should minimize the risks.[29]

The British Thrombolysis Study Group has collected information on over 1000 episodes of peripheral arterial thrombolysis.[30] Their overall results show an amputation-free survival rate of 75% at 30 days, a mortality rate of 12.5%, and an amputation

puncture. Computed tomography or ultrasound imaging are occasionally needed to make the diagnosis. If the risk to life becomes greater than the risk to the leg, it may be necessary to reverse the bleeding tendency caused by thrombolysis. Clotting factors can be given, although cryoprecipitate is the most useful infusion to restore levels of fibrinogen that have been degraded by the lytic agents. Antifibrinolytic drugs such as tranexamic acid may have a role. All fibrinolytic drugs cause abnormalities of coagulation, particularly if continued for many hours.

with survival rate of 12.5%. A multivariate analysis was performed to evaluate factors that affected outcome. Amputation-free survival was improved in patients taking coumadin before the episode, and was poorer in diabetic patients, those who had threatened legs with a neurologic deficit, and those with a short duration of ischemia. Other factors that adversely affected mortality and amputation rates included female gender, a history of ischemic heart disease, and an occlusion due to embolism. In general, amputation rates were higher in patients with a thrombosis and mortality rates were higher in patients with embolism. Amputation rates and mortality were not insubstantial when patients with acute claudication were treated with thrombolysis, and this is no longer recommended.[31]

Using data like these, surgeons and radiologists should be able to start predicting outcomes from intra-arterial thrombolysis for leg ischemia. The Thrombolysis Study Group has used sequential audit data to improve their clinical results with thrombolysis over the last decade. Other pre-treatment assessments such as Physiological and Operative Severity Score for enUmeration of Mortality and morbidity (POSSUM) scoring could also be used to determine outcome for individual patients.[32]

Aspiration embolectomy

The principle of aspiration embolectomy is to remove small fragments of clot percutaneously.[33] The easiest way of doing this is to use a 5F or 7F catheter with the tapered end removed (modified Van Andel predilator). This is passed into the occlusion and pulled back through it. A 50mL syringe is attached to the end of the catheter and aspirated at the time it is withdrawn through the occlusion. The aspirated clot is collected and angiography used to confirm forward flow. Manufacturers have created sets containing all the equipment needed to perform this technique (Cook Single Handed Aspiration Set, Cook, UK). The results in selected patients with small emboli are good. Often, adjuvant thrombolysis is required if larger occlusions are treated. The technique is usefully employed by radiologists when distal embolization occurs during endovascular therapy. It has obvious advantages over conventional surgical embolectomy.

Mechanical thrombectomy

The aim here is to break up thrombus within the vessel and aspirate it percutaneously. All techniques use relatively expensive single-use equipment and are only recommended in fresh occlusions less than 14 days old. There are two different principles. The Amplatz thrombectomy device (Microvena) uses rotational forces, like a whisk, to break up the thrombus into tiny fragments that simply disperse within the circulation. Clinically significant embolization is rare. More popular are the devices that use high-pressure saline jets to create a vortex at the catheter tip, so that thrombus is aspirated into a maceration chamber and then removed through a separate channel. This technique has the hazard that a significant volume of blood can be lost during aspiration of a long occlusion. Current devices include the Hydrolyser (Cordis), Oasis (Boston Scientific), and the Angiojet (Possis). Although the US Food and Drug Administration has approved eight thrombectomy devices for use in occluded hemodialysis grafts, only the Angiojet is licenced for use in peripheral arterial occlusions.

All of these devices have the advantage of immediacy, but in general are used mainly in patients with stable acute ischemia. There are no comparative trials with surgery, or more importantly with thrombolysis. It is often necessary to supplement thrombectomy with further thrombolysis. Large puncture wounds are needed in the groin, and hematoma formation is common. Significant arterial damage is also an occasional complication. However, results comparable with other treatments have been reported in selected patients.[34,35]

SUMMARY

The practical management of ALI remains a challenge, as it involves one of the most complex decision pathways in vascular surgery. A successful outcome depends upon an experienced team (vascular radiologist and surgeon) with access to, and the ability to use, the full range of available techniques. Treatment should be based on the severity of the ischemia rather than the underlying cause.

An arteriogram should be obtained in all patients with a threatened limb, time and availability permitting.

The role of conventional balloon catheter embolectomy is diminishing, due to the proliferation of new percutaneous techniques and the decreasing incidence of cardiac embolism. However, the precise role of each treatment modality remains unclear.

REFERENCES

1. Rutherford RB, Flanigan DP, Gupta SK, et al. Suggested standards for reports dealing with lower extremity ischemia. J Vasc Surg 1986;4:80–94.
2. TransAtlantic Inter-Society Consensus (TASC). Management of peripheral arterial disease (PAD). Eur J Vasc Endovasc Surg 2000;19(Suppl A): S114-43.
3. Campbell WB. Non-intervention and palliative care in vascular patients Br J Surg 2000;87:1601–2.
4. Galland RB, Earnshaw JJ, Baird RN, et al. Acute limb deterioration during intra-arterial thrombolysis. Br J Surg 1993;80:1118–20.
5. Thompson JF, Beard J, Scott DJA, Earnshaw JJ. Intraoperative thrombolysis in the management of thrombosed popliteal aneurysm. Br J Surg 1993;80:858–9.
6. Eyers P, Earnshaw JJ. Acute non-traumatic arm ischaemia. Br J Surg 1998;85:1340–6.
7. Berridge DC, Hopkinson BR, Makin GS. Acute lower limb arterial ischaemia: a role for continuous oxygen inhalation. Br J Surg 1980; 76:1021–3.
8. Blaisdell FW, Steele M, Allen RE. Management of lower extremity arterial ischaemia due to embolism and thrombosis. Surgery 1978; 84:822–34.
9. Campbell WB, Ballard PK. Intra-arterial lignocaine in embolectomy. Br J Surg 1996;83:244.
10. Gwynn BR, Shearman CP, Simms MH. The anatomical basis for the route taken by Fogarty catheters in the lower leg. Eur J Vasc Surg 1987; 1:129–32.
11. Bosma HW, Jorning PJG. Intraoperative arteriography in arterial embolectomy. Eur J Vasc Surg 1990;4:469–72.
12. Beard JD, Nyamekye I, Earnshaw JJ, Scott DJA, Thompson JF. Intra-operative streptokinase: a useful adjunct to balloon catheter embolectomy. Br J Surg 1993;80:21–4.

13. Knaus J, Ris HB, Do D, Stirnemann P. Intraoperative catheter thrombolysis as an adjunct to surgical revascularization for infrainguinal limb threatening ischaemia. Eur J Vasc Surg 1993;7:507–12.

14. Quinones-Baldrich WJ, Baker D, Busuttil RW, Machleder HI, Moore WS. Intraoperative infusion of lytic drugs for thrombotic complications of revascularization. J Vasc Surg 1989;10:408–17.

15. Law MM, Gelabert HA, Colburn MD, Quinones-Baldrich WJ, Ahn SS, Moore WS. Continuous postoperative intra-arterial urokinase infusion in the treatment of no reflow following revascularization of the acutely ischaemic limb. Ann Vasc Surg 1994;8:66–73.

16. Youkey JR, Clagett GP, Cabellon S Jr, Eddleman WL, Salander JM. Rich NM. Thromboembolectomy of arteries explored at the ankle. Ann Surg 1984;199:367–71.

17. Wyffels PL, DeBord JR. Increased limb salvage with distal tibial/peroneal artery thrombectomy/embolectomy in acute lower limb ischaemia. Am J Surg 1990;56:468–75.

18. Wyffels PL, DeBord JR, Marshall JS, Thors G, Marshall WH. Increased limb salvage with intraoperative and postoperative ankle level urokinase infusion in the treatment of no reflow following revascularisation of the acutely ischaemic limb. Ann Vasc Surg 1994;8:66–73.

19. Ernst CB. Fasciotomy in perspective. J Vasc Surg 1989;9:829–30.

20. Hammarsten J, Holm J, Shersten T. Positive and negative effects of anticoagulant treatment during and after arterial embolectomy. J Cardiovasc Surg 1978;19:373–9.

21. Walker PM, Romaschim AD, Davis S, Piovesan J. Lower limb ischemia: phase 1 results of salvage perfusion. J Surg Res 1999;84:193–8.

22. Ljungman C, Adami H-O, Bergqvist D, Sparen P, Bergstrom R. Risk factors for early lower limb loss after embolectomy for acute arterial occlusion: a population-based case-control study. Br J Surg 1991;78:1482–5.

23. Campbell WB, Ridler BM, Szymanska TH. Two year follow-up after acute thromboembolic leg ischaemia: the importance of anticoagulation. Eur J Vasc Endovasc Surg 2000;19:169–73.

24. Connolly SJ. Anticoagulation for patients with atrial fibrillation and risk factors for stroke. BMJ 2000;320:1219–20.

25. Ouriel K. Current status of thrombolysis for peripheral arterial occlusive disease. Ann Vasc Surg 2002;16:797–804.

26. Yusuf SW, Whitaker SC, Gregson RHS, et al. Prospective randomized comparative study of pulse spray and conventional local thrombolysis. Eur J Vasc Endovasc Surg 1995;10:136–41.

27. Armon MP, Yusuf SW, Whitaker SC, Gregson RHS, Wenham PW, Hopkinson BR. Results of 100 cases of pulse spray thrombolysis for acute and subacute leg ischaemia. Br J Surg 1997;84:47–50.

28. Braithwaite BD, Buckenham TM, Galland RB, et al. Prospective randomized trial of high-dose bolus versus low dose tissue plasminogen activator infusion in the management of acute limb ischaemia. Br J Surg 1997;84:646–50.

29. Whitman B, Parkin D, Earnshaw JJ. Management of acute leg ischaemia. In: Beard JD, Murray S, eds. Pathways of care in vascular surgery. Worcester:TFM Publishing; 2002:99–105.

30. Earnshaw JJ, Whitman B, Foy C on behalf of the Thrombolysis Study Group. National Audit of Thrombolysis for Acute Leg Ischaemia (NATALI) database: final clinical analysis. Br J Surg 2003;90:A504–5.

31. Braithwaite BD, Tomlinson MA, Walker SR, et al. Peripheral thrombolysis for acute onset claudication. Br J Surg 1999;86:800–4.

32. Neary B, Whitman B, Foy C, Heather BP, Earnshaw JJ. Value of POSSUM physiology scoring to assess outcome after intra-arterial thrombolysis for acute leg ischaemia. Br J Surg 2001;88:1344–5.

33. Cleveland TJ, Cumberland DC, Gaines PA. Percutaneous aspiration thromboembolectomy to manage the embolic complications of angioplasty and as an adjunct to thrombolysis. Clin Radiol 1994;49:549–52.

34. Kasirajan K, Haskal ZJ, Ouriel K. The use of mechanical thrombectomy devices in the management of acute peripheral arterial occlusive disease. J Vasc Interv Radiol 2001;12:405–11.

35. Morgan R, Belli A-M. Percutaneous thrombectomy: a review. Eur Radiol 2001;12:205-17.

CHAPTER
18

Metabolic and Systemic Consequences of Acute Limb Ischemia and Reperfusion

Shubha Varma, Frank Padberg Jr, Robert W Hobson II, and Walter N Durán

KEY POINTS

- Severe muscle necrosis occurs as a direct result of prolonged ischemia; however, it is the local and systemic injury produced by successful reperfusion that is often a major determinant of outcome for both patient and limb.

- There is extensive experimental research on drugs that might reduce the severity of ischemia reperfusion injury, but none is yet useful clinically.

- Reperfusion injury can be minimized by prompt revascularization.

- Careful observation in patients at risk should enable early identification of compartment syndrome; the diagnosis is mainly clinical but can be confirmed by measuring compartment pressures.

- If compartment syndrome is suspected, prompt and thorough surgical fasciotomy is vital.

- Continued research into the mechanisms of microvascular dysfunction may enable the development of new therapeutic interventions which could be administered at the time of reperfusion, when injury is anticipated.

INTRODUCTION

Acute limb ischemia may result from arterial trauma or thromboembolism. The magnitude of the acute ischemic injury increases proportionally with the duration of ischemia and the amount of tissue affected. Reperfusion contributes to injury of nerve, skeletal muscle, and even remote end organs. The mechanism of injury in reperfusion involves a series of events including inadequate oxygen delivery, reduction in cellular energy stores, accumulation of noxious metabolites and oxygen free radical derived injury.[1] The release of toxic metabolic products into the systemic circulation causes remote organ cellular dysfunction and increases in microvascular permeability and tissue edema. Increased permeability to macromolecules is one of the earliest signs of dysfunction in skeletal muscle. Intravital microscopy techniques indicate that a significant increase in macromolecular transport occurs during the reperfusion phase.[2] The cellular alterations produced by ischemia are exaggerated by reperfusion. Additionally, reperfusion causes new injury due to complex interactions between newly reintroduced molecular oxygen and the cellular metabolic state set up by ischemia.

Significant secondary complications such as tissue necrosis, neuromuscular dysfunction, sepsis, and multisystem organ failure may result following acute arterial ischemia and reperfusion of ischemic skeletal muscle.[3,4] When the increase in permeability occurs within a restricted space, progressive swelling may obstruct venous return, capillary perfusion, and, finally, arterial flow. The combined effect produces ischemic injury to the tissues within that space. This condition, known as compartment syndrome, may be amenable to interventions including mechanical decompression by fasciotomy, or pharmacotherapy designed to prevent or reduce tissue edema.

ETIOLOGY

Ischemia followed by restoration of blood flow precipitates increases in permeability and local edema. The duration of ischemia can often be assessed accurately after trauma but it is often less clear after arterial thromboembolism. Combined arteriovenous injuries are more likely to result in tissue edema, particularly when associated with venous obstruction.

Edema due to reperfusion of an ischemic extremity by embolectomy or arterial reconstruction may develop several hours following revascularization; therefore, monitoring for compartmental hypertension should be a routine part of postoperative evaluation.

Several common clinical situations are typically associated with compartment syndrome (Table 18.1). Examples include popliteal and brachial artery injuries, high velocity injuries with extensive soft tissue damage, and injuries associated with crushing.[5,6,7] The most common non-arterial cause is fracture with secondary hemorrhage within a compartment. In addition, in unusual clinical situations, acute compartmental hypertension may mimic acute arterial ischemia. Examples include prolonged compression of a muscular part, which may result from pressure on the skin during protracted surgery or immobilization.[8–12] Intra-arterial drug injections may produce similar diffuse arterial injury or pseudoaneurysms.[13] A dressing or a plaster cast that is too tight can cause external pressure, as can an eschar from a circumferential burn. Other rare causes of compartment syndrome include massive soft tissue swelling following the bites of poisonous snakes and insects due to release of toxins, unintentional extravascular infusion of intravenous fluids or medications, and iatrogenic compartment syndrome resulting from the prolonged occlusion of the extremity with a tourniquet, or the use of military anti-shock trousers.[14] Unusual causes include phlegmasia cerulea dolens, and malfunctioning pneumatic venous compression boots or intra-aortic balloon counter pulsation devices.[15,16,17]

Causes of compartment syndromes.	
Decreased compartment volume	Closure of fascial defects
	Application of excessive traction
Increased compartment content	Bleeding
	major vascular
	coagulation disorder
	Increased capillary filtration
	bites
	ischemia-reperfusion
	trauma
	intra-arterial drug injection
	cold
	orthopedic injury
	Increased capillary pressure
	acute venous obstruction
	Diminished serum osmolarity
	nephrotic syndrome
	Other causes
	infusion infiltration
	pressure transfusion
	muscular hypertrophy
	popliteal cyst
Externally applied pressure	Tight casts, dressings, or splints
	Increased pressure on limb due
	to prolonged immobilization
	during long surgical procedures
	or after recreational drug use

Table 18.1 Causes of compartment syndromes.

PATHOPHYSIOLOGY

The clinical components of acute limb ischemia may be considered in three broad categories:

- ischemia;
- reperfusion, with its potential systemic effects; and
- local tissue hypertension.

Ischemia

The magnitude of the injury is directly related to the duration of ischemia and the mass of involved tissue, as well as the severity of hypoperfusion. Skeletal muscle can tolerate complete ischemia for 4–6 hours, after which the injury becomes irreversible. In experience from this laboratory, 6 hours of complete ischemia consistently produced necrosis of canine skeletal muscle. This was verified in whole limb preparations with both tourniquet- and multiple ligation-induced ischemia, and with isolated gracilis muscle preparations.[18,19] When ischemia is prolonged, the microvasculature loses its integrity and massive increases in permeability accompany restoration of arterial perfusion.

Reperfusion

The reperfusion phase following ischemia is complex and produces both local metabolic abnormalities and a systemic inflammatory response due to the release and activation of toxic metabolic products. Hemodynamically, reperfusion is characterized by diffuse hyperemic flow to the entire extremity.[19] Clinical mani-

festations include acidosis, hyperkalemia, renal failure, acute respiratory insufficiency, arrhythmias, and neuromotor dysfunction. Acidosis and hyperkalemia result from the washout of accumulated byproducts of anaerobic metabolism. The factors responsible for the development of ischemia-reperfusion (I/R) injury are the toxic metabolites of molecular oxygen, such as superoxide radicals and hydroxyl radicals. The electronic configurations of these free radicals are highly unstable, and they react with other molecules to stabilize themselves; however, in so doing, they cause structural and functional changes in cell membranes and organelles, resulting in their disruption. Many of these reactions result in the release of even more free radicals, which propagate this process.[20]

Specific tissues

Studies of the fundamental mechanisms of reperfusion injury suggest that it is similar in many organs, including the gastrointestinal tract, skin, heart, kidney, and brain. Remote organ injury, including lungs, kidney, heart, gastrointestinal tract, and brain, as a consequence of I/R is a major cause of morbidity and even death from multi-organ failure.

Vulnerability to I/R varies between different organs and tissues, and under different clinical situations. Compared with the extremities, the brain, kidney, and intestine are more susceptible, and shorter periods of ischemia may precipitate the I/R syndrome. The duration of ischemia that can be tolerated is variable, being as short as 3–4 minutes for the brain but up to 40–60 minutes for the kidney. This is partly because these tissues characteristically have a low resistance–high flow circulation with a high metabolic rate. Additionally, acute renal failure may result from myonecrosis following prolonged ischemia, which results in release and entry of myoglobin into the systemic circulation, leading to myoglobinuria.

Within the extremities, the most sensitive tissues are the sensory and motor nerves, followed by skeletal muscle, skin, and bone, which is why a neurosensory deficit is often found in the acutely ischemic leg before muscle paralysis. Bourne and Rorabeck have shown that muscle blood flow and peroneal nerve conduction velocities decreased proportionally with the duration and magnitude of tissue hypertension.[21] Peroneal nerve conduction was lost completely after 30 minutes of complete arterial ischemia. Significant nerve damage is also caused by reperfusion, and was present when pressures of 30–40mmHg were present for 6–12 hours.[12] Ashton et al. have measured critical closing pressures in the capillaries and found they were 21 and 33mmHg in the leg and arm, respectively.[22]

Local tissue hypertension

Compartment syndrome has been described as a clinical condition in which increased pressure within a fascial compartment compromises the circulation and function of the tissues within that space.[11] Increased microvascular permeability promotes local edema. Arteriolar and capillary flow are the most sensitive to changes in compartment pressures. Subcutaneous tissues tolerate uncontrolled edema reasonably well, but when the edema is contained within a fascial compartment, the pressure soon exceeds the intraluminal pressure of the venules, which results in regional venous obstruction. Compartmental pressures as low as 20–40mmHg may cause compromised arterial inflow and tissue ischemia. Early mechanical decompression by fasciotomy is effective in minimizing the secondary local complications of compartment syndrome.

DIAGNOSIS AND MANAGEMENT

Ischemia

Timely recognition of compromised circulation is critical to the successful management of acute leg ischemia, since mortality and amputation rates increase after 6 hours of ischemia.[23] Peripheral arterial flow is occasionally reduced as a compensation for acute blood loss but should return after appropriate resuscitation. Ankle–brachial indices or absolute ankle pressures are useful to determine the degree of arterial insufficiency and can be repeated at regular intervals. Early recognition of ischemia is the first step, followed by expeditious revascularization. Diagnostic arteriography is often unnecessary after trauma, but may be advantageous when clinical evaluation suggests an occlusion proximal to the inguinal ligament or the clavicle. When time is short, or prolonged transport is needed for transfer, temporary bypass using appropriately sized carotid shunts is a valuable tool for diminishing the ischemic interval. This is most useful in war or in trauma surgery.

Reperfusion

Reperfusion after successful revascularization releases toxic metabolites that have accumulated during the ischemia. This reperfusion syndrome is characterized by acidosis, hyperkalemia, myoglobinuria, renal failure, and refractory dysrhythmias.[24,25] The presence of myoglobin stains the urine a dark, reddish color; the urine reacts to hemoglobin when no cells are present on microscopy, and pigmented granular casts are noted in the sediment. Measurement of serum creatinine phosphokinase is a marker of ischemic muscle injury; values in the thousands of units reflect severe muscle injury. Replacement of intravascular volume helps to avoid renal hypoperfusion and increases parenchymal and tubular flow. In addition, intravenous mannitol and alkalinization of the urine can minimize precipitation of myoglobin in the renal tubules.

Acidosis and hyperkalemia contribute to myocardial irritability; specific antiarrhythmic therapy may be supplemented by infusion of dextrose, insulin, and fluids. Pharmacotherapy aimed at prevention and treatment of reperfusion-induced injury continues to be investigated. Additional management options include restricted flow restoration, outflow washout, pre-perfusion agents, and leukocyte depletion.[26–30]

Local tissue hypertension

The clinical diagnosis of compartmental hypertension may be quite subtle, since it is normally determined from non-specific clinical findings. As a result, heightened suspicion and good clinical judgment play a large role in diagnosis. Objective measurement of intracompartment pressures may help to determine the need for surgical intervention. Compartment hypertension commonly has a delayed onset. Pain is an early complaint and is often remarkable because it seems to be out of proportion to the physical findings; however, its absence may be falsely reassuring in a patient with spinal cord injuries or an altered level of consciousness. Severe tenderness and pain on passive stretch are signs of compartment syndrome. Unfortunately, all of these findings are non-specific. On palpation, the muscle compartment may feel tense, and even board-like. Neurologic clinical findings such as hypesthesia, paresthesias, and/or decreased motor function, especially if progressive, are strongly suggestive of compartment syndrome. The earliest abnormality is often numbness in the dorsal web space between the first and second toes; sensory innervation of this anatomic site is distributed through the lateral anterior tibial nerve, a branch of the deep peroneal nerve that exits the anterior compartment. However, in the setting of trauma, these have to be differentiated from direct nerve injuries. Loss of pulses or diminution of arterial Doppler signals constitute a very late sign of compartmental hypertension and indicate pathologic intracompartment pressures in the absence of arterial injury. Changes in venous Doppler signals have been suggested as an early marker, since normal venous pressure is rapidly exceeded in compartmental hypertension.

In general, the sensitivity of clinical examination for diagnosing compartment syndrome of the leg is low (13–19%).[31] The positive predictive value of clinical examination was 11% to 15%, and the specificity and negative predictive value were both 97% to 98%. These findings suggest that the clinical features of compartment syndrome of the lower leg are more useful by their absence in excluding the diagnosis than they are when present in confirming the diagnosis. The probability of compartment syndrome with one clinical sign present was approximately 25%, compared to 93% when three clinical signs were present.[31]

When a patient at risk complains of pain that is suspicious of compartment syndrome, the first step should be to remove all circumferential dressings. If a plaster cast is present, it may be split and removed, or a window cut for additional evaluation. If the clinical findings are convincing, complete fasciotomy should be considered. However, if the diagnosis remains uncertain, determination of compartment pressures may be of value.

COMPARTMENTAL DECOMPRESSION

Measurement of compartment pressures

In patients in whom it is not easy to assess sensorimotor function, measurement of compartment pressures is the best method of diagnosing a compartment syndrome, or to exclude it. Feliciano recommended that compartment pressure measurements be considered routinely in the susceptible patient.[32] Reperfusion edema may develop insidiously and may not be evident immediately. Continuous or repeated pressure measurements may be required in conjunction with clinical evaluation when fasciotomy is not performed initially.

Several different catheters have been used for measurement of intracompartmental pressures. Wick or slit catheters (**Fig. 18.1**) are equally effective in continuous monitoring of compartment pressures. The Stryker (Intra-compartmental pressure monitoring system, Stryker Surgical, Kalamazoo, MI®) needle (**Fig. 18.2A**) is a portable instrument that allows single puncture measurement of compartment pressures at the bedside and is currently the most commonly used method in North America. However, no special equipment is necessary for measuring compartment pressure in intraoperative or critical care settings. A standard intravascular transducer system can be used to determine tissue pressures and the same needle may be used to probe multiple fascial compartments (**Fig. 18.2B**). A decrease in tissue pressure following decompression may also be documented.

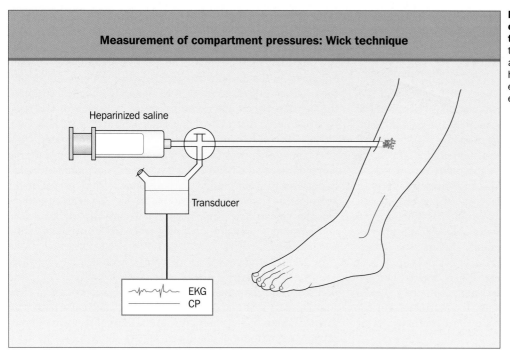

Measurement of compartment pressures: Wick technique

Heparinized saline

Transducer

EKG
CP

Figure 18.1 Measurement of compartment pressures: Wick technique. Continuous monitoring of tissue pressures can be maintained for as long as necessary. This may be helpful in the patient who has an evolving clinical course and whose examination is equivocal.

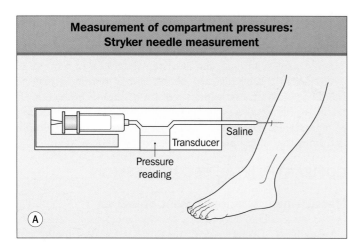

Measurement of compartment pressures: Stryker needle measurement

Saline

Transducer

Pressure reading

(A)

Figure 18.2 Measurement of compartment pressures. (A) The Stryker is a portable instrument that allows single puncture measurement of compartment pressures at the bedside. (B) The standard intravascular transducer system may be used to determine tissue pressures at a given point in time and the same needle may be used to probe multiple fascial compartments.

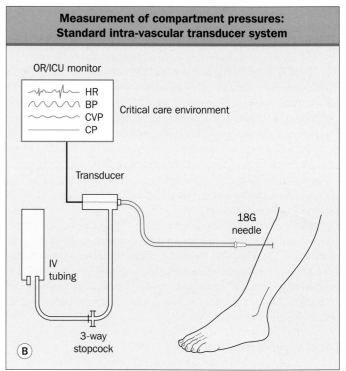

Measurement of compartment pressures: Standard intra-vascular transducer system

OR/ICU monitor

HR
BP
CVP
CP

Critical care environment

Transducer

18G needle

IV tubing

3-way stopcock

(B)

Indications for fasciotomy

Fasciotomy should be considered whenever there is clinical evidence of compartmental hypertension. The clinical findings are often non-specific and, when in doubt, compartment pressures may be measured to support clinical decisions. The final decision to proceed with fasciotomy remains controversial and the decision is based upon clinical judgment and experience.

Based on experimental work, decompressive fasciotomy is recommended when intracompartmental pressure is greater than 30mmHg to 45mmHg. Unfortunately, there is no specific pressure at which compartment syndrome occurs. Matsen et al. demonstrated uniform damage when tissue pressures exceeded these values,[33] but compartment syndrome can occur at pressures as low as 20–30mmHg, without loss of arterial blood flow. The duration of the compartmental hypertension, the systemic hemodynamics of the patient at that time, and the presence of coexisting peripheral vascular disease are factors that may dictate a lower threshold for considering fasciotomy.

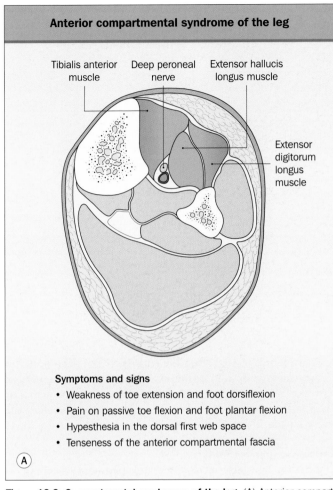

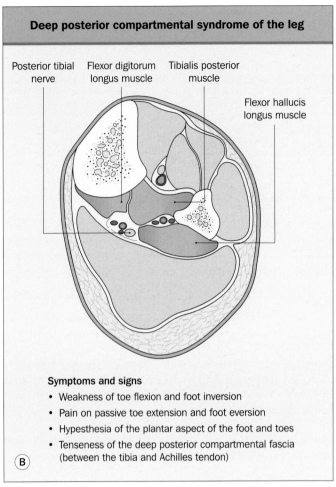

Figure 18.3 Compartmental syndromes of the leg. (A) Anterior compartmental syndrome of the leg. The anterior compartment contains the deep peroneal nerve (DPN) along with three muscles: tibialis anterior (TA), extensor hallucis longus (EHL), and extensor digitorum longus (EDL). (B) Deep posterior compartmental syndrome of the leg. The deep posterior compartment contains the posterior tibial nerve (PTN) as well as three muscles: tibialis posterior (TP), flexor hallucis longus (FHL), and flexor digitorum longus (FDL).

Heppenstall et al. emphasized the concept of compartmental perfusion pressures, defined as the mean systemic arterial pressure minus the compartmental pressure.[34] An increasing compartmental pressure with systemic hypotension can rapidly reduce the CPP to zero. Compartment syndrome is seen frequently when the difference between the mean arterial pressure and the pressure in the involved compartment is less than 40mmHg, and blood flow ceases when the compartmental perfusion pressure is 25mmHg or less.[35]

Common locations and management

The forearm and the lower leg are the usual locations for compartment syndrome. Clinicians should also be aware of its potential to occur at less common sites such as the hand or the foot, or even the shoulder, upper arm, buttock, or thigh. These sites are more typically involved when there is prolonged inadvertent compression of muscle groups, such as when an unattended patient remains collapsed and unconscious for several hours after a stroke or drug overdose. The compression is removed when the affected extremity is moved and reperfusion commences. The compartment syndrome may be more common in the forearm and leg because the compartments in these locations have tighter, better defined fascial boundaries.

Lower extremity

Compartment syndrome may involve all four compartments of the leg. The anterior tibial compartment is most likely to be involved (**Fig. 18.3A**) but significant damage is most common in the deep posterior compartment (**Fig. 18.3B**).[12,13] The incidence of compartment syndrome is higher when arterial and venous injuries are combined, such as after trauma. Once recognized, immediate fasciotomy is indicated for decompression of the muscle compartment, to prevent tissue necrosis and irreversible loss of neuromuscular function.

Anatomic considerations

A major nerve traverses each of the four compartments of the leg (**Fig. 18.4**), the identification of which is important in localizing symptoms. Knowledge of their anatomic course is useful in performing successful uncomplicated fasciotomy. The deep peroneal nerve arises from the common peroneal nerve and traverses the anterior compartment to exit as the anterior tibial nerve. It carries sensory innervation to the dorsum of the foot in the first web space and motor fibers to the forefoot extensors. The superficial peroneal nerve also arises from the common peroneal nerve and exits the lateral compartment at mid-leg; it provides sensory innervation to the medial great toe and the

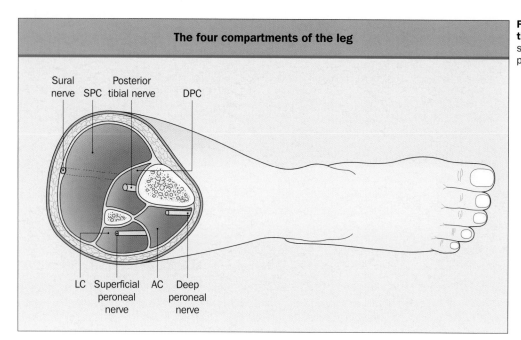

The four compartments of the leg

Sural nerve
SPC
Posterior tibial nerve
DPC
LC
Superficial peroneal nerve
AC
Deep peroneal nerve

Figure 18.4 The four compartments of the leg. Anterior (AC), lateral (LC), superficial posterior (SPC), and deep posterior compartments (DPC).

second, third, and fourth dorsal web spaces. This nerve must be identified during fasciotomy to prevent injury. The posterior tibial nerve forms the nerve of the deep posterior compartment and is responsible for plantar sensation and toe flexion. The superficial posterior compartment contains the gastrocnemius and soleus muscles and is traversed by the sural nerve that provides sensory input to the lateral aspect of the foot.

Operative treatment

Mechanical decompression of established compartmental hypertension is achieved by the release of skin and fascia by incision. When a tense firm fascia is incised in a limb with compartment hypertension, the muscles bulge into the operative field, change color from pale to dusky to bright red, and become soft and pliable. There are three main techniques for decompression of the leg:

- dual-incision fasciotomy;
- single-incision, lateral four-compartment fasciotomy; and
- fibulectomy fasciotomy.

Dual-incision fasciotomy

The authors prefer dual-incision, four-compartment fasciotomy to ensure complete skin and fascial decompression of all leg compartments (**Fig. 18.5**). There is a temptation to reduce the length of the skin incision in the hope of avoiding the need for a skin graft later; however, inadequate fasciotomy is most often the result of inadequate skin or fascial incisions. The initial incision should include skin and subcutaneous tissue down to the fascia. The lateral and anterior fasciotomy is then started in the mid-portion of the leg over the junction of the anterior and lateral compartments, with particular attention to the identification and preservation of the superficial peroneal nerve that exits the fascia at the level of the mid-leg. The fascial incisions are extended from the extensor retinaculum at the ankle to just below the fibular head, using long blunt-tipped scissors. A medial incision is then made in the mid- to distal third of the leg. The saphenous vein is retracted anteriorly and the superficial posterior

compartment is incised along the entire leg. The deep posterior compartment is opened posteromedially, where the superficial posterior muscles form the Achilles tendon and the avascular plane of the posterior intermuscular septum is incised along the entire length of the leg.

Single-incision fasciotomy

The cut for the single-incision four-compartment fasciotomy is made laterally over the posterior fibular border from just below the fibular head to 4cm above the malleolus (**Fig. 18.6**). Anterior and posterior skin flaps are raised and longitudinal incisions are made in the anterior, lateral, and superficial posterior compartments. Retracting the muscles of the lateral compartment anteriorly, the attachments of the soleus to the posterior fibula aid in identification and incision of the deep posterior compartment. Care must be taken to avoid injury to the peroneal and posterior tibial neurovascular bundles, which are located adjacent and medial to the fibula. Some authors have expressed difficulty with this approach when there is severe disruption of tissue planes. In addition, tibial fracture management is difficult through this incision.

Fibulectomy–fasciotomy

Fibulectomy fasciotomy achieves decompression of the posterior and anterior compartments through fibulectomy via the periosteal bed. Fibulectomy must not include the fibular head or the distal 8cm of the fibula, to minimize deformity and to maintain stability of the ankle. Removal of the fibula requires considerably more dissection than the other methods and for this reason it has not been adopted widely. Since equivalent decompression is achieved with the single- and dual-incision techniques, this procedure has not gained widespread acceptance.

Thigh and buttock fasciotomy

Thigh and gluteal compartment syndrome is rare, and seldom recognized. It occurs most commonly in individuals unconscious following ingestion of drugs or alcohol, who remain in one position

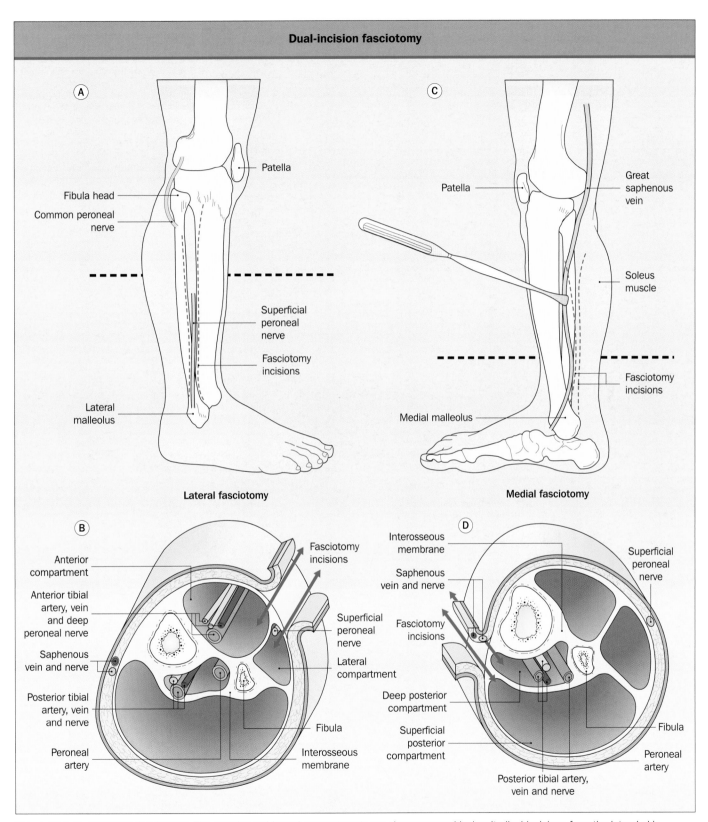

Dual-incision fasciotomy

Ⓐ

Patella

Fibula head

Common peroneal nerve

Superficial peroneal nerve

Fasciotomy incisions

Lateral malleolus

Lateral fasciotomy

Ⓒ

Patella

Great saphenous vein

Soleus muscle

Fasciotomy incisions

Medial malleolus

Medial fasciotomy

Ⓑ

Anterior compartment

Anterior tibial artery, vein and deep peroneal nerve

Saphenous vein and nerve

Posterior tibial artery, vein and nerve

Peroneal artery

Fasciotomy incisions

Superficial peroneal nerve

Lateral compartment

Fibula

Interosseous membrane

Ⓓ

Interosseous membrane

Saphenous vein and nerve

Fasciotomy incisions

Deep posterior compartment

Superficial posterior compartment

Posterior tibial artery, vein and nerve

Superficial peroneal nerve

Fibula

Peroneal artery

Figure 18.5 Dual-incision fasciotomy. The anterior and lateral compartments are decompressed by longitudinal incisions from the lateral skin incision. The superficial peroneal nerve exits the fascia very close to the skin incision (A, B). The superficial and deep posterior compartments are decompressed through longitudinal incisions on the medial aspect of the leg. The greater saphenous vein and nerve are preserved and retracted anteriorly (C, D). Cross-sections are indicated (B, D).

Parafibular fasciotomy (single incision fasciotomy)

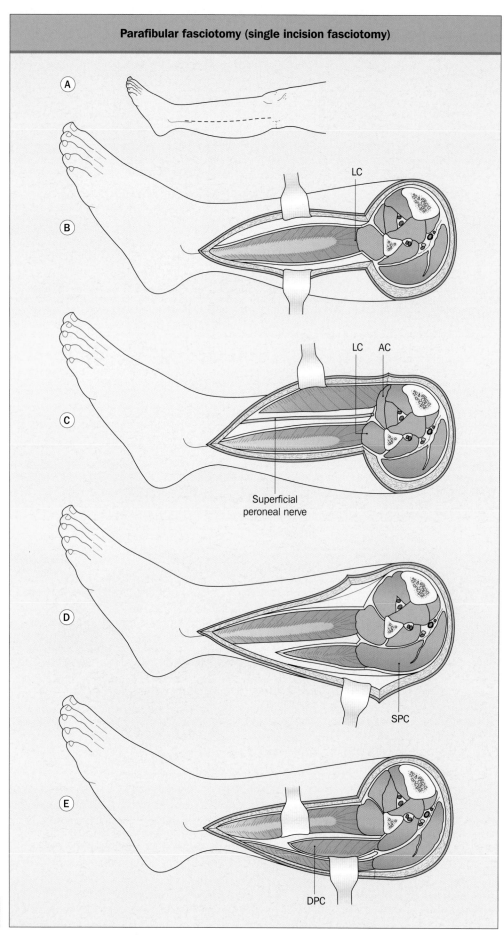

Figure 18.6 Parafibular fasciotomy (single incision fasciotomy).
(A) The skin incision runs along the fibula. (B) The lateral compartment (LC) lies just under the skin. (C) The anterior compartment (AC) is exposed by retracting the anterior skin flap. (D) The superficial posterior compartment (SPC) is exposed by retracting the posterior skin flap. (E) The deep posterior compartment (DPC) is exposed by retracting the lateral compartment anteriorly and the superficial posterior compartment posteriorly and dividing the fibular attachments of the soleus.

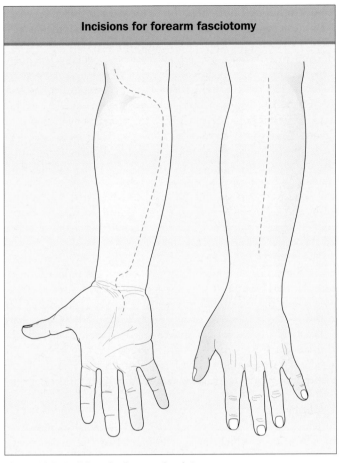

Incisions for forearm fasciotomy

Figure 18.7 Incisions for forearm fasciotomy.

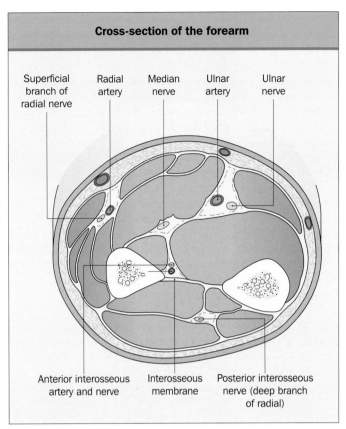

Cross-section of the forearm

Superficial branch of radial nerve

Radial artery

Median nerve

Ulnar artery

Ulnar nerve

Anterior interosseous artery and nerve

Interosseous membrane

Posterior interosseous nerve (deep branch of radial)

Figure 18.8 Cross-section of the forearm.

for a long time. The physiology and manifestations are similar to those in the more common and readily recognized compartment syndromes of the lower leg. The diagnosis is often delayed, resulting in significant morbidity and possible mortality. The mainstay of treatment consists of fasciotomy and debridement.

Decompression of the anterior and posterior compartments of the thigh may be accomplished with full-length incisions. The gluteus is easily decompressed through longitudinal cutaneous incisions. Individual epimysial envelopes may also require decompression incisions.

Arm

Compartment syndromes are uncommon in the arm, and difficult to diagnose. Testing intracompartment pressures may help confirm the diagnosis. The diagnosis should be suspected in children with a supracondylar fracture of the humerus, and following fractures of the forearm, brachial artery puncture, subfascial intravenous infiltrations, crush injuries, extremity replantations and gunshot wounds. The deep volar compartment is most vulnerable as it is supplied by the anterior interosseous artery which has no significant collateral flow.

Technique of fasciotomy

The fasciotomy is performed through the incisions outlined in **Figure 18.7**. Typically, a dorsal and a volar incision are required to decompress the forearm. A curvilinear volar incision allows the release of the flexor compartment. The course of the incision

may be altered to accommodate pre-existing traumatic wounds. In the forearm, the muscles at risk are predominantly located in the volar aspect. Decompressive fasciotomy should relieve the median ulnar and radial nerves and the thumb and finger muscles (**Fig. 18.8**). Although volar release is usually sufficient, dorsal incisions may also be needed. Intraoperative compartment pressure measurement may be valuable in determining the need for a dorsal incision. A longitudinal incision provides release to the extensor compartment. In severe cases, the deep intramuscular fascia enveloping the flexor digitorum superficialis, the flexor digitorum profundus, and the flexor pollicis longus may have to be opened as well. The thick transcarpal ligament is divided distally to perform a carpal tunnel release. The proximal incision should release the lacertus fibrosus, so as to decompress the median nerve at the elbow.

CONTRAINDICATIONS TO REVASCULARIZATION AND COMPLICATIONS

In cases of prolonged and advanced ischemia, tissue necrosis may have already occurred, and revascularization may be contraindicated. Ascertaining the extent of tissue damage is one of the most difficult decisions for a surgeon, especially in a moribund patient with acute ischemia, who cannot give a history as to the duration of the illness. For the patient with a painful, immobile, insensate extremity, functional recovery may be limited by

243

neuropathic pain, weakness, contracture, and loss of protective sensation. Reperfusion following reconstruction and/or fasciotomy may result in the release of toxic metabolites into the systemic circulation and cause myoglobinuric renal failure, systemic inflammatory response syndrome, sepsis, shock, multisystem organ failure, and death. All of these effects are exaggerated in a patient with concomitant hypotension.

The decision to proceed with revascularization and fasciotomy, as opposed to primary amputation, is based primarily on the duration of ischemia and the muscle mass involved. If the duration of profound ischemia is more than 6–12 hours, the likelihood of tissue salvage becomes small and the risk of complications following revascularization becomes proportionately higher. Blaisdell et al. urged restraint when an ischemic leg progressed from 'waxy white' to 'blue mottled', a change indicative of non-viability.[8] However, the systemic effects of I/R are less pronounced when a smaller amount of tissue has been subjected to ischemia. Thus, time alone will not always decide the issue, and the clinician must tailor therapy individually.

Fasciotomy wounds may create new issues related to wound healing in a patient with existing chronic peripheral vascular disease. Thus, co-morbidities predispose to additional complications such as conversion of closed to open fractures, osteomyelitis, delayed wound closure, wound sepsis, bleeding, and cosmetic deformity. Reasons for perceived failure of fasciotomy are related more to associated profound ischemia, delay in fascial decompression, and inadequate fasciotomy. Most patients have few problems with wound healing after fasciotomy, although some will require skin grafts or closure by secondary suture.

MECHANISMS OF MICROVASCULAR DYSFUNCTION AFTER ISCHAEMIA/REPERFUSION

Increased microvascular permeability

One of the key concepts of the structural basis of increased microvascular permeability relates to widening of the intercellular gap junctions due to endothelial cell contraction.[36] The postcapillary venules are the main site of hyperpermeability induced by inflammatory mediators,[37] as studied by electron and fluorescence microscopy. These microvessels are also responsible for the permeability alterations in I/R.

The signaling pathways for inflammatory agents that cause hyperpermeability involve the activation of protein kinase C, activation of nitric oxide synthase (NOS), and synthesis of nitric oxide (NO).[38-43] Reports are consistent with the hypothesis that endothelial NOS (eNOS) activity and release of NO results in activation of soluble guanyl cyclase and synthesis of guanosine 3',5'-cyclic monophosphate (cGMP).[44] cGMP activates the mitogen-activated protein (MAP) kinases p42/44, which are important in the regulation of baseline, as well as agonist-induced permeability.[45] The final step in the sequence of molecular modifications appears to involve proteins located at the cell junctional/cytoskeletal complex. Studies performed mainly in tissue culture have identified vascular endothelial (VE)-cadherin and b-catenins as possibly being key molecules. MAP kinase-induced phosphorylation and disorganization of the VE-cadherin may result in structural changes in the cellular cytoskeleton and hyperpermeability.[46]

Endothelial cell and vascular wall interactions

The xanthine oxidase-containing microvascular endothelial cells, along with neutrophils, are the most probable sources of oxygen-derived free radicals. Ischemia activates a calcium-dependent protease that catalyzes the conversion of xanthine dehydrogenase to its oxidase form. As ischemia continues, adenosine triphosphate is degraded to hypoxanthine, which is then converted to uric acid by xanthine oxidase, along with the production of superoxide anion. Superoxide dismutase converts superoxide anion to hydrogen peroxide, which in the presence of ferric ion produces the hydroxyl radical. The hydroxyl radical is a highly toxic oxidant. Support for the role of oxygen-derived free radicals in the microvascular dysfunction associated with I/R[47,48] comes from the observed efficacy of free radical scavengers in the reduction of the indices of I/R-induced microvascular dysfunction to about half of their unopposed values.

NO, derived from L-arginine, is produced by vascular and perivascular cells and has been implicated in I/R-induced microvascular dysfunction. It may serve as an antiadhesive substance to protect the endothelium against leukocyte adherence.[49] In addition, the uncoupling of NO and formation of peroxynitrite ($ONOO^-$), a powerful reactive oxygen metabolite, leads to the formation of hydroxyl radicals.[50] Peroxynitrite, the reaction product of superoxide and NO, is potentially more harmful than either superoxide or hydroxyl radical, due to its longer half-life.

Leukocytes

Support for the involvement of leukocytes in I/R comes from experiments in which either the animal or the experimental muscle have been rendered leukopenic by radiation, chemical, or physical means.[51,52] Leukopenia decreases the impact of I/R on changes in microvascular permeability by reducing the increase in transport of macromolecules from a sevenfold, down to a twofold increase, compared to that obtained in the untreated ischemic muscle.[51,53] NADPH oxidase, within the leukocytes, converts cytoplasmic NADPH to $NADP^+$, resulting in the formation of superoxide anion and hydrogen peroxide, with subsequent release of hydroxyl radicals. Leukocytes also possess myeloperoxidase, an enzyme that catalyzes a reaction between hydrogen peroxide and chloride to form hypochlorous acid, a powerful oxidant agent. The levels of myeloperoxidase have been found to remain constant during ischemia and to increase at 15 minutes and 1 hour after reperfusion.[54] In addition, activated neutrophils release elastase, collagenase, and cathepsin G – substances that are able to degrade microvascular basement membrane and lead to increases in permeability and cellular dysfunction.

Other chemical mediators and signaling molecules

Calcium ions modulate the activity of leukocytes, as well as the contractile properties of endothelial cells, and play an important role in the pathophysiology of skeletal muscle I/R injury and associated microvascular injury.[54] Thromboxane A_2 (TXA_2) has been implicated in causing microvascular alterations in the lung following reperfusion of ischemic canine hindleg.[52]

Platelet activating factor (PAF) is a vasoconstrictor, a strong promoter of microvascular permeability, and a powerful chemoattractant for neutrophils.[55] The possibility that hydrogen peroxide may be the stimulus for PAF synthesis in I/R is indirectly supported by experiments in which human recombinant superoxide dismutase administered intravenously caused a 30% decrease in neutrophil adherence.[56]

PREVENTIVE STRATEGIES

What can be done to protect organs and tissues from the effects of ischemia and reperfusion injury? Early operation to reduce the duration of ischemia, a temporary bypass shunt to maintain tissue perfusion, and oxygenation and tissue cooling may all be used to decrease metabolic demands. In elective ischemic events such as transplantation, tissue preservation can be enhanced by pre-ischemic interventions. Even in the acute situation, several opportunities present themselves during management of the reperfusion phase. Hypothermic and controlled reperfusion can reduce edema and necrosis.[57] The clinical applicability of biochemical interventions designed to reduce reperfusion-induced injury in end-organs remains unproven. Much experimental work has been done to study pharmacologic intervention for the prevention and treatment of reperfusion-induced injury. The potential beneficial effects of substances such as verapamil, mannitol, prostacyclin, monoclonal antibodies, superoxide dismutase, hetastarch high-molecular-weight carbohydrates, and heparin continue to be investigated. Many of these agents have demonstrated benefits in experimental studies that have not been translated into clinical advantages.

Because leukocyte–endothelium interactions play an important role in bringing about I/R damage,[58,59] these cells and their biochemical processes are possible targets for therapeutic interventions. A major aim is to minimize adhesion of leukocytes to microvascular endothelium.[60] Iloprost, a stable analog of prostacyclin, may ameliorate the impact of I/R by preventing leukocyte adhesion, rather than because of its vasodilating properties.[61,62] Similarly, receptor antagonists to PAF, administered just before reperfusion, effectively inhibit the ability of the phospholipid to recruit leukocytes to the injured area and abrogate their adhesion to the microvascular wall.[60] Reduction or elimination of leukocyte adhesion to endothelium may inhibit the oxidative stress that leads to parenchymal and cellular dysfunction.

Restriction of calcium in reperfusion, either by using entry blockers (such as verapamil)[53] or by administration of low-calcium-modified solutions, may also be a useful way to decrease damage in reperfused muscle and to restore contractile function.[57]

Monoclonal antibodies directed against adhesion molecules on endothelium and/or leukocytes also provide effective protection against experimental I/R damage.[58] The clinical application of these monoclonal antibodies awaits improvement in their design that avoids rendering critically ill patients immunodeficient for a significant interval after treatment. These monoclonal antibodies, and specific receptor blocking agents, work effectively when administered just before reperfusion, and offer the possibility for the development of therapeutic approaches applicable to operations for acute ischemia.

SUMMARY

Ischemic injury to tissues is the primary cause of morbidity and mortality from acute interruption of arterial blood flow. However, the main component of the final injury occurs during reperfusion. Recognition of the severity of ischemia with efficient restoration of limb blood flow is an obvious method for reducing the duration of ischemia. However, intervention at the time of reperfusion offers an additional opportunity, since treatment can be initiated at the time tissue perfusion is restored. The cascade of events that occur after successful revascularization of an ischemic limb may be amenable to innovative interventions. Current investigations are targeted at understanding these cellular mechanisms and interactions in order to develop new therapeutic measures to diminish the detrimental metabolic and systemic consequences of ischemia and reperfusion.

The alert physician is aware of the clinical settings in which compartmental hypertension occurs. The incidence may be much higher than reported because some of the late sequelae, such as joint stiffness, claw toes, or equinus deformity, may be quite subtle. Timely decompressive fasciotomy with adequate incisions may avoid significant and permanent morbidity. In uncertain clinical situations, serial clinical evaluations may facilitate the diagnosis. In patients who are difficult to assess clinically, compartment pressure measurements may resolve the uncertainty. However, the ultimate determination of the need for decompressive fasciotomy arises from the clinician's judgment, as a critical value for compartmental hypertension may vary substantially with different clinical settings. Fasciotomy is often performed too late, and clinicians are advised to err on the side of caution.

REFERENCES

1. Korthuis RJ, Granger DN, Townsley MI, Taylor AE. The role of oxygen-derived free radicals in ischemia-induced increases in canine skeletal muscle vascular permeability. Circ Res 1985;57:599–609.
2. Durán WN, Dillon PK. Effects of ischemia-reperfusion injury on microvascular permeability in skeletal muscle. Microcirc Endothelium Lymphatics 1989;5:223–39.
3. Odeh M. Role of reperfusion induced injury in the pathogenesis of the crush syndrome. N Engl J Med 1991;324:1417–22.
4. Haimovici H. Metabolic complications of acute arterial occlusions and related conditions. Mt Kisco: NY Futura Publishing; 1985
5. Yeager RA, Hobson RW II, Lynch TG, et al. Popliteal and infrapopliteal arterial injuries; differential management and amputation rates. Am Surg 1983;50:155–8.
6. Lim LT, Michuda MS, Flanigan DP, et al. Popliteal artery trauma. 31 cases without amputation. Arch Surg 1980;115:1307–13.
7. Wagner WH, Calkins ER, Weaver FA, et al. Blunt popliteal artery trauma: one hundred consecutive injuries. J Vasc Surg 1988;7:737–48.
8. Blaisdell W, Steele M, Allen RE. Management of acute lower extremity arterial ischemia due to embolism and thrombosis. Surgery 1978; 84:822–34.
9. Yeager RA, Hobson RW II, Padberg FT, et al. Vascular complications related to drug abuse. J Trauma 1986;27: 305–8.
10. Padberg FT, Hobson RW, Lee BC, et al. Femoral pseudoaneurysm from drugs of abuse; ligation or reconstruction? J Vasc Surg 1992; 15:642–8.
11. Matsen FA III, Mubarak SJ, Rorabeck CH. A practical approach to compartment syndromes. Academy of American Orthopedic Surgeons. Instructional Courses Lectures 1983;32:88–113.
12. Mubarak SJ, Hargens A. Compartment syndromes and Volkmann's contracture. Philadelphia: PA Saunders, 1981.

13. Sheridan GW, Matsen FA. Fasciotomy in the treatment of acute compartment syndrome. J Bone Joint Surg 1976; 58A:112–15.

14. Perry MO. Compartment syndromes and reperfusion injury. Surg Clin North Am 1988;68:853–64.

15. Patman RD, Thompson JE, Persson AV. Use and technique of fasciotomy as an adjunct to limb salvage. South Med J 1973;66:1108–16.

16. Werbel GB, Shybut GT. Acute compartment syndrome caused by a malfunctioning pneumatic compression pump. J Bone Joint Surg 1986; 68A:1445–6.

17. Glenville B, Crockett JR, Bennett JG. Compartment syndrome and intraaortic balloon. Thorac Cardiovasc Surg 1986;24:292–4.

18. Franco CD, Hobson RW II, Padberg FT, et al. Hemodynamic changes during canine hindlimb reperfusion; comparison of thigh tourniquet and multiple ligation models. Curr Surg 1987;44:34–7.

19. Padberg FT, Franco CD, Kerr JC, et al. Acute ischemia reperfusion injury in the canine hindlimb. J Cardiovasc Surg 1989;30:925–31.

20. Bulkley GB. The role of oxygen free radicals in human disease processes. Surgery 1983;94:407–11.

21. Bourne RB, Rorabeck CH. Compartment syndromes of the lower leg. Clin Orthop 1989;240:97–104.

22. Ashton H. Critical closing pressures in human vascular beds. Clin Sci 1962;22:79–87.

23. Kendrick J, Thompson BW, Read RC, et al. Arterial embolectomy in the leg. Results in a referral hospital. Am J Surg 1981;142:739–42.

24. Haimovichi H. Metabolic complications of acute arterial occlusions. J Cardiovasc Surg 1979;20:349–57.

25. Presta M, Ragnotti G. Quantification of damage to striated muscle after normothermic or hypothermic ischemia. Clin Chem 1981;27:297–302.

26. Wright JG, Belkin M, Hobson RW II. Hypothermia and controlled reperfusion: two non pharmacologic methods which diminish ischemia reperfusion injury in skeletal muscle. Microcirc Endothelium Lymphatics 1989;53:315–34.

27. Walker PM, Lindsay TF, Labbe A, et al. Salvage of skeletal muscle with free radical scavengers. J Vasc Surg 1987;5:68–75.

28. Keller MP, Hoch JR, Silver D. Urokinase and mannitol modification of skeletal muscle ischemia reperfusion injury. Surg Forum 1991;42:330–2.

29. Blebea J, Kerr J, Hobson RW II. Effect of oxygen free radical scavengers on skeletal muscle ischemia and reperfusion injury. Curr Surg 1987; 44:396–8.

30. Buchbinder D, Karmody A, Leather RD, et al. Hypertonic mannitol: its use in the prevention of revascularization syndrome after acute arterial ischemia. Arch Surg 116:414–21.

31. Ulmer T. The clinical diagnosis of compartment syndrome of the lower leg: are clinical findings predictive of the disorder? J Orthop Trauma 2002;16:572–7.

32. Feliciano DV, Cruse PA, Spjut-Patrinely V, Burch JM, Mattox KL. Fasciotomy after trauma to the extremities. Am J Surg 1988;156:533–6.

33. Matsen FA III, Winquist RA, Krugmire RB. Diagnosis and management of compartment syndrome. J Bone Joint Surg 1980;62A:286–91.

34. Heppenstall RB, Balderston R, Goodwin C. Pathophysiologic effects distal to a tourniquet in the dog. J Trauma 1979;19:234–8.

35. Hartsock LA, O'Farrell D, Seaber AV, Urbaniak JR. Effect of increased compartment pressure on the microcirculation of skeletal muscle. Microsurgery 1998;18:67–71.

36. Suval WD, Duran WN, Boric MP, et al. Microvascular transport and endothelial cell alterations precede skeletal muscle damage in ischemia–reperfusion injury. Am J Surg 1987;154: 211–18.

37. Gawlowski DM, Ritter AB, Duran WN. Reproducibility of microvascular permeability responses to successive topical applications of bradykinin in the hamster cheek pouch. Microvasc Res 1982;24:354–63.

38. Hood JD, Meninger CJ, Ziche M, et al. VEGF upregulates ecNOS message protein, and NO production in human endothelial cells. Am J. Physiol 1998;274:H1054–8.

39. Huang Q, Yuan Y. Interaction of PKC and NOS in signal transduction of microvascular hyperpermeability. Am J Physiol 1997;273:H2442–52.

40. Kobayashi K, Kim D, Hobson RW, et al. Platelet activating factor modulates microvascular transport by stimulation of protein kinase C. Am J Physiol 1994;266:H1214–20.

41. Mayhan WG. Role of nitric oxide in modulating permeability of the hamster cheek pouch in response to adenosine 5' diphosphate and bradykinin. Inflammation 1992;16:295–305.

42. Ramirez, MM, Quardt SM, Kim D, et al. Platelet activating factor modulates microvascular permeability through nitric oxide synthesis. Microvasc Res 1995;50:223–34.

43. Ramirez MM, Kim D, Duran WN. Protein kinase C modulates microvascular permeability through nitric oxide synthase. Am J Physiol 1996; 271:H1702–5.

44. He P, Zeng M, Curry FE. cGMP modulates basal and activated microvessel permeability independently of [Ca 2+]i. Am J Physiol 1998; 274:H1865–74.

45. Varma S, Breslin JW, Lal BK, Pappas PJ, Hobson RW II, Durán WN. P42/44^{MAPK} regulates baseline permeability and cGMP-induced hyperpermeability in endothelial cells. Microvasc Res 2002;63:172–8.

46. Kevil CG, Payne DK, Mire E, Alexander JS. Vascular permeability factor/vascular endothelial cell growth factor-mediated permeability occurs through disorganization of endothelial junctional proteins. J Biol Chem 1998;273:15099–103.

47. Korthuis RJ, Granger DN, Townsley MI, et al. The role of oxygen derived free radicals in ischemia induced increases in canine skeletal muscle vascular permeability. Circ Res 1985;57:599–609.

48. Walker PM, Lindsay TF, Labbe R, et al. Salvage of skeletal muscle with free radical scavengers. J Vasc Surg 1987;5:68–72.

49. Kubes P, Granger DN. Nitric oxide modulates microvascular permeability. Am J Physiol 1992;262:H611–5.

50. Beckman JS, Beckman TW, Chen J, et al. Apparent hydroxyl radical production by peroxynitrite: implications for endothelial cell injury from nitric oxide and superoxide. Proc Natl Acad Sci USA 1990;87:1620–4.

51. Breitbart GB, Dillon PK, Suval WD, et al. Leukopenia reduces microvascular clearance of macromolecules in ischemia reperfusion injury. Curr Surg 1990;47:8–12.

52. Belkin M, Lamorte WL, Hobson RW, et al. The role of leukocytes in the pathophysiology of skeletal muscle ischemic injury. J Vasc Surg 1989; 10:14–19.

53. Klausmer JM, Paterson IS, Valeri CR, et al. Limb ischemia induced increase in permeability is mediated by leukocytes and leukotrienes. Ann Surg 1988;208:755–60.

54. Smith JK, Grisham GB, Granger DN, et al. Free radical defence mechanisms and neutrophils infiltration in postischemic skeletal muscle. Am J Physiol 1989;256:H789–93.

55. Duran WN, Dillon PK. Acute microcirculatory effects of platelet activating factor. J Lipid Mediat 1990;2:S215–27.

56. Kubes P, Suzuki M, Granger DN. Modulation of PAF-induced leukocyte adherence and increased microvascular permeability. Am J Physiol 1990;259:G859–69.

57. Beyersdorf F, Matheis G, Kruger S, et al. Avoiding reperfusion injury after limb revascularization: Experimental observations and recommendations for clinical application. J Vasc Surg1989;9:757–66.

58. Ferrante RJ, Hobson RW II, Miyasaka M, et al. Inhibition of white blood cell adhesion at reperfusion decreases tissue damage in postischemic striated muscle. J Vasc Surg 1996;24:187–93.

59. Belkin M, Lamorte WL, Hobson RW II, et al. The role of leukocytes in the pathophysiology of skeletal muscle ischemic injury. J Vasc Surg 1989;10:14–9.

60. Milazzo VJ, Sabido F, Hobson RW II, et al. Platelet activating factor blockade inhibits leukocyte adhesion to endothelium in ischemia reperfusion. Surg Forum 1992;43;376–8.

61. Blebea J, Cambria RA, Defouw D, et al. Iloprost attenuates the increased permeability in skeletal muscle after ischemia and reperfusion. J Vasc Surg 1990;12:657–66.

62. Belkin M, Wright JG, Hobson RW II. Iloprost infusion decreases skeletal muscle injury after ischemia reperfusion. J Vasc Surg 1990;11:77–83.

CHAPTER

19

Upper Extremity Ischemia: Large Artery Occlusive Disease

Thelinh Nguyen and E John Harris Jr

KEY POINTS

- Atherosclerosis is the most common cause of large artery obstruction in the upper extremities.

- Other upper extremity occlusive disorders include thoracic outlet abnormalities, iatrogenic and non-iatrogenic injuries, Takayasu's arteritis, giant cell arteritis, fibromuscular disease, radiation-induced atherosclerosis obliterans, cardiac embolization, and arterial atheroembolization.

- The left subclavian artery is affected by occlusive disease more frequently than the innominate or common carotid arteries.

- Cardiac catheterization via the brachial artery approach is the most common cause of iatrogenic upper extremity arterial injury.

- Diagnostic evaluation of upper extremity occlusive disease may include physical examination, segmental pressure measurements, duplex ultrasound with color flow scanning, Doppler flow scanning, angiography, echocardiography, computed tomography angiography, or magnetic resonance angiography.

- Direct reconstruction via endarterectomy or aortic arch bypass is the standard treatment for brachiocephalic occlusive diseases.

- Indirect reconstruction of brachiocephalic occlusive disease via extra-anatomic bypasses is typically reserved for patients with multiple co-morbidities.

- Endovascular reconstruction of brachiocephalic occlusive disease is a new treatment modality with a high early success rate but unknown long-term efficacy at this time.

INTRODUCTION

Upper extremity ischemia due to systemic disease is relatively rare compared to symptomatic lower extremity ischemia. However, due to the functional importance of the upper extremities, patients with upper extremity ischemia can be profoundly disabled. Symptoms of upper extremity ischemia range from claudication to necrosis and tissue loss. Unlike lower extremity ischemia, where atherosclerosis is the predominant cause, the causes of upper extremity ischemia are diverse, with atherosclerotic as well as non-atherosclerotic causes. Appropriate diagnosis and treatment are important in relieving symptoms and restoring the quality of life. Upper extremity ischemia is commonly considered in the context of large and small arterial diseases. Large arterial diseases, exclusive of thoracic outlet syndrome, will be addressed in this chapter.

ANATOMY AND PATHOLOGY

The aortic arch typically gives off three branches: the innominate, left carotid, and left subclavian arteries. The innominate artery is unique in that it is essentially the sole supplier of blood to the right side of the brain and the right upper extremity. The innominate artery bifurcates into the right common carotid artery and the right subclavian artery. The anatomy of the right and left subclavian arteries is similar on both sides, with the vertebral, internal mammary, and thyrocervical trunk arteries coming off proximally. As the subclavian artery passes over the first rib, it becomes the axillary artery. The axillary artery has six important branches: the highest thoracic, thoracoacromial, lateral thoracic, subscapular, and anterior and posterior circumflex humeral arteries; all of these vessels can serve as collaterals around the shoulder girdle. As the axillary artery crosses the lower border of the teres major muscle, it becomes the brachial artery. In about 80% of cases, there is one single brachial artery extending to its bifurcation, which is near the radial head. However, in about 20% of cases, there is an additional superficial brachial branch, which begins in the proximal upper arm and courses caudally superficial to the median nerve. A high radial or ulnar artery may originate from the superficial brachial artery. The largest branch of the brachial artery is the deep brachial artery, which usually comes off the main brachial artery just below the teres major muscle level.

Atherosclerotic occlusive disease of the innominate, common carotid, and subclavian arteries is relatively rare compared to that of the carotid bifurcation. Fields and Lemark in a published report on the joint study of extracranial arterial occlusion reported that only 17% of lesions identified on angiography involved the innominate artery and the proximal subclavian artery.[1] The left subclavian artery is more commonly affected than the right subclavian artery. The median ages of patients affected with atherosclerotic occlusive disease of the brachiocephalic arteries range from 50 to 61 years, with a slight male predominance.[2-7] Iatrogenic and non-iatrogenic injuries more commonly involve the axillary, brachial, radial, and ulnar arteries.

PATHOPHYSIOLOGY

Atherosclerosis is the most common cause of large artery occlusion, affecting the innominate, common carotid, and subclavian arteries. Compression of the subclavian artery by bony thoracic outlet abnormalities is another important cause of occlusion, which is easily treatable if recognized. Iatrogenic injuries resulting from cardiac catheterization via the brachial artery, arteriography via direct axillary artery puncture, and arterial monitoring line placement are important causes of upper extremity ischemia. Cardiac catheterization via the brachial artery is the most common iatrogenic cause of upper extremity ischemia, with reported incidences ranging from 0.9% to 4%.[8–10] Non-iatrogenic trauma from blunt or penetrating injuries is another important cause for upper extremity ischemia. Rarer causes include Takayasu's arteritis, giant cell arteritis, fibromuscular disease, radiation-induced atherosclerosis obliterans, cardiac embolization, and arterial atheroembolization.

Hypertension, cholesterol metabolism abnormalities, and diabetes mellitus are usually present in patients with atherosclerotic occlusive disease of the upper extremity. Smoking has been found to be a significant risk factor in patients with brachiocephalic occlusive disease. Not surprisingly, the incidence of concomitant coronary artery disease is also high in patients with atherosclerotic upper extremity ischemia, with reported incidences ranging from 26% to 65%.[3,5–7,11]

CLINICAL PRESENTATIONS

Innominate artery

Occlusive disease of the innominate artery is uncommon. Patients with innominate artery lesions may be asymptomatic or may present with neurologic symptoms, right upper extremity ischemia, or combined neurologic and upper extremity symptoms. Between 5% and 90% of patients with innominate lesions present with neurologic symptoms.[5–7] The neurologic symptoms may be due to anterior (carotid) circulation or posterior (vertebral) circulation problems. Neurologic symptoms from aortic arch branch disease are addressed in Chapter 35.

Between 5% and 63% of patients with innominate lesions present with right upper extremity symptoms.[2,5,6,11] Symptoms range from claudication to tissue loss. Claudication is due to hemodynamically significant stenotic lesions, whereas tissue loss is usually associated with microembolization from ulcerated lesions.

Combined neurologic and upper extremity symptoms occur in 18.4% to 38.5% of patients.[5,11] It is also not unusual for patients with innominate artery occlusive disease to have concomitant disease of the carotid and subclavian arteries as well.

Subclavian artery

Occlusive disease of brachiocephalic arteries affects the subclavian artery more frequently than the innominate or common carotid arteries. The left subclavian artery is affected more frequently than the right. Upper extremity ischemia due to subclavian artery occlusive lesions is rare compared to ischemia of the lower extremities due to occlusive disease, accounting for about 5% of all patients with ischemic limbs.[13–15] Patients who are symptomatic from subclavian lesions may present with exercise-induced arm pain, ischemic rest pain, ulcers, or digital necrosis. The types of symptoms are manifestations of either hemodynamically significant stenoses or occlusion, or atheroembolization from irregular plaques. Upper extremity exertional pain rarely occurs in isolated chronic subclavian lesions, due to the abundant arterial collateral flow of the head, neck, and shoulder. In contrast, atheroemboli from upper extremity arterial lesions

occur more frequently than those from lower extremity arterial lesions, with reported incidences ranging from 37% to 47%.[15,16] Atheroemboli may originate from an ulcerated but not highly stenotic lesion. Patients with atheroemboli may present with palpable radial or ulnar pulses; however, painful discolorations, subungual splinter hemorrhages, or a livedo reticularis pattern may be present in the hands or fingers. Timely diagnosis may further be hampered by the fact that the brachial pressure in the affected arm may not be significantly different from that of the contralateral arm. Patients with suspected atheroembolization require diagnostic arteriography.

Proximal subclavian arterial disease can cause reversal of flow in the ipsilateral vertebral artery, a condition that was first termed 'subclavian steal' by Contorni in 1960.[17] More often than not, subclavian steal is a radiologic finding without significant clinical sequelae, especially in the absence of other concomitant arterial lesions. However, in the presence of concomitant extracranial arterial lesions, symptoms of vertebrobasilar insufficiency and/or upper extremity ischemia can develop. The subject of vertebrobasilar insufficiency is addressed in Chapter 36.

Proximal subclavian stenosis or occlusion can also precipitate myocardial ischemia in patients who have had coronary artery bypass grafting from the internal mammary artery (IMA) to the left anterior descending (LAD) coronary artery due to reversal of flow in the IMA stealing flow from the coronary circulation.

Axillary, brachial, and forearm arteries

Atherosclerosis can affect the axillary, brachial, and forearm arteries. However, embolization, iatrogenic injury, and non-iatrogenic trauma are also important causes of upper extremity ischemia affecting these arteries. Cardiac embolization or arterio-arterial atheroembolization involving upper extremities accounts for about 15% to 30% of all peripheral embolization cases.[18] Cardiac embolization is the most common cause, accounting for about 90% of cases. Arteriosclerotic heart disease, atrial fibrillation, and myocardial infarction are the most common underlying cardiac diseases. The brachial artery is affected in 60% of cases. Emboli typically lodge within the following three locations of the brachial artery: at the area just proximal to the deep brachial artery origin, at the origin of the superior ulnar collateral artery, and at the brachial bifurcation. The axillary and subclavian arteries are involved in about 23% and 12% of embolization cases, respectively.[18] Arterial atheroembolization usually affects the radial and ulnar arteries as well as the more distal digital arteries. Patients with embolic arterial occlusion usually present with the sudden onset of arterial insufficiency. The site of obstruction is frequently detectable by careful physical examination.

Upper extremity ischemia can also be caused by iatrogenic injury to the large arteries. Cardiac catheterization via the brachial artery approach is the most common cause of iatrogenic injury, with reported incidences ranging from 0.9% to 4%.[8,9] Thrombosis of a long arterial segment usually results in acute ischemia. However, short segment arterial thrombosis may instead present with chronic ischemic symptoms, usually brought on by exercise of the limb, without significant acute symptoms.

Iatrogenic axillary injury can be the result of transaxillary arteriography or events such as inadvertent injury to the axillary artery during performance of an axillary block. The incidence of axillary arterial thrombosis following transaxillary arteriography is reported to be 0.8%.[19] Patients may present with ischemic symptoms as well as neurologic symptoms, due to axillary sheath hematoma compressing the adjacent divisions of the brachial plexus. Crutch trauma may also injure the axillary artery.

The incidence of radial artery thrombosis following radial arterial cannulation may be as high as 40%.[20] However, radial arterial cannulation is an uncommon cause of upper extremity ischemia, especially in patients with an intact and non-diseased palmar arch. Severe hand ischemia in patients at risk is reported to range from 0.3% to 0.5%.[21]

Non-iatrogenic injuries from blunt or penetrating trauma are an important cause of upper extremity ischemia.[20,22–26] Series from trauma centers have reported axillary artery involvement in 5% to 9%,[25,26] brachial artery involvement in 30%,[25,26] and radial and ulnar artery involvement in 7% to 20%[25–29] of cases. Physical findings range from an expanding hematoma or hemorrhage at the wound entrance site to extremity ischemia without other significant findings. The presence of distal pulses by no means excludes proximal injury and can be present in 30% of patients with iatrogenic arterial injuries.[27,29–31] Due to its proximity to the axillary vessels, brachial plexus injury may occur concomitantly with arterial injury. In fact, patients with subclinical arterial injury may present with only signs and symptoms of brachial plexus injury. Brachial plexus injury can also be caused by axillary sheath hematoma, which, if unrecognized, can lead to significant long-term morbidity.

DIAGNOSTIC TECHNIQUES

Physical examination remains a standard method for detecting large artery occlusive disease. The carotid, axillary, brachial, radial, and ulnar pulses should be palpated as well as auscultated. The presence of bruits should raise the suspicion of stenotic lesions, or perhaps intimal flaps from arterial dissection. The absence of pulses suggests the presence of more proximal occlusive lesions. The presence of occlusive lesions in the digital arteries with palpable proximal pulses, especially if unilateral, usually suggests arterial embolization from a more proximal source. Although connective tissue disorders can also cause digital arterial occlusive

disease, the process is usually bilateral in such patients. In non-iatrogenic arterial injury, the diagnosis may be obvious, with hemorrhage or expanding hematoma at the injury site, as well as associated bony and soft tissue injuries.

Segmental pressure measurements should be performed in the affected limb and compared to those of the contralateral limb. Normally, the pressure difference between arms should not exceed 15mmHg. Pressure gradients between adjacent vessels of the same arm should also normally be less than 15mmHg.[32] A significant reduction in brachial blood pressure (20mmHg or more) in the affected arm suggests the presence of a proximal (innominate, subclavian, axillary, or upper brachial) lesion. A significant pressure gradient between two adjacent levels in the same arm suggests disease of the intervening segment.

Duplex ultrasound with color flow scanning is a useful non-invasive study to evaluate the arterial system of the upper extremity. Precise anatomic information, including the location and degree of the stenosis and the extent of collateral flow, can be obtained with the B-mode ultrasound component of the duplex ultrasound. Conventional duplex scanning is further enhanced by color flow mapping, which allows easy tracing of the studied vessels. The presence of arterial obstruction or stenosis is easily seen on color flow mapping (**Fig. 19.1**).

Significant information is also obtained from the Doppler flow component of the duplex ultrasound study. A normal Doppler flow signal is biphasic or triphasic, consisting of a rapid rise in velocity to a peak in early systole, followed by an abrupt fall to the baseline value, frequently reversing in early diastole (**Fig. 19.2**). A small forward flow signal may also be present in late diastole. When Doppler flow signals are obtained distal to an obstruction or high-grade stenosis, the signals are significantly attenuated with a slower upslope, a more attenuated peak, and a downslope continuing throughout the diastole (**Fig. 19.3**). The audible signals are now monophasic. Doppler flow signals obtained at or slightly beyond the site of stenosis are noisy, with high frequency flow reflecting the turbulent, high-velocity flow through the stenotic site. Continuous wave Doppler flow study also allows indirect evaluation of arteries that may not be directly accessible by B-mode scanning or duplex ultrasound

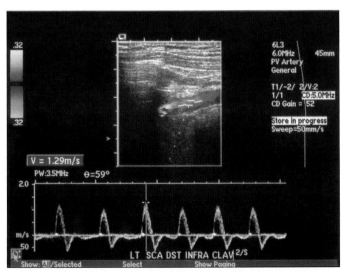

Figure 19.1 Duplex ultrasound with color flow mapping of arterial segments.

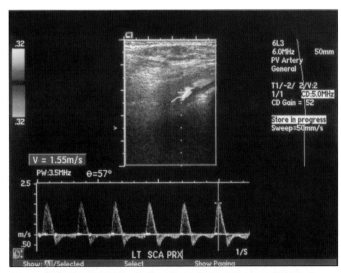

Figure 19.2 Normal triphasic Doppler waveform in a non-diseased arterial segment.

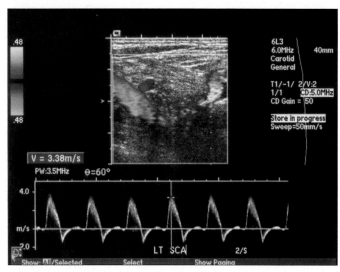

Figure 19.3 Doppler flow signals in a diseased arterial segment. (See text for explanation.)

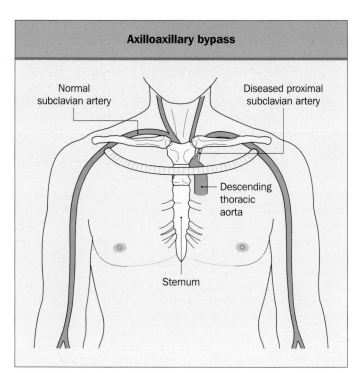

Figure 19.4 Axilloaxillary bypass.

scanning. The subclavian artery is one such example. Normally, the subclavian artery may not be easily visualized by duplex ultrasound scanning, especially at its origin in the thorax or beneath the clavicle. However, the subclavian artery may be indirectly assessed by analyzing Doppler flow patterns in its accessible portions.

Arch aortography with runoff views of the brachiocephalic branches is the gold standard for the diagnosis and localization of upper extremity arterial occlusive disease. Angiography allows the detection of multiple lesions that may be present in 60% to 84% of patients with brachiocephalic occlusive disease.[5,6,7] Angiography is also useful in excluding a proximal arterial embolic source or a proximal arterial dissection.

Echocardiography, especially transesophageal, is useful to identify or detect embolic sources from the heart or from ulcerated atherosclerotic plaques in the aortic arch that may not be detected by conventional arteriography.[33,34]

Computed tomography (CT) angiography and magnetic resonance angiography are promising new non-invasive imaging modalities, especially with three-dimensional reconstruction, which can be applied to patients with brachiocephalic occlusive disease. More and more operations are being performed based solely on CT angiographic images, without adjunctive conventional angiography.[35]

MANAGEMENT

Innominate artery

Surgical intervention is indicated in selected patients with symptomatic occlusive disease, and either neurologic symptoms, upper extremity ischemia, or combined neurologic and upper extremity symptoms. Asymptomatic high-grade lesions (>70% luminal stenosis) or ulcerative lesions with greater then 50% stenosis may possibly benefit from surgical intervention. Surgical options include direct and indirect reconstructions. Direct reconstruction includes innominate endarterectomy or aortic-origin grafting. Indirect reconstructions are performed using extra-anatomic bypasses such as subclavian-subclavian, axillary-

axillary, contralateral carotid-carotid, or carotid-subclavian, or even femoral-axillary bypasses. Reported results in the literature of axilloaxillary artery bypasses are mixed. Lowell and Mills performed a retrospective review of 10 patients at their institution and 253 cases reported in the literature, and found a 5-year patency rate of 90% with minimal complications.[36] Mingoli et al. examined a series of 63 crossover axilloaxillary bypass grafts over a 24-year period and found overall mortality and morbidity rates of 1.6% and 16.1%, respectively. Primary and secondary patency rates at 5 and 10 years in this series were reported to be 86.5% and 82.8% and 88.1% and 84.3%, respectively.[37] However, others have reported less favorable results with axilloaxillary bypasses. Thompson et al. reviewed their series and concluded that axilloaxillary bypasses are prone to thrombosis and skin erosion.[38] Brewster et al. reported a 50% thrombosis rate.[39] Criado recommended against the use of axilloaxillary bypasses, based on their review of the literature.[40]

In general, extra-anatomic bypasses are most appropriately performed in patients with multiple co-morbidities which make them poor operative candidates for direct reconstruction, or in patients with previous median sternotomy or severe chronic obstructive pulmonary disease. Extra-anatomic reconstructions carry some inherent risks. Routing of the graft predisposes patients to skin tunnel erosion and also may complicate the performance of tracheostomy or median sternotomy if these procedures are subsequently needed (**Fig. 19.4**). Extra-anatomic bypasses are also relatively contraindicated in patients with atheroembolism from proximal ulcerative lesions.

Direct reconstruction using innominate endarterectomy (**Fig. 19.5**) is a time-honored, technically demanding operation. Multiple series have shown comparable long-term patency with either endarterectomy or aortic-origin grafting.[11,41] Innominate endarterectomy is limited by the extent of the disease and whether safe clamping of the aortic arch can be performed.

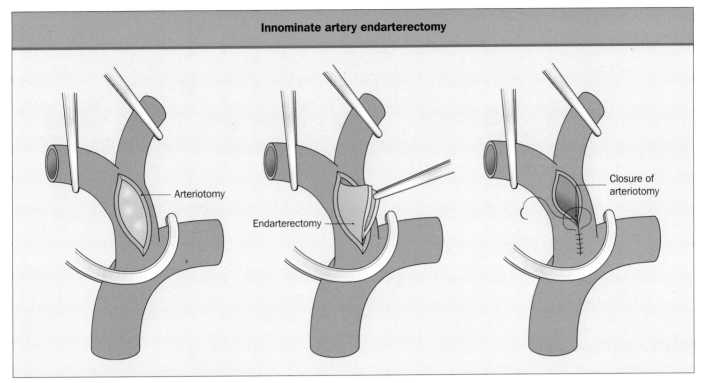

Innominate artery endarterectomy

Arteriotomy

Endarterectomy

Closure of arteriotomy

Figure 19.5 Innominate artery endarterectomy.

Atherosclerosis of the aortic arch at the origin of the innominate artery has been found by some authors to contraindicate for endarterectomy.[2] If the origin of the left carotid artery is close to that of the innominate artery, safe clamping of the proximal innominate artery on the aortic arch may not be feasible.

Direct bypass grafting from the proximal aortic arch is a durable procedure with excellent short-term as well as long-term results. Multiple series have reported early symptom relief in 95% of patients and long-term relief in 87% to 90% of patients.[2–5,11,39,42] Two large series reported primary patency rates of 92.7% to 98.4% at 5 years and 84% to 88% at 10 years.[6,7] Berguer et al. reported a combined death/stroke rate of 16% and an operative mortality rate of 6%.[7] The operative mortality and perioperative stroke/transient ischemic attack rates in the series reported by Kieffer et al. are about 5.4% each.[6] Due to the morbid nature of the procedure, direct reconstruction should only be peformed in symptomatic patients who otherwise are fit for surgery.

Direct aorto-brachiocephalic grafts are performed via a median sternotomy, partial sternotomy, or through an incision in the second or third intercostal space.[43] Dacron or ringed Goretex grafts have been used. Patients with embolization from innominate lesions should have their innominate arteries transected and proximally oversewn to prevent recurrent embolism. The distal anastomosis is performed end to end. Bypass grafting is also preferred over endarterectomy in patients with Takayasu's arteritis or radiation-induced arteritis. Multiple bypasses can be performed at one sitting in patients with multiple lesions (**Fig. 19.6**). Compression by mediastinal structures or the reapproximated sternum may lead to graft failure, venous obstruction, or tracheal obstruction, and is a potential pitfall of this type of bypass grafting, and potentially increased with multiple limbs exiting the mediastinum.[4]

Subclavian artery

Surgical intervention is indicated in patients with symptomatic lesions. Subclavian transposition and carotid subclavian bypass are two operations that have withstood the test of time. Carotid-subclavian bypass (**Fig. 19.7**), a successful and durable extra-anatomic bypass, was first popularized by Diethrich et al. in 1967.[44] Patency rates are generally better with synthetic (Dacron or polytetrafluoroethylene) grafts than with saphenous vein grafts, with reported patency rates of 95% for PTFE, 84% for Dacron, and 65% for vein grafts.[45] Results of carotid-subclavian bypass are excellent. Large series have reported patency rates of 92% to 95% at five years and 83% to 95% at 8 to 10 years. Perioperative complications are low, with reported stroke rates of 0% to 3.2% and mortality rates of 0% to 0.8%.[45–47] For patients with extensive disease of the subclavian artery, carotid-axillary or carotid-brachial bypasses are durable options, with comparable patency rates to those of carotid-subclavian bypass.[48,49]

Subclavian artery transposition (**Fig. 19.8**) onto the common carotid artery has been a successful and durable procedure since its description by Parrott in 1964.[50] Subclavian transposition avoids the need for a synthetic graft. Furthermore, only one anastomosis is required. Subclavian transposition is also very useful in patients with embolization from unstable proximal lesions. The potential disadvantages of this operation are that it requires extensive dissection of the subclavian artery, proximal to the origins of the vertebral and internal mammary arteries, and it can only be performed for very proximal lesions. Subclavian transposition is contraindicated in patients with coronary bypass from the internal mammary artery, as transecting the subclavian artery proximal to the internal mammary artery can precipitate a massive myocardial infarction, unless some form of shunt is used. Results of subclavian transposition are excellent, exceeding those of carotid subclavian

Direct bypass grafting

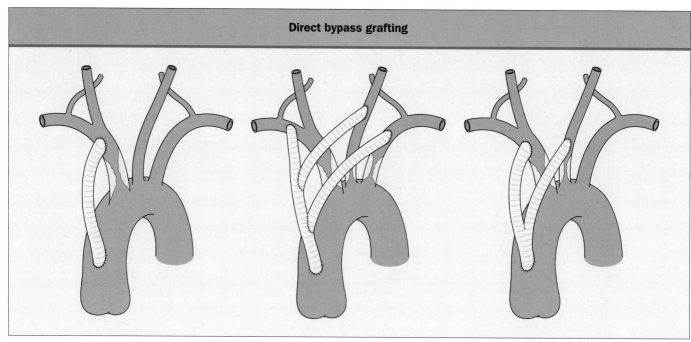

Figure 19.6 Direct bypass grafting.

Carotid-subclavian bypass

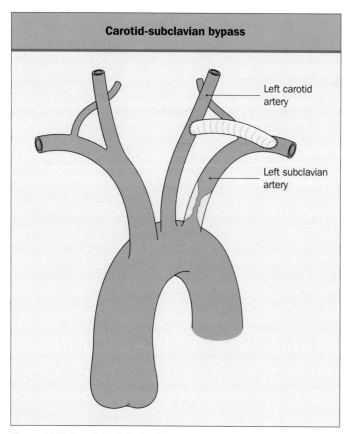

Left carotid artery

Left subclavian artery

Figure 19.7 Carotid-subclavian bypass.

Subclavian artery transposition

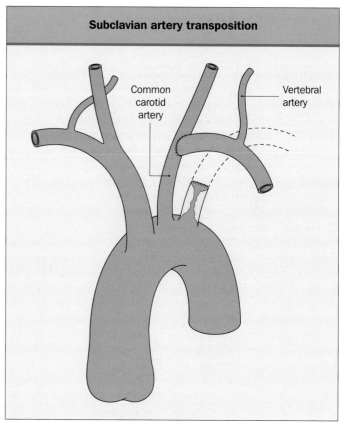

Common carotid artery

Vertebral artery

Figure 19.8 Subclavian artery transposition.

bypass. Most large series reported long-term patency rates of 95% to 100% and a 0% perioperative stroke rate.[50–53]

Axillary and brachial arteries

As mentioned previously, axillary and brachial arteries are mostly affected by embolization and iatrogenic or non-iatrogenic arterial injuries. For embolic lesions, the affected artery can be exposed either via an incision in the upper third of the arm over the bicipital groove or in the antecubital fossa. A transverse arteriotomy is performed to avoid narrowing of the artery at the time of arteriotomy closure. Embolectomy is then performed via the arteriotomy, using a standard technique. Preoperative heparinization should be initiated to prevent propagation of thrombus. Intraoperative arteriography is useful if there is any doubt about the adequacy of the distal thromboembolectomy. Most series report a limb salvage rate of 81% to 100%, with perioperative mortality rates of 0% to 19%, primarily from cardiac disease.[54,55] Thrombolytic therapy may play a role in selected patients with cardiac embolization who present with non-immediately threatening limb ischemia.

Iatrogenic arterial injuries can present in acute or chronic form. Acute ischemia is treated with local exploration of the involved artery followed by thrombectomy, debridement, and primary arteriotomy closure if possible. Again, preoperative heparinization is important in limiting thrombus progression. Segmental resection followed by primary end-to-end anastomosis may be required if the involved artery is significantly damaged. Interposition reversed saphenous vein graft may be needed if there is a long damaged segment of the involved artery. If inadequate blood flow is obtained following thrombectomy, angiography is indicated to rule out proximal dissection. Proximal intimal dissection may be treated with a bypass procedure or endoluminal stenting. Results of surgical intervention for iatrogenic arterial injury are excellent, with reported patency rates of up to 99%.[8,9] Neurologic injury from delayed decompression of axillary sheath hematomas is the main cause of long-term morbidity.

Iatrogenic arterial injury may also cause chronic ischemia if the acute event is not addressed immediately. Symptomatic ischemia, tissue loss, and rest pain are indications for surgical intervention. Bypass using saphenous vein or arm vein is the procedure of choice. Prosthetic conduit may be used if autogenous veins are not available; however, long-term patency of prosthetic conduits remains unknown. The interosseous artery may play an important role in upper extremity revascularization, as it may be the only patent artery distally. Results of surgical bypasses for chronic upper arm ischemia are generally good, with 60% to 90% 2–5-year patency rates.[56,57]

Non-iatrogenic arterial injuries from penetrating or blunt trauma or humeral fractures are also important causes of upper extremity ischemia. Surgical principles include local exposure of the affected artery, fracture stabilization, debridement or resection of the damaged area, and thromboembolectomy followed by primary anastomosis or saphenous vein interposition grafting. Fasciotomy of the forearm may be required for prolonged ischemic time. Results of arterial repair are generally good. Amputation rates, as reported in most series, range from 0% to 10% for axillary arterial injuries and 0% to 2.5% for brachial arterial injuries.[25–27,58] Long-term morbidity is usually caused by associated neurologic injury.

Endovascular management of innominate, subclavian, and axillary arterial occlusive disease

Percutaneous transluminal angioplasty (PTA) is an acceptable treatment modality for selected patients with a symptomatic, high-grade, short, or focal stenosis without severe calcification. PTA can be performed via the femoral or brachial artery approach. Stent placement is indicated for suboptimal angioplasty results and arterial dissection. The technical success rate is high for focal stenotic lesions, with reported technical success rates of 85% to 100%.[59–62] Long or heavily calcified lesions are associated with a lower technical success rate. The technical success rate for complete occlusions is also low, at 46%.[62] Arterial distal embolization, dissection, thrombosis, and bleeding are potential complications. Stent migration and fracture, especially if the stent is placed in the mid- to distal subclavian artery, are other complications. Sullivan et al. reported an overall complication rate of 17.8%, including access site bleeding and distal embolization in 73 subclavian and innominate artery PTA procedures.[61] Embolization following PTA has been reported up to 3 days post PTA.[63] The incidence of transient ischemic attack following PTA has been reported to range from 1% to 9%.[62,64] The incidence of major stroke following brachiocephalic PTA ranges from 0% to 2%.[60,64] Various techniques have been employed to prevent distal cerebral embolization, such as retrograde angioplasty from the common carotid artery[65–67] exposed through a cervical incision and a double balloon technique.[68] With the common carotid artery approach, the angioplasty is performed retrograde through a cervical common carotid arteriotomy, with the distal common carotid artery clamped during the PTA procedure. As technology advances, and the availability of distal protection devices becomes wider, the incidence of distal embolization will undoubtedly decrease.

Reliable long-term patency rates for PTA/stenting have been difficult to determine, since most reports have not been standardized and lack objective long-term follow-up. Huttl et al. recently reported their experience with 89 innominate artery PTA procedures, with short-term primary patency rates of 98% at 6 months.[64] However, no conclusion can be drawn about the long-term patency rate, since this reported rate was calculated over a wide range of 12 to 117 months. For subclavian artery PTA, Henry et al. reported primary and secondary patency rates of 75% and 81%, respectively, at 8 years.[62] Schillinger et al., on the other hand, reported a primary patency rate for subclavian artery PTA of 59% in arteries with stents and 68% in arteries without stents at 4-year follow up.[59] Well-controlled studies are needed to determine the long-term efficacy of these endovascular therapies for brachiocephalic occlusive disease. Undoubtedly, drug-eluting stents, once available, will have a significant impact on the endovascular treatment of brachiocephalic occlusive disease.

SUMMARY

Upper extremity ischemia from large artery occlusive disease, although rare compared to lower extremity ischemia, can cause significant morbidity in afflicted patients. Correct diagnosis and appropriate treatment ensure optimal outcome. For brachiocephalic disease, direct reconstruction is the gold standard. Indirect reconstructions are reserved for patients with multiple co-morbidities which make them poor candidates for median sternotomy or thoracotomy. Percutaneous balloon angioplasty and/or stenting may be appropriate therapy for patients with symptomatic, high-grade, and focal occlusive disease. However, long-term results of angioplasty and/or stenting are not known at this time. Well-controlled, randomized clinical studies are required to evaluate the long-term efficacy of this exciting, yet potentially ineffective technology.

REFERENCES

1. Fields WS, Lemark NA. Joint study of extracranial arterial occlusion: VII. Subclavian steal – a review of 168 cases. JAMA 1972;222:1139–43.
2. Carlson RE, Ehrenfeld WK, Stoney RJ, Wylie EJ. Innominate artery endarterectomy: a 16-year history. Arch Surg 1977;112:1389–93.
3. Vogt DP, Hertzer NR, O'Hara PJ, Beven EG. Brachiocephalic arterial reconstruction. Ann Surg 1982;196:541–52.
4. Crawford ES, Stowe CL, Powers RW Jr. Occlusion of the innominate, common carotid, and subclavian arteries. Long-term results of surgical treatment. Surgery 1983;94:781–91.
5. Reul GJ, Jacobs MJHM, Gregoric ID, et al. Innominate artery occlusive disease: surgical approach and long-term results. J Vasc Surg 1991; 14:405–12.
6. Kieffer E, Sabatier J, Koskas, et al. Atherosclerotic innominate artery occlusive disease. Early and long-term results of surgical reconstruction. J Vasc Surg 1995;21:226–36.
7. Berguer R, Morasch MD, Kline RA. Transthoracic repair of innominate and common carotid artery disease. Immediate and long-term outcome for 100 consecutive surgical reconstructions. J Vasc Surg 1998;27:34–42.
8. Kitzmiller JW, Hertzer NR, Beven EG. Routine surgical management of brachial artery occlusion after cardiac catherization. Arch Surg 1982; 117:1066–71.
9. Kline RM, Hertzer NR, Beven EG, et al. Surgical treatment of brachial artery injuries after cardiac catheterization. J Vasc Surg 1990;12:20–4.
10. Brenner BJ, Couch NP. Peripheral arterial complications of left heart catheterization and their management. Am J Surg 1973;125:521–6.
11. Cherry KJ Jr, McCullough JL, Hallett JW Jr, Pairolero P. Technical principles of direct innominate artery revascularization. A comparison of endarterectomy and bypass grafts. J Vasc Surg 1989;9:718–24.
12. Zelenock GB, Cronenwett JL, Graham LM, et al: Brachiocephalic arterial occlusions and stenoses: Manifestations and management of complex lesions. Arch Surg 1985;120:370–6.
13. Whitehouse WM Jr, Zelenock GB, Wakefield TW, Graham LM, Lindenauer SM, Stanley JC. Arterial bypass grafts for upper extremity ischemia. J Vasc Surg 1986;3:569–73.
14. McCarthy WJ, Flinn WR, Yao JST, et al. Result of bypass grafting for upper limb ischemia. J Vasc Surg 1986;3:741–6.
15. Kadwa AM, Robbs JV. Gangrenous fingers: the tip of the iceberg. J R Coll Surg Edinb 1990;35:71–4.
16. Rapp JH, Reilly LM, Goldstone J, et al. Ischemia of the upper extremity. Significance of proximal arterial disease. Am J Surg 1986;152:122–6.
17. Contorni L. Il circolo collaterale vertebro-vertebrale nella obliterazione dell'arteria succlavia alla sua origine. Minerva Chir 1960;15:268–71.
18. Haimovici H. Cardiogenic embolism of the upper extremity. J Cardiovasc Surg 1982;23:209–13.
19. Hessel SJ, Adams DF, Abrams HL. Complications of angiography. Radiology 1981;138:273–81.
20. Bedford RF, Wollman H. Complications of percutaneous radial-artery cannulation. Anesthesiology 1973;38:228–36.
21. Mozersky DJ, Buckley CJ, Hagood CO, et al. Ultrasonic evaluation of the palmar circulation. Am J Surg 1973;126:810–12.
22. Borman KR, Snyder WH, Weigelt JA. Civilian arterial trauma of the upper extremity. An 11 year experience in 267 patients. Am J Surg 1984; 148:796–9.
23. Katz SG, Kohl RD. Direct revascularization for the treatment of forearm and hand ischemia. Am J Surg 1993;165:312–16.
24. McCroskey BL, Moore EE, Pearce WH, et al. Traumatic injuries of the brachial artery. Am J Surg 1988;156:553–5.
25. Drapanas T, Hewitt RL, Weichert RF, et al. Civilian vascular injuries: a critical appraisal of three decades of management. Ann Surg 1970; 172:351–60.
26. Perry MO, Thal ER, Shires GT. Management of arterial injuries. Ann Surg 1971;173:403–8.
27. Bole PV, Purdy RT, Munda RT, et al. Civilian arterial injuries. Ann Surg 1976;183:13–23.
28. Hardy JD, Raju S, Neely WA, et al. Aortic and other arterial injuries. Ann Surg 1975;181:640–53.
29. Sitzman JV, Ernst CB. Management of arm arterial injuries. Surgery 1984;

30. Rutherford RB. Diagnostic evaluation of extremity vascular injuries. Surg Clin North Am 1988;68:683–91.
31. Smith RF, Elliott JP, Hageman JH, et al. Acute penetrating arterial injuries of the neck and limbs. Arch Surg 1974;109:198–205.
32. Sumner DS, Lambeth A, Russell JB. Diagnosis of upper extremity obstructive and vasospastic syndromes by Doppler ultrasound, plethysmography, and temperature profiles. In: Puel P, Boccalon H, Enjalbert A, eds. Hemodynamics of the limbs 1. Toulouse, France: GEPESC; 1979:365–73.
33. Weinberger J, Azhar S, Danisi F, et al. A new noninvasive technique for imaging atherosclerotic plaque in the aortic arch of stroke patients by transcutaneous real-time B-mode ultrasonography: an initial report. Stroke 1998;29: 673–6.
34. Laperche T, Laurian C, Roudaut R, Steg PG. Mobile thromboses of the aortic arch without aortic debris. A transesophageal echocardiographic finding associated with unexplained arterial embolism: the Filiale Echocardiographic de la Societe Francaise de Cardiologie. Circulation 1977;96:288–94.
35. Carpenter JP, Holand GA, Golden MA, et al. Magnetic resonance angiography of the aortic arch. J Vasc Surg 1997;25:145–51.
36. Lowell RC, Mills JL. Critical evaluation of axilloaxillary artery bypass for surgical management of symptomatic subclavian and innominate artery occlusive disease. Cardiovasc Surg 1993;1:530–5.
37. Mingoli A, Sapienza P, Feldhaus RJ, et al. Long term results and outcomes of crossover axilloaxillary bypass grafting: a 24-year experience. J Vasc Surg 1999;29:894–901.
38. Thompson BW, Read RC, Campbell GS. Operative correction of proximal blocks of the subclavian or innominate arteries. J Cardiovasc Surg 1980; 21:125–30.
39. Brewster DC, Moncure AC, Darling RC, Ambrosino JJ, Abbott WM. Innominate artery lesions: problems encountered and lessons learned. J Vasc Surg 1985;2:99–112.
40. Criado FJ. Extrathoracic management of aortic arch syndrome. Br J Surg 1982;69:45–51.
41. Carlson RE, Ehrenfeld WK, Stoney RJ, Wylie EJ. Innominate artery endarterectomy: A 16-year history. Arch Surg 1977;112:1389–93.
42. Ligush J JR, Criado E, Keagy BA. Innominate artery occlusive disease: management with central reconstructive techniques. Surgery 1997; 121:556–62.
43. Takach TJ, Reul GJ, Cooley DA. Transthoracic reconstruction of the great vessels using minimally invasive technique. Tex Heart Inst J 1996; 23:284–8.
44. Diethrich EB, Garrett HE, Ameriso J, Crawford ES, el-Bayar M, De Bakey ME. Occlusive disease of the common carotid and subclavian arteries treated by carotid-subclavian bypass: analysis of 125 cases. Am J Surg 1967;114:800–8.
45. Law MM, Colburn MD, Moore WS, Quinones-Baldrich WJ, Machleder HI, Gelabert HA. Carotid-subclavian bypass for brachiocephalic occlusive disease: choice of conduit and long-term follow-up. Stroke 1995; 26:1565–71.
46. Perler PA, Williams GM. Carotid-subclavian bypass: a decade of experience. J Vasc Surg 1990;12:716–23.
47. Vitti MJ, Thompson BW, Read RC, Gagne PJ, Barone GW, Barnes RW, Eidt JF. Carotid-subclavian bypass: a twenty-two-year experience. J Vasc Surg 1994;20:411–8.
48. Criado FJ, Queral LA. Carotid-axillary artery bypass: a ten-year experience. J Vasc Surg 1995;22:717–22.
49. Gupta A, Rubin J. Carotid brachial bypass for treating proximal upper-extremity arterial occlusive disease. Am J Surg 1994; 168:210–13.
50. Parrott JC. The subclavian steal syndrome. Arch Surg 1964;88:661–5.
51. Kretschmer G, Teleky B, Marosi L, et al. Obliterations of the proximal subclavian artery: to bypass or to anastomose? J Cardiol Surg 1991; 32:334–9.
52. Sandmann W, Kniemeyer HW, Jaeschock R, Hennerici M, Aulich A. The role of subclavian-carotid transposition in surgery for supra-aortic occlusive disease. J Vasc Surg 1987;5:53–8.

96:895–901.

53. Sterpetti AV, Schultz RD, Farina C, Feldhaus RJ. Subclavian artery revascularization: a comparison between carotid-subclvian artery bypass and subclavian-carotid transposition. Surgery 1989;106:624–32.
54. Banis JC, Rich N, Whelan TJ. Ischemia of the upper extremity due to noncardiac emboli. Am J Surg 1977;134:131–9.
55. James EC, Khuri NT, Fedde CW, Gardner RJ, Tarnay TJ, Warden HE. Upper limb ischemia resulting from arterial thromboembolism. Am J Surg 1979;137:739–44.
56. Brunkwall J, Berqvist D, Bergentz SE. Long-term results of arterial reconstruction of the upper extremity. Eur J Vasc Surg 1994;8:47.
57. Mesh CL, McCarthy WJ, et al. Upper extremity bypass grafting: a 15 year experience. Arch Surg 1993;128:795–801.
58. Borman KR, Snyder WH, Weigelt JA. Civilian arterial trauma of the upper extremity: an 11 year experience in 267 patients. Am J Surg 1984;148:796–9.
59. Schillinger M, Haumer M, Schillinger S, Ahmadi R, Minar E. Risk stratification for subclavian artery angioplasty: is there an increased rate of restenosis after stent implantation? J Endovasc Ther 2001;8:550–7.
60. Gonzales A, Gil-Peralta A, Gonzalez-Marcos JR, Mayol A. Angioplasty and stenting for total symptomatic atherosclerotic occlusion of the subclavian or innominate arteries. Cerebrovasc Dis 2002;13:107–13.
61. Sullivan TM, Gray BH, Bacharach JM, et al. Angioplasty and primary stenting of the subclavian, innominate, and common carotid arteries in 83 patients. J Vasc Surg 1998; 28:1059–65.
62. Henry M, Armor M, Henry I, et al. Percutaneous transluminal angioplasty of the subclavian arteries. J Endovasc Surg 1999;6:33–41.
63. Sawada M, Hashimoto N, Nishi S, Akiyama Y. Detection of embolic signals during and after percutaneous transluminal angioplasty of subclavian and vertebral arteries using transcranial Doppler ultrasonography. Neurosurgery 1997;41:535–40.
64. Huttl K, Nemes B, Simonffy A, Entz L, Berczi V. Angioplasty of the innominate artery in 89 patients: experience over 19 years. Cardiovasc Intervent Radiol 2002; 25:109–14.
65. Levien LJ, Benn CA, Veller MG, Fritz VU. Retrograde balloon angioplasty of brachiocephalic or common carotid artery stenoses at the time of carotid endarterectomy. Eur J Vasc Endovasc Surg 1998;15:521–7.
66. Ruebben A, Tettoni S, Muratore P, et al. Feasibility of intraoperative balloon angioplasty and additional stent placement of isolated stenosis of the brachiocephalic trunk. J Thorac Cardiovasc Surg 1998; 115:1316–20.
67. Merlo M, Conforti M, Apostolou D, Carignanno G. Surgical and endovascular treatment of stenosis of the innominate artery. Minerva Cardioangiol 1999;47:49–54.
68. Korner M, Baumgartner I, Do DD, et al. PTA of the subclavian and innominate arteries: long-term results. Vasa 1999;28:117–22.

CHAPTER

20

Upper Extremity Ischemia: Small Artery Occlusive Disease

James M Edwards and Scott Musicant

KEY POINTS

- Raynaud's syndrome is defined as episodic digital ischemia in response to cold or emotional stress.

- Most patients have normal digits between attacks.

- Raynaud's syndrome may be due to fixed obstruction or episodic vasospasm.

- Raynaud's syndrome is associated with autoimmune diseases.

- Evaluation by the vascular laboratory is useful.

- Initial therapy consists of cold avoidance.

- Medication therapy comprises calcium channel blockers and angiotension-converting enzyme inhibitors.

- Tissue loss is rare, and best treated conservatively.

- Most patients do not develop progressive hand ischemia.

INTRODUCTION

Upper extremity ischemia accounts for less that 5% of patients presenting to a vascular surgeon for evaluation of digital ischemia, with the vast majority of patients in most practices presenting with leg ischemia secondary to atherosclerosis. Patients with upper extremity occlusive disease usually present with Raynaud's syndrome. Raynaud's syndrome is defined as intermittent digital ischemia occurring in response to cold or emotional stress. Most patients describe tri-color changes, with the fingers initially turning white, then blue or purple, and finally red after rewarming. The physiologic sequence responsible for these color changes is as follows:

- the initial pallor is caused by digital ischemia;
- the cyanosis occurs when blood initially returns to the digit and becomes deoxygenated; and
- the rubor upon rewarming occurs as the result of reactive hyperemia.

It is clear that there is a subgroup of Raynaud's patients who do not have the classic tri-color changes, including a small group of patients who have no color changes at all. These patients appear to be otherwise indistinguishable from those patients with color changes. In most patients, the digits are normal between attacks. Raynaud's syndrome may be due to an intrinsic abnormality in the digital blood vessels, sympathetic nervous system, or the thermoregulatory system; or secondary to an associated disease, as will be discussed later in this chapter. Patients with intrinsic abnormalities often have a lifelong history of Raynaud's

syndrome, and may be regarded as otherwise normal individuals who are hypersensitive to cold. Longstanding tradition differentiates Raynaud's patients into those with 'Raynaud's disease' and those with 'Raynaud's phenomenon', where disease refers to patients with episodic digital ischemia in the absence of a diagnosed associated disease, and phenomenon describes those patients with a diagnosed associated disease.[1] We feel that this classification is not useful for several reasons. First, the most commonly associated diseases, the connective tissue diseases, may not become clinically apparent until years after the onset of Raynaud's syndrome, meaning patients may be shifted from one group to another without a change in clinical condition. Secondly, this division does not address the underlying digital artery pathology that may be present.[2,3] Since the presence or absence of arterial pathology or associated disease are the primary and perhaps only objective data available on patients with Raynaud's syndrome, we have suggested grouping Raynaud's patients on this basis. We now term all patients with digital ischemia as having Raynaud's syndrome and subcategorize patients by the presence or absence of associated disease and arterial occlusive disease. The division of numbers between patients with Raynaud's secondary to intrinsic abnormalities and patients with Raynaud's secondary to an associated disease is unclear and depends on referral patterns (primary care practice versus a tertiary referral practice). In this chapter we will discuss the pathophysiology and classification of Raynaud's syndrome, the mechanisms of vasospasm thought to be important in Raynaud's syndrome, the wide variety of connective tissue disorders and small vessel diseases which may be associated with Raynaud's syndrome, and our clinical approach to patients who present with Raynaud's syndrome.

PATHOPHYSIOLOGY

The pathophysiologic mechanism(s) underlying Raynaud's syndrome remain unknown despite over a century of study.[4,5] While it is clear that many patients with Raynaud's syndrome have been diagnosed with a wide variety of disease states which may have a causative casual relationship to the vasospasm, most patients with Raynaud's syndrome do not have an associated disease.[6] The associated disease states, often a variety of autoimmune diseases, share a common feature of small artery arteriopathy and frequently extensive occlusive disease of palmar and digital arteries.

Multiple abnormalities involving the sympathetic nervous system,[7,8] the digital blood vessels themselves,[5] altered sensitivities and numbers of alpha-[9,10] and beta-[11] adrenoceptors, and vasoactive peptides including calcitonin gene-related peptide[12-14] and endothelin[15-17] have been postulated over the last century to explain Raynaud's syndrome. There is also evidence that suggests involvement of both local factors[18] and alterations in the function of the sympathetic nervous system.[19] Our understanding of the basic physiology of blood vessel contraction and relaxation is becoming more and more complex, and it is increasingly clear that the pathophysiologic mechanisms responsible for Raynaud's syndrome are variable and probably overlapping, and likely differ from patient to patient.

Diagnostic criteria and patient classification

While we currently have no way of determining the exact mechanism(s) of vasospasm in a given patient, our experience indicates that patients with Raynaud's syndrome can readily be separated into groups on an objective basis. As noted above, we divide patients into four groups based on the presence or absence of arterial obstructive disease and the presence or absence of an associated disease. Division of patients into groups based on the presence or absence of arterial obstructive disease results in two groups, which we have termed vasospastic and obstructive. These two groups appear to have significantly different pathophysiologic mechanisms underlying the symptoms observed clinically.

Patients with vasospastic Raynaud's syndrome have normal digital artery pressure at rest. As a result of cold or emotional stress, these patients experience an abnormally forceful contraction of digital artery smooth muscle, leading to palmar and digital artery closure. This results in profound, albeit temporary, digital ischemia and pallor. Again, the pathophysiologic mechanism of this abnormally forceful contraction is not known, and may vary between patients, or even between vasospastic episodes. Upon rewarming or relief of stress, the vasoconstriction ceases and the digits return to normal.

Patients with obstructive Raynaud's syndrome have either palmar and digital artery occlusive disease, proximal obstruction of the large arteries of the upper extremity, or a combination of the two, which results in decreased resting digital blood pressure. These patients usually have relatively normal appearing fingers at rest, but may have symptomatic digital ischemia or tissue loss under non-stressed conditions. With cold or emotional stress, a normal (or abnormal) vasoconstrictive response of the digital artery smooth muscle overcomes the decreased intraluminal distending pressure and causes arterial closure with subsequent symptoms. With this mechanism, there is no need to hypothesize an abnormally forceful vasoconstrictive response in these patients, but we suspect that there is overlap between mechanisms such that a number of patients experience both an abnormally forceful contractile response and palmar–digital artery obstructive disease.

The proposed pathophysiologic mechanisms are shown diagrammatically in **Figure 20.1**. The purely vasospastic patient has a normal digital pressure at room temperature that falls rapidly after a critical temperature is reached. The obstructive patient begins at a lower baseline arterial pressure, and the hypothermia-induced pressure decline parallels that of normal individuals until arterial closure occurs. If an obstructive disease patient also has a vasospastic component, the resulting curve is a combination of the two.

A small number of diseases, including the autoimmune connective tissue diseases, Buerger's disease, and hypersensitivity angiitis, have a predilection for damaging the small vessels of

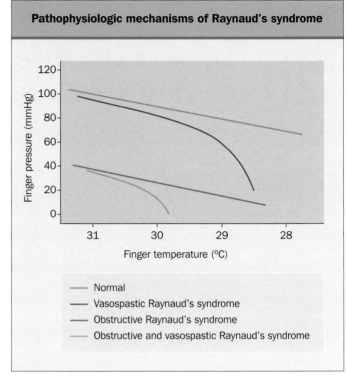

Figure 20.1 Pathophysiologic mechanisms of Raynaud's syndrome. Finger blood pressure response to digital cooling in normals decreases gradually with decreasing finger temperature. Finger blood pressure response to digital cooling in patients with obstructive disease also decreases gradually with decreasing temperature, but reaches zero. Finger blood pressure response to digital cooling in patients with either vasospastic disease alone or both obstructive and vasospastic disease decreases gradually until a critical temperature is reached, at which time it decreases rapidly to zero.

the extremities, primarily the fingers and to a lesser extent the toes. The reason these diseases predispose to damage of distal extremity vessels is not known, but thermally sensitive antigen–antibody reaction with immune complex deposition has been postulated. Curiously, the digits are the coolest part of the body and this finding may explain why the process primarily occurs in the digits.

The number of disease entities associated with upper extremity digital ischemia is legion. In the next section, we will briefly present the clinical and laboratory features of the most frequently encountered small vessel arteriopathies of common clinical importance.

COMMON SMALL VESSEL ARTERIOPATHIES ASSOCIATED WITH UPPER EXTREMITY ISCHEMIA

Scleroderma

The connective tissue disease most commonly identified in patients with Raynaud's syndrome is scleroderma. Scleroderma (progressive systemic sclerosis) is a generalized disorder of connective tissue, the microvasculature, and the small arteries.[20] The name scleroderma is derived from the Greek for 'hard skin'. Scleroderma has a female:male ratio of about 3:1 and the incidence is approximately ten per million population per year in the USA. There are an estimated 50 000 patients with scleroderma in the USA. Cutaneous involvement in scleroderma is almost universal. The clinical course of scleroderma is characterized by progressive scarring and small vessel occlusions in the skin, gastrointestinal tract, kidneys, lungs, and heart. Raynaud's syndrome is present in 80–97% of patients with scleroderma. In our experience, the Raynaud's syndrome usually begins as the vasospastic type, but may progress to the obstructive type over time in a subgroup of patients. Again in our experience, it is the most frequent underlying conditions identified in patients presenting with digital ulceration.

Scleroderma patients may be divided into those who present with involvement of primarily the skin of the hands, forearms, and face (limited involvement group) and those who present with diffuse cutaneous and visceral involvement (diffuse involvement). The first group, which represents about one-half of the total, often present with finger swelling and longstanding Raynaud's syndrome. Because of the usual delay in presentation to a physician, these patients in the limited involvement group are older than those in the diffuse involvement group. The limited involvement group appears to have a relatively benign course with prolonged survival in comparison to the diffuse involvement group. This limited cutaneous involvement syndrome has been termed 'CREST' (for calcinosis, Raynaud's syndrome, esophageal dysmotility, sclerodactyly, and telangiectasias), although many patients with limited involvement do not manifest all these features.

Patients in the diffuse involvement group tend to be younger and usually present soon after development of symptoms of generalized skin involvement or arthritis. The skin involvement is often progressive and most severe in the upper arms and the trunk. Renal involvement is frequent in patients with diffuse scleroderma.

Patients with scleroderma may also be divided into subgroups based on the presence or absence of specific antibodies. Patients with limited involvement often have a positive anticentromere antibody, while those patients with diffuse involvement are more likely to have antibodies to topoisomerase I (anti-Scl-70).

Although the pathophysiologic mechanisms of scleroderma are still being elucidated, the damage seen in scleroderma is likely mediated through cytotoxic antibodies to the endothelium.[21,22] Histopathologic features of scleroderma include a vasculitis of the small arteries, with fibrinoid necrosis and concentric thickening of the intima with deposition of layers of mucopolysaccharides. The cellular infiltrates seen on histopathology are composed of T-cells. Capillary abnormalities may be seen in patients with scleroderma, using nailfold microscopy.[23] These abnormalities include giant capillary loops and capillary dropout. On electron microscopy, these capillaries exhibit thickened basement membranes and endothelial damage.[24]

Systemic lupus erythematosus

While systemic lupus erythematosus (SLE) occurs most frequently in females of childbearing age, approximately 10% of patients are male and cases of SLE have been reported in all age groups.[25] The pathophysiology of SLE remains unknown; however, the damage to the affected organs appears caused primarily by immune complex deposition. Abnormalities in apoptosis have also been postulated in SLE.[26] The diagnosis of SLE is made primarily on a clinical basis since the available laboratory

tests in patients with SLE, such as screening for antinuclear antibody (ANA), though quite sensitive, are not specific.[27] The clinical criteria include fevers, arthralgias, skin rash, Raynaud's syndrome, and nephritis.

The pathologic lesions of SLE typically involve small arteries and capillaries and occur throughout the vascular system. The lesions in the small arteries are characterized by necrosis of all or part of the vessel wall, fibroblastic hyperplasia of the intima or media, and occlusive fibrin deposits. Raynaud's syndrome is one of the most frequent clinical manifestations of SLE, with as many as 80% of patients reporting this symptom. In most patients this is a nuisance condition, but a small number develop significant digital arteriopathy with resulting digital artery occlusion, digital ischemia, and, in the extreme, digital ulceration and gangrene.[28]

Rheumatoid arthritis

Rheumatoid arthritis is a chronic inflammatory joint disease. Afflicted patients have a progressive and inflammatory synovitis with resulting destruction of the articular cartilage, the joint, and surrounding structures. The etiology of rheumatoid arthritis is unknown but it likely results from immune-mediated damage. Most patients have the *HLA-DRW-4* allele and it has been theorized that this marks a genetic predisposition which, in response to an unknown stimulus such as infection, leads to immune complex deposition and resulting inflammation. The diagnosis is made on the basis of clinical and laboratory findings, the most important of which is the presence of rheumatoid factor, an IgM immune globulin. Rheumatoid factor is present in the majority of patients with rheumatoid arthritis, and almost all patients with extra-articular involvement have rheumatoid factor.

While rheumatoid arthritis invariably involves the joints, a subgroup of patients have extra-articular involvement of the skin, eyes, lungs, spleen, and arteries.[29] Several types of vasculitis have been described in patients with rheumatoid arthritis, the most severe of which is termed rheumatoid vasculitis, a systemic process involving both arteries and veins.[30]

The pathologic lesions found in rheumatoid vasculitis include intimal proliferation with vessel occlusion, medial necrosis, and obliterative fibrosis.[31] The clinical manifestations of vasculitis include Raynaud's syndrome with or without digital gangrene, polyneuropathy, purpura, cutaneous gangrene and ulceration, and, rarely, involvement of the systemic arteries, including the coronary and visceral arteries. The diagnosis of rheumatoid vasculitis is made by biopsy together with clinical and laboratory findings.

Sjögren's syndrome

Sjögren's syndrome is characterized by dry eyes and a dry mouth (keratoconjunctivitis sicca and xerostomia). Sjögren's syndrome may be primary or secondary to another connective tissue disease, usually scleroderma, rheumatoid arthritis, or SLE.[32] The diagnosis of Sjögren's syndrome is made primarily on clinical grounds and may be confirmed by buccal salivary gland biopsy.

Sjögren's syndrome may be associated with a small vessel arteriopathy, which may be divided into acute necrotizing, leukocytoclastic, and lymphocytic vasculitis.[33] The necrotizing form involves small and medium-sized arteries, while the others involve capillaries and venules. The vasculitic lesions usually appear several years after diagnosis and may involve the fingers, with resulting ulceration. This diagnosis of vasculitis in Sjögren's syndrome requires biopsy.

Mixed and undifferentiated connective tissue disease

Mixed connective tissue disease (MCTD) and undifferentiated connective tissue disease (UCTD) are terms used to denote a group of disease states that are clearly autoimmune but do not fall into a named disease category. Patients with UCTD may have symptoms including Raynaud's syndrome, isolated kerato-conjunctivitis sicca, unexplained polyarthritis, or at least three connective tissues disorder manifestations such as myalgias, rash, pleuritis, pericarditis, etc.[34] While this is a diagnosis of exclusion, it represents a sufficiently large subset of patients with connective tissue disease that it is a widely accepted diagnostic condition. MCTD clinically presents as an overlap syndrome with features of two or more connective tissue diseases such as SLE, rheumatoid arthritis, or scleroderma.[35] Patients characteristically have high titers of antibodies to an extractable nuclear antigen consisting of ribonucleic acid and protein (RNP). Patients with either MCTD or UCTD may have a diffuse vasculitis, and in our experience these two groups account for a small but significant proportion of patients with severe digital ischemia and digital ulceration.

Buerger's disease

Buerger's disease (thromboangiitis obliterans) describes a clinical syndrome characterized by the occurrence of segmental thrombotic occlusions of the small and medium-sized arteries.[36] The lower extremities are most frequently involved, but upper extremity involvement with resulting Raynaud's syndrome and digital ischemia occurs in as many as 50% of these patients. Ischemic digital ulcerations are frequent. While the existence of Buerger's disease has been questioned by some experts, most accept the currently used objective diagnostic criteria.[36] Buerger's disease classically occurs in young male smokers and is frequently associated with both migratory thrombophlebitis and Raynaud's syndrome. The diagnostic criteria include:

- age less than 45 years;
- tobacco abuse;
- exclusion of other diseases with similar clinical findings;
- normal arteries proximal to the popliteal or brachial arteries; and
- documentation, by objective means, of digital arterial occlusion.[37]

Buerger's disease has also been reported after prolonged marijuana use.[38]

The pathologic lesion of Buerger's disease, in the acute stage, is one of neutrophilic inflammation with preservation of the internal elastic lamina.[39] In contrast, in most immune arteritides and in atherosclerosis, there is disruption of the internal elastic lamina. Other distinguishing features include preservation of the arterial wall, and lack of vascular wall calcification, aneurysms, and atheroma. Later, the lesions have a predominance of mononuclear cells and occasional giant cells. Late lesions are characterized by intense perivascular fibrosis.

The natural history of Buerger's disease is one of progression of disease, with major lower extremity amputation in 20–30% of patients. Interestingly, life expectancy does not appear to be significantly shortened, probably reflecting the typical absence of significant cardiac, cerebral, and visceral vessel disease in these patients. The cornerstone of treatment of Buerger's disease is cessation of smoking. With this, most lesions will heal with simple conservative therapy.

Vibration arterial injury

The finding of Raynaud's syndrome associated with long-term use of vibrating tools was first described nearly a century ago.[40,41] The first reported patients were stonecutters, but since that time this association has been confirmed in a variety of frequent tool users, including welders/grinders in shipyards, timber fellers, and, most recently, in windshield-replacement technicians in the autoglass industry.[42] The condition has been termed vibration white finger. The pathophysiologic mechanism of vibration white finger is not known, but it is clear that kinetic energy imparted to the small vessels and nerves of the hand by vibrating tools with power in certain frequency bands is harmful. This appears to be a cumulative trauma disorder – that is, the damage accumulates and progresses over time. Early on, these patients have vasospastic Raynaud's syndrome, but in the late stage, usually after decades of vibrating tool use, digital artery occlusive disease is seen.[43]

Hypersensitivity angiitis

We have used the term hypersensitivity angiitis to describe a group of patients characterized by an unusual but similar disease process. Such patients typically present with the acute onset of significant digital ischemia, usually with ischemic ulceration, and yet have no demonstrable underlying condition such as a connective tissue disease or embolic source.[44] We have hypothesized that these patients have experienced digital artery occlusions on the basis of immune-mediated arterial wall injury, although we have no objective evidence to support this hypothesis. In some patients, one can identify a potentially responsible drug or environmental agent that may have served as the inciting factor, but in over 50% of patients, no such association is present. We have noted that the palmar and digital arterial injury and occlusion in these patients appears to be a one-time event, quite unlike the ongoing small vessel arteriopathic injury seen in patients with connective tissue diseases. In our experience, patients with hypersensitivity angiitis do not have further episodes of digital ischemia and their clinical course is one of progressive improvement without recurrence.

Fibromuscular disease

The presence of fibromuscular disease (FMD) involving the forearm, palmar, and digital arteries has been described.[45,46] This small group of patients often present with significant finger ischemia as a result of arterial embolization and occlusion. We have postulated that the condition known as 'hypothenar hammer' syndrome, in which patients have the acute onset of hand ischemia after using the heel of their hand as a hammer, is actually not due only to repetitive trauma but acts in susceptible individuals on the substate of an underlying lesion or FMD. We base the hypothesis on the fact that most of these patients have an abnormal palmar artery on the opposite (non-traumatized) side and the pathologic appearance of resected aneurysms is consistent with FMD.[46] This hypothesis is presently unconfirmed.

55

Malignancy

Raynaud's syndrome has been reported in association with a number of different malignancies.[47–49] Although the mechanism of the digital artery occlusions in these patients is unknown, it appears related to tumor-based immunologic processes, including probably both small vessel arteritis and immune complex deposition, possibly including cryoglobulins. Spontaneous improvement with successful treatment of the tumor has been reported.

Frostbite

Freeze injury of the small vessels of the digits results in Raynaud's syndrome. Mild frostbite usually results in vasospastic Raynaud's syndrome, while significant freezing injury may result in occlusive disease of the digital arteries.

CLINICAL PRESENTATION AND DIAGNOSTIC EVALUATION

The usual clinical presentation of Raynaud's syndrome is a young female experiencing episodic finger color changes in response to cold or emotional stress; nonetheless, in our tertiary referral center, we often see patients of all ages who present with a wide spectrum of digital ischemia. This spectrum spans patients presenting with only nuisance vasospastic symptoms to those with severe acute or chronic digital ischemia including the presence of digital gangrene or ulceration. All patients undergo a complete history and physical examination with specific attention to signs and symptoms of underlying connective tissue diseases. Our basic evaluation consists of the clinical laboratory tests and non-invasive vascular studies listed in **Table 20.1**. If this initial battery of tests is non-diagnostic and the patients have significant obstructive disease by vascular laboratory criteria or have digital ulceration, further testing to determine the presence of a hypercoagulable state is conducted. The hypercoagulable screening battery consists of:

- antithrombin III, protein C, and protein S levels;
- tests for the presence of anticardiolipin and antiphospholipid (lupus inhibitor) antibodies;
- lipoprotein (a) levels in patients with hyperlipidemia; and
- tests for familial hypercoagulable states such as factor V Leiden.

Multiple non-invasive vascular laboratory tests have been suggested for the objective diagnosis of Raynaud's syndrome. In our experience, the ischemic digital hypothermic challenge test as described by Nielsen and Lassen has the highest sensitivity and specificity for the diagnosis of Raynaud's syndrome.[50,51] A photograph of the machine used to perform the test is shown in **Figure 20.2** and a diagrammatic representation of the test results is shown in **Figure 20.3**. An objective test is primarily necessary for research purposes, since treatment of Raynaud's syndrome is not curative but only for symptomatic benefit. If the machine for the digital hypothermic challenge test is not available, finger temperature recovery after ice water immersion may be used. Normal individuals will recover to pre-immersion temperature levels in 5min. The sensitivity of the finding of prolonged temperature recovery after ice water immersion is near 100%, but the specificity is only about 50%, with many otherwise normal individuals testing positive. A diagrammatic representation of normal and abnormal temperature recovery after ice water immersion is shown in **Figure 20.4**.

Evaluation of Raynaud's syndrome.

Vascular laboratory:
- Finger pressures
- Finger photoplethysmographic waveforms
- Cold challenge test (Nielsen test – digital hypothermic challenge test)

Basic clinical laboratory:
- Complete blood count
- Erythrocyte sedimentation rate
- Antinuclear antibodies
- Rheumatoid factor

Additional tests in select cases:
- Hypercoagulable screening:
  - protein C
  - protein S
  - antithrombin III
  - lupus anticoagulant
  - anticardiolipin and antiphospholipid antibodies
  - lipoprotein (a)
  - factor V Leiden
- Thyroid panel

Table 20.1 Evaluation of Raynaud's syndrome.

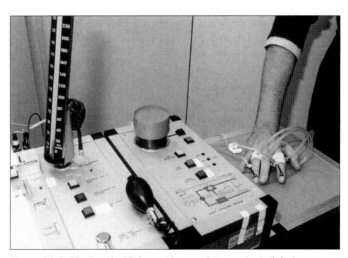

Figure 20.2 Medimatic SP-2 machine used to conduct digital hypothermic challenge test.

Three digital photoplethysmography (PPG) patterns are frequently observed in patients with Raynaud's syndrome (**Fig. 20.5**). The first is a normal pattern, pulsatile with a sharp upstroke. Patients with vasospastic Raynaud's syndrome may have a 'peaked pulse' with the addition of a second smaller peak just after the peak upstroke, apparently related to increased arterial resistance or elasticity.[52] Patients with obstructive Raynaud's syndrome have dampened waveforms with delayed upstroke (>0.2s). It is important to remember that PPG waveforms are qualitative, not quantitative, and that the height of the wave is not important, just the shape and upstroke time. Additionally,

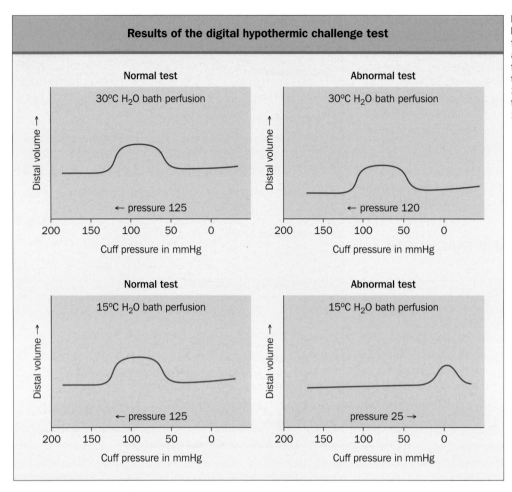

Figure 20.3 Results of the digital hypothermic challenge test. As the finger cuff is slowly released, there is an upstroke in the recording pen as finger pressure is reached. A normal test response has similar pressures at 30°C and 15°C. In an abnormal test, the 30°C pressure is normal, but the 15°C finger pressure is reduced.

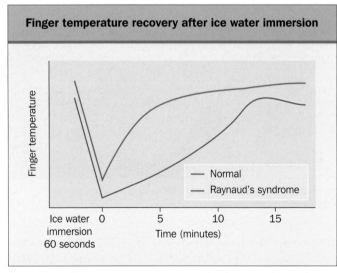

Figure 20.4 Finger temperature recovery after ice water immersion. A normal response to ice water immersion is recovery to baseline temperature in less than 5 min. In an abnormal response, finger temperature recovery takes more than 5 min.

normal patients and those with vasospastic Raynaud's syndrome will have digital blood pressures within 20 torr of brachial pressure, while patients with obstructive Raynaud's syndrome will have digital blood pressures below this level.

We have found that a combination of finger PPG waveforms, digital blood pressures, and the digital hypothermic challenge test provides reliable data concerning the status of the digital arteries (patent or occluded) and the sensitivity of the arteries to cold.

We now reserve arteriography for those patients with unexplained digital artery occlusions in an asymmetric distribution (e.g. several digits on one hand only) to rule out a surgically correctable proximal lesion. Thus, a patient with diffuse occlusions of all fingers of both hands and a high titer ANA would not have arteriography, while a patient with the acute onset of ischemia of two fingers of one hand would undergo arteriography as well as echocardiography. When ordering and performing arteriography, the entire upper extremity circulation from the aortic arch to the fingertips should be visualized. Additionally, both upper extremities should be imaged. Magnification hand views are also useful. We have found that cut-film arteriography offers better resolution than digital imaging. The presence of significant bilateral occlusive disease, which may be seen even in patients with unilateral symptoms, is an indication of a systemic disease state rather than an embolic source. An example of hand arteriography in a patient with multiple digital and palmar arterial occlusions is shown in **Figure 20.6**. Such findings are seen in the multitude of patients with small artery occlusive disease and are not helpful in establishing a specific diagnosis.

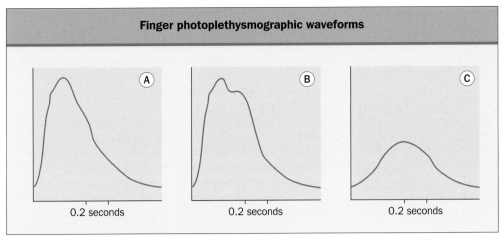

Finger photoplethysmographic waveforms

0.2 seconds   0.2 seconds   0.2 seconds

Figure 20.5 Finger photoplethysmographic (PPG) waveforms. (A) Normal PPG waveform. (B) 'Peaked pulse' pattern often seen in vasospastic Raynaud's. (C) Obstructive pattern.

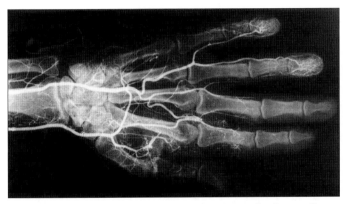

Figure 20.6 Arteriogram from a patient with obstructive Raynaud's syndrome.

TREATMENT

The vast majority of patients with Raynaud's syndrome are best managed by cold and tobacco avoidance without the need for medication. Several medications have been shown in randomized trials to be beneficial in the treatment of Raynaud's syndrome. The most effective drug treatment to date has been the calcium channel blocker nifedipine.[53,54] The administration of 30mg/day of the extended-release formulation will relieve or improve symptoms in about one-half the patients with vasospastic Raynaud's syndrome. Losartan, an angiotensin II type 1 receptor antagonist, has been demonstrated to be effective in patients with Raynaud's syndrome in randomized trials,[55] although in our experience the results are not as dramatic as those seen with nifedipine. Fluoxetine, a selective serotonin reuptake inhibitor, has shown benefit in a double-blind randomized controlled trial[56] but we have no clinical experience with it. Thymoxamine, which is not available in the USA, has been shown to be effective in a small trial.[57]

Unfortunately, the results in patients with obstructive Raynaud's syndrome are less satisfying. Since this group of patients probably does not have abnormal contraction of the digital arteries in response to cold, pharmacologic intervention is predictably less effective. About 20–30% of patients do not tolerate nifedipine because of headache, ankle swelling, or a diffuse feeling of lassitude. Thus, drug therapy of Raynaud's

syndrome appears effective in about one-half the small number of patients requiring such. Other drugs that have been used in the treatment of Raynaud's syndrome include reserpine, captopril,[58] guanethidine, niacin, omega-3 fatty acids, and dibenzyline.

Thoracic sympathectomy has been used both for the treatment of digital artery vasospasm and as an adjunct for healing of digital ischemic ulceration. As a treatment for vasospasm, thoracic sympathectomy is almost always initially successful, but the symptoms of vasospasm invariably return, usually within 3 to 6 months. We have performed thoracic sympathectomy for hyperhidrosis in patients with concomitant Raynaud's syndrome and have noted a lifelong cessation of sweating but the rapid recurrence of Raynaud's attacks. The underlying pathophysiologic basis for this differential remains unknown but probably relates to incomplete sympathectomy. Thoracic sympathectomy as an adjunctive measure for the treatment of digital ulceration is unproven. Our results without sympathectomy in 100 patients with digital ulceration[28] were as good or better than those reported with sympathectomy.[59,60] Patients with digital ulceration have obstructed digital arteries and are most likely already maximally vasodilated; thus, sympathectomy is unlikely to improve blood flow. While sympathectomy is now often performed via a thoracoscopic approach, there is no evidence that this is any more effective than sympathectomy via thoracotomy.

Other treatments that have been reported for the treatment of severe Raynaud's syndrome include spinal cord stimulation,[61] biofeedback,[53] and periarterial digital sympathectomy.[62] None has been shown to be effective in well-designed controlled trials.

Our current recommendation for patients with severe digital ischemia and ulceration is local cleansing and debridement with simple soap and water washing, and antibiotics as needed. Medical therapy with nifedipine or losartan is also used if tolerated, but without proven benefit for ulcer healing. Resectional debridement of the ulcers is frequently needed, including local resection of protruding phalangeal bone tips, but major amputations to the metacarpophalangeal joint are rarely required. We no longer perform thoracic sympathectomy for digital ulceration. With this regimen, our ulcer healing rates without recurrence are approximately 90%, although the time to healing is often many months. We have also noted that ulcers that appear in the late fall and winter may not resolve until months after the onset of warmer weather in the spring. **Figure 20.7** demonstrates healing of a significant digital ulcer with this treatment regimen.

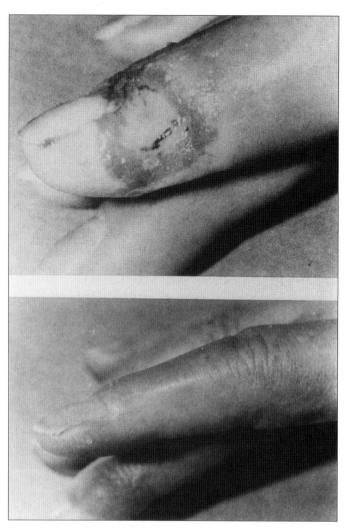

Figure 20.7 Healing of a significant digital ulcer with the treatment regimen outlined in this chapter.

had a clinic devoted to Raynaud's syndrome patients at the Oregon Health Sciences University for over 30 years and have enrolled over 1300 patients. All of these patients have been prospectively evaluated with a number of serologic, radiologic, and non-invasive vascular laboratory tests, both to evaluate the Raynaud's syndrome and to detect the presence of an associated disease process.

In our review of the overall group of patients, we divided patients into four groups based on the presence or absence of occlusive disease or associated disease.[66] Patients without evidence of occlusive disease or an associated disease had a low incidence of progression to developing an associated disease, similar to that seen in the general population (2% in 10 years). Patients with occlusive disease but without evidence of an associated disease were unlikely to develop evidence of an associated disease (8.5% in 10 years) but had a 48% risk of ulcer occurrence. Patients with an associated disease but without evidence of obstructive disease had a moderate risk of developing ulcers (15.5% at 10 years) as well as progression to the presence of occlusive disease. Patients with both occlusive disease and an associated disease were the most likely to develop new or recurrent ulcers (56%). Amputation was uncommon in all groups. Curiously, patients appeared to have their most severe symptoms at the time of presentation. Only about 50% of patients presenting with digital ulceration had recurrent ulcers.

We have also reviewed our experience with the subgroup of patients who presented with severe finger ischemia and ischemic digital ulceration.[28,67] Severe digital ischemia with ulceration is limited to patients with small vessel occlusions caused by a variety of diseases, most often the digital arteriopathy of connective tissue disease. In 100 patients with ischemic finger ulceration, 54% had a connective tissue disease, most frequently scleroderma, and the remainder had a variety of other conditions including Buerger's disease, hypersensitivity angiitis, and atherosclerosis. All patients with recurrent ulceration in our series suffered from a connective tissue disease.

SUMMARY

Raynaud's syndrome is a condition characterized by episodic digital ischemia in response to cold or emotional stress. In the great majority of patients, it is a nuisance condition that can be treated by cold and tobacco avoidance. A few patients will have symptoms that require treatment with vasodilators, and an even smaller number of patients, all of whom have palmar and digital artery obstruction, will have ischemic digital ulceration.

The small vessel arteriopathies are a frequent cause of digital arterial damage that may result in severe digital ischemia and, in some cases, digital ulceration. The diagnosis of the underlying disease is made on the basis of clinical and laboratory findings. Regardless of the underlying disease process, satisfactory healing of digital ulceration from small vessel arteriopathies can be expected with conservative therapy, although recurrence can be expected in approximately 50% of patients if the underlying disease process is ongoing.

To date, ulcer recurrences have been limited to those patients with connective tissue disease who have ongoing digital artery damage from an associated small vessel arteriopathy. Treatment of the diseases causing the small vessel arteriopathy is beyond the scope of this chapter. While controlling the associated disease will not have any curative effect on the digital arterial obstruction, the arrest or attenuation of the vasculitis associated with many of these diseases may prevent progression of digital ischemia in this patient group.

PROGNOSIS

Since Allen and Brown's pivotal publication in 1932,[1] dividing Raynaud's syndrome into Raynaud's phenomenon and Raynaud's disease based on the presence or absence of an associated disease, a great deal of interest has focused on the incidence and the subsequent development of such associated diseases in patients presenting with Raynaud's syndrome.[2,63–65] We have

REFERENCES

1. Allen E, Brown G. Raynaud's disease: a critical review of minimal requisites for diagnosis. Am J Med Sci 1932;83:187–200.
2. Priollet P, Vayssairat M, Housset E. How to classify Raynaud's phenomenon: long-term follow-up study of 73 cases. Am J Med 1987;83:494–8.
3. Weiner ES, Hildebrandt S, Senecal JL, et al. Prognostic significance of anticentromere antibodies and anti-topoisomerase I antibodies in Raynaud's disease. A prospective study. Arthritis Rheum 1991;34:68–77.
4. Raynaud M. On local asphyxia and symmetrical gangrene of the extremities. In: Selected monographs. London:New Sydenham Society; 1888.
5. Lewis T, Pickering G. Observations upon maladies in which the blood supply to the digits ceases intermittently or permanently and upon bilateral gangrene of the digits: Observations relevant to so-called 'Raynaud's disease'. Clin Sci 1934;1:327–66.
6. Edwards JM, Porter JM. Associated diseases with Raynaud's syndrome. Vasc Med Rev 1990;1:51–8.
7. de Takats G, Fowler EF. The neurogenic factor in Raynaud's phenomenon. Surgery 1962;51:9–18.
8. Ekenvall L, Lindblad LE. Is vibration white finger a primary sympathetic nerve injury? Br J Ind Med 1986;43:702–6.
9. Edwards JM, Phinney ES, Taylor LM Jr, Keenan EJ, Porter JM. Alpha2-adrenergic receptor levels in obstructive and spastic Raynaud's syndrome. J Vasc Surg 1987;5:38–45.
10. Freedman RR, Subhash SC, Desai N, Wenig P, Mayes M. Increased alpha-adrenergic responsiveness in idiopathic Raynaud's disease. Arthritis Rheum 1989;32:61–5.
11. Brotzu G, Susanna F, Roberto M, Palmina P. Beta-blockers: a new therapeutic approach to Raynaud's disease. Microvasc Res 1987;33:283–8.
12. Bunker CB, Terenghi G, Springall DR, Polak JM, Dowd PM. Deficiency of calcitonin gene-related peptide in Raynaud's phenomenon. Lancet 1990;336:1530–3.
13. Terenghi G, Bunker CB, Liu YF, et al. Image analysis quantification of the peptide-immunoreactive nerves in the skin of patients with Raynaud's phenomenon and systemic sclerosis. J Pathol 1991;164:245–52.
14. Bunker CB, Goldsmith PC, Leslie TA, Hayes N, Foreman JC, Dowd PM. Calcitonin gene-related peptide, endothelin-1, the cutaneous microvasculature and Raynaud's phenomenon. Br J Dermatol 1996; 134:399–406.
15. Cimminiello C, Milani M, Uberti T, Arpaia G, Perolini S, Bonfardeci G. Endothelin, vasoconstriction, and endothelial damage in Raynaud's phenomenon. Lancet 1991;337:114–5.
16. Zamora MR, O'Brien RF, Rutherford RB, Weil JV. Serum endothelin-1 concentrations and cold provocation in primary Raynaud's phenomenon. Lancet 1990;336:1144–7.
17. Freedman RR, Girgis R, Mayes MD. Abnormal responses to endothelial agonists in Raynaud's phenomenon and scleroderma. J Rheumatol 2001; 28:119–21.
18. Lewis T, Landis EM. Observations upon the vascular mechanism in acrocyanosis. Heart 1930;15:229–46.
19. de Trafford JC, Roberts VC. Thermal entrainment. In: Cooke E, Nicolaides A, Porter J, eds. Raynaud's syndrome. London: Med-Orion; 1991:111–23.
20. Geppert T. Clinical features, pathogenic mechanisms, and new developments in the treatment of systemic sclerosis. Am J Med Sci 1990; 299:193–209.
21. Kahaleh MB, Sherer GK, Leroy ED. Endothelial injury in scleroderma. J Exp Med 1979;149:1326–35.
22. Silveri F, De Angelis R, Poggi A, et al. Relative roles of endothelial cell damage and platelet activation in primary Raynaud's phenomenon (RP) and RP secondary to systemic sclerosis. Scand J Rheumatol 2001; 30:290–6.
23. Mariq HR, Spencer-Green G, Leroy EC. Skin capillary abnormalities as indicators of organ involvement in scleroderma (systemic sclerosis), Raynaud's syndrome and dermatomyositis. Am J Med 1976;61:862–70.
24. Fleischmajer R, Perlish JS, Shaw KV, et al. Skin capillary changes in early systemic sclerosis. Arch Dermatol 1976;112:1553–7.
25. Grishman E, Spiera H. Vasculitis in connective tissue disease, including hypocomplementemic vasculitis. In: Churg A, Churg J, eds. Systemic vasculitides. New York:Igaku Shoin; 1991:273–92.
26. Gordon C, Salmon M. Update on systemic lupus erythematosus: autoantibodies and apoptosis. Clin Med 2001;1:10–4.
27. Tan EM, Cohen AS, Fries JF, et al. The 1982 revised criteria for the clasification of systemic lupus erythematosus. Arthritis Rhem 1982; 25:1271–7.
28. Mills JL, Friedman EI, Taylor LM Jr, Porter JM. Upper extremity ischemia caused by small artery disease. Ann Surg 1987;206:521–8.
29. Ragan C, Farrington E. The clinical features of rheumatoid arthritis. JAMA 1967;181:663–7.
30. Panush RS, Katz P, Longlry S, et al. Rheumatoid vasculitis: survival and associated risk factors. Medicine 1986;65:365–75.
31. Bywaters EGL. Peripheral vascular obstruction in rheumatoid arthritis and its relationship to other vascular disorders. Ann Rheum Dis 1957; 16:84–103.
32. Talal N. Sjogren's syndrome and connective tissue diseases associated with other immunologic disorders. In: McCarty DJ, ed. Arthritis and allied conditions, 11th edn Baltimore, MD:Williams & Wilkins; 1985:1197–213.
33. Tsokos M, Lazarou SA, Moutsopoulos HM. Vasculitis in Sjogren's syndrome. Histologic classification and clinical presentation. Am J Clin Pathol 1987;88:26–31.
34. Alarcon GS, Williams GV, Singer JZ, et al. Early undifferentiated connective tissue disease. I. Early clinical manifestation in a large cohort of patients with undifferentiated connective tissue diseases compared to cohorts of well established connective tissue disease. J Rheumatol 1991;18:1332–9.
35. Sharp GC, Irwin WS, Tan ES, et al. Mixed connective tissue disease – an apparently distinct rheumatic disease syndrome associated with a specific antibody to an extractable nuclear antigen (ENA). Am J Med 1972;52:149–59.
36. Mills JL, Porter JM. Buerger's disease (thromboangiitis obliterans). Ann Vasc Surg 1992;5:570–2.
37. Mills JL, Taylor LM Jr, Porter JM. Buerger's disease in the modern era. Am J Surg 1987;154:123–9.
38. Schneider HJ, Jha S, Burnand KG. Progressive arteritis associated with cannabis use. Eur J Vasc Endovasc Surg 1999;18:366–7.
39. Shionoya S, Ban I, Nakata Y, et al. Diagnosis, pathology, and treatment of Buerger's disease. Surgery 1974;75:695–700.
40. Loriga G. Pneumatic tools: occupation and health. Boll Inspett Labor 1911;2:35.
41. Hamilton A. A study of spastic anemia in the hands of stonecutters. Effect of the air hammer on the hands of the stonecutters. US Bureau Labor Stat Bull 1918;236:53–66.
42. McLafferty RB, Edwards JM, Ferris BL, et al. Raynaud's syndrome in workers who use vibrating pneumatic air knives. J Vasc Surg 1999; 30:1–7.
43. Schatz IJ. Occlusive disease of the hand due to occupational trauma. N Engl J Med 1963;268:281–4.
44. Baur GM, Porter JM, Bardana EJ Jr, Wesche DH, Rösch J. Rapid onset of hand ischemia of unknown etiology. Ann Surg 1977;186:184–9.
45. Edwards JM, Antonius JI, Porter JM. Critical hand ischemia caused by forearm fibromuscular dysplasia. J Vasc Surg1985;2:459–63.
46. Ferris BL, Taylor LM Jr, Oyama K, et al. Hypothenar hammer syndrome: proposed etiology. J Vasc Surg 2000;31:104–13.
47. Friedman SA, Bienenstock H, Richter IH. Malignancy and arteriopathy. Angiology 1969;20:136–43.
48. Vayssairat M, Fiessinger JN, Bordet F, Housset E. Rapports entre necroses digitales du membre superieur et affections malignes. Nouv Presse Med 1978;7:1279–82.
49. Taylor LM Jr, Hauty MG, Edwards JM, Porter JM. Digital ischemia as a manifestation of malignancy. Ann Surg 1987;206:62–8.

50. Nielsen SL, Lassen NA. Measurement of digital blood pressure after local cooling. J Appl Physiol 1977;43:907–10.

51. Gates KH, Tyburczy JA, Zupan T, Baur GM, Porter JM. The non-invasive quantification of digital vasospasm. Bruit 1984;8:34–7.

52. Sumner DS, Strandness DE Jr. An abnormal finger pulse associated with cold sensitivity. Ann Surg 1972;175:294.

53. Kiowski W, Erne P, Buhler FR. Use of nifedipine in hypertension and Raynaud's phenomenon. Cardiovasc Drugs Ther 1990;Suppl 5:935–40.

54. Anonymous. Comparison of sustained-release nifedipine and temperature biofeedback for treatment of primary Raynaud phenomenon. Results from a randomized clinical trial with 1-year follow-up. Arch Intern Med 2000;160:1101–8.

55. Dziadzio M, Denton CP, Smith R, et al. Losartan therapy for Raynaud's phenomenon and scleroderma: clinical and biochemical findings in a fifteen-week, randomized, parallel-group, controlled trial. Arthritis Rheum 1999;42:2646–55.

56. Coleiro B, Marshall SE, Denton CP, et al. Treatment of Raynaud's phenomenon with the selective serotonin reuptake inhibitor fluoxetine. Rheumatology 2001;40:1038–43.

57. Grigg MJ, Nicolaides AN, Papadakis K, Wolfe JH. The efficacy of thymoxamine in primary Raynaud's phenomenon. Eur J Vasc Endovasc Surg 1989;3:309–13.

58. Aikimbaev KS, Oguz M, Ozbek S, Demirtas M, Birand A, Batyraliev T. Comparative assessment of the effects of vasodilators on peripheral vascular reactivity in patients with systemic scleroderma and Raynaud's phenomenon: color Doppler flow imaging study. Angiology 1996;47:475–80.

59. Machleder HI, Wheeler E, Barber WF. Treatment of upper extremity ischemia by cervico-dorsal sympathectomy. Vasc Surg 1979; 13:399–404.

60. Dale WA. Occlusive arterial lesions of the wrist and hand. J Tenn Med Assoc 1964;57:402–6.

61. Neuhauser B, Perkmann R, Klingler PJ, Giacomuzzi S, Kofler A, Fraedrich G. Clinical and objective data on spinal cord stimulation for the treatment of severe Raynaud's phenomenon. Am Surg 2001; 67:1096–7.

62. McCall TE, Petersen DP, Wong LB. The use of digital artery sympathectomy as a salvage procedure for severe ischemia of Raynaud's disease and phenomenon. J Hand Surg [Am] 1999;24:173–7.

63. Harper F, Mariq H, Turner R, Lidman R, Leroy E. A prospective study of Raynaud phenomenon and early connective tissue disease. Am J Med 1982;72:883–8.

64. Kallenberg CG, Wouda AA, The TH. Systemic involvement and immunologic findings in patients presenting with Raynaud's phenomenon. Am J Med 1980;69:675–80.

65. Velayos E, Roginson H, Porciuncula F, Masi A. Clinical correlation analysis of 137 patients with Raynaud's phenomenon. Am J Med Sci 1970;262:347–56.

66. Landry GJ, Edwards JM, McLafferty RB, Taylor LM Jr, Porter JM. Long-term outcome of Raynaud's syndrome in a prospectively analyzed patient cohort. J Vasc Surg 1996;23:76–86.

67. McLafferty RB, Edwards JM, Taylor LM Jr, Porter JM. Diagnosis and long-term clinical outcome in patients diagnosed with hand ischemia. J Vasc Surg 1995;22:361–9.

CHAPTER
21

Thoracic Outlet Syndrome

David A Rigberg and Julie A Freischlag

KEY POINTS

- The thoracic outlet is a limited space through which a large number of important structures must traverse (subclavian artery and vein, brachial plexus).

- The form of thoracic outlet syndrome (TOS) depends on the structure compressed: arterial, venous (axillo-subclavian thrombosis), or nerve (neurogenic).

- Neurogenic is the most common form, and generates a considerable amount of controversy regarding both its diagnosis and treatment.

- Usually, excision of the first rib decompresses the thoracic outlet, regardless of the form of TOS.

- The presentation of the vascular forms can be dramatic. Neurogenic TOS presents with pain and paresthesias that can be a diagnostic challenge.

- History and physical examination are the cornerstones of diagnosis. Ancillary testing is helpful mostly for excluding other conditions.

- Arteriography and venography play important roles in the arterial and venous forms.

- Treatment is conservative for most patients (physical therapy), but a significant number have symptoms that persist. Surgical decompression is warranted in these cases.

- Both the transaxillary and supraclavicular approaches to first-rib excision are used, and there are benefits and limitations to each approach.

- Well-performed clinical outcomes studies are needed to objectively assess the results of first-rib resection in these patients.

INTRODUCTION

The thoracic outlet syndrome (TOS) describes a spectrum of symptoms and signs which are all related to the passage of key anatomic structures through a narrow aperture on their way to the distal upper extremity. The colorful descriptions of patients suffering from some form of this disorder date back thousands of years, with some authors going so far as to attribute Abraham's sparing of his son Isaac to an acute TOS.[1] This syndrome is manifest in three main forms, based on the specific structures compressed: neurogenic, venous, and arterial. There is considerable controversy regarding the diagnosis, and some would even argue the existence of the most common, neurogenic, form. The objective findings in the other two variants

preclude this discussion. Nonetheless, there continues to be a large patient population presenting with a constellation of symptoms attributable to TOS, and the vascular surgeon should be able to recognize and treat the various forms of this disorder.

Several early anatomists, most notably Galen, described the presence of cervical ribs, and this structure was considered the key etiologic agent as physicians first gained an appreciation for compressive symptoms of the thoracic outlet. In 1821, Sir Astley Cooper related this structure to the development of ischemic fingers secondary to subclavian artery compression. Twenty years later, Gruber published what is still considered the definitive classification of cervical ribs. In 1861, Coote demonstrated the development of a subclavian artery aneurysm in a patient with a cervical rib. He then went on to resect the rib via a supraclavicular approach. Both Mayo and Halsted published reports on subclavian aneurysms related to TOS, with Mayo describing a first-rib exostosis as the cause. Mention should be made at this point of the work of Paget and Schroetter, who, in 1875, simultaneously published their findings of axillo-subclavian venous thrombosis in what has become known as the Paget–Schroetter syndrome, or effort thrombosis.

By the early 20th century, physicians were incriminating the cervical rib not only as a cause of vascular complications, but for neurogenic symptoms as well. Keene in 1907 presented his series of TOS patients, the majority of whom had neurogenic complaints. At about the same time, however, Branwell published descriptions of TOS patients who had neither cervical ribs nor any identifiable first-rib anomalies. As early as 1910, Murphy was performing excision of normal first ribs for what had become known as 'cervical rib syndrome'. Law's descriptions of ligamentous attachments to cervical rib, followed by Adson and Coffey's publications in 1927 on dividing the anterior scalene muscle, helped to shift the focus away from the cervical rib. The 'scalenus anticus syndrome', described in the late 1930s by both Naffziger and DeBakey, was treated for a time by scalenectomy. This operation, which involved dividing the muscle in the neck, did not prove to be particularly effective, and even when initially successful had a high rate of recurrence.

In the early 1950s, following work by Telford and Stopford describing the bony confines provided by the normal first rib, attention shifted, so that compression between the clavicle and first rib was considered the culprit. This was termed the costo-clavicular syndrome, and led briefly to the use of claviculectomy, described by Rosati and Lord, as the treatment of choice. Because it is disfiguring, the operation was usually performed bilaterally, to maintain symmetry. It was not particularly effective, and soon fell out of favor.

The major shift in our modern conception of TOS occurred in 1956, with Peet's coining of the term TOS and his description of a therapeutic exercise program, essentially the first physical therapy for TOS.[2] The term was used again by Standeven and Rob 2 years later, and encompassed all of the previous 'anatomic' terms used for this set of symptoms. This also coincided with the therapeutic focus shifting to the first rib, and it was in 1962 that Clagett presented his high thoracoplasty for first-rib resection, an operation requiring the division of the trapezius and rhomboid muscles.[3] Roos, in 1966, described what has become for many the modern treatment of choice for TOS, the transaxillary first-rib resection.[4] This operation was fashioned after the transaxillary sympathectomy, and first-rib resection by this route offered reasonable exposure and minimal morbidity, especially when compared to previously employed techniques. Gol's infraclavicular approach was described a year later, but operative exposure was difficult and required a large, cosmetically displeasing scar. This operation never gained widespread use.

ANATOMY

The limited space and large number of important structures that must traverse the neck and chest areas on their way to the upper arm make the thoracic outlet an area like no other in the body. Although there are several anatomic anomalies that predispose or directly cause compression to the neural, venous, or arterial structures within its confines, the normal anatomy itself does not leave much room for stress positioning.

Definitions may vary from author to author, but it is generally accepted that the thoracic outlet is the area from the edge of the first rib extending medially to the upper mediastinum and superiorly to the 5th cervical nerve. The clavicle and subclavius muscles can be pictured as forming a roof, while the superior surface of the first rib forms the floor. Machleder's description of the thoracic outlet as a triangle with its apex pointed towards the manubrium is helpful in visualizing the three dimensional orientation of the structures, as well as the dynamic changes that can lead to injury.[5] In this model, the clavicle and its under-lying subclavius muscle and tendon form the superior limb, while the base is the first thoracic rib. The point at which these two structures 'overlap' medially can be pictured as the fulcrum of a pair of scissors that open and close as the arm moves, potentially causing compression of the thoracic outlet contents (**Fig. 21.1**).

Although most TOS symptoms are related to nerve compression, almost any structure that travels through the thoracic outlet can be involved (**Fig. 21.2**). Moving from medially to laterally, one first encounters the exiting of the subclavian vein, usually positioned adjacent to the region where the first rib and clavicular head fuse to form a fibrocartilaginous joint with the manubrium. Immediately lateral to the vein is the anterior scalene muscle, which inserts onto a prominence on the first rib. Lateral to this site is the subclavian artery, so that the anterior scalene muscle lies between the subclavian artery and vein, with the artery deep, lateral and somewhat cephalad. The brachial plexus is the next structure encountered. The C4–C6 roots are superiorly oriented, and the C7–T1 roots inferior. As shall be seen, this arrangement has important implications for the symptom constellation in neurogenic TOS. Posterior and lateral to the plexus, there is a generally rather broad attachment of the middle scalene to the first rib. This is an area of particular

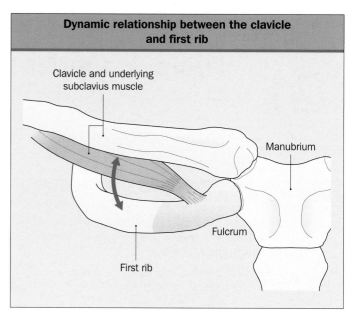

Figure 21.1 Dynamic relationship between the clavicle and first rib. Note the potential for impingement of structures with movement of the arm.

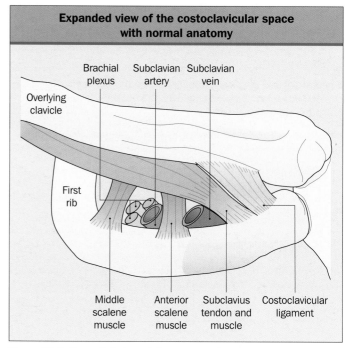

Figure 21.2 Expanded view of the costoclavicular space with normal anatomy.

importance during operative decompression of the thoracic outlet, for it is here that the long thoracic nerve can be inadvertently injured as it travels to the serratus anterior muscle (**Fig. 21.3**).

Other structures encountered in the thoracic outlet include the phrenic and dorsal scapular nerves, the stellate ganglion, the thoracic duct, and the cupola of the lung. The phrenic nerve lies between the prescalene fat pad and the anterior scalene muscle. Compression of this structure does not generally occur, but it can be injured during supraclavicular approaches and must be

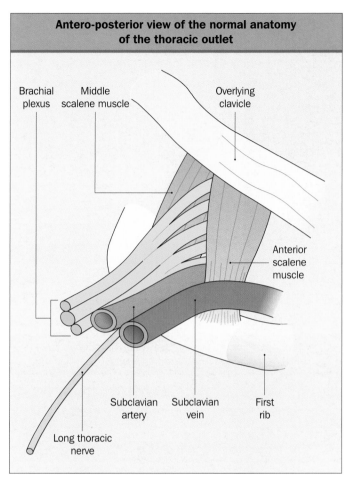

Figure 21.3 Antero-posterior view of the normal anatomy of the thoracic outlet. Note the course of the long thoracic nerve and the potential for injury to the nerve during operations in this area.

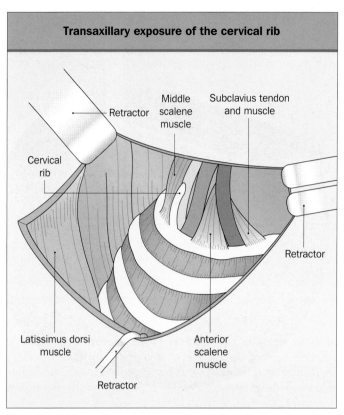

Figure 21.4 Transaxillary exposure of the cervical rib. Note the impingement on the brachial plexus as well as the cervical rib's origin from the first rib. The middle scalene muscle is displaced laterally and is intimately associated with the cervical rib.

left intact while the underlying scalene muscle is dissected. The dorsal scapular nerve comes off the brachial plexus on its way to innervate the medially inserting muscles of the scapula (rhomboids and levator scapulae). It is usually neither involved nor encountered. The stellate ganglion is found along the sympathetic chain. This structure can be involved in compression and occasionally a cervicothoracic sympathectomy is part of the treatment plan for TOS. The thoracic duct may be encountered if a left supraclavicular approach is undertaken, and care must be taken not to injure it or to ligate it if injury occurs. Finally, one must watch for pleural injury in any approach to TOS, and be prepared to evacuate pneumothoraces when indicated.

PATHOPHYSIOLOGY

Once the normal anatomy of the thoracic outlet is appreciated, it becomes clear that any structure that intrudes into, or otherwise limits, the aperture of this region predisposes the nerves, arterial, and venous structures to compression. Although there are specific anatomic configurations that favor the development of each form of TOS, they are not entirely specific, and considerable overlap can occur. In addition to the obvious gross consequences of injury to the contents of the thoracic outlet, there are histologic and biochemical changes observed in the

involved tissues. These serve to stress the uniqueness of the outlet's configuration, and offer objective support to the chronicity of many of these injuries.

The cervical rib is the most obvious bony abnormality contributing to TOS, and autopsy studies indicate that roughly 0.5% of the general population have this structure[6] (**Figs 21.4 & 21.5**). Series from the USA generally report 10% of TOS patients with cervical ribs, although others have reported up to 65%. Authors in the European literature report closer to 25%. The reason for this discrepancy is not known. Cervical ribs can be completely formed or rudimentary. In the latter case, there is almost always a compressive band of tissue extending to the first rib. As they project from transverse processes, cervical ribs displace involved structures forward. The subclavian artery is particularly vulnerable to damage in this configuration, and some authors feel that arterial changes secondary to TOS rarely occur in the absence of a cervical rib.

There are a number of other bony abnormalities found in association with TOS. Post-traumatic changes following clavicular or first-rib fractures are commonly reported, with callous formation at the clavicle and pseudoarthroses of the first rib. Elongated C7 transverse processes are also occasionally seen. These changes can frequently be appreciated radiographically.

The majority of TOS cases are associated with some form of soft tissue anomaly. Work by Juvonen, Raymond and others led

269

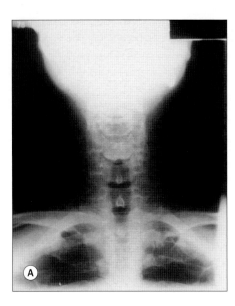
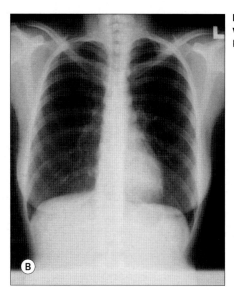

Figure 21.5 Bilateral cervical ribs in a patient with symptoms of neurogenic TOS. (A) In neutral position and (B) with arms partially abducted.

to appreciation of the multiple forms. However, the classification system of Roos is the most thorough, with ten distinct anomalies with several subtypes described based on intra-operative observations.[7] Type I is the previously mentioned incomplete cervical rib, with a band passing under the T1 nerve on its way to attachment on the first rib. Type II is essentially an abortive cervical rib with a band to the first rib. Type III is an accessory muscle found between the neck and tubercle of the first rib that separates the T1 nerve and subclavian artery. Type IV is a large middle scalene muscle compressing the T1 nerve root. This appears to be the most common variant presenting with ulnar symptoms. There is also a variant in which the muscle pins the nerve to the vertebral body.

The type V lesion essentially describes the presence of a scalenus minimus muscle (**Fig. 21.6**). This can attach to either the first rib behind the scalene tubercle or, as in the type VI lesion, to the endothoracic fascia covering the cupola of the lung. Type VII is a band extending anteriorly from the middle scalene to either the costal cartilages or the sternum. Type VIII is a similar lesion, but the band passes directly under the subclavian vein on its way to its costocartilage attachment site. This lesion, not surprisingly, is associated with Paget–Schroetter syndrome. The type IX anomaly is a web filling the inner curve of the first rib, and type X, which is quite unusual, is a double band attached to the cupola which arises from a cervical rib, attaches to the first rib, and then sends a limb from this point to either costocartilage or sternum.

As would be expected, these anomalies frequently occur in association with one another, and do not tend to be symmetrical. There are several other muscular anomalies, mostly involving thickened muscle branches encompassing nerves; one such example is slips of anterior scalene between the C5–C7 nerve roots, or even a bulky muscle anteriorly displacing the nerves. There have been reports of these muscle fibers becoming incorporated into the epineurium of these nerves as well. One particularly interesting configuration is when a fibrous band stretches over the proximal C5 nerve. Muscular spasm of the neck and shoulder can then lead to direct compression, with upper cord symptoms.

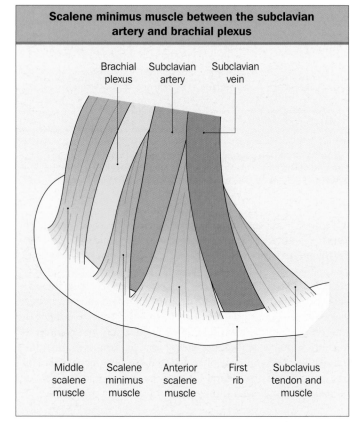

Scalene minimus muscle between the subclavian artery and brachial plexus

Brachial plexus — Subclavian artery — Subclavian vein

Middle scalene muscle — Scalene minimus muscle — Anterior scalene muscle — First rib — Subclavius tendon and muscle

Figure 21.6 Scalene minimus muscle between the subclavian artery and brachial plexus. This is a type V Roos deformity.

In addition to these anatomic arrangements, hypertrophy of the normal musculature or tendons has been implicated in TOS. For example, some authors report a link between Paget–Schroetter syndrome and subclavius tendon hypertrophy, particularly in the presence of an enlarged insertion tubercle (**Fig. 21.7**). Others have implicated a role for the pectoralis minor muscle. Another scenario involves the weight lifter, frequently a young man, with hypertrophied scalene musculature. There have been

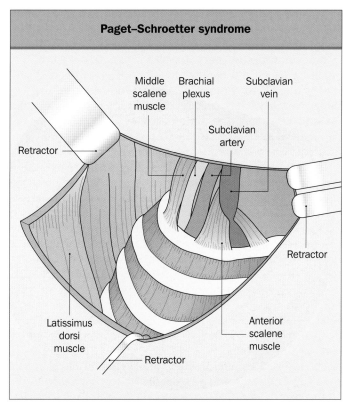

Paget–Schroetter syndrome

Middle scalene muscle

Brachial plexus

Subclavian vein

Subclavian artery

Retractor

Retractor

Latissimus dorsi muscle

Retractor

Anterior scalene muscle

Figure 21.7 Paget–Schroetter syndrome. Transaxillary exposure of the thoracic outlet demonstrating a subclavian vein compressed by subclavius and anterior scalene muscles. These are originating from first rib exostosis. This is one of several configurations that can be associated with Paget–Schroetter syndrome.

anatomic studies documenting the compression of the subclavian vein by this muscle into the costoclavicular notch. This has clear implications for axillo-subclavian vein thrombosis.

Trauma in general is implicated in the pathogenesis of neurogenic TOS, particularly localized to the neck and shoulder. Hyperextension, or whiplash, injuries occur in this patient population with some frequency. Neurogenic TOS can also be seen with repetitive motion type injuries. In Sander's review of operative TOS patients, 86% had a history of trauma.[8] This percentage is considerably higher than that cited in many other reports, but stresses the role that trauma can play in the disorder. Chronic trauma, such as that associated with poor posture, has also been implicated. This is termed the 'pectoralis minor syndrome', and the symptoms can be reproduced with an external compression of the pectoralis musculature.[9]

In a large series of patients, Machleder determined the etiology for operative cases of TOS when approached via a transaxillary incision.[10] Interestingly, no anatomic defect was visualized in 34%. This stands in contrast to other studies in which defects were almost always found. Cervical ribs were found in 8.5%, 10% had a scalenus minimus muscle, 19.5% had a defect in the subclavius tendon or its insertion, 43% had a developmental or insertional defect in the scalene musculature, and 7.5% had anatomic configurations whose developmental history was unclear.

As mentioned previously, there are histologic and biochemical changes in the tissues involved with TOS. Work by Sanders et al. demonstrated inflammation surrounding compressed

nerve trunks.[11] This inflammation could cause direct irritation of the nerve trunks, or set up a perineural inflammatory process leading to vasospasm in the vasa nervorum. Histologic changes in both the mesoneurium and endoneurium of involved nerves have been described, and the local formation of edema and adhesions is frequently observed.

At the molecular level, there have been several reports of the transition from type 2 to type 1 muscle fibers in TOS. Sanders and others have published on this topic, and Machleder and colleagues' studies clearly demonstrated this phenomenon.[12] Briefly, most skeletal muscle fibers are the quick-reacting type 2 fibers that have reactivity with phosphorylase and myosin ATPase. The slower, type 1 fibers have an increased oxidative capacity and a pronounced, slow tonic contractile pattern. Immunohistochemical analysis shows greater numbers of type 1 fibers in the anterior scalene muscle of TOS patients than in any other kind of tissue. The signaling required for this transition is not completely understood, but it does provide a molecular backdrop to the gross changes seen in TOS.

CLINICAL PRESENTATIONS OF DIFFERENT FORMS OF TOS

Neurogenic TOS
The typical case

A 25-year-old office worker presented with moderate pain and weakness of her right upper extremity that started around her shoulder and seemed to spread up her back and arm. These symptoms worsened with activity, especially with elevation of her arm. Medical history was otherwise unremarkable. Physical examination revealed no muscle atrophy of either upper extremity. The elevated arm stress test (EAST) was positive, as was Adson's test. Further testing was not undertaken at this time.

Based on this information, the patient was referred for an 8-week course of physical therapy. Although she was able to complete this program, her symptoms continued and were interfering with her performance at work and in her daily activities.

The patient was sent for a scalene block. This test was positive, and she was offered therapy in the form of transaxillary first-rib resection. She accepted this treatment option.

The patient was taken to the operating room, where the transaxillary approach was used to expose the first rib and contents of the thoracic outlet. The rib was excised uneventfully, and the patient tolerated the procedure without any problems. Her discharge home occurred on postoperative day 3.

The patient followed up in the office, and noted that her symptoms had gradually improved. At 3 months postoperatively, she is almost completely free of symptoms, and has noted that she is now more easily able to perform her job and to undertake her daily routine.

Patients can present with the symptoms of neurogenic TOS at any age, although the usual case involves a young to middle-aged adult with no other major health issues. When confronted by the pediatric or younger teenage patient with purely neurogenic symptoms, most authors recommend a period of waiting to see if growth will allow the symptoms to abate. The neurogenic symptoms can range in severity from nuisance to severely debilitating pain. Motor effects are seen, and although gross dysfunction of the upper extremity is unusual, a degree of weakness is not. This occasionally manifests as a decrease in grip strength. Gilliat and colleagues' description of classic neurogenic TOS with muscle wasting in the hand is not common.[13]

The pain may originate anywhere in the upper extremity, but the most common site is the back of the shoulder. The suprascapular portion of the trapezius may be involved. From the shoulder, pain can spread up the ipsilateral extremity, along the back or neck, or even up the face. This situation can lead to hemicranial headaches that can be labeled as migraines.

Arm pain can be generalized or localized to a particular nerve distribution. When localized, ulnar symptoms tend to be the most common, leading to difficulties with the ring and small fingers. Many authors report that these 'lower plexus' (C8–T1) symptoms are more common than 'upper' (C5–C7) manifestations.

Patients may report pain at rest that is not relieved by positioning. However, the typical patient will report that stress positioning exacerbates symptoms. This is particularly the case with work-related situations. People who must perform tasks with elevated arms or hold their arms in other awkward positions note they are no longer able to perform these tasks. Examples include waitresses, mechanics, and truck drivers. With prolonged stress positioning, patients may report finger discoloration, coolness of the extremity, or even swelling. Activities such as driving an automobile may precipitate numbness and tingling in the fingers.

Patients will often report that their symptom complex onset followed a specific traumatic event. Direct injury to the chest wall or shoulder can also precipitate symptoms, particularly if associated with a clavicular fracture or an acromioclavicular joint dislocation. Whiplash-type injuries are associated with TOS. Even a relatively minor injury can 'unmask' the syndrome in a previously completely asymptomatic individual. In other patients, symptoms may result from repetitive-type injuries, such as seen with pitchers and other athletes.

Patients complain of a broad spectrum of symptoms. A review of several series reveals that the most common finding is some form of paresthesia, which occurs in over 90% of patients. This is followed by upper limb pain, which is reported almost as frequently. The incidence of suprascapular pain is roughly 80%. The occurrence of headaches varies widely, although some studies report them in as many as 65% of patients.[14]

Two unusual presenting symptoms should be mentioned. First, ipsilateral hyperhidrosis can occur, and the proximity of the sympathetic chain to the other involved structures explains this phenomenon. The hyperhidrosis of TOS always occurs in association with other complaints.

Second, a 'pseudo' anginal syndrome has been described, in which patients complain of symptoms consistent with coronary artery disease.[15] Interestingly, many of these patients do not have the usual upper extremity symptoms with their initial presentation, leading to delay in diagnosis. The more common symptoms frequently develop over time, eventually leading to the diagnosis of TOS.

Venous TOS: Paget–Schroetter syndrome
The typical case
A 19-year-old college baseball player presented with the sudden onset of severe, uniform swelling of his pitching arm 2 days after a game. The patient denied having any other trauma or sustaining

any injury during the game. He also denied having any other medical problems. Physical examination revealed a swollen, somewhat red extremity with normal pulses at the wrist. Examination was otherwise unremarkable.

The patient had a duplex ultrasound which suggested subclavian thrombosis. Prompt venography was confirmatory and the patient underwent catheter-directed fibrinolysis of the clot using tissue plasminogen activator (tPA), with full resolution. He underwent transaxillary first-rib excision during the same hospitalization and was discharged home on warfarin.

The patient had a normal venogram 2 weeks after surgery, and was maintained on warfarin for 12 weeks. At that time, the patient was symptom free, and there have been no recurrent episodes of arm swelling.

Paget–Schroetter syndrome (axillo-subclavian vein thrombosis or 'effort' thrombosis) usually presents suddenly in a previously healthy patient with no symptoms of neurogenic TOS. Typically, the patient is a young athlete or worker participating in a sport or job that requires prolonged or repetitive stressful positioning of the arm. Examples include baseball players, swimmers, weight lifters, volleyball players, and mechanics. This presentation is dramatic compared to neurogenic TOS, and patients promptly seek medical attention.

The involved extremity often has a degree of discoloration, from rubor to cyanosis. The redness may be confused with the erythema of an infection, leading to a delay in diagnosis. Physical examination may reveal the presence of dilated collateral veins around the shoulder and upper arm. The remainder of the physical examination is normal at this point.

If the condition is left untreated, the swelling will resolve over the course of days or weeks. The patient will note a return to their normal state at rest, but that they are unable to use their arm for any period of time, particularly in a stressed (abducted, externally rotated) position. The collateral channels that develop and allow the swelling to abate are almost never adequate to accommodate the increased venous return that occurs with activity.

An alternative presentation is in association with an acute traumatic injury. Typically, the patient has an injury to the shoulder area. After a few days, some degree of ipsilateral arm swelling occurs. The natural history of these two variants is the same, reflecting the fact that the injury most likely contributed to compression in the thoracic outlet, so that the thrombosis associated with injury is really the same insult seen in 'spontaneous' thrombosis.

As mentioned previously, symptoms of neurogenic TOS are not usually associated with Paget–Schroetter syndrome. Although not common, ipsilateral sympathetic hyperactivity is not rare in this setting.

Arterial TOS
The typical case
A 42-year-old woman complained of a several month history of vague right arm symptoms, including periods of cold-intolerance, swelling, and Raynaud's phenomenon.

Plain radiographs revealed a right cervical rib and digital plethysmography showed obstructive waveforms in multiple fingers at the right hand.

Angiography revealed emboli obstructing digital arteries in the ipsilateral hand and post-stenotic dilatation of the subclavian artery when her arm was in the neutral position. A clear area of arterial compression was demonstrated when the patient's arm was abducted during angiography.

The patient underwent cervical rib resection and interposition grafting of the injured portion of the subclavian artery via a supraclavicular approach. Cervicothoracic sympathectomy was also performed. The patient recovered from the operation without complication. At follow-up, she was found to be symptom-free.

Because subclavian artery compression can lead to a number of injuries, its presentation is the most varied of the three forms of TOS. Damage to the subclavian artery itself can lead to anything from a small stenosis to aneurysm formation or complete occlusion. Each of these can then have its own sequelae secondary to embolization or thrombosis, or the extremely rare rupture of a subclavian aneurysm.

Patients are not infrequently misdiagnosed with collagen vascular disease because of the cold-sensitivity, Raynaud's phenomenon, and other symptoms. These patients may go on to have frank ischemic conditions of the hands, with paronychial ulcers or fingertip gangrene. If the subclavian artery is completely occluded, patients may present with early fatigue of the involved side. This can be in the form of crampy pain with exercise and has led to the term 'arm claudication'.

As with Paget–Schroetter syndrome, arterial TOS is not usually accompanied by symptoms of the neurogenic form. This probably contributes to the difficulty in making this diagnosis.

DIAGNOSIS

As the majority of cases of TOS present with neurogenic symptoms, it is the diagnosis of this form of the syndrome that will be addressed first. There is no generally accepted battery of tests that must be performed to confirm the presence of TOS. Most surgeons routinely dealing with the disorder require, at a minimum, a physical examination consistent with the symptoms, cervical films to rule out disc disease, and a chest radiograph to visualize any bony abnormalities one may encounter. The diagnostic evaluation varies among specialists, and the need for invasive or costly tests is an area of considerable debate.

History and physical examination

An extensive history should be elicited from the patient, including any injuries as well as the patient's occupation. Activities that worsen and improve the discomfort or other symptoms should be ascertained. In conjunction with a good history, most cases of TOS are diagnosed on the basis of physical examination. In addition, the physical examination plays an important role in excluding other conditions. A thorough examination should focus not only on the site of complaints, but also on other areas commonly involved in neurologic conditions. This includes the general appearance of the patient and other signs of symptom impact. Note should be made of symmetry of the muscle groups of the shoulders and upper extremities. Serratus anterior atrophy is occasionally present with TOS, as demonstrated by a winged scapula. Although cervical symptoms are common with TOS, limited cervical range of motion is not and there should not be excessive tenderness over the vertebral bodies. The presence of either of these suggests an alternative diagnosis. Deep-tendon reflexes, grip strength, and pulses should

be routinely assessed. Palmar hyperhidrosis should be noted if present. Machleder points out that, even in neurogenic TOS, changes in pulses can sometimes be readily detected (personal communication). Specific provocative neurologic maneuvers, such as downward compression of the head to rule out cervical disc disease, can be utilized when necessary. After this general neurologic assessment, tests more specific for the presence of thoracic outlet compression can be performed.

Patients with TOS generally do not have obvious muscle atrophy, and in fact have nearly normal gross baseline sensory and motor examinations. However, useful information can still be obtained if one uses an organized approach. Initial palpation of the structures of the chest wall, cervical area, and shoulder can be useful before undertaking provocative testing. The region overlying the anterior scalene muscle is frequently exquisitely tender in the face of brachial plexus entrapment or irritation. In addition, percussion of the clavicle can reproduce pains and paresthesias in TOS patients. These simple maneuvers should be performed before more complex maneuvering of the patient, which may cloud later findings.

The most commonly utilized provocative test for neurogenic TOS is the elevated arm stress test (EAST), originally described by Roos in 1966.[16] In the test, the patient is asked to completely elevate the shoulders and arms ('hold-up position') and then to repeatedly clench and unclench his or her hands (**Fig. 21.8**). This positioning is designed to constrict the costoclavicular space, and according to many reports will bring on weakness and paresthesias in the ulnar and median nerve distributions in patients with TOS within 3 minutes. Its proponents argue that it is specific for TOS and that the time of symptom onset correlates with the severity of TOS. In addition, it is felt by many that the test is good for reproducing the symptoms that patients suffer while using their upper extremities at work. Attention should also be given to the color of the hands during the EAST, as one may become pale and ischemic if arterial compromise is involved.

This test is not without its detractors. Although anecdotally reported to have excellent specificity, a study from 1985 found a positive test in over 80% of patients with carpal tunnel syndrome (CTS), and an earlier study by this same group found a positive EAST in almost all healthy asymptomatic individuals, although they did note that the positive tests occurred earlier in patients with TOS.[17] Additionally, some authors question the anatomic basis for the test, particularly how clenching and unclenching of the hand can lead to stress of the brachial plexus.[18]

Closely related to the EAST is the abduction and external rotation (AER) test (**Fig. 21.9**). The arm is abducted and rotated and held in that position. This test works by a similar mechanism, and likewise produces the weakness and numbness seen with EAST in a similar distribution, namely the C8 to T1 fibers supplying the median and ulnar nerves. In addition, one can sometimes detect a bruit below the lateral portion of the clavicle, which is attributable to partial compression of the axillary artery. Both of these tests appear particularly suited to work-related and repetitive motion associated TOS.[19]

There are several variants and positional tests that can be utilized, each with its own benefits and shortcomings. The 'Military brace' position can often reproduce TOS symptoms in patients with the disorder. The shoulders are braced backward

Elevated arm stress test position

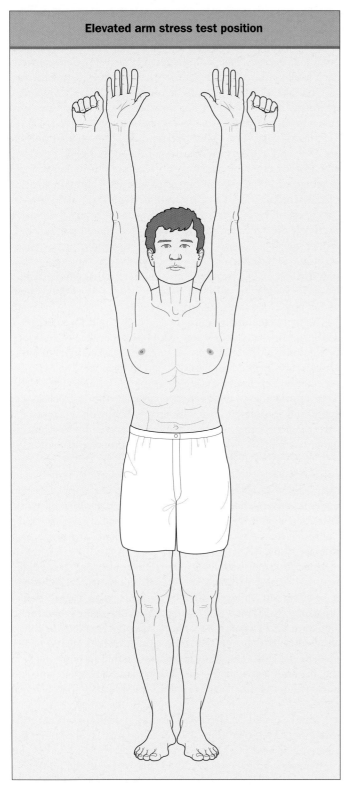

Abduction and external rotation test

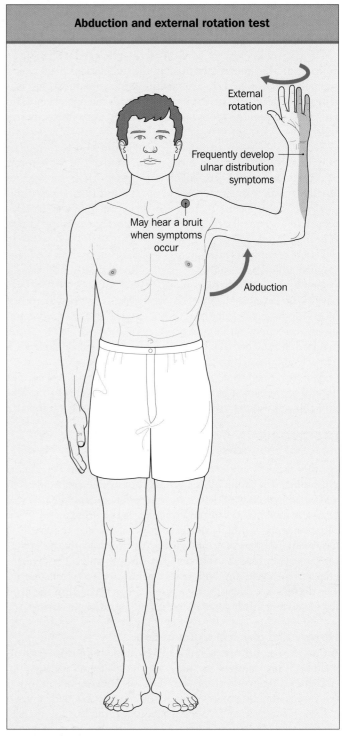

External rotation

Frequently develop ulnar distribution symptoms

May hear a bruit when symptoms occur

Abduction

Figure 21.9 Abduction and external rotation test (AER). The patient may be asked to clench and unclench the fist. A bruit is sometimes heard over the lateral aspect of the clavicle (axillary artery).

Figure 21.8 Elevated arm stress test (EAST) position. The fists are repeatedly clenched and unclenched, usually for 3min, or less if the symptoms start earlier. The costoclavicular space is narrowed via this maneuver (see Fig. 21.1).

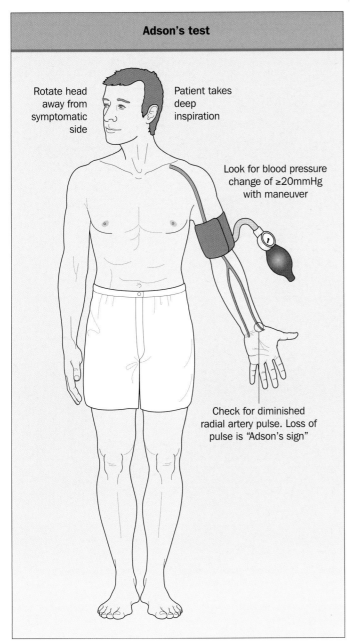

Adson's test

Rotate head away from symptomatic side

Patient takes deep inspiration

Look for blood pressure change of ≥20mmHg with maneuver

Check for diminished radial artery pulse. Loss of pulse is "Adson's sign"

Figure 21.10 Adson's test. This test is notoriously insensitive, with only about 3% of patients with thoracic outlet syndrome demonstrating loss of the radial pulse. Changes in blood pressure can add to the sensitivity, but this test is infrequently helpful.

and downward, effectively causing a narrowing of the thoracic outlet. Symptoms will arise within 2 minutes in a susceptible patient. The upper limb tension test (ULTT) uses graduated tension to test for irritation of the brachial plexus by extending the forearm with the shoulder abducted and externally rotated. Other tests include the timed Morley and Eden studies.

Additional information can be gained by adding pulse examination to the above tests. The original Adson's test consisted of assessment of the radial pulse following rotation of the neck to the contralateral side and deep inspiration (**Fig. 21.10**). 'Adson's sign' is the subsequent loss of the radial pulse. This test is notoriously insensitive, and has been reported to be positive in fewer than 3% of TOS patients.[20] In 1945, Wright described the

hyperabduction position, which is also of little clinical utility, given its positive result in most healthy individuals. However, measurements that quantify blood pressure are more sensitive, and a drop of 20mmHg after movement from the neutral position, or the same pressure difference from one extremity to the other, is frequently present in TOS. These tests are facilitated by using the Doppler probe. Additional positioning tests can also be used with simultaneous pulse assessment, including both the costoclavicular and anticus maneuvers. Of note, the cutaneous color changes associated with stress positioning do not correlate well with the presence of TOS.[21] None of the aforementioned tests is pathognomonic, but the presence of one or more of them can help to support the diagnosis of TOS.

Objective testing
Neurogenic form

The cervical spine film and chest radiograph are the most important objective studies needed in making the diagnosis of TOS. Clearly, cervical disease must be excluded as a cause of neurologic symptoms, and the bony abnormalities of TOS (cervical ribs, elongated C7 transverse processes, fractures with exostosis or callous formation) can be appreciated on plain chest films. The use of magnetic resonance imaging and computed tomography is advocated by some, but the utility of these studies is unproven.

The use of objective neurodiagnostic tests for TOS has met with some success, although it continues to be an area of considerable controversy. Perhaps the main criticism of these tests is that they only tend to be positive in patients with advanced disease, in whom history and physical examination should be sufficient. Thus, no less an authority than Roos suggests that they offer 'little definitive diagnostic information' and that one 'still must rely on careful history and physical…'[22] All of this reflects the fact that most electrophysiologic tests evaluate larger myelinated nerve fibers, rather than the smaller fibers whose injury mediates the pain associated with TOS. A recent study by Franklin and co-authors found that, of 158 TOS patients, only 7.6% had abnormalities in their electrodiagnostic tests.[14] Nonetheless, they can still aid in making the diagnosis of TOS and in excluding other conditions.

Neurophysiologic testing came to the forefront in the early 1960s, but the anatomic constraints of attempting to measure changes across the brachial plexus have always made its application in this position difficult. After Jebsen published the results of conduction velocity testing for the ulnar nerve in 1968, Urschel investigated its potential in the diagnosis of TOS. Hongladarom subsequently applied F-wave studies to the field in 1976, and Glover did the same with somatosensory evoked potentials in 1981. The application of neurophysiologic testing has continued to evolve, and modifications in techniques have improved sensitivity and specificity.

Nerve conduction studies can offer limited information in the workup of TOS, and can show evidence of CTS, either alone or in conjunction with the double-crush syndrome; approximately 20% of patients with TOS can also have CTS. Conduction studies do not offer definitive diagnostic information as specific for TOS. To measure velocities usefully, the nerve must be stimulated proximal to the potential point of injury. For compression at the thoracic outlet, this could mean stimulation at the roots, a site not conducive to easy testing. Several authors have described their experience using ulnar conduction velocity from Erb's point (above the clavicle and lateral to the insertion of the sternocleidomastoid muscle) to the elbow to assess TOS, but this technique has been criticized.[18] However, if there is severe disease with concomitant axonal damage, changes in ulnar action potentials can be demonstrated. A reasonable approach to conduction studies includes sensory testing of the median and ulnar nerves at the wrist to screen for CTS and TOS, respectively. The addition of motor nerve conduction velocities can be considered if additional information is needed to rule out CTS or ulnar entrapment neuropathy. However, no specific motor pathways for demonstrating TOS have been determined.

Electromyography may provide objective data supporting the diagnosis of TOS, although, again, this is in a setting of advanced disease. This study can demonstrate spontaneous firing of acutely denervated muscle fibers (positive sharp waves, fibrillation potentials), but this is not the usual clinical situation for TOS. Rather, after reinnervation, prolonged and irregular potentials are seen. Because this is a reflection of previous denervation injury, many of these patients will have atrophy of the involved muscle groups, and the electromyogram (EMG) can confirm injury of the lower trunk of the brachial plexus. However, in patients without evidence of atrophy, this test is not likely to reveal such findings. Standard EMG tests are negative in greater than 50% of TOS patients.[23] However, these tests can be used to examine the paraspinal muscles, which can be important in ruling out radiculopathy as the cause of the patient's symptoms.

Electromyography has an additional role which bears mentioning, that of being an adjunct to needle placement for scalene block. This test has utility as a predictor of surgical outcome for neurogenic TOS, with relaxation of the anterior scalene muscle approximating the decompression achieved with first-rib resection/scalenectomy. Improper needle placement can confuse the results of this test or cause injury, particularly to the brachial plexus itself or even the sympathetic ganglia at that level. Patients are given a series of injections of either lidocaine or saline, after which pain with provocative maneuvers is assessed (generally via the EAST). Jordan and Machleder reported on 122 patients in whom this technique was used and found a 90% positive predictive value for correlation with the clinical diagnosis of TOS.[24] In addition, for patients undergoing first-rib resection for TOS, those with a positive scalene block had a much greater chance of a good outcome (94%) than those with a negative preoperative scalene block (50%). This test can be positive with other disorders, particularly radiculopathies, but is another useful adjunct, not only in the diagnosis of TOS but also in estimating likelihood of surgical benefit.

F-wave studies are an attractive concept for evaluating TOS because they allow for distal propagation of the stimulus back to the spinal cord, thus crossing the brachial plexus and obviating the need for proximal nerve access. In this technique, nerve stimulation at the wrist leads not only to an immediate action potential in the affected muscle groups, but also to this proximal propagation with a concomitant reflection from the cord leading to a secondary action potential. This returning potential is the F-wave. Generally, multiple trials are recorded, and the shortest period between percutaneous stimulus and the secondary response is taken as the latency. This period is delayed if the nerve fibers are damaged, and this can be seen with TOS. There are additional parameters that can be assessed, but it is not clear

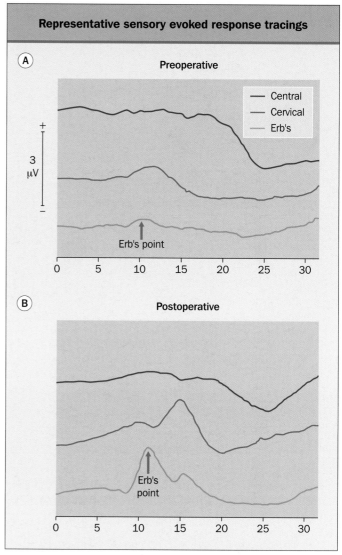

Figure 21.11 Representative sensory evoked response tracings, preoperatively (A) and postoperatively (B). The improved amplitude at Erb's point, recorded over the brachial plexus, is often seen when preoperative blunting is present. This tracing is from a patient with lower (ulnar) symptoms.

if these add any relevant information to TOS evaluations. It should also be noted that these tests tend to be poorly tolerated by many patients and it is prudent to avoid their use unless other tests have proved unrewarding and further diagnostic information is required.

Somatosensory evoked potentials (SSEPs) can play a role in the workup of TOS. Since 1979, when Siivola showed that multiple position recordings could be used to help locate peripheral nerve deficits related to the brachial plexus, the technique has been refined and applied to TOS.[25] Currently, assessment of the ulnar and median nerves can be used for evidence of their compression at the thoracic outlet. These studies, when abnormal, tend to show lower plexus injury (ulnar) with normal median function. This is seen primarily as a blunting of the Erb's point peak[26] (**Fig. 21.11**). Several studies have documented abnormal SSEPs with TOS. Machleder and colleagues showed that 74% of their patients carrying a clinical diagnosis of TOS had abnormal evoked responses.[27] Furthermore, when these patients were studied following operative decompression of their thoracic outlets, over 90% had a correlation between improved symptoms and normalization of their SSEPs. Other series have shown 45–70% of patients with TOS demonstrate corresponding SSEP changes. Increases in the sensitivity of these tests can be achieved with provocative maneuvers, such as arm positioning, although these maneuvers can also cause SSEP changes in patients with no clinical evidence of TOS. As with other forms of TOS testing, most of the patients with abnormal SSEPs will also have an abnormal physical examination and other electrophysiologic examinations. As with these other tests, SSEPs can be used to diagnose other processes causing the patient's symptoms.

Venous TOS: Paget–Schroetter syndrome

In the TOS patient who presents with upper extremity swelling, the diagnosis of axillo-subclavian vein thrombosis is suggested by the physical examination and history. Assessment of the venous system is usually initiated with non-invasive duplex ultrasonography and dynamic phlebography. Provocative positioning, such as external rotation and abduction, can increase the sensitivity of these tests. Other authors describe a two-position technique, with the arms adducted fully and then by 90 degrees. It is not clear at this time how useful magnetic resonance venography is for axillo-subclavian evaluation. It does appear to have the same anatomic limitation as duplex scanning, with poor quality of images in the retroclavicular space.

Most patients go on to have a diagnostic venogram, which is the gold standard for thrombosis in this location (**Fig. 21.12**). In the acute setting, lytic therapy is then administered. Although venography confirms the diagnosis of thrombosis, the occasional patient will require further clarification as to its cause. Neurogenic symptoms are usually not present; limb swelling, pain, and bluish discoloration are the usual findings.

Arterial TOS

As previously discussed, there can be a number of symptoms and signs as a consequence of arterial involvement in TOS. Physical examination can reveal a pulsatile mass in the supraclavicular fossa, but this is not a consistent finding. Clearly, the diagnostic algorithm is not straightforward. Patients should initially be evaluated with bilateral digital plethysmography, segmental arterial pressures, and upper extremity duplex examination. Unilateral digital artery obstruction should always prompt a search for a proximal arterial embolic source. Arteriography is required (**Fig. 21.13**) when arterial compression is suspected; imaging should include an arch study as well as the subclavian and axillary arteries. Frequently, arterial compression can be better demonstrated if the arm is abducted 90 degrees, and most studies are obtained with the arms in both neutral and abducted positions. When distal embolization is suspected, angiography should include magnified studies of the digital arteries at the hand.

TREATMENT

The vast majority of patients with neurogenic TOS in all likelihood go undiagnosed, and thus receive no therapy. This reflects the range of severity inherent in the spectrum of symptoms associated with TOS. For those who seek medical intervention,

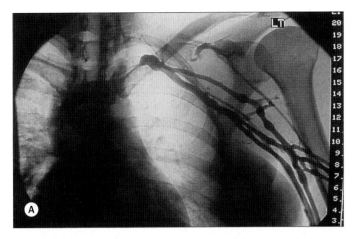
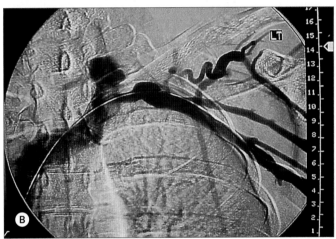

Figure 21.12 Venography and Paget–Schroetter syndrome. (A) Pre-treatment venogram from a patient with axillo-subclavian thrombosis (Paget–Schroetter syndrome). This patient underwent lysis and a venogram (B) was obtained. This therapy was followed by transaxillary first-rib resection.

it is clear that most have substantial improvement without operation. Although the numbers are controversial and dependent upon the modalities utilized to make the diagnosis, over 95% of patients avoid operation. There is currently considerable debate surrounding neurogenic TOS surgery, with several groups reporting no long-term benefit from operation compared to physical therapy. Nonetheless, most surgeons with considerable experience with neurogenic TOS report good surgical results with appropriately selected patients.

Before embarking on a treatment plan for a patient with a secure diagnosis of TOS, it is important to consider the variant of the syndrome being addressed. This discussion will start with the neurogenic form, which we have already noted as the most common. Differences in treatments for the other forms will follow.

Neurogenic TOS

For many surgeons, referral patterns are such that patients have already failed conservative therapy before seeking further consultation. It is important for surgeons to be aware of this selection bias. It is also important to have an algorithm for conservative treatment so that the correct patients are selected for operation. Recent reports suggest that a minimum of

277

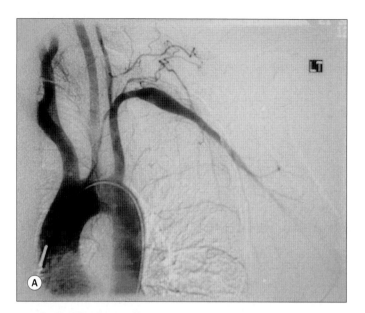

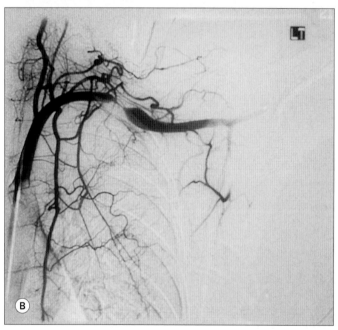

Figure 21.13 Arteriograms showing arterial changes in thoracic outlet syndrome. (A) A subclavian aneurysm at the site of the thoracic outlet is shown. (B) When the arm is abducted into a stressed position, a tight stenosis proximal to the area of dilatation is revealed.

6 weeks of physical therapy is required before its effects can be evaluated. It is also vital that the correct program is utilized, as it has been recognized that inappropriate physical therapy can worsen TOS symptoms. In general, these programs are designed to relax muscle groups that tighten the thoracic outlet, while conditioning those that open it. Aligne and Barral thus described a program in which the trapezius, levator scapulae, and sternocleidomastoid muscles are strengthened and the middle scalene, subclavius, and pectoralis muscles relaxed.[28] These goals can be met via many different protocols, usually with a combination of supervised and at-home exercises.

Other, non-surgical interventions are available. Following the concept of diagnostic scalene blocks, attempts have been made at therapeutic blockade of the scalene muscles. Steroid injection has not been successful, and early attempts at using botulinum toxin were complicated by dysphagia in as many as 20% of attempts. However, recent work by Jordan and co-authors demonstrated that electrophysiologic and fluoroscopic guidance of needle placement decreased the incidence of dysphagia and relieved symptoms for a mean duration of 88 days.[29] This technique may prove to be a useful tool, either in relieving symptoms in the preoperative period or in allowing the patient to tolerate an extended period of physical therapy or other adjustments, such as in their ergonomics at work.

Transaxilliary first-rib resection

When a symptomatic patient who has sought treatment fails to improve with physical therapy, surgical intervention is warranted. The initial operative treatment is most commonly trans-axillary first-rib resection (**Fig. 21.14**). The patient is placed in the lateral decubitus position, with the head neutral. No paralytic agents are used. A variety of devices are available for elevation of the arm on the operative side, all of which should allow for easy lowering of the extremity intermittently throughout the case, to facilitate periods of increased arterial inflow and decreased tension on stretched nerves. The incision is placed between the pectoralis major and the latissimus dorsi in the lower aspect of the axilla. Dissection is carried out, with care taken to identify intercostal brachial cutaneous nerves. These structures should be avoided and preserved when possible, but it is preferable to sacrifice them than to leave them injured and subject the patient to possible causalgic pain. Care must be taken in the region of the posterior scalene muscle to identify the long thoracic nerve, as injury with resulting winged scapula has been reported when this structure aberrantly passes closer to the mid-axillary line.

After the connective tissue over the thoracic outlet has been opened using blunt techniques with a peanut, the subclavian vein and artery, anterior scalene muscle, and lower trunk of the brachial plexus can be identified and cleared (**Fig. 21.15**). The anterior scalene muscle is now carefully separated from the subclavian vessels, and its attachment to the first rib can be divided. The subclavius tendon is also divided. Before the rib can be removed, further attachments between it and the middle scalene and first intercostal muscle must be released with particular care taken not to injure the T1 nerve. A right-angled rib shear is next positioned posteriorly over the first rib, so that it approaches the transverse process of T1. Anteriorly, the rib is divided almost at the level of the costal cartilage. Following removal of the rib, considerable care must be taken to smooth the posterior stump to prevent any subsequent T1 injury. At this point, any further encountered anomalies (fibromuscular bands, scalenus minimus muscles) should be resected. Cervical ribs are resected in a similar fashion to the first rib, requiring division of their attachments to the middle scalene and inter-costal muscles.

Before closure, the wound is irrigated and inspected for a pleural leak. In the presence of a leak, a small chest tube can be used for pleural drainage. This can usually be removed the following day. A postoperative chest radiograph is obtained. Most patients are discharged to home on postoperative day 1 or 2. Careful follow-up and physical therapy are also employed in the early postoperative period.

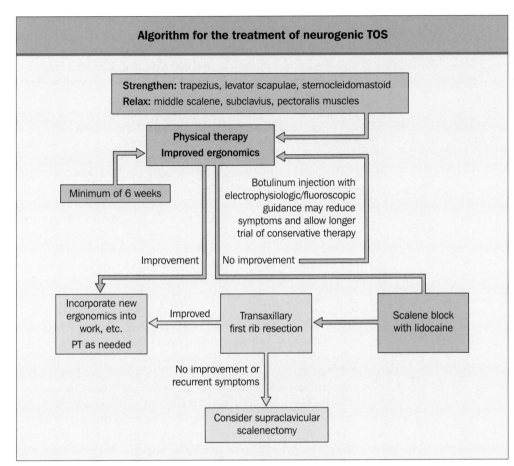

Algorithm for the treatment of neurogenic TOS

Strengthen: trapezius, levator scapulae, sternocleidomastoid
Relax: middle scalene, subclavius, pectoralis muscles

Physical therapy
Improved ergonomics

Minimum of 6 weeks

Botulinum injection with electrophysiologic/fluoroscopic guidance may reduce symptoms and allow longer trial of conservative therapy

Improvement — No improvement

Incorporate new ergonomics into work, etc. PT as needed

Improved — Transaxillary first rib resection — Scalene block with lidocaine

No improvement or recurrent symptoms

Consider supraclavicular scalenectomy

Figure 21.14 Algorithm for the treatment of neurogenic thoracic outlet syndrome. Some surgeons prefer a supraclavicular scalenectomy as the initial route of intervention. This can be done with, or without first-rib resection.

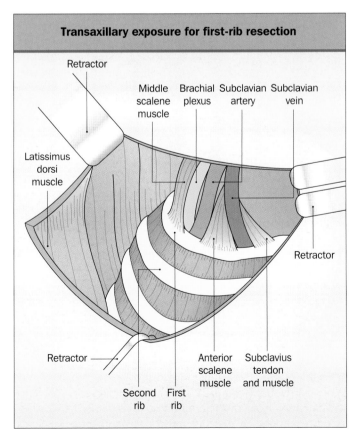

Transaxillary exposure for first-rib resection

Retractor

Middle scalene muscle — Brachial plexus — Subclavian artery — Subclavian vein

Latissimus dorsi muscle

Retractor

Retractor — Anterior scalene muscle — Subclavius tendon and muscle

Second rib — First rib

Figure 21.15 Transaxillary exposure for first-rib resection.

Supraclavicular scalenectomy

There are three situations in which scalenectomy is considered for TOS. Firstly, when the patient's symptoms are particularly suggestive of upper brachial plexus involvement (as opposed to the more common lower plexus), as has been described by Roos, it is reasonable to use an approach in which these nerves can be more directly decompressed. Secondly, the operation can be employed for patients who have undergone transaxillary operation but now have upper plexus symptoms. Thirdly, there are surgeons who feel that the supraclavicular approach is as effective as the transaxillary operation and that it is safer. Thus, they use this approach routinely. The first rib can also be resected as a component of this procedure, although some argue that it cannot be done with the same margins as the transaxillary approach.

As with the transaxillary approach, no paralytic agents are used, so that nerve function can be assessed intraoperatively. The patient is placed in the semi-Fowler position, with the head turned away from the operative side. An incision is placed two fingerbreadths above the clavicle, extending from the external jugular vein to the sternocleidomastoid muscle. This muscle is subsequently mobilized medially, while the omohyoid muscle must usually be transected. The scalene fat pad is carefully divided, taking care to avoid the underlying phrenic nerve. This structure must be protected throughout the course of the operation (**Fig. 21.16**). Underlying the nerve is the anterior scalene muscle. This is divided inferiorly at its insertion on the first rib. There are usually adhesions between the muscle and the subclavian artery and brachial plexus components that also

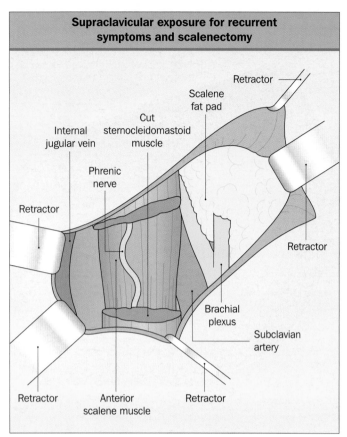

Supraclavicular exposure for recurrent symptoms and scalenectomy

Retractor

Scalene
fat pad

Cut
Internal   sternocleidomastoid
jugular vein   muscle

Phrenic
nerve

Retractor

Retractor

Brachial
plexus

Subclavian
artery

Retractor   Anterior   Retractor
scalene muscle

Figure 21.16 Supraclavicular exposure for recurrent symptoms and scalenectomy.

must be freed, and the origin end of the muscle is divided medially to expose the C5–C7 roots. The area between the C7 root and the subclavian artery is next cleared, including the division of a subclavius minimus muscle, if present. At this point, the C5 roots should be completely cleared and tested using a nerve stimulator, although several authors have noted that is often difficult to assess the T1 nerve root in this manner.

If the operation is to include first-rib resection, the middle scalene muscle must be divided. The rib is divided posteriorly and a finger used to dissect it from the pleura while elevating the divided end. The subclavian artery must be freed from the anterior portion of the rib before it can be divided and carefully extracted.

Irrigation is placed in the wound to assess for pleural leak. If present, the soft closed suction drain can be positioned so that the tip drains the pleural space. Otherwise, the drain can be placed to drain the wound. A postoperative chest radiograph is obtained, and the patient is usually discharged home within 1 or 2 days.

Thoracoscopic first-rib resection has been reported but has not gained widespread acceptance, as some authors question the benefits versus the transaxillary approach. Nonetheless, this operation is offered at several centers, and it remains to be seen what place it will have in the treatment of TOS.[30]

Venous TOS or Paget–Schroetter syndrome

Unlike the elective nature of neurogenic TOS therapies, venous occlusion at the thoracic outlet should be treated expeditiously.

Although this disease was once treated with anticoagulation and arm elevation, therapeutic protocols now stress the importance of dissolving the clot, maintaining patency of the axillo-subclavian veins, and correcting any anatomic abnormalities contributing to the thrombosis. Once the diagnosis has been established, the patient should undergo catheter-directed fibrinolysis of the clot. Streptokinase, urokinase, and tPA have all been used in the past, and the agent employed is institution dependent. A recent trial by Gelabert and colleagues compared tPA and urokinase in this setting and suggested similar results.[31] In addition to the clot-directed therapy, patients are heparinized and then placed on oral coumadin. Work by Perler and Mitchell, later supported by that of Machleder and Kunkle, demonstrated that a period of 1–3 months of anticoagulation allowed for intimal healing of the damaged vein before the patient was taken for definitive surgery in the form of first-rib resection.[32–34] Following surgery, the vein is again assessed. If residual stricture exists, the patient undergoes further catheter-based treatment.

The above protocol and variants of it have been widely adopted at centers treating Paget–Schroetter syndrome. However, in order to decrease the period of disability between the initial lysis and the definitive operation, some authors have advocated first-rib resection during the initial hospitalization. The UCLA group recently reported a series of patients treated in this fashion, and noted no increased morbidity compared to those patients undergoing delayed operation.[35] In particular, none of the theoretical concerns for bleeding following thrombolytic instillation were observed, nor were there particular technical problems secondary to the inflammation associated with the venous thrombosis. Although no randomized, prospective trial has yet compared these two protocols, it is likely that a number of centers will adopt a policy of early surgical intervention.

A brief mention should be made regarding complicated venous injuries in the setting of TOS. Angioplasty for residual stricture appears to work quite well in this setting, following correction of the anatomic problems, although stenting has not been particularly useful. Meier reported on the high incidence of stent deformity in the setting of TOS, even after first-rib resection.[36] Nonetheless, some authors continue to utilize stents for post-operative venous strictures. Finally, there are cases in which the vein is so severely damaged that the only operative repair that can be performed is a jugular-subclavian turndown or bypass. This procedure is rarely indicated, and only if the patient has continued severe symptoms of venous hypertension.

For patients with thrombus that resists thrombolysis, there is usually a component of chronic disease. Machleder observed that these patients may in fact have intermittent periods of clot propagation for which their collaterals are not adequate to compensate.[37] It is during these times that there is 'acute' swelling. It is not clear what the ideal treatment should be in this situation. If the patient has resolution of the acute symptoms, observation with anticoagulation is a reasonable option. For symptomatic patients, some surgical or endovascular procedure tailored to the particular problem is warranted.

Arterial TOS

As previously discussed, there are a number of arterial problems that can arise from thoracic outlet obstruction, although they are not common. Clearly, the urgency of intervention depends on the severity of the problem, with ischemia clearly dictating

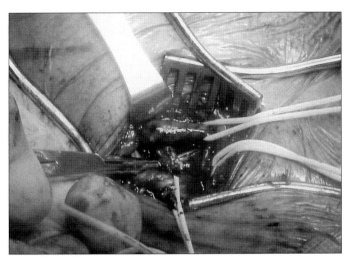

Figure 21.17 Supraclavicular exposure of a subclavian artery aneurysm and cervical rib. Vessel loops are around the artery and the right angle clamp is partially elevating the cervical rib.

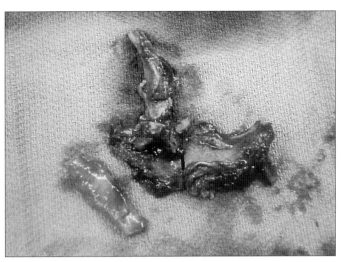

Figure 21.18 Specimen from first-rib resection and repair of subclavian artery aneurysm. This lesion was approached via the supraclavicular route. The aneurysm, cervical rib, and first rib are shown.

an expeditious approach. For most, transaxillary first-rib resection followed by arterial repair remains the treatment of choice. If there is a cervical rib, it needs to be removed as well. The area of arterial involvement is usually the retroscalene subclavian to pre-pectoral region of the axillary artery. In patients with distal embolization, surgical thrombectomy or catheter-based thrombolysis is usually necessary before addressing the source.

Aneurysms secondary to TOS are usually treated no differently than such lesions when due to atherosclerosis, namely resection and graft reconstruction. This also holds true for axillo-subclavian post-stenotic dilatation and obstruction. These operations are described elsewhere in this text, so only a few points will be made about them here. Standard approaches are utilized, with a high anterior thoracotomy for proximal lesions on the left, and median sternotomy for the right. For more distal lesions, a variety of clavicular incisions may be utilized (**Figs 21.17 & 21.18**). Graft material is a matter of surgeon's preference, but it is clear that synthetic material, and vein and arterial grafts have all been used with success in this position. Postoperative anticoagulation is not usually indicated, and patients tend to do well if the thoracic outlet is adequately decompressed and the vessel is no longer subjected to trauma.

An additional consideration in these patients is the presence of reflex sympathetic dystrophy, causalgia, or other autonomic dysfunction. Cervicodorsal or cervicothoracic sympathectomy is offered to these patients and can often be performed at the time of the arterial repair by standard approaches. Alternatively, this operation can be performed at a separate setting via a thoracoscopic route if its need is not clear. It should also be noted that these same symptoms can occur in patients with primary neurogenic TOS if the sympathetic nerves in the inferior trunk of the brachial plexus are involved. These patients can also be treated by sympathectomy if necessary.

Finally, patients with arterial consequences of TOS can have diverse complications. Machleder has reported an embolizing aneurysm of the posterior humeral circumflex artery necessitating aneurysm excision and cephalic vein bypass of the distal common and posterior humeral circumflex artery to the anterior humeral circumflex artery.[37] Clearly, the variety of problems arising from arterial involvement in TOS leads to the most varied presentations, and concomitantly to the most varied therapies.

Recurrent TOS
Recurrence of TOS following operative intervention is not uncommon. Published series have reported rates as low as 2.2%, but most range from 15% to 20%.[38–41] Defining recurrence in this situation is frequently difficult, because it is not always clear that the patient's symptoms ever improved. Symptoms tend to be similar to the original complaints, with paresthesias of the hand and pain of the neck and shoulder being the most common manifestations. The etiology of recurrence is usually not clear, although postoperative scarring is considered to be one of the main culprits. Several studies have looked at the implications of a long posterior first-rib stump, but there is little correlation with return of symptoms. Other reported etiologies include middle scalene reattachment, calcified rib masses, and missed cervical ribs or cervical rib stumps. Some authors have drawn a distinction between a spontaneous recurrence, attributable to scar, and a recurrence secondary to a traumatic insult. In the latter situation, the patient again tends to have the original symptoms, despite the fact that the thoracic outlet has already been decompressed. A whiplash-type injury frequently occurs in this scenario.

The workup for recurrence is essentially the same as for untreated disease. Special emphasis should be placed on ruling out other causes, as a percentage of patients failing treatment will have done so on the basis of a faulty diagnosis. Iatrogenic injury to the plexus, CTS, tendonitis, cervical arthritis, or spine injury must be sought before treatment for the recurrence is started. A conservative plan is initially undertaken, although the overwhelmingly positive response seen with physical therapy in TOS patients who avoid the original operation is not reproduced here. If conservative methods fail, reoperation is considered, although it should be noted that only a 50% improvement rate is quoted for these patients.

Although clinical practices vary, many surgeons have adopted an algorithm for reoperation. If the original operation was via a transaxillary approach, a supraclavicular approach is taken. Care is taken to identify any remaining first rib, and to resect it all the way to the transverse process. If the patient's original operation did not include first-rib resection, it is removed now. Most surgeons also add some form of neurolysis to the reoperation, whereby the scar around the nerves is carefully removed. Some surgeons remove the middle scalene during the course of re-exploration. If the supraclavicular approach has already been used, the transaxillary approach is utilized for the second operation. Again, care is taken to remove the entire first rib, any remaining attachments, and scar tissue. Neurolysis can also be performed via this route, with some authors preferring it to the supraclavicular approach, particularly when ulnar symptoms predominate.

Several methods have been tried to prevent the formation of scar tissue and adhesions following thoracic outlet decompression, particularly in the face of reoperation. After clearing the nerve roots, they are usually covered with the overlying adipose tissue, although the benefit of this technique has never been documented. Similarly, care is taken to replace the scalene fat pad, but this does not appear to influence the formation of scar tissue. Attempts to control scarring with the administration of exogenous agents, including steroids, have also been disappointing. Sheets of polytetrafluoroethylene (PTFE) have been used to cover the nerves, but this technique has been abandoned by most surgeons, and probably leads to additional scar tissue formation. The use of hyaluronic acid gels showed some promise several years ago, but it is not clear whether these products are particularly helpful and they are not approved by the US Food and Drug Administration for this use.

COMPLICATIONS

Any structure encountered in the dissection for first-rib resection is a potential site of injury. The catastrophic complications of brachial plexus injury, subclavian artery, and subclavian vein injury occur infrequently. Concern about brachial plexus injury dates back to the early days of first-rib resection. Particularly in the neurology literature, this has been a controversial topic. For a number of years, there were only a few case reports of plexus injuries. However, Dale in 1982 published the results of a survey of thoracic surgeons performing first-rib resections, in which 273 injuries were discovered, 19% of which were permanent.[42] While this study certainly suggested underreporting of this complication, reports of plexus injuries remained low, although not the almost negligible rate that had been accepted.

What is most notable about the publications that followed is that no mention was made of the incidence of this injury. Wilbourn in 1988 reported on eight patients with plexus injuries from the Cleveland Clinic.[43] They underwent first-rib resection some time between 1974 and 1983, but the total number of procedures performed is not given. Likewise, Horowitz reported on four cases of plexus injury, but no figures are given regarding the number of procedures performed from which these patients were derived.[44] The same can be said of the four cases reported by Cherington et al. in 1986.[45] In several large recent surgical series, most notably that of Roos, the incidence of such injuries is very low (0–2%). In the UCLA experience, there have been no such injuries. It is fair to say that plexus injuries certainly do occur, but that the risk of the injury must be weighed against the possible benefits of the procedure.

Another issue regarding plexus injuries is that of retraction. It is highly likely that most of the neurologic injuries were related to stretching of the perineurium with resultant ischemia. During the transaxillary approach, a considerable amount of stretch is applied to the arm, and most surgeons relieve the traction intermittently to allow blood flow. This may not necessarily be the case when an assistant is retracting. Specialized retraction systems, such as the Machleder retractor, allow for periods of extremity relaxation with easy repositioning to continue the procedure.

The incidence of major arterial or venous injury during first-rib resection is also difficult to determine. It is clear that these injuries can and do occur, and that they demand immediate attention. In a review of 2445 cases, Roos reported only three instances of major injuries of this nature (0.12%).[46] In all three cases, the patients had full recovery. Delayed bleeding, usually from a small subclavian branch or intercostal artery, is also seen. Roos reported seven cases in the same series (0.2%). The patients also had complete recovery. In the review by Green et al. of 136 patients, there were no major vascular injuries.[47] The UCLA group reported one such injury in an operative series spanning over 10 years.

Injuries to other nerves occur, particularly the long thoracic nerve. Roos reported a 0.12% incidence, with two of the patients having complete recoveries and one lost to follow up. In Sharp and colleagues' series of 36 patients, there was one such injury.[48] Most of these injuries tend to be temporary, but permanent winged scapula can occur. Phrenic injuries are not common and are more associated with the anterior approach, particularly with reoperative cases. Most of these injuries result in temporary, subclinical diaphragmatic paralysis, although complete division with permanent injury is possible.

The most common nerve injury is not a true complication, but a by-product of the operation: division of intercostal brachial cutaneous branches leading to cutaneous numbness. This occurs to some extent in most patients, not unlike that which occurs with axillary dissection for other disease states. It is usually well tolerated and resolves.

Reports of patients with postoperative causalgia or other pains are also difficult to place into clinical perspective. In most series, they are unusual. Significant causalgia is usually attributed to brachial plexus injury, and thus should parallel the incidence of this injury. In the Washington State Workers' Compensation Study, 6% of patients were reported to have causalgia, and 13% had 'other pains'.[16] It is not clear what these represented. Green's series of 136 cases included three patients with some form of postoperative vasospasm.[47] Finally, postoperative Horner's syndrome occurs in between 0.5% and 2% of patients in most series. In almost all reported cases, it is self-limiting.

Entry into the pleural space occurs in as many as 30% of cases. This is usually recognized and easily evacuated at the time of operation, without the need for a chest tube. The highest reported incidence of postoperative pneumothorax is 5%.

As mentioned previously, there are reports of injuries to all of the structures encountered during first-rib resection. Thus, supraclavicular approaches can lead to thoracic duct or even recurrent laryngeal nerve injury, although these injuries are rare. The risk of complications is increased with reoperative surgery. Many structures tend to be adherent in a particular pattern during these procedures, for example the subclavian artery to the anterior scalene muscle. Care must be taken in these cases to identify all structures adequately.

PROGNOSIS

For the majority of patients with TOS, the prognosis is excellent, with improvement in symptoms following physical therapy or other adjustments in their working postures or activities. However, for the patients with more debilitating symptoms that require surgical intervention, the long-term prognosis is not clear. In addition, it is difficult to objectively study the outcomes following surgery for neurogenic TOS. A variety of endpoints have been examined, but no prospective outcomes-based study of operation for TOS has been published. Such a study is currently in progress at the authors' institution. Nonetheless, reported results vary widely.

There are several series with recurrence rates between 15–20% following first-rib resection either by the transaxillary or supraclavicular route. Sanders reported a similar range, and noted that the vast majority of these occur within 2 years of the initial operation.[11] In this same study, it was reported that the subjectively determined immediate postoperative success rate of 84% decreased to 59% at 2 years, 69% at 5 years, and to as low as 41% at the 10–15-year interval using life-table analysis. Reoperation for these patients resulted in improvement, so that at the 5–10-year interval, 86% of patients still were reporting subjective benefits from their procedures. Patients with symptoms that were persistent, rather than recurrent, also tended to fare worse following reoperation.

The study by Sharp and authors focused on patients' ability to return to work following TOS surgery, noting that 80% of the patients in their study were able to do so, and that 85% of the patients subjectively described their outcomes as good to excellent.[48] As was noted previously, employment and disability issues complicate outcomes in TOS. In the Washington State Workers' Compensation Study, 40% of postoperative TOS patients were still not working 2 years after their operations; this percentage was actually worse at 5 years (44%).[16] Interestingly, the conservatively treated patients in this study did better in this regard, although this was a retrospective study, in which the cohorts were not particularly well matched. Numerous other studies have shown worse outcomes when the patients have work-related or legal issues related to their TOS.[49]

Other factors predicting outcome following TOS surgery have been studied. Trauma as the event precipitating TOS is associated with poor outcomes in several series, but not in others.[47,50] In addition, preoperative depression has also been linked to worse outcome. In a report by Axelrod et al., those patients with preoperative depression were more likely to have continued functional and vocational disability following operation.[51] This study combined pre- and postoperative interviews, psychological evaluations, and patient examinations, with an overall 67% of patients subjectively reporting 'good or average' outcome. At an average of 47 months' follow-up, 64% of patients were satisfied with their outcomes and 69% reported they would undergo operation again, if faced with the same symptoms. Eighteen percent of the patients considered themselves disabled.

In one of the largest series of TOS patients, Roos reported that in 1844 transaxillary first-rib resections, 90% of patients

were able to return to performing tasks they had been unable to perform preoperatively. In addition, 97% said that they would recommend rib resection to other patients with symptoms of TOS. There was a 5% recurrence, which was better than the 19% seen with scalenectomy (although this was without rib resection). Green also reported higher recurrence following the anterior approach, although other authors have reported that the two approaches yielded equivalent recurrence rates.[47]

The prognosis for untreated axillo-subclavian venous thrombosis was one of progressive disability. Even after the institution of immobilization and anticoagulation, a study in 1970 revealed that 75% of patients had poor outcomes.[52] Following modern treatment protocols, most patients are able to resume normal activities, which is of particular importance in this group of predominantly young and otherwise healthy patients. The most important factor is the time to treatment following thrombosis, with most treatment failures occurring in the face of delays. As far as long-term results are concerned, Feugier and colleagues reported that all treated patients were asymptomatic at an average follow-up of 45 months.[53] These authors found that, if treated expeditiously, with complete recanalization of the vein and removal of the compressive rib, long-term sequelae are not common. However, if this cannot be accomplished, repeated venous problems occur, and can lead to debilitating situations.

The prognosis for patients with arterial involvement in TOS is highly variable, depending on the pattern of disease. Again, if the compressive element of the process is adequately dealt with, the issue becomes the arterial repair itself. The data for subclavian artery repairs can be found elsewhere, but is generally good. Likewise, the outcomes from the infrequently required sympathectomy parallel those for reflex-sympathetic dystrophy when performed in appropriately selected patients.

SUMMARY

Neurogenic TOS is a controversial diagnosis and, despite over a century of treatment plans, there is still no universal acceptance of the diagnosis in many cases – or, for that matter, the treatment. At the center of the controversy is the lack of objective tests for the most commonly diagnosed neurogenic form of the syndrome. Although physical maneuvers and data from scalene blocks can certainly support the diagnosis, it remains a clinical diagnosis in the absence of vascular involvement.

Likewise, assessing the outcomes of intervention for the neurogenic form of the syndrome is difficult and is an area of debate. Studies have shown conflicting results, with patients reporting dissatisfaction with their first-rib resection but a willingness to undergo the operation again if the same symptoms were to develop contralaterally. Although an oversimplification, most surgical series reflect fairly high patient satisfaction, while reviews by other specialists tend to be less positive.

It is clear that outcomes data will be of great value in this debate. First-rib surgery is, for the most part, patient driven. Many of these patients have dealt with their symptoms for prolonged periods of time with no relief. They are therefore more than willing to undergo surgery because nothing else has worked. Quality of life data from these patients will help surgeons decide the extent to which our interventions are actually helping these people.

REFERENCES

1. Roos DB, Edgar J. Poth Lecture. Thoracic outlet syndromes: update 1987. Am J Surg 1987;154:568–73.
2. Peet RM, Hendricksen JD, Anderson TP, et al. Thoracic outlet syndrome: evaluation of the therapeutic exercise program. Mayo Clin Proc 1956; 31:281–7.
3. Clagett OT. Presidential address: research and prosearch. J Thorac Cardiovasc Surg 1962;44:153–66.
4. Roos DB. Transaxillary approach for first rib resection to relieve thoracic outlet compression syndrome. Ann Surg 1966;163:354.
5. Machleder HI. Vascular disorders of the upper extremity, 3rd edn. Armonk, New York: Futura Publishing Company, Inc; 1998.
6. Roos DB. Historical perspectives and anatomic considerations. Thoracic outlet syndrome. Semin Thorac Cardiovasc Surg 1996;8:183–9.
7. Roos DB. Congenital anomalies associated with thoracic outlet syndrome: anatomy, symptoms, diagnosis and treatment. Am J Surg 1976;132:771–8.
8. Sanders RJ, Haug CE, Pearce WH, et al. Recurrent thoracic outlet syndrome. J Vasc Surg 1990;12:390–400.
9. Nakada T, Knight RT, Mani RL. Intermittent venous claudication of the upper extremity: the pectoralis minor syndrome. Ann Neurol 1982; 11:433–4.
10. Machleder HI. Thoracic outlet syndromes: new concepts from a century of discovery. Cardiovasc Surg 1994;2:137–45.
11. Sanders RJ, Jackson CGR, Baushero N, et al. Scalene muscle abnormalities in traumatic thoracic outlet syndrome. Am J Surg 1990;159:231–6.
12. Machleder HI, Moll F, Verity A. The anterior scalene muscle in thoracic outlet compression syndrome. Arch Surg 1986;121:1141–4.
13. Gilliat RW, LeQuesne PM, Logue V, et al. Wasting of the hand associated with a cervical rib or band. J Neurol Neurosurg Psychiatry 1970;33:615–24.
14. Franklin GM, Fulton-Kehoe D, Bradley C, et al. Outcome of surgery for thoracic outlet syndrome in Washington State Workers' Compensation. Neurology 2000;54:1252–7.
15. Urschel HC Jr, Razzuk MA, Hyland JW, et al. Thoracic outlet syndrome masquerading as coronary artery disease. Ann Thorac Surg 1973; 16:239–48.
16. Roos DB, Owens JC. Thoracic outlet syndrome. Arch Surg 1966; 93:71–4.
17. Costigan DA, Wilbourn AJ. The elevated arm stress test; specificity in the diagnosis of thoracic outlet syndrome. Neurology 1985;35(Suppl 1):74–5.
18. Wilbourn AJ. Thoracic outlet syndrome is overdiagnosed. Muscle Nerve 1999;22:130–6.
19. Toomingas A, Nilsson T, Hagberg M, et al. Predictive aspects of the abduction external rotation test among male industrial and office workers. Am J Ind Med 1999;35:32–42.
20. Roos DB. The place for scalenectomy and first-rib resection in thoracic outlet syndrome. Surgery 1982;92:1077–85.
21. Abe M, Katsuaki I, Nishida J. Diagnosis, treatment and complications of thoracic outlet syndrome. J Orthop Sci 1999;4:66–9.
22. Roos DB. Thoracic outlet syndrome is underdiagnosed. Muscle Nerve 1999;22:126–9.
23. Smith T, Trojaborg, W. The diagnosis of thoracic outlet syndrome: value of sensory and motor conduction studies and quantitative electromyography. Arch Neurol 1987;44:1161–3.
24. Jordan SE, Machleder HI. Diagnosis of thoracic outlet syndrome using electrophysiologically guided anterior scalene blocks. Ann Vasc Surg 1998;12:260–4.
25. Siivola J, Myllyla VV, Sulg I, et al. Brachial plexus and radicular neurography in relation to cortical evoked responses. J Neurol Neurosurg Psychiatry 1979;42:1151–8.
26. Siivola J, Sulg I, Pokela R. Somatosensory evoked responses as a diagnostic aid in thoracic outlet syndrome (a preoperative study). Acta Chir Scand 1982;148:647–52.
27. Machleder HI, Mill F, Nuwer M, et al. Somatosensory evoked potentials in the assessment of thoracic outlet compression syndrome. J Vasc Surg 1987;6:177–84.
28. Aligne C, Barral X. Rehabilitation of patients with thoracic outlet syndrome. Ann Vasc Surg 1992;6:381–9.
29. Jordan SE, Ahn SS, Freischlag JA. Selective botulinum chemo-denervation of the scalene muscles for treatment of neurogenic thoracic outlet syndrome. Ann Vasc Surg 2000;14:365–9.
30. Ohtsuka T, Wolf RK, Dunsker SB. Port-access first-rib resection. Surg Endosc 1999;13:940–942.
31. Gelabert HA, Freischlag JA, Angle N. Comparison of retavase and urokinase for management of spontaneous subclavian vein thrombosis. J Vasc Surg 2003 (submitted).
32. Perler BA, Mitchell SE. Percutaneous transluminal angioplasty and transaxillary first rib resection. A multidisciplinary approach to the thoracic outlet syndrome. Am Surg 1986;52:485–8.
33. Machleder HI. Evaluation of a new treatment strategy for Paget–Schroetter syndrome: spontaneous thrombosis of the axillary-subclavian vein. J Vasc Surg 1993;17:305–17.
34. Kunkel JM, Machleder HI. Treatment of Paget–Schroetter syndrome. A staged, multidisciplinary approach. Arch Surg 1989;124:1153–8.
35. Angle N, Gelabert HA, Farooq MM, et al. Safety and efficacy of early surgical decompression of the thoracic outlet for Paget–Schroetter syndrome. Ann Vasc Surg 2001;15:37–42.
36. Meier GH, Pollak JS, Rosenblatt M, et al. Initial experience with venous stents in exertional axillary-subclavian vein thrombosis. J Vasc Surg 1996;24:974–83.
37. Machleder HI. Vascular disorders of the upper extremity, 3rd edn. Armonk, New York: Futura Publishing Company, Inc; 1998:217–8.
38. Lindgren KA, Leino E, Lepantalo M, et al. Recurrent thoracic outlet syndrome after first rib resection. Arch Phys Med Rehabil 1991; 72:208–10.
39. Roos, DB. Recurrent thoracic outlet syndrome after first rib resection. Acta Chir Belg 1980;79:363–72.
40. Sessions RT. Recurrent thoracic outlet syndrome: causes and treatment. South Med J 1982;75:1453–61.
41. Sanders RJ, Monsour JW, Gerber FG, et al. Scalenectomy versus first rib resection for treatment of the thoracic outlet syndrome. Surgery 1979;85:109–21.
42. Dale WA. Thoracic outlet compression syndrome. Arch Surg 1982; 164:149–53.
43. Wilbourn AJ. Thoracic outlet syndrome surgery causing severe brachial plexopathy. Muscle Nerve 1988;11:66–74.
44. Horowitz SH. Brachial plexus injuries with causalgia resulting from transaxillary rib resection. Arch Surg 1985;120:1189–91.
45. Cherington M, Happer I, Machanic B, et al. Surgery for thoracic outlet syndrome may be hazardous to your health. Muscle Nerve 1986;9:632–4.
46. Roos DB. Thoracic outlet nerve compression. In: Rutherford RB, ed. Vascular surgery, 3rd edn. Philadelphia:WB Saunders Co; 1989:858–75.
47. Green RM, McNamara J, Ouriel K. Long-term follow-up after thoracic outlet decompression: an analysis of factors determining outcome. J Vasc Surg 1991;14:739–46.
48. Sharp WJ, Nowak LR, Zamani T, et al. Long-term follow-up and patient satisfaction after surgery for thoracic outlet syndrome. Ann Vasc Surg 2001;15:32–6.
49. Lepantalo M, Lindgren KA, Leino E, et al. Long-term outcome after resection of the first rib for thoracic outlet syndrome. Br J Surg 1989;76:1255–6.
50. Sanders RJ, Pearce WH. The treatment of thoracic outlet syndrome; a comparison of different operations. J Vasc Surg 1989;10:626–32.
51. Axelrod DA, Proctor MC, Geisser ME, et al. Outcomes after surgery for thoracic outlet syndrome. J Vasc Surg 2001;33:1220–5.
52. Tilney ML, Griffiths HJ, Edwards EA. Natural history of major venous thrombosis of the upper extremity. Arch Surg 1970;101:792–6.
53. Feugier P, Aleksic I, Salari R, et al. Long-term results of venous revascularization for Paget–Schroetter syndrome in athletes. Ann Vasc Surg 2001;15:212–8.

CHAPTER

22

Acute and Chronic Arterial Mesenteric Ischemia

Thomas C Bower

KEY POINTS

- Acute mesenteric ischemia (AMI) is most often caused by emboli from the heart or in-situ thrombosis secondary to an underlying atherosclerotic lesion.

- Diagnosis of AMI requires a high index of clinical suspicion. Patients have abdominal pain out of proportion to physical findings. Early diagnosis is vital, as the mortality from this problem remains high.

- Outcomes following operative treatment of chronic mesenteric ischemia have improved over the years. There is controversy regarding the need for single versus multiple vessel reconstruction and the preference for antegrade versus retrograde bypass. Choice of operation should be individualized, based on patient age, risk, and anatomy.

- The role of endovascular treatment for either acute or chronic mesenteric ischemia is yet to be defined.

The diagnosis and management of patients with acute (AMI) or chronic (CMI) mesenteric arterial ischemia is challenging. Surgical results for patients treated with CMI have improved, but there has been little advance in the early diagnosis and treatment of patients with AMI.[1–24]

This chapter will review the classification, etiology, clinical presentation, diagnosis, and treatment for patients with AMI and chronic mesenteric ischemia. The management of patients with non-occlusive mesenteric ischemia will not be discussed. Much of the information in this chapter is based on Mayo Clinic experience, as well as selected comparative data from the literature.

ACUTE MESENTERIC ISCHEMIA

The etiology of AMI is primarily due to arterial obstruction.[11,12,25] Emboli usually originate in the heart but may come from proximal aortic aneurysms or atherosclerotic lesions.[11,12] Typically, the proximal small bowel is spared but the remainder of the small intestine and proximal colon are ischemic because the embolus occludes the superior mesenteric artery (SMA) a few centimeters beyond its origin, sparing the proximal branches.[11]

Acute thrombosis of the SMA is often secondary to an underlying proximal atherosclerotic lesion.[11] Dissections or aneurysms are rare causes. Most of the small bowel and colon are ischemic in various proportions, depending on the status of the collateral circulation.[11]

Clinical presentation

Most patients are in the sixth or seventh decade of life.[11,12,25] The patients have a history of severe abdominal pain out of proportion to their physical examination findings. The overwhelming majority (95%) have abdominal pain for a median of 24 hours prior to presentation.[12] The remaining few present in extremis with acidosis and shock. Nausea and diarrhea are the next most common symptoms and are present in 30–40% of patients. Blood per rectum is rare and occurs in about 15% of patients.[12]

There is no specific laboratory abnormality that is 100% specific for AMI. Leukocytosis, lactic acidosis, seromuscular enzyme levels, and phosphate abnormalities are the most common findings but are noted late in the course of the acute episode.[25]

Acute mesenteric ischemia occurs more often in women than in men. The mean age of patients is 67 years but AMI may be seen over a wide age range. Mesenteric artery thrombosis occurs in 64% of patients, embolism in 28%, and non-occlusive mesenteric ischemia in the remaining 8%. Atherosclerosis in other vascular beds is common, regardless of etiology. Patients with embolic occlusion of the SMA are older than those with thrombosis and have atrial fibrillation or ventricular arrhythmias more often. Patients with SMA thrombosis are more often female and over one-half have a history of chronic abdominal pain and weight loss consistent with CMI.[12]

Diagnosis

The key to diagnosis is a high index of clinical suspicion.[11,12,25] Diagnosis is confirmed by arteriography.[11] In some cases, because of the lack of a specific pattern to the pain, computed tomographic (CT) imaging is obtained. Whether the study is performed with standard cross-sectional or angiographic imaging, diagnosis can be made on the basis of this study alone.[12,26,27] In our experience, approximately 60% of patients with AMI have CT scan abnormalities, including bowel dilatation, wall thickening, pneumatosis intestinalis, and filling defects in the proximal SMA.[12]

Arteriography of an embolic occlusion shows a cutoff or meniscus sign several centimeters beyond the origin of the SMA. The middle colic artery is often spared and delayed images will show refilling of the distal SMA branches. Patients with in-situ thrombosis of the SMA usually have non-visualization of this artery. The other major mesenteric arteries may be stenotic and intestinal collaterals may be well-developed (e.g. meandering mesenteric artery) in patients with chronic symptoms. The SMA trunk beyond the occlusion is usually seen on delayed views but there is a paucity of contrast in the distal arcades.[11,28]

Treatment

Acute mesenteric ischemia is a surgical emergency. Patients with abdominal pain or other risk factors suggestive of AMI should undergo arteriography prior to operation if there is no evidence of peritonitis or shock. Patients with rebound tenderness, abdominal rigidity, severe acidosis, or shock should undergo immediate operation.[11,12] Operation should not be delayed in these latter circumstances.

Since the mortality rate for patients treated operatively for AMI is high,[1–12] selected patients may be candidates for other therapies. Thrombolysis followed by balloon angioplasty or stent placement of the stenotic artery at the time of arteriography is a reasonable option if diagnosis is made early, the patient is hemodynamically stable, there are no signs of peritonitis, and the thrombus burden is small.[11,12,29–31] Failure of thrombolytic therapy or a worsening clinical status warrants operation.[11] If therapy is successful, we still favor laparotomy, since the extent and degree of intestinal ischemia cannot be accurately predicted by physical examination, laboratory studies, or diagnostic tests. Only eight patients with AMI were treated with endovascular techniques at the Mayo Clinic in 1999.[12] Six had transcatheter vasodilator therapy for non-occlusive mesenteric ischemia. Of the two who had balloon angioplasty or catheter-directed thrombolysis, one required laparotomy. Whether percutaneous techniques will lower the mortality and morbidity is yet to be determined.[11,12]

Operative treatment of AMI is dictated by the appearance of the intestine and the status of blood flow within the SMA. The goals of therapy include restoration of SMA blood flow and resection of non-viable bowel.[11] Importantly, the severity of ischemia to the bowel may be masked by its appearance. The bowel may be dull gray in color, lack peristalsis, or have patchy areas of cyanosis.[11] There is no palpable SMA pulse at the base of the mesentery in patients with SMA thrombosis. A patient with an embolus may have a water-hammer pulse in the proximal artery but an absent pulse distally. Foul-smelling fluid or perforation is seen in advanced cases of ischemia. Extensive microemboli will produce multiple patchy areas of ischemia throughout the entire small and large intestine and infarcts of the solid organs.[11]

Methods to restore blood flow to the SMA are dependent on operative findings and the preoperative arteriogram, if one was obtained. The SMA is isolated at the base of the mesentery, with the transverse colon retracted superiorly and the small intestine retracted toward the right side except for the distal duodenum/proximal jejunum.[11] If the artery is soft, it is opened transversely. Fogarty catheters (number 2, 3, or 4) are passed proximally and distally in the artery to extract the embolic material and thrombus (**Figs 22.1 & 22.2**). Passage of the Fogarty catheter into the main divisions of the artery must be performed with care to avoid perforation of these segments. The artery should be opened longitudinally if clinical findings or the arteriogram suggests in-situ thrombosis or if there is palpable atherosclerotic disease in the SMA.[11] Longitudinal arteriotomies can be closed with a patch of saphenous vein, bovine pericardium, or synthetic material if excellent inflow is achieved. Transverse arteriotomies are closed primarily.

A bypass to the artery is required if there is poor inflow. The bypass may be performed retrograde from the infrarenal aorta or iliac artery, or antegrade from the supraceliac aorta.[11,12] The

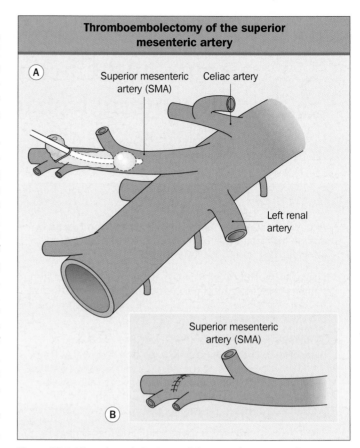

Figure 22.1 Thromboembolectomy of the superior mesenteric artery. Performed through a transverse incision (A). The incision is closed primarily (B).

group from Portland, Oregon, has championed the use of a retrograde graft from the distal infrarenal aorta or proximal common iliac artery which is then looped in a C-fashion so that the distal anastomosis of the graft is in an antegrade position vis-à-vis the SMA.[11,32] This graft may minimize the chance of kinking or buckling, which is a problem with retrograde grafts performed in other orientations.[11,32] A bifurcated graft from the supraceliac aorta is used to reconstruct both the celiac artery and the SMA in stable patients with clear occlusive disease of both arteries.[12] However, celiac reconstruction should follow that of the SMA in this circumstance. We have preferred the use of prosthetics but have used saphenous vein in patients with gross contamination of the peritoneal cavity. Thromboendarterectomy of the celiac artery and SMA is rarely performed in the acute setting because the exposure is time-consuming and the technique is demanding.[33]

Once blood flow is restored, an assessment of bowel viability is necessary. Clinical examination is helpful but less reliable than other techniques. The presence of pulses in the distal mesenteric arcades, return of peristalsis and normal color to the bowel, and audible Doppler flow on the mesenteric and antimesenteric borders of the intestine are encouraging signs.[11,34] Intravenous fluorescein with ultraviolet imaging is useful. Uniform perfusion under an ultraviolet lamp indicates viable bowel, whereas patchy or no perfusion indicates ischemic, non-viable bowel.[11,12,34,35] Our preference has been to perform a second-look procedure in all but the rarest of cases, as we have had some patients who remain

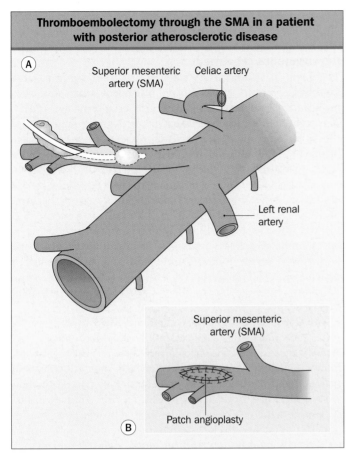

Thromboembolectomy through the SMA in a patient with posterior atherosclerotic disease

(A) Superior mesenteric artery (SMA) Celiac artery

Left renal artery

Superior mesenteric artery (SMA)

Patch angioplasty

(B)

Figure 22.2 Thromboembolectomy through the superior mesenteric artery in a patient with posterior atherosclerotic disease. The artery is opened longitudinally (A) and closed with either an autogenous or prosthetic patch (B).

hemodynamically stable despite progressive bowel ischemia. The decision to perform a second-look procedure is made at the first operation and is performed within the first 12–24 hours.[11,12]

A few patients with advanced cases of intestinal ischemia may remain hemodynamically unstable en route to the operating room, even with aggressive fluid resuscitation. Abdominal exploration often reveals large segments of severely ischemic or gangrenous bowel. If a decision is made to attempt revascularization, these patients benefit from clamping of the venous outflow of the gangrenous segments with bowel clamps prior to isolation of the SMA. This reduces the washout of toxins into the portal circulation and may improve hemodynamics as restoration of blood flow to the SMA proceeds.

Forty-three of 58 patients with AMI treated at the Mayo Clinic had revascularization of the SMA.[12] The others could not be revascularized because of the extent of gangrenous bowel. Bypass grafting was performed in 22 patients, thromboembolectomy in 19, endarterectomy in five, and reimplantation in two. Eleven had patch angioplasty of the SMA. Seventeen of 22 patients with SMA bypass had polyester grafts, of which 10 were bifurcated. The other five patients had vein grafts. Inflow was from the supraceliac aorta in 15 patients and from the infrarenal aorta in seven. Only 23 patients (40%) had second-look procedures but almost one-half of the patients had additional bowel resected.[12]

The mortality rate from AMI is high (24–96%) and has changed little over the years.[1–12] In the Mayo Clinic report, the 30-day mortality rate was highest for patients with non-occlusive AMI (80%) but was 31% and 32% for patients with SMA embolism or thrombosis, respectively.[12] Major complications can be expected in one-half to three-quarters of patients, with respiratory failure and multi-organ system failure being most common.[12] Factors associated with increased mortality rate include multi-system organ failure (67%), recurrent mesenteric thrombosis during the same hospitalization (50%), and age over 70 years (40%). Long-term survival was only 59% at 1 year and 32% at 2 years. Over one-third of patients died from recurrent mesenteric ischemia during late follow-up.[12]

CHRONIC MESENTERIC ISCHEMIA

In 1936, Dunphy correlated fatal intestinal infarction and obstruction of the intestinal arteries to clinical histories of chronic recurrent abdominal pain.[36] Of 12 patients who died of intestinal infarction, seven (58%) had a history of recurrent abdominal pain which preceded the fatal event by weeks, months, or years.

Atherosclerotic disease of the mesenteric arteries usually affects their origins. The prevalence of disease ranges from 6–10% in random autopsy studies to 14–24% of patients undergoing aortography.[23,25,37] Usually, at least two of the three intestinal arteries must be either occluded or tightly stenotic to cause symptoms because of the rich collateral network between the celiac, SMA, inferior mesenteric artery (IMA), and hypogastric arteries.[18,23] We have treated several patients, however, with SMA disease alone who had relief of symptoms after single-vessel reconstruction.[24] Importantly, these patients had poorly developed collaterals between their mesenteric arteries.

The natural history of asymptomatic patients found to have high-grade stenoses or occlusions of one or more visceral arteries is not well established. Data published by Thomas et al., from the University of Kansas, provide some insight.[37] They reviewed 980 aortograms between 1989–1995 and found 60 patients (6%) who had significant visceral artery disease. Fifteen of these had involvement of all three visceral vessels. Four of the 15 patients (27%) developed symptoms over a mean follow-up of 2.6 years and one died from intestinal infarction.[37] If others confirm the findings of Thomas and colleagues, asymptomatic patients with significant three-vessel involvement may require operative intervention, or at least very close follow-up.[23] Intestinal ischemia or infarction has occurred after aortic reconstructions in patients who had no visceral ischemic symptoms preoperatively but in whom there was documented visceral artery stenosis or occlusion.[23] Reconstruction of the SMA, reimplantation of the IMA, or hypogastric artery revascularization is necessary in such cases.[23]

Clinical presentation

The typical patient with CMI is between the ages of 40 and 70 years and is more often female. The classic symptoms include abdominal pain, weight loss, and 'food fear'.[23,24] Pain is often post-prandial and begins within 10–30 minutes of meals. It is usually mid-abdominal in location, crampy, and lasts from minutes to hours.[14,23,25] Recent data from the Mayo Clinic documented abdominal pain in 97% and weight loss in 94% of 98 patients operated.[24] Mean duration of symptoms prior to operation was 15 months, but ranged from 1 month to 5 years.

At times, the clinical presentation is less specific. Vague mid-abdominal or epigastric pain, nausea, vomiting, or a change in bowel habits may be present without a classic postprandial component to the pain.[24] Additionally, almost 10% of our patients had diffuse small ulceration in the stomach or proximal duodenum, liver function abnormalities, or scattered patchy areas of ischemia in the colon as the initial presenting features.

The most common associated findings include a history of smoking or hypertension.[18,23,24] Two-thirds of patients will have had symptomatic disease in other vascular beds, including the coronary, cerebrovascular, renal, or peripheral circulations.[23,24] Physical examination findings include a reduction in peripheral pulses or bruits. An abdominal bruit is present in approximately 50% of patients.[24] Muscle wasting or inanition are seen in severe cases.[23]

Diagnosis

Diagnosis of CMI is suggested by the clinical history and examination and confirmed by a variety of studies including duplex ultrasonography, magnetic resonance angiography (MRA), CT angiography, or bi-plane aortography.[25] Tests of intestinal absorptive and excretory function have not been useful.[15,25]

Duplex ultrasonography has been used to screen patients with abdominal pain or an epigastric bruit. The group at the Oregon Health Sciences University have used peak systolic velocity (PSV) in the SMA of >275cm/s and in the celiac artery exceeding 200cm/s to indicate stenoses of 70% or more.[25,38] While these velocities were initially derived from a retrospective comparative analysis of duplex scan and aortography, they were later confirmed in a blinded prospective study of 100 patients. A PSV >275cm/s, as an indicator of ≥ 70% SMA stenosis, had a sensitivity of 92%, specificity of 96%, positive predictive value of 80%, and a negative predictive value of 99%. A PSV of 200cm/s in the celiac artery as a predictor of a ≥ 70% stenosis had somewhat lower values.[25,38] End-diastolic flow velocities of 45cm/s or higher in the SMA and reversal of blood flow in the hepatic and splenic arteries also indicate significant lesions in these vessels.[39,40] Preprandial versus postprandial blood flow velocities are not specific enough to distinguish physiologically appropriate from inappropriate blood flow responses.[25]

MRA and CT angiography are used to study patients with visceral or renal artery stenoses. Even though the software has improved, we still prefer bi-plane aortography as the preoperative imaging test of choice. Bi-plane views of the aorta define the location, severity, and extent of visceral artery involvement, identify the presence of concomitant lesions in the renal or iliac arteries, and indicate the suitability of the supraceliac or infra-renal aorta as inflow sites.[23,33] While extensive intestinal collaterals may be evident on arteriography, the presence or absence of a collateral network cannot be used as the only means of determining hemodynamic significance of visceral artery lesions.[25] Arteriography in 98 patients operated at the Mayo Clinic for CMI over the last 10 years showed occlusion or critical stenosis (70–99%) of the SMA in 92%, the celiac artery in 83%, and of both arteries in 78%.[24]

Other, more common conditions such as pancreatic cancer may have similar clinical presentations. Therefore, preoperative

tests such as CT, upper and lower gastrointestinal endoscopy, or ultrasonography are necessary.[23–25]

Percutaneous treatment

Treatment of visceral artery stenoses and short segment occlusions by balloon angioplasty or stent placement is attractive, since many of the patients with CMI are older and malnourished.[23] Recurrent stenosis has been the bane of this technique because the atherosclerotic lesions are an extension of intra-aortic plaque.[21,41–43] Tegtmeyer and Selby have summarized clinical series to address the issue of recurrent stenosis with balloon angioplasty.[43] The majority of patients reviewed had non-orificial lesions. Initial technical success and relief of symptoms occurred in 80%. Thirty-five patients were followed for a mean of 28 months. Eight patients (29%) required repeat angioplasty or operation for recurrent symptoms. The rate of recurrent stenosis increased at longer follow-up intervals. Less than one-half of patients who had initial success and were followed for at least 12 months had a durable result.[23,43] Others have reported similar experiences.[23,42]

The use of an endovascular stent may help to improve the recurrence rate, similar to patients treated for orificial renal artery stenoses. A recent review, from the Cleveland Clinic, still found a higher symptomatic recurrence rate at 3 years in patients who had angioplasty and stenting compared to those who underwent open conventional repair.[21] These authors suggested that low-risk patients be treated by operation because of better durability and long-term symptom relief. Endovascular treatment should be reserved for older, high-risk patients.[21,24] The role of angioplasty or stenting as a 'diagnostic' maneuver for patients with vague symptoms and moderate visceral artery stenoses of only one or two arteries is yet to be defined.

Surgical treatment

Open surgical repair for patients with symptomatic CMI is offered to low-risk patients, especially those age 70 years or younger.[13–24] A number of operative techniques can be used to perform either single or multiple vessel reconstructions in an antegrade or retrograde fashion. Each technique has its own advantages and disadvantages. There is controversy regarding the number of visceral vessels reconstructed, which artery is the most important to revascularize, and the configuration of the graft.[23,24,33]

Bypass grafting

Reconstruction of the celiac artery and the SMA with a bifurcated prosthetic graft originating from the supraceliac aorta is performed in over 80% of our patients.[24] The others have had either single-vessel reconstruction to the SMA or all three mesenteric arteries reconstructed by endarterectomy.[18,24]

The operation is performed through an upper midline or bilateral subcostal incision. The lesser omentum is opened and the left lobe of the liver is retracted after division of the left triangular ligament. The esophagus is retracted toward the patient's left side with a nasogastric tube in place, and the stomach is gently retracted caudally. The diaphragmatic crura are divided and the supraceliac aorta is dissected free to allow performance of the proximal graft anastomosis. Usually, only the celiac trunk and proximal hepatic and splenic arteries need isolation, but with more extensive disease, the common hepatic artery may require dissection toward the origin of the gastro-duodenal artery. The left gastric artery is often quite small and can be divided without sequelae. This generally allows a better configuration of the celiac graft limb and makes tunneling of the SMA graft behind the pancreas easier.[33]

The SMA may be exposed above or below the pancreas, depending on the extent of disease and the patient's anatomy. As much as 3–4cm of the SMA may be dissected free by mobilization of the superior border of the pancreas. Otherwise, the artery is isolated at the base of the mesentery beyond the ligament of Treitz, in a similar way to exposure discussed for patients with AMI.[33]

Patients are given heparin and mannitol, and in some cases also receive dopamine or furosemide. We prefer the use of two cross-clamps on the aorta rather than a partial occlusion clamp, as we feel it affords better exposure for the proximal aortic-graft anastomosis. A straight or angled aortic clamp (Cherry supraceliac clamp®) and a Wylie hypogastric clamp® work well. Placed appropriately, occlusion of the lumbar vessels is achieved as well. A vertical or slightly oblique aortotomy is made. A 12mm × 7mm knitted polyester graft is sewn end-to-side to the aorta with permanent suture. Aortic cross-clamp time rarely exceeds 20 minutes and most often ranges from 12–15 minutes. The risk of renal ischemia or distal microembolization is low when patients are properly selected and have a relatively disease-free supraceliac aorta.[33]

The celiac artery anastomosis is performed end-to-end, most often with a tongue of graft extending onto one of the two major branch arteries, usually the hepatic. The anastomosis to the SMA is done in an end-to-end fashion when performed above the pancreas but in an end-to-side fashion when the anastomosis is performed at the base of the mesentery (**Fig. 22.3**).[33] In the latter case, it is important to relax retraction on the mesentery when cutting the graft to length, to avoid graft angulation or kinking. This same relaxation is necessary for estimating graft length with retrograde bypass.

Supraceliac-origin grafts are a poor choice in patients with compromised cardiac or pulmonary function or those with extensive atherosclerosis or circumferential calcification of the supraceliac aorta. In these cases, infrarenal sources of inflow are preferred.[23,33]

The infrarenal aorta is an excellent inflow source and has been preferred by the group from the Oregon Heath Sciences University.[23,32] The infrarenal aorta may be replaced, if diseased, by a prosthetic graft followed by retrograde reconstruction of the SMA.[23,33] In general, we reconstruct only one artery if a retrograde graft is used. The proximal anastomosis is performed to the anterolateral wall of the aorta and can be done with either two cross-clamps or partial occlusion clamps, depending on the aortic size and the presence of atherosclerosis or calcification within that segment.[33] The Oregon group prefers the anastomosis at the distal infrarenal aorta or the infrarenal aorta–right common iliac artery junction.[23,32] The key to performance of the distal anastomosis is fashioning the graft in such a way that the SMA assumes a nearly anatomic position. This reduces the chances of graft elongation, angulation, or kinking. If a short retrograde graft is performed, the distal anastomosis is often carried out first, followed by the aortic graft anastomosis (**Fig. 22.4**). The Portland group has favored a C-shaped graft, fashioned in such a way that the distal anastomosis to the SMA

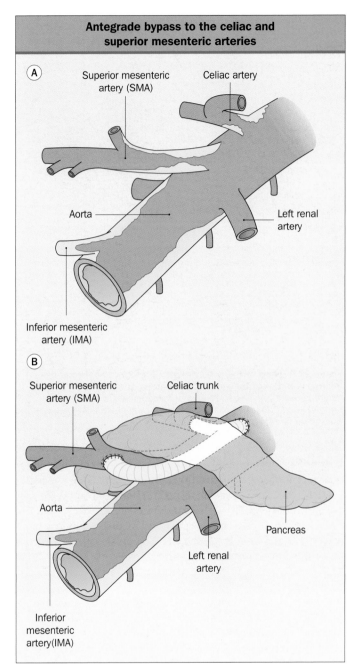

Figure 22.3 Antegrade bypass to the celiac and superior mesenteric arteries. Illustration of a patient with chronic mesenteric ischemia and high-grade stenoses of the celiac and superior mesenteric arteries (A). The patient was reconstructed with a bifurcated synthetic graft taken from the supraceliac aorta. The celiac anastomosis is performed end-to-end and the SMA anastomosis is performed end-to-side. The latter graft limb is tunneled behind the pancreas.

allows for antegrade blood flow from the graft.[23,32] Although we have no experience with this technique, the Portland group has had excellent results and few graft failures.

In our most recent retrospective review, retrograde grafts have worked as well as antegrade grafts, although the former patients were older and had reduced life spans.[24,33] There is a subset of patients with extensive circumferential calcification of the entire abdominal aorta but in whom the common iliac arteries are soft and good donor vessels. Either the right or left

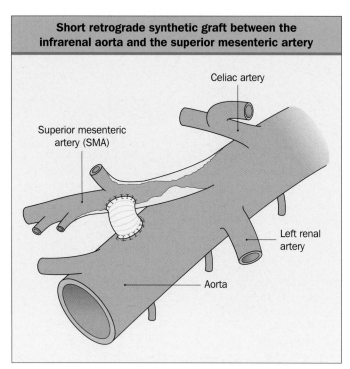

Short retrograde synthetic graft between the infrarenal aorta and the superior mesenteric artery

Celiac artery

Superior mesenteric artery (SMA)

Left renal artery

Aorta

Figure 22.4 Short retrograde synthetic graft placed between the infrarenal aorta and the superior mesenteric artery (SMA). The graft length is usually 1–1.5cm. The distal anastomosis to the SMA is performed first, followed by the aortic anastomosis to allow return of the SMA to its normal anatomic position.

common iliac artery can be chosen for inflow, depending on the orientation of that artery to the more normal anatomic position of the SMA.[33] Two-vessel reconstructions can be performed with retrograde grafts by doing a side-to-side anastomosis to the SMA and an end-to-side anastomosis to the common hepatic artery. The graft may be passed on top of or beneath the pancreas and curved in a C-fashion towards the hepatic artery.

Endarterectomy

Transaortic endarterectomy of the mesenteric arteries may be preferred to other techniques of revascularization when there is bacterial contamination or perforated bowel, previous abdominal irradiation changes, extensive abdominal wall hernias, or other hostile conditions.[33] Our preference is to approach the paravisceral aorta through full-length midline abdominal or subcostal incisions. These incisions carry lower pulmonary morbidity than a thoraco-abdominal approach in these nutritionally depleted patients.

Nonetheless, thoracoabdominal incision may be useful for patients whose body habitus makes a purely abdominal approach difficult.[16,33,44] Those with narrow costal margin flares, rib cages that lie close to the iliac crest, or those who are truly obese may benefit from this exposure. An abdominal incision alone in such patients is suboptimal. Access to the origins of the visceral arteries is restricted, there is poor orientation from which to perform the endarterectomy, and it is difficult to adequately retract the costal margins.[33]

A medial visceral rotation is performed but the left kidney is left in its bed.[33,44] Dissection of the SMA can be carried out over several centimeters. A longitudinal or trap door aortotomy is performed after the patient has been given heparin and diuretics, and supraceliac and infrarenal aortic clamps have been placed.

An endarterectomy of the paravisceral aorta, including the celiac artery and SMA, is effected. The endarterectomy ends at the renal artery orifices. In rare patients in whom there are symptomatic renal artery stenoses, the aortotomy can be extended into the infrarenal aorta and the specimen can include the renal arteries as well. The distal endpoint may require tacking sutures to avoid aortic dissection. The aortotomy is closed longitudinally and rarely requires a patch (**Fig. 22.5**). Endarterectomy of the celiac artery usually has an endpoint at its bifurcation, whereas SMA disease may extend beyond the limits that ostial endarterectomy allows. In this case, the aortotomy is closed, flow restored to the distal aorta and celiac artery, and a completion endarterectomy of the SMA is effected.[33] The SMA may be opened transversely or longitudinally, depending on the extent of residual distal disease. If a longitudinal incision is made, it is closed with a prosthetic or vein patch.[33]

We now routinely use intraoperative duplex scan to assess the technical outcomes of the reconstruction. A widely patent visceral artery reconstruction imaged by duplex scan has reduced the number of early postoperative graft failures at our institution.

Postoperative management

Patients are monitored in an intensive care unit for 1–3 days. Patients with severe ischemia preoperatively or a prolonged intraoperative course often have major fluid shifts during this interval. Maintaining a core temperature >35°C is critical to minimizing massive third-space fluid accumulation and cardiac arrhythmias. Patients may 'third-space' fluid because of loss of autoregulation of the arterioles, so it is common for patients to require fluid boluses over the first 48 hours. However, persistent hypotension, tachycardia, leukocytosis, reduction in urine output with elevated bladder pressures, or an increase in abdominal pain may suggest a graft occlusion, ischemic intestine, or an abdominal compartment syndrome.[23,45] Arteriography and/or abdominal re-exploration is needed to exclude graft occlusion or intestinal infarction.

Return of oral intake varies by individual but may be prolonged. Thus, total parenteral nutrition may be required. The 'food fear' which many patients experience preoperatively does not resolve quickly after operation, as it is often a 'learned behavior'[23] Finally, the absorptive capacity of the gut changes and patients often experience diarrhea over the first few postoperative weeks. Medications which slow bowel motility or help to thicken the stools are often necessary.

Outcomes

The mortality rate for patients undergoing reconstruction for CMI has improved over the years. In a recent report from the Mayo Clinic, three patients died within 30 days of operation, giving a mortality rate of 3.1% and an overall in-hospital mortality rate of 5.1%. Cardiac ischemia accounted for 60% of these deaths and all patients who died were older than 70 years.[24] The reduction in mortality is likely to be due to patient selection, choice of reconstruction, improved anesthesia techniques and critical care, and a focus on reconstruction of the mesenteric disease alone and avoidance of extensive non-essential aortic reconstructions.[23,24,33] In contrast to our earlier experience, where concomitant aortic or renal revascularization was associated with a 19% mortality,[18] current results suggest that concomitant aortic procedures do not increase morbidity and mortality, provided

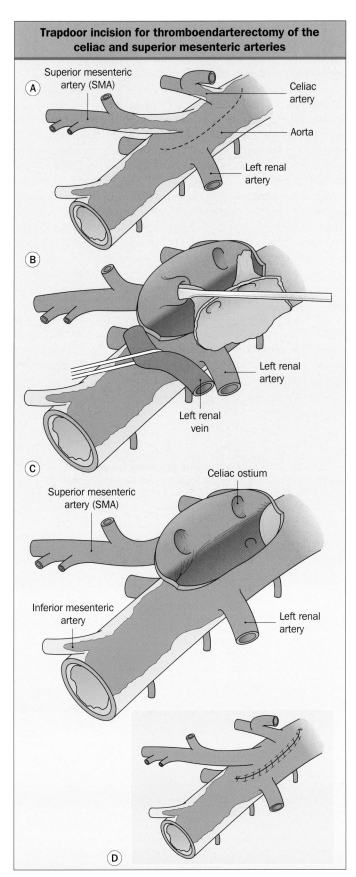

Trapdoor incision for thromboendarterectomy of the celiac and superior mesenteric arteries

(A) Superior mesenteric artery (SMA); Celiac artery; Aorta; Left renal artery

(B) Left renal artery; Left renal vein

(C) Superior mesenteric artery (SMA); Celiac ostium; Inferior mesenteric artery; Left renal artery

(D)

Figure 22.5 **Trapdoor incision for thromboendarterectomy of the celiac and superior mesenteric arteries carried out after medial visceral rotation.** The aortotomy can be made longitudinally or in a trap-door fashion (A). The endarterectomy is performed using an eversion technique (B). Distal tacking sutures are placed (C). The aortotomy is closed primarily (D).

that they are confined to the infrarenal aorta and are performed to provide a source of inflow.[24] The most common early postoperative complications at our institution have been respiratory insufficiency requiring tracheostomy and cardiac problems, primarily myocardial infarction. Renal failure has occurred in only one patient over the past 10 years.[24]

Successful long-term outcome is based on graft patency, relief of symptoms, and long-term survival. Assurance of graft patency begins in the operating room. We employ two methods to assess the graft. The first is electromagnetic flow measurements. Blood flows of ≥ 600ml/min have been a predictor of long-term patency in our experience.[24,33] Most grafts will have blood flow measurements ranging between 500–1000ml/min.[23] It is important that blood flow measurements be made with no retraction on the viscera or the grafts. Secondly, intraoperative duplex scan has been excellent in assessing technical defects either at the graft-arterial anastomoses or within the graft itself.[24,33] Excellent early and long-term patency has been documented with either bifurcated or single-limb reconstruction, or grafts placed in an antegrade or retrograde position.[23,24,32]

We currently reimage the mesenteric grafts between 6–12 months postoperatively and then on an annual basis, unless symptoms warrant. This practice was begun in recent years. In our most recent review, restenosis of the celiac or SMA graft limb occurred in 11 of 93 survivors.[24] Three had restenosis or occlusion of both graft limbs and all underwent revision. Five patients had stenosis of the celiac limb. All of these had bifurcated grafts and none needed reintervention. Three other patients developed stenosis of the SMA graft. One of these patients had a single graft to the SMA with moderate stenosis but was asymptomatic. The other two had bifurcated grafts and one patient underwent revision for symptoms. Reintervention was reserved for symptomatic patients. Such patients typically had stenosis or occlusion of both limbs of a bifurcated graft or of a single graft to the SMA.[24]

Six patients developed recurrent symptoms during follow-up.[24] All had abdominal pain and two developed weight loss. Four of these patients had stenosis or occlusion of an SMA graft, and the other two had patent grafts and normal findings on endoscopic and radiologic evaluation of the gastrointestinal tract. The latter two were treated expectantly and one patient later developed Crohn's disease. Two patients with graft stenosis underwent percutaneous angioplasty with symptom relief. The two with occluded SMA graft limbs were reoperated. One had thrombectomy and patch angioplasty of the graft and the other underwent a redo two-vessel reconstruction after an initial attempt at angioplasty failed. Both patients had relief of symptoms. Late pain relief was documented in 74 of 80 patients queried (93%) and weight gain was noted in 61 of 71 patients (86%) who had documented reference to weight change in the analysis. Symptom recurrent-free survival in the Mayo Clinic study was 98% at 90 days, 95% at 1 year, and 92% at 5 years.[24]

The most common cause of late death was cardiac. Two patients died of bowel infarction. Survival was 83% at 1 year, 62% at 5 years, and 55% at 8 years, all significantly worse than an age- and sex-matched, control population. Survival was unaffected by the number of vessels bypassed or by graft orientation, even though patients with retrograde grafts were older (mean age 75 years) than those with antegrade grafts (mean age 65 years).[24]

SUMMARY

Management of patients with AMI and CMI remains challenging. The mortality rate for patients with AMI remains high because there has been little improvement in the ability to diagnose and treat these patients in an early phase of the ischemic process. A high index of clinical suspicion is important to make an early diagnosis and to initiate therapy before bowel ischemia reaches an advanced stage. Operative treatment is dictated based on the etiology of the problem and the intraoperative findings. Generally, if a bypass is needed, single limb reconstructions are performed to the SMA with the orientation of the graft dictated by the patient's clinical condition and the extent of aortic disease. The use of thrombolytic therapy and balloon angioplasty or stent placement of offending lesions is intriguing, but additional clinical data will be necessary to determine the role of these therapies.

Our management of patients with CMI has evolved over the years. The operation should focus on mesenteric artery revascularization as the primary goal and should avoid extensive aortic or renal artery reconstruction in all but the fewest of cases. This approach has clearly lowered our mortality rate. However, infrarenal aortic replacement, if needed for inflow, can be safely carried out. Certainly, patient selection, preoperative cardiac evaluation and treatment, and improvement in anesthesia and intensive care monitoring have all contributed to a lower mortality rate as well. Older, high-risk patients may be best served by interventional techniques, although data to support this approach are few. If operative repair is necessary in this group, single-vessel reconstruction to the SMA may be preferable.

We believe that it is no longer necessary to revascularize all three mesenteric arteries.[24] However, we continue to favor antegrade two-vessel reconstruction to the superior mesenteric and the celiac arteries in selected patients because of the excellent durability and symptom-free survival. Since mesenteric disease involves multiple arteries, there may be some margin of safety in a two-vessel reconstruction if one limb occludes or becomes stenotic during follow-up.[24] Reconstruction of the SMA alone is certainly preferable for patients who present with acute-on-chronic mesenteric ischemia and for older, high-risk patients.[23] Retrograde versus antegrade reconstruction is not as important as careful patient selection and attention to detail during the operation to avoid technical pitfalls.

Since CMI is rare, it is unlikely that controlled clinical trials will be able to determine the importance of any one single variable in treatment.[33] Choice of operation should be dictated based on age, co-morbid conditions, and a detailed assessment of the aortic and visceral artery anatomy.

REFERENCES

1. Ottinger LW. The surgical management of acute occlusion of the superior mesenteric artery. Ann Surg 1978;188:721–31.
2. Wilson C, Gupta R, Gilmour DG, et al. Acute superior mesenteric ischemia. Br J Surg 1987;74:279–81.
3. Boley SJ, Feinstein FR, Sammartano R, et al. New concepts in the management of emboli of the superior mesenteric artery. Surg Gynecol Obstet 1981;153:561–9.
4. Hertzer NR, Beven EG, Humphries AW. Acute intestinal ischemia. Am Surg 1978;44:744–9.
5. Batellier J, Kieny R. Superior mesenteric artery embolism: eighty-two cases. Ann Vasc Surg 1990;4:112–6.
6. Lazaro T, Sierra L, Gesto R, et al. Embolization of the mesenteric arteries: surgical treatment in twenty-three consecutive cases. Ann Vasc Surg 1986;1:311–5.
7. Smith S, Patterson LT. Acute mesenteric infarction. Am J Surg 1976; 42:562–7.
8. Stoney RJ, Cunningham CG. Acute mesenteric ischemia. Surgery 1993; 114:489–90.
9. Konturek A, Cichon S, Gucwa J, et al. Acute intestinal ischemia in material of the III Clinic of General Surgery Collegium Medicum at the Jagellonian University. Przegl Lek 1996;53:719–21.
10. Mamode N, Pickford I, Leiberman P. Failure to improve outcome in acute mesenteric ischemia: seven year review. Eur J Surg 1999; 165:203–8.
11. Taylor LM, Moneta GL, Porter JM. Treatment of acute intestinal ischemia caused by arterial occlusions. In: Rutherford RB, ed: Vascular surgery, 5th edn. Philadelphia, PA:WB. Saunders; 2000:1512–8.
12. Park WM, Gloviczki P, Cherry KJ, et al. Contemporary management of acute mesenteric ischemia: factors associated with survival. J Vasc Surg 2002:35:445–52.
13. Zelenock GB, Graham LM, Whitehouse WM, et al. Splanchnic arteriosclerotic disease and intestinal angina. Arch Surg 1980;115:497–501.
14. Olofsson PA, Connelly DP, Stoney RJ. Surgery of the celiac and mesenteric arteries. In: Haimovici H, ed: Vascular surgery: principles and techniques. Norwalk, Connecticut:Appleton Lange; 1989:750–62.
15. Marston A. Chronic intestinal ischemia. In: Marston A, ed. Vascular disease of the gastrointestinal tract: pathophysiology, recognition and management. Baltimore, MD:Williams and Wilkens; 1986:116–42.
16. Cunningham CG, Reilly LM, Rapp JH, et al. Chronic visceral ischemia. Ann Surg 1991;214:276–88.
17. Rapp JH, Reilly LM, Qvarfordt PG, et al. Durability of endarterectomy and antegrade grafts in the treatment of chronic visceral ischemia. J Vasc Surg 1986;3:799–806.
18. McAfee MK, Cherry KJ, Naessens JM, et al. Influence of complete revascularization on chronic mesenteric ischemia. Am J Surg 1992; 164:220–4.
19. Moawad J, McKinsey JF, Wyble CW, et al. Current results of surgical therapy for chronic mesenteric ischemia. Arch Surg 1997;132:613–9.
20. Matero RB, O'Hara PJ, Hertzer NR, et al. Elective surgical treatment of symptomatic chronic mesenteric occlusive disease: early results and late outcomes. J Vasc Surg 1999;29:821–32.
21. Kasirajan K, O'Hara PJ, Gray BH, et al. Chronic mesenteric ischemia: open surgery versus percutaneous angioplasty and stenting. J Vasc Surg 2001;33:63–7.
22. Cho JS, Carr JA, Jacobsen G, et al. Long-term outcome following mesenteric artery reconstruction: a 37-year experience. J Vasc Surg 2002;35:453–60.
23. Taylor LM, Moenta GL, Porter JM. Treatment of chronic visceral ischemia. In: Rutherford RB, ed. Vascular surgery, 5th edn. Philadelphia, PA:WB Saunders; 2000:1532–41.
24. Park WM, Cherry KJ, Chua HK, et al. Current results of open revascularization for chronic mesenteric ischemia: a standard for comparison. J Vasc Surg 2002;35:853–9.
25. Moneta GL. Diagnosis of intestinal ischemia. In: Rutherford RB, ed. Vascular surgery, 5th edn. Philadelphia, PA:WB Saunders; 2000:1501–10.
26. Czerny M, Trubel W, Claeys L, et al. Acute mesenteric ischemia. Zentralbl Chir 1997;122:538–44.
27. Fock CM, Kullnig P, Ranner G, et al. Mesenteric arterial embolism: the value of emergency CT in diagnostic procedure. Eur J Radiol 1994; 18:12–4.
28. Clark RA, Gallant TE. Acute mesenteric ischemia: angiographic spectrum. Am J Roentgenol 1984;142:555–62.

29. Gallego AM, Ramirez P, Rodriquez JM, et al. Role of urokinase in the superior mesenteric artery embolism. Surgery 1996;120:111–3.

30. van Deinse WH, Zawacju JK, Phillips D. Treatment of acute mesenteric ischemia by percutaneous transluminal angioplasty. Gastroenterology 1986;91:475–8.

31. McBride KD, Gaines PA. Thrombolysis of a partially occluded superior mesenteric artery thromboembolus by streptokinase. Cardiovasc Intervent Radiol 1994;17:164–6.

32. Foley MI, Moneta GL, Abou-Zamzam AM, et al. Revascularization of the superior mesenteric artery alone for treatment of intestinal ischemia. J Vasc Surg 2000;32:37–47.

33. Cherry KJ. Visceral revascularization for chronic visceral ischemia: transabdominal approach. In: Geroulakos G, Cherry KJ, eds. Disease of the visceral circulation. New York, NY:Arnold Publishing; 2002:94–100.

34. Ballard JL, Stone WM, Hallett JW, et al. A critical analysis of adjuvant techniques used to assess bowel viability in acute mesenteric ischemia. Am Surg 1993;59:309–11.

35. Bergman RT, Gloviczki P, Welch TJ, et al. The role of intravenous fluorescein in the detection of colon ischemia during aortic reconstruction. Ann Vasc Surg 1992;6:74–9.

36. Dunphy JE. Abdominal pain of vascular origin. Am J Med Sci 1936;192:109.

37. Thomas JH, Blake K, Pierce GE, et al. The clinical course of asymptomatic mesenteric arterial stenosis. J Vasc Surg 1998;27:840–4.

38. Moneta GL, Lee RW, Yeager RA, et al. Mesenteric duplex scanning: a blinded prospective study. J Vasc Surg 1993;17:79.

39. Bowersox JC, Zwolak RM, Walsh DB, et al. Duplex ultrasonography in the diagnosis of celiac and mesenteric artery occlusive disease. J Vasc Surg 1991;14:780.

40. LaBonbard FE, Musson A, Bowersox JC, et al. Hepatic artery duplex as an adjunct in the evaluation of chronic mesenteric ischemia. J Vasc Tech 1992;16:7.

41. Matsumoto AH, Tegtmeyer CJ, Fitzcharles EK, et al. Percutaneous transluminal angioplasty of visceral arterial stenoses: results and long-term clinical follow-up. J Vasc Interv Radiol 1995;6:165–74.

42. Allen RC, Martin GH, Rees RC, et al. Mesenteric angioplasty in the treatment of chronic mesenteric ischemia. J Vasc Surg 1996;24:415–23.

43. Tegtmeyer CJ, Selby JB. Balloon angioplasty of the visceral arteries (renal and mesenteric circulation): indications, results and complications. In: Moore WS, Ahn SS, eds. Endovascular surgery. Philadelphia, PA:WB Saunders; 1989:223–57.

44. Reilly LM, Ramos TK, Murray SP, et al. Optimal exposure of the proximal abdominal aorta. A critical appraisal of transabdominal medial visceral rotation. J Vasc Surg 1994;19:375–90.

45. Gewertz BL, Zarins CK. Postoperative vasospasm after antegrade mesenteric revascularization: a report of three cases. J Vasc Surg 1991;14:382–5.

CHAPTER
23

Mesenteric Venous Thrombosis

Rainier V Aquino and Robert Y Rhee

KEY POINTS

- Mesenteric venous thrombosis (MVT) is an uncommon but potentially lethal form of mesenteric ischemia secondary to thrombosis of the porto-mesenteric venous system.

- Signs and symptoms of MVT are typically non-specific.

- A high index of suspicion is necessary, particularly in those patients with a prior history of coagulation abnormalities.

- The diagnostic test of choice is computed tomographic scanning. Early diagnosis is crucial for patient survival.

- Confirmation of MVT warrants immediate anticoagulation therapy.

- Peritonitis on presentation mandates immediate surgical exploration to rule out ischemic bowel.

- Second-look laparotomy should be performed liberally.

- If there are no contraindications, anticoagulation therapy should be continued indefinitely after the acute episode.

INTRODUCTION

Mesenteric venous thrombosis (MVT) is an uncommon form of mesenteric ischemia. It was first described by Elliot[1] in 1895 as intestinal gangrene resulting from 'thrombosis of the porto-mesenteric venous system'. This disorder is potentially lethal, with associated mortality rates of 15–40%.[2–5] Warren and Eberhard's historic report[6] in 1935 characterized MVT as a distinct clinical entity and emphasized its lethality, reporting a mortality rate of 34% following intestinal resection for thrombosed veins in the mesentery of the bowel. MVT comprises only 2–15% of all acute mesenteric ischemic cases reported in the literature.[7,8] Autopsy analysis reported 0.2–2% of the population having MVT.[6,8] However, its true incidence is not known since MVT may not be suspected on presentation. Abdu et al.[2] reported 372 total cases in the literature, identified from 1911 to 1984. The Mayo Clinic series[9] identified 72 cases from 1972 to 1993, comprising 6.2% of 1167 patients treated for mesenteric ischemic disorders during that time period. In a study by Ottinger and Austen,[8] MVT comprised only 0.006% of hospital admissions and less than 2% of autopsy cases. Intestinal infarction associated with MVT is estimated to be less than 1 in 1000 laparotomies for the acute abdomen.[10] Most recently, Morasch et al.[11] reported 31 cases of MVT over a 14-year period.

ANATOMY AND PATHOLOGY

The porto-mesenteric venous system comprises the portal, superior mesenteric, inferior mesenteric, and splenic veins (**Fig. 23.1**). The junction or confluence of the superior mesenteric and splenic veins forms the portal vein, posterior to the neck of the pancreas. The portal vein ascends superiorly and posterior to the first part of the duodenum at the level of the second lumbar vertebra. The portal vein is fairly large, 1–3cm in diameter, and varies from 5 to 8cm in length. It terminates into the left and right branches at the level of the porta hepatis. The portal vein typically passes behind the hepatic artery and the bile duct in the hepatoduodenal ligament. The inferior mesenteric vein arises from the splenic vein posterior to the mid body of the pancreas, prior to the junction of the superior mesenteric and splenic vein. For MVT, the typical distribution of thrombi in the porto-mesenteric venous system, based on findings from the Mayo series, is shown in **Figure 23.2**.

ETIOLOGY AND PATHOPHYSIOLOGY

Mesenteric venous thrombosis can be classified into primary and secondary. Primary MVT is defined as idiopathic, spontaneous thrombosis of the mesenteric veins not associated with any disease processes.[12] The incidence of primary MVT has decreased substantially over the past decade because of improvement in diagnosis and recognition of previously unknown circulating anticoagulants. An autopsy series reported by Johnson and Baggenstoss[13] identified 99 cases of MVT. There were only eight patients (12.4%) who did not have identifiable etiologic factors associated with MVT.

Secondary MVT, representing most of the reported cases in the literature, is associated with known conditions which predispose the mesenteric venous system to a thrombotic process (**Table 23.1**). Abdu et al.[2] found that 81% of cases of MVT were secondary or related to an underlying condition. Multiple hypercoagulable conditions are reported in the literature associated with secondary formation of mesenteric venous disease, the most common being polycythemia vera. Others report induced hypercoagulable conditions, most notably neoplastic diseases and heparin-induced thrombocytopenia (HIT).[11] Hassan[14] and Nesbitt & Deweese[15] have cited oral contraceptive use associated with MVT. Other hematologic disorders reported to be associated with MVT comprise protein C and S deficiency, antithrombin III deficiency, dysfibrinogenemia, abnormal plasminogen, thrombocytosis, sickle cell disease, the *20210A* allele of the prothrombin gene, and the factor V Leiden mutation.[11,16–20] In the Mayo series,[9] 42% had a documented hypercoagulable disorder, with polycythemia vera being the most common.

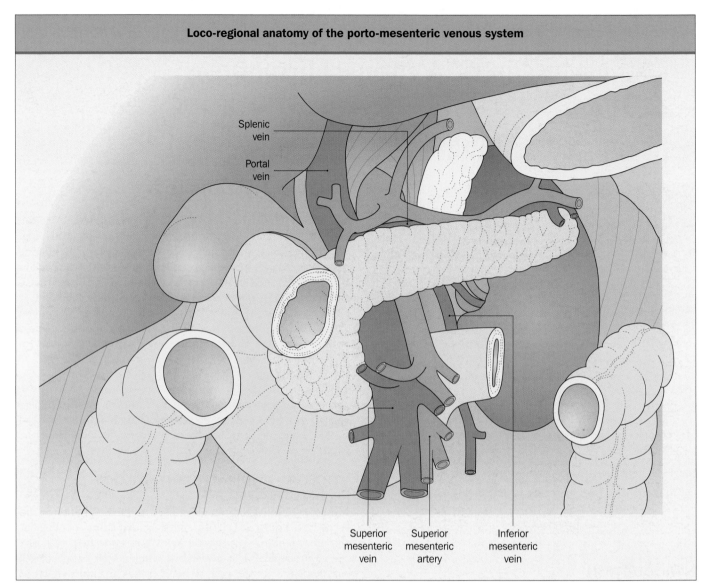

Loco-regional anatomy of the porto-mesenteric venous system

Splenic vein

Portal vein

Superior mesenteric vein

Superior mesenteric artery

Inferior mesenteric vein

Figure 23.1 Loco-regional anatomy of the porto-mesenteric venous system.

Morasch et al.[11] reported that 56% of patients with MVT were found to have an identifiable coagulopathy. The true incidence of hypercoagulability associated with MVT is likely to be higher than that reported currently in the literature as, prior to the last decade, many of these patients may not have been appropriately screened for any hypercoaguable conditions.[3,11]

CLINICAL PRESENTATION

Acute MVT
Although patients with acute MVT present with clinical findings similar to patients with acute mesenteric arterial ischemia, the symptoms and signs are much more subtle and can be misleading. Like acute mesenteric arterial ischemia, the delay in diagnosis is still frequent and is a significant contributory factor to the mortality rate of 13–50% reported in the literature.[2–5,21,22] Typically, patients with acute MVT may present with pain out of proportion to physical findings, plus nausea and vomiting, with or without diarrhea. The pain may be diffuse, intermittent,

lasting for several days or even weeks. Mathews & White[23] found that about 50% of patients had experienced pain from 5 days to as much as 30 days prior to seeking evaluation, and as many as 27% reported having had pain for more than 1 month. In the Mayo series (**Table 23.2**),[9] abdominal distention was the most frequent sign of acute MVT, albeit present in only 43% of patients. Only four of 53 patients presented with symptoms of less than 24 hours' duration. Seventy-five percent of the patients had had symptoms present for more than 48 hours at the time of diagnosis, signifying the frequency in delay of diagnosis. Peritonitis was present in only a little over one-third of patients and fever in 25%. In the most recent report, Morasch et al.[11] found that only 16% of their patients had severe peritonitis. Abdu et al.[2] found that the only true constant finding of MVT was pain out of proportion to the physical findings, with slow progression, often with steady low-grade symptoms for more than 48 hours. Prior medical history or familial-related history of hypercoagulable syndromes associated with presenting complaints of abdominal pain may help suggest the diagnosis.[20]

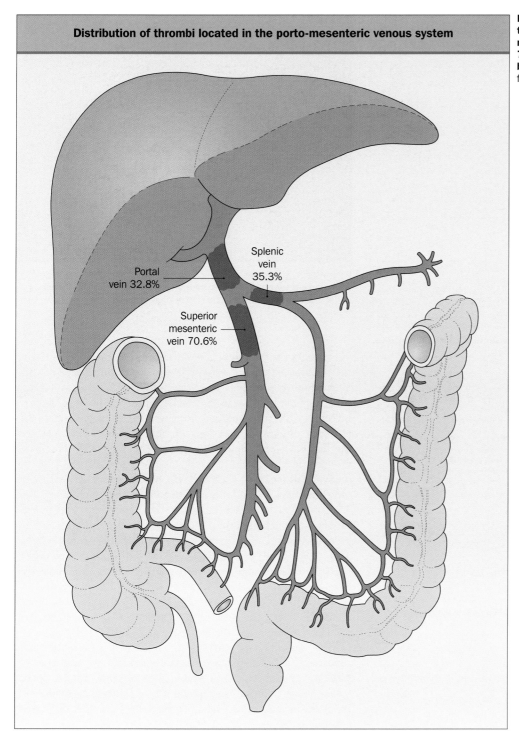

Distribution of thrombi located in the porto-mesenteric venous system

Splenic
vein
35.3%

Portal
vein 32.8%

Superior
mesenteric
vein 70.6%

Figure 23.2 The distribution of thrombi located in the porto-mesenteric venous system based on 72 patients treated at the Mayo Clinic between 1972 and 1993. (Adapted from Rhee et al.[9])

Morasch et al.[11] found that 42% of patients in their series had some form of factor deficiency associated with hypercoagulability. Similarly, the Mayo series reported 42%.[9]

Chronic MVT

Presentations with the chronic form vary widely, from subtle abdominal findings to asymptomatic. This is particularly true with patients who have incidental findings on abdominal computed tomography (CT) scan for another pathologic process unrelated to chronic MVT.

DIAGNOSTIC TECHNIQUES

Laboratory tests

As in other mesenteric ischemic disorders, laboratory tests are not helpful in making the diagnosis of acute MVT – they can neither confirm nor exclude it – and should be used for screening purposes only. In fact, Boley et al.[5] reported that a white blood cell (WBC) count greater than 12 (10×10^9/L) and bandemia were present in only two-thirds of their patients. The Mayo series[9] reported elevated WBC counts in 49% of patients. Other

Conditions associated with mesenteric venous thrombosis.
Hypercoagulable states
Polycythemia vera
Antithrombin III deficiency
Protein C and S deficiency
20210A allele of the prothrombin gene
Factor V Leiden gene mutation
Oral contraceptive use
Heparin-induced thrombocytopenia
Lupus anticoagulant
Neoplasms
Previous abdominal surgery
Previous MVT
Smoking
Previous DVT
Alcohol abuse
Cirrhosis

Table 23.1   Conditions associated with mesenteric venous thrombosis.

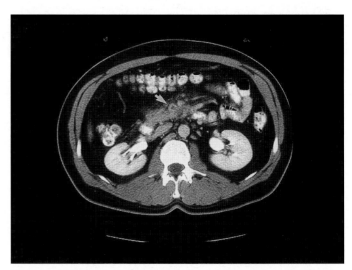

Figure 23.3 Abdominal computed tomography (CT) scan of a patient with acute mesenteric venous thrombosis. Arrow shows the thrombus in the superior mesenteric vein. (From Rhee et al.[9])

Symptoms of acute mesenteric venous thrombosis.	
Symptoms	*No. of patients (%)*
Abdominal pain	44 (83)
Anorexia	28 (53)
Diarrhea	23 (43)
Nausea and vomiting	22 (42)
Upper GI bleeding	15 (28)
Lower GI bleeding	12 (23)
Constipation	7 (13)

Table 23.2 Symptoms of acute mesenteric venous thrombosis. GI, gastrointestinal. (Adapted from Rhee et al.[9])

biochemical variables such as serum lactate and amylase are not elevated in most patients.

Radiographic diagnosis

Prior to the advent of CT, the diagnosis of MVT had been difficult to establish objectively. Plain abdominal radiographs demonstrate evidence of ischemic bowel in less than 5% of patients. In general, abdominal X-rays are non-specific and of little use in the diagnostic process. Venous-phase mesenteric angiography was then the preferred non-operative method for diagnosing MVT.[10] Most reports at that time diagnosed MVT at laparotomy or autopsy. Since then, owing to improved image resolution of CT scanning and magnetic resonance imaging (MRI) with gadolinium, the disease process is diagnosed more readily.

Computed tomography is the diagnostic test of choice in acute MVT.[24] Harward et al.[3] reported a 90% sensitivity in the

10 patients they studied. The most common positive finding is the demonstration of thrombus in the superior mesenteric vein, as shown in **Figure 23.3**. Associated findings which may suggest MVT include bowel wall thickening, pneumatosis, and 'streaky' mesentery. Portal or mesenteric venous gas strongly suggests the presence of bowel infarction. Combining bowel ischemia and the presence of venous thrombosis, the sensitivity of CT in showing an abnormality was 100% in the Mayo series.[9] In the study by Morasch et al.,[11] CT was considered diagnostic in 18 of 20 patients (90%) who underwent the test, including 15 of 15 (100%) who presented with abdominal pain or diarrhea. Similarly, Vogelzang et al.[25] diagnosed MVT using CT in all 14 patients studied.

Duplex ultrasonography and MRI are promising modalities. Duplex ultrasonography can be diagnostic only if obtained early. The Mayo study[9] pointed to an 80% overall sensitivity demonstrating either a thrombus or absence of flow in the mesenteric veins. However, in chronic presentations, the sensitivities are not as high because of the extensive collateralizations.

MRI, although expensive, is also very sensitive. Gehl et al.[26] reported 100% sensitivity in diagnosing MVT with the use of MRI in 115 patients. Improved image resolution of high-speed CT scanning and use of gadolinium as a contrast agent in MRI for more accurate visceral evaluation improve the diagnostic capabilities in detecting MVT.

MANAGEMENT: ACUTE MVT

There are various therapies for MVT, including surgical resection of bowel, lytic therapy, and medical management (**Table 23.3**). All patients require resuscitation and antibiotic coverage. Anticoagulation should be instituted to limit thrombosis as well as to prevent recurrence. The sole objective of surgical therapy is to prevent or limit bowel gangrene. Patients who present with peritonitis should undergo immediate surgical exploration. Without findings of peritonitis, radiographic assessment may be warranted to delineate further abdominal pathology. In the

		Management and early mortality of 195 patients with acute mesenteric venous thrombosis.				
Author (year)	No. of patients	Bowel resection	Laparotomy only	Non-operative	Anticoagulation	Mortality No. (%)
Sack & Aldrete (1982)[4]	9	9	0	0	6	2 (22)
Wilson et al. (1987)[20]	16	10	3	3	6	8 (50)
Clavien & Harder (1988)[22]	12	12	0	0	12	5 (42)
Harward et al. (1989)[3]	16	5	0	11	7	3 (19)
Levy et al. (1990)[28]	21	19	2	2	17	8 (38)
Grieshop et al. (1991)[34]	15	5	0	10	9	2 (13)
Boley et al.(1992)[5]	22	22	0	0	22	7 (32)
Rhee et al. (1994)[9]	53	30	4	19	33	14 (27)
Morasch et al. (2001)[11]	31	8		14	19	7 (23)
Total	**195**	**120**	**9**	**59**	**131**	**56 (29)**

Table 23.3 Management and early mortality of 195 patients with acute mesenteric venous thrombosis.

Mayo series,[9] 64% (34/53) of patients with acute MVT eventually required abdominal exploration. Morasch et al.[11] reported a total of ten patients (32%) ultimately required exploration. Features of MVT include edema of the mesentery and cyanotic discoloration of the involved bowel. Infarction from MVT commonly involves the middle segment of the small intestine: the colon is usually not affected. Duodenal involvement suggests that bowel infarction is not venous in origin. The sites of thrombosis in most patients are located in the smaller, distal mesenteric veins. Once the diagnosis is made, either intraoperatively or preoperatively with radiographic assessments, immediate anticoagulation should be started. The risk of bleeding complications may be increased in the perioperative period. However, the benefit decreases the risk of re-thrombosis and ultimately improves survival.[9]

At operation, minimal bowel resection and liberal use of second-look laparotomy after 24 hours is the primary goal. Up to 90% of patients present with transmural necrosis, with bowel perforation present in 20% of cases. The length of bowel resection can be fairly extensive. If initial infarction is extensive, limited resection is recommended. Recurrent infarction from repeated venous thrombosis involves the area adjacent to the bowel anastomosis in 60% of patients.[10] If any doubt remains about bowel viability, a second look is certainly warranted. In most situations, a diverting ileostomy or colostomy may be preferred, although primary repair is possible in stable patients with local confined intestinal infarction. Intraoperative assessment of intestinal viability with Wood's light illumination and/or Doppler may be difficult in this situation.[10] Thus, second-look procedures should be used liberally.

Thrombectomy of the superior mesenteric vein has been previously described.[9,11,27] The vein is typically to the right of the artery. Access is standard and is obtained by lifting the transverse colon superiorly, displacing the small intestines to the right, and dividing the ligament of Treitz. Inahara[27] describes a linear venotomy, proximal thrombectomy, and removal of small clots of the distal venous mesentery by 'milking' the veins of the bowel and mesentery. Fogarty catheters are also used to retrieve thrombi. Because of the high failure rate of mesenteric venous thrombectomy, we do not advocate this treatment in any situation. In fact, most patients have such diffuse MVT with distal extent that a venous thrombectomy of the superior mesenteric vein does very little in relieving the venous congestion in the mesentery.

The use of thrombolytic therapy in this setting is controversial. Reports of thrombolysis[11,28–31] have described limited success, although the hemorrhagic complications make the option less appealing. Recently, Train et al.[32] described successful treatment of MVT by intra-arterial lytic therapy. Intra-mesenteric venous lytic therapy using urokinase for MVT has also been reported.[33] Although these anecdotally reported cases are limited and no long-term follow-up data are available, this modality may represent the only option in selected cases.

Medical therapy

Non-operative medical management with anticoagulation and observation constitutes treatment of those patients who have not developed peritonitis, those with no evidence of ongoing bowel necrosis, and those with incidental findings of venous thrombosis on radiographic studies. Boley and colleagues[5] suggest that anticoagulation should be started at the time of diagnosis and maintained lifelong to decrease the incidence of recurrence unless there are significant risks of bleeding complications due to portal venous hypertension.

Anticoagulation therapy

The required course of anticoagulation is not known. Current recommendations suggest that anticoagulation should be continued indefinitely unless contraindications prevent use. Primary mesenteric ischemia should be treated with indefinite anticoagulation since the source may be an undefined or yet undetected anticoagulation factor. Patients with secondary mesenteric ischemic disorders should also receive indefinite anticoagulation therapy, although consideration for the etiology should be considered.

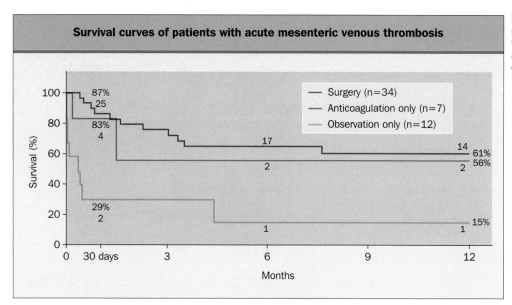

Figure 23.4 Survival curves of acute mesenteric venous thrombosis treated with surgery and anticoagulation, anticoagulation alone, and observation. (Adapted from Rhee et al.[9])

PROGNOSIS: ACUTE MVT

The natural history of MVT is not known. The 30-day mortality remains high (13–15%) and can be as high as 50%. Morasch et al.[11] reported a 30-day mortality of 23%, with only two patients dying of massive bowel infarction. **Figure 23.4** depicts the survival curves of acute MVT for the Mayo series.[9] In that series, prolonged hospitalization was observed in patients who presented with peritonitis and required bowel resection. Mean stay for acute MVT was beyond 22 days, ranging from 1 to 98 days. Thirty-eight percent (20/53) of the patients presenting with acute MVT ultimately died due to disease progression. Anticoagulation was found to be the factor that altered *early* survival in that series. *Late* survival of acutely presenting patients with MVT was consistently poor. Patients treated surgically and with anticoagulation had improved survival. In a review of the international literature by Abdu et al.,[2] similar benefits were seen for those without surgery, although not as good as surgery with anticoagulation. The recurrence rate of acute MVT is generally high.[9,11] Most occur during the same hospitalization or within 30 days. Anticoagulation alone appears to have a higher recurrence rate than surgery with anticoagulation.[9] The cause of the MVT does not appear to affect survival.

CHRONIC MVT

Presentation may vary from vague abdominal pain or abdominal distention to being completely asymptomatic. Mild leukocytosis may be the only significant laboratory finding in these patients, but was present in less than half of patients in the Mayo series.[9]

The incidental finding of a thrombosed mesenteric venous system is not uncommon, in particular during evaluation of other abdominal pathology. In most cases of chronic MVT, collateral venous circulation is usually sufficient to maintain adequate drainage of the affected bowel.[9] Prognosis, however, is determined by the underlying abdominal disease, and late survival appears to be better than in those patients who present with acute MVT.[9]

SUMMARY

MVT is an uncommon yet important cause of visceral ischemia. Suspicion should be very high, particularly in those patients with prior histories of hypercoagulable disorders. Operative therapy is necessary to assure that the intestinal ischemia from venous thrombosis has not progressed to transmural infarction. If not, observation and anticoagulation therapy is appropriate. Lifelong anticoagulation therapy is necessary to decrease the frequency of recurrences.

The overall outcome for those patients who present acutely, still remains fairly poor. The 30-day mortality rate is high and is comparable to that for its arterial counterpart causing visceral ischemia. Despite adequate anticoagulation and disease awareness, the recurrence rate is also high. Long-term prognosis for acute MVT, too, is poor. Overall outcome is much better for the chronic form of MVT and appears to be determined by the underlying disease process. Unfortunately, as reflected in the international literature published over the past 20 years, there has been only a slight improvement in overall survival in those patients who suffer from MVT.

REFERENCES

1. Elliot JW. The operative relief of gangrene of intestine due to occlusion of the mesenteric vessels. Ann Surg 1895;21:9–23.
2. Abdu R, Zakhour BJ, Dallis DJ. Mesenteric venous thrombosis – 1911 to 1984. Surgery 1987;101:383–8.
3. Harward TRS, Green D, Bergan JJ, Rizzo RJ, Yao JST. Mesenteric venous thrombosis. J Vasc Surg 1989;9:328–33.
4. Sack J, Aldrete JS. Primary mesenteric venous thrombosis. Surg Gynecol Obstet 1982;154:205–8.
5. Boley SJ, Kaleya RN, Brandt LJ. Mesenteric venous thrombosis. Surg Clin North Am 1992:72:183–201.
6. Warren S, Eberhard TP. Mesenteric venous thrombosis. Surg Gynecol Obstet 1935;61:102.

7. Kairaluoma MI, Karkola P, Heikkinen E, et al. Mesenteric infarction. Am J Surg 1977;133:188–93.

8. Ottinger LW, Austen WG. A study of 136 patients with mesenteric infarction. Surg Gynecol Obstet 1967;124:251–61.

9. Rhee RY, Gloviczki P, Mendonca CT, et al. Mesenteric venous thrombosis: still a lethal disease in the 1990s. J Vasc Surg 1994;20:688–97.

10. Kazmers A. Intestinal ischemia caused by venous thrombosis. In: Rutherford RB, ed. Vascular surgery, 5th edn. Philadelphia:WB Saunders; 2000:1524–31.

11. Morasch MD, Ebaugh JL, Chiou AC, Matsumura JS, Pearce WH, Yao JS. Mesenteric venous thrombosis: a changing clinical entity. J Vasc Surg 2001;34:680–4.

12. Kitchens CS. Evolution of our understanding of the pathophysiology of primary mesenteric venous thrombosis. Am J Surg 1992;163:346–8.

13. Johnson CC, Baggenstoss AH. Mesenteric vascular occlusion. I. Study of 99 cases of occlusion of the veins. Proc Staff Meet Mayo Clinic 1949; 24:628.

14. Hassan HA. Oral contraceptive-induced mesenteric venous thombosis with resultant intestinal ischemia. J Clin Gastroenterol 1999;29:90–5.

15. Nesbit RR Jr, Deweese JA. Mesenteric venous thrombosis and oral contraceptives. South Med J 1977;70:360–2.

16. Bontempo FA, Hassett AC, Faruki H, et al. The Factor V Leiden mutation: spectrum of thrombotic events and laboratory evaluation. J Vasc Surg 1997;25:271–5.

17. Inagaki H, Sakakibara O, Miyaika H, et al. Mesenteric venous thrombosis in familial free protein S deficiency. Am J Gastroenterol 1993; 88:134–8.

18. Ostermiller W Jr, Carter R. Mesenteric venous thrombosis secondary to polycythemia vera. Am Surg 1969;35:407.

19. Tollefson DFJ, Friedman KD, Marlar RA, et al. Protein C deficiency: a cause of unusual or unexplained thrombosis. Arch Surg 1988;123:881–4.

20. Wilson C, Walker ID, Davidson JF, et al. Mesenteric venous thrombosis and antithombin III deficiency. J Clin Pathol 1987;40:906–8.

21. Carr N, Jamison MH. Superior mesenteric venous thrombosis. Br J Surg 1981;68:343–4.

22. Clavien PA, Harder F. Mesenteric venous thrombosis. Helv Chir Acta 1988;55:29–34.

23. Mathews JE, White RR. Primary mesenteric venous occlusive disease. Am J Surg 1971;122:579–83

24. Rahmouni A, Mathieu D, Golli M, et al. Value of CT and sonography in the conservative management of acute splenoportal and superior mesenteric venous thrombosis. Gastrointest Radiol 1992;17:135–40.

25. Vogelzang RL, Gore RM, Anschuetz SL, Blei AT. Thrombosis of the splanchnic veins: CT diagnosis. Am J Roentgenol 1988;150:93–6.

26. Gehl HB, Bohndorf K, Klose KC, et al. Two-dimensional MR angiography in the evaluation of abdominal veins with gradient refocused sequences. J Comput Assist Tomogr 1990;14:619–24.

27. Inahara T. Acute superior mesenteric venous thrombosis treatment by thrombectomy. Ann Surg 1971;174:956–61.

28. Levy PJ, Krausz MM, Manny J. The role of second-look procedure in improving survival time for patients with mesenteric venous thrombosis. Surg Gynecol Obstet 1990;170:287–91.

29. Bilbao JI, Rodriguez-Cabello J, Longo J, et al. Portal thrombosis: percutaneous transhepatic treatment with urokinase – a case treated with thombectomy. Surgery 1974;76:286.

30. Robin, P, Gurel Y, Lang M, et al. Complete thrombolysis of mesenteric vein occlusion with recombinant tissue-type plasminogen activator. Lancet 1988;1:1391.

31. Miller VE, Berland LL. Pulsed doppler duplex sonography and CT of portal vein thrombosis. Am J Roentgenol 1985;145:73–6.

32. Train JS, Ross H, Weiss JD, Feingold ML, Khoury-Yacoub A, Khoury PT. Mesenteric venous thrombosis: successful treatment by intraarterial lytic therapy. J Vasc Interv Radiol 1998;9:461–4.

33. Poplausky MR, Kaufman JA, Geller SC, Waltman AC. Mesenteric venous thrombosis treated with urokinase via the superior mesenteric artery. Gastroenterology 1996;110:1633–5.

34. Grieshop RJ, Dalsing MC, Cikrit DF, et al. Acute mesenteric venous thrombosis: revisited in a time of diagnostic clarity. Am Surg 1991; 57:573–8.

CHAPTER

24 Pathophysiology of Renovascular Hypertension

Stephen C Textor

KEY POINTS

- 'Renovascular hypertension' refers to de-novo development or acceleration of hypertension produced by high-grade vascular renal artery stenosis.

- Activation of the renin-angiotensin system occurs when renal artery perfusion falls.

- Mechanisms of sustained hypertension differ between one- and two-kidney forms of renovascular hypertension, depending upon the ability of the contralateral kidney to excrete sodium.

- Sustained rises in arterial pressure and vascular resistance develop despite a fall in renin activity, corresponding to recruitment of alternative pressor systems.

- Medical treatment of systemic hypertension may reduce post-stenotic renal perfusion pressures to levels prone to induce 'ischemic nephropathy'.

- Ischemic nephropathy refers to intrarenal tissue injury resulting from reduced renal perfusion.

- Renal injury beyond arterial stenosis results from oxidative stress, proinflammatory cytokine release, and disturbances of fibrotic mechanisms.

- The severity of renal injury appears to be modified by interactions with other factors including age, dyslipidemias, and atheroembolic disease.

INTRODUCTION

'Renovascular hypertension' refers to the syndrome of elevated arterial blood pressure produced by reduced kidney perfusion. A wide variety of lesions affecting the kidney vasculature can produce this syndrome, which remains among the most common forms of secondary hypertension. Understanding the pathways by which vascular compromise to the kidney affects both blood pressure and renal function is important for clinicians caring for such patients. Rapid advances in medical therapy, vascular imaging, and interventional strategies make it more important than ever to grasp the mechanisms by which changes in renal perfusion modify both kidney function and hemodynamics.

The importance of vascular lesions in the kidney in regulating systemic blood pressure is a seminal observation made almost 70 years ago in experiments performed in dogs.[1] When these observations were extended to humans, renovascular hypertension became a prototype for a 'secondary' cause of hypertension for which specific intervention and potential surgical cure could be considered. Many investigators view these studies as the first to

establish the central role of the kidney in overall regulation of blood pressure.

Most renovascular hypertension is the result of atherosclerotic lesions. These lesions often are located at the ostium or early portion of the main renal artery. A smaller number are related to fibromuscular lesions of the main and segmental renal arteries, and additional cases of renal artery distortion result from extrinsic lesions, such as tumors and cysts. Understanding the interaction of pre-existing cardiovascular risk, including hypertension, hyperlipidemia, and diabetes, in the pathogenesis of clinical renovascular hypertension, therefore, is essential. One result of improved antihypertensive therapy has been a shift to greater concern for preservation of renal function in patients with renovascular disease. It should be emphasized that mechanisms leading to renovascular hypertension may differ from those leading to parenchymal renal injury, so-called 'ischemic nephropathy'.[2] The term 'ischemic' itself may not be strictly correct. Unlike the heart or brain, the kidney is vastly over-supplied with blood, consistent with its filtration function. Under normal circumstances, less than 10% of renal blood flow is needed for metabolic support. Renal vein oxygen tension remains high. In fact, reduced glomerular filtration in stenotic kidneys reduces oxygen consumption, leading to higher than baseline venous oxygen tension.[3] Furthermore, measurement of venous erythropoietin levels show no evidence of stimulation despite major activation of the renin–angiotensin system and reduced renal perfusion.[4]

Nonetheless, some conditions of vascular compromise are associated with reduced glomerular volume, tubular atrophy, and interstitial fibrosis. At some point, restoring renal blood flow no longer restores glomerular filtration or function of the kidney.[2] Because refractory hypertension is no longer the primary reason for considering renal revascularization, it is important to understand the structural ramifications of reduced blood flow to the kidney.

DIAGNOSTIC CRITERIA

For more than a century, the kidney has been recognized as a source of pressor materials. Identification of components of the renin–angiotensin system has provided a crucial link to under-standing these systems. Circulating renin is derived primarily from the kidney in response to a reduction of renal perfusion pressure detected by loss of afferent arteriolar stretch.[5,6] Renin itself has biological activity directed mainly to the enzymatic release of angiotensin I from its circulating substrate, angiotensinogen, in plasma and possibly other sites. Two further peptides are cleaved from angiotensin I through the action of angiotensin-converting enzyme (ACE) to produce angiotensin II. Generation

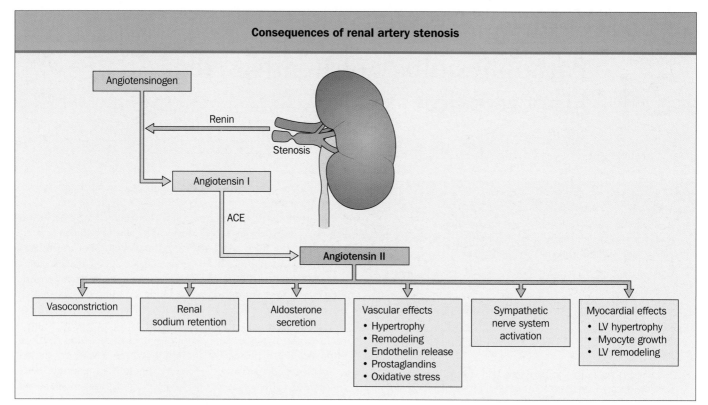

Figure 24.1 Consequences of renal artery stenosis. Reduction of perfusion pressure to the kidney leads to release of renin from juxtaglomerular cells in the afferent arteriole. This leads to a cascade eventually amplifying the signal to produce both local and systemic angiotensin II, whose actions are complex. Angiotensin II raises arterial pressure by direct vascular effects and by changing renal sodium homeostasis, in addition to having wide effects on other pressor systems, fibrosis, and remodeling. ACE, angiotensin-converting enzyme; LV, left ventricular.

of angiotensin II in plasma occurs mainly during passage through the lung. Hence, the signal of reduced kidney pressures is amplified and transmitted to release of a major vasopressor system which acts throughout the body, accounting for one key mechanism by which renovascular hypertension develops.

The importance of the renin–angiotensin system in renovascular hypertension cannot be overemphasized. Experimental models of two-kidney, one-clip renovascular hypertension can be prevented so long as this system is blocked by inhibition of ACE.[7] The actions of angiotensin II are manifold and widespread, as indicated in **Figure 24.1**. Activation of this pressor system from a local signal within the kidney provides a means of signaling the entire organism to increase vascular resistance, to retain sodium, and to stimulate aldosterone, all of which are systemic effects. Further studies indicate that complex interactions between angiotensin II and tissue and cellular systems occur, leading to vascular remodeling, left ventricular hypertrophy, and activation of fibrogenic mechanisms. Complex interactions between angiotensin and other vasoactive systems combine to produce sustained elevations of vasomotor tone. These are mediated by sympathetic nerve traffic, endothelin, nitric oxide, and generation of oxygen free radicals.[8–12]

DIFFERENCES BETWEEN ONE-KIDNEY AND TWO-KIDNEY RENOVASCULAR HYPERTENSION

Experimental studies of renovascular hypertension identify important differences between one- and two-kidney models

(**Fig. 24.2**). These studies indicate that two-kidney, one-clip hypertensive models present a paradigm of renovascular hypertension, with activation of restorative pressor mechanisms in the 'affected' kidney which tend to be counterbalanced by a normal 'contralateral' kidney. The release of renin from the affected side produces elevated arterial pressures, sodium retention in the underperfused kidney, and, under some circumstances, reduced renal blood flow and glomerular filtration in the affected kidney.[13] The contralateral kidney is exposed to elevated arterial pressures. As a result, release of renin is suppressed in the contralateral kidney, which is undergoing 'pressure natriuresis' and enhanced urinary excretion of sodium. The contralateral kidney, then, tends to work continually against the sodium-retaining actions of the post-stenotic kidney. The resulting profile then can be established by comparing the function and hormonal status of one kidney as compared with the other. The hallmark of such an arrangement is a persistently elevated level of renin and angiotensin II, dependence of systemic hypertension on the pressor action of angiotensin II, and side-to-side differences during comparative studies of renal blood flow, sodium excretion, and glomerular filtration. Side-to-side differences have been employed in a variety of pre-interventional functional studies to predict the likelihood of blood pressure benefit or 'cure' of renovascular hypertension.[14–16]

By contrast, one-kidney, one-clip hypertension represents a model reflecting the situation of the entire renal mass (both kidneys or a solitary functioning kidney) being affected by vascular occlusive disease. Although initial underperfusion of the kidney

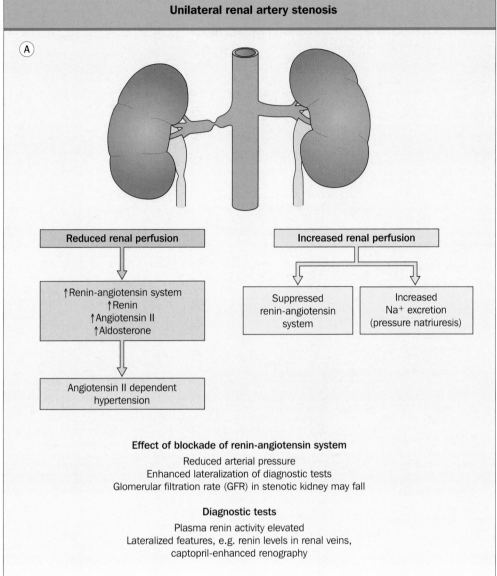

Unilateral renal artery stenosis

Ⓐ

| Reduced renal perfusion | | Increased renal perfusion |

↑Renin-angiotensin system
↑Renin
↑Angiotensin II
↑Aldosterone

Suppressed
renin-angiotensin
system

Increased
Na+ excretion
(pressure natriuresis)

Angiotensin II dependent
hypertension

Effect of blockade of renin-angiotensin system
Reduced arterial pressure
Enhanced lateralization of diagnostic tests
Glomerular filtration rate (GFR) in stenotic kidney may fall

Diagnostic tests
Plasma renin activity elevated
Lateralized features, e.g. renin levels in renal veins,
captopril-enhanced renography

Figure 24.2 Differences between unilateral (two-kidney, one-clip) and bilateral (one-kidney, one-clip) renovascular hypertension. These figures illustrate the differences observed in models whereby a normal contralateral kidney is present or not. When two kidneys are present, differences in sodium excretion and renin activation favor angiotensin-dependent hypertension and lateralization of diagnostic tests (e.g. renal vein renin determinations). When both kidneys (or the entire renal mass, such as a solitary functioning kidney) are affected by vascular stenosis, sodium retention and volume expansion eventually suppress renin release, obscuring the role of the renin–angiotensin system (see text). (Modified from Textor.[13])

activates the renin–angiotensin system as with two-kidney models, the one-kidney model does not have a 'normal' contralateral kidney. Sodium-retaining mechanisms are activated and produce positive volume status, finally returning renal perfusion pressures nearly to normal. As a result, plasma renin activity falls and arterial pressure is not dependent upon the pressor effects of angiotensin II.[17] Volume expansion is critical, as the dependence of hypertension upon angiotensin can be demonstrated only after sodium depletion.[18] Side-to-side comparisons cannot be made in this form of renovascular hypertension.

Many human clinical disease situations appear more closely to approximate the one-kidney, one-clip model of hypoperfusion of the entire mass than the two-kidney model. This may be the case even when main renal artery stenosis affects only one kidney. It may be argued that small vessel changes in an otherwise normal contralateral kidney lead to volume retention and mask the angiotensin-II-dependent status of two-kidney, one-clip forms of human hypertension in some instances.

PREVALENCE AND INCIDENCE

As with other vascular occlusive lesions, clinicians recognize that simply finding a renal artery stenosis (RAS) does not establish its functional significance. Imaging studies during coronary and peripheral angiography indicate that at least moderate RAS (>50%) can be identified in 20–30% of patients with atherosclerosis elsewhere.[19,20] Earlier autopsy studies indicated that hypertensive individuals had some degree of RAS in nearly 60% of cases. Because mortality rates from stroke and cardiovascular disease continue to fall in western countries,[21] the prevalence of high-grade atherosclerotic renal artery lesions developing in older individuals appears to be increasing. As a result, most cases of renovascular hypertension develop gradually and are superimposed upon essential hypertension. Some authors suggest that up to 14–20% of patients reaching end-stage renal disease (ESRD) have renovascular disease as the primary etiologic factor.[22] Remarkably, fibromuscular diseases which activate

305

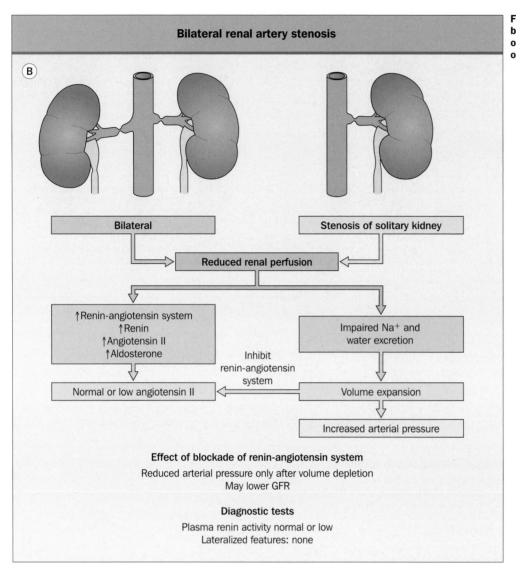

Figure 24.2 (*Cont'd*) Differences between unilateral (two-kidney, one-clip) and bilateral (one-kidney, one-clip) renovascular hypertension.

pressor mechanisms and produce renovascular hypertension in younger individuals rarely produce renal parenchymal injury unless total occlusion develops. This observation has led some to suggest that other factors related to age and other diseases, such as nephrosclerosis and/or diabetes, may be required for irreversible tissue injury to occur (**Fig. 24.3**).

The physiologic effects of renal artery lesions can vary widely, as illustrated in **Figure 24.4**. Many are 'incidental' lesions with no significant hemodynamic effect.

Studies of vascular occlusion in which cross-sectional lumen was measured with latex cast indicate that detectable changes in either blood flow or pressure can be identified only after more than 70–80% lumen obstruction occurs (**Fig. 24.5**).[23] When enough obstruction is present to reduce distal pressures, it is considered 'critical' renal artery stenosis. Hence, identification of a renal artery lesion alone is rarely enough to determine its role in a given patient. Once a gradient is established with reduced renal perfusion, a sequence of events (see below) ensues to restore renal perfusion pressure at the expense of elevated systemic arterial pressures.

An important corollary of this observation is that renal perfusion is generally normal in untreated, early renovascular

hypertension. Hence, the pressor effects of the post-stenotic kidney restore blood flow and renal functional capacity, albeit at the expense of systemic hypertension. Progressive vascular obstruction, however, triggers further reduction to the kidney and further pressure elevation, which if unchecked can produce malignant-phase hypertension.[24,25]

A second corollary is that medical therapy of systemic hypertension with critical renovascular disease reduces perfusion to the post-stenotic kidney. This can lead to activation of counter-regulatory mechanisms, making antihypertensive therapy less effective, and in some situations to critical loss of blood flow in the affected kidney, leading to irreversible renal injury, which some have labeled 'ischemic nephropathy'.[26]

CLINICAL APPLICATION OF RENAL PHYSIOLOGY IN RENOVASCULAR HYPERTENSION

A large body of experimental and clinical investigation has been directed toward determining the functional significance of renal artery disease. Studies using split renal function measurements obtained with ureteral catheters demonstrate that reduced renal

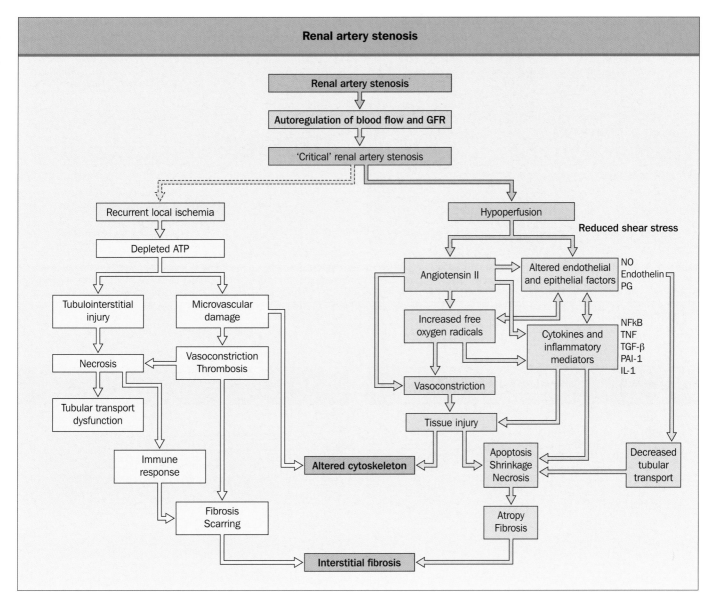

Figure 24.3 Renal artery stenosis. Summary of mechanisms by which 'critical' renal artery stenosis can produce both local hypoperfusion and activation of mechanisms inducing tissue injury. Alterations of endothelial function, oxidative stress, and cytokine production have been demonstrated and favor interstitial fibrosis, despite oversupply of oxygenated blood to the kidney as a whole. GFR, glomerular filtration rate; IL-1, interleukin-1; NO, nitric oxide; PAI-1, plasminogen activator inhibitor-1; PG, prostaglandins; TGF-β, transforming growth factor-beta; TNF, tumor necrosis factor. (From Lerman & Textor[49] with permission.)

perfusion is associated with sodium avidity and reduced free water clearance. Eventually, plasma flow and glomerular filtration fall in the affected kidney.[14,15,27] As a general principle, the more clear the differences between the stenotic and contralateral kidney, the more likely that surgical revascularization will improve (or cure) high blood pressure. Demonstrating significant abnormalities in the non-stenotic kidney, such as reduced renal blood flow, is considered a marker for likely failure to reverse hypertension.[28]

Subsequent studies have built upon these principles. Measurement of renal vein renin levels and measurement of differential renal function by isotope renography are more recent clinical examples of identifying hemodynamically significant renal artery lesions using physiologic probes. Measurement of circulating plasma renin activity, both before and after administration of an agent that blocks the conversion of angiotensin I to angiotensin II,

has been used to establish 'renin-dependency' of hypertension and to identify candidates for renovascular intervention.[29,30]

For many reasons, these studies are less commonly performed today than before. A major limitation is the relatively poor performance of these measurements as predictors of either renovascular disease or the response to renal revascularization when extended to wider populations.[31] In general, the predictive value of lateralizing studies has been most useful when the study is positive, i.e. when substantial lateralization is present.[32,33] They have been far less useful when negative, as reflected by the observation that despite no lateralization of renal vein renin determinations, more than 50% of subjects undergoing revascularization had a positive clinical outcome.[34,35] While this is less than the 93% likelihood of benefit with strongly lateralizing study, failure to lateralize such a study leads to an unacceptably high rate of missed disease.

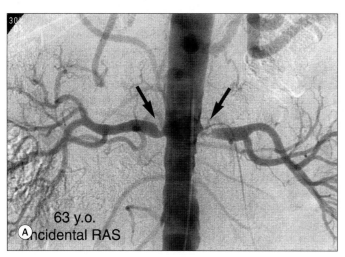

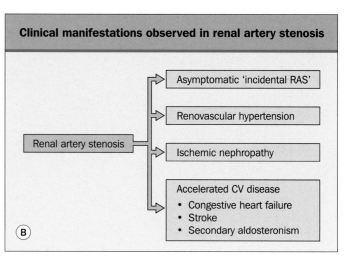

Figure 24.4 Renal artery lesions. (A) Aortogram from a patient with moderate hypertension and normal renal function, demonstrating the potential for 'incidental' renal artery stenosis to be detected during angiography performed for other reasons. (B) Spectrum of clinical manifestations observed with varying degrees of renal artery stenosis. These range from 'incidental' lesions with minimal hemodynamic effects to advanced renal failure and accelerated cardiovascular risk from congestive heart failure and stroke. Clinicians face the challenge of identifying the role of such lesions in individual patients.

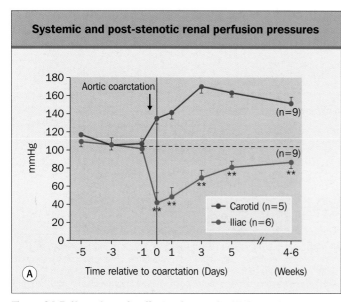

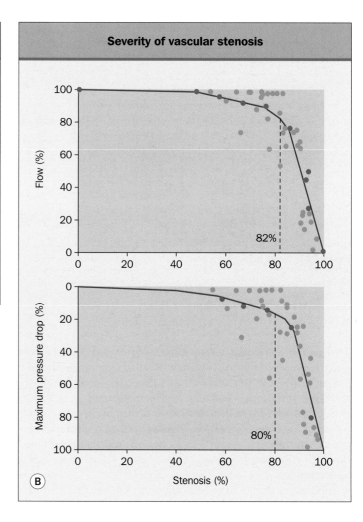

Figure 24.5 Hemodynamic effects of stenosis. (A) Systemic and post-stenotic renal perfusion pressures measured after placement of an aortic clip between the renal arteries. The rise in systemic arterial pressure allows preservation of renal perfusion pressure to near normal levels. (B) Severity of vascular stenosis (as determined by latex casts of blood vessel lumen) and the measured blood flow and pressure drop in artery. These observations indicate that only when lumen obstruction exceeds 70–80% are hemodynamic effects sufficient to compromise flow. Many less severe lesions produce no clinical effects (see text). (Modified from May et al[23] with permission).

Why are physiologic tests prone to underestimate the importance of renal artery disease? Among several reasons, it is clear that detecting the role of activation of the renin–angiotensin system is dependent upon the testing conditions, particularly the level of sodium intake and balance. Many antihypertensive medications strongly affect circulating levels. In general, high sodium intake and sympatholytic medications, including beta-blockers, suppress activation of renin release. Hence, maneuvers such as sodium depletion, diuretic administration, and administration of potent vasodilators such as nitroprusside and hydralazine have been applied as diagnostic tools to enhance identification of RAS.[36,37] Another reason measurement of circulating renin does not correlate well with outcomes of revascularization may be its interaction and recruitment of additional pressor mechanisms.

Other pressor mechanisms and phases of renovascular hypertension

Reduced renal perfusion activates other mechanisms related to renal and systemic hemodynamics. Recent reviews of this subject emphasize the complex interactions and sequence of vascular changes developing over time.[6]

Sympathetic nervous tone is increased during reduced renal perfusion,[38] as is production of the potent vasoconstrictor, endothelin.[39] It is clear that mechanisms beyond the direct pressor actions of angiotensin II modulate vascular tone and blood pressure.[40] Recent data indicate that low-dose angiotensin II is capable of altering the level of oxidative 'stress' in the microvasculature. These changes shift production of oxidative metabolites from vasodilating forms, including nitric oxide, to active vasoconstrictors, including oxygen free radicals and isoprostanes (**Fig. 24.6**).[41]

The degree to which these mechanisms participate in developing renovascular hypertension varies over time. The precise role of each at any point is difficult to determine. Studies of experimental renovascular hypertension indicate that the effects of stenosis undergo a series of transitions starting from an early phase with elevated angiotensin II and prompt reversal of hypertension after removal of the lesion.[42] Later, renal artery clip hypertension is associated with lower angiotensin II levels, despite sustained hypertension. This phase remains amenable to reversal of hypertension after removal of the vascular lesion. Eventually, however, a late phase develops with sustained hypertension, normal levels of renin and angiotensin II, and no response to removal of the clip lesion. This important observation suggests that mechanisms sustaining arterial hypertension sometimes undergo a transition to an irreversible stage.

Whether such a set of transitional stages (**Fig. 24.7**) applies in human renovascular hypertension is not well understood. This paradigm has been invoked to explain treatment failures, although the date of onset of renovascular hypertension only rarely can be established with certainty. Although the single best predictor of a favorable response to renal revascularization has been 'short duration' of hypertension (when known), clinicians are aware of patients with sustained, long-term hypertension which can be reversed with successful restoration of blood flow.[43]

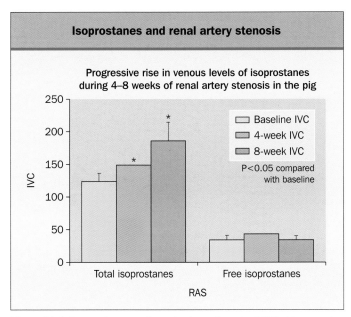

Figure 24.6 Isoprostanes and renal artery stenosis (RAS). Measured levels of isoprostanes, a marker of oxidative stress, at 1 and 2 months after inducing renovascular hypertension in a pig model. The sustained rise in arterial pressure induced by progressive renal artery disease was associated with increased oxidative stress and production of pressor oxidative metabolites even after circulating levels of renin activity had returned to normal. Additional mechanisms are recruited over time, which produce reduced renal blood flow and activate intrarenal tissue injury.

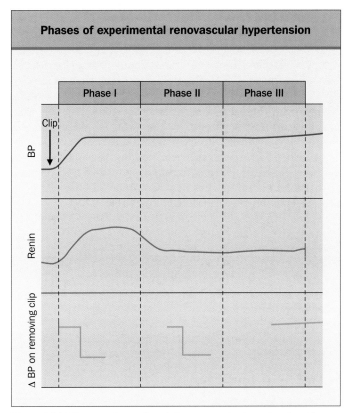

Figure 24.7 Phases of experimental renovascular hypertension. There is transition from an early 'renin-dependent' but reversible phase to finally a stage that is neither 'renin-dependent' nor reversible. These phases are difficult to define in clinical practice, but highlight the recruitment of non-angiotensin-dependent mechanisms sustaining renovascular hypertension during the long term. (From Brown et al.[42])

Prognosis

A major consideration in both diagnosis and management of RAS is the potential for progressive renal artery occlusion. **Table 24.1** summarizes some of the potential syndromes associated with renovascular disease. Many of these reflect the tendency of atherosclerotic disease to progress over time, leading to different clinical manifestations. Rates of progression are highly variable. Recent Doppler ultrasound studies indicate that atherosclerotic disease can progress with demonstrably greater velocities in nearly 50% of subjects starting with high-grade lesions (>60% stenosis) over a period of between 3 and 5 years.[44] When the severity of stenosis advances, the chances for loss of renal volume ('atrophy') increase, as does the likelihood of arterial occlusion, fibrosis, and irreversible parenchymal injury (**Fig. 24.8**).

One major concern is the progression to involvement of the total renal mass, either as bilateral RAS or stenosis to a solitary functioning kidney. In this instance, mechanisms identified under one-kidney, one-clip models come into play. Furthermore, the potential for clinical volume expansion, rapid changes in arterial pressure, and diastolic dysfunction associated with rapid rises in afterload become relevant. Sudden changes in circulatory congestion, out of proportion to systolic left ventricular function, result in 'flash pulmonary edema'. This can be abrogated by successful renal revascularization and should be considered in this clinical circumstance.[45]

THE ROLE OF THE RENIN–ANGIOTENSIN SYSTEM IN MAINTAINING GLOMERULAR FILTRATION

Angiotensin-converting enzyme inhibitors (and angiotensin II receptor blockers) now are administered widely for reasons beyond treatment of high blood pressure. They have established survival benefits in the treatment of congestive cardiac failure, recurrent myocardial infarction, and proteinuric renal diseases, including diabetic nephropathy. One result of these trends is that many individuals with unsuspected renal artery disease are being treated with agents capable of blocking the pathophysiologic pathways associated with renovascular hypertension. It is important to recognize the effects this may have upon both development and presentation of renal arterial disease (**Fig. 24.9**).

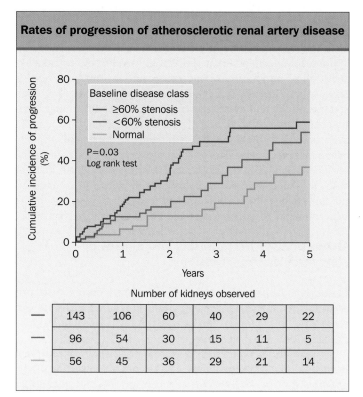

Rates of progression of atherosclerotic renal artery disease

Number of kidneys observed

143	106	60	40	29	22
96	54	30	15	11	5
56	45	36	29	21	14

Figure 24.8 Rates of progression of atherosclerotic renal artery disease. Serial ultrasound measurements at 6-month intervals demonstrate the potential for renal artery atherosclerosis to develop to more severe vascular occlusion. Progression was defined as a rise in Doppler velocity by 100cm/s. A total of 170 patients with 295 target vessels were studied prospectively between 1990 and 1997. Those most likely to progress had the most severe (>60%) stenosis from the outset. Factors predictive of disease progression included systolic blood pressure levels, ankle–brachial index and diabetes. (Modified from Caps et al.[44])

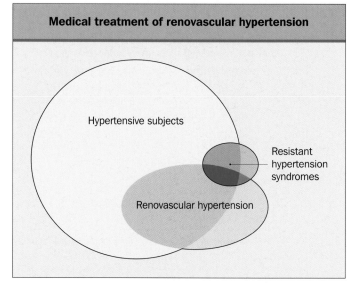

Medical treatment of renovascular hypertension

Figure 24.9 Medical treatment of renovascular hypertension. It is likely that many patients with renal artery stenosis, including some with true renovascular hypertension, are never identified. It is a subgroup of patients with clinically refractory hypertension or other syndromes (see Fig. 24.7) who are more fully evaluated. This overlap increases with the wider administrations of agents that block the renin–angiotensin system, such as angiotensin-converting enzyme inhibitors and angiotensin II receptor blockers.

Syndromes of renovascular disease.
Paroxysmal hypertension
Treatment-resistant hypertension
Bilateral disease/solitary functioning kidney • Progressive renal failure in treated HTN • Renal failure limiting antihypertensive therapy • Pulmonary vascular congestion: 'flash' pulmonary edema • End-stage renal disease

Table 24.1 Syndromes of renovascular disease. Many patients with moderate renovascular hypertension are never identified until complications arise. These may take the form of 'treatment-resistant' hypertension or syndromes of deteriorating kidney function or circulatory congestion.

One of the prominent intrarenal effects of angiotensin is the preferential constriction of efferent arteriolar tone at the glomerulus. Normally, the afferent arterioles preceding the glomerulus are capable of sufficient autoregulation to preserve glomerular capillary blood flows and pressure over a wide range of conditions. Hence, transcapillary pressures, which determine the amount of filtrate formed as plasma traverses the glomerular capillaries, are high enough to generate adequate urine formation. There is little dependence upon efferent arteriolar resistance in this situation. However, when afferent pressures are reduced from pre-glomerular vascular disease, the transcapillary pressure gradient becomes dependent upon increased efferent resistance. Filtration then depends upon the presence of angiotensin II under these conditions, particularly when sodium intake is low. Blockade of the renin–angiotensin system, with administration of either ACE inhibitors or angiotensin receptor blockers, has the potential to reduce transcapillary filtration pressures further. This leads to abrupt loss of glomerular filtration, so-called 'functional acute renal insufficiency' (**Fig. 24.10**).[46,47]

This post-glomerular hemodynamic effect is the basis for identification of major changes in the isotope renogram after administration of captopril, for stimulation of renal vein renins, and for reduction of proteinuria in patients with renal failure. It is also the basis for early decrements in glomerular filtration after starting these agents, particularly when high-grade RAS is present and affecting the entire renal mass.

Clinicians must be attuned to the possibility of this loss of glomerular filtration rate (GFR) and understand its significance. A major fall in GFR should alert the physician to the possibility of bilateral disease or a solitary functioning kidney and highlight the need to define the circulation precisely. Glomerular filtration will recover if angiotensin effect and/or adequate pre-glomerular pressures are restored. A minor decrement in GFR may be difficult to detect, particularly since the contralateral kidney can increase filtration.[48]

MECHANISMS OF TISSUE INJURY IN RENOVASCULAR DISEASE

The pathways by which fibrogenic injury causes scarring of the kidney are complex and not fully understood. Proposed mechanisms include those summarized in **Figure 24.3**.[49] Some of these derive from recurrent episodes of local ischemic injury.

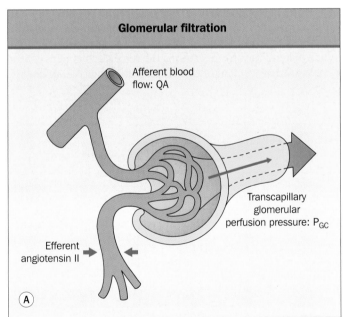

Glomerular filtration

Afferent blood flow: QA

Transcapillary glomerular perfusion pressure: P_GC

Efferent angiotensin II

(A)

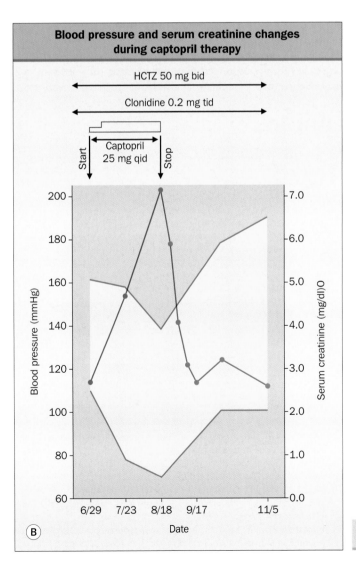

Blood pressure and serum creatinine changes during captopril therapy

HCTZ 50 mg bid

Clonidine 0.2 mg tid

Captopril 25 mg qid

Start Stop

Blood pressure (mmHg)

Serum creatinine (mg/dl)O

6/29 7/23 8/18 9/17 11/5

Date

(B)

Figure 24.10 Blockade of the renin–angiotensin sytem in the kidney. (A) Schematic of the glomerulus, illustrating the role of angiotensin II in maintaining efferent vascular tone and transcapillary filtration pressure. Removal of efferent vascular tone by blockade of the renin–angiotensin system may reduce filtration pressure and lower the glomerular filtration rate (GFR). When the entire renal mass is affected by renal artery stenosis, this effect can produce a 'functional acute renal insufficiency'. This is usually reversible upon withholding blockade of angiotensin. (B) Example of acute renal insufficiency induced by blockade of angiotensin in a patient with renal artery stenosis and renovascular hypertension. The rise in serum creatinine can be associated with preserved blood flow and thereby reflects primarily reduced filtration pressure. Such examples provide evidence that filtration can depend upon angiotensin II under certain conditions and provide an impetus for restoring the renal blood supply by renal revascularization.

Blood pressures vary greatly during circadian cycles and in response to antihypertensive therapy. Post-stenotic pressures may fall periodically to such low levels that mechanisms of acute ischemia supervene, leading to altered cytoskeleton, depletion of ATP sources, and local necrosis. Although these periods may be temporary and lead to restoration of function via normal repair processes, long-term activation of local cytokines may produce an environment favorable to scarring. Such a sequence has been established for other models of acute injury, such as glycerol-induced acute tubular necrosis.[50]

The roles of angiotensin and altered endothelial function in reduced perfusion are extremely complex. Angiotensin II is known to stimulate cellular hypertrophy and hyperplasia.[51] It is capable of activating local inflammatory and fibrogenic responses in a variety of models of tissue injury. Infusion of angiotensin II leads to parenchymal renal injury with focal and segmental glomerulosclerosis.[52] Blockade of angiotensin receptors and/or ACE inhibition in several experimental models diminish cell proliferation and infiltration of mononuclear cells, which triggers extracellular matrix proteins and nephrosclerosis.[53]

The vascular endothelium is a source of multiple vasoactive mediators, including endothelin and nitric oxide. Nitric oxide is recognized as a potent modulator of smooth muscle growth, mesangial cell hypertrophy and hyperplasia, and the extracellular matrix. Reduced renal perfusion leads to reduced shear stress on the vascular wall. Shear stress is a major stimulus for nitric oxide; hence, nitric oxide is diminished in the post-stenotic kidney. This allows intrarenal vasoconstrictors, including angiotensin II and other locally produced materials such as thromboxane and endothelin, to predominate. Endothelin has a wide variety of effects and is particularly potent within the kidney. It activates genes related to growth and differentiation and can be stimulated by local cytokines, such as thrombin and transforming growth factor-beta (TGF-β), interleukin-1, and tumor necrosis factor (TNF). As noted above, a change in the balance of these species can lead to production of oxygen-radical generating systems, in preference to oxygen-radical scavenging systems. This is termed 'oxidative stress' and itself can promote formation of vasoactive mediators and inflammatory cytokines.[54]

SUMMARY

Major reductions in mortality rates from coronary and cerebrovascular disease over the last three decades have given rise to longer lifespans and an aging US population. One result of these changes is a larger number of individuals reaching the seventh, eighth, and ninth decades of life and delayed onset of vascular disease. The mean age of interventional and surgical patient series is increasing. It is essential for clinicians to recognize that the syndromes of renovascular hypertension and ischemic nephropathy can develop at any age. They are more common now among older subjects than ever before. Advances in our understanding of these disorders and the antihypertensive agents available provide a wider set of options regarding effective blood pressure control. As a result, physicians must recognize the factors predisposing to disease progression and the limitations of medical management for each patient. Understanding the pathways by which vascular disease progresses to produce syndromes which benefit most from restoring the renal circulation is central to optimal management of the patient with renovascular disease.

REFERENCES

1. Goldblatt H, Lynch J, Hanzal RE, Summerville WW. Studies on experimental hypertension. I. The production of persistent elevation of systolic blood pressure by means of renal ischemia. J Exp Med 1934; 59:347–79.
2. Textor SC, Wilcox CS. Renal artery stenosis: a common, treatable cause of renal failure? Annu Rev Med 2001;52:421–42.
3. Nielsen K, Rehling M, Henriksen JH. Renal vein oxygen saturation in renal artery stenosis. Clin Physiol 1992;12:179–84.
4. Jensen G, Bjorck S, Nielsen OJ, Volkmann R, Aurell M. Diagnostic use of renal vein erythropoietin measurements in patients with renal artery stenosis. Nephrol Dial Transplant 1992;7:400–5.
5. Cowley AW, Roman RJ. The role of the kidney in hypertension. JAMA 1996;275:1581–9.
6. Romero JC, Feldstein AE, Rodriguez-Porcel MG, Cases-Amenos A. New insights into the pathophysiology of renovascular hypertension. Mayo Clin Proc 1997;72:251–60.
7. DeForrest JM, Knappenberger RC, Antonaccio MJ, Ferrone RA, Creekmore JS. Angiotensin II is a necessary component for the development of hypertension in the two-kidney, one clip rat. Am J Cardiol 1982;49:1515–7.
8. Ruiz-Ortega M, Gomez-Garre D, Alcazar R, et al. Involvement of angiotensin II and endothelin in matrix protein production and renal sclerosis. J Hypertens 1994;12(Suppl):S51–8
9. Romero JC, Reckelhoff JF. Role of angiotensin and oxidative stress in essential hypertension. Hypertension 1999;43:943–9.
10. Herizi A, Jover B, Bouriquet N, Mimran A. Prevention of the cardiovascular and renal effects of angiotensin II by endothelin blockade. Hypertension 1998;31:10–4.
11. Faria FA, Salgado MC. Facilitation of noradrenergic transmission by angiotensin in hypertensive rats. Hypertension 1992;19(Suppl 2):II30–5
12. DiBona G. Central sympathoexcitatory actions of angiotensin II: role of type 1 angiotensin II receptors. J Am Soc Nephrol 1999;10:S90–4.
13. Textor SC. Renovascular hypertension. In: Johnson RJ, Feehally J, eds. Comprehensive clinical nephrology. London:Mosby; 2000:41.1–41.12.
14. Stamey TA, Nudelman JJ, Good PH, et al. Functional characteristics of renovascular hypertension. Medicine 1961;40:347–94.
15. Howard JE, Berthrong N, Gould D, Yendt ER. Hypertension resulting from unilateral renovascular disease and its relief by nephrectomy. Bull Johns Hopkins Hosp 1954;94:51–74.
16. Safian RD, Textor SC. Medical progress: renal artery stenosis. N Engl J Med 2001;344:431–42.
17. Gavras H, Brunner HR, Vaughan ED, Laragh JH. Angiotensin-sodium interaction in blood pressure maintenance of renal hypertensive and normotensive rats. Science 1973;180:1369–70.
18. Gavras H, Brunner HR, Thurston H, Laragh JH. Reciprocation of renin dependency with sodium-volume dependency in renal hypertension. Science 1975;188:1316–7.
19. Olin JW, Melia M, Young JR, Graor R, Risius B. Prevalence of atherosclerotic RAS in patients with atherosclerosis elsewhere. Am J Med 1990;88:46N–51N.
20. Rihal CS, Textor SC, Breen JF, et al. Incidental renal artery stenosis among a prospective cohort of hypertensive patients undergoing coronary angiography. Mayo Clin Proc 2002;77:309–16.
21. Schneider E, Guralnik J. The aging of America: impact on health care costs. JAMA 1990;263:2335–40.
22. Scoble JE, Hamilton G. Atherosclerotic renovascular disease: remediable cause of renal failure in the elderly. BMJ 1990;300:1670–1.
23. May AG, Van de Berg L, DeWeese JA, et al. Critical arterial stenosis. Surgery 1963;54:250–9.
24. Dzau VJ, Siwek LG, Rosen S, et al. Sequential renal hemodynamics in

experimental benign and malignant hypertension. Hypertension 1981; 3:63–8.

25. Textor SC, Smith-Powell L. Post-stenotic arterial pressure, renal haemodynamics and sodium excretion during graded pressure reduction in conscious rats with one- and two-kidney coarctation hypertension. J Hypertens 1988;6:311–9.

26. Jacobson HR. Ischemic renal disease: an overlooked clinical entity. Kidney Int 1988;34:729–43.

27. Textor SC, Novick A, Mujais SK, et al. Responses of the stenosed and contralateral kidneys to (Sar-1, Thr-8) AII in human renovascular hypertension. Hypertension 1983;5:796–804.

28. Palmer JM. Prognostic value of contralateral renal plasma flow in renovascular hypertension. JAMA 1971;217:794–802.

29. Mueller FB, Sealey JE, Case DB, et al. The captopril test for identifying renovascular disease in hypertensive patients. Am J Med 1986;80:633–44.

30. Vaughan ED Jr, Buhler FR, Laragh JH, Sealey JE, Baer L, Bard RH. Renovascular hypertension: renin measurements to indicate hypersecretion and contralateral suppression, estimate renal plasma flow and score for surgery. Am J Med 1973;55:402–14.

31. Elliot WJ, Martin WB, Murphy MB. Comparison of two non-invasive screening tests for renovascular hypertension. Arch Intern Med 1993; 153:755–64.

32. Grim CE, Weinberger MH. Diagnosis of renovascular hypertension: the case for renin assays. In: Narins RG, ed. Controversies in nephrology and hypertension. New York:Churchill Livingstone; 1984:109–22.

33. Luscher TF, Greminger P, Kuhlmann U, Stiegenthaler W, Largiader F, Vetter W. Renal venous renin determinations in renovascular hypertension. Nephron 1986;44:17–24.

34. Mann JFE. The diagnosis of renovascular hypertension: state of the art 1995. Nephrol Dial Transplant 1995;10:1285–6.

35. Marks LS, Maxwell MH, Varady PD. Renovascular hypertension: does the renal vein renin ratio predict operative results? J Urol 1976;115:365–8.

36. Hunt JC, Sheps SG, Harrison EG, Strong CG, Bernatz PE. Renal and renovascular hypertension: a reasoned approach to diagnosis and management. Arch Intern Med 1974;133:988–99.

37. Strong CG, Hunt JC, Sheps SG. Renal venous renin activity. Enhancement of sensitivity of lateralization by sodium depletion. Am J Cardiol 1971;27:602–11.

38. Kooner JS, Peart WS, Mathias CJ. The sympathetic nervous system in hypertension due to unilateral renal artery stenosis in man. Clin Auton Res 1991;1:195–204.

39. Hunley TE, Kon V. Endothelin in ischemic acute renal failure. Curr Opin Nephrol Hypertens 1997;6:394–400.

40. Dohi Y, Criscione L, Luscher TF. Renovascular hypertension impairs formation of endothelium-derived relaxing factors and sensitivity to endothelin-1 in resistance arteries. Br J Pharmacol 1991;104:349–54.

41. Lerman LO, Nath KA, Rodriguez-Porcel M, Krier JD, Schwartz RS, Napoli C. Increased oxidative stress in experimental renovascular hypertension. Hypertension 2001;37:541–6.

42. Brown JJ, Davies DL, Morton JJ, et al. Mechanism of renal hypertension. Lancet 1976;1:1219–21.

43. Hughes JS, Dove HG, Gifford RW, et al. Duration of blood pressure elevation in accurately predicting cure of renovascular hypertension. Am Heart J 1981;101:408–13.

44. Caps MT, Perissinotto C, Zierler RE, et al. Prospective study of atherosclerotic disease progression in the renal artery. Circulation 1998;98:2866–72.

45. Bloch MJ, Trost DW, Pickering TG, Sos TA, August P. Prevention of recurrent pulmonary edema in patients with bilateral renovascular disease through renal artery stent placement. Am J Hypertens 1999;12:1–7.

46. Hall JE, Guyton AC, Jackson TE, Coleman TG, Lohmeier TE, Trippodo NC. Control of glomerular filtration rate by renin-angiotensin system. Am J Physiol 1977;233:F366–72.

47. Hricik DE, Browning PJ, Kopelman R, Goorno WE, Madias NE, Dzau VJ. Captopril-induced functional renal insufficiency in patients with bilateral renal-artery stenosis or renal-artery stenosis in a solitary kidney. N Engl J Med 1983;308:377–81.

48. Textor SC, Tarazi RC, Novick AC, Bravo EL, Fouad FM. Regulation of renal hemodynamics and glomerular filtration in patients with renovascular hypertension during converting enzyme inhibition with captopril. Am J Med 1984;76:29–37.

49. Lerman L, Textor SC. Pathophysiology of ischemic nephropathy. Urol Clin North Am 2001;28:793–803.

50. Nath KA, Croatt AJ, Haggard JJ, Grande JP. Renal response to repetitive exposure to heme proteins: chronic injury induced by an acute insult. Kidney Int 2000;57:2423–33.

51. Neyses L, Nouskas J, Luyken J, et al. Induction of immediate-early genes by angiotensin II and endothelin-1 in adult rat cardiomyocytes. J Hypertens 1993;11:927–34.

52. Zou LX, Imig JD, von Thun AM, Hymel A, Ono H, Navar LG. Receptor-mediated intrarenal angiotensin II augmentation in angiotensin II-infused rats. Hypertension 1996;28:669–77.

53. Geiger H, Fierlbeck W, Mai B, et al. Effects of early and late antihypertensive treatment on extracellular matrix proteins and mononuclear cells in uninephrectomized SHR. Kidney Int 1997;51:750–61.

54. Napoli C, Lerman LO. Involvement of oxidation-sensitive mechanisms in the cardiovascular effects of hypercholesterolemia. Mayo Clin Proc 2001;76:619–31.

313

CHAPTER
25 Evaluation of Renovascular Hypertension

Thomas T Terramani and Elliot L Chaikof

KEY POINTS

- Systemic hypertension affects 20% of the adult population.

- Renal artery occlusive disease is present in 5% of the hypertensive population.

- A high index of suspicion along with careful history and clinical examination will continue to provide the initial guidepost in determining whether additional anatomic or functional studies are warranted.

- Duplex, CT, MR, and conventional angiography all have inherent strengths and weaknesses in the evaluation of renal artery disease.

- Bilateral renal artery disease limits the usefulness of all functional studies of renovascular hypertension.

INTRODUCTION

Systemic hypertension affects roughly 20% of the adult population. Renovascular hypertension caused by atherosclerosis or fibromuscular dysplasia of the main renal artery remains the most common treatable form of secondary hypertension, accounting for up to 5% of the hypertensive population. Perhaps of equal significance, renovascular disease may be an important cause of renal insufficiency in up to 15% of patients with dialysis-dependent end-stage renal disease.[1,2] Thus, the primary motivation for screening symptomatic patients for renovascular occlusive disease and for pursuing catheter- or surgical-based interventions is the benefit derived from improved control of hypertension and preservation of renal function.

However, renal revascularization by either modality is not without risk. Moreover, while recent reviews have documented that renal revascularization improves blood pressure control in the majority of treated patients, there has been a noticeable decline in reported cure rates for hypertension, with a significant proportion of patients unable to obtain substantial benefit. For example, in areas of renal scarring, renin synthesis may be heterogeneous if glomerular perfusion is compromised from an adjacent area of infarction. Therefore, correction of renal artery stenosis (RAS) may not improve hypertension in a case where hyperrenin production varies at the inter-nephron level. Overall, significant uncertainty remains in predicting which patients are most likely to benefit from intervention, and further refinement of diagnostic tools is certainly required. Despite these current challenges, efforts to identify whether an occlusive lesion of the renal artery is both hemodynamically and functionally significant remains the best mechanism for optimizing the success of any intervention.

IDENTIFYING SUSCEPTIBLE PATIENT POPULATIONS

All patients with hypertension should have a careful history taking and physical examination, along with urinalysis and measurement of serum electrolytes and creatinine. Serum electrolytes may be helpful if primary hyperaldosteronism is suspected as the cause of the hypertension, and serum creatinine may indicate the presence of concomitant ischemic nephropathy. In short, the diagnosis of renovascular disease should be entertained in any patient who exhibits acute worsening of previously well-controlled hypertension, malignant hypertension, or new-onset hypertension after the age of 55 years. Likewise, significant asymmetry in kidney size, unexplained renal dysfunction, or a deterioration of renal function that is precipitated by angiotensin-converting enzyme (ACE) inhibitors should also initiate an evaluation for renovascular disease. Clinical predictors of renovascular hypertension are summarized in **Table 25.1**. Notably, the incidence of renal artery occlusive disease (>50% luminal stenosis) may be as a high as 20% among patients with clinical evidence of peripheral vascular,[3] coronary artery,[4] and aortoiliac disease.[5] As one might expect, the utility and predictive value of non-invasive diagnostic screening improves when applied to symptomatic patients at greatest risk. In general terms, non-invasive tests for evaluating renovascular disease can be subdivided into anatomic and physiologic studies.

DIAGNOSTIC ANATOMIC STUDIES

The development of an ideal screening study for renovascular disease has been driven by a desire to obtain a non-invasive and cost-effective tool that has both a high level of specificity and sensitivity, as well as an attendant low complication rate. While a perfect diagnostic study does not exist, many of the objectives of an ideal test are being approached by the three commonly available non-invasive screening techniques that assess renal artery anatomy: renal duplex ultrasonography (RDU), computed tomography angiography (CTA), and magnetic resonance angiography (MRA). Significantly, none of these imaging modalities require a procedural change in hypertensive medication or diet.

Renal duplex ultrasonography

Renal artery duplex combines B-mode imaging with Doppler ultrasound velocity measurements of blood flow. In addition, a measure of kidney size, as well as an assessment of intrinsic small

Clinical predictors of renovascular hypertension.
Predictors of hypertension
Accelerated or malignant hypertension (any age group)
Acute onset or worsening of hypertension (any age group)
Severe hypertension in a child or young adult (suggestive of FMD)
Severe hypertension at >50 years of age (suggestive of atherosclerosis)
Onset of hypertension before age 20 or after age 55
Hypertension refractory to three or more antihypertensive agents
Predictors of impaired excretory renal function
Impairment of renal function associated with ACE inhibitor therapy
Hypertension with unexplained impairment of renal function
Unilateral reduction in kidney size
Sudden worsening of renal function in a hypertensive patient
Unexplained azotemia
Other risk factors or potential indicators of renovascular disease
Unexplained congestive heart failure or acute pulmonary edema
Epigastric abdominal or flank bruit
Hypertensive retinopathy
Atherosclerotic disease in other arterial beds (carotid, coronary, extremity)
Unexplained hypokalemia in a hypertensive patient

Table 25.1 Clinical predictors of renovascular hypertension.
ACE, angiotensin-converting enzyme; FMD, fibromuscular dysplasia.

Criteria for significant (>60%) renal artery stenosis.
Renal artery peak systolic velocity >180cm/s
Ratio of the renal artery peak systolic velocity to aorta peak systolic velocity >3.5
Turbulent flow in the poststenotic area of the renal artery
Arterial occlusion is indicated by the failure to obtain a Doppler signal from an imaged (B-mode) renal artery

Table 25.2 Criteria for significant (>60%) renal artery stenosis.

proximal high-grade stenosis can often be inferred by identifying a *tardus* or *parvus* waveform in the distal vessels. Duplex criteria for defining RAS are summarized in **Table 25.2**.

Since the mere presence of a stenosis does not ensure that treatment will lead to a clinical response, recent investigations have sought to identify duplex criteria for predicting a positive outcome after renal artery intervention. Radermacher and associates[9] have proposed the use of a renal artery resistance index (RI) where:

$$RI = (1 - [\text{end-diastolic velocity/maximal systolic velocity}]) \times 100$$

In a prospective analysis of 138 patients who underwent renal artery angioplasty or surgery, a renal resistance index of greater than 80 reliably identified patients who did not respond to renal artery revascularization by an improvement in renal function, blood pressure, or kidney survival.[9] While a potentially useful tool, the renal artery resistance index may be falsely elevated in patients with decreased cardiac output.

Although duplex imaging continues to play an important role in screening for clinically significant renovascular disease, it bears emphasis that if the clinical index of suspicion remains high, further imaging studies should be pursued despite a negative duplex scan. Indeed, a recent meta-analysis of 63 studies demonstrated that both CTA and MRA were associated with a better diagnostic yield and accuracy than renal duplex scanning.[10]

Computed tomography angiography

In prospective comparisons with conventional angiography, CTA has proven to be a reliable and accurate modality for evaluating the presence of renovascular disease.[11,12] With appropriate contrast administration and image reconstruction, CTA can be expected to detect a luminal stenosis of >50% with a sensitivity and specificity of 89% and 98%, respectively. An evolving technology is electron beam CT scanners, which enable quantification of intrarenal hemodynamics and segmental nephron dynamics, and renal function.[13] Therefore, this developing technology may provide both anatomic and functional information regarding a RAS lesion. Nonetheless, helical or spiral CTA is inapplicable for patients with marginal renal function, and, as previously implied, adequate bolus, appropriate injection-to-scan delay, and suitable acquisition properties, such as collimation, acquisition time, pitch, and reconstruction interval, are critical for an optimal study. Additional limitations include the presence of arterial wall calcification, a lengthy post-procedure processing time, and the potential for inadequate visualization of accessory renal arteries.

vessel renovascular disease, can be obtained. However, an inability to accurately identify multiple or accessory renal arteries, as well as lesions in the distal branches, are acknowledged limitations of duplex scanning. This can result in up to a 20% false-negative rate when the main renal artery is found to be normal, despite the presence of an undetected significant stenosis in an accessory artery.[6] A further drawback comprises prolonged examination times, which may approach 45 to 60 minutes, with body habitus an important determinant of the level of technical difficulty. While widespread experience remains limited, the continued development of intravenous ultrasound contrast agents might prove to be an important adjunct in enhancing diagnostic accuracy and reducing technical difficulty of duplex ultrasound.

Characteristically, renal artery duplex imaging is performed after an overnight fast, to minimize the presence of bowel gas and abdominal distention. The entire length of the renal artery is examined, with an increase in velocity indicative of a significant stenosis. In this regard, two recent reports have demonstrated that a peak systolic velocity above 180–200cm/s is a reliable indicator of a stenosis that exceeds 60%, with greater than 90% sensitivity.[7,8] Analysis of the acceleration time, acceleration index, and waveform pattern can also provide a measure of the significance of a stenotic lesion. For example, the presence of a

CTA is clearly less operator-dependent than ultrasound and the technology is continuing to improve.

Magnetic resonance imaging/angiography

The use of the gadolinium-enhanced gradient echo technique has improved the accuracy of MRA, which does not require either ionizing radiation or a nephrotoxic contrast agent. Moreover, MRA can be safely performed in the presence of significant renal insufficiency. Validation studies for MRA have reported sensitivities of >95% and specificities of >90%.[14,15] In addition, MRA is superior to duplex ultrasound in visualizing accessory renal arteries.[16] Significantly, MRA may also play a role in the physiologic assessment of renovascular disease by determining gadolinium clearance (glomerular filtration) and renal artery blood flow.[17,18] In this regard, a recent report demonstrated that MR-based measurements of renal artery flow relative to renal parenchymal volume were predictive of clinical outcome after renal artery angioplasty.[19] Notably, MRA is associated with a high sensitivity or few false-negatives, lending itself as an important tool for screening for RAS. Nonetheless, differentiating between a moderate and severe stenosis may be difficult and MRA is contraindicated for patients with claustrophobia, pacemakers, or other non-MRA-compatible metallic implants.

Contrast angiography

Contrast angiography remains the gold standard for documenting an anatomic lesion of the renal artery. It provides an excellent means to assess the presence of multiple renal arteries, and pressure gradients can be obtained to document whether a lesion may be hemodynamically significant. Typically, a stenosis is considered significant if there is a diameter reduction of greater than 50% or if the peak systolic blood pressure gradient exceeds 15%. Angiography can also be used to evaluate renal dimensions, as well as the presence of associated aneurysmal and occlusive disease of the aorta. All of this information may be important in the decision for and selection of an interventional plan. Established drawbacks of angiography, however, include procedural expense, puncture site complications, contrast-induced nephrotoxicity, and renal artery embolization. In this respect, the Cooperative Study of Renovascular Hypertension demonstrated a mortality rate of 0.11%, a major morbidity rate of 1.2%, and a minor morbidity rate of 2.7% following conventional angiography in 2374 patients.[20] As anticipated, patients at greatest risk of contrast-induced nephrotoxicity were those with diabetes and renal insufficiency. Minimizing contrast load, selective use of carbon dioxide[21] or gadolinium,[22] as well as hydration and prophylaxis with oral acetylcysteine (600mg twice daily), initiated 24 hours prior to the study and continued for an additional 24 hours,[23] all assist in reducing the incidence of this complication.

In summary, conventional angiography remains an important component for identifying a potentially treatable lesion, especially when clinical suspicion remains and other non-invasive diagnostic modalities have proven inadequate or technically incomplete.

DIAGNOSTIC FUNCTIONAL STUDIES OF HISTORIC SIGNIFICANCE

The development of studies to assess the functional significance of a renovascular lesion has been primarily motivated by an effort to select physiologically and anatomically significant lesions in which therapeutic intervention would have the greatest likelihood of achieving a beneficial clinical outcome.

Intravenous pyelography (IVP)

Rapid-sequence IVP was widely used in the 1960s and 1970s as a screening test for RAS by detecting differences in kidney size, delay in contrast agent appearance in the caliceal system, and a persistent nephrogram with hyperconcentration of contrast agent on delayed images.[24] The high incidence of false-positive and false-negative studies, especially among patients with bilateral disease, along with a significant contrast load requirement, dampened the early enthusiasm for this approach.

Peripheral plasma renin activity

Renin levels in the peripheral venous blood have been measured in an effort to detect a hyperrenin state due to renovascular disease. Unfortunately, plasma renin activity may be suppressed by a high salt intake and antihypertensive drug therapy, and has a known diurnal variation.[25] Thus, this test is associated with a low sensitivity and specificity and has no role in the evaluation of renovascular hypertension.

Split renal function studies

Split renal function studies measure the excretory capacity of each kidney by selective ureteral catheterization. In principle, the presence of RAS results in a reduction of renal blood flow with an increase in reabsorption of sodium and water in the affected kidney. As a consequence, the presence of a functionally significant lesion is suspected if urine flow is reduced by 40–60%, urinary sodium concentration is decreased by 15%, or the concentration of non-reabsorbable substances is increased by 50–100%.[26] The invasive nature of this test has limited its current use in clinical practice.

DIAGNOSTIC FUNCTIONAL STUDIES IN CURRENT USE

Captopril renography (CRS)

Captopril renography, also known as ACE inhibitor scintigraphy, is the only imaging modality that directly tests for the presence of renovascular hypertension. This examination consists of two sequential renograms prior to and following administration of an ACE inhibitor, and provides a comparative measurement of renal artery blood flow and excretion. When an ACE inhibitor is administered, the synthesis of angiotensin II is reduced, diminishing efferent arteriole vasoconstriction and thus causing a decrease in the glomerular filtration pressure. The reduction in the glomerular filtration rate results in a decrease in renal uptake of the filtered radioactive tracer, either technetium-99m diethylenetriaminepentaacetic acid (99mTc-DTPA) or mercaptoacetyltriglycine (99mTc-MAG3), with a delay in tubular transit time. In a collected series of 12 reports, the sensitivity and specificity of CRS in detecting RAS was 92.5% and 92.2%, respectively.[27] Details of a proposed system for grading the probability of functionally significant renovascular disease are detailed elsewhere.[28–30] CRS is an ideal test in young to middle-aged patients with normal renal function and unilateral disease. However, accuracy is reduced by the presence of renal insufficiency or bilateral RAS, and in patients on chronic ACE inhibitors or angiotensin II receptor blockers. Additionally, adequate hydration together with the cessation of diuretics, ACE inhibitors, and angiotensin II receptor blockers is required at least 3 to 7 days prior to the study.

Stimulated plasma renin activity (captopril test)

While random plasma renin levels are of limited diagnostic value, the measurement of serum plasma renin activity after captopril dosing does improve the diagnostic sensitivity and specificity of this test.[31,32] Typically, testing is performed 1 hour after an oral dose of 25mg of captopril or 15 minutes after an intravenous dose of 0.04mg/kg of enalapril maleate. The captopril test reportedly can detect both unilateral and bilateral RAS. Its limitations are reduced utility in patients with azotemia and the need to stop all ACE inhibitors and angiotensin II receptor antagonists prior to testing.

Renal vein renin assays

Renal vein renin assays may occasionally be helpful in assessing the functional significance of a RAS. In their original report, Vaughan and associates[33] measured renal vein renin secretion in patients with unilateral RAS and found increased secretion of renin by the affected kidney together with suppressed secretion in the contralateral kidney. This test has a high specificity but a low sensitivity in predicting an improvement or cure after intervention.[34,35] Specifically, this study is generally unreliable in the presence of bilateral renal artery disease or a solitary kidney. Its widespread use has also been limited by its expense and need for selective renal vein catheterization. It is also necessary for patients to stop all antihypertensives for 5 to 7 days and limit sodium intake to less than 2g per day for 2 weeks prior to the study. If hypertension is poorly controlled, bed rest may be required along with a calcium channel blocker and/or a diuretic.

CURRENT RECOMMENDATIONS

Renovascular hypertension is a potentially curable disease, but a single screening method does not exist that is capable of identifying those lesions in which percutaneous or operative treatment will predictably lead to either cure or an improvement in clinical status. Therefore, at this time, it remains difficult to advocate widespread screening for renovascular disease in all patients who present with hypertension. A high index of suspicion among patients at risk along with a careful history and clinical examination will continue to provide the initial guidepost in determining whether additional anatomic or functional studies are warranted. Should further evaluation be deemed appropriate, RDU and MRA are the best available screening methods for detecting RAS. In assessing the physiologic significance of a unilateral lesion, we currently utilize captopril renography. However, we believe that as MRA technology evolves, with anticipated reductions in costs and improvements in its ability to obtain both anatomic and functional information, it may supplant other studies as the acknowledged primary screening method for renovascular disease. Finally, it is important to note an exception to these guidelines. In a patient in whom there is a strong suspicion of fibromuscular dysplasia, we would proceed directly to contrast angiography, which provides the best information for a process that may be difficult to detect by ultrasonography or MRA and most commonly affects the mid to distal renal arteries and accessory branches.

REFERENCES

1. O'Neil EA, Hansen KJ, Canzanello VJ, Pennell TC, Dean RH. Prevalence of ischemic nephropathy in patients with renal insufficiency. Am Surg 1992;58:485–90.
2. Rimmer JM, Gennari FJ. Atherosclerotic renovascular disease and progressive renal failure. Ann Intern Med 1993;118:712–9.
3. Wachtell K, Ibsen H, Olsen MH, et al. Prevalence of renal artery stenosis in patients with peripheral vascular disease and hypertension. J Hum Hypertens 1996;10:83–5.
4. Harding MB, Smith LR, Himmelstein SI, et al. Renal artery stenosis: prevalence and associated risk factors in patients undergoing routine cardiac catheterization. J Am Soc Nephrol 1992;2:1608–16.
5. Miralles M, Corominas A, Cotillas J, Castro F, Clara A, Vidal-Barraquer F. Screening for carotid and renal artery stenoses in patients with aortoiliac disease. Ann Vasc Surg 1998;12:17–22.
6. Zierler RE. Is duplex scanning the best screening test for renal artery stenosis? Semin Vasc Surg 2001;14:177–85.
7. Hua HT, Hood DB, Jensen CC, Hanks SE, Weaver FA. The use of colorflow duplex scanning to detect significant renal artery stenosis. Ann Vasc Surg 2000;14:118–24.
8. Motew SJ, Cherr GS, Craven TE, et al. Renal duplex sonography: main renal artery versus hilar analysis. J Vasc Surg 2000;32:462–9; 469–71.
9. Radermacher J, Chavan A, Bleck J, et al. Use of Doppler ultrasonography to predict the outcome of therapy for renal-artery stenosis. N Engl J Med 2001;344:410–7.
10. Vasbinder GB, Nelemans PJ, Kessels AG, Kroon AA, de Leeuw PW, van Engelshoven JM. Diagnostic tests for renal artery stenosis in patients suspected of having renovascular hypertension: a meta-analysis. Ann Intern Med 2001;135:401–11.
11. Elkohen M, Beregi JP, Deklunder G, Artaud D, Mounier-Vehier C, Carre AG. A prospective study of helical computed tomography angiography versus angiography for the detection of renal artery stenoses in hypertensive patients. J Hypertens 1996;14:525–8.
12. Kim TS, Chung JW, Park JH, Kim SH, Yeon KM, Han MC. Renal artery evaluation: comparison of spiral CT angiography to intra-arterial DSA. J Vasc Interv Radiol 1998;9:553–9.
13. Romero JC, Lerman LO. Novel noninvasive techniques for studying renal function in man. Semin Nephrol 2000;20:456–62.
14. Bakker J, Beek FJ, Beutler JJ, et al. Renal artery stenosis and accessory renal arteries: accuracy of detection and visualization with gadolinium-enhanced breath-hold MR angiography. Radiology 1998;207:497–504.
15. De Cobelli F, Vanzulli A, Sironi S, et al. Renal artery stenosis: evaluation with breath-hold, three-dimensional, dynamic, gadolinium-enhanced versus three-dimensional, phase-contrast MR angiography. Radiology 1997;205:689–95.
16. De Cobelli F, Venturini M, Vanzulli A, et al. Renal arterial stenosis: prospective comparison of color Doppler US and breath-hold, three-dimensional, dynamic, gadolinium-enhanced MR angiography. Radiology 2000;214:373–80.
17. Grist TM. Magnetic resonance angiography of renal artery stenosis. Am J Kidney Dis 1994;24:700–12.
18. Niendorf ER, Grist TM, Lee FT Jr, Brazy PC, Santyr GE. Rapid in vivo measurement of single-kidney extraction fraction and glomerular filtration rate with MR imaging. Radiology 1998;206:791–8.
19. Binkert CA, Debatin JF, Schneider E, et al. Can MR measurement of renal artery flow and renal volume predict the outcome of percutaneous transluminal renal angioplasty? Cardiovasc Intervent Radiol 2001; 24:233–9.
20. Oliva VL, Soulez G, Lesage D, et al. Detection of renal artery stenosis with Doppler sonography before and after administration of captopril: value of early systolic rise. AJR Am J Roentgenol 1998;170:169–75.

21. Schreier DZ, Weaver FA, Frankhouse J, et al. A prospective study of carbon dioxide-digital subtraction vs standard contrast arteriography in the evaluation of the renal arteries. Arch Surg 1996;131:503–7; discussion 507–8.

22. Matchett WJ, McFarland DR, Russell DK, Sailors DM, Moursi MM. Azotemia: gadopentetate dimeglumine as contrast agent at digital subtraction angiography. Radiology 1996;201:569–71.

23. Tepel M, van der Giet M, Schwarzfeld C, Laufer U, Liermann D, Zidek W. Prevention of radiographic-contrast-agent-induced reductions in renal function by acetylcysteine. N Engl J Med 2000;343:180–4.

24. Bookstein JJ, Abrams HL, Buenger RE, et al. Radiologic aspects of renovascular hypertension. 2. The role of urography in unilateral renovascular disease. JAMA 1972;220:1225–30.

25. Rossi GP, Pavan E, Chiesura-Corona M, et al. Renovascular hypertension with low-to-normal plasma renin: clinical and angiographic features. Clin Sci (Lond) 1997;93:435–43.

26. Dossetor JB, Fam W, Gutelius JR, Turgeon-Knaack C, Morehouse DD. Differential renal function studies in the diagnosis of renal hypertension. Can Med Assoc J 1970;102:500–4.

27. Taylor A. Functional testing: ACEI renography. Semin Nephrol 2000; 20:437–44.

28. Oei HY. Captopril renography. Early observations and diagnostic criteria. Am J Hypertens 1991;4(12 Pt 2):678S–684S.

29. Nally JV Jr, Chen C, Fine E, et al. Diagnostic criteria of renovascular hypertension with captopril renography. A consensus statement. Am J Hypertens 1991;4(12 Pt 2):749S–752S.

30. Taylor A, Nally J, Aurell M, et al. Consensus report on ACE inhibitor renography for detecting renovascular hypertension. Radionuclides in Nephrourology Group. Consensus Group on ACEI Renography. J Nucl Med 1996;37:1876–82.

31. Muller FB, Sealey JE, Case DB, et al. The captopril test for identifying renovascular disease in hypertensive patients. Am J Med 1986;80:633–44.

32. Frederickson ED, Wilcox CS, Bucci M, et al. A prospective evaluation of a simplified captopril test for the detection of renovascular hypertension. Arch Intern Med 1990;150:569–72.

33. Vaughan ED Jr, Buhler FR, Laragh JH, Sealey JE, Baer L, Bard RH. Renovascular hypertension: renin measurements to indicate hypersecretion and contralateral suppression, estimate renal plasma flow, and score for surgical curability. Am J Med 1973;55:402–14.

34. Sellars L, Shore AC, Wilkinson R. Renal vein renin studies in renovascular hypertension – do they really help? J Hypertens 1985;3:177–81.

35. Pickering TG, Sos TA, Vaughan ED Jr, et al. Predictive value and changes of renin secretion in hypertensive patients with unilateral renovascular disease undergoing successful renal angioplasty. Am J Med 1984;76:398–404.

CHAPTER
26 Treatment of Renovascular Disease

Treatment of Renovascular Disease: Medical Therapy

Paul N Harden

KEY POINTS

- Atherosclerotic renal artery disease is common in arteriopaths.

- Vascular co-morbidity and mortality is high.

- Two year mortality is greater than many cancers at 38%.

- Tight lipid and blood pressure control should be standard therapy.

- Cardioprotective medical therapy should be utilized where possible.

- Angiotensin Converting Enzyme Inhibitors and Angiotensin II Receptor blocking agents are the antihypertensive therapy of first choice and can be used safely to control blood pressure in most cases.

- Non-pharmacological measures should be applied to reduce cardiovascular risk, e.g. smoking cessation, weight reduction.

- No direct evidence for benefit of medical therapy on clinical outcomes in renovascular disease, although most patients have systemic arterial disease meriting medical modulation of cardiovascular risk factors.

- Interventional radiological therapy is of controversial benefit in most cases: Trial outcomes are awaited.

INTRODUCTION

Atherosclerotic renal artery stenosis (ARAS) is an important rare cause of hypertension and is increasingly recognized as a cause of progressive renal insufficiency.[1] The proximal part (first 10mm) of the renal artery and the adjacent aorta (**Fig. 26a.1**) are primarily involved in 85% of cases;[2] thus, the disease should be more correctly termed aorto-renal atheroclerotic disease. The aorta is always diffusely involved with atherosclerotic disease, except in the extremely rare case of fibromuscular dysplasia causing more distal renal artery stenosis, which is frequently multiple (**Fig. 26a.2**). Progressive renal damage may also result from cholesterol embolization from the aorta or proximal renal artery,[3] and disease of intermediate and small renal vessels.

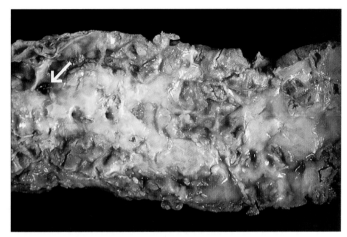

Figure 26a.1 Generalized aortic atheroma associated with circumferential stenosis of the right renal artery with patent Palmaz stent (arrow).

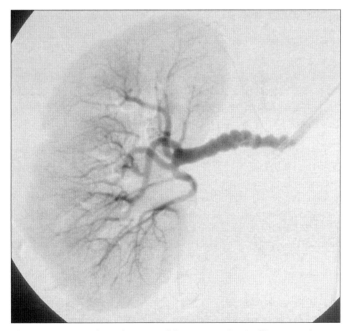

Figure 26a.2 Multiple distal arterial stenoses due to fibromuscular dysplasia shown on selective renal angiography.

Atherosclerotic renovascular disease (ARVD) is associated with systemic vascular disease[4] and commonly coexists with significant coronary, carotid, or peripheral arterial disease.[5] The heavy burden of generalized atherosclerosis results in a high mortality rate – ranging from 29.7% at 3 years[4] to 38% at 2 years[5] – predominantly due to fatal cardiac events. The absolute risk of

Medical therapeutic approaches to atherosclerotic renal artery disease.
• Blood pressure control
• Lipid-lowering therapy
• Antiplatelet agent
• Cessation of tobacco smoking

Table 26a.1 Medical therapeutic approaches to atherosclerotic renal artery disease.

concomitant cardiovascular disease is heavily influenced by risk factors including age, gender, blood pressure (BP), and serum lipids.[6]

Medical treatment aims to prevent or retard further progression of atherosclerosis locally in the aorto-renal arterial tree and systemically, to minimize the risks of progressive renal ischemia and mortality. Moreover, aggressive medical therapy has been shown to cause regression of atherosclerosis in other vascular beds.[7] Cardiovascular risk factor modification including effective BP control is the cornerstone of current therapeutic strategies (**Table 26a.1**). This chapter will outline the therapeutic approaches currently available that should be applied to all patients with ARVD irrespective of whether revascularization is performed.

MEDICAL THERAPEUTIC OPTIONS

Medical therapy is targeted at modification of atherogenic risk factors (**Table 26a.1**).

Hypertension

Persistent uncontrolled hypertension is an important cause of increased cardiovascular morbidity and mortality.[8,9] A kidney supplied by a normal renal artery in unilateral ARVD will be at risk of progressive end-organ damage due to hypertension. Hypertensive renal damage may result whenever glomeruli are subjected to elevated perfusion pressures, which can occur even in the presence of a functionally insignificant proximal ARAS. Once the ARAS exceeds 70%, perfusion of the distal glomeruli is reduced, resulting in the production of renin by the juxta-glomerular apparatus and activation of the renin–angiotensin system (**Fig. 26a.3**). The resultant angiotensin II causes efferent arteriolar constriction to preserve glomerular perfusion and filtration, together with systemic vasoconstriction, with resultant renovascular hypertension. Angiotensin-converting enzyme inhibitors (ACEIs) and angiotensin II receptor blocking agents (ARBs) are effective and safe antihypertensive agents in renovascular disease (**Fig. 26a.3**) while total glomerular filtration is not critically dependent on renal perfusion maintained by the activated renin–angiotensin system.[4,10,11] There are potentially additional beneficial effects of ACEIs in ARAS, as these agents cause reduced proteinuria[12] and reduced glomerular scarring in a variety of renal diseases.[13,14] Introduction of these agents has greatly improved target BP control in renovascular hypertension: 35.3% achieved a target BP <140/90mmHg and 57.4% a BP <160/95mmHg, exceeding the national average of 24% of patients with treated essential hypertension in the USA who achieve target BP.[15] Caution and close clinical supervision is

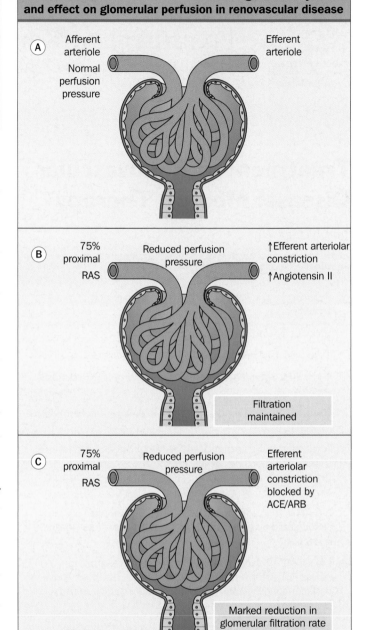

Figure 26a.3 Activation and blockade of the Renin-Angiotensin System and effect on glomerular perfusion in renovascular disease. (A) Normal renal perfusion. (B) Maintenance of glomerular perfusion by Angiotensin II mediated efferent arteriolar constriction when renal artery perfusion is reduced in significant renal artery disease. (C) Adverse effect of ACE/ARB on renal perfusion in significant proximal renovascular disease.

required in patients with renal failure (baseline serum creatinine >130μmol/L; glomerular filtration rate <70mL/min). Serial serum creatinine and potassium levels should be monitored before and 5 and 10 days after initiation of ACEIs or ARBs and thereafter every 4–6 months at clinical review. An initial rise in the serum creatinine of >15% is suspicious of functional renal artery disease, and the ACEI or ARB should be discontinued.[16] An acute deterioration in renal function can also occur in individuals with stable subcritical renal artery disease on ACEIs who develop dehydration with intravascular volume depletion

Range of antihypertensives, with details of mode of action.			
Drug class – example	*Mode of action*	*Key side effects*	*Dose in CRF*
Beta-blocker – atenolol, metoprolol	Selective beta$_1$-blockade	Lethargy, bronchospasm	50% decrease
Alpha-blocker – doxazosin	Postsynaptic alpha-blockade	Edema, orthostatic hypotension	Nil
Calcium channel antagonist – nifedipine, amlodipine	Blockade of T-type channel	Edema, headaches	Nil
ACEI – enalapril, lisinopril	Inhibit ACE	Raised K^+, cough	Caution, watch K^+
ARB – losartan	Block angiotensin II receptors	Raised K^+	Caution, watch K^+
Diuretic – furosemide	Natriuresis	Hyperuricemia, hyperglycemia	Increased doses

Table 26a.2 Range of antihypertensives, with details of mode of action. ACE, angiotensin-converting enzyme; ACEI, ACE inhibitor; ARB, angiotensin II receptor blocking agent; K^+, potassium.

due to gastrointestinal fluid losses or excessive use of diuretic therapy.[16] Patients with atherosclerotic renal artery disease taking ACEIs or ARBs should be advised to withhold these drugs at times of gastrointestinal disturbances and seek medical advice early. The acute deterioration in renal function is usually reversible with adequate fluid repletion and temporary suspension of the ACEI/ARB. Once renal function has recovered following the acute episode, the ACEI/ARB can usually be safely re-introduced with close monitoring of serum creatinine and potassium. Recurrent acute renal insufficiency would suggest the development of critical renal artery stenosis, requiring further investigation and contraindicating ACEI/ARB use.

Frequently, more than one agent will be required to achieve target BP control. A loop diuretic is an effective adjuvant to ACEI/ARB therapy, through promotion of increased sodium excretion in the nephron. Loop diuretics have a good dose–response curve in progressive renal failure, while thiazide diuretics are less effective in moderate-to-severe chronic renal failure. The range of antihypertensives that can be employed, with details of mode of action, are shown in **Table 26a.2**. Beta-adrenoreceptor blockers can be used in the absence of critical peripheral vascular disease, and may have a beneficial effect on cardiac function in the presence of concurrent myocardial damage. Doses should be reduced in elderly patients or those with renal failure due to impaired excretion.

Non-pharmacologic measures of BP reduction should be actively employed, but are rarely sufficient alone in achieving target BP control.[17] Targeted weight reduction to a body mass index corrected for age should be encouraged, coupled with reduction of salt intake, moderation of alcohol consumption and increased regular exercise. It is essential to involve a dedicated dietician in the multidisciplinary team.

Target blood pressure

Many studies have demonstrated a reduction in cardiovascular morbidity and mortality achieved by good BP control.[18] Consensus groups in Europe and North America have developed target BP levels for the treatment of hypertension.[19,20] These targets (**Table 26a.3**) are derived from the treatment of essential hypertension but are likely to have at least an equal beneficial effect in renovascular hypertension. Generalized atherosclerotic disease is associated with stiffening of the major arterial tree, with reduced compliance and an increased incidence of systolic hypertension.

Guidelines for the treatment of hypertension.

1. Joint British Recommendations

Lifestyle targets for all patients:
Stop smoking
Increase aerobic exercise
Moderate alcohol intake
BMI <25kg/m^2 is desirable
Make healthier food choices

Target blood pressure:
<140mmHg systolic and <85mmHg diastolic
(diabetic: <130mmHg systolic and <80mmHg diastolic)

Target lipids:
Total cholesterol <5mmol/L: LDL cholesterol <3mmol/L

Cardioprotective drug treatment:
Aspirin, 75mg daily, for all patients
Beta-blockers post MI for >3 years
Statins at doses used in clinical trials
ACEIs in heart failure post MI or ejection fraction <40%
Anticoagulants – large anterior infarcts, severe heart failure

2. US Guidelines: Joint National Committee

	Blood pressure (systolic/diastolic) (mmHg)		
	130–139/85–89	140–159/90–99	>160/100
Risk group A*	Modify lifestyle	Modify lifestyle	Drug therapy
Risk group B†	Modify lifestyle	Modify lifestyle up to 6 months	Drug therapy
Risk group C†	Drug therapy	Drug therapy	Drug therapy

* Risk group A: no risk factors, target organ damage, or complications
† Risk group B: at least one risk factor; no target damage or complications
† Risk group C: target organ damage/complications +/– diabetes

Table 26a.3 Guidelines for the treatment of hypertension.
ACEIs, angiotensin-converting enzyme inhibitors; BMI, body mass index; LDL, low-density lipoprotein; MI, myocardial infarction.

First-line therapy should include an ACEI or ARB, with a loop diuretic if required. This regimen is well tolerated in the majority of patients with subcritical ARAS and may control BP alone. Many patients with ARAS are elderly and therefore more susceptible to postural hypotension, which can limit the use of vasodilating agents. Frequently, these arteriopaths have concurrent coronary artery disease, which may require specific therapy with selective β-blockade, nitrate, and calcium-channel blockade. All of these agents have useful antihypertensive properties that will contribute to target BP control. Individuals who continue to have poor BP control despite the use of three or four antihypertensive agents may have poor drug compliance or, rarely, require the addition of centrally acting antihypertensives. Refractory hypertension is seldom controlled by revascularization procedures[21] unless a critical level of stenosis has developed causing ipsilateral impairment of glomerular filtration and resultant intolerance of ACEIs and ARBs. In this specific circumstance, successful revascularization can afford the safe re-introduction of ACEIs or ARBs with effective BP control.[11]

Lipid-lowering therapy

Patients with atherosclerotic renal artery disease have a high incidence of coexisting ischemic heart disease, cerebrovascular disease, and peripheral vascular disease. Compelling evidence from large multicenter trials of control of total and low-density lipoprotein (LDL) cholesterol with lipid-lowering therapy shows a significant reduction in secondary cardiovascular events and mortality.[22,23] However, no direct evidence supports an effect of lipid control on the progression of renal artery disease; tight control of total and LDL cholesterol is justified to reduce cardiovascular morbidity and mortality. Hemorrhage into unstable atheromatous plaques may result in rupture, surface thrombosis, and a reduction of functional vessel diameter. There is a pool of lipid in atheromatous plaques that is amenable to removal with lipid-lowering therapy.[24] Target cholesterol levels have been set in Europe[25] and North America (**Table 26a.3**). The majority of patients with renal artery disease have elevation of total cholesterol and the LDL fraction, with a detrimentally low high-density lipoprotein (HDL) fraction,[26] except in individuals with coexisting diabetes mellitus, who often have hypertriglyceridemia. Dietary modification is rarely successful, as rigorous dietary compliance can only reduce cholesterol levels by 10%. The majority of patients will require specific drug therapy to achieve target cholesterol levels.

Hydroxymethylglutaryl (HMG) CoA reductase inhibitors effectively reduce total and LDL cholesterol, with some increase in HDL cholesterol, and have a lesser effect on the reduction of triglycerides. HMG-CoA reductase inhibitors (statins) promote stabilization of atherosclerotic plaques by multiple effects, including inhibition of cholesterol synthesis in hepatocytes, inhibition of proliferation of vascular smooth muscle cells and fibroblasts, and suppression of inflammation.[27] Statins are well tolerated, although rarely they are hepatotoxic and can cause myositis. It is recommended to check serum liver enzyme levels at baseline and 2 weeks after initiation of therapy; statins should be discontinued if there is a greater than threefold rise in liver enzymes. The dose should be titrated upwards at monthly intervals until the target total and LDL cholesterol levels are achieved or the maximum daily dose is reached. Statins are potent, with an average cholesterol-lowering potential of 20–30% over baseline levels. Rarely, a fibrate is required when hypertriglyceridemia is the predominant lipid abnormality; these agents can also provoke myositis and should be used with caution in patients with chronic renal failure.

Antiplatelet therapy

Platelet activation is implicated in the pathogenesis of atherosclerosis and is associated with elevated serum levels of thromboglobulin and P-selectin.[28] Atheromatous plaques in renal artery disease, fibrinogen, and damaged endothelial cells may trigger or promote the formation of platelet thrombi, which in turn promote the local release of inflammatory cytokines and chemoattractants. Elevated fibrinogen levels correlate with the severity of peripheral vascular disease and angina.[29] Antiplatelet therapy has been shown to reduce risk of secondary events in patients with ischemic heart disease[30] and carotid arterial disease. There are no trials to directly support a beneficial effect of antiplatelet therapy on progression of renal arterial disease. However, the close association of significant coronary and peripheral vascular disease merits the administration of antiplatelet therapy in the majority of cases.

Smoking cessation

An active policy of facilitating smoking cessation should be encouraged in all patients with renovascular disease as an important means of reducing cardiovascular risk and reducing progression of generalized atherosclerosis.

Other cardiovascular risk factors

Elevated levels of serum homocysteine have been associated with cardiovascular risk and have been demonstrated in renovascular patients. Homocysteine levels can be reduced using oral folic acid,[31] although no trial data are available on outcome of reduced homocysteine levels in renal artery disease. Increasingly, generalized atherosclerosis is considered as a systemic inflammatory disease with associated elevation of inflammatory markers, including C-reactive protein.[32] A reduction in the levels of acute-phase proteins was observed in patients treated with statins and is associated with improved cardiovascular outcomes.[33] Despite much active research interest, there is no evidence to date for the use of anti-inflammatory therapy. Recently, intra-arterial recombinant basic fibroblast growth factor (FGF-2) has been shown to significantly increase peak walking time at 90 days in patients with moderate-to-severe peripheral vascular disease.[34] It is not clear whether targeted angiogenesis could improve renal ischemia in atherosclerotic renal artery disease.

THERAPEUTIC OPTIONS

All patients with atherosclerotic renal artery disease should have a thorough clinical assessment of total burden of atherosclerotic disease and appropriate cardiovascular risk factor modification. Frequently, a multidisciplinary team approach is required, with active contributions from clinicians managing cardiac, renal, neurological, and peripheral vascular disease. It is important that there is close coordination between these services to optimize holistic care, preferably with a lead clinician in a specialized vascular risk clinic.

Macrovascular renovascular disease has been shown to progress in studies utilizing sequential angiography or Doppler ultrasound; 10% of renal artery stenoses >60% occluded over 2 years on sequential Doppler studies[35] and 14% of renal artery stenoses >75% occluded over 2 years at repeat angiography.[36] Risk of progression has encouraged many centers to undertake surgical or radiologic intervention to preserve vessel patency,[37,38] although only very limited trial evidence is available to support intervention for the control of renovascular hypertension[22] and none for preservation of renal function. The natural history of ARVD is poorly understood, with a variable decline in glomerular filtration demonstrated in a group of patients with renal artery stenosis >50% bilaterally or in a solitary functioning kidney.[4] Randomized controlled trial evidence is urgently required to assess whether interventions can influence the progression of ARVD and improve clinical outcomes. There is now overwhelming clinical evidence that good BP and lipid control can markedly improve clinical outcomes in cardiovascular disease, which contraindicates randomized studies in patients with ARVD given the high proportion of such with cardiovascular co-morbidity meriting control of cardiovascular risk factors. It is essential that randomized studies are undertaken to examine the therapeutic impact and indications of revascularization procedures and assess the potential benefit of additional therapy to control newly recognized cardiovascular risk factors.

REFERENCES

1. Mailloux LU, Napolitano B, Bellucci AG, et al. Renal vascular disease causing end-stage renal disease; incidence, clinical correlates and outcomes: a 20 year clinical experience. Am J Kidney Dis 1994;24:622–9.
2. Greco BA, Breyer JA. Atherosclerotic ischemic renal disease. Am J Kidney Dis 1997;29:176–87.
3. Meyrier A, Buchet P, Simon P, et al. Atheromatous renal disease. Am J Med 1988;85:139–46.
4. Chabova V, Schirger A, Stanson AW, McKusick MA, Textor SC. Outcomes of atherosclerotic renal artery stenosis managed without revascularization. Mayo Clin Proc 2000;75:437–44.
5. Baboolal K, Evans C, Moore RH. Incidence of end-stage renal disease in medically treated patients with severe bilateral atherosclerotic renovascular disease. Am J Kidney Dis 1998;31:971–7.
6. Anderson KV, Odell PM, Wilson PWF, Kannel WB. Cardiovascular disease risk profiles. Am Heart J 1991;121:293–8.
7. Loscalzo J. Regression of coronary atherosclerosis. N Engl J Med 1990;323:337–9.
8. MacMahon S, Peto R, Cutler J, et al. Blood pressure, stroke, and coronary heart disease. Part 1. Prolonged differences in blood pressure: prospective observational studies corrected for the regression dilution bias. Lancet 1990;335:754–74.
9. SHEP Cooperative Research Group. Prevention of stroke by antihypertensive drug treatment in older persons with isolated systolic hypertension. Final results of the Systolic Hypertension in the Elderly Program (SHEP). JAMA 1991;265:3255–64.
10. Textor SC. ACE inhibitors in renovascular hypertension. Cardiovasc Drugs Ther 1990;4:229–35.
11. Goldsmith DJA, Reidy J, Scoble J. Renal arterial intervention and angiotensin blockade in atherosclerotic nephropathy. Am J Kidney Dis 2000;36:837–43.
12. Lewis EJ, Hunsicker LG, Bain RP, Rohde RD. The effect of angiotensin-converting enzyme inhibition on diabetic nephropathy. N Engl J Med 1993;329:1456–62.
13. Maschio G, Alberti D, Janin G, et al. Effect of the angiotensin-converting enzyme inhibitor benazepril on the progression of chronic renal insufficiency. N Engl J Med 1996;334:939–44.
14. Reggenenti P, Perna A, Gherardi G, et al. Renoprotective properties of ACE-inhibition in non-diabetic nephropathies with non-nephrotic proteinuria. Lancet 1999;354:359–64.
15. JNC-VI. The sixth report of the Joint National Committee on Prevention. Institutes of Health; 1997; NIH publication 98-4080.
16. Kalra PA, Kumwenda M, MacDowall P, Roland MO. ACE-inhibitor usage and monitoring in general practice: the need for guidelines to prevent renal failure. BMJ 1999;318:234–7.
17. Alderman MH. Non-pharmacological treatment of hypertension. Lancet 1994;344:307–11.
18. Hansson L, Zanchetti A, Carruthers SG, et al. Effects of intensive blood pressure lowering and low-dose aspirin in patients with hypertension. Principal results of the Hypertension Optimal Treatment (HOT) randomised trial. Lancet 1998;351:1755–62.
19. Ramsay LE, Williams B, Johnston JD, et al. British Hypertension Society guidelines for hypertension management 1999: summary. BMJ 1999;319:630–5.
20. Joint National Committee on detection, evaluation and treatment of high blood pressure. Sixth report (JNC-VI). Arch Intern Med 1997;157:2413–46.
21. van Jaarsveld BC, Krijnen P, Pieterman H, et al. The effect of balloon angioplasty on hypertension in atherosclerotic renal artery stenosis. N Engl J Med 2000;342:1007–14.
22. LaRosa JC, He J, Vupputuri S. Effect of statins on risk of coronary disease: meta-analysis of randomized controlled trials. JAMA 1999;282:2340–6.
23. West of Scotland Coronary Prevention Group. West of Scotland coronary prevention study: identification of high-risk groups and comparison with other cardiovascular intervention trials. Lancet 1996;348:1339–42.
24. Brown BG, Zhou XQ, Sacco DE, Albers JJ. Lipid lowering and plaque regression. New insights into plaque disruption and clinical events in coronary artery disease. Circulation 1993;87:1781–91.
25. Joint British recommendations on prevention of coronary heart disease in clinical practice: summary. British Cardiac Society, British Hyperlipidaemia Association, British Hypertension Society, British Diabetic Association. BMJ 2000;320:705–8.
26. Scoble JE, deTakats D, Ostermann ME, et al. Lipid profiles in patients with atherosclerotic renal artery stenosis. Nephron 1999;83:117–21.
27. Rosenson RS, Tangney CC. Anti-atherothrombotic properties of statins: implications for cardiovascular event reduction. JAMA 1998;279:1643–50.
28. Wu KK. Platelet activation mechanisms and markers in arterial thrombosis. J Intern Med 1996;239:17–34.
29. Fowkes FGR, Lowe GDO, Housley E, et al. Cross-linked fibrin degradation products, progression of peripheral vascular arterial disease, and risk of coronary heart disease. Lancet 1993;342:84–6.
30. Antiplatelet Trialists' Collaboration. Secondary prevention of vascular disease by prolonged anti-platelet treatment. BMJ (Clin Res Ed) 1988;296:320–31.
31. Hankey GJ, Eikelboom JW. Homocysteine and vascular disease. Lancet 1999;354:407–13.
32. Stenvinkel P, Heimburger O, Paultre F, et al. Strong association between malnutrition, inflammation, and atherosclerosis in chronic kidney failure. Kidney Int 1999;55:1899–911.
33. Ridker PM, Rifai N, Pfeffer MA, et al. Long-term effects of pravastatin on plasma concentration of C-reactive protein. The Cholesterol and Recurrent Events (CARE) Investigators. Circulation 1999;100:230–5.
34. Lederman RJ, Mendelsohn FO, Anderson RD, et al. Therapeutic angiogenesis with recombinant fibroblast growth factor-2 for intermittent claudication (the Traffic study): a randomised trial. Lancet 2002;359:2053–8.
35. Zierler RE, Bergelin RO, Davidson RC, et al. A prospective study of disease progression in patients with atherosclerotic renal artery stenosis. Am J Hypertens 1996;9:1055–61.
36. Schreiber MJ, Pohl MA, Novick AC. The natural history of atherosclerotic and fibrous renal artery disease. Urol Clin North Am 1984;11:383–92.
37. Harden PN, MacLeod MJ, Rodger RSC, et al. Effect of renal artery stenting on progression of renovascular renal failure. Lancet 1997;349:1133–6.
38. Plouin PF, Chantellier G, Darne B, et al. Blood pressure outcome of angioplasty in atheromatous renal artery stenosis: a randomised trial. Essai Multicentrique Medicaments vs Angioplastie (EMMA) Study Group. Hypertension 1998;31:823–9.

Treatment of Renovascular Disease: Endovascular Therapy

Jonathan G Moss

KEY POINTS

- Renal artery stenosis is divided into atheromatous and non-atheromatous etiologies.

- Atheromatous lesions are ten times more prevalent than non-atheromatous lesions.

- Percutaneous transluminal angioplasty (PTA) is the procedure of choice for non-atheromatous lesions.

- The improvement of blood pressure control in non-atheromatous lesions is good-to-excellent following PTA.

- The majority of atheromatous lesions are ostial in nature.

- Stents have a higher technical success rate compared with PTA in atheromatous ostial lesions (AHA: A).

- Stents have a higher patency rate compared with PTA in atheromatous ostial lesions (AHA: A).

- Improvement of blood pressure control in atheromatous lesions following PTA is marginal but may reduce the drug burden for the patient (AHA: B).

- Results in atheromatous patients with renal insufficiency following PTA or stenting are variable, with no consensus.

- Two randomized controlled trials are looking at stenting versus medical treatment in renal insufficiency.

INTRODUCTION

Renal artery stenosis (RAS) is an anatomic description of a lesion that may lead to a variety of pathophysiologic disease processes or simply exist as a silent lesion throughout life. To add more confusion, the disease entities hypertension, renal insufficiency, and pulmonary edema are common and have a myriad of etiologies, only one of which is RAS. It is often difficult to determine how much contribution the RAS is making to the symptomatology, if any.

Renal artery stenosis is caused by either atheromatous disease (of the aorta) or a variety of disparate entities, which include fibromuscular disease, neurofibromatosis, and Takayasu's arteritis, to name but a few. Fibromuscular disease usually affects young females and children and the presenting feature is hypertension. It is very rare for renal function to be impaired. The lesions almost never involve the renal artery ostium but predominate in the mid to distal main vessel and can extend out to the first- and second-order side branches. Although rare, the arteritides are rewarding to treat, usually responding well to percutaneous transluminal angioplasty (PTA), with 10-year cumulative patency of 87% and cure rates for hypertension approaching 50%.[1,2]

Atherosclerotic renal artery stenosis (ARAS) is a common disorder, prevalent in the population of patients encountered with coronary, carotid, and peripheral vascular disease. Although much of the original research focused on renovascular hypertension, there has been a renewed interest focusing on renal impairment. ARAS is now the commonest cause of end-stage renal failure (ESRF) in patients aged over 60 years on renal replacement therapy, accounting for at least 25% of this group.[3] ARAS is known to be a progressive disorder, with a cumulative incidence of progression to occlusion of 5% per annum in stenoses ≥ 60%.[4] Renal revascularization by either an endovascular or open surgical method has the potential to alter this process and prevent progression to ESRF. Two randomized controlled trials (RCTs) in the UK (ASTRAL) and Holland (STAR) are comparing renal stenting with best medical treatment to test this hypothesis and should report in 5 years.

TECHNIQUE

Non-atheromatous lesions

These lesions invariably respond to simple PTA; thus, stenting will not be described here.

Non-branch lesions

These are usually relatively simple to treat. Initially, a flush abdominal aortogram is performed via a transfemoral approach. If the angulation of the renal artery is severe, one may wish to consider accessing the vessel from a left brachial or radial approach, although in the author's experience this is only required in 10% of cases. Having administered intravenous heparin, the renal artery should be catheterized with an appropriately shaped 4–5F catheter. From a femoral approach, the most useful configuration is the 'reverse curve' or 'shepherd's crook', such as the Sos Omni (Angiodynamics, USA) (**Fig. 26b.1A**). Occasionally, the femoro-visceral or 'cobra shape' catheter is a useful alternative (**Fig. 26b.1B**). Having selected the renal artery, an antispasmodic drug should be administered (e.g. glycerol trinitrate, 150–500µg) to prevent renal spasm. A selective angiogram is then performed, which is important, as distal branch vessel disease may be present that was not apparent on the flush aortogram study. The stenosis is crossed atraumatically with a 0.035in guidewire, keeping the tip under constant fluoroscopic view. The guidewire should only be advanced a couple of centimeters beyond the lesion, as very distal guidewire placement can invoke spasm and even perforate

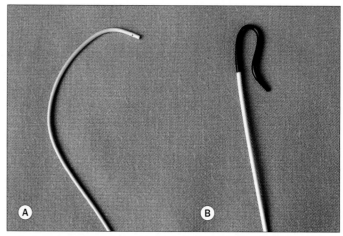

Figure 26b.1 Catheters. (A) Sos Omni. (B) Femoro-visceral.

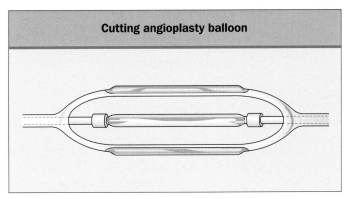

Cutting angioplasty balloon

Figure 26b.2 Cutting angioplasty balloon with three blades attached at 120° intervals.

the kidney. The TAD11 wire (Boston Scientific, USA) is very useful as it has a soft, atraumatic, 0.018in platinum tip but a relatively stiff 0.035in shaft, which provides the necessary support for the balloon catheter. In addition, this wire can be pre-shaped to suit the anatomy and also has an 'LOC extension' option, which simply screws onto the end of the guidewire and converts it to a 260cm working length for an arm approach. If the lesion is difficult to cross (which can occur in the classic 'string of beads' appearance), then changing to one of the hydrophilic wires is usually successful. The stenosis should be dilated with a short (2cm) balloon, the diameter matching that of the normal renal artery. Some of the arteritides can be very resistant to PTA and it may be necessary to use high-pressure balloons. Another alternative is a cutting balloon, which has recently become available and licensed for renal use (Boston Scientific, USA). This consists of three blades attached to the balloon surface at 120° intervals (**Fig. 26b.2**). The blades are protected by the wrap of the balloon material, permitting atraumatic passage across the stenosis. As the balloon is inflated, the exposed blades relieve

the 'hoop stress' by making three small controlled incisions into the vessel wall. The expanded balloon then flattens or dilates the cut area with the minimal amount of trauma. (**Fig. 26b.3**). These cutting balloons are available in diameters up to 6mm and can be used as a 'precut' for vessels larger than this, allowing the introduction of an appropriate sized conventional balloon.

Finally, when dilating the beaded type of fibromuscular lesion, the angiographic appearance may not change very much following PTA, but, usually, measurement of the pressure gradient will demonstrate a marked improvement (**Fig. 26b.4**).

Branch lesions

These are more complex and technically demanding. The basic principles still apply and the pharmacology is identical to that in the previous section. The small-platform 0.014–0.018in balloon systems should be used together with a guiding catheter. The smaller wires are less traumatic to smaller vessels, and the balloons on 3–4F shafts are far less likely to 'dotter' the lesion. A guiding catheter with an integral dilator (Cordis, Miami, USA) avoids the need to place a sheath and helps minimize the access puncture site size. The shape of the guiding catheter will depend on the local anatomy but a 65cm renal double curve (RDC) is the most useful from the groin and a 90cm multipurpose shape from the arm. A twin-port Tuohy–Borst adaptor will also be needed. If possible, the guiding catheter should be placed in the proximal renal artery, then the appropriate balloon and wire are placed and the lesion crossed. The second balloon and wire are then placed in a 'kissing' manner. Prior to inflating the balloons, one must check the measurements and ensure that the main vessel proximal to the branch is not smaller in diameter than the sum of both balloon diameters (**Fig. 26b.5**). If this is the situation, then the balloons must only be inflated individually. Contrast can be injected through the guiding catheter at any stage to check position and post-PTA appearances. Once again, if required, cutting balloons can be used, but should not be placed in a 'kissing' fashion as they can burst the adjacent balloon.

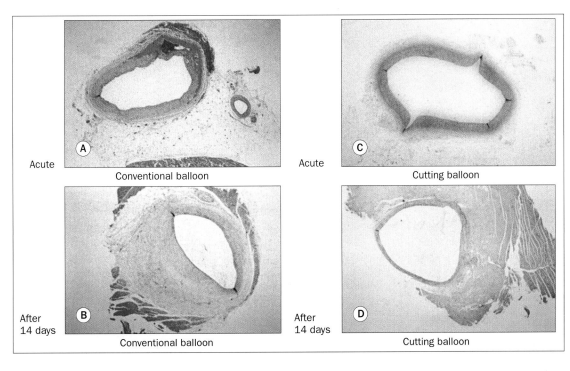

Acute — Conventional balloon

After 14 days — Conventional balloon

Acute — Cutting balloon

After 14 days — Cutting balloon

Figure 26b.3 Percutaneous transluminal angioplasty (PTA). Photomicrographs of an artery having undergone PTA with a standard balloon (A,B) and a cutting balloon (C,D).

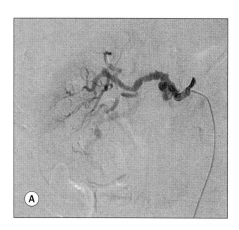 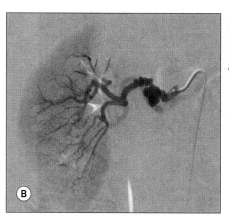

Figure 26b.4 Beaded type of fibromuscular lesion. (A) Angiogram showing classic 'string of beads' appearance. (B) Following PTA, there is no angiographic improvement but the pressure gradient dropped from 44mmHg to 5mmHg.

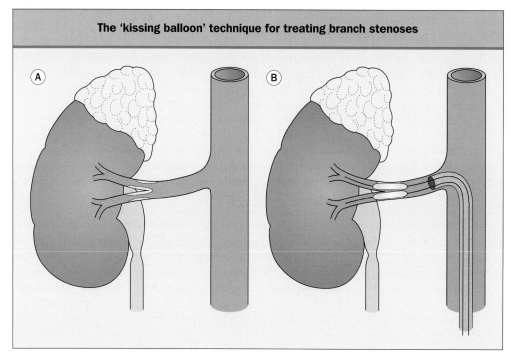

The 'kissing balloon' technique for treating branch stenoses

Figure 26b.5 The 'kissing balloon' technique for treating branch stenoses. Two small-platform balloons are simultaneously placed through a guiding catheter and inflated.

An alternative to the small-platform systems is the 'balloon on a wire'. Originally introduced by Tegtmeyer, they are very torquable and offer a low profile (0.035in), but have to some extent been superseded by the small-platform systems.

Atheromatous lesions

These lesions differ from the non-atherosclerotic lesion in that the vast majority are ostial, which is defined as lying within 10mm of the opacified aortic wall on an arteriogram.[5] Even when such lesions appear to be non-ostial on angiography, studies using computed tomography (CT) angiography have shown that they are in fact ostial.[5] A randomized trial[6] (see following section) has demonstrated a clear technical advantage of stenting over PTA for these lesions; thus, only stenting will be described here.

Pre-stenting assessment

The following are desirable prior to the procedure:

- non-invasive imaging – magnetic resonance angiography (MRA);
- adequate hydration; and
- renoprotective drugs, e.g. acetylcysteine.

Gadolinium-enhanced three-dimensional MRA should now be considered the norm for assessing renal arteries in atheromatous patients. Good accurate images can be obtained in both the transverse and coronal planes with no risk of contrast nephropathy or cholesterol embolization previously seen with catheter angiography. In addition, renal size can be assessed and other pathologies detected.[7,8] The transverse images are useful in that the angle of origin of the renal arteries can be measured and this angle reproduced on the angiographic 'c-arm' so that the ostium is seen in profile, ensuring accurate stent placement (**Fig. 26b.6**).[9]

It is important that patients with impaired renal function are not dehydrated prior to stenting or PTA, as this increases the susceptibility to iodinated contrast nephropathy. A randomized trial has shown that intravenous infusion of 0.45% saline (at 100–150mL/hour) for 12 hours before and 12 hours after intervention reduces the incidence of contrast nephropathy.[10] Furthermore, a recent RCT has shown a renoprotective benefit following the prophylactic administration of acetylcysteine (1200mg before and after iodinated contrast administration).[11] Acetylcysteine appears to work by improving renal hemodynamics and having

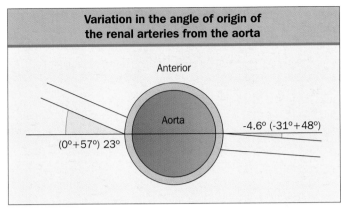

Figure 26b.6 Variation in the angle of origin of the renal arteries from the aorta. The right arises anterior to the mid-coronal plane (0 to 57 degrees). The left is more variable and can arise either side of the mid-coronal plane (–31 to +48 degrees).

antioxidant properties. Other drugs such as fenoldopam are currently under investigation.

Finally, it should be remembered that the best way to avoid iodinated contrast nephropathy is to avoid the use of such contrast altogether. It is now perfectly possible to place a renal stent using either carbon dioxide exclusively or with 5–10cm^3 of iodinated contrast at the most.[12] Gadolinium is another alternative contrast agent with no nephrotoxicity, but is considerably more expensive.[13]

Renal stenting technique
There are two different methods in use: the first uses conventional 0.035in guidewire technology (standard platform, **Fig. 26b.7**), whereas the more recent small-platform systems use 0.014–0.018in guidewires. Both will be described.

Standard platform
Depending on the pre-procedural imaging, a decision has to be made whether to use a femoral or brachial approach. Recently, a radial artery approach has been described.[14] Each has its advocates, and the advantages and disadvantages are shown in **Table 26b.1**. The author's preference is to use the femoral route unless the caudal angulation is severe and/or the iliac anatomy hostile. Once the access vessel has been catheterized, heparin (3000–5000IU) is administered intravenously. The 'c-arm' should be rotated to profile the renal artery ostium as dictated on the MRA images. A 5F reverse curve catheter (Sos Omni, Angiodynamics, USA) is reformed in the infrarenal aorta and a Bentson guidewire (Boston, USA) used with the catheter to selectively cross the stenotic vessel. A small amount of contrast or CO_2 may be necessary to locate the artery. Once the wire is across the lesion, the catheter is gently withdrawn, which advances it across the stenosis. At this stage, a proprietary vasodilator (e.g. glycerol trinitrate, 150–500μg) is given through the catheter into the renal circulation to minimize the risk of spasm. A selective renal angiogram is then performed. If this shows severe intrarenal disease, then the procedure should probably be abandoned, as it is very unlikely that revascularization will bring

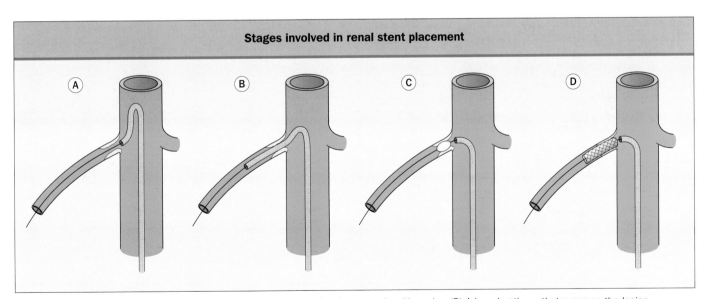

Figure 26b.7 Stages involved in renal stent placement. (A) Crossing the stenosis with a wire. (B) Advancing the catheter across the lesion. (C) Balloon dilatation. (D) Stent deployment.

Route	Angulation	Distance to vessel	Diameter of access vessel	Aortic plaque	Access vessel damage
Femoral	+	++	+++	+	++
Arm	+++	+	++	++	+

Table 26b.1 Pros and cons of a femoral versus arm approach for renal angioplasty and stenting.

329

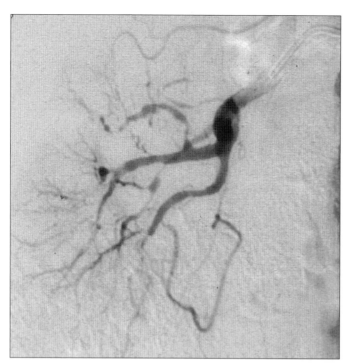

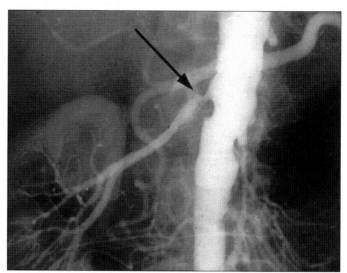

Figure 26b.9 Six-month angiogram showing restenosis of the original lesion due to the stent not adequately covering the renal ostium (arrow). This was treated by placing a second stent.

Figure 26b.8 Angiogram showing severe intrarenal small vessel disease not suitable for revascularization.

about any therapeutic benefit (**Fig. 26b.8**). At present, MRA is not usually able to accurately image the intrarenal circulation.

A tapered TAD11 guidewire (Boston Scientific, USA) is then placed through the catheter across the lesion. This tapered guide-wire has a soft atraumatic 0.018in tip and a stiff 0.035in shaft, which provides support for the balloon catheter, yet minimizes spasm in the renal branch vessels. The stenosis is either fully dilated (6–7mm) or predilated (3–4mm) using a short tipped (2cm) balloon. Predilatation may produce less atheroembolization than full dilatation, but this has not yet been proven. A renal stent (**Table 26b.2**) is then placed using either a 7–8F RDC guiding catheter or a 45cm-long 6F sheath. Both will provide support and allow small volumes (5mL) of contrast to be injected to ensure accurate placement. It is not necessary – and undesirable – to access the other groin to inject large volumes of

contrast through a pigtail catheter. One should ensure that the renal ostium is fully covered, which necessitates leaving approximately 1–3mm of stent protruding into the aorta. **Figure 26b.9** shows a restenosis caused by inadequate covering of the ostium due to incorrect 'c-arm' angulation. Stent diameter should match the normal vessel and the length should be just enough to cover the stenosis (usually 15–18mm).

If using a brachial approach, the following equipment should be available:

- 90cm sheath *or* 90cm multipurpose shape guiding catheter;
- exchange length wires (260cm) *or* use LOC extension on TAD11 wire; and
- 120cm shaft balloons.

Small-platform systems
These have emerged over the last 5 years as a spinoff from the cardiology market and are gaining in popularity. Although there are theoretical advantages over the conventional systems, these have not been proven in the atherosclerotic renal artery territory.

Renal stents available in the EEC (standard and small platform).				
Manufacturer	Standard platform	Working lengths/Sheath size	Small platform	Working lengths/Sheath size
Cordis	Palmaz Genesis 0.035in	80cm, 135cm 6F–7F**	Palmaz Genesis 0.018in	80cm, 135 cm 5F–6F**
Medtronic	Bridge Extra Support 0.035in	75cm, 120cm 7F	Bridge X3 0.018in	75cm, 120cm 6F
Guidant	n/a	n/a	Herculink Plus 0.014in	80cm, 135cm 5F or 6F**
Jomed	Jostent renal 0.035in	75cm 6F	n/a	n/a
Bard	Saax renal 0.035in	75cm, 120cm 6F	n/a*	n/a*
*The Saax stent (Bard, UK) can be hand crimped onto a low-platform balloon which will fit through a 5F sheath				
**Where two sheath sizes are quoted, the largest only applies to the 6.5–7mm diameter stents				

Table 26b.2 Renal stents available in the EEC (standard and small platform).

Potential advantages of small-platform systems include:
- less traumatic 0.014–0.018in guidewires;
- less traumatic 3.5F shaft balloons;
- superior trackability;
- smaller puncture site (5F sheath or 7F guide catheter);
- small 3mm predilatation; and
- rapid exchange systems, avoiding need for long wires.

It is assumed that these smaller systems cause less risk of atheroembolism and reduce local groin complications. They may be particularly advantageous when using a brachial or radial approach. Most of the evidence is anecdotal and comes from the carotid territory, where it is relatively easy to measure atheroembolic events using transcranial Doppler.

The technique is basically the same as for the standard-platform systems, except that having crossed the lesion with the low-profile wire, the stenosis is predilated to 3mm prior to placing the stent. The correct choice of guidewire is important with these systems and some of the recommended choices are shown in **Table 26b.3**.

Troubleshooting
Although most renal arteries are relatively straightforward to stent, some can be exceedingly difficult and, on occasion, impossible.

The wire will not cross the stenosis
1. A curved hydrophilic wire should be tried. These should be used with great care as they can easily dissect the vessel without the operator being aware.
2. A different access approach can be tried (usually the left brachial).
3. Change the catheter shape.
4. Try a 0.014–0.018in guidewire.

Nothing will follow the wire
1. Try a 4F hydrophilic cobra catheter (Terumo, Japan).
2. Try a 4F Van Andel tapered catheter (Cook, UK).
3. If not already using a guiding catheter, use one for extra support.
4. Use a small-platform system.

Post procedure
A 6F sheath and an 8F guiding catheter both make the same size hole in the access vessel, i.e. 8F. A closure device should be strongly considered, particularly if the patient is hypertensive and/or has renal impairment (which increases the bleeding time), to prevent groin complications. It may not be necessary to use a closure device with the small-platform systems.

Guidewires for renal angioplasty and stenting.		
Manufacturer	Standard platform	Small platform
Boston Scientific	TAD 11 0.035in	Platinum Plus 0.018in
Cordis		SV-5 0.018in
Guidant		Spartacore 0.014in 130, 190, 300cm

Table 26b.3 Guidewires for renal angioplasty and stenting.

Intravenous hydration should be continued for 12 hours and blood pressure and renal function carefully monitored for 24–48 hours. The real risk of labile blood pressure swings and temporary renal deterioration make daycase renal stenting an unrealistic option in most circumstances.

Antiplatelet therapy (aspirin, 75–325mg daily) should be routinely given on a lifelong basis. If the patient is intolerant to aspirin, then clopidogrel (75mg daily) can be used.

Restenosis
Restenosis following renal stenting is much less common than after PTA and occurs in 15% of stents at 6 months, as determined by angiography. Its treatment is more difficult, however, and there is no consensus regarding the optimal approach. The pathologic process is neointimal hyperplasia. In general, simple PTA of this tissue leads to suboptimal results, due to recoil. Recently, cutting balloons have been advocated as an alternative, but there are insufficient data to make any firm recommendation on their use.[15]

SELECTION OF THERAPY
Arteritides
These patients are often young females with hypertension and normal renal function. Although an abdominal bruit may be present, most of the renal artery lesions are detected on conventional catheter angiography. Selective views may be necessary to detect subtle branch lesions. The decision to offer the patient PTA should be a team judgment, involving the blood pressure physician, vascular radiologist, and vascular surgeon. Although the pharmacologic control of hypertension has improved over the last 20 years, the potential of PTA to cure hypertension makes a strong case for intervention. However, occasionally, the distribution and number of lesions may make PTA hazardous, and the risk of causing permanent renal damage must be balanced against the potential benefits. In these circumstances, the decision should be made on an individual patient basis and will depend on factors that include the center's experience and results. The results of PTA are good, with 10-year cumulative patency rates of 87%; up to 50% of patients are cured of their hypertension, with the remainder having a reduced drug burden and improved blood pressure control.[1,2] If, however, the patient is asymptomatic, a more expectant policy can be adopted. Although fibromuscular disease has been reported to progress in up to a third of patients, occlusion and loss of renal function is very rare. There may be an argument for routine follow-up and possibly imaging, but prophylactic PTA is difficult to justify.

Takayasu's arteritis is a non-specific inflammatory disease which mainly affects large arteries such as the aorta and its main branches, including the renal artery. It is the most common cause of renovascular hypertension in India and China, in contrast to Western countries. The majority of patients can be managed medically with corticosteroids, monitoring disease activity using the erythrocyte sedimentation rate (ESR). When in the chronic inactive stage, renovascular hypertension can be successfully managed by PTA, with good clinical results.[16]

Atheromatous disease
The selection of patients for treatment by revascularization in this group is difficult and still very contentious. Widely differing

views are held, ranging from those who rarely advocate stenting to those who treat all lesions. Several small recent RCTs have helped the decision-making a little, although many questions still remain, particularly regarding renal insufficiency.

The goals of therapy are to improve or cure hypertension and/or improve or prevent deterioration in renal function. It is easiest to look at these two objectives separately.

Hypertension

Evidence

Three RCTs have compared revascularization (essentially PTA) with best medical treatment.[17–19] The trials were small: the largest recruited 106 patients. Many patients were excluded before randomization, and slow recruitment restricted patient numbers. Blood pressure is notoriously difficult to measure and reproduce, and the three trials used different measurement criteria. All reported only short-term results (3–54 months). Of the total 210 patients, only two were treated with stents. Patient crossover from one arm to the other was frequent and occurred in 44% in the largest trial. None of these trials produced any good evidence to support the routine use of angioplasty in the treatment of hypertension, although there was some reduction in the drug burden in the PTA arm in all three studies. This limited benefit was countered by the complications of PTA, which included one nephrectomy. However, the confidence limits in all these trials was wide and consequently they had little power to detect moderate but potentially worthwhile benefits. A much larger trial would be required to answer this question for certain. These impressions have been supported by a recent meta-analysis conducted by the University of Birmingham Clinical Trials Unit.[20]

There is a growing consensus that hypertension is rarely, if ever, cured by PTA or stenting in ARAS and that a slight reduction in either blood pressure or drug medication is the best that can be hoped for. Therefore, revascularization is best reserved for patients with poorly controlled hypertension in spite of maximum drug treatment or in those who cannot take the appropriate medications due to side effects.

Renal insufficiency

The aim of treatment in this group is to improve or stabilize renal function. Even slowing the rate of deterioration is of benefit, as it may delay or prevent the need for renal replacement therapy.[21]

Once patients have reached ESRF, recoverable renal function following revascularization is very uncommon. A rare exception to this is the patient who presents in acute renal failure with bilateral renal artery occlusions but at least one reasonable-sized kidney (**Fig. 26b.10**). Provided the occlusion can be crossed and stented, there is at least a 50% chance of regaining sufficient function to obviate the need for dialysis. If the lesion cannot be stented, then a surgical bypass should be considered if the patient is fit.[22] Although hugely rewarding for both doctor and patient, these are rare situations. Renal arteries usually progress to occlusion in a very insidious asymptomatic way, with permanent loss of renal mass and function.[23] It is not clear at what stage in the progressive stenotic process one should intervene. Two recent publications have failed to demonstrate any relationship between the severity of stenosis and renal function.[24,25] Strandness et al. were the first to accurately measure this process and showed that renal arteries with ≥ 60% stenosis have a cumulative risk of

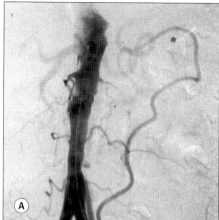

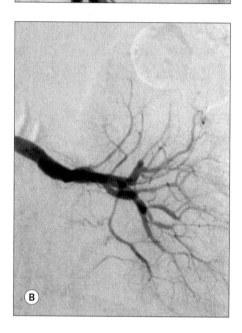

Figure 26b.10 Renal insufficiency. (A) Bilateral renal artery occlusion presenting with acute renal failure. (B) The left renal artery was stented and renal function recovered, allowing the patient to discontinue dialysis.

occlusion of 5% per year.[4] This is much less than was originally postulated from retrospective cohort studies. It is possible that the widespread use of statins and other lipid-lowering agents in atherosclerotic disease has modulated the disease process in recent years.

The best indications for renal stenting comprise:

- difficult-to-control hypertension in spite of full medical treatment, or intolerance to the drugs;
- angiotensin-converting enzyme (ACE) inhibitor-induced renal insufficiency, with a good clinical indication to remain on ACE inhibitors;
- rapidly deteriorating renal function;
- acute renal failure with renal artery occlusion and a good-sized kidney
- flash pulmonary edema.

Uncertain indications for renal stenting include:
- stable but impaired renal function;
- moderately severe hypertension;
- stenosis in a single kidney (other kidney not functioning);
- bilateral high-grade stenoses; and
- patients with high-grade stenoses undergoing coronary surgery.

Evidence

The evidence here is less clear-cut than for hypertension. Although all the three blood pressure RCTs measured renal function in a variety of different ways, none was powered to detect an improvement in renal function.[17–19] Two of the trials excluded patients with moderate to severe renal impairment. None of the trials showed any clear benefit for PTA in terms of serum creatinine or creatinine clearance. Because of the weak power of the studies, however, it is possible that a modest but important benefit from PTA was not detected. Stents were only used in 1% of the revascularized patients. A much larger study is needed, and the ASTRAL and STAR trials are currently randomizing 1150 patients between stenting with best medical treatment versus best medical treatment alone. The primary outcome measure is renal function and the trials should report in approximately 5 years time.

The decision to treat should be made by a multidisciplinary team involving the nephrologist or blood pressure physician, vascular radiologist, and surgeon. The risks of damaging the kidney should be balanced against the perceived benefits, which should be realistic. Until the ASTRAL and STAR trials report, patients should understand that the evidence for revascularization remains weak.

Endovascular or surgical revascularization?

Only one RCT (AHA: A) has compared PTA with surgical (mainly endarterectomy) revascularization.[26] This small study (n=58) found that the technical success rate was higher in the surgical group (97% versus 83%) and the primary 2-year patency superior (96% versus 75%). However, the secondary patency rates were similar, and the authors suggested that PTA should be the first-choice treatment, provided adequate surveillance and reintervention was available. This trial (1993) predated the stent era.

Angioplasty or stents?

A single RCT (AHA: A) compared PTA with stenting in 85 patients with ostial lesions.[6] The technical success rate of stents was superior to that of PTA (88% versus 55%) and primary 6-month patency was likewise superior (75% versus 29%). The trial was stopped following an interim analysis of the data. The clinical outcomes in the two groups were similar, although the study was not powered to detect differences in blood pressure or renal function. The results of this trial came as no surprise to many radiologists, who recognized the poor technical results that PTA gave when dealing with ostial disease, which is due to recoil of the aortic plaque.[27]

Stents or surgery?

There are no trials to answer this question and it seems doubtful there ever will be, as the two treatments are so different in nature that patient recruitment would be very difficult. Although it is unlikely that the patency rates of any endovascular technique will match those of surgical reconstruction, the increased morbidity and mortality of surgery will restrict its use to the young and fit with a long life expectancy. These patients are uncommon in the atherosclerotic renovascular field. A rare indication for surgery is a stent technical failure, which most commonly occurs when attempting to treat complete occlusions. It is possible that some complications such as cholesterol embolization may be less common with a surgical revascularization, as there is usually no instrumentation of the lesion.

COMPLICATIONS

The endovascular approach offers some obvious advantages over a conventional surgical reconstruction, which include the avoidance of a general anesthetic and the morbidity associated with an abdominal incision in what is often a high-risk population with other co-morbid vascular disease. However, it would be naïve to assume that that an endovascular procedure is risk-free.

The literature quotes complications rates ranging from 0% to 66% for renal PTA/stenting. Most of the series are retrospective and there are no agreed reporting standards or definitions. It has been suggested to classify complications as:

- major – serious complications requiring active management;
- minor – complications which usually require expectant observation only; and
- radiologic – technical – complications occurring during the procedure which produce no adverse clinical symptoms.[28]

It is difficult to compare the complication rates with surgical series as these usually report events up to 30 days whereas radiologic papers often report complications within a shorter time window. In the single RCT (AHA: A) comparing surgery with PTA,[23] the major complication rate following PTA was 17%, versus 31% following surgery, with minor complications in 48% of the PTA group versus 7% in the surgical group. These differences were not statistically significant. The Dutch RCT (AHA: A) comparing PTA with stenting reported a 39% complication rate following PTA compared with 43% following stenting.[6] Although most of these complications were minor and groin related, more serious complications such as vessel rupture and cholesterol embolization can have grave consequences for the patient.

Table 26b.4 shows complications compiled from 10 published PTA and 14 published stent studies. There is no difference between the complications rates of PTA and stenting. Many complications can be avoided by good technique and treated by endovascular methods (**Table 26b.5**). Surgical salvage should be rarely required and often is too late to save a kidney, due to the relatively short warm ischemic time of this organ (approximately 90min).

Perforation of the renal artery is a dreaded complication but can usually be treated either by simple balloon tamponade or by placing a stent graft (**Fig. 26b.11**).

Deterioration in renal function (usually temporary) is one of the commonest complications. It is usually due to the effects of iodinated contrast and appears in the first 24–48 hours (**Fig. 26b.12**). Efforts to minimize this have been discussed previously, but once it does occur, supportive treatment usually suffices. Only about 1% of cases require dialysis, although their outcome is poor. More worrying is cholesterol atheroembolism, which occurs either due to simple catheter manipulation in the aorta, crossing the stenosis, or balloon inflation and stent placement. The onset is more insidious (over 1–3 weeks) (**Fig. 26b.13**) and may be associated with an elevated ESR, eosinophilia, and the typical livedo reticularis skin rash. Atheroembolism is probably more common than previously thought and will often go undetected in patients with a normal contralateral kidney and/or normal renal function. It should be remembered that

Complications of renal artery angioplasty and stenting.

Complication	PTRA (n = 675 procedures)		Stents (n = 512 patients)	
	n (%)	Mortality	n (%)	Mortality
Major				
Permanent renal insufficiency	2 (0.3)		10 (1.9)	
Renal artery occlusion	1 (0.15)		5 (1)	
Renal artery damage	10 (1.5)		4 (0.8)	2 (†)
Segmental infarct embolization	2 (0.3)		7 (1.4)	
Retroperitoneal hematoma	5 (0.75)		7 (1.4)	
Groin complications	8 (1.2)		10 (2)	1 (†)
MI/stroke	6 (0.8)	1 (†)		
Other	3 (0.4)		2 (0.4)	
Total	47 (7)		45 (8.8)	
Minor				
Temporary renal insufficiency	25 (3.7)		16 (3.1)	
Segmental infarct	6 (0.9)			
Retroperitoneal hematoma	1 (0.15)		1 (0.2)	
Groin complications	8 (1.2)		14 (2.7)	
Other	4 (0.46)		8 (1.6)	
Total	44 (6.5)		39 (7.6)	
Radiologic	1 (0.15)		33 (6.4)	

Table 26b.4 Complications of renal artery angioplasty and stenting. Compilation of published results from 10 percutaneous transluminal renal angioplasty (PTRA) and 14 stent series.

one has to lose about 50% of the renal functional mass before the serum creatinine begins to rise above normal levels. However, once renal function does deteriorate following cholesterol embolization, the prognosis is guarded and little can be done beyond general supportive measures. Some patients will progress to ESRF as a result. Attempts to reduce the incidence of athero-embolism lie with the so-called protection devices, which consist of either temporary occlusion balloons or filter membranes. Designed for the carotid artery, they are at present far from ideal for the renal artery owing to difficult angulation and geometry. There is some limited experience in the literature to support their use.[29] Macro cholesterol embolization rarely occurs and can be treated by aspiration thrombectomy.

Management and prevention of endovascular complications.

Complication	Prevention	Treatment
Groin related	Small-platform systems Closure devices	Supportive Thrombin injection
Contrast nephropathy	Minimize contrast load Use CO_2 Acetylcysteine	Supportive
Cholesterol embolization	Minimize manipulations Small-platform systems Protection devices	Supportive
Renal artery perforation	Correct balloon size	Balloon tamponade Covered stent (Jomed, UK)
Retroperitoneal bleed (perirenal)	Avoid stiff-tipped guidewire Avoid distal guidewire placement	Supportive

Table 26b.5 Management and prevention of endovascular complications.

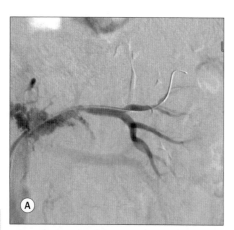
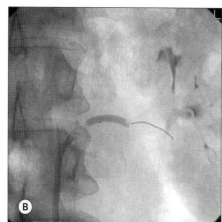
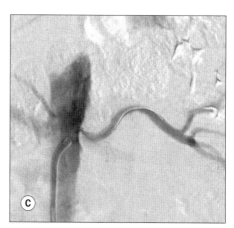

Figure 26b.11 Perforation of a renal artery following PTA (A). Balloon tamponade for 5 minutes (B) achieved vascular stasis (C).

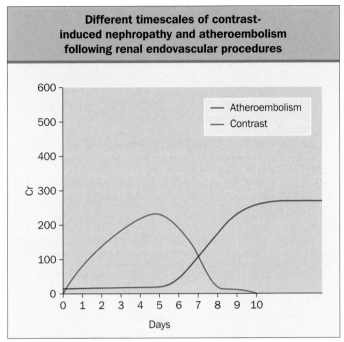

Figure 26b.12 Different timescales of contrast-induced nephropathy and atheroembolism following renal endovascular procedures.

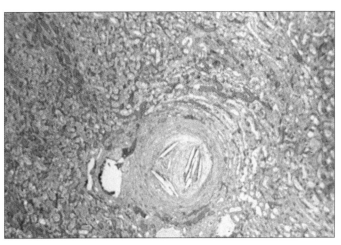

Figure 26b.13 Photomicrograph of a renal biopsy, showing cholesterol crystals in a medium-sized arteriole.

SUMMARY

Atherosclerotic renovascular disease is a complex multifactorial entity. It is naïve to think of it as being simply due to a flow-limiting stenosis which can be treated by revascularization. Atheroembolism, small vessel atheroma, and hypertensive nephropathy often coexist. The three randomized hypertension trials comparing PTA with medical treatment have been difficult to conduct, are small, and have not demonstrated much useful gain from PTA other than a possible drug-sparing effect with the risk of the complications of PTA. Research has now turned toward renal function and as to whether revascularization can influence this disease process.

Two RCTs (ASTRAL in the UK and STAR in Holland) are currently comparing stenting plus best medical treatment with best medical treatment alone. These should report in approximately 5 years time.

The preferred method of revascularization – endovascular versus surgical – remains contentious and it seems unlikely there will be much enthusiasm for an RCT to answer this question. The perceived advantages of an endovascular approach seem obvious to many, particularly in the aging high-risk vasculopath. The Dutch RCT has demonstrated the technical superiority of stents over PTA in ostial lesions, and stenting has become the standard endovascular technique in those undergoing renal revascularization for atherosclerotic disease.

REFERENCES

1. Tegtmeyer CJ, Selby JB, Hartwell GD, Ayers C, Tegtmeyer V. Results and complications of angioplasty in fibromuscular disease. Circulation 1991;83(2 Suppl):I155–61.
2. Tegtmeyer CJ, Matsumoto AH, Angle JF. Percutaneous transluminal angioplasty in fibrous dysplasia and children. In: Novick A, Scoble J, Hamilton G, eds. Renal vascular disease, 1st edn. London:WB Saunders; 1996:363–83.
3. Mailloux LU, Napolitano B, Bellucci AG, et al. Renal vascular disease causing end-stage renal disease, incidence, clinical correlates and outcomes: a 20 year clinical experience. Am J Kidney Dis 1994;24:622–9.
4. Zierler RE, Bergelin RO, Isaacson JA, Strandness DE Jr. Natural history of atherosclerotic renal artery stenosis: a prospective study with duplex ultrasonography. J Vasc Surg 1994;19:250–8.
5. Kaatee R, Beek FJA, Verschuyl EJ, et al. Atherosclerotic renal artery stenosis: ostial or truncal? Radiology 1996;199:637–40.
6. Van de ven PJG, Kaatee R, Beutler JJ, et al. Arterial stenting and balloon angioplasty in ostial atherosclerotic renovascular disease: a randomised trial. Lancet 1999;353:282–6.
7. Roditi G. Contrast-enhanced magnetic resonance angiography. Br J Surg 2002;89:817–20.
8. Weigner M, Pruessmann KP, Kassner A, et al. Contrast-enhanced 3D MRA using SENSE. J Magn Reson Imaging 2000;12:671–7.
9. Verschuyl E-J, Kaatee R, Beek FJA, et al. Renal artery origins: best angiographic projection angles. Radiology 1997;205:115–20.
10. Solomon R, Werner C, Mann D, D'Elia J, Silva P. Effects of saline, mannitol and furosemide on acute decreases in renal function induced by radiocontrast agents. N Engl J Med 1994;331:1416–20.
11. Tepel M, van der Giet M, Schwarzfeld C, Laufer U, Liermann D, Zidek W. Prevention of radiographic contrast agent induced reductions in renal function by acetylcysteine. N Engl J Med 2000;343:180–4.
12. Spinosa DJ, Matsumoto AH, Angle JF, et al. Safety of CO_2^- and gadodiamide-enhanced angiography for the evaluation and percutaneous treatment of renal artery stenosis in patients with chronic renal insufficiency. AJR Am J Roentgenol 2001;176:1305–11.
13. Reyes R, Carreira JM, Pardo MD, et al. Utility of gadolinium as a contrast medium in endovascular therapeutic procedures. Radiologia 2001;43:435–8.
14. Kessel DO, Robertson I, Patel JV. Transradial renal artery intervention. Cardiovasc Intervent Radiol 2003;26:146–9.
15. Munneke GJ, Engelke C, Morgan RA, Belli A-M. Cutting balloon angioplasty for resistant renal artery in-stent restenosis. J Vasc Interv Radiol 2002;13:327–31.
16. Tyagi S, Singh B, Kaul UA, et al. Balloon angioplasty for renovascular hypertension in Takasayu's arteritis. Am Heart J 1993;125:1386–93.

17. Plouin P-F, Chatellier G, Darne B, et al. Blood pressure outcome of angioplasty in atherosclerotic renal artery stenosis. Hypertension 1998; 31:823–9.
18. Webster J, Marshall F, Abdalla M, et al. Randomised comparison of percutaneous angioplasty vs continued medical therapy for hypertensive patients with atheromatous renal artery stenosis. J Hum Hypertens 1998;12:329–35.
19. Van Jaarsveld BC, Krijnen P, Pieterman H, et al. The effects of balloon angioplasty on hypertension in atherosclerotic renal artery stenosis. N Engl J Med 2000;342:1007–14.
20. Ives N, Wheatley K, Gray R. Continuing uncertainty about the value of revascularisation in atherosclerotic renovascular disease: a meta-analysis of previous trials. 5th UK Renovascular Forum, Glasgow, 2001 (Abstr).
21. Harden PN, Macleod MJ, Rodger RSC, et al. Effect of renal artery stenting on progression of renovascular renal failure. Lancet 1997;349:1133.
22. Schefft P, Novick AC, Stewart BH, et al. Renal revascularisation in patients with total occlusion of the renal artery. J Urol 1980;124:184–6.
23. Guzman RP, Zierler RE, Isaacson JA, Bergelin RO, Strandness DE Jr. Renal atrophy and arterial stenosis: a prospective study with duplex ultrasound. Hypertension 1994; 23:346–50.
24. Suresh M, Laboi P, Mamtora H, Kalra PA. Relationship of renal dysfunction to proximal arterial disease severity in atherosclerotic renovascular disease. Nephrol Dial Transplant 2000;15:631–6.
25. Farmer CKT, Cook GJR, Reidy J, Scoble J. Individual kidney function in atherosclerotic renovascular disease is not related to the presence of renal artery stenosis. Nephrol Dial Transplant 1999;14:2880–4.
26. Weibull H, Bergqvist D, Bergentz S-E, et al. Percutaneous transluminal renal angioplasty versus surgical reconstruction of atherosclerotic renal artery stenosis: a prospective randomised study. J Vasc Surg 1993; 18:841–52.
27. Cicuto KP, McLean GK, Oleaga JA, et al. Renal artery stenosis: anatomical classification for percutaneous transluminal angioplasty. AJR Am J Roentgenol 1981;137:599–601.
28. Beek FJA, Kaatee R, Beutler JJ, et al. Complications during renal artery stent placement for atherosclerotic ostial stenosis. Cardiovasc Intervent Radiol 1997;20:184–90.
29. Henry M, Klonaris C, Henry I, et al. Protected renal stenting with the PercuSurge Guardwire device: a pilot study. Journal Endovasc Ther 2001;8:227–37.

Treatment of Renovascular Disease: Surgical Therapy

Matthew S Edwards, Gregory S Cherr, and Kimberley J Hansen

KEY POINTS

- Atherosclerotic renovascular disease may be clinically silent or may contribute to severe, secondary hypertension and renal insufficiency (i.e. *ischemic nephropathy*).
- Advanced age, severe hypertension, and rapidly deteriorating renal function are markers of increased risk for the presence of atherosclerotic renal artery disease.
- Greater than 95% of hemodynamically significant atherosclerotic renal artery lesions are ostial (i.e. aortic in origin).
- Intervention for atherosclerotic renal artery disease should be considered only in patients with evidence of physiologically significant lesion(s) (producing severe hypertension with or without renal insufficiency).
- A beneficial blood pressure response can be expected in approximately 85% of selected patients treated with surgical renal artery repair.
- A beneficial renal function response can be expected in approximately 60% of selected patients with ischemic nephropathy treated with surgical renal artery repair.
- Improved renal function after operation is the principal determinant of dialysis-free survival, with improved survival demonstrated only among patients with improved renal function.
- Percutaneous transluminal renal artery angioplasty (PTRA), with or without endoluminal stenting, for ostial renal artery atherosclerosis produces inferior renal functional response compared with surgical renal artery repair.
- Surgical reconstruction following failed PTRA frequently requires branch artery exposure and repair.
- Renal artery repair combined with elective aortic surgery should be reserved for patients with severe hypertension with or without renal insufficiency.

INTRODUCTION

The introduction of new, more potent antihypertensive agents and percutaneous endovascular techniques has influenced surgical intervention for atherosclerotic renovascular disease.[1] Many physicians currently limit surgical intervention to:

- severe hypertension despite maximal medical therapy;
- failures or disease patterns not amenable to percutaneous transluminal renal artery angioplasty (PTRA); or
- renovascular disease associated with excretory renal insufficiency (i.e. *ischemic nephropathy*).

As a result, the patient population selected for operative management is characterized by ostial renal artery atherosclerosis (85%) superimposed on diffuse extrarenal atherosclerotic disease (95%) in combination with renal insufficiency.[1-3]

Although there are several operative methods that can correct atherosclerotic renal artery disease, no single technique predominates. Optimal methods of renal reconstruction vary with the patient, the pattern of renal artery disease, and the clinical significance of associated aortic lesions.

PREVALENCE, EVALUATION AND DIAGNOSIS

Renovascular disease accounts for approximately 3% of hypertension within the general population and as many as 5–10% of incident cases of dialysis-dependence among patients over the age of 65.[4] Although its prevalence in patients with mild hypertension (diastolic blood pressure <95mmHg) is low, renovascular disease is a frequent etiologic factor in patients with severe hypertension. Among patients aged ≥ 60 years with diastolic blood pressure ≥ 110mmHg, approximately 50% have significant renal artery stenosis or occlusion. When associated with an elevated serum creatinine (SCr), the prevalence increases to 70%, with half of these patients demonstrating bilateral renal artery disease.

These data suggest the probability of finding clinically significant renal artery disease correlates with the patient's age, the severity of hypertension, and the presence and severity of renal insufficiency. With this in mind, one should search for renovascular disease in all persons with severe hypertension, especially when this is found in combination with excretory renal insufficiency.

A non-invasive screening test that accurately identifies renal artery disease in all individuals does not yet exist.[5] Currently available tests can be characterized broadly as functional or anatomic. With the exception of captopril renography, studies that rely on activation of the renin–angiotensin axis have been associated with an unacceptable rate of false-negative results. Current isotope renography utilizes a variety of radiopharmaceuticals before and after exercise or angiotensin-converting enzyme (ACE) inhibition. However, the methods employed and the criteria for interpretation have been continuously modified in an effort to improve their sensitivity and specificity.[6]

Consequently, direct screening methods are preferable.[7] Renal duplex sonography is the preliminary study of choice for both renovascular hypertension and ischemic nephropathy. Through continued improvements in software and probe design, renal duplex has proven an accurate method to identify hemodynamically significant renal artery occlusive disease, with a 91% sensitivity, 96% specificity, and 92% overall accuracy.[8,9] The examination poses no risk to residual excretory renal function, and overall accuracy is not affected by concomitant aortoiliac disease. In addition, preparation is minimal (an overnight fast), and there is no need to alter antihypertensive medications.

Previous results suggest that a negative renal duplex effectively excludes ischemic nephropathy since the primary consideration is global renal ischemia based on main renal artery disease to both kidneys. However, when renal duplex is used to screen for renovascular hypertension, multiple or polar renal arteries and their associated disease pose a potential limitation. Despite enhanced recognition of multiple arteries provided by Doppler color-flow, only 40% of these accessory renal vessels are currently identified by renal duplex examination. Consequently, our group proceeds with conventional angiography when hypertension is severe or poorly controlled, despite a negative duplex result.

When a unilateral renal artery lesion is confirmed by angiography, its functional significance should be defined. Both renal vein renin assays (RVRA) and split renal function studies have proven valuable in assessing the functional significance of renovascular disease. RVRA should demonstrate a ratio of renin activity exceeding 1.5:1.0 between involved and uninvolved sides before a diagnosis of renovascular hypertension is established. Unfortunately, neither functional study has great value when severe bilateral disease or disease to a solitary kidney is present. Therefore, the decision for empiric intervention is based on the severity of the renal artery lesions, the severity of hypertension, and the degree of associated renal insufficiency. In this latter instance, issues determining recovery of excretory renal function in patients with ischemic nephropathy remain ill defined. Our center's experience with over 210 patients having severe hypertension and preoperative SCr ≥ 1.8mg/dL has demonstrated a significant association between an improved renal function response after operative intervention and the site of renal artery disease, the extent of renovascular repair, and the rate of decline in preoperative renal function.[1,2,10–13] Global renal disease submitted to complete renal artery repair after rapid decline in excretory renal function is associated with the best opportunity for recovery of renal function.[10,11,13] Moreover, improved renal function after operation is the primary determinant of dialysis-free survival.[13]

Management of renal artery disease discovered incidentally during evaluation of aneurysmal or occlusive disease of the abdominal aorta is controversial. In this setting, the surgeon must address the need for additional diagnostic study and the decision of whether to perform combined aortic and renal artery reconstruction. In the following discussion, combined management of aortic and renal artery disease will be considered as either a prophylactic or empiric procedure.

The term *prophylactic repair* describes renal revascularization that is performed prior to any pathologic or clinical sequelae related to the lesion. By definition, therefore, the patient considered for prophylactic renal artery repair has neither hypertension nor reduced renal function. Correction of the renal artery lesion in this setting assumes that a significant percentage of these asymptomatic patients will survive to the point that the renal lesion will cause hypertension or renal dysfunction. Furthermore, prophylactic intervention assumes that pre-emptive correction is necessary to prevent a clinically adverse event for which the patient either cannot be treated or where re-operative treatment would be unduly hazardous.

Data regarding the frequency of anatomic progression of renovascular disease are summarized in **Table 26c.1**. In patients with hypertension, ipsilateral progression of renal artery lesions occurred in 44%. Among patients prospectively randomized to medical management, progression to total occlusion occurred in 12%. However, among these latter patients, only one (3%) had loss of a previously reconstructible renal artery.[14] In the absence of hypertension, one has to assume that the renal artery lesion must progress anatomically to become functionally significant (i.e. produce hypertension). Based on the preceding data, progression

Angiographic progression of renal artery atherosclerosis.					
Reference	Mean follow-up (months)	No.	Ipsilateral lesions Percent exhibiting progression	Percent progressing to occlusion	Contralateral lesions Percent exhibiting progression
82,83	29–35	85	44	16	–
14	28	35	–	12	17

Table 26c.1 Angiographic progression of renal artery atherosclerosis. (From Edwards MS, Hansen KJ. Combined aortorenal reconstruction. In: Green RM, ed. Complex aortic surgery. New York:Marcel Dekker [Forthcoming].)

of a renal artery lesion to produce renovascular hypertension could be expected in approximately 44% of normotensive patients. If one also assumes that the subsequent development of renovascular hypertension is managed medically, then the next consideration is the frequency of decline in renal function. Among 30 patients with renovascular hypertension (i.e. renal artery lesions with severe hypertension and lateralizing functional studies) randomized to medical management, significant loss of renal function, manifest by at least a 25% decrease in estimated glomerular filtration rate (EGFR), occurred in 40% of patients during a follow-up period of 15–24 months.[14] These patients were considered failures of medical management and submitted to operative renal artery repair. However, 13% of those patients who were subsequently submitted to operation continued to exhibit progressive deterioration in renal function. Therefore, of the patients with renovascular hypertension randomized to medical management, only 36% had potentially preventable loss of renal function by means of an earlier operation. Novick et al.[15] have reported that among patients who demonstrate a decline in kidney function during medical management, 67% of properly selected patients will have renal function restored by renal artery repair.

The relevance of these issues to prophylactic renal revascularization can be demonstrated by considering 100 hypothetical patients without hypertension who have an unsuspected renal artery lesion detected by angiography prior to aortic repair (**Table 26c.2**). If the renal artery lesion is not repaired prophylactically, 44 patients may eventually develop renovascular hypertension. Sixteen (36%) of these 44 patients may experience a preventable reduction in renal function during follow-up. However, delayed operation would restore function in 11 (67%) of these 16 patients. In theory, therefore, only five of these 100 hypothetical patients would receive *unique benefit* from prophylactic intervention.

This unique benefit should be considered in terms of the associated morbidity and mortality of combined aortorenal repair. The operative mortality associated with the surgical treatment of isolated renal artery disease at our institution is 1.6%; however, combined aortorenal reconstruction is associated with a 5.3% perioperative mortality.[16] If direct aortorenal methods of reconstruction are employed in conjunction with intraoperative completion duplex sonography, the early technical failure rate is approximately 0.8%, with 3.6% late failure on follow-up. In all, early and late failures of reconstruction can be expected in 4–5% of renal artery repairs.[3] Therefore, adverse results could be

Comparison of risk to benefit of prophylactic renal revascularization in 100 hypothetical normotensive patients.	
Benefit/Risk	No. of patients
Benefit	
Progression to RVH (44/100 or 44%)	44
RVH patients who lose renal function (16/44 or 36%)	16
Renal function restored by later operation (11/16 or 67%)	11
Renal function not restored by later operation (5/16 or 33%)	5
Unique benefit	5 patients
Risk	
Operative mortality (5.3%)	5
Early technical failure (0.8%)	1
Late failure of revascularization (3.6%)	4
Adverse outcome	10 patients

Table 26c.2 Comparison of risk to benefit of prophylactic renal revascularization in 100 hypothetical normotensive patients. RVH, renovascular hypertension. (From Edwards MS, Hansen KJ. Combined aortorenal reconstruction. In: Green RM, ed. Complex aortic surgery. New York:Marcel Dekker [Forthcoming].)

expected in nine or ten of these 100 hypothetical patients after combined aortorenal repair.

In this hypothetical group of 100 normotensive patients, prophylactic renal artery surgery combined with aortic repair would probably provide unique benefits in five patients but would probably produce an adverse outcome in ten patients. Based on available data, we find no justification for prophylactic renal artery surgery either as an independent procedure or as a procedure performed in combination with aortic repair. These conclusions are supported by the retrospective experience reported by Williamson et al.[17]

In contrast to prophylactic renal revascularization, empiric renal artery repair is appropriate under select circumstances.

The term *empiric repair* implies that hypertension and/or renal dysfunction are present, although a causal relationship between the renal artery lesion and these clinical sequelae has not been established by functional studies.

Repair of unilateral renal artery disease may be appropriate as a combined aortorenal procedure in the absence of functional studies (i.e. RVRA) when:

- hypertension is severe;
- the patient is without significant risk factors for operation; and
- the probability of technical success is greater than 95%.

In these circumstances, correction of a renal artery lesion may be justified in order to eliminate all possible causes of hypertension and renal dysfunction. However, because the probability of blood pressure benefit is lower in such a patient, morbidity from the procedure must also be predictably low.

When a patient has bilateral renal artery stenoses and hypertension, the decision to combine renal artery repair with correction of the aortic disease is based on severity of the hypertension and the renovascular lesions. If the renal artery lesions consist of severe disease on one side and only mild or moderate disease on the contralateral side, then the patient is treated as if only a unilateral lesion exists. If both lesions are only moderately severe (65% to 80% diameter-reducing stenosis), then renal revascularization is undertaken only if the hypertension is severe. In contrast, if both renal artery lesions are severe (>80% stenosis) and the patient has drug-dependent hypertension, bilateral simultaneous renal revascularization is performed. Hypertension secondary to severe bilateral renal artery stenoses is often particularly severe and difficult to control. Furthermore, at least mild excretory renal insufficiency is often present. Since renal insufficiency usually parallels the severity of hypertension, a patient who presents with severe renal insufficiency but only mild hypertension usually has renal parenchymal disease. Characteristically, renovascular hypertension associated with severe renal insufficiency or dialysis-dependence is also associated with very severe bilateral stenoses or total renal artery occlusions. When considering combined repair of incidentally defined renal artery disease with correction of aortic disease, one should evaluate the clinical status with respect to this characteristic presentation. In such situations, combined renal artery repair at the time of aortic surgery is indicated to improve excretory renal function, with beneficial blood pressure response a secondary goal. Such indications appear justified in light of the observed increase in dialysis-free survival associated with improved renal function despite the increased morbidity and mortality of a combined aortorenal procedure in this patient population.

MANAGEMENT OPTIONS

In recent years, optimal management of renal artery disease has become increasingly controversial. In the absence of prospective randomized trials, advocates of medical management, PTRA with endoluminal stenting or operative management cite selective clinical data to support their views. A majority of the medical community evaluate patients for renovascular disease only when medications are not tolerated or hypertension remains severe and uncontrolled. The study by Hunt & Strong[18] remains the most informative study available to assess the comparative value of medical therapy and operation. In their non-randomized study, the results of operative treatment in 100 patients was compared with the results of drug therapy in 114 similar patients. After 7 to 14 years of follow-up, 84% of the operated group were alive, as compared with 66% in the drug therapy group. Of the 84 patients alive in the operated group, 93% were cured or significantly improved, compared with 16 (21%) of the patients alive in the drug therapy group. Death during follow-up was twice as common in the medically treated group as in the surgically managed group. Antihypertensive agents in current use provide improved blood pressure control compared with those in this earlier era. However, additional data regarding medical therapy for renovascular hypertension suggest that a decrease in kidney size and renal function occur despite satisfactory blood pressure control.[14]

In patients with functionally significant renal artery lesions and severe hypertension, the detrimental changes that occur during medical therapy alone, combined with the excellent contemporary results of operative management, argue for an aggressive attitude toward renal artery intervention.[1,2] The authors' indications for operation include all patients with severe, difficult-to-control hypertension. This includes patients with complicating factors such as branch lesions and extrarenal vascular disease and patients with associated cardiovascular disease that would be improved by blood pressure reduction. Age, type of lesion, medical co-morbidity, and aortic disease must be considered in selecting patients for open surgical or endovascular management.

Percutaneous transluminal angioplasty with and without stenting (see also p. 333)

Experience with the liberal use of PTRA has helped to clarify its role as a therapeutic option in the treatment of renovascular hypertension. Like operative repair, accumulated data argue for its selective application. In this regard, PTRA of non-ostial atherosclerotic lesions and medial fibroplasia of the main renal artery yields blood pressure results comparable to the results of operative repair. In contrast, suboptimal lesions for PTRA include congenital lesions, fibrodysplastic lesions involving renal artery branches, ostial atherosclerotic lesions, and renal artery occlusions. In each instance, these lesions are associated with inferior results and increased risk of complications.

A review of published reports over the past 12 years documenting blood pressure and renal function after PTRA for atherosclerotic renovascular disease revealed angiographic success in 86% of cases and a beneficial blood pressure response in 65% of patients. Thirty-two percent of patients with pre-existing renal insufficiency experienced improved excretory renal function while 51% remained unchanged and 17% had worsened renal function. Major complications were observed in 12% of patients and restenosis was observed in 25% of treated arteries at 6- to 12-month follow-up intervals (**Table 26c.3**).[19–33]

In an effort to improve upon the outcome of angioplasty, endoluminal stenting has been combined with PTRA. Although no stent has been approved for renal use in the USA, the most common indications for the employment of such appear to be:

- elastic recoil of the vessel immediately after angioplasty;
- renal artery dissection after angioplasty; and
- restenosis after angioplasty.

Results after primary percutaneous transluminal renal artery angioplasty for atherosclerotic renal artery stenosis.

Reference	No. of patients	Technical success	No. of patients with renal dysfunction	Renal function response			Hypertension response			Restenosis	Major complications
				Improved	Unchanged	Worsened	Cured	Improved	Failed		
Canzanello (1989)[19]	100	73%	66		52%	48%		59%	41%	19%	20%
Klinge (1989)[20]	134	78%	n/r	n/r	n/r	n/r	11%	78%	10%	16%	11%
Baert (1990)[21]	165	83%	n/r	n/r	n/r	n/r	32%	36%	32%	10%	11%
Tykarski (1993)[22]	26	81%	16	69%	31%	0%	45%	35%	20%	15%	n/r
Weibull (1993)[23]	29	83%	n/r	21%	75%	4%	13%	71%	17%	25%	17%
Losinno (1994)[24]	153	95%	59	27%	67%	6%	12%	51%	37%	n/r	8%
Rodriguez-Perez (1994)[25]	37	78%	n/r	No change in mean SCr			3%	80%	17%	11%	8%
Bonelli (1995)[26]	190	82%	n/r	No change in mean SCr			8%	62%	30%	10%	23%
Hoffman (1998)[27]	50	58%	36	44%	23%	33%	3%	64%	32%	27%	14%
Klow (1998)[28]	295	92%	n/r	No change in mean SCr			5%	59%	31%	40%	8%
Zuccala (1998)[29]*	99	92%	33	39%	50%	11%	18%	44%	48%	17%	8%
Paulsen (1999)[30]	135	90%	79	23%	56%	21%	6%	41%	53%	45%	9%
van de Ven (1999)[31]	41	57%	22	18%	55%	27%	5%	44%	51%	48%	29%
Baumgartner (2000)[32]	33	95%	107	33%	42%	25%		43%	57%	35%	3%
Van Jaarsveld (2000)[33]	56	91%	n/r	No change in mean SCr			7%	61%	32%	48%	5%
TOTALS	1543	86%	418	32%	51%	17%	11%	54%	35%	25%	12%

*All diabetic patients

Table 26c.3 Results after primary percutaneous transluminal renal artery angioplasty for atherosclerotic renal artery stenosis. n/r, not reported; SCr, serum creatinine.

Recently, primary stenting of atherosclerotic renal artery disease has been widely applied. Review of published reports of percutaneous renal artery stenting reveals no clinical improvement beyond PTRA alone, with 61% of atherosclerotic patients experiencing blood pressure benefit while 25% experienced improvement in renal function. Restenosis was observed in 18% of patients at variable follow-up intervals (**Table 26c.4**).[31,32,34–54] Review of PTRA and endoluminal stenting for ostial atherosclerosis of the renal artery demonstrated similar results. When renal artery stenting was applied to ostial atherosclerotic renal artery stenosis in patients with ischemic nephropathy, only 18% experienced improvement in excretory renal function while 17% had worsened renal function. Restenosis was observed in 21% of patients (**Table 26c.5**).[31,32,34,38–41,46,48,49,51,52,54] These results are inferior to those in selected patients treated surgically. Consequently, for the majority of patients with ostial atherosclerosis in combination with renal insufficiency, we believe operative repair remains the best treatment. Nevertheless, the decision for interventional therapy for atherosclerotic renovascular disease must be individualized. In this regard, significant and independent predictors of accelerated death on follow-up (i.e. clinical congestive heart failure, long-standing diabetes mellitus, uncorrectable azotemia) are considered before any intervention is made.

Operative management
General issues
The presence of hypertension is considered a prerequisite for renal artery intervention. In general, functional studies are used to guide the management of unilateral lesions. Empiric renal artery repair is performed without functional studies when hypertension is severe, renal artery disease is bilateral, or the patient has ischemic nephropathy.[1,2,13] Accordingly, prophylactic renal artery repair in the absence of hypertension, whether as an isolated procedure or combined with aortic reconstruction, is not recommended. During surgical reconstruction, all hemodynamically significant renal artery disease is corrected in a single operation, with the exception of disease requiring bilateral ex-vivo reconstructions, which are staged. Having observed beneficial blood pressure and renal function response regardless of kidney size or histologic pattern on renal biopsy, nephrectomy is reserved for unreconstructable renal artery disease to a non-functioning kidney (i.e. ≤ 10% function by renography).[3,10,11,13] Direct aortorenal reconstructions are preferred over indirect methods

Results after primary renal artery stent placement for atherosclerotic renal artery stenosis.

Reference	Patients	Technical success	No. of patients with renal dysfunction	Renal function response			Hypertension response			Restenosis	Major complications
				Improved	Unchanged	Worsened	Cured	Improved	Failed		
Rees (1991)[34]	28	96%	14	35%	36%	29%	11%	53%	36%	39%	18%
Wilms (1991)[35]	10	80%	1	0%	100%	0%	30%	40%	30%	22%	18%
Kuhn (1991)[36]	8	92%	n/r	n/r	n/r	n/r	22%	34%	44%	17%	13%
Joffre (1992)[37]	11	91%	4	50%	50%	0%	27%	64%	9%	18%	13%
Hennequin (1994)[38]	15	100%	6	20%	40%	40%	7%	93%	0%	27%	19%
Raynaud (1994)[39]	15	100%	7	0%	43%	57%	7%	43%	50%	13%	13%
MacLeod (1995)[40]	28	100%	16	25%	75%		0%	40%	60%	17%	19%
van de Ven (1995)[41]	24	100%	n/r	33%	58%	8%	0%	73%	27%	13%	13%
Dorros (1995)[42]	76	100%	29	28%	28%	45%	6%	46%	48%	25%	11%
Henry (1996)[43]	55	100%	10	20%	80%		18%	57%	24%	9%	3%
Iannone (1996)[44]	63	99%	29	36%	46%	18%	4%	35%	61%	14%	32%
Harden (1997)[45]	32	100%	32	35%	35%	29%	n/r	n/r	n/r	13%	19%
Blum (1997)[46]	68	100%	20	0%	100%	0%	16%	62%	22%	17%	0%
Boisclair (1997)[47]	33	100%	17	41%	35%	24%	6%	61%	33%	0%	21%
Rundback (1998)[48]	45	94%	45	18%	53%	30%	n/r	n/r	n/r	26%	9%
Fiala (1998)[49]	21	95%	9	0%	100%	0%		53%	47%	65%	19%
Dorros (1998)[50]	163	99%	63	No mean change in SCr			1%	42%	57%	n/r	14%
Tuttle (1998)[51]	120	98%	74	16%	75%	9%	2%	46%	52%	14%	4%
Gross (1998)[52]	30	100%	12	55%	27%	18%	0%	69%	31%	13%	n/r
Henry (1999)[53]	200	99%	48	29%	67%	4%	19%	61%	20%	11%	2%
Rodriguez-Lopez (1999)[54]	108	98%	32	No mean change in SCr			13%	55%	32%	26%	12%
van de Ven (1999)[31]	40	88%	29	17%	55%	28%	15%	43%	42%	14%	30%
Baumgartner (2000)[32]	64	95%	n/r	33%	42%	25%		43%	57%	28%	9%
TOTALS	1257	98%	497	25%	56%	19%	10%	51%	39%	18%	11%

Table 26c.4 Results after primary renal artery stent placement for atherosclerotic renal artery stenosis. n/r, not reported; SCr, serum creatinine.

since concomitant disease of the celiac axis is present in 40–50% of patients and bilateral repair is required in half.[1,3] Failed renal artery repair is associated with a significantly increased risk of dialysis-dependence.[3] To minimize these failures, intraoperative duplex is utilized to evaluate the technical results of surgical repair.[55]

Preoperative preparation

Antihypertensive medications are reduced during the preoperative period to the minimum necessary for blood pressure control. Patients requiring large doses of multiple medications will often have reduced requirements while hospitalized at bed rest. If continued therapy is required, vasodilators and selective β-adrenergic blocking agents are the agents of choice. If the diastolic blood pressure exceeds 120mmHg, operative treatment is postponed until the pressure is brought under control. In

this instance, the combination of intravenous nitroprusside and esmolol is administered in an intensive care setting.

Operative techniques

A variety of operative techniques have been used to correct renal artery atherosclerosis. From a practical standpoint, three basic operations have been most frequently utilized:

- aortorenal bypass;
- renal artery thromboendarterectomy; and
- renal artery reimplantation.

Although each method may have its proponents, no single approach provides optimal repair for all types of renal artery disease. Aortorenal bypass, preferably with saphenous vein, is probably the most versatile technique; however, thromboendarterectomy is especially useful for ostial atherosclerosis involving

Results after primary renal artery stent placement for ostial atherosclerotic renal artery stenosis.

Reference	No. of patients with ostial lesions	No. of patients with renal dysfunction	Renal function response			Hypertension response			Restenosis
			Improved	Unchanged	Worsened	Cured	Improved	Failed	
Rees (1991)[34]	28	14	36%	35%	29%	11%	54%	36%	39%
Hennequin (1994)[38]	7	2	0%	50%	50%	0%	100%	0%	43%
Raynaud (1994)[39]	4	3	0%	33%	67%	0%	50%	50%	33%
MacLeod (1995)[40]	22	13	15%	85%		0%	31%	69%	20%
van de Ven (1995)[41]	24	n/r	33%	58%	8%	0%	73%	27%	13%
Blum (1997)[46]	68	20	0%	100%	0%	16%	62%	22%	17%
Rundback (1998)[48]	32	32	16%	53%	31%	n/r	n/r	n/r	26%
Fiala (1998)[49]	21	9	0%	100%	0%		53%	47%	65%
Tuttle (1998)[51]	129	74	16%	75%	9%	2%	46%	52%	14%
Gross (1998)[52]	30	12	55%	27%	18%	0%	69%	31%	12%
Rodriguez-Lopez (1999)[54]	82	n/r	No change in mean SCr			13%	55%	32%	26%
van de Ven (1999)[31]	40	29	17%	55%	28%	15%	43%	42%	14%
Baumgartner (2000)[32]	21	n/r	33%	42%	25%	43%	57%		20%
TOTALS	508	208	18%	65%	17%	7%	53%	40%	21%

Table 26c.5 Results after primary renal artery stent placement for ostial atherosclerotic renal artery stenosis. n/r, not reported; SCr, serum creatinine. (From Hansen KJ, Cherr GS, Edwards MS. Management of atherosclerotic renovascular disease. In: Pearce WH, Yao JST, eds. Advances in vascular surgery. Chicago:Precept Press; 2001:209–18.)

multiple renal arteries. When the artery is sufficiently redundant, reimplantation is probably the simplest technique and one particularly appropriate for combined repairs of aortic and renal pathology.

Certain measures are used in almost all renal artery operations. Mannitol is administered intravenously in 12.5g doses early, and repeated before and after periods of renal ischemia, up to a total dose of 1g per kilogram patient body weight. Just prior to renal artery occlusion, 100 units of heparin per kilogram body weight is given intravenously, and systemic anticoagulation is verified by activated clotting time. Unless required for hemostasis, protamine is not routinely administered for reversal of heparin at the completion of the operation.

Mobilization and dissection

A xiphoid-to-pubis midline abdominal incision is made for operative repair of atherosclerotic renal artery disease. The last 1–2cm of the proximal incision coursing to one side of the xiphoid is important in obtaining full exposure of the upper abdominal aorta and renal branches. Some form of fixed mechanical retraction is also advantageous, particularly when combined aortorenal procedures are required. Otherwise, extended flank and subcostal incisions are reserved for ex-vivo reconstructions or splanchnorenal bypass.

When the supraceliac aorta is utilized as an inflow source for aortorenal bypass, an extended flank incision is useful. With the flank elevated, the incision extends from the semilunar line into the flank, bisecting the abdominal wall between the costal margin and iliac crest. A visceral mobilization allows access to

the renal vasculature and the aortic crus. If necessary, the crus can be divided and an extrapleural dissection of the descending thoracic aorta can provide access to the T9–T10 thoracic aorta for proximal control and anastomosis.

When the midline xiphoid-to-pubis incision is used, the posterior peritoneum overlying the aorta is incised longitudinally and the duodenum is mobilized at the ligament of Treitz (**Fig. 26c.1**). During this maneuver, it is important to identify visceral collaterals which course at this level. Finally, the duodenum is reflected to the patient's right, to expose the left renal artery. By extending the posterior peritoneal incision to the left along the inferior border of the pancreas, an avascular plane posterior to the pancreas can be entered (**Fig. 26c.1**) to expose the entire renal hilum on the left.

This exposure is of special significance when there are distal renal artery lesions to be managed (**Fig. 26c.2A**). The left renal artery lies behind the left renal vein. In some cases, the vein can be retracted cephalad to expose the artery; in other cases, caudal retraction of the vein provides better access. Usually, the gonadal and adrenal veins, which enter the left renal vein, must be ligated and divided to facilitate exposure of the distal artery. Frequently, a lumbar vein enters the posterior wall of the left renal vein, and it can be easily avulsed unless special care is taken while mobilizing the renal vein (**Fig. 26c.2B**). The proximal portion of the right renal artery can be exposed through the base of the mesentery by ligating two or more pairs of lumbar veins and retracting the left renal vein cephalad and the vena cava to the patient's right (**Fig. 26c.2C**). However, the distal portion of the right renal artery is best exposed by mobilizing the duodenum and right

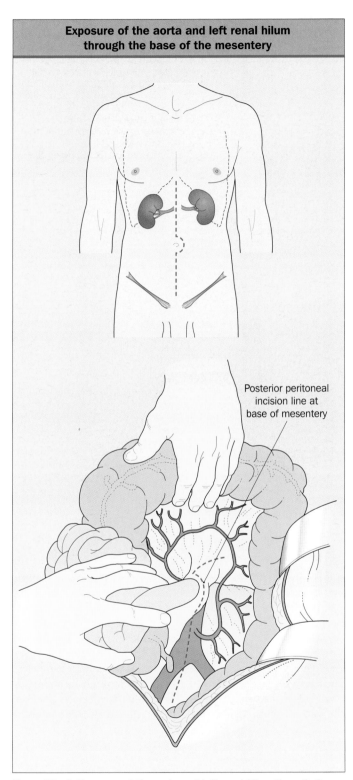

Exposure of the aorta and left renal hilum through the base of the mesentery

Posterior peritoneal incision line at base of mesentery

Figure 26c.1 Exposure of the aorta and left renal hilum through the base of the mesentery. Extension of the posterior peritoneal incision to the left, along the inferior border of the pancreas, provides entry to an avascular plane behind the pancreas. This allows excellent exposure of the entire left renal hilum as well as the proximal right renal artery.

colon medially. Then, the right renal vein is mobilized and usually retracted cephalad in order to expose the artery (**Fig. 26c.3**).

Exposure of the distal right renal artery is achieved by hepatic and duodenal mobilization. First, the hepatic flexure is mobilized at the peritoneal reflection. With the right colon retracted medially and inferiorly, a Kocher's maneuver mobilizes the duodenum and pancreatic head to expose the inferior vena cava and right renal vein. Typically, the right renal artery is located just inferior to the accompanying vein, which can be retracted superiorly to provide best exposure. Though accessory vessels may arise from the aorta or iliac vessels at any level, all arterial branches coursing anterior to the vena cava should be considered accessory renal branches and carefully preserved (**Fig. 26c.3**).

When bilateral renal artery lesions are to be corrected in combination with aortic reconstruction, these exposure techniques can be modified. Extended exposure may be provided by mobilizing the base of the small bowel mesentery to allow complete evisceration of the entire small bowel, and ascending and transverse colon. For this extended exposure, the posterior peritoneal incision begins with division of the ligament of Treitz and proceeds along the base of the mesentery to the cecum and then up the lateral gutter to the foramen of Winslow (**Fig. 26c.4**). The inferior border of the pancreas is fully mobilized to enter a retropancreatic plane, thereby exposing the aorta to a point above the superior mesenteric artery. Through this modified exposure, simultaneous bilateral renal endarterectomies, aortorenal grafting, or renal artery attachment to the aortic graft can be performed with wide visualization of the entire area.

Aortorenal bypass

Three types of materials are available for aortorenal bypass:

- autologous saphenous vein;
- autologous hypogastric artery; and
- synthetic prosthetic.

The decision as to which graft should be used depends on a number of factors. We use the saphenous vein preferentially. However, if the vein is small (<4mm in diameter) or sclerotic, the hypogastric artery or a synthetic prosthesis may be preferable. A 6mm, thin-walled polytetrafluoroethylene (PTFE) or Dacron polyester graft is satisfactory when the distal renal artery is of large caliber (≥ 4mm).

When an end-to-side renal artery bypass is used, the anastomosis between the renal artery and the graft is performed first (**Fig. 26c.5A**). Silastic slings can be used to occlude the renal artery distally. This method of vessel occlusion is especially applicable to this procedure. In contrast to vascular clamps, these slings are essentially atraumatic to the delicate renal artery and avoid the presence of clamps in the operative field. Furthermore, when tension is applied to the slings, they lift the vessel out of the retroperitoneal soft tissue for better visualization. The length of the arteriotomy should be at least three times the diameter of the smaller conduit, to guard against late suture-line stenosis (**Fig. 26c.5B**). A 6-0 or 7-0 polypropylene suture is employed with loop magnification. After the renal artery anastomosis is completed, the occluding clamps and slings are removed from the artery rand a small bulldog clamp is placed across the vein graft adjacent to the anastomosis. The aortic anastomosis is then performed (**Fig. 26c.5C**) after removing an ellipse of the anterolateral aortic wall. If the graft is too long, kinking of the vein and subsequent thrombosis may result. In this instance,

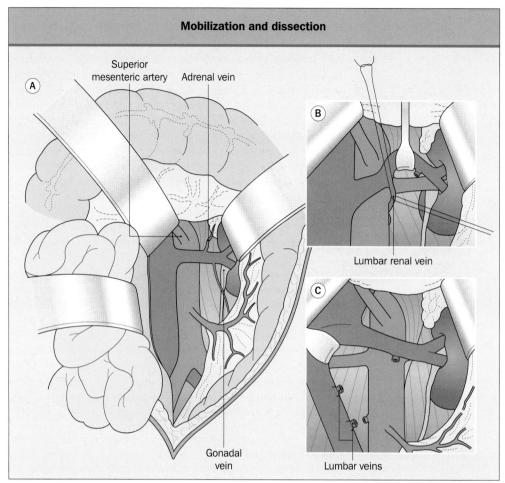

Mobilization and dissection

(A)
Superior
mesenteric artery   Adrenal vein

(B)

Lumbar renal vein

(C)

Gonadal
vein   Lumbar veins

Figure 26c.2 Mobilization and dissection. (A) Exposure of the proximal right renal artery through the base of the mesentery. (B) Mobilization of the left renal vein by ligation and division of the adrenal, gonadal, and lumbar-renal veins allows exposure of the entire left renal artery to the hilum. (C) Two pairs of lumbar vessels have been ligated and divided to allow retraction of the vena cava to the right, revealing adequate exposure of the proximal renal artery.

the aortic anastomosis should be taken down and revised after appropriate orientation of the graft. In the majority of instances, an end-to-end anastomosis between the graft and the renal artery provides a better reconstruction (**Fig. 26c.5D**). We routinely employ end-to-end renal artery anastomosis when combining aortic replacement with renal revascularization. In this circumstance, the proximal anastomosis is performed first and the distal renal anastomosis performed second, to limit renal ischemia. Regardless of the type of distal anastomosis, the proximal aortorenal anastomosis is best performed after excision of an ellipse of aortic wall. This is especially important when the aorta is relatively inflexible due to atherosclerotic involvement.

Thromboendarterectomy

In some cases of bilateral atherosclerotic occlusions of the renal artery origins, simultaneous bilateral endarterectomy may be the most applicable procedure. Endarterectomy may be either transaortic or transrenal. In the latter instance, the aortotomy is made transversely and is carried across the aorta and into the renal artery to a point beyond the visible disease (**Fig. 26c.6A**). With this method, the distal endarterectomy can be assessed and tacked down with mattress sutures under direct vision if necessary. Following completion of the endarterectomy, the arteriotomy is closed. In most patients, this closure is performed with a Dacron patch to ensure that the proximal renal artery is

widely patent (**Fig. 26c.6B,C**). In the majority of instances, the transaortic endarterectomy technique is used. The transaortic method is particularly applicable in patients with multiple renal arteries that demonstrate orificial disease. Transaortic endarterectomy is performed through a longitudinal aortotomy with sleeve endarterectomy of the aorta and renal arteries (**Fig. 26c.7**). When combined aortic replacement is planned, the transaortic endarterectomy is performed through the transected aorta (**Fig. 26c.8**). When using the transaortic technique, it is important to mobilize the renal arteries extensively, to allow eversion of the vessel into the aorta. This allows the distal endpoint to be completed under direct vision.

Renal artery reimplantation

After the renal artery has been dissected from the surrounding retroperitoneal tissue, the vessel may be somewhat redundant. When the renal artery stenosis is orificial and there is sufficient vessel length, the renal artery can be transected and reimplanted into the aorta at a slightly lower level. The renal artery must be spatulated and a portion of the aortic wall removed as in renal artery bypass.

Splanchnorenal bypasses

Splanchnorenal bypass and other indirect procedures have received increased use as an alternative method for renal revascularization.[56]

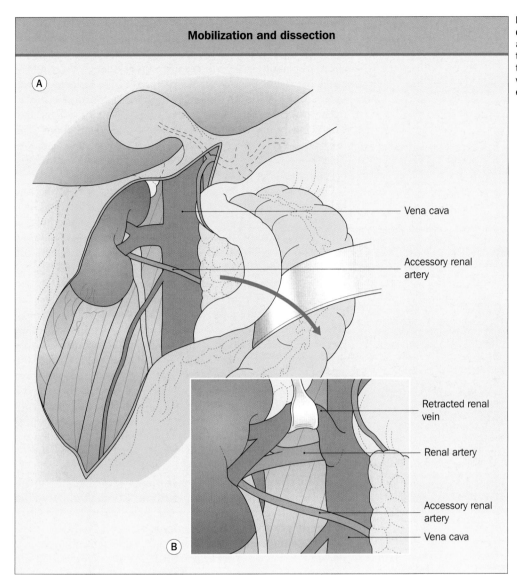

Mobilization and dissection

Vena cava

Accessory renal artery

Retracted renal vein

Renal artery

Accessory renal artery

Vena cava

Figure 26c.3 Mobilization and dissection. (A) Not uncommonly, an accessory right renal artery arises from the anterior aorta and crosses anterior to the vena cava. (B) The right renal vein is typically mobilized superiorly for exposure of the distal renal artery.

In general, we do not believe that these procedures are comparable with direct reconstructions, but they are useful in a selected subgroup of high-risk patients.

Hepatorenal bypass
A right subcostal incision is used to perform the hepatorenal bypass.[56] The lesser omentum is incised to expose the hepatic artery both proximal and distal to the gastroduodenal artery (**Fig. 26c.9**). Next, the descending duodenum is mobilized by Kocher's maneuver, the inferior vena cava is identified, the right renal vein is identified, and the right renal artery is encircled where it is found, either immediately cephalad or caudad to the renal vein.

A greater saphenous vein graft is usually used to construct the bypass. The hepatic artery anastomosis of the vein graft can be placed at the site of the amputated stump of the gastroduodenal artery; however, this vessel may serve as an important collateral for intestinal perfusion. Therefore, the proximal anastomosis is usually made to the common hepatic artery. After completion of this anastomosis, the renal artery is transected and brought

anterior to the vena cava for anastomosis end-to-end to the graft (**Fig. 26c.10**).

Splenorenal bypass
Splenorenal bypass can be performed through a midline or a left subcostal incision. The posterior pancreas is mobilized by reflecting the inferior border cephalad. A retropancreatic plane is developed and the splenic artery mobilized from the left gastroepiploic artery to the level of its branches. The left renal artery is exposed cephalad to the left renal vein after division of the adrenal vein. After the splenic artery has been mobilized, it is divided distally, spatulated, and anastomosed end-to-end to the transected renal artery (**Fig. 26c.11**).

Ex-vivo reconstruction
In part, operative strategy for renal artery branch vessel repair is determined by the required exposure and anticipated period of renal ischemia. When reconstruction can be accomplished with less than 30 minutes of ischemia, an in-situ repair is undertaken without special measures for renal preservation. When longer

345

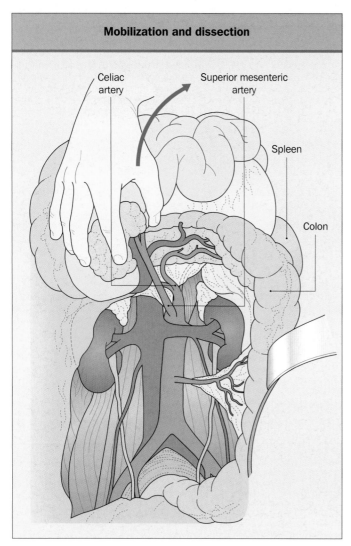

Mobilization and dissection

Celiac artery

Superior mesenteric artery

Spleen

Colon

Figure 26c.4 Mobilization and dissection. For complex bilateral renal artery reconstruction, wide exposure can be obtained with mobilization of the cecum and ascending colon. The entire small bowel and right colon are then mobilized to the right upper quadrant and placed on to the chest wall. Division of the diaphragmatic crura exposures the origin of the mesenteric vessels.

periods of ischemia are anticipated, one of two techniques for hypothermic preservation of the kidney are considered:

• renal mobilization without renal vein transection; and
• ex-vivo repair and anatomic replacement in the renal fossa.

For atherosclerotic renovascular disease, these techniques are most commonly required after failure or complications of PTRA.

Ex-vivo management is necessary when extensive exposure is required for extended periods. This includes:

• patients with fibromuscular dysplasia (FMD) and aneurysms or stenoses involving renal artery branches;
• patients with FMD and renal artery dissection and branch occlusion;
• patients with congenital arteriovenous fistulae of renal artery branches requiring partial resection; and
• patients with degeneration of previously placed grafts to the distal renal artery.

Several methods of ex-vivo hypothermic perfusion and reconstruction are available. A midline xiphoid-to-pubis incision is used for most renovascular procedures and is preferred when autotransplantation of the reconstructed kidney or combined aortic reconstructions are to be performed. For isolated branch renal artery repairs, an extended flank incision is made parallel to the lower rib margin and carried to the posterior axillary line. This is our preferred approach for ex-vivo reconstructions. The ureter is always partially mobilized, but left intact, and an elastic sling or non-crushing clamp is placed around the ureter to prevent collateral perfusion and subsequent renal rewarming.

Gerota's fascia is opened with a cruciate incision and the kidney is mobilized and the renal vessels divided (**Fig. 26c.12A**). The kidney is placed on the abdominal wall and perfused with a chilled renal preservation solution. Continuous perfusion during the period of total renal ischemia is possible with perfusion pump systems, and may be superior for prolonged renal preservation. However, simple intermittent flushing with a chilled preservation solution provides equal protection during the shorter periods (2–3 hours) required for ex-vivo dissection and branch renal artery reconstructions. For this technique, we refrigerate the preservative overnight, add the additional components immediately before use to make up a liter of solution, and hang the chilled (5–10°C) solution at a height of at least 2 meters. Three to five hundred milliliters of solution are flushed through the kidney immediately after its removal from the renal fossa until the venous effluent is clear. As each anastomosis is completed, the kidney is perfused with an additional 150–200mL of solution. Besides maintaining satisfactory hypothermia, periodic perfusion demonstrates suture-line leaks, which are repaired prior to reimplantation. In addition to perfusion, surface hypothermia is used during ex-vivo renal artery reconstruction. Our method of surface hypothermia consists of the following steps. We place liter bottles of normal saline solution in ice slush overnight. When we elevate the kidney, we place it in a watertight plastic sheet, which serves as a barrier from which excess saline solution can be suctioned. Laparotomy pads are placed over the kidney, keeping it cool and moist by a constant drip of the chilled saline solution. With this technique, we can maintain renal core temperatures at 10–15°C throughout the period of reconstruction. Autotransplantation to the iliac fossa is unnecessary for most ex-vivo reconstructions. Reduction in the magnitude of the operative exposure, manual palpation of the transplanted kidney, and ease of removal when treatment of rejection fails are all practical reasons for placing the transplanted kidney into the recipient's iliac fossa, but none of these advantages apply to the patient requiring autogenous ex-vivo reconstruction. In this latter patient group, the factors most important relate to those improving the long-term patency after renal artery repair. Because many ex-vivo procedures are performed in relatively young patients, the durability of operation must be measured in terms of decades. For this reason, attachment of the kidney to the iliac arterial system within or below sites that are susceptible to subsequent atherosclerotic occlusive disease subjects the repaired vessels to atherosclerotic disease that may threaten their long-term patency. Moreover, subsequent management of peripheral vascular disease may be complicated by the presence of the autotransplanted kidney. Finally, if the kidney is replaced in the renal fossa and the renal artery graft is properly attached to the aorta at a proximal infrarenal site, the result should mimic that of the standard

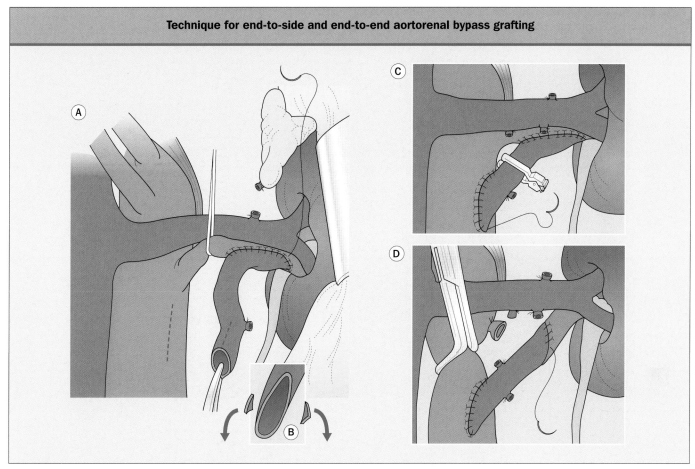

Technique for end-to-side and end-to-end aortorenal bypass grafting

Figure 26c.5 Technique for end-to-side (A–C) and end-to-end (D) aortorenal bypass grafting. The length of arteriotomy is at least three times the diameter of the artery, to prevent recurrent anastomotic stenosis. For the anastomosis, 6/0 or 7/0 monofilament polypropylene sutures are used in continuous fashion, under loupe magnification. If the apex sutures are placed too deeply or with excess advancement, stenosis can be created, posing a risk of late graft thrombosis.

aortorenal bypass and thus carry a high probability of technical success and long-term durability.

For replacement of the kidney in its original site, a large vascular clamp is placed to partially occlude the vena cava where it is entered by the renal vein. An ellipse of vena cava containing the entrance site of the renal vein is then excised, and the kidney is removed for ex-vivo perfusion and reconstruction (**Fig. 26c.12A**). When the renal artery–graft anastomoses are completed and the kidney is replaced in its bed, the ellipse of vena cava is reattached (**Fig. 26c.12B**). This technique protects against stenosis of the renal vein anastomosis. The renal artery graft is then attached to the aorta in the standard manner (**Fig. 26c.12C**).

Intraoperative duplex sonography

Provided the best method of reconstruction is chosen for renal artery repair, the short course and high blood flow rates characteristic of renal reconstruction favor their patency. Consequently, flawless technical repair plays a dominant role in determining postoperative success. The negative impact of technical errors unrecognized and uncorrected at operation is implied by the fact that we have observed no late thromboses of renovascular reconstruction completely free of disease after one year.

Intraoperative assessment of most arterial reconstructions has been made by intraoperative angiography. This method has serious limitations, however, when applied to upper aortic and branch aortic reconstruction. At these locations, intraoperative angiography requires additional suprarenal or supraceliac aortic occlusion. The study obtained provides static images in the absence of pulsatile blood flow and provides anatomic evaluation in only one projection.[57,58] In addition, arteriolar vasospasm in response to cross-clamp ischemia and contrast injection may falsely suggest distal vascular occlusion. Finally, coexisting renal insufficiency is frequently present, increasing the risk of postoperative contrast nephropathy.

These risks and the inherent limitations of completion angiography are not demonstrated by intraoperative duplex sonography.[55] Because the ultrasound probe can be placed immediately adjacent to the vascular repair, high carrying frequencies may be used which provide excellent B-scan detail sensitive to <1mm anatomic defects. Once imaged, defects can be viewed in a multitude of projections during conditions of uninterrupted, pulsatile blood flow. Intimal flaps not apparent during static conditions are easily imaged while avoiding the adverse effects of additional renal ischemia. In addition to excellent anatomic

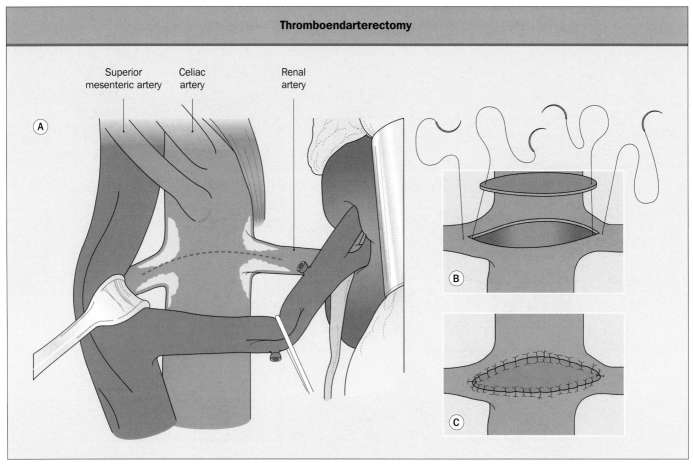

Thromboendarterectomy

Superior
mesenteric artery

Celiac
artery

Renal
artery

Figure 26c.6 Thromboendarterectomy. (A) Exposure of the juxtarenal aorta and renal arteries in preparation for transrenal endarterectomy. (B) Transverse aortotomy is used in some instances, being certain to carry the incision out on to the renal artery to a point beyond the stenosis. (C) Following completion of the endarterectomy, the arteriotomy is usually closed with a Dacron patch angioplasty to ensure that the newly repaired renal artery is left widely patent.

detail, important hemodynamic information is obtained from the spectral analysis of the Doppler-shifted signal proximal and distal to the imaged defect.[55] Freedom from static projections, the absence of potentially nephrotoxic contrast material or additional ischemia, and the hemodynamic data provided by Doppler spectral analysis make duplex sonography a very attractive intraoperative method to assess renovascular repairs.

In order to realize the advantages of intraoperative duplex, close cooperation between the vascular surgeon and the vascular technologist is required for accurate intraoperative assessment. Although the surgeon is responsible for manipulating the probe head to acquire optimal B-scan images of the vascular repair at likely sites of technical error, proper power and time gain adjustments are best made by an experienced technologist. Close cooperation is likewise required to obtain complete pulse-Doppler and color-flow sampling associated with abnormalities on B-scan. While the surgeon images areas of interest at an optimal insonation angle, the technologist sets the Doppler sample depth and volume and estimates blood flow velocities from the Doppler spectrum analysis. Finally, the participation of the vascular technologist during intraoperative assessment enhances his or her ability to obtain satisfactory surveillance duplex studies during follow-up. Our technique of intraoperative

assessment with the routine participation of a vascular technologist has yielded a scan time of 7 to 10 minutes and a 98% study completion rate.[55,57]

Currently, we use a 15.0/7.0mHz compact linear array probe with Doppler color flow designed specifically for intraoperative assessment. The probe is placed within a sterile sheath with a latex tip containing sterile gel. After the operative field is flooded with warm saline, B-scan images are first obtained in longitudinal projection. Care is taken to image the entire upper abdominal aorta and renal artery origins along the entire length of the repair. All defects seen in longitudinal projection are imaged in transverse projection to confirm their anatomic presence and to estimate associated luminal narrowing. Doppler samples are then obtained just proximal and distal to imaged lesions in longitudinal projection, determining their potential contribution to flow disturbance. Our criteria for major B-scan defects associated with ≥ 60% diameter-reducing stenosis or occlusion have been validated in a canine model of graded renal artery stenosis (**Table 26c.6**).

We have studied 249 renal artery repairs with anatomic follow-up evaluation.[59] Intraoperative assessment was normal in 157, while 84 (35%) repairs demonstrated one or more B-scan defects. Twenty-five of these defects (10%) had focal increases

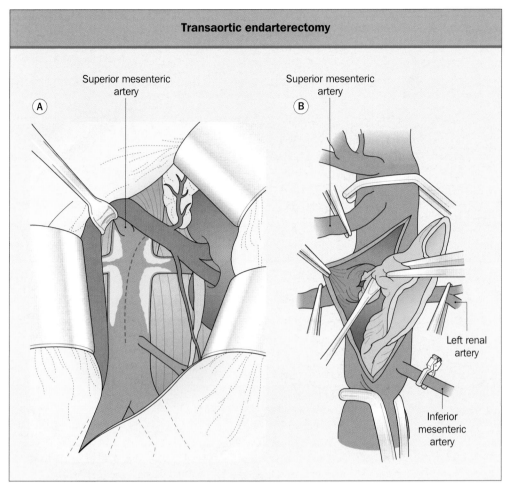

Transaortic endarterectomy

A

Superior mesenteric artery

B

Superior mesenteric artery

Left renal artery

Inferior mesenteric artery

Figure 26c.7 Transaortic endarterectomy. Exposure for a longitudinal transaortic endarterectomy is through the standard transperitoneal approach. The duodenum is mobilized from the aorta laterally in standard fashion or, for more complete exposure, the ascending colon and small bowel are mobilized. (A) Dotted line shows the location of the aortotomy. (B) The plaque is transected proximally and distally, and with eversion of the renal arteries, the atherosclerotic plaque is removed from each renal ostium. The aortotomy is typically closed with a running 4/0 or 5/0 polypropylene suture.

Intraoperative Doppler velocity criteria for renal artery repair.	
B-scan defect	*Doppler criteria*
Minor	
<60% diameter-reducing stenosis	PSV from entire artery <2.0m/s
Major	
≥60% diameter-reducing stenosis	Focal PSV ≥2.0m/s *and* distal turbulent waveform
Occlusion	No Doppler-shifted signal from renal artery B-scan image
Inadequate study	Failure to obtain Doppler samples from entire arterial repair

Table 26c.6 Intraoperative Doppler velocity criteria for renal artery repair. (From Hansen KJ, Benjamin ME, Dean RH. Renal artery disease: management options. In: Gewertz BL, Schwartz LB, eds. Surgery of the aorta and its branches. Philadelphia:WB Saunders; 2000:272–87.)

in estimated peak systolic velocity of ≥ 2.0m/s with turbulent distal waveform and were defined as major. Each major B-scan defect prompted immediate operative revision, and in each case a significant defect was discovered. B-scan defects defined as minor were not repaired. At 12-month follow-up, renal artery patency free of critical stenosis was demonstrated in 97% of normal studies, 100% of minor B-scan defects, and 88% of revised major B-scan defects, providing an overall patency of 97%. Among the five failures with normal B-scan studies, three occurred after ex-vivo branch renal artery repair.

RESULTS OF OPERATIVE REPAIR

Demographics and perioperative management

From January 1987 through December 1999, 626 patients had operative renal artery repair at our center.[2] Five hundred patients underwent repair for atherosclerotic renovascular disease, while 126 patients were treated for non-atherosclerotic renovascular disease, including congenital lesions, renal artery aneurysms, and FMD.

Among atherosclerotic patients, there were 254 women and 246 men, with a mean age of 65 ± 9 years. Their mean blood

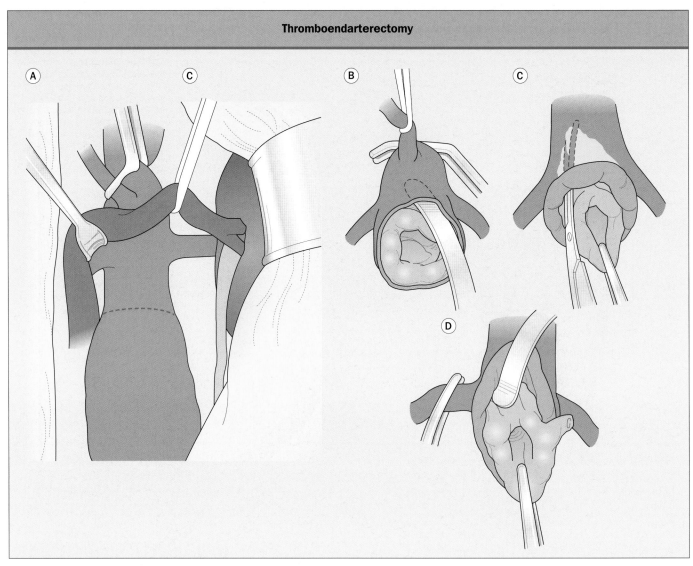

Thromboendarterectomy

Figure 26c.8 Thromboendarterectomy. For aortic repair combined with bilateral ostial stenosis of the renal arteries, thromboendarterectomy is most commonly performed through the divided aorta.

pressure was 200 ± 35/104 ± 21mmHg, with a mean duration of hypertension of 10 years. Preoperative mean and median SCr was 2.6mg/dL and 1.7mg/dL, respectively, with a mean EGFR of 40.5 ± 23.2mL/min/m². As a group, patients with atherosclerosis had widespread disease, with 70% demonstrating at least one manifestation of cardiac disease, including either angina, prior myocardial infarction, left ventricular hypertrophy, or a prior coronary artery intervention. Thirty-two percent demonstrated a prior history significant for transient ischemic attack, cerebrovascular infarct, or carotid endarterectomy. Overall, 90% of patients exhibited some clinical manifestation of extrarenal atherosclerosis. Finally, as evidenced by an SCr of 1.8 mg/dL or greater, 49% were considered to have ischemic nephropathy, including 40 patients who were dialysis-dependent.

Angiography demonstrated significant (≥ 80% ostial stenosis or occlusion) unilateral renal artery disease in 41% of patients and bilateral disease in 59% of patients with atherosclerotic renovascular disease. The vast majority of stenotic lesions (>95%)

were ostial and renal artery occlusions were noted in 31% of patients. Twenty-six percent of patients had abdominal aortic aneurysms and 51% demonstrated severe aortoiliac occlusive disease.

Among 720 renal artery reconstructions, aortorenal bypass was performed in 384 instances, with 204 vein grafts, 159 PTFE, and 21 Dacron prosthetic grafts (**Table 26c.7**). Splanchnorenal bypass was performed in 13 instances. Renal artery reimplantation was performed in 56 instances, while renal artery thromboendarterectomy was performed in 267 instances. Revascularization was combined with aortic or mesenteric reconstruction in 41% of patients. There were a total of 56 nephrectomies for a total of 776 kidneys which underwent operation.

Operative morbidity and mortality

Perioperative morbidity occurred in 81 patients (16%). These morbid events included myocardial infarction (15 patients), stroke (five patients), significant arrhythmia (22 patients), and

Summary of operative management (n = 500 patients).	
Procedure	Number of kidneys
Aortorenal bypass	384
Vein	204
PTFE	159
Dacron	21
Splanchnorenal bypass	13
Reimplantation	56
Endarterectomy	267
Nephrectomy	56
Primary	13
Contralateral	43
Total kidneys operated	**776**

Table 26c.7 Summary of operative management (n = 500 patients). PTFE, polytetraflouroethylene. (From Cherr et al.[2])

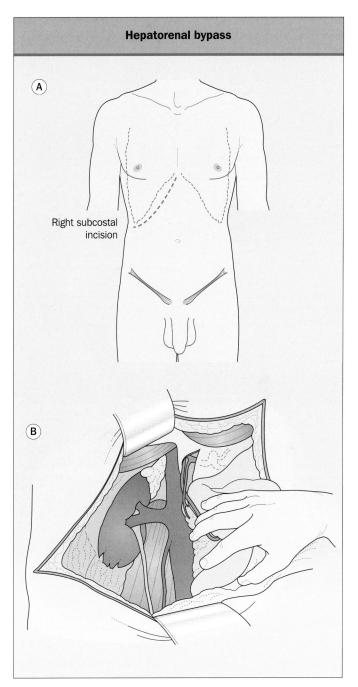

Figure 26c.9 Hepatorenal bypass. In preparation for extra-anatomic reconstruction of the right renal artery, the common hepatic artery and proximal gastroduodenal artery are exposed in the hepatoduodenal ligament. Exposure would typically be through a right subcostal skin incision.

pneumonia (36 patients). Five patients had worsening renal function after operation that resulted in permanent dialysis-dependence within 1 month of surgery. The mean preoperative SCr and EGFR for these five patients were 3.4mg/dL and 20.2ml/min/m^2, respectively. Nine patients on dialysis prior to renal revascularization continued to require renal replacement therapy after operation.

Perioperative mortality, defined as in-hospital death or death within 30 days of surgery, occurred in 23 patients (4.6%). All but one death occurred following bilateral renal artery reconstruction or renal reconstruction combined with simultaneous aortic or mesenteric artery repair. Mortality following isolated renal artery repair (0.8%) differed significantly from mortality following combined or bilateral repair (6.9%). Perioperative mortality demonstrated significant and independent associations with advanced age and clinical congestive heart failure.

Blood pressure response

Using previously published criteria,[3] blood pressure measurements and medication requirements at least 1 month after operative intervention were used to define blood pressure response. Among all surgical survivors, 85% were cured or improved, while 15% were considered failed (**Table 26c.8**). When compared with blood pressure improved or failed, blood pressure cured was significantly and independently associated with an improved dialysis-free survival. Although improved blood pressure was associated with significant postoperative decreases in blood pressure and medication requirements (205/107mmHg versus 147/81mmHg and 2.8 versus 1.7, respectively), these differences were not associated with increased dialysis-free survival. Product-limit estimates of dialysis-free survival according to postoperative blood pressure response are depicted in **Figure 26c.13**.

Renal function response

Considering all surgical survivors, renal function increased significantly after operation (preoperative versus postoperative mean EGFR, 41.1 ± 23.9mL/min/m^2 versus 48.2 ± 25.5mL/min/m^2; p<0.0001). For individual patients, a significant change in excretory renal function was defined as a change in EGFR of ≥ 20% obtained at least 3 weeks after repair. Patients were classified as improved if they were removed from dialysis or if their EGFR increased by ≥ 20%. Patients were considered worsened if their EGFR decreased by ≥ 20%. All others were considered unchanged. Fifty-eight percent of patients with ischemic nephropathy (preoperative SCr ≥ 1.8mg/dL) were

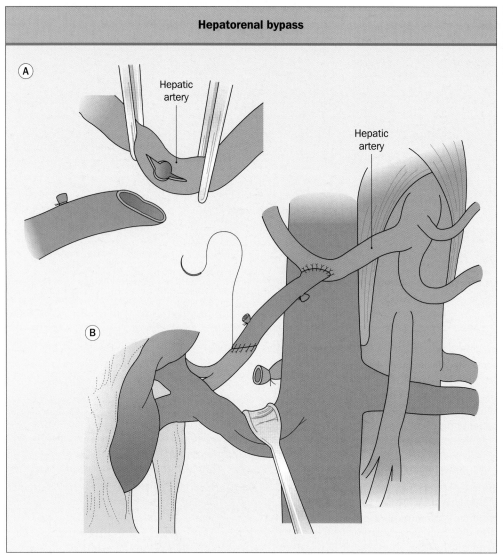

Hepatorenal bypass

(A)

Hepatic artery

Hepatic artery

(B)

Figure 26c.10 Hepatorenal bypass.
The reconstruction is completed using a saphenous vein interposition graft between the side of the hepatic artery (A) and the distal end of the transected right renal artery (B).

Blood pressure response to operation (n = 472 patients).					
Response*	Number of patients (%)	Preoperative blood pressure (mmHg)	Postoperative blood pressure (mmHg)	Preoperative number of medications	Postoperative number of medications
Cured	57 (12)	195 ± 35/103 ± 22	137 ± 16[†]/78 ± 9[†]	2.0 ± 1.1	0 ± 0[†]
Improved	345 (73)	205 ± 35/107 ± 21	147 ± 21[†]/81 ± 11[†]	2.8 ± 1.1	1.7 ± 0.8[†]
Failed	70 (15)	182 ± 30/87 ± 13	158 ± 28[†]/82 ± 12[‡]	2.0 ± 0.9	2.0 ± 0.9
All	472 (100)	201 ± 35/104 ± 22	148 ± 22[†]/81 ± 11[†]	2.6 ± 1.1	1.6 ± 0.9[†]
*See text for definition [†] p<0.0001 compared with preoperative value [‡] p = 0.001 compared with preoperative value					

Table 26c.8 Blood pressure response to operation (n = 472 patients). Blood pressures and medications are mean ± standard deviation. (From Cherr et al.[2])

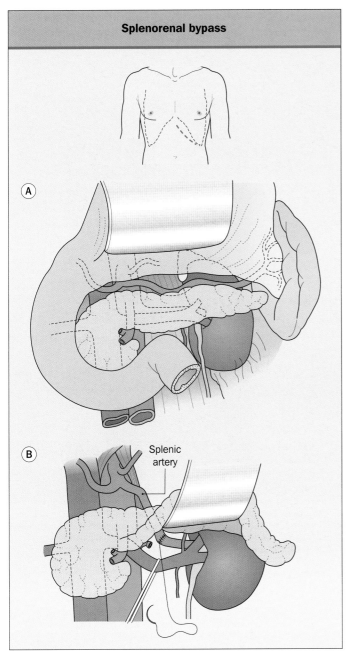

Splenorenal bypass

(A)

(B)

Splenic
artery

Figure 26c.11 Splenorenal bypass. (A) Exposure of the left renal hilum in preparation for splenorenal bypass. (B) The pancreas has been mobilized along its inferior margin and retracted superiorly to reveal the posterior surface. The transected splenic artery is tunneled behind the pancreas and anastomosed end-to-end to the transected left renal artery. A splenectomy is not routinely performed.

improved, including 28 patients who were removed from dialysis. Thirty-five percent remained unchanged, while 7% had worsened renal function.[2,13] The proportion of patients improved increased with increasing severity of preoperative renal dysfunction, with 70% of dialysis-dependent patients removed from dialysis (**Table 26c.9**). This association with increased preoperative SCr and improved postoperative renal function was significant (p<0.0001).

Significance of blood pressure and renal function benefit

Progression to death or dialysis demonstrated significant associations with both preoperative parameters and postoperative blood pressure and renal function response. Preoperative factors significantly and independently associated with death or dialysis included diabetes mellitus, severe aortic occlusive disease, poor renal function, and high systolic blood pressure. Significant and independent associations were noted for blood pressure cured compared with blood pressure improved or worsened. Moreover, improved postoperative renal function demonstrated significant and independent associations with increased dialysis-free survival compared with renal function unchanged. The relationship between each category of renal function response and dialysis-free survival demonstrated significant interactions with preoperative renal function. For patients with renal function unchanged, an increased risk of death or dialysis was observed for patients with poor preoperative renal function. For patients worsened, an increased risk of death or dialysis was significant for those with preoperative renal function at median values of EGFR or greater. These significant and independent interactions are shown for predicted dialysis-free survival according to postoperative renal function response in **Figure 26c.14**.

COMBINED AORTIC AND RENAL RECONSTRUCTION

To assess the management philosophy of combined repair described above, we reviewed the subset of 133 patients who had combined aortic and renovascular procedures at our center from January 1987 through July 1995.[16] Patients requiring extra-anatomic or ex-vivo renal artery reconstruction, or repair combined with supraceliac, thoracic, thoracoabdominal, or extra-anatomic aortic repair were excluded, as were patients with ruptured aneurysms. Aortic replacements (29% tube grafts; 71% bifurcated grafts) were combined with unilateral renal artery repair in 63 (47%) patients; 70 (53%) had bilateral repair. These combined aortorenal procedures were compared with results from 182 consecutive patients who had isolated in-situ repair for atherosclerotic renovascular disease and 562 patients who underwent isolated elective aortic reconstruction during this same period.

Perioperative mortality after combined repair was 5.3%, which differed significantly from that observed for the 'renal surgery alone' group (1.6%) and the 'aortic surgery alone' group (0.7%).

Regarding blood pressure response – defined using blood pressure measurements and medication requirements at least 8 weeks after operation – 2% of surgical survivors in the combined group were considered cured, 63% were improved, and 35% demonstrated no beneficial blood pressure response. Based on at least a 20% change in SCr, excretory renal function was improved in 33% of patients with combined repair, while 53% had no change and 14% were worsened. These results compare favorably with other large series of combined aortorenal repair (**Table 26c.10**).[16,60–77] Compared with renal artery repair alone, however, both blood pressure benefit (63% versus 95%; p<0.001) and renal function response (33% versus 58% improved; p=0.01) were significantly decreased. These differences suggest that simultaneous aortic and renal artery repair should only be performed empirically for strong clinical indications. Prophylactic repair

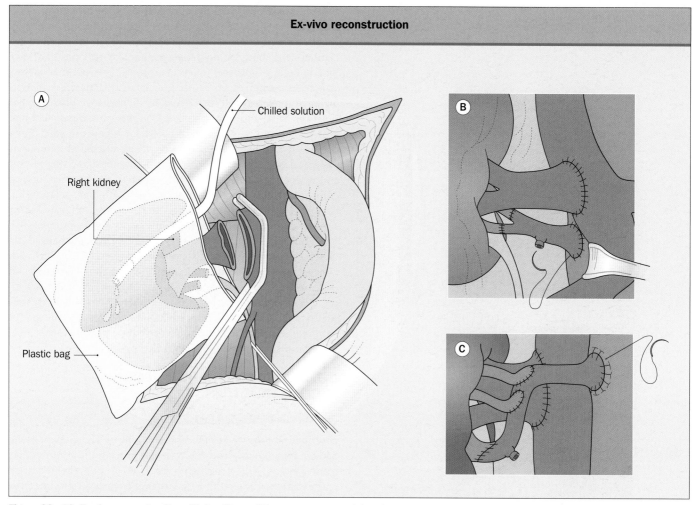

Figure 26c.12 Ex-vivo reconstruction. (A) An ellipse of the vena cava containing the renal vein origin is excised by placement of a large partially occluding clamp. After ex-vivo branch repair, the renal vein can then be reattached without risk of anastomotic stricture. (B) The kidney is repositioned in its native bed after ex-vivo repair. Gerota's fascia is reattached to provide stability to the replaced kidney. Arterial reconstruction can be accomplished via end-to-end anastomoses – as in (B) – or occasionally with a combination of end-to-end and end-to-side anastomoses (C).

Renal function response versus preoperative serum creatinine (SCr) (n=469 patients).					
Renal function response*	Preoperative SCr			Dialysis-dependent	Total
	<1.8mg/dL	1.8–2.9mg/dL	≥3.0mg/dL		
Improved (%)	71 (29%)	75 (54%)	29 (58%)	28 (76%)	203 (43%)
No change (%)	142 (58%)	52 (38%)	17 (34%)	9 (24%)	220 (47%)
Worse (%)	31 (13%)	11 (8%)	4 (8%)	0 (0%)	46 (10%)
*See text for definition					

Table 26c.9 Renal function response versus preoperative serum creatinine (SCr) (n=69 patients). (From Cherr et al.[2])

Comparison of major series reporting combined aortorenal reconstruction.								
Reference	Year	Mean age (years)	No. of patients	Unilateral reconstruction	Bilateral reconstruction	Hypertension benefit	Perioperative mortality	Renal function benefit
Perry[60]	1984	n/r	60	n/r	n/r	50%	5%	n/r
Sterpetti[61]	1986	62	39	64%	36%	66%	10%	n/r
Tarazi[62]	1987	63	89	63%	37%	58%	10%	n/r
O'Mara[63]	1988	67	32	0%	100%	90%	3%	n/r
Atnip[64]	1990	66	27	79%	21%	64%	10%	n/r
Allen[65]	1993	66	102	83%	17%	86%	5%	n/r
McNeil[66]	1994	64	101	64%	36%	74%	1%	n/r
Chaikof[67]	1994	66	50	34%	66%	50%	2%	42%
Huber[68]	1995	n/r	56	n/r	n/r	n/r	9%	n/r
Brothers[69]	1995	63	70	59%	41%	n/r	16%	n/r
Cambria[70]	1995	68	100	82%	18%	68%	7%	50%
Dougherty[71]	1995	67	52	36%	64%	70%	0%	n/r
Clair[72]	1995	68	39	21%	79%	83%	5%	19%
Benjamin[16]	1996	63	133	47%	53%	63%	5%	33%
Chaikof[73]	1996	63	32	66%	34%	47%	3%	n/r
Ballard[74]	1996	68	50	n/r	n/r	34%	10%	n/r
Kulbaski[75]	1998	63	43	53%	47%	50%	5%	n/r
Taylor[76]	2000	64	31	61%	39%	90%	6%	n/r
Hassen-Khodja[77]	2000	67	39	69%	31%	61%	3%	57%

Table 26c.10 Comparison of major series reporting combined aortorenal reconstruction. n/r, not reported. (From Edwards MS, Hansen KJ. Combined aortorenal reconstruction. In: Green RM, ed. Complex aortic surgery. New York:Marcel Dekker [Forthcoming].)

of clinically silent disease is not supported by these results or available natural history data.

OPERATIVE FAILURES AND CONSEQUENCES OF SECONDARY REPAIR

A renal artery repair will eventually fail in approximately 5% of patients. Blood pressure response after secondary operative intervention is often equivalent to that observed among patients with primary operative intervention only. However, patients requiring secondary renal artery intervention have a significantly greater risk of worsened renal function (40% versus 13%), including eventual dialysis-dependence (35% versus 4%). Furthermore, patients requiring secondary intervention demonstrate decreased dialysis-free survival.

Our experience with failed renal artery repairs reinforces two important issues. First, significant hypertension is considered a prerequisite for renovascular intervention.[2,13,16] The irretrievable loss of excretory renal function observed after failed renal artery repair supports the view that renal revascularization should be performed for clear clinical indications, not as a 'prophylactic' procedure in the absence of either hypertension or renal insufficiency. Second, the direct aortorenal reconstructions in

these patients are characterized by their short length and high blood flow, favoring prolonged patency. Early failures of repair reflect errors in surgical technique or operative judgment.

The use of PTRA after failed renal artery intervention has proved disappointing. In the case of failed operative repair, the technical challenges posed by secondary operative intervention may make PTRA appealing. Although widely applied to a variety of renal artery lesions, little information is available regarding the immediate or long-term results of PTRA after failed operative intervention.[78,79,80] Given this paucity of data, secondary operative intervention should be considered the preferred, albeit challenging, method of remedial management.

SURGERY AFTER FAILED PTRA

With these results in mind, we recently reviewed our experience with 32 consecutive atherosclerotic patients repaired after a prior failed PTRA (F-PTRA).[81] We examined the influence of failure of PTRA on methods of secondary surgical management, and blood pressure and excretory renal function response to operation.

Twenty-five patients had unilateral and seven had bilateral PTRA (including two solitary kidneys). Prior to PTRA, 31 patients

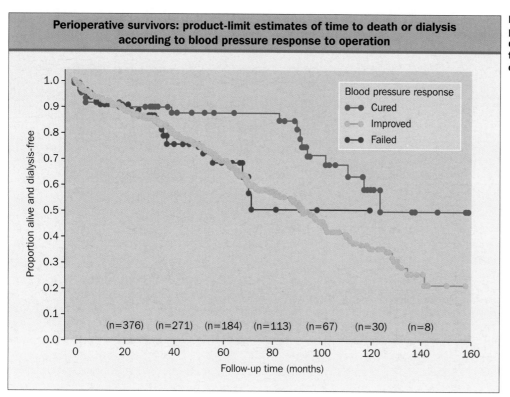

Figure 26c.13 Perioperative survivors: product-limit estimates of time to death or dialysis (n = 472) according to blood pressure response to operation. (From Cherr et al.[2])

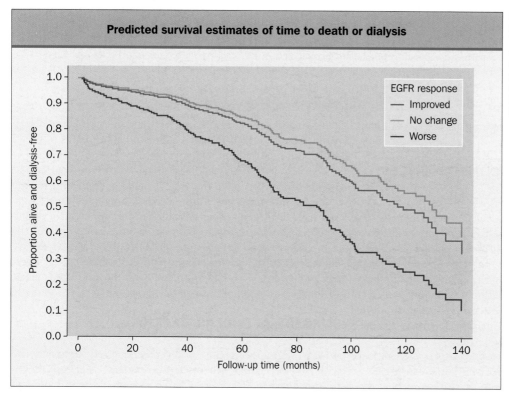

Figure 26c.14 Predicted survival estimates of time to death or dialysis. The interaction between preoperative estimated glomerular filtration rate (EGFR) and renal function response for dialysis-free survival was significant and independent. Preoperative EGFR = 38mL/min/m**2 (median). (From Cherr et al.[2])

had significant hypertension (mean blood pressure, 188 ± 32/ 102 ± 15mmHg) and 19 patients had ischemic nephropathy (mean SCr, 2.0 ± 1.3mg/dL; range, 1.3–6.6mg/dL). Twenty patients had ischemic nephropathy after F-PTRA (mean SCr, 2.0 ± 0.8mg/dL; range, 1.3–4.1mg/dL [excluding two patients dialysis-dependent]). Excluding the three emergency operative procedures, the interval between F-PTRA and surgical repair ranged from 3 weeks to 12 years (mean, 24.8 ± 32.6 months; median, 9 months).

Secondary operative repair was considered complicated by F-PTRA in 19 patients (59%). In all, four nephrectomies were required. Bilateral procedures were performed in 20 patients. Aortorenal bypass was performed most commonly. Renal artery reimplantation, renal artery thromboendarterectomies, and combined aortic reconstruction were other successful options.

Blood pressure response

Among the 28 operative survivors with atherosclerotic renovascular disease and hypertension repaired after F-PTRA, 7% were considered cured, 50% were improved, and 43% were considered failed. Compared with patients treated by operative repair only, F-PTRA was associated with significantly decreased blood pressure benefit (57% versus 89% benefited; p<0.001).

Renal function response

Among operative survivors with preoperative renal insufficiency, 41% were considered improved and 59% were unchanged. Compared with patients treated with operative repair only, the proportion of patients with improved renal function after surgery was similar (p = 0.804).

CONCLUSIONS

With proper patient selection and preparation, operative repair of atherosclerotic renovascular disease results in both blood pressure and renal function benefit. Improvement in renal function is associated with a significant increase in dialysis-free survival independent of other co-morbidities. The application of intra-operative duplex to assess renal artery reconstruction has resulted in long-term primary patency exceeding 96%. However, when failure of operative repair does occur, eventual renal function is worsened, culminating in an increased risk of dialysis-dependence and death.

Percutaneous transluminal angioplasty with or without stenting offers similar blood pressure benefit as operative repair for non-ostial atherosclerotic lesions of the main renal artery. However, for ostial lesions, especially in the presence of ischemic nephropathy, PTRA with or without endoluminal stenting yields inferior renal function benefit. The common practice of reporting unchanged renal function as 'preserved' after PTRA may be misleading. Patients with ischemic nephropathy unchanged after surgical intervention remain at increased risk for eventual dialysis-dependence and death.[2,10,13] In addition, the requirements of operative reconstruction after a failed angioplasty are not insignificant. Our experience demonstrates increased complexity of repair as well as an inferior blood pressure benefit. Whether renal function can be considered improved relative to initial function remains unclear. For these reasons, we recommend operative repair of ostial atherosclerosis and renal artery occlusion associated with severe hypertension and renal insufficiency.

REFERENCES

1. Hansen KJ, Starr SM, Sands RE, et al. Contemporary surgical management of renovascular disease. J Vasc Surg 1992;16:319–31.
2. Cherr GS, Hansen KJ, Craven TE, et al. Surgical management of atherosclerotic renovascular disease. J Vasc Surg 2002;35:236–45.
3. Hansen KJ, Deitch JA, Oskin TC, et al. Renal artery repair: consequence of operative failures. Ann Surg 1998;227:678–90.
4. Mailloux LU, Napolitano B, Bellucci AG, Vernace M, Wilkes BM, Mossey RT. Renal vascular disease causing end stage renal disease, incidence, clinical correlates, and outcomes: a twenty year clinical experience. Am J Kidney Dis 1994;24:622–9.
5. Svetkey LP, Bollinger RR, Kotman PE, et al. Prospective analysis of strategies for diagnosing renovascular hypertension. Hypertension 1989; 14:242–57.
6. Nally JV Jr, Chen CC, Skakianakis G, et al. Diagnostic criteria of renovascular hypertension with captopril renography: a consensus statement. Am J Hypertens 1991;4:749S–752S.
7. Dean RH, Benjamin ME, Hansen KJ. Surgical management of renovascular hypertension. Curr Probl Surg 1997;34:209–308.
8. Hansen KJ, Tribble RW, Reavis S, et al. Renal duplex sonography: evaluation of clinical utility. J Vasc Surg 1990;12:227–36.
9. Motew SJ, Cherr GS, Craven TE, et al. Renal duplex sonography: main renal artery versus hilar analysis. J Vasc Surg 2000;32:462–71.
10. Dean RH, Tribble RW, Hansen KJ, et al. Evolution of renal insufficiency in ischemic nephropathy. Ann Surg 1991;213:446–55.
11. Hansen KJ, Thomason RB, Craven TE, et al. Surgical management of dialysis-dependent ischemic nephropathy. J Vasc Surg 1995;21:197–209.
12. Hansen KJ, Benjamin ME, Appel RG, et al. Renovascular hypertension in the elderly: results of surgical management. Geriatr Nephrol Urol 1996;6:3–34.
13. Hansen KJ, Cherr GS, Craven TE, et al. Management of ischemic nephropathy: dialysis-free survival after surgical repair. J Vasc Surg 2000;32:472–82.
14. Dean RH, Kieffer RW, Smith BM, et al. Renovascular hypertension: anatomic and renal function changes during drug therapy. Arch Surg 1981;116:1408–15.
15. Novick AC, Pohl MA, Schreiber M, et al. Revascularization for preservation of renal function in patients with atherosclerotic renovascular disease. J Urol 1983;129:907–12.
16. Benjamin ME, Hansen KJ, Craven TE, et al. Combined aortic and renal artery surgery: a contemporary experience. Ann Surg 1996; 233:555–65.
17. Williamson WK, Abou-Zamzam AM, Moneta GL, et al. Prophylactic repair of renal artery stenosis is not justified in patients who require infrarenal aortic reconstruction. J Vasc Surg 1998;28:14–22.
18. Hunt JC, Strong CG. Renovascular hypertension. Mechanisms, natural history and treatment. Am J Cardiol 1973;32:562–74.
19. Canzanello JC, Millan VG, Spiegel JE, et al. Percutaneous transluminal renal angioplasty in management of atherosclerotic renovascular hypertension: results in 100 patients. Hypertension 1989;13:163–72.
20. Klinge J, Mali WP, Puijlaert CB, et al. Percutaneous transluminal renal angioplasty: initial and long-term results. Radiology 1989;171:501–6.
21. Baert AL, Wilms G, Amery A, et al. Percutaneous transluminal renal angioplasty: initial results and long-term follow-up in 202 patients. Cardiovasc Intervent Radiol 1990;13:22–8.
22. Tykarski A, Edwards R, Dominiczak AF, et al. Percutaneous transluminal renal angioplasty in the management of hypertension and renal failure in patients with renal artery stenosis. J Hum Hypertens 1993; 7:491–6.

23. Weibull H, Bergqvist D, Bergentz SE, et al. Percutaneous transluminal renal angioplasty versus surgical reconstruction of renal artery stenosis: a prospective randomized study. J Vasc Surg 1993;18:841–50.

24. Losinno F, Zuccala A, Busato F, et al. Renal artery angioplasty for renovascular hypertension and preservation of renal function: long-term angiographic and clinical follow-up. Am J Radiol 1994;162:853–7.

25. Rodriguez-Perez JC, Plaza C, Reyes R, et al. Treatment of renovascular hypertension with percutaneous transluminal angioplasty: experience in Spain. J Vasc Interv Radiol 1994;5:101–9.

26. Bonelli FS, McKusick MA, Textor SC, et al. Renal artery angioplasty: technical results and clinical outcomes in 320 patients. Mayo Clin Proc 1995;70:1041–52.

27. Hoffman O, Carreres T, Sapoval MR, et al. Ostial renal artery stenosis: immediate and mid-term angiographic and clinical results. J Vasc Interv Radiol 1998;9:65–73.

28. Klow N-E, Paulsen D, Vatne K, et al. Percutaneous transluminal renal artery angioplasty using the coaxial technique: ten years of experience from 591 procedures in 419 patients. Acta Radiol 1998;39:594–603.

29. Zuccala A, Losinno F, Zucchelli A, Zuchelli PC. Renovascular disease in diabetes mellitus: treatment by percutaneous transluminal renal angioplasty. Nephrol Dial Transplant 1998;13:26–9.

30. Paulsen D, Klow NE, Rogstad B, et al. Preservation of renal function by percutaneous angioplasty in ischemic renal disease. Nephrol Dial Transplant 1999;14:1454–61.

31. van de Ven PJ, Kaatee R, Beutler JJ, et al. Arterial stenting and balloon angioplasty in ostial atherosclerotic renovascular disease. A randomised trial. Lancet 1999;353:282–6.

32. Baumgartner I, von Aesch K, Do DD, et al. Stent placement in ostial and non-ostial atherosclerotic renal arterial stenoses: a prospective follow-up study. Radiology 2000;216:498–505.

33. van Jaarsveld BC, Krijnen P, Pieterman H, et al. The effect of balloon angioplasty on hypertension in atherosclerotic renal artery stenosis: Dutch Renal Artery Stenosis Intervention Cooperative Group. N Engl J Med 2000;342:1007–14.

34. Rees CR, Palmaz JC, Becker GJ, et al. Palmaz stent in atherosclerotic stenosis involving the ostia of the renal arteries: preliminary report of a multicenter study. Radiology 1991;181:507–14.

35. Wilms GE, Peene PT, Baert AL, et al. Renal artery stent placement with use of the Wallstent endoprosthesis. Radiology 1991;179:457–62.

36. Kuhn FP, Kutkuhn B, Torsello G, et al. Renal artery stenosis: preliminary results of treatment with the Strecker stent. Radiology 1991;180:367–72.

37. Joffre F, Rousseau H, Bernadet P, et al. Midterm results of renal artery stenting. Cardiovasc Intervent Radiol 1992;15:313–8.

38. Hennequin LM, Joffre FG, Rousseau HP, et al. Renal artery stent placement: long term results with the Wallstent endoprosthesis. Radiology 1994;191:713–9.

39. Raynaud AC, Beyssen BM, Turmel-Rodrigues LE, et al. Renal artery stent placement: immediate and midterm technical and clinical results. J Vasc Interv Radiol 1994;5:849–58.

40. MacLeod M, Taylor AD, Baxter G, et al. Renal artery stenosis managed by Palmaz stent insertion: technical and clinical outcome. J Hypertens 1995;13:1791–5.

41. van de Ven PJG, Beutler JJ, Kaatee R, et al. Transluminal vascular stent for ostial atherosclerotic renal artery stenosis. Lancet 1995; 346:672–4.

42. Dorros G, Jaff M, Jain A, et al. Follow-up of primary Palmaz–Schatz stent placement for atherosclerotic renal artery stenosis. Am J Cardiol 1995;75:1051–5.

43. Henry M, Amor M, Henry I, et al. Stent placement in the renal artery: three-year experience with the Palmaz stent. J Vasc Interv Radiol 1996;7:343–50.

44. Iannone LA, Underwood PL, Nath A, et al. Effect of primary balloon expandable renal artery stents on long-term patency, renal function, and blood pressure in hypertensive and renal insufficient patients with renal artery stenosis. Cathet Cardiovasc Diagn 1996;37:243–50.

45. Harden PN, MacLeod MJ, Rodger RSC, et al. Effect of renal artery stenting on progression of renovascular renal failure. Lancet 1997; 249:1133–6.

46. Blum U, Krumme B, Flugel P, et al. Treatment of ostial renal artery stenosis with vascular endoprostheses after unsuccessful balloon angioplasty. N Engl J Med 1997;336:459–65.

47. Boisclair C, Therasse E, Oliva VL, et al. Treatment of renal artery angioplasty failure by percutaneous renal artery stenting with Palmaz stents: midterm technical and clinical results. AJR Am J Roentgenol 1997;168:245–51.

48. Rundback JH, Gray RJ, Rozenblit G, et al. Renal artery stent placement for the management of ischemic nephropathy. J Vasc Interv Radiol 1998;9:413–20.

49. Fiala LA, Jackson MR, Gillespie DL, et al. Primary stenting of atherosclerotic renal artery ostial stenosis. Ann Vasc Surg 1998;12:128–33.

50. Dorros G, Jaff M, Mathiak L, et al. Four-year follow-up of Palmaz-Schatz stent revascularization as treatment for atherosclerotic renal artery stenosis. Circulation 1998;98:642–7.

51. Tuttle KR, Chouinard RF, Webber JT, et al. Treatment of atherosclerotic ostial renal artery stenosis with the intravascular stent. Am J Kidney Dis 1998;32:611–22.

52. Gross CM, Kramer J, Waigand J, et al. Ostial renal artery stent placement for atherosclerotic renal artery stenosis in patients with coronary artery disease. Cathet Cardiovasc Diagn 1998;45:1–8.

53. Henry M, Amor M, Henry I, et al. Stents in the treatment of renal artery stenosis: long-term follow-up. J Endovasc Surg 1999;6:42–51.

54. Rodriguez-Lopez JA, Werner A, Ray LI, et al. Renal artery stenosis treated with stent deployment: indications, technique, and outcome for 108 patients. J Vasc Surg 1999;29:617–24.

55. Hansen KJ, O'Neil EA, Reavis SW, et al. Intraoperative duplex sonography during renal artery reconstruction. J Vasc Surg 1991;14:364–74.

56. Moncure AC, Brewster DC, Darling RC, et al. Use of the splenic and hepatic arteries for renal revascularization. J Vasc Surg 1986;2:196–203.

57. Goldstone J. Intraoperative assessment of renal and visceral arterial reconstruction using doppler and duplex imaging. In: Ernst CB, Stanley JC, eds. Current therapy in vascular surgery, 2nd edn. Philadelphia:Decker, 1991:872.

58. Okuhn SP, Reilly LM, Bennett JR, et al. Intraoperative assessment of renal and visceral artery reconstruction: the role of duplex scanning and spectral analysis. J Vasc Surg 1987;5:137–47.

59. Hansen KJ, Reavis SW, Dean RH. Duplex scanning in renovascular disease. Geriatr Nephrol Urol 1996;6:89.

60. Perry MO, Silane MF. Management of renovascular problems during renal operations. Arch Surg 1984;119:681–5.

61. Sterpetti AV, Schultz RD, Feldhaus RJ, et al. Aortic and renal atherosclerotic disease. Surg Gynecol Obstet 1986;163:54–9.

62. Tarazi RY, Hertzer NR, Beven EG, et al. Simultaneous aortic reconstruction and renal revascularization: risk factors and late results in eighty-nine patients. J Vasc Surg 1987;5:707–14.

63. O'Mara CS, Maples MD, Kilgore TL, et al. Simultaneous aortic reconstruction and bilateral renal revascularization. J Vasc Surg 1988;8:357–66.

64. Atnip RG, Neumeyer MM, Healy DA, et al. Combined aortic and visceral arterial reconstruction: risks and results. J Vasc Surg 1990;12:705–15.

65. Allen BT, Rubin BG, Anderson CB, et al. Simultaneous surgical management of aortic and renovascular disease. Am J Surg 1993;166:726–33.

66. McNeil JW, String ST, Pfeiffer RB. Concomitant renal endarterectomy and renal reconstruction. J Vasc Surg 1994;20:331–7.

67. Chaikof EL, Smith RB, Salam AA, et al. Ischemic nephropathy and concomitant aortic disease: a ten year experience. J Vasc Surg 1994; 19:135–48.

68. Huber TS, Harward TRS, Flynn TC, et al. Operative mortality rates after elective infrarenal aortic reconstructions. J Vasc Surg 1995;22:287–94.

69. Brothers TE, Elliott BM, Robison JG, et al. Stratification of mortality risk for renal artery surgery. Am Surg 1995;61:45–51.

70. Cambria RP, Brewster DC, Italien GL, et al. Simultaneous aortic and renal artery reconstruction: evolution of an eighteen year experience. J Vasc Surg 1995;21:916–25.

71. Dougherty MJ, Hallett JW, Naessens J, et al. Renal endarterectomy vs. bypass for combined aortic and renal reconstruction: is there a difference in clinical outcome? Ann Vasc Surg 1995;9:87–94.

72. Clair DG, Belkin M, Whittemore AD, Mannick JA, Donaldson MC. Safety and efficacy of transaortic renal endarterectomy as an adjunct to aortic surgery. J Vasc Surg 1995;21:926–34.

73. Chaikof EL, Smith RB, Salam AA, et al. Empiric reconstruction of the renal artery: long-term outcome. J Vasc Surg 1996;24:406–14.
74. Ballard JL, Hieb RA, Smith DC, et al. Combined renal artery stenosis and aortic aneurysm: treatment options. Ann Vasc Surg 1996;10:361–4.
75. Kulbaski MJ, Kosinski AS, Smith RB, et al. Concomitant aortic and renal artery reconstruction in patients on an intensive antihypertensive medical regimen: long-term outcome. Ann Vasc Surg 1998;12:270–7.
76. Taylor SM, Langan EM, Snyder BA, Cull DL, Sullivan TM. Concomitant renal revascularization with aortic surgery: are the risks of the combined procedures justified? Am Surg 2000;66:768–72.
77. Hassen-Khodja R, Sala F, Declemy S, Bouillane PJ, Batt M. Renal artery revascularization in combination with infrarenal aortic reconstruction. Ann Vasc Surg 2000;14:577–82.
78. Libertino JA, Beckmann CF. Surgery and percutaneous angioplasty in the management of renovascular hypertension. Urol Clin North Am 1994;21:235–43.
79. Novick AC. Percutaneous transluminal angioplasty and surgery of the renal artery. Eur J Vasc Surg 1994;8:1–9.
80. Erdoes LS, Berman SS, Hunter GC, et al. Comparative analysis of percutaneous transluminal angioplasty and operation for renal revascularization. Am J Kidney Dis 1996;27:496–503.
81. Wong JM, Hansen KJ, Oskin TC, et al. Surgery after failed percutaneous renal artery angioplasty. J Vasc Surg 1999;30:468–83.
82. Wollenweber J, Sheps SG, Davis GD. Clinical course of atherosclerotic renovascular disease. Am J Cardiol 1968;21:60–71.
83. Schreiber MJ, Phol MA, Novick AC. The natural history of atherosclerotic fibrous renal artery disease. Urol Clin North Am 1984;11:383–92.

CHAPTER
27
Hemodialysis Access: Placement and Management of Complications

Peter J Mackrell, David L Cull, and Christopher G Carsten III

KEY POINTS

- The Committee on Reporting Standards of the Society of Vascular Surgery and the American Association for Vascular Surgery has developed a nomenclature system for arteriovenous (AV) access procedures.

- A long-term strategy that plans for multiple access procedures should be developed for each patient.

- Vascular access practice patterns are driven primarily by physician and facility preference, not patient factors, which results in significant regional variation in vascular access management.

- Duplex ultrasonography can assess the arterial inflow, determine the diameter and quality of the superficial veins of the extremity, and confirm patency of the central veins, which can be helpful for selecting the most appropriate site for AV access placement.

- Autogenous AV accesses require fewer interventions to maintain long-term patency compared to non-autogenous AV accesses.

- Surgeons who provide vascular access should have a number of autogenous and non-autogenous AV access procedures in their surgical armamentarium and should understand the advantages and disadvantages of each.

- Prophylactic intervention on AV accesses with functional deterioration identified by surveillance testing can extend access survival.

INTRODUCTION

Chronic hemodialysis became feasible as a treatment for end-stage renal disease in 1960 after Quinton and Scribner devised the external shunt which provided repetitive access to the circulation. The subsequent development of vascular access techniques and devices now permit patients to be maintained on dialysis for decades. The ideal vascular access system provides:

- reliable, repetitive access to the circulation;
- flow rates sufficient to deliver efficient dialysis;
- prolonged patency; and
- low rate of complications.

Despite advances in vascular access over the past 40 years, the significant morbidity and cost associated with the establishment and maintenance of vascular access in the hemodialysis patient population reflects how far we are from achieving the 'ideal' vascular access system. Hemodialysis access failure is the most frequent cause of hospitalization and is responsible for the greatest number of hospitalized days for the patient on hemodialysis.[1] Vascular access establishment and maintenance accounts for nearly 17% of total Medicare spending for hemodialysis patients in the USA.[2] It is ironic that the ability to provide vascular access, so crucial to the development of chronic dialysis 40 years ago, is responsible for much of the cost and morbidity associated with dialysis today.

A technological breakthrough that will significantly reduce the morbidity and cost associated with vascular access does not appear to be on the horizon. The methods and devices available today for vascular access are fundamentally the same as those available 20 years ago. With this realization in mind, recent efforts have focused on developing algorithms to better define patient selection criteria for each access method and surveillance techniques to identify the failing vascular access. Vascular access for hemodialysis is obtained by one of the following methods:

- placement of a temporary or permanent double lumen central venous catheter;
- creation of an autogenous arteriovenous (AV) access (native or natural fistula); or
- placement of a non-autogenous AV access (bridge AV graft).

Although the most appropriate access option for a particular patient is dependent on a number of factors such as patient age, co-morbid diseases, vascular anatomy, previous access procedures, and timing of hemodialysis, several generalizations regarding each access method can be made (**Table 27.1**).

Studies have shown considerable geographic variation in the pattern of vascular access method use in the USA. Using random national samples of patients from the US Renal Data System, Hirth demonstrated a trend away from autogenous AV access use in the USA in the 1990s and large regional variations in the relative use of autogenous and non-autogenous AV accesses.[3] For example, the utilization of prosthetic AV accesses ranged from 23% in New England to 85% in the southeastern USA. These variations were not due to differences in patient demographics such as older patient age, gender, presence of diabetes mellitus, peripheral vascular disease, or obesity which might favor prosthetic AV access placement, but rather due to variations in practice patterns across the USA.

Dialysis registries also show large geographical variations in vascular access practice patterns worldwide.[4–8] These variations were recently demonstrated by results of the Dialysis Outcomes and Practice Patterns Study (DOPPS), which noted strikingly different rates of autogenous AV access utilization among hemodialysis patients in the USA compared to Europe. This study also showed the use of dialysis catheters was significantly more common in the USA (**Table 27.2**). There are differences in patient characteristics between the US and European hemodialysis

Dialysis access method: advantages and disadvantages.

Method	Advantages	Disadvantages
Dialysis catheter	• Easily inserted and removed • Immediately available for use • Hemodynamic effects of AV shunt (heart failure, steal) do not occur • Placement possible in nearly all patients	• Highest risk for infection • Incites central venous thrombosis or stenosis that may preclude use of extremities for AV access • Inconsistently provides blood flow rates adequate for optimum dialysis
Autogenous AV access	• Fewer secondary procedures required to maintain equivalent patency • Resistant to infection	• More difficult to cannulate • Early failure rate higher compared with bridge grafts • Requires prolonged maturation period • Hemodynamic effects (heart failure, steal) may occur • Anatomy may preclude procedure in some patients
Non-autogenous (prosthetic) AV access	• Available for use in 2–3 weeks • Easy to cannulate • Superior early technical success in patients with small or diseased vasculature • Placement possible in most patients	• Infection often requires removal • Hemodynamic effects (heart failure, steal) may occur • Multiple secondary procedures usually required to maintain patency

Table 27.1 Dialysis access method: advantages and disadvantages.

Vascular access method among hemodialysis patients in Europe and the USA.*

	Access method for all (prevalent) hemodialysis patients			Access method for new (incident) hemodialysis patients		
	Autogenous	Non-autogenous	Catheters	Autogenous	Non-autogenous	Catheters
USA	24%	58%	17%	15%	24%	60%
Europe	80%	10%	8%	66%	2%	31%
*Dialysis Outcomes and Practice Patterns Study[9]						

Table 27.2 Vascular access method among hemodialysis patients in Europe and the USA.*

population, with prosthetic AV access placement being favored in the US; however, after adjusting for these factors, autogenous AV access use was still much higher in Europe than the USA.[9] These studies have shown that, although vascular access method selection is associated with particular patient characteristics, facility preferences and established vascular access practice patterns appear to be important determinants of the type of access given to patients.

NOMENCLATURE FOR AV ACCESS

Although extensive literature has been published on the patency and complications of hemodialysis access procedures, it is difficult to compare outcomes because of the wide variety of access materials, locations, risk factors, and quality of inflow and outflow vessels. Many terms are used inconsistently to describe various configurations of AV access. The Committee on Reporting Standards of the Society of Vascular Surgery and the American Association for Vascular Surgery recently published reporting standards for surgical access placement and its revision. This document also provides standardized definitions related to AV access procedures[10], the nomenclature recommended by this report is used throughout this chapter.

- *Autogenous AV access*: an access created by a connection between an artery and a vein, whereby the vein serves as an accessible conduit. This type of access was previously referred to as a native or natural fistula.
- *Non-autogenous AV access*: an access created by connecting an artery to a vein with a graft. This access can be divided into prosthetic (e.g. polytetrafluoroethylene, Dacron) and biograft (e.g. bovine heterograft, human umbilical vein).
  In terms of written descriptions, the arterial site of the AV access is reported first, followed by a hyphen and then the venous outflow site. In situations where the arterial location may be ambiguous (e.g. brachial artery), a broader anatomic reference is included, such as forearm or upper arm (e.g. prosthetic brachial-antecubital forearm loop access).
- *Transposition*: used when the peripheral portion of the vein is moved from its original position (usually to a more superficial tunnel) and connected to the artery. The more central portion of the vein remains intact in its native location (e.g. autogenous brachial-basilic transposition).
- *Translocation*: describes a vein that has been disconnected both proximally and distally and is placed in a position remote from its origin (e.g. autogenous brachial-cephalic saphenous vein looped translocation).
- *Looped and straight*: refer to the course of the conduit.

- *Primary patency*: the interval from the time of access placement until any intervention designed to maintain or re-establish patency or functionality.
- *Assisted primary patency*: the interval from the time of access placement until access thrombosis, including intervening manipulations, such as balloon angioplasty, designed to maintain the functionality of a patent access.
- *Secondary patency*: the interval from the time of access placement until access abandonment, including intervening manipulations, such as thrombectomy, designed to re-establish functionality in thrombosed access.

SITE SELECTION

The surgeon must consider numerous factors when planning dialysis access placement. Patients with end-stage renal disease often have co-morbid diseases, such as coronary artery disease, peripheral vascular disease, and diabetes mellitus, that may increase the risk of surgery and adversely affect the long-term function of the access. The patient's medical condition should be optimized prior to surgery. In situations where the patient's medical condition is tenuous, it is best to allow the patient to dialyze via a dialysis catheter until the patient is stabilized and the operation can be performed safely.

A major determinant of AV access success is the size and quality of the arterial inflow and venous outflow. The arterial inflow should be evaluated by obtaining a history to elicit symptoms of arterial insufficiency. The axillary, brachial, radial, and ulnar pulses should be carefully palpated and the upper extremity blood pressures should be compared. Competence of the palmar arch is assessed with the Allen's test. If a lower extremity access is planned, the femoral, popliteal, and pedal pulses are palpated. If there is doubt as to the adequacy of the donor artery inflow or runoff, duplex ultrasonography may be helpful in clarifying the anatomy. In selected patients, an arteriogram that shows the entire arterial anatomy of the limb may be necessary.

The venous outflow is assessed by history and physical examination. A history of thrombophlebitis, central venous catheterization, or placement of pacemaker wires via the subclavian vein, or findings on physical examination of arm edema or prominent venous pattern of the shoulder and chest wall, should alert the surgeon to the possibility of central venous stenosis or occlusion. These findings should prompt preoperative imaging with venography. The size and quality of the superficial veins are determined by carefully palpating the veins with and without a tourniquet on the upper arm. If the vein cannot be visualized because of overlying subcutaneous fat, the superficial veins should be assessed with duplex ultrasonography. The technique for upper extremity duplex ultrasound vein mapping and criteria for selection of superficial veins for autogenous AV access creation have been reported by Silva et al.[11] A tourniquet is placed on the arm and the superficial veins are insonated with a 5MHz or 7MHz scanning probe. Veins are assessed for compressibility and diameter. Patency of the axillary and subclavian veins are also confirmed with the study. A superficial vein diameter exceeding 2.5mm without segmental stenosis or occlusion is considered suitable for autogenous AV access creation.

An important factor to be considered when determining the optimal site for access placement is the influence of that site selection on subsequent access procedures. Each access procedure invariably fails and it is possible that some patients will outlive their available access sites. The ill-timed use of an access site may compromise future use of other sites in that extremity when the access fails. The surgeon should therefore develop a long-term strategy for each patient that plans for multiple access procedures.

Although access procedures of the proximal extremity tend to have longer patency than those placed distally, the access should be placed as distally in the extremity as practical. This practice will preserve more sites in the limb for subsequent access procedures. Additionally, the more distally placed access procedures are associated with fewer hemodynamic complications such as arterial steal and congestive heart failure. Should surgical intervention for steal or infection become necessary, accesses located in the distal extremity are more easily treated than those located proximally. The order of preference for AV access placement using the new and traditional nomenclature is shown in **Table 27.3**.

AUTOGENOUS AV ACCESS

Autogenous radial-cephalic direct wrist access (radiocephalic fistula, Brescia-Cimino fistula)
General considerations
The radial-cephalic direct wrist access is often referred to as the 'gold standard' for hemodialysis access because its creation is associated with a low complication rate and excellent long-term patency for those patients who develop a mature access. The major limitation of the access is its relatively high early failure rate, which has been reported in up to 50% of cases. Early failure is more common in patients with diabetes mellitus and in elderly, female, and obese patients. Patients with cephalic veins measuring less than 2.5mm by preoperative vein mapping with duplex ultrasonography are also less likely to develop a mature access. As the demographics of the hemodialysis population shift to older and sicker patients, fewer are considered candidates for this access. The benefits of the radial-cephalic direct wrist access probably warrant consideration of its creation in the majority of patients who are referred for vascular access months in advance of the anticipated need for dialysis. Failure of the access in this situation doesn't 'burn any bridges' for subsequent access procedures and may result in dilatation of the more proximal vein, thereby increasing success of subsequent procedures if the access fails.[12]

For patients who are referred late for vascular access, a more selective approach is necessary. The likelihood of successful access maturation based on patient factors and vein size, and the risk of prolonged dialysis catheter use while awaiting maturation, must be considered. Patency for the autogenous radial-cephalic direct wrist access ranges between 56% and 79% at 1 year (**Table 27.4**).[13-17]

Technique
The radial-cephalic direct wrist access procedure involves creation of an anastomosis between the radial artery and the cephalic vein at the wrist. A number of anastomotic configurations have been described; however, the end-of-vein to side-of-artery anastomosis is most commonly used because it provides superior

363

Order of preference for AV access placement.		
	New nomenclature	*Traditional nomenclature*
First choice	Autogenous radial-cephalic direct wrist access Autogenous posterior radial branch-cephalic direct access	Brescia-Cimino fistula Snuffbox fistula
Second choice	Autogenous radial-basilic forearm transposition Autogenous ulnar-basilic forearm transposition Autogenous radial-cephalic forearm transposition Autogenous ulnar-cephalic forearm transposition Autogenous brachial-cephalic direct access	Superficial forearm vein transposition Superficial forearm vein transposition Superficial forearm vein transposition Superficial forearm vein transposition Brachiocephalic fistula
Third choice	Prosthetic radial-antecubital forearm access Prosthetic brachial-antecubital forearm loop access Autogenous brachial-basilic upper arm transposition	Forearm straight bridge AV graft Forearm loop bridge AV graft Basilic vein transposition
Fourth choice	Prosthetic brachial-axillary upper arm access Prosthetic axillary-axillary upper arm access	Upper arm straight bridge AV graft Upper arm loop bridge AV graft
Fifth choice	Prosthetic popliteal-greater saphenous straight access Prosthetic femoral-greater saphenous looped access Autogenous popliteal-superficial femoral transposition	Thigh straight bridge AV graft Thigh looped bridge AV graft Superficial femoral vein transposition
Sixth choice	Prosthetic brachial-axillary chest access Prosthetic brachial-internal jugular access Prosthetic axillary-axillary chest loop access Prosthetic axillary-internal jugular chest loop access Prosthetic axillary-axillary straight chest loop access	Brachioaxillary straight bridge AV graft Brachiojugular straight bridge AV graft Axilloaxillary loop bridge AV graft Axillojugular loop bridge AV graft Axilloaxillary straight bridge AV graft
Seventh choice	Prosthetic axillary-femoral access	Axillofemoral bridge AV graft

Table 27.3 Order of preference for AV access placement.

Summary of results of wrist direct AV access.						
				Cumulative patency		
Study	*Study design*	*n*	*1 year*	*2 years*	*3 years*	*Infection*
Wolowczyk 2000[14]	Retrospective SBDA	210	65%	58%	55%	0%
Golledge 1999[15]	Retrospective RCDA	107	70%	63%	—	—
Burger 1995[16]	Prospective RCDA	208	79%	68%	59%	—
Leapman 1996[17]	Retrospective RCDA	150	56%	50%	45%	—
Palder 1985[13]	Retrospective RCDA	99	65%	50%	—	1%

Table 27.4 Summary of results of wrist direct AV access. RCDA, radial-cephalic direct AV access; SBDA, snuffbox radial-cephalic direct AV access.

blood flow rates compared to the end-to-end anastomosis and minimizes the risk of venous hypertension associated with the side-to-side anastomosis.

In most instances, the operation is performed with local anesthesia. A transverse incision is made over the radial artery and cephalic vein at the level of the head of the radius. The cephalic vein is mobilized for 3–4cm. To achieve adequate mobilization, it may be necessary to ligate and divide several venous tributaries. To prevent inadvertent twisting of the vein, the anterior surface is carefully marked with ink prior to transection. A superficial sensory branch of the radial nerve lies lateral to the brachioradialis muscle. Injury to this nerve during dissection should be avoided. The radial artery is exposed by longitudinally incising the deep forearm fascia over the arterial

pulse. A 2cm length of artery is mobilized. The cephalic vein is ligated as far distally as possible, divided, and the proximal vein is gently flushed with heparinized saline. If the vein does not flush easily, it is probed with a 2.5mm coronary artery dilator. An inability to advance the dilator should prompt an intraoperative venogram prior to performing the vascular anastomosis. A stenosis of the cephalic vein, if identified, should be corrected. If the location or length of a venous stenosis precludes revision, an alternative site for vascular access should be considered. After administration of systemic heparin, fine vascular clamps are applied to the artery. The pneumatic tourniquet can be used to avoid clamp injury to the vessel.[18] The vein is spatulated for approximately 5mm. If the venous anatomy permits, a side tributary of the vein can be used to create a patch-like end of

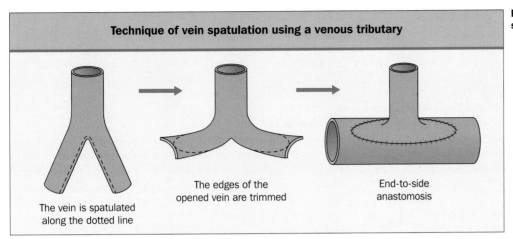

Figure 27.1 Technique of vein spatulation using a venous tributary.

Technique of vein spatulation using a venous tributary

The vein is spatulated
along the dotted line

The edges of the
opened vein are trimmed

End-to-side
anastomosis

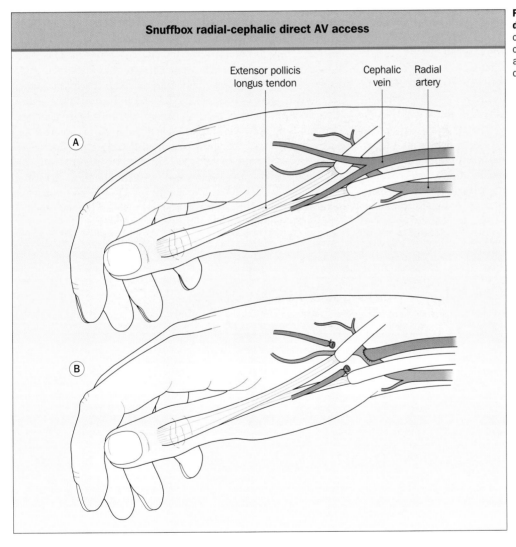

Figure 27.2 Snuffbox radial-cephalic direct AV access. (A) Before access construction and (B) after access construction, showing the cephalic vein[1] and the radial artery[2] between the dissected extensor pollicis tendons.[3]

Snuffbox radial-cephalic direct AV access

Extensor pollicis
longus tendon

Cephalic
vein

Radial
artery

A

B

the vein. (**Fig. 27.1**) A 5mm arteriotomy is made and the anastomosis is performed in the standard fashion using a continuous running 6-0 polypropylene suture. Following release of the vascular clamps, an easily palpable thrill over the cephalic vein is expected. A weak or absent thrill is indicative of either anastomotic stenosis or arterial spasm. Proximal obstruction of the vein is suspected if a strong pulse in the fistula is present. If an abnormality is suspected, an intraoperative fistulogram should be obtained.

An alternative exposure of the radial artery and cephalic vein for fistula creation is in the anatomic snuffbox. A longitudinal incision is made between the tendons of the extensor pollicis longus and brevis. At this location, the cephalic vein and the radial artery are in close proximity to one another. The cephalic vein is mobilized. The radial artery lies beneath a fascial layer, which must be incised. The same anastomotic technique described for standard radial-cephalic direct wrist access creation is used (**Fig. 27.2**).

365

Autogenous brachial-cephalic direct access (brachiocephalic fistula)

General considerations

The brachial-cephalic direct access is often referred to as a 'secondary' vascular access procedure. This label is meant to emphasize the status of the radial-cephalic direct wrist access as the 'gold standard' for access procedures. Unfortunately, this label tends to minimize significant advantages of the brachial-cephalic direct access over other access procedures. First of all, owing to the larger artery and vein at the antecubital fossa, the early failure rate is lower and the blood flow rate is greater with this access compared to the autogenous wrist accesses. Secondly, the effect of age, female gender, and diabetes mellitus do not appear to negatively impact the maturation of upper arm autogenous accesses. Consequently, the percentage of dialysis patients who are candidates for autogenous AV access creation can be significantly increased if the upper arm autogenous AV access procedures are considered.

Like the direct wrist AV accesses, the brachial-cephalic direct access is resistant to infection. The patency for the brachial-cephalic direct AV access ranges between 70% and 84% at 1 year (**Table 27.5**).[19–23] The disadvantages of the brachial-cephalic direct access include a slightly greater incidence of arterial steal compared to the wrist accesses. Also, the access may not be accessible in obese patients with significant subcutaneous fat overlying the cephalic vein in the upper arm. The risk of arterial steal may be minimized by limiting the arterial anastomosis to 5mm. The authors have salvaged many brachial-cephalic direct accesses that lie too deep with an operation called the fistula elevation procedure. Using local anesthesia, the access is mobilized from the antecubital fossa to the proximal upper arm. The subcutaneous fat is closed beneath the access with interrupted 3-0 polyglycolic suture. The skin is closed with a running subcuticular closure with 4-0 polyglycolic suture. After healing, the fistula is accessed directly through the cicatrix which overlies the AV access (**Fig. 27.3**).[24]

Technique

The operation is performed using local anesthesia. A 6cm transverse incision is made approximately one finger breadth distal to the antecubital crease. The superficial veins in the antecubital fossa are exposed. The superficial venous anatomy of the antecubital fossa is variable (**Fig. 27.4**). There are often several vein sites that can be used for the venous anastomosis. The most appropriate site is determined by the vein size, quality, and position relative to the artery. If the anatomy permits, a venous tributary can be spatulated, creating a vein patch which can be incorporated into the arterial anastomosis (**Fig. 27.1**). The brachial artery lies beneath the bicipital aponeurosis. This fascia is incised transversely. The brachial artery is dissected for a distance of approximately 3cm. Care is taken to avoid injury to the median nerve, which lies medial and posterior to the artery. After systemic heparin is administered, the vessels are clamped. The vein is marked with ink to prevent rotation, transected, and gently flushed with heparinized saline. If the surgeon perceives any resistance to flow while flushing the vein, the patency and quality of the proximal vein must be investigated as described previously. The arteriovenous anastomosis is limited to approximately 5mm in length and is completed with a 6-0 polypropylene continuous running suture.

Summary of results of brachial–cephalic direct AV access.

Study	Study design	n	Cumulative patency			Infection
			1 year	2 years	3 years	
Dunlop 1986[19]	Retrospective	81	70%	57%	—	2%
Sparks 1997[20]	Retrospective	111	—	80%	—	—
Livingston 1999[21]	Retrospective	39	70%	—	—	2%
Bender 1995[22]*	Retrospective	73	84%	78%	78%	1%
Ascher 2001[23]	Retrospective	109	72%	—	—	0%
*Patency not defined						

Table 27.5 Summary of results of brachial–cephalic direct AV access.

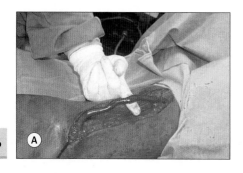

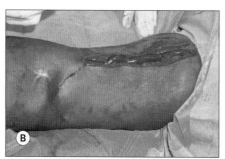

Figure 27.3 Fistula elevation procedure. (A) The brachial-cephalic direct AV access is mobilized. (B) The subcutaneous tissue is approximated beneath the AV access. A subcuticular closure is used to approximate the skin over the access.

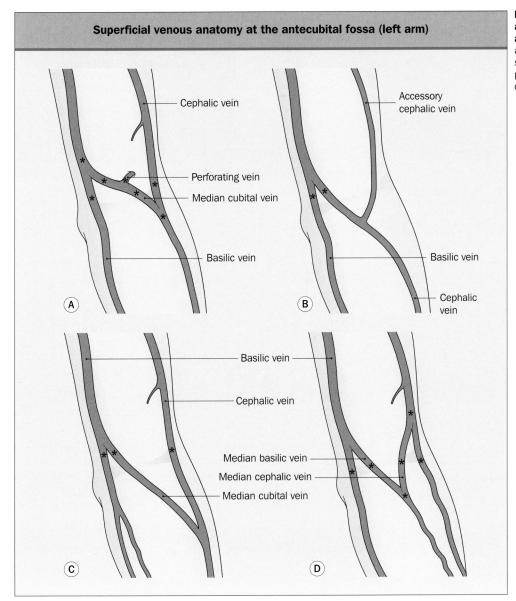

Superficial venous anatomy at the antecubital fossa (left arm)

Figure 27.4 Superficial venous anatomy at the antecubital fossa (left arm). (A) Standard superficial venous anatomy. (B–D) Variations in the superficial venous anatomy. *denotes possible venous sites for autogenous direct AV access creation.

Occasionally, preoperative vein mapping or physical examination will identify a large, patent cephalic vein in the upper arm immediately above thrombosed or sclerotic veins in the antecubital fossa. This finding often occurs after a forearm prosthetic AV access thrombosis. The technique for creating a brachial-cephalic direct access in this situation is modified. Longitudinal incisions over the cephalic vein and the brachial artery proximal to the antecubital crease are made. The cephalic vein and brachial artery are mobilized. The cephalic vein is ligated distally and transected. The vein is tunneled subcutaneously to the brachial artery. An end-to-side anastomosis is constructed as described previously (**Fig. 27.5**).

AUTOGENOUS TRANSPOSITION AV ACCESSES
These comprise:

- forearm vein transposition;
- brachial-basilic transposition (basilic vein transposition); and
- popliteal-superficial femoral transposition.

General considerations
The transposition procedures are considered as secondary, or, as in the case of the popliteal-superficial femoral transposition, tertiary vascular access procedures. This is because the operations are more extensive and require more time to perform than other autogenous AV access procedures and most prosthetic AV access procedures. Each of the procedures requires long incisions to expose and mobilize the vein. The vein is transposed to a more superficial position through a subcutaneous tunnel. An end-to-side anastomosis is created between the vein and an inflow artery. Although the authors use local anesthesia in the majority of cases for forearm and brachial-basilic transpositions, many prefer axillary block for anesthesia. Epidural or general anesthesia is required for the popliteal-superficial femoral transposition.

The brachial-basilic transposition was first described over 25 years ago by Dahger. The basilic vein is usually of greater diameter than the cephalic vein and is rarely damaged by previous venopuncture because of its deep location in the upper arm. Several studies have shown superior patency and resistance

367

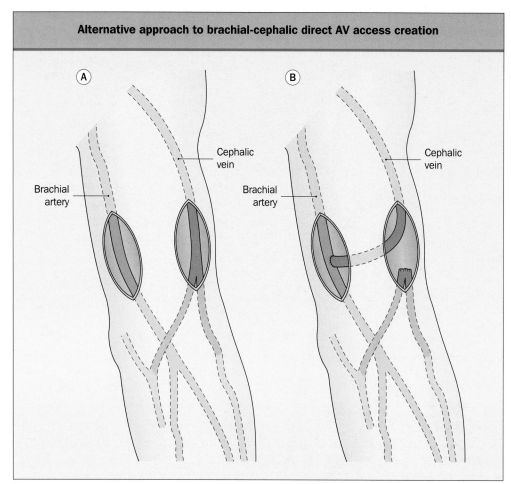

Alternative approach to brachial-cephalic direct AV access creation

(A)

(B)

Cephalic
vein

Cephalic
vein

Brachial
artery

Brachial
artery

Figure 27.5 Alternative approach to brachial-cephalic direct AV access creation if the superficial veins in the antecubital fossa are sclerotic or thrombosed. (A) Brachial artery and cephalic vein in the distal upper arm are exposed. (B) Cephalic vein is transected distally and tunneled subcutaneously to the brachial artery.

Summary of results of brachial–basilic transposition.

| Study | Study design | # Patients | | Cumulative patency | | | | Infection | |
| | | | | 1 year | | 2 years | | | |
		BBT	PTFE	BBT	PTFE	BBT	PTFE	BBT	PTFE
Coburn 1994[25]	Retrospective BBT vs PTFE	59	47	90%	87%	86%	64%*	3%	16%
Rivers 1993[27]	Retrospective BBT	65	—	—	—	49%	—	2%	—
Matsuura 1998[26]	Retrospective BBT vs PTFE	30	68	88%	78%	70%	51%*	0%	10%
Oliver 2001[28]	Retrospective BBT vs PTFE	59	82	65%	63%	—	—	2%	13%*
Murphy 2000[29]	Retrospective BBT	61	—	55%	—	35%	—	4%	—
Ascher 2001[23]	Retrospective BBT	63	—	70%	—	—	—	0%	—
*Differences are statistically significant									

Table 27.6 Summary of results of brachial–basilic transposition. BBT, brachial-basilic transposition; PTFE, polytetrafluoroethylene AV access.

to infection of the brachial-basilic transposition compared to prosthetic AV accesses (**Table 27.6**).[23,25–29] The major criticism of the brachial-basilic transposition is that it utilizes a proximal upper extremity vein which may preclude use of veins more distally in the arm for forearm prosthetic AV access placement if the brachial-basilic transposition fails. It is the authors' experience, and has been reported by others, that a failed brachial-basilic transposition does not preclude subsequent forearm or upper arm prosthetic AV access placement. The cephalic, brachial, and axillary veins usually remain patent and can be utilized for venous outflow of other AV access procedures in the extremity. Also, due to the large size of the basilic vein, the procedure has been associated with an increased incidence of arterial steal compared to the other upper extremity AV access procedures.

The authors believe that the advantages of the brachial-basilic transposition of enhanced patency and resistance to infection warrants its use in preference to forearm prosthetic AV access placement if two criteria are met. The first criterion is that preoperative vein mapping indicates that the basilic vein is of adequate size and quality for use. The size of the vein at the level of the antecubital fossa is important because extensive branching of the vein can occur, rendering it too small for use. The vein diameter should exceed 2.5mm by duplex ultrasound vein mapping. Also, in approximately 5% of cases, the basilic vein empties into the brachial vein at the mid-upper arm rather than at the axilla. This anatomic variation usually precludes the procedure because there is inadequate length of vein to transpose and may be identified preoperatively with duplex ultrasonography. The second criterion is that the patient's medical condition must permit the more extensive procedure required to perform the operation.

Recently, Silva et al. reported the results of a technique for transposing veins in the forearm for autogenous AV access creation, similar to the brachial-basilic transposition.[30] The procedure is used when preoperative vein mapping indicates that a forearm vein is of adequate caliber (>2.5mm) and quality for fistula creation; however, the vein lies too deep to facilitate easy needle cannulation.

Technique
The technique of forearm vein transposition is shown in **Figure 27.6**. In Silva and colleagues' series of 89 patients who underwent the procedure, the primary cumulative patency rate was 84% at 1 year and 69% at 2 years.[30]

Recently, two reports have been published describing the technique of autogenous AV access construction with transposed superficial femoral vein.[31,32] Due to the extensive nature of the procedure, the indications for the procedure are limited. The authors of the present chapter have utilized the procedure in young patients in whom all upper extremity sites for AV access have been exhausted. To have an adequate length of vein for needle cannulation after vein transposition, the vein must be mobilized from the popliteal fossa to its origin at the common femoral vein, and the patient must be thin. The incidence of symptoms of significant venous hypertension of the lower extremity is infrequent; however, it is important that the profunda vein be preserved. The cumulative patency in a limited series of 25 patients reported by Gradman et al. was 73% at 1 year.[31] The procedure is associated with major wound complications in nearly one-third of patients and is also associated with a high incidence of arterial steal. The length of the arterial anastomosis must be limited to minimize the risk of steal.

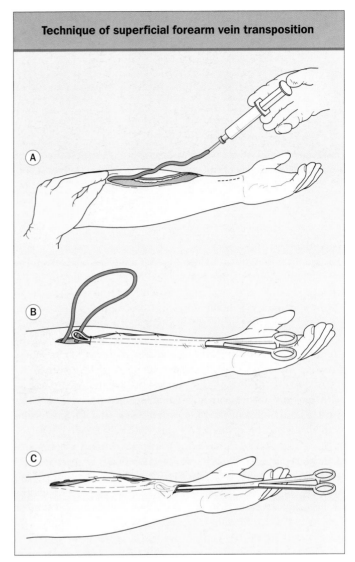

Technique of superficial forearm vein transposition

Figure 27.6 Technique of superficial forearm vein transposition. (A) Complete dissection of vein and dilatation with heparinized saline solution; separate radial artery incision marked. (B) Construction of subcutaneous tunnel. (C) Vein transposed through mid-forearm volar subcutaneous tunnel to the radial artery.

BRACHIAL-BASILIC TRANSPOSITION
General considerations
The major consideration concerns the anatomy; the basilic vein courses along the ulnar aspect of the forearm, passing 1–2cm anterior to the medial epicondyle. The vein converges with the median cubital vein above the antecubital crease. The basilic vein usually lies in the deep subcutaneous tissue at the antecubital crease and pierces the brachial fascia in the distal third of the upper arm; however, occasionally it lies beneath the fascia at the antecubital crease. In the upper arm, the basilic vein parallels and is superficial to the course of the brachial artery in the bicipital groove. Proximally, it drains into the axillary vein.

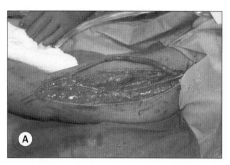
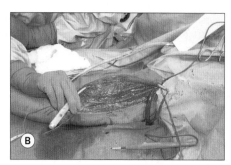
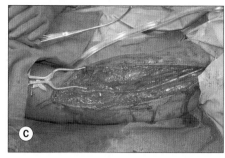

Figure 27.7 Technique of brachial-basilic transposition. (A) Basilic vein mobilized from the proximal forearm to its junction with the axillary vein. (B) Subcutaneous tunnel is created over the anterior upper arm. (C) Basilic vein is brought through the tunnel and anastomosed end-to-side to the brachial artery.

Technique

The vein is exposed through an incision which extends from the antecubital crease to the axilla. This dissection is begun in the mid-upper arm and proceeds distally. At the confluence of the basilic and median cubital veins, the incision and dissection proceeds along the larger of the two veins to the antecubital crease. It may be necessary to extend the dissection to the proximal forearm to achieve adequate mobilization in obese patients. Mobilization of the basilic vein is carried proximally to its junction with the axillary vein. Venous tributaries are ligated with fine silk suture and divided. There may be several large, short venous branches between the basilic and brachial veins which need to be divided and closed with 6-0 polypropylene suture. Care is taken to avoid injury to the medial antebrachial cutaneous nerve, which is a sensory nerve that is draped over the basilic vein. The brachial artery is exposed proximal to its entry into the antecubital fossa. Exposure of the artery can usually be accomplished through the same incision used to mobilize the vein. The basilic vein is transected and gently flushed with heparinized saline. A gently curving subcutaneous tunnel is created with a tunneling device over the anterior upper arm. The basilic vein is brought through this tunnel. Care is taken to avoid twisting or kinking the vein during tunneling. Systemic heparin is administered. An end-to-side anastomosis is created using 6-0 polypropylene suture. To minimize the risk of steal, the length of the arteriotomy is limited to 5mm. The wound is closed in two layers (**Fig. 27.7**).

NON-AUTOGENOUS AV ACCESS

General considerations

The prosthetic AV access is the most common access utilized for dialysis in the USA. Studies indicate a trend toward increased utilization of this access in recent years. There are several reasons for its popularity. Prosthetic AV access procedures are simple to perform. Because the access can be constructed between nearly any artery and vein that are in reasonable proximity to one another, there are usually several options available for prosthetic AV access placement in the dialysis patient. Only occasionally does one encounter a patient in whom no site for prosthetic AV access placement is available. The early failure rate of prosthetic AV accesses is generally less than that of autogenous accesses. Prosthetic AV accesses can be cannulated in 2–3 weeks rather than the minimum 6–8 weeks required for autogenous AV access maturation. Finally, prosthetic AV accesses are often preferred in dialysis units because they are easier to cannulate than autogenous accesses. Despite these advantages, efforts are underway in the USA and Canada to reverse the trend of increased use of prosthetic AV accesses, because studies indicate greater morbidity associated with prosthetic AV accesses compared to autogenous AV accesses.[1,33]

Prosthetic AV access construction is performed by tunneling a graft subcutaneously between an artery and a vein, then creating an end-to-side anastomosis between the graft and the vessels. The graft is placed in either a straight or a U (loop) configuration. The straight graft configuration is used if the artery and vein are separated by some distance (**Fig. 27.8**). The U or loop configuration is used if the sites of the arterial and venous anastomoses to the graft are adjacent to one another (**Fig. 27.9**). Studies which have examined the effect of graft configuration on patency suggest the loop configuration is superior to the straight configuration. However, it is unclear from these studies whether these differences are related to the graft configuration or to the size of the inflow artery.[34–36] The loop configuration does have the advantage of providing more graft area for needle cannulation, which may reduce the incidence of local complications related to repeated needle sticks at the same site on the graft.

A number of biologic and synthetic conduits have been used to construct AV accesses. The requirements of such a conduit are that it be non-antigenic and have a non-thrombogenic luminal surface. It should be resistant to infection. Needle puncture sites should seal quickly. The conduit should have desirable handling characteristics. Thrombectomy should be easily accomplished if the conduit thromboses. None of the conduits currently available satisfy all these requirements (**Table 27.7**).[37–52]

Expanded polytetrafluoroethylene (ePTFE) has become the most widely used conduit for prosthetic AV access construction because it most closely satisfies the criteria for an ideal conduit. PTFE is non-thrombogenic, non-antigenic, and handles well. With time, a stable pseudointimal layer develops on the luminal surface of the graft, and the exterior surface of the graft becomes 'incorporated' by connective tissue ingrowth. The PTFE graft is easily punctured. The holes created with the dialysis needles heal with connective tissue ingrowth. In contrast to biologic conduits, PTFE grafts are available in a variety of sizes.

The PTFE graft most often employed for hemodialysis access has a uniform luminal diameter of 6mm. Eight-millimeter grafts are sometimes used for prosthetic AV accesses placed in the proximal upper extremity or the thigh. Although the larger graft

Upper extremity straight prosthetic AV accesses

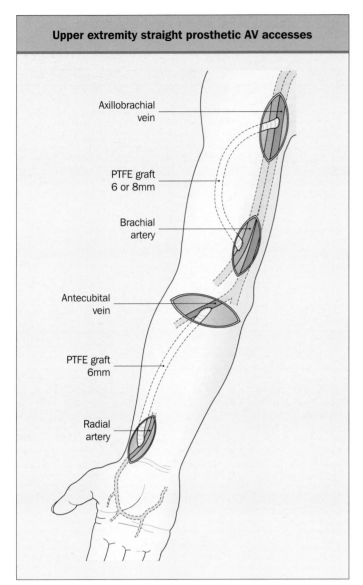

Figure 27.8 Upper extremity straight prosthetic AV accesses.

Upper extremity loop prosthetic AV accesses

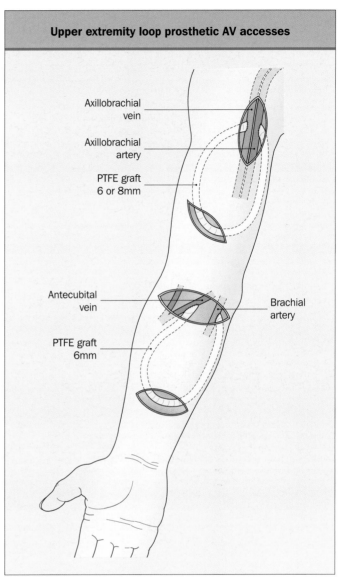

Figure 27.9 Upper extremity loop prosthetic AV accesses.

provides greater flow rates, it is associated with an increased risk of hemodynamic complications such as arterial steal or congestive heart failure.

Several modifications of the geometric configuration of PTFE grafts have been developed to increase patency and reduce complications. One such modification, the tapered or stepped PTFE graft, is narrowed at the arterial end. By reducing flow at the arterial limb of the graft, it was hoped that arterial steal would be minimized and flow dynamics within the graft would diminish venous stenosis and increase graft patency. Recent studies, however, have failed to demonstrate a benefit of the tapered graft configuration over the standard non-tapered graft.[53,54] Attempts to alter the flow dynamics at the venous end of the graft with a prefabricated hood or the addition of a venous cuff have not resulted in improved patency rates over the standard graft.[53,55] Although numerous structural modifications of the PTFE graft have been developed, several of which are currently being marketed, none of these changes has been shown to reduce complications or enhance patency compared to the standard PFTE graft.[56–61] Several studies have suggested that

prosthetic accesses with PTFE can be accessed immediately after implantation if necessary.[62–64] Despite these studies, however, most surgeons delay initial cannulation for 2 to 3 weeks after implantation until early graft incorporation has occurred, to reduce the likelihood of local complications of perigraft hematoma or seroma. The results of prosthetic AV access with PTFE for the upper and lower extremities and chest wall are shown in **Table 27.8**.[25,26,34,43,44,58,65–69]

Technique for prosthetic upper extremity AV access placement

The majority of prosthetic upper extremity AV accesses are placed with local or regional anesthesia. Rarely is general anesthesia necessary. Four sites for prosthetic upper extremity AV accesses are commonly used (**Figs 27.8 & 27.9**):

- radial artery to antecubital vein forearm straight access;
- brachial artery to antecubital vein forearm looped access;
- brachial artery to axillary vein upper arm straight access; and
- axillary artery to axillary vein upper arm looped access.

Conduits utilized for arteriovenous access.			
Conduits	Advantages	Disadvantages	References
Polytetrafluoroethylene (PTFE)	• Non-antigenic • Patency exceeded only by natural fistulae • Good handling characteristics • Easy to thrombectomize • Easy to cannulate	• Risk of infection higher compared with biologic grafts	
Bovine carotid heterograft	• Patency equivalent to PTFE • Good handling characteristics	• Increased incidence of aneurysm and graft degeneration • Increased cost • Increased risk of infection?	(37–40)
Autologous saphenous vein	• Patency equivalent to PTFE • Resistant to infection	• Difficult to cannulate • Vein harvest increases operative complexity and hospitalization • Sacrifices potential conduit for coronary or limb bypass	(41–43)
Homologous saphenous/ superficial femoral vein	• Patency equivalent to PTFE • Resistant to infection?	• Increased cost • Increased incidence of aneurysm and graft degeneration • Immunogenicity may preclude transplantation	(44–46)
Human umbilical vein	• None	• Increased cost • Increased incidence of aneurysm and graft degeneration? • Experience with graft for AV access limited	(47,48)
Dacron	• Excellent tissue ingrowth • Patency equivalent to PTFE?	• More difficult to cannulate • Experience with graft for AV access limited • Thrombectomy difficult	(49–52)

Table 27.7 Conduits utilized for arteriovenous access.

Results of prosthetic AV access using PTFE.									
Author	Location	Study design	n	Primary patency		Secondary patency		Infection	Steal
				1 year	2 years	1 year	2 years		
Lenz[58]	FA-L	Prospective	56	49%	38%	92%	59%	2%	?
Rizzuti[34]	FA-L	Retrospective	111	—	—	80%	70%	10%	
Rizzuti[34]	FA-S	Retrospective	68	—	—	70%	47%	—	
Bosman[44]	FA	Retrospective	67	40%	—	63%	—	13%	
Steed[65]	UA	Retrospective	20	84%	67%	—	—	10%	
Staramos[66]	UA	Retrospective	64	—	—	80%	64%	—	
Coburn[25]	T	Retrospective	47	70%	49%	87%	64%	16%	8%
Matsuura[26]	T	Retrospective	68	68%	46%	78%	51%	10%	
Khadra[67]	BJ	Retrospective	74	—	—	74%	63%	16%	3%
Bhandari[43]	AA, AJ	Retrospective	49	—	—	85%	82%	35%	
Vega[68]		Retrospective	51	57%	43%	74%	63%	2%	
McCann[69]		Retrospective	40	63%	43%	85%	68%	3%	

Table 27.8 Results of prosthetic AV access using PTFE. AA, axillary-axillary; AJ, axillary-internal jugular; BJ, brachial-jugular; FA-L, forearm loop; FA-S, forearm straight; T, thigh; UA, upper arm.

A transverse incision is used to expose the brachial artery and veins in the antecubital fossa. A longitudinal incision is used to expose the radial artery and vessels of the upper arm. The artery and vein are mobilized for a distance of 3–4cm. The authors use a 6mm standard PTFE graft for the majority of prosthetic accesses placed in the upper extremity. The graft is advanced through a superficial subcutaneous tunnel using a graft tunneler such as the Kelly-Wick tunneling device. The tunneled graft should be readily palpable beneath the skin. If the graft lies too deeply it will be difficult to cannulate. The graft, however, should lie below the dermis, for if it is too superficial, wound complications may result. A counter-incision is necessary to place the graft in the loop configuration. The graft is first passed through a tunnel from the artery and brought out the counter-incision. The graft is then passed through another tunnel from the counter-incision to the vein. A wide loop is created to prevent the graft from kinking. The guideline on the graft is used during tunneling to prevent graft twisting. To reduce the risk of infection, the graft should not touch the skin at any time during the procedure. The patient is heparinized. Atraumatic vascular clamps are placed proximally and distally on the artery. A 6mm arteriotomy is made. The angle of the graft to the artery is slightly less than 90 degrees. An end-to-side anastomosis is performed with a continuous 5-0 or 6-0 monofilament suture. Prior to completing the anastomosis, a cushioned clamp is placed across the graft and the arterial clamps are flashed to flush air and thrombus from the artery. After the anastomosis is completed the arterial clamps are released and flow is re-established to the hand. Either atraumatic vascular clamps or silastic vessel loops are used to obtain proximal and distal control of the vein. A venotomy approximately 1cm in length is made. The adequacy of the venous outflow is confirmed by inserting a 3mm probe into the vein and gently advancing it proximally. If the vein does not accommodate the probe or if the probe cannot be advanced, an alternative vein should be used for the venous anastomosis. The graft is beveled to a length that precisely matches that of the venotomy. An end-to-side anastomosis is performed with a continuous 5-0 or 6-0 monofilament suture.

Technique for prosthetic lower extremity access placement

The sites most commonly used for prosthetic access placement in the lower extremity are:

- femoral artery to greater saphenous or femoral vein loop AV access; and
- popliteal artery to greater saphenous or femoral vein straight AV access (**Fig. 27.10**).

A regional anesthesia technique is usually used. The femoral artery and greater saphenous vein are exposed using a single longitudinal groin incision that is positioned over the femoral pulse. The proximal superficial femoral artery and greater saphenous vein near the saphenofemoral junction are mobilized for a distance of 3–4cm. The superficial femoral artery is the preferred site for arterial inflow because graft complications such as arterial steal or graft infection are more easily treated than grafts arising from the common femoral artery. The common femoral artery, however, is used as inflow if significant occlusive disease is present in the superficial femoral artery. The preferred site for the venous anastomosis is the saphenous vein. Alter-

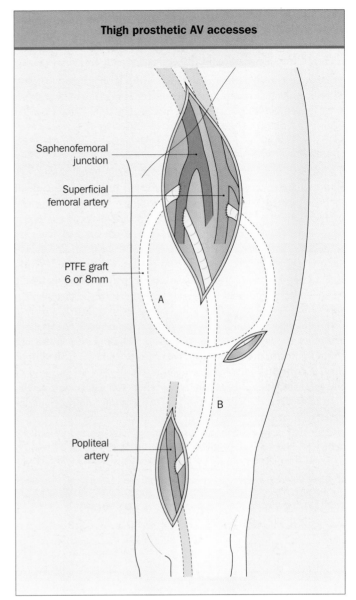

Figure 27.10 Thigh prosthetic AV accesses. (A) Prosthetic femoral-saphenous loop AV access. (B) Prosthetic popliteal-saphenous straight AV access.

natively, the superficial femoral or common femoral vein can be used, as dictated by the venous anatomy. The same tunneling technique described for prosthetic forearm loop AV access placement is used for prosthetic thigh AV access placement. Although some surgeons use an 8mm PTFE graft for thigh AV access, the authors use a 6mm graft to minimize the risk of arterial steal.

Exposure of the popliteal artery for prosthetic popliteal-greater saphenous straight access placement is obtained using a longitudinal incision on the distal medial thigh. The sartorius muscle is reflected posteriorly and the popliteal artery is identified as it emerges from the adductor hiatus. The graft is tunneled from the popliteal artery to the saphenofemoral junction in a curvilinear course over the anterior thigh. This course provides a long straight segment of graft that can be easily cannulated with the patient's extremity in a comfortable position.

Technique of prosthetic chest wall/cervical AV access placement

The sites most commonly used for prosthetic AV access placement on the chest wall and the cervical region are:

- axillary artery to ipsilateral axillary vein loop access;
- axillary artery to contralateral axillary vein straight access;
- axillary artery to ipsilateral internal jugular vein straight access; and
- brachial artery to ipsilateral internal jugular vein access (**Figs 27.11 and 27.12**).

These procedures are usually performed using general anesthesia. The axillary artery and vein are exposed using a longitudinal incision positioned approximately one finger breadth below the inferior border of the clavicle. The fibers of the pectoralis major muscle are split. The axillary vein lies below the muscle. The vein is mobilized for a distance of approximately 5 or 6cm. To achieve adequate mobilization it may be necessary to ligate and divide several venous tributaries and to divide part of the pectoralis minor muscle. A fascial layer beneath the axillary vein separates the vein from the axillary artery. The axillary artery pulse is often not palpable until this fascial layer is divided. The axillary artery is mobilized by a distance of 3–4cm. Loop grafts are tunneled using the technique described previously. The venous limb is positioned laterally on the chest wall. The venous end of the graft is directed centrally rather than at a right angle to the vein or toward the extremity. This orientation facilitates endovascular intervention should the graft thrombose.

The graft can be tunneled subcutaneously from the axillary artery to the contralateral axillary vein. If the internal jugular vein is selected as the outflow site the graft is tunneled anterior to the clavicle.

RESULTS OF AUTOGENOUS AND NON-AUTOGENOUS ARTERIOVENOUS ACCESS

Although there is substantial literature which shows that the failure rate of non-autogenous AV accesses is higher than that of autogenous AV accesses,[25,26,70–74] other studies have shown the overall patency of autogenous AV accesses to be inferior or equivalent to non-autogenous AV accesses.[13,75] As a result of these conflicting reports, objective measures of access outcome, such as patency or adequacy of dialysis, often play a smaller role in access selection than physician preference. Hodges et al. recently identified several factors responsible for these conflicts.[75] First of all, there are no large, prospective, randomized studies comparing results of autogenous to non-autogenous AV accesses. Second, the access literature lacks a standard reporting method that allows comparison of access technique. For example, studies may exclude the early autogenous AV access failures or those that do not mature from patency analysis. Other studies report AV accesses that remain patent but not usable for successful hemodialysis. These, less strict definitions of success tend to favor results toward the autogenous AV access procedures. Finally, studies often fail to differentiate primary and secondary patency data.[75] Patency results for each of the autogenous and non-autogenous AV access procedures is shown in **Tables 27.4, 27.5, 27.6,** and **27.8.** Patency was clearly defined in each of the studies referenced in the tables.

Despite these limitations of the vascular access literature, there is compelling evidence that autogenous AV accesses have

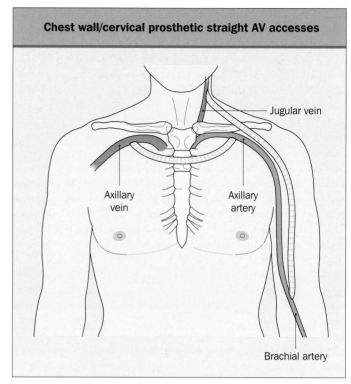

Chest wall/cervical prosthetic straight AV accesses

Jugular vein

Axillary vein

Axillary artery

Brachial artery

Figure 27.11 Chest wall/cervical prosthetic straight AV accesses.

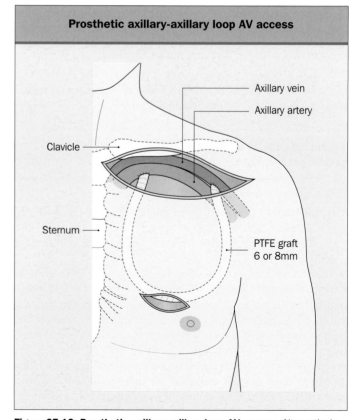

Prosthetic axillary-axillary loop AV access

Axillary vein

Axillary artery

Clavicle

Sternum

PTFE graft 6 or 8mm

Figure 27.12 Prosthetic axillary-axillary loop AV access. Alternatively the venous limb can be tunneled over the clavicle and anastomosed to the jugular vein.

better long-term patency rates and require fewer interventions to maintain patency than non-autogenous AV accesses.[70–72] Autogenous AV accesses also are less likely to become infected than non-autogenous AV accesses.

To change practice patterns and obtain improved patient outcomes, the National Kidney Foundation initiated the Dialysis Outcome Quality Initiative (NKF-DOQI) to create literature-based clinical practice guidelines in nephrology for the USA. Practice guidelines for vascular access are included in this document. The DOQI guidelines have established a goal that a minimum of 50% of new accesses placed in the US are autogenous.[1] Similar guidelines have been developed in Canada; these have recommended that 60% of the hemodialysis population have an autogenous AV access.[33]

Recently, several authors have reported strategies or algorithms for maximizing autogenous AV access utilization to achieve the DOQI guideline benchmark.[76–78] These algorithms have emphasized the following:

- preoperative upper extremity vein assessment with duplex ultrasonography;
- use of the cuffed dialysis catheter as a bridge to autogenous AV access maturation;
- use of 'secondary' AV access procedures such as the brachial-cephalic direct access or venous transposition procedures;
- revision of failing autogenous AV accesses; and
- re-evaluating the patient for autogenous AV access creation after previous access failure.

POSTOPERATIVE MANAGEMENT

The vein must dilate and the vein wall thicken (arterialize) before the fistula can be used for hemodialysis. A minimum of 6 to 8 weeks is required for autogenous AV access 'maturation' to occur. Needling the access before it has matured risks hematoma formation, fistula injury, and thrombosis. Maturation may be enhanced by having the patient regularly exercise the hand by squeezing a rubber ball. Patients are instructed to notify the surgeon immediately if they develop numbness or pain of the hand which may be symptoms of arterial steal. Failure to promptly recognize and correct significant arterial steal can result in permanent neurologic injury. The patient is also instructed on how to regularly palpate the access for presence of a thrill. Loss of the thrill usually indicates that the access has thrombosed. Early thrombectomy and revision may salvage the access.

Greater skill is required to access an autogenous AV access than a prosthetic AV access. Infiltration and thrombosis often occur when the dialysis needle punctures the back wall of the access. The surgeon should communicate directly with the dialysis nurse on when the access is ready to be cannulated. It is advisable that initial access cannulation be performed by an experienced dialysis nurse.

PEDIATRIC DIALYSIS ACCESS

Every year, 13 children per million of the US population develop chronic renal failure.[79] Although this translates into a relatively small number of children each year who require dialysis access, considerable time and resources are consumed in planning and providing their access. The small number of pediatric patients with renal failure also means that single institutions rarely have a large experience with providing access for children. Thus, there are few large series available in the literature that report results of pediatric dialysis access. Those series that are published tend to be single institutional retrospective reviews acquired over many years. Consequently, there are few level I data available to guide planning of dialysis access in children.

Children have been successfully dialyzed since the mid-1950s. Initially, children were dialyzed using separate arterial and venous catheters or a single catheter positioned in the inferior vena cava via the saphenous vein. With time, the management of children with chronic renal failure began to more closely parallel that of adults.

The ultimate therapy for a child with chronic renal failure is kidney transplantation. Children who undergo transplantation have fewer hospitalizations, improved quality of life, and improved growth characteristics compared to children who undergo dialysis. Unfortunately, the 5-year transplant graft survival rate is as low as 38% in certain pediatric populations.[79] Thus, many children with transplants will ultimately present with failed grafts needing dialysis access.

Peritoneal dialysis is the most common method of dialysis in the pediatric population. It is utilized in 95% of infants requiring dialysis.[80] Peritoneal dialysis is preferred in the pediatric population for the following reasons:

- establishing a functional peritoneal dialysis access is easier than hemodialysis access;
- peritoneal dialysis is more convenient for families who live a long distance from the dialysis center;
- growth of the child may be superior compared to the situation with hemodialysis;
- school attendance is not interrupted by dialysis center schedules;
- frequent needle sticks are avoided; and
- fewer fluid and dietary limitations are necessary.[79,81]

Despite these advantages, there are no data supporting the physiologic superiority of peritoneal dialysis over hemodialysis in the pediatric population.

Peritoneal dialysis is performed using cuffed or non-cuffed catheters that are placed surgically or percutaneously within the peritoneal cavity. Non-cuffed catheters can be placed percutaneously at the bedside and utilized immediately. Since they are associated with an increased incidence of infectious and thrombotic complications, the non-cuffed catheters are considered only a temporary means for dialysis access. The cuffed dialysis catheters require surgical placement. They have single or double cuffs that are positioned in the subcutaneous tissue of the abdominal wall. The double cuff peritoneal dialysis catheter may have a lower infection rate compared to the single cuff catheter.[82] A number of techniques for peritoneal dialysis catheter placement have been described which may affect catheter survival and influence infection rates.[83,84]

Hemodialysis is performed via a central venous dialysis catheter, an autogenous direct AV access, or a non-autogenous AV access. The method of hemodialysis access used is often dictated by the clinical situation and institutional preference. Dialysis catheters are utilized for hemodialysis access in 60–75% of the pediatric patient population.[83,84] These cuffed silastic catheters are placed in the internal jugular, subclavian, or femoral vein percutaneously or by surgical cutdown. If the cutdown method is used, hemostatic control of the vessel is obtained by placing a pursestring suture around the catheter rather than placing ligatures proximal and distal to the vessel puncture site. By avoiding the use of ligatures, the vessel may remain patent after catheter removal, potentially preserving a site for future dialysis access. A number of series have demonstrated the superiority of the right internal jugular vein for dialysis catheter placement in adults; however, such data are lacking in the pediatric literature.[84] In fact, the North American Pediatric Renal Transplant Cooperative Study showed that the subclavian vein was chosen for 77% of percutaneously placed catheters, whereas only 15% of catheters were placed in the jugular vein.[83] Despite the lack of data in the pediatric population regarding catheter site complications, the high incidence of central venous stenosis associated with subclavian venous catheters in adults is a cause for concern and should be considered when planning catheter-based hemodialysis access in children. Infection and thrombosis are the major complications associated with hemodialysis catheters in children.[85] Nearly half of the dialysis catheters placed in the pediatric population become non-functional or infected within 1 year. Catheters that provide poor flow rates or occlude may be salvaged with catheter exchange over a guidewire. Infection, manifesting as either exit-site drainage or bacteremia, may be treated initially with antibiotics in stable patients. In cases where the tunnel or exit site is not involved, catheter salvage has been reported with guidewire exchange in conjunction with intravenous antibiotics.[86]

The autogenous AV access is considered the optimal access for hemodialysis in the pediatric patient population. Originally described for use in adults by Brescia in 1966, the radial-cephalic direct AV access was soon utilized in the pediatric population. Although its early use was limited to larger children, modern microsurgical techniques have allowed for the successful creation and use of the access in children who weigh less than 10 kilograms.[87] Ulnar-basilic direct AV access and radial-basilic transposed AV access procedures have been utilized in the pediatric population.[88,89] Davis reported 2-year patency rates of 83% for the brachial-basilic transposition AV access in pediatric patients.[90] The same considerations and diagnostic modalities used to select the appropriate hemodialysis access in the adult are employed in the child. The techniques used for AV access placement in the child are the same as those in the adult, with two important exceptions. Arteriovenous access creation is facilitated in the pediatric patient by the use of microsurgical techniques using microsurgical instruments and adequate magnification. The arteriovenous anastomosis is performed with 8-0 to 10-0 polypropylene suture. Also, to minimize vessel dissection and vasospasm, vascular control is obtained with use of a sterile tourniquet.[91]

The reported patency rates for AV accesses in the pediatric population vary widely and are mostly retrospective reviews of limited series.[81,83,85,88–90] Secondary patency rates as high as 85% at 12 months are reported for autogenous AV accesses.[89] Lerner reported a median survival for autogenous AV accesses of 805 days.[83] The patency rates of autogenous AV accesses in children weighing more than 15kg was 70% at 48 months in a series reported by Bagolan et al.[91] The patency of autogenous AV accesses in children in Lumsden and colleagues' series, however, was only 6 months compared to 11 months for prosthetic AV accesses placed in the upper arm.[85]

In conclusion, the pediatric patient presents significant challenges for the surgeon tasked to provide dialysis access. The ultimate goal in all of these patients is renal transplantation. For small children in whom vascular access is more difficult, peritoneal dialysis is advisable. Peritoneal dialysis also affords older children a more normal lifestyle, allowing them to participate more readily in school and other activities. Hemodialysis can be provided with percutaneously or surgically placed catheters; however, infectious and thrombotic complications are common. Ideally, pediatric patients needing hemodialysis should be considered for an autogenous AV access placed as distally as possible in the extremity. If the superficial vasculature is unsuitable for an autogenous AV access, a prosthetic AV access can be placed with acceptable results.

HEMODIALYSIS CATHETERS

According to the Dialysis Outcome Quality Initiative (DOQI) guidelines, less than 10% of the dialysis population should be maintained on chronic hemodialysis via a dialysis catheter for more than 3 months.[1] To achieve this goal, adequate planning on the part of the primary care physician, the nephrologist, and the surgeon is required. Patients at risk for development of end-stage renal disease should be identified and referred to a nephrologist to maximize medical management, and to a surgeon for evaluation and placement of permanent access. Every effort should be made to provide a functioning autogenous or non-autogenous AV access prior to the initiation of hemodialysis. This ideal, however, is often not realized, and a significant number of patients with end-stage renal disease will require hemodialysis via a dialysis catheter.

Dialysis catheters can be used immediately after their placement for hemodialysis. The uncuffed dialysis catheter is generally reserved for situations where the anticipated need for hemodialysis is for less than 3 weeks. Cuffed dialysis catheters can be utilized from several months to years if necessary. Patients who require dialysis via a dialysis catheter usually fall into one of several categories. Those with access malfunction or infection may need a short-term method of dialysis, which can be provided with an uncuffed catheter until the access is revised or the infection cleared. Patients with acute renal failure in whom recovery of renal failure is uncertain are best dialyzed with a cuffed dialysis catheter. If permanent dialysis becomes necessary, an autogenous or non-autogenous AV access can be placed and the dialysis catheter used until the AV access is ready for cannulation. Cuffed dialysis catheters are also utilized in patients with chronic renal insufficiency who present with an acute exacerbation of their renal failure and require urgent hemodialysis. The cuffed catheter is used as a bridge for dialysis until permanent access is available. Finally, patients who have exhausted all peripheral sites for AV access, or with poor cardiac output or hypercoagulable disorders, in whom AV access cannot be maintained can be dialyzed long term with a cuffed dialysis catheter.

The veins commonly used for dialysis catheter insertion are the internal jugular vein, external jugular vein, subclavian vein, femoral vein, and inferior vena cava. The right internal jugular vein is the most ideal vein for dialysis catheter insertion, for the following reasons:

- it has the straightest course to the superior vena cava and right atrium, which is the target for the tip of the catheter;
- the anatomic landmarks identifying its location are easily identified; and
- tunneling of the cuffed catheter to an infraclavicular position allows for maximum patient mobility and comfort.[1,92,93]

The left internal jugular vein is the second choice for dialysis catheter insertion. It is associated with lower catheter flow rates and higher rates of catheter malfunction compared to the right internal jugular vein.[1,92,93] The left internal jugular venous catheter also places the left upper extremity at risk for venous outflow obstruction, since the catheter crosses the innominate vein and can precipitate its stenosis or occlusion. The subclavian vein should be used for dialysis catheter placement only if absolutely necessary, because of the significant rate of central venous stenosis associated with its use. Studies have shown that up to 50% of patients who have had central venous access via the subclavian vein will develop a significant stenosis, potentially rendering the ipsilateral upper extremity unusable for AV access placement.[94–97] The femoral vein is easily accessible and frequently used for temporary catheter placement; however, it is associated with a significantly higher rate of infection than internal jugular or subclavian venous catheters. Dialysis catheters placed via the femoral vein must be at least 19cm long to prevent recirculation.[98] If the internal jugular and subclavian veins have been exhausted, however, the femoral vein can be used for cuffed dialysis catheter placement.[99,100] The translumbar approach to the inferior vena cava is used for dialysis catheter placement when all other peripheral and central sites for catheter insertion have been exhausted. Catheters placed via this approach have a higher incidence of catheter dislodgement and infection than other sites, and are technically more difficult to place.[101,102]

Cuffed dialysis catheters are inserted either percutaneously or by surgical cutdown. If a surgical cutdown technique is used, hemostasis should be obtained by placing a pursestring suture in the vessel around the catheter, rather than placing proximal and distal ligatures, which precludes the future use of the vessel for dialysis access when the catheter is removed. The percutaneous placement of dialysis catheters may be performed blindly using only anatomic landmarks. Although this is the traditional method taught to most surgeons, ultrasound guidance offers significant advantages to blind placement. Patients with end-stage renal disease often have had multiple catheters placed previously, and one or more of the access veins may be thrombosed.[103,104] Thrombosis of the internal jugular, external jugular, and femoral veins are easily identified with ultrasonography. Ultrasonography can also identify variations of the venous anatomy that can occur

in 26–35% of patients.[105,106] A recent study showed that ultrasound guidance decreases the number of punctures required, decreases the time required, and improves the success rate of dialysis catheter placement.[107] Current DOQI guidelines recommend the use of ultrasound guidance for cuffed dialysis catheter placement.[1]

The uncuffed dialysis catheters are stiffer than cuffed dialysis catheters. When placed from the jugular or subclavian approach, the tip of the uncuffed catheter should be positioned in the superior vena cava rather than the right atrium, to minimize the risk of cardiac perforation. Uncuffed catheters placed in the femoral vein should be left in for no more than 5 days and the patients should be kept at bed rest.

Insertion of the cuffed dialysis catheters is more technically challenging than that of the uncuffed catheters. To place a cuffed dialysis catheter via the internal jugular vein, the patient's neck and chest are prepared and draped. Intravenous antibiotics are administered preoperatively. Sterile insonation gel is placed on the neck. The ultrasound probe is covered with a sterile sheath and used to visualize the internal jugular vein. Local anesthesia is infiltrated over the vein. The ultrasound image is used to guide a large-gauge needle into the vein. A flexible guidewire is inserted through the needle using the Seldinger technique. A 1–2cm incision is made at the guidewire insertion site in the neck. Another 1cm incision is made in the chest in the lateral infraclavicular region. The dialysis catheter is passed through a subcutaneous tunnel from the chest incision to the neck. The tract into the jugular vein is serially dilated over the guidewire, followed by placement of the dilator/introducer complex. The wire and dilator are removed. The catheter is inserted through the introducer sheath, and the sheath is peeled away. Air embolism during the procedure is prevented by maintaining the patient in a 'head down' position. The procedure is performed with fluoroscopic guidance to confirm accurate positioning of the catheter tip. Optimal flow rates are obtained with the catheter tip positioned in the right atrium.[92] The course of the catheter must be inspected with fluoroscopy to insure that the catheter is not kinked (**Fig. 27.13**). If the catheter is of the 'stepped tip' design, care must be taken to orient the longer venous limb along the outer curve of the catheter (**Table 27.9**). The early catheter failure rate most often is due to technical problems, such as kinks in the course of the catheter or catheter tip malposition.[103–108] The DOQI guidelines recommend that early failure rates not exceed 5%.[1]

Complications of dialysis catheters can be categorized as 'early' or 'late' (**Table 27.10**). Aside from mechanical failure, the early complications include pneumothorax, arterial puncture/laceration,

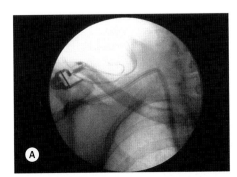

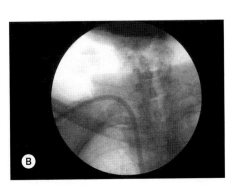

Figure 27.13 Dialysis catheter. (A) Radiograph of a kinked, tunneled dialysis catheter. (B) Radiograph of a dialysis catheter tunneled correctly.

Tips for tunneled dialysis catheter placement via the internal jugular or subclavian vein.

- Venous access is obtained using ultrasound guidance
- The patient is positioned 'head down' to prevent air embolism
- The catheter position is confirmed with fluoroscopy at the time of insertion
- The catheter tip is positioned in the right atrium
- The 'stepped tip' catheter is oriented with the longer limb (venous limb) along the outer curve

Table 27.9 Tips for tunneled dialysis catheter placement via the internal jugular or subclavian vein.

Complications of central venous catheterization.

Early complications	Late complications
• Mechanical obstruction of the catheter	• Infection
• Pneumothorax	• Catheter thrombosis
• Arterial puncture/laceration	• Central venous stenosis/occlusion
• Hematoma	• Endocarditis/metastatic infection
• Hemothorax/hemomediastinum	• Catheter fracture/embolization
• Thoracic duct injury	• Catheter dislodgement
• Nerve injury	
• Cardiac arrhythmia	
• Cardiac perforation	
• Air embolism	

Table 27.10 Complications of central venous catheterization.

hematoma, and air embolism. These early complications may be decreased if the catheter is placed using ultrasound guidance.[107]

Infection is one of the most serious late complications and is a primary reason for catheter loss. In a large prospective study, dialysis catheter related bacteremia occurred once every 256 catheter days.[109] Retrospective studies have reported catheter-associated bacteremia rates ranging from 0.72 to 5.5 episodes per 1000 catheter-days.[110,111] Catheter infection may present in one of four fashions:

- exit-site infection;
- tunnel infection;
- bacteremia; or
- systemic sepsis.

The management of each of these is somewhat different.

Exit-site infections represent infections between the Dacron cuff and the skin, and present with redness, crusting, and an exudate. Blood cultures are negative. Local wound care with topical antibiotics is often sufficient to clear the infection. If the infection fails to respond to local measures then parenteral antibiotic therapy may be necessary.

Tunnel tract infection and catheter-related bacteremia are more difficult to treat. Intravenous antibiotic therapy alone is associated with a low rate of catheter salvage and a significant incidence of metastatic infection.[109,112] This is probably related to poor antibiotic penetration of the fibrin sheath that forms on the catheter. The definitive treatment for tunnel tract infection

and catheter-related bacteremia is catheter removal and intravenous antibiotics. The catheter access site can be salvaged with guidewire exchange of the catheter in patients who rapidly respond to intravenous antibiotics by becoming afebrile and who do not develop other signs of systemic sepsis. If the exit site and the tunnel do not show evidence of active infection, the catheter can be removed and replaced over a guidewire using the same tunnel. Catheters that have erythema and tenderness along the tunnel tract or those that have exit-site infection with bacteremia can also undergo guidewire exchange; however, a new tunnel and exit site must be created. The steps of this procedure are:

- cut down on the catheter at its insertion in the jugular vein in the neck;
- divide the catheter;
- remove the subcutaneous catheter and cuff;
- cover the old exit site with an occlusive dressing;
- tunnel a new catheter through an uninfected field;
- insert a guidewire through the central portion of the catheter;
- remove the remainder of the old catheter, leaving the guidewire in place; and
- place the new catheter through the introducer sheath as previously described.

All patients treated with catheter exchange require at least 3 weeks of culture-directed antibiotic therapy and should be monitored for evidence of recurrent infection.[113] In one report, 83% of these catheter infections were successfully treated with antibiotics and guidewire exchange of the catheter; this is similar to the results achieved with catheter removal and subsequent replacement using a new site.[113,114]

Catheters should be removed and temporary access utilized in patients who present with signs of systemic sepsis or who fail to respond to antibiotic therapy. A cuffed catheter can be inserted at a new site after the patient has been afebrile for 48–72 hours and when blood cultures are negative. Although the majority of catheter infections are caused by gram-positive organisms, gram-negative and mixed flora infections are not infrequent.[111] According to the DOQI guidelines, the target rate of infection for cuffed dialysis catheters should be less than 10% at 3 months and less than 50% at 1 year.[1]

Catheter malfunction is a common problem associated with dialysis catheters. The catheter patency rate varies widely in the literature and may be affected by the type of catheter placed and its tip configuration.[110,112,115,116] Retrospective data suggest that catheters with both side and end holes have improved patency rates.[110] Although a recent randomized, prospective study found improved catheter survival with a 'split-tip' compared to a 'step-tip' design, others found no difference in survival between three catheter types.[117,118] Currently, there is insufficient evidence to support the use of one catheter over another.[1]

Late catheter occlusion is most often caused by thrombus formation within the tip of the catheter or formation of a sleeve of fibrin that envelops the catheter. Thrombus formation may be related to inadequate heparinization of the catheter following use.

A chest radiograph is obtained in patients with catheter occlusion to exclude the possibility of kinking of the catheter or catheter tip malposition. Once excluded, thrombolytic agents have proven beneficial in restoring the patency of occluded catheters. Both urokinase and tissue plasminogen activator (t-PA) have been used to restore catheter patency; however, in a blinded, randomized, prospective trial, t-PA was found to be superior to urokinase.[119] Several protocols have been used. The usual dose of t-PA is 2mg, which is allowed to dwell in the catheter for 2 hours.[120]

If thrombolysis fails to re-establish catheter patency, radiologic stripping of the catheter to remove the pericatheter fibrin sheath may be successful. A nitinol gooseneck snare is introduced through the femoral vein to snare the catheter and strip the sheath. Symptomatic embolization related to catheter stripping is rare. The initial success of this procedure is reported to be 94–100%.[103,121] Failure of this method mandates catheter replacement which often can be accomplished with a guidewire exchange.

Although dialysis catheters provide an invaluable method of access in a difficult group of patients, they are at best a secondary form of access. Efforts should be made to limit the duration of dialysis catheter use by promptly providing patients with a functioning autogenous or non-autogenous AV access.

COMPLICATIONS OF AV ACCESS

Thrombosis

Thrombosis is the most common complication associated with AV access and is the most common cause for access abandonment. There are multiple etiologies for access thrombosis, including systemic hypotension, poor arterial inflow, hypercoagulability, access infection, central venous stenosis or occlusion, and external compression of the access. The most common etiology of access thrombosis for both autogenous and prosthetic AV accesses is the development of a venous stenosis. A venous stenosis has been identified after thrombectomy of prosthetic AV accesses in more than 90% of cases.[122] The majority of the venous stenoses that develop in prosthetic AV accesses occur within 1 cm of the venous anastomosis (**Fig. 27.14**).[123] The stenosis is often found more centrally in autogenous AV accesses near areas of vein bifurcation, pressure points, and venous valves.[1] Histopathologic examination of the wall of stenotic veins removed from failing dialysis accesses has revealed progressive intimal smooth muscle cell proliferation and extracellular matrix secretion.[124] The etiology for the development of the venous stenosis after access placement is probably related to venous trauma from one or all of the following:

- compliance mismatch between the prosthetic graft and the vein;
- the effect of increased blood pressure in the venous system;
- injury related to the AV anastomosis creation; and
- turbulent blood flow within the vein.[125]

Historically, treatment of access thrombosis involved abandonment of the access, with placement of a new access in a different anatomic location. This approach, however, quickly exhausts venous sites for hemodialysis. Over time, both surgical and percutaneous methods have been developed to salvage thrombosed AV accesses. The treatment of a thrombosed AV access involves the following steps:

- removal of the thrombus from the access;
- fistulography to identify the cause for access failure; and
- correction of the underlying access or venous outflow stenosis.

Surgical thrombectomy of an AV access is accomplished by exposing a segment of the access and mechanically removing the

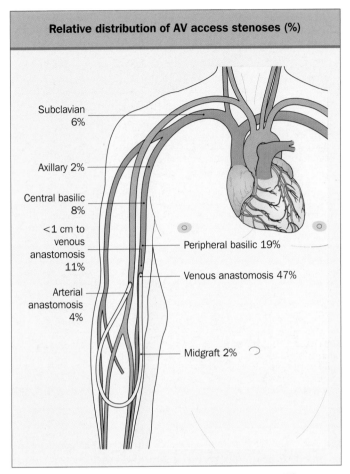

Figure 27.14 Relative distribution of AV access stenoses (%).

thrombus with a Fogarty embolectomy catheter. The technical success of surgical thrombectomy ranges between 82% and 94%.[126–129]

Several percutaneous techniques have been developed to restore AV access patency. Continuous infusion of thrombolytic agents into the access was used initially; however, the technical success of this method was inferior to surgical thrombectomy, required prolonged infusion times, and was associated with bleeding complications.[130] To shorten infusion times, a number of methods have been developed to mechanically disrupt the thrombus, thus exposing a greater surface area of thrombus to the thrombolytic agent. These include pharmacomechanical methods of 'lacing' the thrombus with a high dose of thrombolytic agent, or forcefully injecting it into the thrombus (the 'pulse-spray' technique). Others have reported the use of external massage, balloon maceration, and balloon clot displacement to disrupt the thrombus prior to infusion of the thrombolytic agent. The addition of pharmacomechanical and mechanical methods of thrombus disruption has resulted in much lower infusion times and technical success rates that are equivalent to surgical thrombectomy.[131,132]

More recently, percutaneous techniques have been developed to mechanically remove thrombus from AV accesses without thrombolytic agents. These techniques involve the use of thrombectomy devices that strip or pulverize the thrombus, which can then be aspirated out of the access or flushed into the venous

							Primary patency		
Study	Study design	Indication	Access type	Method	n	Technical success	1 month	6 months	12 months
Schwartz[126]	Retrospective	Thrombosis	Prosthetic	Surg T/Rev	24	87%	60%%	30%	13%
Dougherty[142]	Prospective/ Randomized	Thrombosis	Prosthetic	Surg T/Rev PMT/BA	41 39	— —	— —	— —	26% 14%
Marston[129]	Prospective/ Randomized	Thrombosis	Prosthetic	Surg T/Rev PMT/BA	56 59	82% 71%	61% 44%	34% 11%	24% 9%
Trerotola[133]	Retrospective	Thrombosis	Prosthetic	MT/BA	34	94%	56%	20%	0
Overbosch[135]	Retrospective	Thrombosis	Prosthetic/ Autogenous	MT/BA	65	89%	71%	36%	—
Brooks[143]	Prospective/ Randomized	Malfunction	Prosthetic	Surg Rev PTA	19 24	— —	— —	68% 34%	62% 24%
Lumsden[144]	Retrospective	Malfunction	Prosthetic	PTA	40	—	76%	27%	10%
Beathard[137]	Retrospective	Malfunction	Prosthetic/ Autogenous	PTA	285	—	91%	61%	38%

Table 27.11 Results of treatment for failing and failed AV access. MT/BA, percutaneous mechanical thrombectomy/balloon angioplasty; PMT/BA, pharmacomechanical thrombectomy/balloon angioplasty; PTA, percutaneous transluminal angioplasty; Surg Rev, surgical revision; Surg T/Rev, surgical thrombectomy/revision.

system. Advocates for these devices claim that their use avoids the cost and risk associated with thrombolytic agents. The technical success rates reported with these devices are similar to those achieved with surgical thrombectomy and pharmaco-mechanical thrombolysis.[128,129,133–135]

Although the initial technical success of both the surgical and percutaneous methods for restoring access patency approximate 90%, the long-term patency rates are poor for access thrombectomy alone without intervention. Since 90% of all access thromboses are associated with a hemodynamically significant stenosis, it is mandatory that all thrombosed accesses undergo fistulography and repair of any identified stenosis.[136] Failure to do so leads to high early failure rates. Stenoses that are identified by fistulography undergo either surgical revision or balloon angioplasty.

Most studies that report results of balloon angioplasty for AV access stenosis do not stratify patients based on lesion characteristics; however, short segment and anastamotic stenoses appear to respond better to balloon angioplasty than long-segment stenoses or occlusions.[137]

Intravascular stents have been used to treat access-related stenosis. Several reports have examined the use of stents as a means of salvage of a failed angioplasty, particularly for lesions with significant elastic recoil. These reports have shown patency rates similar to balloon angioplasty.[138,139] Reports comparing balloon angioplasty alone and balloon angioplasty with stenting as primary treatment of venous stenoses have shown no improvement in patency and increased cost with stenting.[140,141] At the present time, stenting of access-related stenoses should not routinely be used. Stenting may be helpful in situations where balloon angioplasty has failed and the position of the access is not favorable for surgical revision, such as an access located in the proximal upper arm.

The majority of series that have reviewed results for surgical thrombectomy and revision of failed AV accesses report outcomes as cumulative patency from initial access placement rather than primary patency from access revision. The studies that have reported primary patency results for the surgical and percutaneous management of failed AV accesses have not demonstrated clear superiority of one method over the other (Table 27.11).[126,129,133,135,137,142–144]

Proponents of the percutaneous methods for the management of AV access thrombosis emphasize that these techniques are less invasive than surgical thrombectomy and revision. The procedures are performed on an outpatient basis in the radiology suite, which is often more accessible than the operating theater. Since the percutaneous methods treat the stenosis with dilatation rather than bypass, vein is preserved for future access revision or placement. A potential risk of percutaneous intervention, particularly for the mechanical thrombectomy techniques, is the embolism of disrupted thrombus into the pulmonary circulation. Lung perfusion scans after percutaneous thrombectomy have shown that a high percentage of these patients have detectable emboli.[145] Although fatal pulmonary emboli have been reported, the majority of these are not clinically significant and their relevance is unclear.[145,146] It has been the authors' practice to surgically revise those accesses that fail balloon angioplasty early or those that have long-segment venous stenoses or occlusion which do not respond well to balloon angioplasty. The DOQI guidelines concluded that there was no clear superiority between surgical revision and percutaneous intervention and that treatment should be based on each institution's expertise and available facilities.[1]

If fistulography fails to identify a stenosis, another etiology for access thrombosis must be considered. Dialysis personnel and records should be queried to determine if the thrombotic episode could be caused by hypotension or excessive post-dialysis needle site compression. Recurrent episodes of access thrombosis can be caused by an underlying hypercoaguable disorder. These include protein C or S deficiency, antithrombin III deficiency, factor V Leiden mutation, and the presence of anticardiolipin antibodies. Patients with these disorders or in whom a cause for access failure cannot be determined are treated with chronic oral anticoagulation.

Thrombosis of autogenous AV accesses may present differently than non-autogenous AV accesses. The volume of thrombus in an autogenous access can vary. There may be only a short segment that is thrombosed at the site of stenosis. With time, the thrombus can propagate and lead to full-length occlusion. If the thrombosis is detected before propagation has occurred, the access may be salvaged with revision. A short-segment occlusion near the arteriovenous anastomosis may be revised, with creation of a new arteriovenous anastomosis more proximally on the artery and vein. Long-segment occlusions can be difficult to thrombectomize and may have to be abandoned. Percutaneous methods of treatment for failing AV fistulas have been reported, with reasonable results.[147,148]

Infection

Access infection accounts for 20% of all hemodialysis-related complications and is a major cause of morbidity and mortality in the dialysis patient population. It results in up to 10% of all death in these patients, ranking second only to cardiovascular disease as the most common cause of death.[149]

Multiple systemic and local factors are responsible for the high incidence of infection noted in these patients. The adverse effects of uremia and chronic renal failure on the immune system are well documented. Studies have demonstrated decreased phagocytosis and cellular killing by polymorphonuclear cells and inhibited lymphocyte transformation in patients with chronic renal failure.[150,151]

Access infections which occur in the immediate postoperative period are most often caused by a break in sterile technique that leads to bacterial seeding of the graft. An infection remote to the surgical site can also lead to early graft seeding. Meticulous intraoperative technique and use of prophylactic antibiotics have reduced the incidence of early graft infection to less than 4%.[152]

Wounds heal poorly in patients on chronic hemodialysis. In the setting of a recent access placement, poor healing can lead to wound breakdown and graft exposure. Excessive edema can also lead to breakdown of incisions as well as blistering and cellulitis. Seroma or hematoma increase the potential for postoperative wound and graft infection.

Infections that occur after initial wound healing and graft incorporation are usually related to local graft manipulation, in particular recurrent needle cannulation. Puncture of the skin during access cannulation is a potential source of bacterial introduction. Poor hemostasis following needle removal can lead to hematoma or pseudoaneurysm formation and subsequent infection. Access thrombectomy or revision also presents an opportunity for graft contamination and infection.

The majority of vascular access infections are caused by bacteria that comprise normal skin flora. *Staphylococcus aureus* is the most common pathogen cultured from infected AV access wounds. The high rate of *S. aureus* infections may in part be due to patient and dialysis staff colonization, which occurs in 60% of

patients on chronic hemodialysis and 30% of the dialysis staff. This compares to a colonization rate of 10–14% in the general population.[153]

The AV access method and location play a significant role in the incidence of access infection. The incidence of infection ranges between 0% and 5% for autogenous AV accesses and between 6% and 35% for non-autogenous AV accesses.[23,25–29,43,67] Accesses located in the thigh position are associated with a higher rate of infection than those located in the upper extremity or thoracic position.[43,67]

An infected dialysis access can present with a variety of signs and symptoms. Local signs of infection include erythema, warmth, and tenderness over the access. Autogenous AV accesses tend to manifest infection only as cellulitis, whereas non-autogenous AV accesses usually present with perigraft fluid, fluctuance over the graft, or a draining sinus. *Staphylococcus epidermidis* may cause a chronic, indolent graft infection. Patients with grafts infected with *S. epidermidis* present with perigraft fluid or anastomotic pseudoaneurysms and may exhibit no other manifestations of infection. Access infection may also be complicated by the development of distant sites of infection or systemic sepsis syndrome. Endocarditis, osteomyelitis, septic arthritis, and septic pulmonary emboli have all been reported in conjunction with AV access infection.[154]

The diagnosis of access-related infections relies heavily on clinical judgment. Blood cultures or local fluid cultures are obtained to determine responsible pathogens and to confirm the success of treatment. Cultures are often negative, particularly if antibiotics are started before blood cultures are obtained. Once a treatment course has been completed, blood cultures should be repeated because a continued positive culture is highly predictive of infection recurrence.[149] Duplex ultrasonography of the access can identify perigraft fluid or pseudoaneurysm, which may be suggestive of access infection.

Treatment of access-related infection begins with antibiotics. Due to the high percentage of cultures that are positive for methicillin-resistant *S. aureus*, most authors recommend empiric treatment with vancomycin.[149,153] An antibiotic effective against gram-negative organisms is also added initially. Once cultures return, antibiotic therapy is tailored appropriately. If no gram-positive organisms are present, or if methicillin-sensitive organisms are found, the vancomycin should be stopped to minimize development of resistant organisms. The optimal duration of antibiotic therapy is not well defined by the literature, and recommendations vary depending on the extent of infection.

Autogenous AV access infections usually present with cellulitis that can be effectively treated with antibiotics alone. Infected pseudoaneurysms or abscesses that directly involve the vein require ligation or segmental bypass of the access.

Non-autogenous AV access infection may be localized to a segment of the graft or may involve the entire graft. Graft removal offers the best chance for complete eradication of the infection; however, since sites for vascular access are limited, the decision to remove an infected access requires careful consideration. Early infection that develops before tissue ingrowth into the graft occurs usually involves the entire graft, and treatment mandates complete graft excision. Successful graft salvage of localized infections with incision and drainage, long-term antibiotics, and wound packing has been reported.[155] This treatment modality may result in wound contraction and fixation

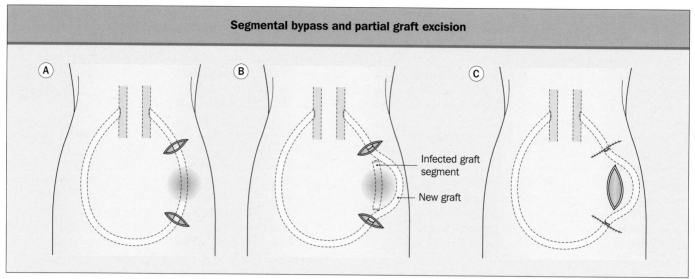

Segmental bypass and partial graft excision

Infected graft segment

New graft

Figure 27.15 Technique of segmental bypass and partial graft excision for localized prosthetic AV access infection. (A) Graft is exposed proximal and distal to the infected graft segment at sites remote from the infection. (B) The ends of the infected graft segment and tunnel are oversewn. A graft is tunneled through clean tissue planes around the infected graft segment and sewn end-to-end to the old graft. (C) The incisions are closed and dressed. The infected graft segment is excised and the open wound is packed.

of the graft at or above skin level, precluding any chance for wound epithelialization and long-term cure. Coverage of exposed AV graft segments has been achieved with skin or muscle flaps.[156,157] These techniques are reported as isolated cases, with no large series.

Another treatment for localized graft infection is segmental bypass and partial graft excision. The procedure is performed by making a cutdown on the graft proximal and distal to the infected graft segment at sites that appear remote from the infection. The graft at each of these sites is assessed for infection. If the graft is unincorporated or if perigraft fluid is present at either of these sites, the graft is completely excised. If the graft is well incorporated and does not appear infected, it is divided and the ends of the infected graft segment and tunnel are oversewn. Graft continuity is restored with an interposition graft that is tunneled through clean tissue planes around the infected graft segment. The interposition graft is sewn end to end to the old graft. The incisions are closed and covered with an occlusive dressing. The infected graft segment is excised and the open wound is packed. If there is an adequate length of the initial graft remaining to allow cannulation away from the new graft segment, the graft can be used immediately (**Fig. 27.15**). Schwab et al. reviewed 17 patients treated with this technique and reported a 94% late graft salvage rate, with no perioperative deaths and no major morbidity.[158]

Aneurysm and pseudoaneurysm

Long-term AV access use can be complicated by formation of pseudoaneurysms. Less commonly, true aneurysmal dilatation of the access can occur. Pseudoaneurysm formation is most often due to poor technique in cannulating the access, whether it be from repeated needle sticks in a limited area of the access or from poor hemostasis after needle removal. Although there is little scientific evidence to support it, prosthetic AV accesses are generally not cannulated for 2 weeks after placement, to minimize the risk for pseudoaneurysm formation due to lack of graft incorporation into the surrounding soft tissue.

Infection may occur either as a primary cause for development of an AV access pseudoaneurysm or as a later secondary event. Distinguishing between a sterile and infected pseudoaneurysm can be difficult, as the local effects of a pseudoaneurysm on skin temperature and color can mimic changes secondary to infection. Other complications of aneurysms include thrombosis and rupture.

Most small, asymptomatic aneurysms do not require treatment. Treatment becomes mandatory for larger aneurysms that appear at risk for rupture and for aneurysms complicated by thrombosis or infection. If the skin overlying an aneurysm becomes ulcerated or ischemic, surgical revision or ligation of the access is indicated. Sterile pseudoaneurysms of a prosthetic AV access can be locally excised and the graft repaired. Multiple pseudoaneurysms in close proximity may require partial graft excision and interposition bypass. Infected pseudoaneurysms can be treated with segmental bypass and partial excision, as described previously, with good result.[158] There have been case reports of percutaneously placed stent-grafts across sterile pseudoaneurysms.[159,160] Results of these reports have generally been poor, with the majority developing recurrent pseudo-aneurysms or graft thrombosis. At the present time, open repair remains the primary treatment.

High-output congestive heart failure

An AV access can have marked effects on the cardiovascular system. The establishment of a high flow connection between the arterial and venous systems causes an immediate and significant drop in peripheral arterial resistance. To maintain blood pressure, the body responds with an increase in cardiac output by increasing heart rate and stroke volume. Although this response is well tolerated in the majority of patients, congestive heart failure may occur in patients who have poor cardiac reserve. Today's dialysis machines require flow rates up to 600mL/min. Flow rates in this range rarely cause cardiac failure, except in the patient with minimal cardiac reserve. AV access flow rates in excess of 1000mL/min are generally required for cardiac failure to ensue. Such high flow rates are more commonly encountered when the larger vessels of the upper arm or proximal thigh are used for AV access, rather than the smaller vessels of the forearm.

Since congestive heart failure related to volume overload, anemia, severe hypertension, and cardiac dysfunction occurs frequently in the dialysis patient population, the role of the AV access is often overlooked as a potential cause of congestive heart failure. By recognizing those patients at risk for development of access-related congestive heart failure and utilizing appropriate diagnostic maneuvers and testing, the clinician can identify those patients who may benefit from correction or removal of the access.

Decreased cardiac reserve must be present to develop symptoms. Patients at risk include those with coronary artery disease, severe hypertension, and hypertrophic cardiomyopathy.[161] Systemic hypertension may increase flow through the low-resistance access and exacerbate the stress on the heart.

Diagnosis requires documentation of a drop in cardiac output with fistula compression. In patients with congestive heart failure secondary to an AV access, the pre-compression volume of flow through the access is usually greater than the subsequent drop in cardiac output with compression of the access.[161]

Although ligation of the access is the most definitive treatment, there are reports of successful treatment of access-related congestive heart failure with banding or narrowing of the access, which reduces AV shunting.[162] Flow through the access can be assessed as it is narrowed. The goal is to decrease the flow rate to less than 1000mL/min, as measured by intraoperative or postoperative duplex examination.

Vascular steal

Extremity ischemia after creation of an AV access is uncommon. This complication more frequently occurs with accesses that are located in the proximal extremity, such as the upper arm or thigh. It is also more commonly seen with prosthetic than autogenous AV accesses. Patients with diabetes mellitus who have atherosclerotic occlusive disease are especially susceptible to access-related ischemia.

Vascular steal is caused by a drop in distal perfusion pressure to the extremity, resulting from creation of a proximal low-resistance AV shunt. The difference in resistance between the shunt and the runoff bed can cause reversal of flow in the native artery distal to the access that shunts blood away from the distal extremity. In patients who have adequate flow through collaterals, this flow reversal does not result in the development of symptomatic steal. In patients with vascular occlusive disease or in those patients in whom the access flow rate is high, collateral flow can be inadequate, resulting in the development of signs and symptoms of limb ischemia. Reversal of blood flow does not necessarily result in symptoms, as studies have shown that clinically silent retrograde flow occurs in up to 67% of autogenous radial-cephalic AV accesses and in 86% of prosthetic upper arm AV accesses.[163] Ischemia can occur without flow reversal as well, especially in cases of severe peripheral occlusive disease and from embolic events.

Patients with vascular steal may present with a variety of symptoms, ranging from hand coolness or paresthesias that occur only during dialysis, to severe ischemia with tissue necrosis. Patients may complain of pain, stiffness, or swelling of the

fingers, or hand weakness. On examination, the fingers may be cool, with delayed capillary refill and decreased sensation. A radial pulse is usually absent. Compression of the access may result in relief of symptoms and return of a radial pulse, and is diagnostic of access-related vascular steal. Objective documentation of steal can be obtained in the vascular laboratory by demonstrating augmentation of digital pressures and pulse volume recordings with access compression. Duplex ultrasonography can also identify retrograde flow in the runoff artery distal to the AV access, which becomes antegrade with access compression.

Treatment is based on the severity of symptoms and the anatomy. Mild symptoms that occur early after access placement are observed and treated conservatively. Most will resolve with time.[164] Patients who present with severe acute limb-threatening ischemia are best treated with access ligation. Those patients who develop progressive moderate to severe symptoms are evaluated to determine the etiology of the ischemia. Duplex ultrasonography and, in selected cases, arteriography can identify inflow arterial occlusive disease, which contributes to distal ischemia after access placement in 20–30% of cases.[165] Vascular steal caused by a stenosis of the arterial inflow to the access can often be treated with balloon angioplasty, endarterectomy, or arterial bypass. Vascular steal following creation of an autogenous radial-cephalic AV access may be treated by ligation of the radial artery distal to the AV anastomosis. The success of this treatment requires that the arterial inflow be normal, and the ulnar artery and palmar arch be patent. This treatment will be unsuccessful in patients who rely solely on the radial artery for hand perfusion. Various techniques have been developed for the prevention or treatment of vascular steal; these increase flow resistance in the AV access, to increase distal arterial perfusion. Access banding, plication, or use of tapered interposition grafts have all been used to increase the flow resistance through the access.[164,166,167] This approach to the treatment of vascular steal has met with limited success. It is difficult to objectively determine intraoperatively the degree of graft narrowing necessary to relieve symptoms of ischemia but at the same time maintain access patency. An alternative method for treating access-related vascular steal is the distal revascularization with interval ligation procedure (DRIL) procedure described by Schanzer et al.[169] The procedure increases collateral circulation to the ischemic limb by the creation of a bypass from the artery proximal to the AV access to the artery distal to the access. To prevent retrograde arterial flow, the native artery is ligated between the access and the distal anastomosis of the bypass (**Fig. 27.16**). This procedure has been effective in relieving symptoms of limb ischemia in more than 90% of patients with access-related vascular steal.[164,168,169]

Peripheral neuropathy

Placement of a vascular access can lead to peripheral neuropathy. The etiology for this complication is multifactorial and includes ischemia, venous hypertension, and local compression. As with ischemic complications, the presenting symptoms can vary widely. The diagnosis and treatment depend on the severity of symptoms and the underlying causative factors.

Ischemic monomelic neuropathy

Ischemic monomelic neuropathy (IMN) is characterized by pain, weakness, and paralysis of the muscles of the forearm and

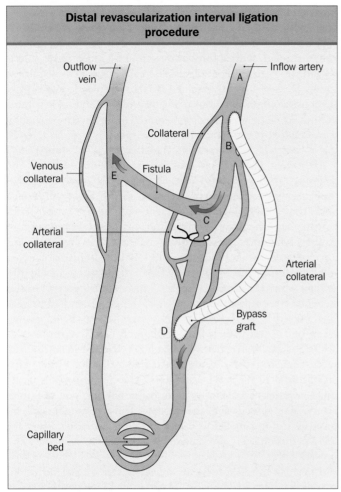

Distal revascularization interval ligation procedure

Outflow vein

Inflow artery

A

Collateral

B

Venous collateral

Fistula

E

Arterial collateral

C

Arterial collateral

Bypass graft

D

Capillary bed

Figure 27.16 Technique of distal revascularization interval ligation (DRIL) procedure. A critical component of technical success is the location of the bypass origin in relation to the origin of the access. This distance should be at least 3cm. A ligature is placed around the artery just distal to the access to prevent retrograde flow.

hand that develops minutes to hours after placement of an antecubital AV access. Sensory loss may also be present. In contrast to access-related vascular steal, which results in global ischemia of the distal extremity, IMN results in ischemia isolated to the nerves, and develops in the immediate postoperative period. It is probably caused by nerve ischemia in the vascular 'watershed area' for the radial, ulnar, and median nerves at the antecubital fossa.

IMN is a rare complication of AV access creation, although the actual incidence is probably under-reported in the literature.[170] Patients at risk are older and almost exclusively have diabetes mellitus. Patients who have pre-existing peripheral neuropathy and peripheral vascular disease are prone to this complication. It only occurs with accesses placed at the antecubital position.

The classic presentation of IMN is the development of weakness of all or most of the muscles of the forearm and hand, paresthesias, and numbness along the distribution of the radial, ulnar, and median nerves. There are usually minimal findings of distal limb ischemia. Generally, the hand is warm and a radial pulse is present. Objective examination of distal perfusion generally reveals a digital pressure greater than 50mmHg and a digital-brachial index less than 0.3. Nerve conduction studies show

axonal loss and reduced motor and sensory nerve conduction velocities of the radial, ulnar, and median nerves.[171]

Treatment requires immediate access ligation, with restoration of distal perfusion. Even with prompt action, neurologic deficits may not be reversible.[171,172] Due to the low incidence of IMN, and because many of the symptoms are confused with routine postoperative complaints, the diagnosis of IMN is often delayed. The routine performance of a thorough neurologic examination in the perioperative period may distinguish those patients with localized pain or single nerve dysfunction due to edema or compression from those patients with IMN.

Local compression and carpal tunnel syndrome

A postoperative fluid collection, such as a seroma, hematoma, or abscess, can cause nerve compression and result in neuropathy. Motor and sensory deficits in the distribution of a single nerve, combined with the presence of a local fluid collection adjacent to the nerve, make it straightforward to distinguish this entity from IMN or vascular steal. The treatment involves decompression of the space-occupying fluid collection. If the diagnosis is established and the nerve decompressed promptly, full recovery of neurologic function is likely.

A pathologic entity which has been described but is not fully understood is access-related carpal tunnel syndrome. Multiple causes for the syndrome have been proposed, including elevated venous pressure, vascular steal leading to ischemia of the median nerve, and thickening of the flexor synovium. The diagnosis can be confirmed by demonstrating decreased median nerve conduction velocities across the carpal ligament. Successful treatment of the syndrome has been reported with release of the carpal ligament.[172]

SURVEILLANCE OF AV ACCESS

The poor results associated with the treatment of a thrombosed AV access, combined with the fact that most access thromboses are associated with a venous stenosis, has led to the development of surveillance protocols to identify dysfunctional grafts for intervention prior to thrombosis. These programs are predicated on the assumption that prophylactic AV access intervention for stenosis prior to access thrombosis will increase the longevity of the access. Schwab et al. showed that prophylactic AV access intervention in patients with elevated venous line pressure results in fewer thrombotic episodes compared to those patients who do not undergo intervention.[173] Others have also shown that intervention prior to thrombosis extends access survival.[137,174]

While physical findings such as extremity edema, prolonged post-dialysis bleeding, and changes in the characteristics of the access thrill can be helpful in predicting access dysfunction, most screening programs to identify hemodynamically significant stenosis have relied on more objective methods such as calculation of access flow rates, increased urea recirculation rates, high venous line pressures, and duplex ultrasonography. There are advantages and disadvantages to each of these surveillance methods (**Table 27.12**). Low access blood flow rates or a downward trend in flow rates have been shown to be reliably predictive of access thrombosis, and at this time appear to be the preferred method, if available at a given institution, for

Methods of access surveillance: advantages and disadvantages.		
Methods	Advantages	Disadvantages
Flow rate measurement	• Most predictive of access failure • Serial measurements obtainable	• Not available at all institutions • Duplex methods not performed in dialysis unit and requires experienced technologist
Venous pressure measurement	• Performed in the dialysis unit • Inexpensive • Serial measurements easily obtained	• Unable to detect inflow and in-graft stenosis • Significant overlap between venous pressures obtained in failing and normal grafts
Urea recirculation measurement	• Serial measurements easily obtained • Performed in the dialysis unit	• Relatively late predictor access dysfunction • Threshold value for intervention is not well defined
Duplex ultrasonography	• Accurate in identifying >50% stenosis • Serial measurements easily obtained	• Duplex methods not performed in dialysis unit and requires experienced technologist • Not shown to reliably predict access failure

Table 27.12 Methods of access surveillance: advantages and disadvantages.

access surveillance.[1,175,176] Calculation of access blood flow rates can be accomplished through Doppler-derived calculations after access interrogation by duplex ultrasound. Duplex-based calculation of access flow rates requires specialized technical skills and is best accomplished in a vascular laboratory. Use of one of several ultrasonic dilution techniques can also be used to calculate flow rates. These techniques are carried out using the arterial and venous hemodialysis lines and thus do not require a separate trip to a vascular laboratory. The calculation of urea recirculation rates and the assessment of venous line pressures can be carried out during dialysis and followed serially. An increased urea recirculation rate is a relatively late indicator of access stenosis and has had mixed results in predicting access failure.[176–179] Static or dynamic venous pressure elevations are predictive of outflow stenosis and risk of access thrombosis; however, inflow and in-graft stenosis may occur without causing an increase in venous pressures.[173] Color flow duplex ultrasonography has been used as a screening tool to identify hemodynamically significant access stenosis. Studies that have correlated color flow duplex ultrasonography with angiography have demonstrated it to be accurate in identifying hemodynamically significant AV access stenoses.[144,180] It has not been conclusively shown, however, that intervention on prosthetic AV accesses with a stenosis identified with duplex ultrasonography will extend access function. Lumsden et al. found no difference in long-term patency rates between treatment and observation groups of patients shown to have greater than 50% stenosis in functioning PTFE grafts;[144] however, none of the grafts in this study had any prior evidence of dysfunction. Therefore, the significance of a stenosis identified without associated evidence of access dysfunction remains unclear, and routine duplex screening without assessment for concomitant graft dysfunction is not currently recommended.

SUMMARY

The substantial cost and morbidity associated with the maintenance of hemodialysis access will continue to stimulate industry, managed care providers, and researchers to solve the vexing problem of AV access failure. The population-based studies that show reduced morbidity associated with autogenous AV accesses, and significant regional variations in autogenous access utilization, are likely to prompt managed care providers to exert pressure to increase their placement. The DOQI guideline goals stating that 50% of patients starting dialysis have an autogenous access placed and that 40% of the hemodialysis population be dialyzed via an autogenous access may be a benchmark used by managed care.

Further work is needed to define the role of AV access surveillance. Methods that directly measure AV access blood flow seem to hold the greatest promise. However, currently, the cost-effectiveness of implementing a surveillance program for the entire dialysis population has not been established. Although surveillance can detect AV access stenosis and can significantly improve access patency, this improved patency is obtained at the cost of many additional procedures. Perhaps the cost-effectiveness of surveillance will be achieved by developing methods of identifying and surveying only those patients at greatest risk for AV access failure.

Industry continues to modify the structure and configuration of PTFE and to develop new biomaterials for AV access use in an attempt to create the ideal conduit. The limitations of currently available prosthetic conduits are:

• a susceptibility to infection;
• an inability to cannulate the access immediately after implantation; and
• a propensity for development of stenosis at or near the venous anastomosis.

The development of new biomaterials with improved perigraft tissue ingrowth, perhaps with concomitant advances in gene therapy and the use of vascular endothelial growth factors, may result in methods to increase graft endothelialization, thereby reducing access infection and stenosis.

Recent innovations that reduce stent restenosis following coronary angioplasty are being investigated to determine if they are effective in blocking the venous hyperplastic response responsible for 80–90% of AV access thromboses. Rapamycin, a macrolide antibiotic, and paclitaxel, a new type of anticancer agent, have been shown to inhibit vascular smooth muscle cell

385

proliferation and migration. These drugs can be bonded to vascular stents. In limited trials, these drug eluting stents have been effective in preventing the restenosis associated with standard coronary angioplasty and stenting. Brachytherapy has also been shown to prevent restenosis after coronary angioplasty and stenting. Currently, catheter-based systems are being developed to deliver radiation to blood vessels. Limited trials are underway to determine if the drug eluting stents or brachytherapy will prevent the venous stenosis associated with AV access. Although the results that have been achieved thus far in the coronary circulation with these modalities are a cause for optimism, the pathophysiology associated with myointimal hyperplasia in the coronary arteries following angioplasty is quite different to that associated with AV accesses. The stimulus to smooth muscle cell proliferation is presumably over after the initial injury with coronary balloon angioplasty, whereas the stimulus to smooth muscle cell proliferation in AV accesses is ongoing. It remains to be seen whether these innovative technologies that have shown promise in the coronary circulation will result in enhanced survival of AV accesses.

REFERENCES

1. National Kidney Foundation. K/DOQI Clinical Practice Guidelines For Vascular Access, 2000. Am J Kidney Dis 2001;37(Suppl 1):S137–81.
2. USRDS 1997 Annual Data Report. X. The economic cost of ESRD vascular access procedures and medicare spending for alternative modalities of treatment. Am J Kidney Dis 1997;30:S160–77.
3. Hirth RA, Turenne MN, Woods JD, et al. Predictors of type of vascular access in hemodialysis patients. JAMA 1996;276:1303–8.
4. Besarab A. Vascular access in Europe and the US: striking contrasts. Contemp Dialysis Nephrol 1999;20:22–8.
5. Rodriguez JA, Lopez J, Cleries M, et al. Vascular access for hemodialysis: an epidemiological study of the Catalan Renal Registry. Nephrol Dial Transplant 1999;14:1651–7.
6. Quarello F, Forneris G, Bocro R, et al. Vascular access for chronic hemodialysis: current status and new directions in the Piedmont. Minerva Urol Nephrol 1998;50:9–15.
7. Bonucchi D, D'Amelio A, Capelli G, et al. Management of vascular access for dialysis: an Italian survey. Nephrol Dial Transplant 1999; 14:2116–8.
8. Ezzahiri R, Lemson MS, Kitslaar PJEHM, et al. Hemodialysis vascular access and fistula surveillance methods in the Netherlands. Nephrol Dial Transplant 1999;14:2110–5.
9. Pisoni RL, Young EW, Dykstra DM, et al. Vascular access use in Europe and the United States: results from the DOPPS. Kidney Int 2002;61:305–16.
10. Sidawy AN, Gray R, Besarab A, et al. Recommended standards for reports dealing with arteriovenous hemodialysis accesses. J Vasc Surg 2002; 35:603–10.
11. Silva MB Jr, Hobson RW II, Pappas PJ, et al. A strategy for increasing use of hemodialysis access procedures: impact of preoperative non-invasive evaluation. J Vasc Surg 1998;27:302–8.
12. Keoghane SR, Kar Leow C, Gray DWR. Routine use of arteriovenous fistula construction to dilate the venous outflow prior to insertion of an expanded polytetrafluoroethylene (PTFE) loop graft for dialysis. Nephrol Dial Transplant 1993;8:154–6.
13. Palder SB, Kirkman RL, Whittemore AD. Vascular access for hemodialysis: patency rates and results of revision. Ann Surg 1985; 202:235–9.
14. Wolowczyk L, Williams AJ, Donovan KL, et al. The snuffbox arteriovenous fistula for vascular access. Eur J Vasc Endovasc Surg 2000; 19:70–6.
15. Golledge J, Smith CJ, Emery J, et al. Outcome of primary radiocephalic fistula for haemodialysis. Br J Surg 1999;86:211–6.
16. Burger H, Kluchert BA, Kootstra G, et al. Survival of arteriovenous fistulas and shunts for haemodialysis. Eur J Surg 1995;161:327–34.
17. Leapman SB, Boyle M, Pescovitz MD, et al. The arteriovenous fistula for hemodialysis access: gold standard or archaic relic? Am Surg 1996; 62:652–7.
18. Dickson CS, Gregory RT, Parent FN, et al. A new technique for hemodialysis access surgery: use of the pneumatic tourniquet. Ann Vasc Surg 1996;10:373–7.
19. Dunlop MG, Mackinlay JY, Jenkins AM. Vascular access: experience with the brachiocephalic fistula. Ann R Coll Surg Engl 1986;68:203–6.
20. Sparks SR, VanderLinden JL, Gnanadev DA, Smith JW, Bunt TJ. Superior patency of perforating antecubital vein arteriovenous fistulae for hemodialysis. Ann Vasc Surg 1997;11:165–7.
21. Livingston CK, Potts JR. Upper arm arteriovenous fistulas as a reliable access alternative for patients requiring chronic hemodialysis. Am Surg 1999;65:1038–42.
22. Bender MHM, Bruyninckx CMA, Gerlag PGG. The Gracz arteriovenous fistula evaluated. Results of the brachiocephalic elbow fistula in haemodialysis angio-access. Eur J Vasc Endovasc Surg 1995;10:294–7.
23. Ascher E, Hingorani A, Gunduz Y, et al. The value and limitations of the arm cephalic and basilic vein for arteriovenous access. Ann Vasc Surg 2001; 15:89–97.
24. Cull DL, Taylor SM, Carsten CG, et al. The fistula elevation procedure: a valuable technique for maximizing arteriovenous fistula utilization. Ann Vasc Surg 2002;16:85–8.
25. Coburn MC, Carney WI Jr. Comparison of basilic vein and polytetrafluoroethylene for brachial arteriovenous fistula. J Vasc Surg 1994; 20:896–902.
26. Matsuura JH, Rosenthal D, Clark M, et al. Transposed basilic vein versus polytetrafluoroethylene for brachial-axillary arteriovenous fistulas. Am J Surg 1998;176:219–21.
27. Rivers SP, Scher LA, Sheehan E, et al. Basilic vein transposition: an underused autologous alternative to prosthetic dialysis angioaccess. J Vasc Surg 1993;18:391–7.
28. Oliver MJ, McCann RL, Indridason OS, et al. Comparison of transposed brachiobasilic fistulas to upper arm grafts and brachiocephalic fistulas. Kidney Int 2001;60:1532–9.
29. Murphy GJ, White SA, Knight AJ, et al. Long-term results of arteriovenous fistulas using transposed autologous basilic vein. Br J Surg 2000;87:819–23.
30. Silva MB, Hobson RW, Pappas PJ, et al. Vein transposition in the forearm for autogenous hemodialysis access. J Vasc Surg 1997;26:981–8.
31. Gradman WS, Cohen W, Hagi-Aghaii M. Arteriovenous fistula construction in the thigh with transposed superficial femoral vein: our initial experience. J Vasc Surg 2001;33:968–75.
32. Jackson MR. The superficial femoral-popliteal vein transposition fistula: description of a new vascular access procedure. J Am Coll Surg 2000; 191:581–4.
33. Ethier JH, Lindsay RM, Barre PE, et al. Clinical practice guidelines for vascular access. Canadian Society of Nephrology. J Am Soc Nephrol 1999;10 (suppl 1):S297–S305.
34. Rizzuti RP, Hale JC, Burkart TE. Extended patency of expanded polytetrafluoroethylene grafts for vascular access using optimal configuration and revisions. Surg Gynecol Obstet 1988;166:23–7.
35. Lazarides MK, Iatrou CE, Karanikas IO, et al. Factors affecting the lifespan of autologous and synthetic arteriovenous access routes for hemodialysis. Eur J Surg 1996;162:297–301.
36. Hylander B, Fernstrom A, Swedenborg J. Interposition graft fistulas for hemodialysis. Acta Chir Scand 1988;154:107–10.
37. Hurt AV, Batello-Cruz M, Skipper BJ, et al. Bovine carotid artery heterografts versus polytetrafluoroethylene grafts. Am J Surg 1983; 146:844–7.

38. Lilly L, Ngheim D, Mendez-Picon G, et al. Comparison between bovine heterografts and expanded PTFE grafts for dialysis access. Am Surg 1980; 46:694–6.

39. Butler HG, Baker LD, Johnson JM. Vascular access for chronic hemodialysis: polytetrafluoroethylene (PTFE) versus bovine heterografts. Am J Surg 1977;134:791–3.

40. Reese JC, Esterl R, Lindsey L, et al. A prospective randomized comparison of bovine heterografts versus Impra grafts for chronic hemodialysis. In: Henry ML, Fergusen RM, eds. Vascular access for hemodialysis III. Chicago:WL Gore & Associates, Inc and Precept Press; 1993:57–163.

41. May J, Harris J, Fletcher J. Long-term results of saphenous vein graft arteriovenous fistulas. Am J Surg 1980;140:387–90.

42. Jenkins AM, Buist TAS, Glover SD. Medium-term follow-up of forty autogenous vein and forty polytetrafluoroethylene (Gore-Tex) grafts for vascular access. Surgery 1980;88:667–72.

43. Bhandari S, Wilkinson A, Sellors L. Saphenous vein forearm grafts and Gore-Tex thigh grafts as alternative forms of vascular access. Clin Nephrol 1995;44:325–8.

44. Bosman PJ, Blankestign PJ, van der Graaf Y, et al. A comparison between PTFE and denatured homologous vein grafts for hemodialysis access: a prospective randomized multicentre trial. Eur J Vasc Endovasc Surg 1998;16:126–32.

45. Matsuura JH, Johansen KH, Rosenthal D, et al. Cryopreserved femoral vein grafts for difficult hemodialysis access. Ann Vasc Surg 2000; 14:50–5.

46. Bolton W, Cull DL, Taylor SM, et al. The use of cryopreserved femoral vein grafts for hemodialysis access in patients at high risk for infection: a word of caution. J Vasc Surg 2002;36:464–8.

47. Dardik H, Ibrahim IM, Dardik I. Arteriovenous fistulas constructed with modified human umbilical cord vein graft. Arch Surg 1976; 111:60–2.

48. Karkow WS, Cranley JJ, Cranley RD, et al. Extended study of aneurysm formation in umbilical vein grafts. J Vasc Surg 1986;4:486–92.

49. Jamil Z, O'Donnell JA, Merk EA, Hobson RW. A comparison of knitted Dacron velour and bovine heterograft for hemodialysis access. J Surg Res 1979;26:423–9.

50. Burdick JF, Scott W, Cosimi AB. Experience with Dacron graft arteriovenous fistulas for dialysis access. Ann Surg 1978;187:262–6.

51. Levowitz BS, Flores L, Dunn I, et al. Prosthetic arteriovenous fistula for vascular access in hemodialysis. Am J Surg 1976;132:368–72.

52. Farmer DL, Goldstone J, Lim RC, et al. Failure of glow-discharge polymerization onto woven Dacron to improve performance of hemodialysis grafts. J Vasc Surg 1993;18:570–6.

53. Hiranaka T. Tapered and straight grafts for hemodialysis access: a prospective, randomized, comparison study. In: Henry ML, ed. Vascular access for hemodialysis VII. Chicago:WL Gore & Associates, Inc and Precept Press; 2001:219–24.

54. Shaffer D. A prospective randomized trial of 6-mm versus 4–7-mm PTFE grafts for hemodialysis access in diabetic patients. In: Henry ML, Ferguson RM, eds. Vascular access for hemodiaysis V. Chicago:WL Gore & Associates, Inc and Precept Press; 1997:91–4.

55. Lemson MS, Tordoir JH, van Det RJ, et al. Effects of a venous cuff at the venous anastomosis of polytetraflurorethylene grafts for hemodialysis vascular access. J Vasc Surg 2000;32:1155–63.

56. Coyne DW, Lowell JA, Windus DW, et al. Comparison of survival of an expanded polytetrafluoroethylene graft designed for early cannulation to standard wall polytetrafluoroethylene grafts. J Am Coll Surg 1996;183:401–5.

57. Almonacid PJ, Pallares EC, Rodriguez AQ, et al. Comparative study of use of Diastat versus standard wall PTFE grafts in upper arm hemodialysis access. Ann Vasc Surg 2000;14:659–62.

58. Lenz BJ, Veldenz HC, Dennis JW, et al. A three-year follow-up on standard versus thin wall ePTFE grafts for hemodialysis. J Vasc Surg 1998;28:464–70.

59. Kaufman JL, Garb JL, Berman J, et al. A prospective comparison of two expanded polytetrafluoroethylene grafts for linear forearm hemodialysis: does the manufacturer matter? J Am Coll Surg 1997;185:74–9.

60. Tordoir JH, Hofsba L, Leunisson KM, et al. Early experience with stretch polytetrafluoroethylene grafts for hemodialysis access surgery: results of a prospective randomized study. Eur J Vasc Endovasc Surg 1995;9:305–9.

61. Bourquelot P, Stolba J, Cheret P, et al. Carbon-PTFE versus standard-PTFE A-V bridge grafts for chronic hemodialysis. In: Henry ML, Ferguson RM, eds. Vascular access for hemodialysis IV. Chicago: WL Gore & Associates, Inc and Precept Press; 1995:303–7.

62. Jaffers G, Angstadt JD, Bowman JS III. Early cannulation of plasma TFE and Gore-Tex grafts for hemodialysis: a prospective randomized study. Am J Nephrol 1991;11:369–73.

63. Haag BW, Paramesh V, Roberts T. Early use of polytetrafluoroethylene grafts for hemodialysis access. In: Sommer BG, Henry ML, eds. Vascular access for hemodialysis II. Chicago:WL Gore & Associates, Inc and Precept Press; 1990:173–8.

64. Hakaim AG, Scott TE. Durability of early prosthetic dialysis graft cannulation: results of a prospective nonrandomized clinical trial. J Vasc Surg 1997;25:1002–6.

65. Steed DL, McAuley CE, Rault R, et al. Upper arm graft fistula for hemodialysis. J Vasc Surg 1984;1:660–3.

66. Staramos DN, Lazarides MK, Tzilalis VD, et al. Patency of autologous and prosthetic arteriovenous fistulas in elderly patients. Eur J Surg 2000; 166:777–81.

67. Khadra MH, Dwyer AJ, Thompson JF. Advantages of polytetrafluoroethylene arteriovenous loops in the thigh for hemodialysis access. Am J Surg 1997;73:280–3.

68. Vega D, Polo JR, Polo J, et al. Brachial-jugular expanded PTFE grafts for dialysis. Ann Vasc Surg 2001;15:553–6.

69. McCann RL. Axillo-axillary (necklace) grafts for hemodialysis access. In: Henry ML, ed. Vascular access for hemodialysis VI. Chicago: WL Gore & Associates Inc and Precept Press; 1999:197–202.

70. Woods JD, Turenne MN, Strawderman RL, et al. Vascular access survival among incident hemodialysis patients in the United States. Am J Kidney Dis 1997;30:50–7.

71. Churchill DW, Taylor DW, Cook RJ. Canadian Hemodialysis Morbidity Study. Am J Kidney Dis 1992;19:214–34.

72. Gibson KD, Gillen DL, Caps MT, et al. Vascular access survival and incidence of revisions: a comparison of prosthetic grafts, simple autogenous fistulas, and venous transposition fistulas from the United States Renal Data System Dialysis Morbidity and Mortality Study. J Vasc Surg 2001;34:694–700.

73. Kheriakian GM, Roedersheimer LR, Arbaugh JJ, et al. Comparison of autogenous fistula versus expanded polytetrafluoroethylene graft fistula for angioaccess in hemodialysis. Am J Surg 1986;152:238–43.

74. Chazan JA, London MR, Pono LM. Long-term survival of vascular accesses in a large chronic hemodialysis population. Nephron 1995; 69:228–33.

75. Hodges TC, Fillinger MF, Zwolak RM, et al. Longitudinal comparison of dialysis access methods: risk factors for failure. J Vasc Surg 1997; 26:1009–19.

76. Ascher E, Gade P, Hingorami A, et al. Changes in the practice of angioaccess surgery: impact of dialysis outcome and quality initiative recommendations. J Vasc Surg 2000;31:84–92.

77. Beathard GA. Strategy for maximizing the use of arteriovenous fistulae. Semin Dial 2000;13:291–9.

78. Miller A, Holzenbein TJ, Gottlieb MN, et al. Strategies to increase the use of autogenous arteriovenous fistula in end-stage renal disease. Ann Vasc Surg 1997;11:397–405.

79. United States Renal Data System: USRDS 1999Annual Data Report. The National Institutes of Health, National Institute of Diabetes and Digestive and Kidney Diseases, Bethesda, MD, 1999.

80. Beanes SR, Kling KM, Fonkalsrud EW, et al. Surgical aspects of dialysis in newborns and infants weighing less than 10 kilograms. J Pediatr Surg 2000;35:1543–8.

81. Bunchman TE. Pediatric hemodialysis: lessons from the past, ideas for the future. Kidney Int 1996;49:S64–7.

82. Stone MM, Fonkalsrud EW, Salusky IB, Takiff H, Hall T, Fine RN. Surgical management of peritoneal dialysis catheters in children: five-year experience with 1,800 patient-month follow-up. J Pediatr Surg 1986;21:1177–81.

83. Lerner GR, Warady BA, Sullivan EK, et al. Chronic dialysis in children and adolescents. Pediatr Nephrol 1999;13:404–7.

84. Warady BA, Bunchman TE. An update on peritoneal dialysis and hemodialysis in the pediatric population. Curr Opin Pediatr 1996; 8:135–40.

85. Lumsden AB, MacDonald MJ, Allen RC, et al. Hemodialysis access in the pediatric patient population. Am J Surg 1994;168:197–201.

86. Sharma A, Zilleruelo G, Abitbol C, et al. Survival and complications of cuffed catheters in children on chronic hemodialysis. Pediatr Nephrol 1999; 13:245–8.

87. Bourquelot P, Wolfeler L, Lamy L. Microsurgery for haemodialysis distal arteriovenous fistulae in children weighing less than 10 kg. Proc Eur Dial Transplant Assoc 1981;18:537–41.

88. Sanabia J, Polo JR, Morales MD, et al. Microsurgery in gaining paediatric vascular access for haemodialysis. Microsurgery 1993;14:276–9.

89. Brittinger WD, Walker G, Twittenhoff WD, et al. Vascular access for hemodialysis in children. Pediatr Nephrol 1997;11:87–95.

90. Davis JB, Howell CG, Humphries AL Jr. Hemodialysis access: elevated basilic vein arteriovenous fistula. J Pediatr Surg 1986;21:1182–3.

91. Bagolan P, Spagnoli A, Ciprandi G, et al. A ten-year experience of Brescia-Cimino arteriovenous fistula in children: technical evolution and refinements. J Vasc Surg 1998;27:640–4.

92. McLaughlin K, Jones B, Mactier R, et al. Long-term vascular access for hemodialysis using silicon dual-lumen catheters with guidewire replacement of catheters for technique salvage. Am J Kidney Dis 1997;29:553–9.

93. Oliver MJ, Edwards LJ, Treleaven DJ, et al. Randomized study of temporary hemodialysis catheters. Int J Artif Organs 2002;25:40–4.

94. Schillinger F, Schillinger D, Montagnac R, et al. Post-catheterization vein stenosis in haemodialysis: comparative angiographic study of 50 subclavian and 50 internal jugular accesses. Nephrol Dial Transplant 1991;6:722–4.

95. Surratt RS, Picus D, Hicks ME, et al. The importance of preoperative evaluation of the subclavian vein in dialysis access planning. AJR 1991; 156:623–5.

96. Hernandez D, Diaz F, Rufino M, et al. Subclavian vascular access stenosis in dialysis patients: natural history and risk factors. J Am Soc Nephrol 1998; 9:1507–10.

97. Barrett N, Spencer S, McIvor J, et al. Subclavian stenosis: a major complication of subclavian dialysis catheters. Nephrol Dial Transplant 1988;3:423–5.

98. Kelber J, Delmez JA, Windus DW. Factors affecting delivery of high-efficiency dialysis using temporary vascular access. Am J Kidney Dis 1993; 22:24–9.

99. Montagnac R, Bernard C, Guillaumie J, et al. Indwelling silicone femoral catheters: experience of three haemodialysis centres. Nephrol Dial Transplant 1997;12:772–5.

100. Weitzel WF, Boyer CJ, El-Khatib MT, et al. Successful use of indwelling cuffed femoral vein catheters in ambulatory hemodialysis patients. Am J Kidney Dis 1993;22:426–9.

101. Biswal R, Nosher JL, Siegel RL, et al. Translumbar placement of paired hemodialysis catheters (Tesio catheters) and follow-up in 10 patients. Cardiovasc Intervent Radiol 2000;23:75–8.

102. Lund GB, Trerotola SO, Scheel PJ Jr. Percutaneous translumbar inferior vena cava cannulation for hemodialysis. Am J Kidney Dis 1995;25:732–7.

103. Suhocki PV, Conlon PJ Jr, Knelson MH, et al. Silastic cuffed catheters for hemodialysis vascular access: thrombolytic and mechanical correction of malfunction. Am J Kidney Dis 1996;28:379–86.

104. Lund GB, Trerotola SO, Scheel PF, et al. Outcome of tunneled hemodialysis catheters placed by radiologists. Radiology 1996; 198:467–72.

105. Lin BS, Kong CW, Tarng DC, et al. Anatomical variation of the internal jugular vein and its impact on temporary haemodialysis vascular access: an ultrasonographic survey in uraemic patients. Nephrol Dial Transplant 1998; 13:134–8.

106. Forauer AR, Glockner JF. Importance of US findings in access planning during jugular vein hemodialysis catheter placements. J Vasc Interv Radiol 2000;11:233–237.

107. Lin BS, Huang TP, Tang GJ, et al. Ultrasound-guided cannulation of the internal jugular vein for dialysis vascular access in uremic patients. Nephron 1998;78:423–8.

108. Obialo CI, Conner AC, Lebon LF. Tunneled hemodialysis catheter survival: comparison of radiologic and surgical implantation. ASAIO J 2000;46:771–4.

109. Marr KA, Sexton DJ, Conlon PJ, et al. Catheter-related bacteremia and outcome of attempted catheter salvage in patients undergoing hemodialysis. Ann Intern Med 1997;127:275–80.

110. Meester JD, Vanholder R, De Roose J, et al. Factors and complications affecting catheter and technique survival with permanent single-lumen dialysis catheters. Nephrol Dial Transplant 1994;9:678–83.

111. Saad TF. Bacteremia associated with tunneled, cuffed hemodialysis catheters. Am J Kidney Dis 1999;34:1114–24.

112. Moss AH, Vasilakis C, Holley JL, et al. Use of silicone dual-lumen catheter with a dacron cuff as a long-term vascular access for hemodialysis patients. Am J Kidney Dis 1990;16:211–5.

113. Robinson D, Suhocki P, Schwab SJ. Treatment of infected tunneled venous access hemodialysis catheters with guidewire exchange. Kidney Int 1998; 53:1792–4.

114. Tanriover P, Carlton D, Saddekni S, et al. Bacteremia associated with tunneled dialysis catheters: comparison of two treatment strategies. Kidney Int 2000;57:2151–5.

115. Tesio F, De Baz H, Panarello G, et al. Double catheterization of the internal jugular vein for hemodialysis: indications, techniques, and clinical results. Artif Organs 1994;18:301–4.

116. Trerotola SO, Shah H, Johnson M, et al. Randomized comparison of high-flow versus conventional hemodialysis catheters. J Vasc Interv Radiol 1999;10:1032–8.

117. Trerotola SO, Kraus M, Shah H, et al. Randomized comparison of split tip versus step tip high-flow hemodialysis catheters. Kidney Int 2002; 62:282–9.

118. Richard HT III, Hastings GS, Boyd-Kranis RL, et al. A randomized, prospective evaluation of the Tesio, Ash Split, and Opti-flow hemodialysis catheters. J Vasc Interv Radiol 2001;12:431–5.

119. Haire WD, Arkinson JB, Stephens LC, et al. Urokinase versus recombinant tissue plasminogen activator in thrombosed central venous catheters: a double-blinded, randomized trial. Thromb Haemost 1994; 72:543–7.

120. Daeihagh P, Jordan J, Chen GJ, et al. Efficacy of tissue plasminogen activator administration on patency of hemodialysis access catheters. Am J Kidney Dis 2000;36:75–9.

121. Crain MR, Mewissen MW, Ostrowski GJ, et al. Fibrin sleeve stripping for salvage of failing hemodialysis catheters: technique and initial results. Radiology 1996;198:41–4.

122. Beathard GA. Mechanical versus pharmacomechanical thrombolysis for the treatment of thrombosed dialysis access grafts. Kidney Int 1994;45:1401–6.

123. Kanterman RY, Vesely TM, Pilgrim TK, et al. Dialysis access grafts: anatomic location of venous stenosis and results of angioplasty. Radiology 1995;195:135–9.

124. Swedberg SH, Brown BG, Sigley R. Intimal fibromuscular hyperplasia at the venous anastomosis of PTFE grafts in hemodialysis patients. Clinical, immunocytochemical, light, and electron microscopic assessment. Circulation 1989;80:1726–36.

125. Krysl J, Kumpe DA. Failing and failed hemodialysis access sites: management and percutaneous catheter methods. Semin Vasc Surg 1997; 10:175–83.

126. Schwartz CJ, McBrayer CV, Sloan JH, et al. Thrombosed dialysis grafts: comparison of treatment with transluminal angioplasty and surgical revision. Radiology 1995;194:337–41.

127. Schuman E, Quinn S, Standage B, et al. Thrombolysis versus thrombectomy for occluded hemodialysis grafts. Am J Surg 1994;167:473–6.

128. Uflacker R, Rajagopalan PR, Vujic I, et al. Treatment of thrombosed dialysis access grafts: randomized trial of surgical thrombectomy versus mechanical thrombectomy with the Amplatz device. J Vasc Interv Radiol 1996;7:185–92.

129. Marston WA, Criado E, Jaques PF, et al. Prospective randomized comparison of surgical versus endovascular management of thrombosed dialysis access grafts. J Vasc Surg 1997;26:373–80.

130. Gray RJ. Percutaneous intervention for permanent hemodialysis access: a review. J Vasc Interv Radiol 1997;8:313–27.

131. Berger MF, Aruny JE, Skibo LK. Recurrent thrombosis of polytetra-fluoroethylene dialysis fistulas after recent surgical thrombectomy and salvage by means of thrombolysis and angioplasty. J Vasc Interv Radiol 1994;5:725–30.

132. Valji K, Bookstein JJ, Roberts AC, et al. Pulse-spray pharmaco-mechanical thrombolysis of thrombosed hemodialysis access grafts: long-term experience and comparison of original and current techniques. Am J Roentgenol 1995;164:1495–500.

133. Trerotola SO, Lund GB, Scheel PJ Jr, et al. Thrombosed dialysis access grafts: percutaneous mechanical declotting without urokinase. Radiology 1994;191:721–6.

134. Sofocleous CT, Cooper SG, Schur I, et al. Retrospective comparison of the Amplatz thrombectomy device with modified pulse-spray pharmacomechanical thrombolysis in the treatment of thrombosed hemodialysis access grafts. Radiology 1999;213:561–7.

135. Overbosch EH, Pattynama PM, Aarts HJ, et al. Occluded hemodialysis shunts: Dutch multicenter experience with the hydrolyser catheter. Radiology 1996;201:485–8.

136. Beathard GA, Welch BR, Maidment HJ. Mechanical thrombolysis for the treatment of thrombosed hemodialysis access grafts. Radiology 1996; 200:711–6.

137. Beathard GA. Percutaneous transvenous angioplasty in the treatment of vascular access stenosis. Kidney Int 1992;42:1390–7.

138. Patel RI, Peck SH, Cooper SG, et al. Patency of wallstents placed across the venous anastamosis of hemodialysis grafts after percutaneous recanalization. Radiology 1998;209:365–70.

139. Hood DB, Yellin AE, Richman MF, et al. Hemodialysis graft salvage with endoluminal stents. Am Surg 1994;60:733–7.

140. Hoffer EK, Sultan S, Herskowitz MM, et al. Prospective randomized trial of a metallic intravascular stent in hemodialysis graft maintenance. J Vasc Interv Radiol 1997;8:965–73.

141. Quinn SF, Schuman ES, Demlow TA, et al. Percutaneous transluminal angioplasty versus endovascular stent placement in the treatment of venous stenoses in patients undergoing hemodialysis: intermediate results. J Vasc Interv Radiol 1995;6:851–5.

142. Dougherty MJ, Calligaru KD, Schindler N, et al. Endovascular versus surgical treatment for thrombosed hemodialysis grafts: a prospective randomized trial. J Vasc Surg 1999;30:1016–23.

143. Brooks JL, Sigley RD, May KJ, et al. Transluminal angioplasty versus surgical repair for stenosis of hemodialysis grafts. Am J Surg 1987; 153:530–1.

144. Lumsden AB, MacDonald MJ, Kikeri D, et al. Prophylactic balloon angioplasty fails to prolong patency of expanded polytetrafluoroethylene arteriovenous grafts: results of a prospective randomized study. J Vasc Surg 1997;26:382–92.

145. Swan TL, Smyth SH, Ruffenach SJ, et al. Pulmonary embolism following hemodialysis access thrombolysis/thrombectomy. J Vasc Interv Radiol 1995; 6:683–6.

146. Smits HF, Van Rijk PP, Van Isselt JW, et al. Pulmonary embolism after thrombolysis of hemodialysis grafts. J Am Soc Nephrol 1997;8:1451–61.

147. Lay JPY, Ashleigh RJ, Tranconi L, et al. Result of angioplasty of Brescia-Cimino haemodialysis fistulae: medium-term follow-up. Clin Radiol 1998; 53:608–11.

148. Manninen HI, Kaukanen ET, Ikaheimo R, et al. Brachial arterial access: endovascular treatment of failing Brescia-Cimino hemodialysis fistulas – initial success and long-term results. Radiology 2001; 218:711–8.

149. Sexton DJ. Vascular access infections in patients undergoing dialysis with special emphasis on the role and treatment of *staphylococcus aureus*. Infect Dis Clin North Am 2001;15:731–42.

150. Alexiewicz JM, Smogorzewski M, Fadda GZ, et al. Impaired phago-cytosis in dialysis patients; studies on mechanisms. Am J Nephrol 1991; 11:102–11.

151. Pederson JO, Knudsen F, Nielsen AH, Grunnet N. The ability of uremic serum to induce neutrophil chemotaxis in relation to hemodialysis. Blood Purif 1987; 5:24–8.

152. Albers FJ. Clinical considerations in hemodialysis access infection. Adv Ren Replace Ther 1996;3:208–17.

153. Kudva A, Hye RJ. Management of infectious and cutaneous compli-cations in vascular access. Semin Vasc Surg 1997;10:184–90.

154. Butterly DW, Schwab SJ. Dialysis access infections. Curr Opin Nephrol Hypertens 2000;9:631–5.

155. Bhat DJ, Tellis VA, Kohlberg WI, et al. Management of sepsis involving polytetrafluoroethylene grafts for hemodialysis access. Surgery 1980; 87:445–50.

156. Tellis VA, Weiss P, Matas AJ. Skin-flap coverage of polytetra-fluoroethylene vascular access graft exposed by previous infection. Surgery 1988;103:118–21.

157. McKenna PJ, Leadbetter MG. Salvage of chronically exposed Gore-Tex vascular access grafts in the hemodialysis patient. Plast Reconstr Surg 1988; 82:1046–9.

158. Schwab DP, Taylor SM, Cull DL, et al. Isolated arteriovenous dialysis access graft segment infection: the results of segmental bypass and partial graft excision. Ann Vasc Surg 2000;14:63–6.

159. Hausegger KA, Tiessenhausen K, Klimpfinger M, et al. Aneurysms of hemodialysis access grafts: treatment with covered stents: a report of three cases. Cardiovasc Intervent Radiol 1998;21:334–7.

160. Sapoval MR, Turmel-Rodrigues LA, Raynaud AC, et al. Cragg covered stents in hemodialysis access: initial and midterm results. J Vasc Interv Radiol 1996;7:335–42.

161. Engelberts I, Tordoir JH, Boon ES, et al. High-output cardiac failure due to excessive shunting in a hemodialysis access fistula: an easily overlooked diagnosis. Am J Nephrol 1995;15:323–6.

162. Tzanakis I, Hatziathanassiou A, Kagia S, et al. Banding of an over-functioning fistula with a prosthetic graft segment. Nephron 1999; 81:351–2.

163. Miles AM. Vascular steal syndrome and ischaemic monomelic neuropathy: two variants of upper limb ischemia after hemodialysis vascular access surgery. Nephrol Dial Transplant 1999;14:297–300.

164. Rivers SP, Scher LA, Veith FJ. Correction of steal syndrome secondary to hemodialysis access fistulas: a simplified quantitative technique. Surgery 1992;112:593–7.

165. Wixon CL, Mills JL, Berman SS. Distal revascularization-interval ligation for maintenance of dialysis access and restoration of distal perfusion in ischemic steal syndrome. Semin Vasc Surg 2000;13:77–82.

166. West JC, Bertsch DJ, Peterson SL, et al. Arterial insufficiency in hemodialysis access procedures: correction by banding technique. Transplant Proc 1991;23:1838–40.

167. Rosental JJ, Bell DD, Gaspar MR, et al. Prevention of high flow problems of arteriovenous grafts: development of a new tapered graft. Am J Surg 1980; 140:231–3.

168. Berman SS, Gentile AT, Glickman MH, et al. Distal revascularization-interval ligation for limb salvage and maintenance of dialysis access in ischemic steal syndrome. J Vasc Surg 1997;26:393–404.

169. Schanzer H, Skladany M, Haimov M. Treatment of angioaccess-induced ischemia by revascularization. J Vasc Surg 1992;16:861–6.

170. Hye RJ, Wolf YG. Ischemic monomelic neuropathy: an under-recognized complication of hemodialysis access. Ann Vasc Surg 1994; 8:578–82.

171. Miles AM. Upper limb ischemia and vascular access surgery: differ-ential diagnosis and management. Semin Dial 2000;13:312–5.

172. Redfern AB, Zimmerman NB. Neurologic and ischemic complications of upper extremity vascular access for dialysis. J Hand Surg 1995; 20:199–204.

173. Schwab SJ, Raymond JR, Saeed M, et al. Prevention of hemodialysis fistula thrombosis. Early detection of venous stenosis. Kidney Int 1989;36:707–11.

174. Sands JJ, Miranda CL. Prolongation of hemodialysis access survival with elective revisions. Clin Nephrol 1995;44:329–33.

175. Back MR, Bandyk DF. Current status of hemodialysis access grafts. Ann Vasc Surg 2001;15:491–502.

176. May RE, Himmelfarb J, Yenicesu M, et al. Predictive measures of vascular access thrombosis: a prospective study. Kidney Int 1997; 52:1656–62.

177. Windus DW, Audrain J, Vanderson R, et al. Optimization of high-efficiency hemodialysis by detection and correction of fistula dysfunction. Kidney Int 1990;38;337–41.

178. Daniels ID, Berlyne GM, Barth RH. Blood flow rates and access recirculation in hemodialysis. Int J Artif Organs 1992;15:470–4.

179. Strauch BS, O'Connell RS, Geoly KL, et al. Forecasting thrombosis of vascular access with Doppler color flow imaging. Am J Kidney Dis 1992; 19:554–7.

180. Middleton WD, Picus DD, Marx MV, et al. Color Doppler sonography of hemodialysis vascular access: comparison with angiography. Am J Radiol 1989;152:633–9.

CHAPTER

28

Pathophysiology and Natural History of Abdominal Aortic Aneurysms

Andrew W Hoel and Robert W Thompson

KEY POINTS

- Risk factors associated with abdominal aortic aneurysm (AAA) disease include age over 65 years, male gender, hypertension, family history of aortic aneurysm, cigarette smoking, chronic obstructive pulmonary disease, atherosclerosis, and peripheral arterial disease.

- Aneurysm pathophysiology is characterized by chronic transmural inflammation, destructive remodeling of the extracellular matrix, depletion of vascular smooth muscle cells, and redistribution of hemodynamic stresses on the vessel wall.

- The inflammatory infiltrate in AAAs is composed primarily of mononuclear phagocytes; these cells are likely stimulated by proinflammatory mediators of chemotaxis and immune activation, including chemokines, cytokines, hypoxia, and the products of matrix degradation. Circumstantial evidence indicates that infectious agents (i.e. *Chlamydia pneumoniae*) may possibly play a role, at least in some patients.

- Smooth muscle cell depletion in the wall of the aneurysmal aorta probably plays a prominent role in progression of disease, by reducing the capacity for fibrous remodeling of the extracellular matrix in response to injury.

- Aneurysms are characterized microscopically by destruction of the medial elastic fibers and disordered (compensatory) remodeling of the extracellular matrix, which is likely mediated by a spectrum of proteolytic enzymes, particularly members of the matrix metalloproteinase (MMP) family.

- The biomechanical forces on the aortic wall are dramatically altered in aneurysm formation, resulting in increased local wall stress which may significantly increase the risk of aneurysm rupture.

- The diagnosis of an AAA is notoriously difficult by history and physical examination alone. Abdominal imaging (i.e. ultrasound or computed tomography) provides a very sensitive and specific means of detecting aneurysms in virtually all patients. Ultrasound screening can detect AAAs in their earliest stages, but the overall cost-effectiveness of this approach remains controversial in the absence of proven therapies for small asymptomatic AAAs.

- The risk of aneurysm rupture is significant in patients with aortic diameter greater that 5.5cm and that risk increases disproportionately for AAAs larger in diameter. Despite many advances in resuscitation and surgical critical care, the mortality rate for ruptured AAAs remains very high.

- Two recent population-based studies have shown no clear survival benefit for repair of aneurysms less than 5.5cm in diameter, provided adequate patient follow-up by imaging surveillance can be maintained.

- Regardless of aneurysm size or the treatment selected, the life expectancy of patients with AAAs is significantly decreased in comparison with age- and gender-matched controls.

INTRODUCTION

Abdominal aortic aneurysms (AAAs) represent a chronic degenerative disease with life-threatening implications. AAAs are currently thought to be caused by a localized form of arterial wall injury superimposed on degenerative changes related to age, hemodynamics, systemic risk factors, and a genetically determined predisposition, but the exact nature or sequence of these events is unknown. Once the aneurysmal process affects a given segment of the aorta, destructive remodeling of the aortic wall as well as longitudinal extension occur. Several distinct interrelated processes contribute to the pathologic changes observed in AAAs. The most important of these include chronic inflammation, destructive remodeling of the extracellular matrix, and depletion of vascular smooth muscle cells (SMC). Progression of these changes results in segmental aortic dilatation and alterations in vessel geometry. These changes are accompanied by redistribution of hemodynamic wall stresses and diminished tensile strength, thereby increasing the potential for rupture. Thus, the natural history of aneurysmal disease generally involves progressive structural deterioration, gradual expansion, and eventual rupture.

The purpose of this chapter is to summarize basic knowledge regarding the pathophysiology of aneurysmal degeneration, to review our current understanding of the natural history of AAAs, and to assess how these insights might eventually lead to alternative forms of treatment than those currently available.[1]

PATHOPHYSIOLOGY

Aortic wall structure

The normal aorta is a large fibroelastic conduit that must sustain a continuous mechanical load over a lifetime of hemodynamic stress. The functional requirements of the aortic wall include resilience to cyclic deformation, resistance to structural failure, and durability over the lifespan of the organism. These unique demands are met by the biomechanical properties attributable to elastin and collagen, the fibrillar matrix proteins found in the aortic media and adventitia.

Biophysical interactions between elastin and collagen determine how the aortic wall functions under hemodynamic stress. The distensible elastic fibers of the aortic media are thought to be responsible for load bearing under most physiologic conditions, whereas adventitial collagen acquires load-bearing functions at higher pressures or in settings where elastin fails.[2] Early experimental studies demonstrated that enzymatic treatment of arteries with elastase leads to arterial dilatation and stiffening at physiologic pressures, whereas treatment with collagenase leads to arterial rupture with little dilatation.[3] These findings fostered the notion that mechanical failure or degradation of elastin is a key step in the development of aneurysmal dilatation but that mechanical failure or degradation of collagen is ultimately required for aneurysm rupture.[2,4]

Etiology

Demographic risk factors associated with aortic aneurysm disease include aging, male gender, hypertension, cigarette smoking, chronic obstructive pulmonary disease (COPD), atherosclerosis, and peripheral arterial disease.[5,6] Although AAAs are often considered an end-stage manifestation of complicated atherosclerosis, the actual cause of aortic aneurysms remains unknown. The pathology of AAAs involves a transmural degenerative process usually localized to a specific arterial segment, whereas atherosclerosis is a more diffuse disease of the intima that affects vessels throughout the arterial tree. Additionally, AAAs involve the entire circumference of the aorta, whereas atherosclerotic plaques typically develop in a highly eccentric manner. Since atherosclerosis in the infrarenal aorta is usually located along the posterior wall, it remains uncertain how this process might lead to the circumferential degeneration seen in AAAs. Nonetheless, it is possible that aneurysms represent an extreme, uncontrolled form of expansive arterial remodeling, a process frequently associated with eccentric atheroma in smaller arteries.[7] The specific relationship between atherosclerosis and aneurysmal degeneration is further confounded by the observation that several strong risk factors for atherosclerosis, such as diabetes, hyperlipidemia, and homocystinemia, do not appear to be significantly associated with AAAs.

Patients with degenerative AAAs often exhibit a familial pattern of disease, with 15–20% of patients having a positive family history.[8-12] AAAs are also occasionally associated with aneurysms in other sites, especially the popliteal arteries. These observations have raised the possibility that AAAs might arise, at least in some patients, through an inherited genetic predisposition. Despite enthusiasm for identifying the genetic basis for familial aggregation of AAAs, this problem has presented a significant challenge to traditional genetic approaches. The reasons for this difficulty include the fact that AAAs occur primarily in

the elderly, they are likely multifactorial (polygenetic) in nature, and construction of family pedigrees is frustrated by inaccurate data in previous generations. The fundamental genetic aspects of degenerative AAAs are therefore still an open question, but remain under active investigation.[13-20]

Hemodynamic factors have long been implicated in the degenerative arterial remodeling associated with AAAs, particularly in their predilection for the infrarenal aorta. The infrarenal aorta is subject to greater turbulence and pulsatile hemodynamic stresses than other regions of the aorta, due in part to its peculiar location with respect to the mesenteric and renal artery branches and the reflection of pressure waves from the iliac bifurcations. The infrarenal aorta is also subject to a substantial increase in flow and shear stress during exercise, which may actually serve to protect against aneurysmal degeneration. Loss of this factor in sedentary elderly individuals may therefore contribute to development of AAAs.

Clinical patterns of disease suggest that the infrarenal aorta is structurally predisposed toward aneurysmal degeneration. Studies on matrix proteins have revealed that the elastin content of the aorta progressively diminishes as one travels from the ascending aorta to the iliac arteries, with a prominent decrease occurring several centimeters below the renal arteries. This is accompanied by a corresponding decrease in medial thickness and the number of elastic lamellae. The physical properties of the infrarenal aorta therefore exhibit less elasticity than more proximal segments. These features are further compounded by a decrease in aortic elastin that normally occurs with aging and an impaired capacity for elastic fiber synthesis that is exhibited in the adult. Finally, unlike the thoracic aorta, the infrarenal aorta is normally devoid of vasa vasorum, indicating that nutrient supply to the tunica media is dependent on diffusion from the lumen. With the development of intimal thickening or atherosclerotic plaques that might compromise nutrient diffusion, ischemia within the outer media may potentiate the regional predisposition to aneurysm formation.

Pathobiology

Most investigations on human AAAs involve examination of aortic wall tissue obtained at the time of surgical repair or at autopsy ('end-stage' disease). Such studies are limited inherently by the advanced stage of disease from which the tissue is obtained, yet numerous and essential insights into the pathophysiology of human AAAs have been obtained by this approach. Moreover, knowledge of the changes present in established human AAAs has guided the development of representative animal models, which have been fruitful in advancing our understanding of disease mechanisms and in testing hypotheses regarding potential therapeutic strategies.

As noted earlier, the histopathology of established AAAs is dominated by chronic inflammation, destruction of the elastic lamellae, and depletion of medial smooth muscle. These processes are closely interrelated, and together they account for the progressive tissue degeneration that results in aortic dilatation. Consequently, aneurysmal degeneration exhibits an inherent balance between favorable and unfavorable processes. Like most chronic pathobiologic conditions, a sustained imbalance in these competitive interactions results in disease progression. Knowledge of the pathophysiologic factors that promote and suppress aneurysmal disease is therefore crucial to understanding how the disease progresses differently between individual patients and how the disease might be modulated differently in the same patient at different periods in time. Knowledge of these variables is also necessary to eventually harness biologic mechanisms that might be used to protect the aortic wall from further degeneration, an essential step in devising new therapeutic strategies.

Chronic inflammation

The inflammatory response in AAAs is usually transmural and circumferential in distribution, with cellular infiltrates most often located within the outer media and adventitia.[21] These cells are distributed in variable patterns, with enormous heterogeneity between specimens from different patients and between different regions of the same specimen, and they range from scattered inflammatory cells within an amorphous media to dense focal aggregates resembling lymphoid tissue.[22] Patients with the subset of lesions known as 'inflammatory AAAs' represent one extreme of this variability, in which the aortic wall is characterized by a thick sheet of mononuclear inflammatory cells surrounded by a dense fibrotic reaction that extends well into the periaortic retroperitoneal tissues. In the vast majority of AAAs, the inflammatory response appears to be consistently dominated by infiltrating monocytes/macrophages, B-lymphocytes, plasma cells, and T-lymphocytes (including both CD4$^+$ and CD8$^+$ T-cells), whereas polymorphonuclear neutrophils (PMNs) are only rarely observed.[23]

The factors responsible for initiating the chronic inflammatory response in AAAs are not yet known but may include an extension of intimal atherosclerosis into the tunica media, release of biologically active products derived from matrix degradation, local production of chemotactic cytokines (chemokines) and proinflammatory cytokines, and an immune response targeting either infectious agents or cellular and structural components of the outer aortic wall. Peptide fragments derived from the degradation of extracellular matrix components, including elastin, laminin, and fibronectin, may have a particularly important influence on inflammatory cell recruitment and function in the degenerating aortic wall. Thus, soluble elastin-derived peptides (EDPs) released within human AAA tissue can subsequently attract mononuclear phagocytes through interactions with the 67kD cell surface elastin-binding protein found on inflammatory cells, thereby providing a plausible molecular mechanism to explain the location, extent, and chronicity of the inflammatory response that accompanies aneurysmal degeneration.[24] In the experimental setting, local release of EDPs following transient aortic perfusion with elastase may explain the induction of monocytic inflammation and aneurysmal development.[25]

Several members of the chemokine family are known to be elevated in human and experimental AAA tissues, such as interleukin-8 (IL-8), monocyte chemoattractant protein-1 (MCP-1), and RANTES (Regulated on Activation Normal T-cell Expressed and Secreted).[26,27] The potent chemotactic properties of these small proteins suggest that they likely play an important role in the recruitment and retention of inflammatory cells, especially monocytes and T-lymphocytes. Some of these chemokines may play an additional role as co-stimulatory molecules, which may facilitate local immune responses within AAA tissue.

A host of proinflammatory cytokines have also been proposed to have a major role in AAAs, both in facilitating leukocyte recruitment and by acting in concert to amplify inflammatory cell activities. In particular, tissues from human and experimental AAAs produce abundant amounts of prostaglandin E$_2$ (PGE$_2$), tumor necrosis factor-alpha (TNF-α), interleukin-1beta (IL-1β), and interleukin-6 (IL-6), as well as highly reactive oxygen- and nitrogen-derived free radicals.[28-33] Each of these mediators may augment chronic inflammation and tissue injury, in part by inducing the expression of specific matrix-degrading proteinases. Oxidative stress may be a particularly important factor in the microenvironment of the aneurysm wall, with the reactive species produced being capable of causing both direct and indirect tissue damage.[33-38]

Growing evidence suggests that the immune response contributes to the pathogenesis of AAAs, either helping to initiate the disease or as a secondary factor that may amplify and sustain local inflammation. Several studies have demonstrated herpesviruses and *Chlamydia pneumoniae* in up to 30–50% of human AAA tissues, and anti-chlamydial antibodies are detected frequently in patients with AAAs.[39,40] Although aneurysms can obviously arise in the absence of these micro-organisms and the high incidence of chlamydial infection in the general population (up to 80%) makes it difficult to draw any firm conclusions about its causative role in cardiovascular disease, the immune response to this ubiquitous infection may augment cellular inflammatory responses within aneurysm tissue.[41-43]

Another intriguing possibility is that chronic cellular and humoral immune responses, perhaps initially targeting chlamydia or other organisms, may extend eventually to other aortic wall components. This may include structurally important extracellular matrix proteins through the processes of epitope spreading and molecular mimicry, thereby providing another explanation for the localization of the inflammatory response to the elastic media in AAAs. This is especially pertinent in light of recent studies in mice, which suggest that the elastic media of the great vessels may be an immune-privileged site normally resistant to lymphocyte infiltration.[44] Because it has been demonstrated clearly that antibodies isolated from human AAA tissue exhibit reactivity for naturally occurring matrix proteins, the autoimmune phenomena may contribute to aneurysmal disease, at least in some patients.[45]

Conventional wisdom predicts that the immune response in AAAs is fundamentally detrimental. Thus, antibodies directed against normal components of the aortic wall would be expected to amplify inflammatory cell destruction of structural connective tissue through T-cell production of proinflammatory (Th-1) cytokines capable of activating macrophages (i.e. TNF-α, IL-1β, and interferon-gamma), and through immune-mediated cytotoxicity causing apoptosis of normal vascular wall cell types (i.e. vascular SMC). Recent evidence challenges this view, however, since CD4$^+$ T-cells within aneurysmal tissue can also produce a spectrum of anti-inflammatory (Th-2) cytokines, such as interleukin-4 (IL-4) and interleukin-10 (IL-10).[46,47] These immunomodulatory cytokines can inhibit macrophage activation and expression of connective tissue proteinases, thereby suppressing tissue degeneration, and their elevated expression in human AAAs suggests the presence of endogenous mechanisms to counter aneurysmal degeneration.[48,49] These observations indicate that better understanding of the specificity of the immune response in AAAs may be a key area for further research, to determine both how this response varies between different patients and how pharmacologic manipulation might be used to enhance responses that favor stabilization of the aneurysm wall.

Experimental studies using animal models have been extremely valuable in demonstrating the functional importance of chronic inflammation in AAAs. Thus, the elastase-induced model of AAAs in rats has been used to demonstrate that inflammation correlates with aneurysm formation and that treatment with corticosteroids effectively suppresses aneurysmal dilatation and reduces aortic wall elastin degradation.[50,51] Further studies have shown similar effects using anti-CD18 (pan-leukocyte) antibodies, cytokine antagonists, and non-steroidal anti-inflammatory drugs (NSAIDs).[52–55]

Disordered remodeling of the extracellular matrix

A second pathologic feature of AAAs is pronounced destruction of medial elastic fibers. Because the structural failure of medial elastin is considered the primary event in aneurysm formation and because elastin is normally an extraordinarily stable protein, accelerated enzymatic degradation of elastic fibers has long been suspected to be an early and critical process in AAAs. The loss of elastin in AAA tissue also promotes a shift in tensile wall stress from elastic fibers to medial and adventitial collagen. Not surprisingly, AAAs are often accompanied by a variable degree of collagenous fibrosis in the media and adventitia, which may be a valuable compensatory response to accommodate increased structural demands. Indeed, human and experimental AAAs are associated with an increased expression of procollagen mRNA, and type III collagen content is increased significantly in human aneurysm tissue.[56–60] Degradation of elastin and collagen is associated closely with the chronic inflammatory response and is likely dependent on increased local production of elastin- and collagen-specific proteinases. Consequently, a great deal of investigative effort has been directed toward identifying the specific enzymes responsible for these events.

Abundant evidence indicates that connective tissue remodeling in AAAs is mediated largely by matrix metalloproteinases (MMPs), a superfamily of enzymes involved in normal development and wound healing, as well as a variety of pathologic conditions.[61] Members of the MMP family share several basic structural features, including a zinc-binding active site, an amino-terminal propeptide domain, and several additional domains that determine the substrate specificity of individual enzymes. MMP production is regulated at the level of gene transcription. Rather than being stored within cells, most MMPs are secreted as soluble zymogens that require post-translational activation in the extracellular space. Although the actual in-vivo mechanisms are unknown, extracellular activation of proMMPs can occur through limited proteolytic cleavage of the propeptide domain by other enzymes, such as plasmin, urokinase-type plasminogen activator, or other MMPs, by binding to cell membrane proteins with enzymatic activity, or by oxidative modification and auto-activation. Like many enzymes secreted in association with chronic inflammation, the activity of MMPs is also modulated by interaction with naturally occurring proteinase inhibitors, such as plasma alpha-2-macroglobulin and an associated family of at least four specific tissue inhibitors of metalloproteinases (TIMPs). Local expression of MMPs and pericellular proteolysis may therefore provide tissues with a high degree of spatial and temporal regulation over extracellular matrix degradation, while

the concomitant secretion of TIMPs may serve to prevent more widespread tissue destruction.

Four members of the MMP family can effectively degrade insoluble elastin fibers, including the 72kD and 92kD gelatinases (MMP-2 and MMP-9, respectively), matrilysin (MMP-7), and macrophage elastase (MMP-12).[61] MMP-9 is expressed prominently in chronic inflammatory conditions and has attracted particular interest with respect to AAAs. It has activity against insoluble elastin fibers and is the most abundant elastolytic proteinase produced by human AAA tissues. Studies utilizing substrate gel zymography, immunoblotting, and enzyme-linked immunosorbent assays (ELISAs) have demonstrated that MMP-9 is increased to a greater extent in AAAs than in atherosclerotic occlusive disease, and it is expressed abundantly at the site of tissue damage by aneurysm-infiltrating macrophages.[62] MMP-9 synthesis in AAA tissue is correlated with increased aneurysm diameter, and elevated circulating levels of MMP-9 are often found in patients with AAAs.[63,64] Additional studies reveal increased expression of macrophage elastase (MMP-12) in human AAAs.[22] MMP-12 is localized prominently to residual elastin fiber fragments within aneurysm tissue by immunohistochemistry, a pattern quite distinct from other elastolytic MMPs. The elevated production of MMP-12 and its unique localization to fragmented aortic elastin suggest a role for this enzyme in aneurysmal degeneration. Finally, other MMPs, such as gelatinase A (MMP-2) and stromelysin (MMP-3), may also participate in aneurysmal disease. MMP-2 may be particularly important since it can degrade both elastin and interstitial collagen, is expressed and bound by vascular SMC as well as macrophages, and is increased in human AAAs, especially in association with the insoluble extracellular matrix.[65]

Studies using small animal models of AAAs have helped define the importance of MMPs in aneurysmal degeneration.[66,67] Transient aortic perfusion with pancreatic elastase, topical administration of calcium chloride, or decellularized rat aortic xenografts can induce the sequential production of several different metalloproteinases within the aorta, with increased production of endogenous proteinases being correlated temporally with the onset of aortic wall inflammation and dilatation.[68–70] The first demonstration that pharmacologic inhibition of MMPs can suppress aneurysmal degeneration *in vivo* arose through studies in the elastase-induced rat model of AAAs, where Petrinec et al. used the antibiotic doxycycline as a non-selective MMP antagonist.[71] Equivalent aneurysm-suppressing effects were observed subsequently in the same animal model using a series of non-antibiotic chemically modified tetracyclines, as well as additional agents capable of antagonizing MMP activity, such as direct-acting hydroxamate-based MMP inhibitors.[72–74] In addition, MMP inhibition has the potential to suppress aneurysm rupture, using local overexpression of the TIMP-1 gene in the rat xenograft model of AAAs.[70]

Inducible animal models of AAAs have also been applied to mice with targeted gene deficiencies, in order to elucidate the molecular mediators of aneurysmal degeneration with greater specificity. The first example of this approach was to apply the elastase-induced model of AAAs to mice with deletion of the MMP-9 gene, with these mice exhibiting a significant suppression of aneurysmal dilatation as compared with wild-type controls.[75] While this reduction in AAAs was associated with preservation of the medial elastic lamellae, inflammatory cell infiltration into the aortic wall was not suppressed. This finding supports the notion that MMP-9 plays a critical function in AAAs related to its matrix-degrading enzymatic activities. By subjecting mice to lethal irradiation and bone marrow reconstitution prior to elastase perfusion, it was also shown that the 'aneurysm-resistant' phenotype of MMP-9-deficient animals can be altered to an 'aneurysm-susceptible' phenotype after transplantation with marrow from wild-type mice. Conversely, 'aneurysm-susceptible' wild-type animals can be converted to an 'aneurysm-resistant' phenotype after transplantation with marrow from MMP-9-deficient mice. These observations indicate that inflammatory cell production of MMP-9 plays an indispensable role in aneurysmal degeneration induced by elastase perfusion, perhaps by acting as a direct enzymatic mediator of elastin degradation.

More recent studies using the calcium chloride-induced model of AAAs confirm the importance of both MMP-9 and MMP-2 in AAAs, demonstrating suppression of aneurysm development in MMP-2-deficient mice to an extent equivalent to that observed in MMP-9-deficient animals.[76] Moreover, because reinfusion of wild-type macrophages does not rescue the 'aneurysm-resistant' phenotype of MMP-2-deficient mice, production of MMP-2 by aortic wall SMC and fibroblasts appears to be as necessary for aneurysm formation as macrophage expression of MMP-9. Taken together, the concepts emerging from these experimental studies are that aneurysms evolve through a dynamic sequence of changes involving stimulation of resident mesenchymal cells and recruitment of mononuclear phagocytes to promote transmural aortic wall inflammation, followed by localized upregulation of MMPs (and other proteinases), to cause progressive degradation and remodeling of medial elastin and collagen.

Smooth muscle cell depletion

Although the events responsible for precipitating aneurysm rupture are not well understood, this catastrophic event represents the end result of biomechanical factors acting on a marginally compensated aortic wall over time. It is also evident that tensile wall stress is increased markedly in aneurysmal tissues and that collagen fibers prevent aortic rupture at these extremes.[77] Specific factors involved in this process may include an insufficient increase in aortic wall collagen content to counteract the increase in structural demands, production of altered or distorted collagen fibers with diminished tensile strength, or accelerated collagen degradation. Like fibroblasts within a wound under tension, vascular SMC undergo proliferation and increased production of extracellular matrix protein, particularly collagen, when subjected to cyclic strain. This suggests that SMC within the wall of an aortic aneurysm might provide an important source of increased collagen production, and that strain-induced alterations in SMC might serve to stabilize the aneurysm wall. Recent evidence indicates that connective tissue repair is critical in preventing aortic rupture during development of experimental AAAs, and clinical studies indicate that collagen metabolism is sufficiently active in aneurysm tissue to produce elevated levels of procollagen peptides, a biochemical marker of collagen production, in the circulation of patients with AAAs.[78–80]

While increased proteolytic activity is accepted as a major factor in the pathogenesis of AAAs, impaired connective tissue repair may also be critical, either in the gradual progression of disease or in precipitating aneurysm rupture. Several recent studies have emphasized that depletion of medial SMC may be a previously overlooked factor in aneurysmal degeneration. Medial SMCs in AAAs thereby bear markers of apoptosis and frequently express molecular signals capable of initiating cell death, suggesting that the induction of SMC apoptosis may underlie depletion of this cell population in aneurysm tissue.[81,82] An additional possibility is that SMC depletion might involve a process of replicative senescence, whereby a cell population exhausts its replicative capacity over time and can no longer sustain proliferation.[83] Aneurysmal disease may therefore represent an example of 'localized' aging, in which tissue-specific processes lead to accelerated replicative SMC senescence, contributing to selective medial SMC depletion.

In a recent study designed to examine the hypothesis that vascular SMC might exert a protective effect against inflammation and proteolysis in the rat xenograft model of AAAs, Allaire et al. used decellularized aortic grafts seeded with vascular SMC to demonstrate that viable SMC prevent aneurysm formation, elastin degradation, and infiltration by monocyte-macrophages.[84] This protective effect was associated with a shift in the balance of proteolytic activities throughout the aortic wall, suggesting that SMC also exert paracrine effects on other cell types within the adventitia. These findings thereby provide novel experimental evidence to support the view that medial SMC perform critical protective functions during aneurysmal degeneration, and that depletion of medial SMC is a major pathophysiologic mechanism in the progression of aneurysmal disease.

Biomechanics

Understanding how molecular and cellular changes influence tissue structure and function lies at the heart of the interface between biomechanics and molecular cell biology, an emerging area that has provided additional clues to the pathophysiology of aneurysmal degeneration. One factor influencing biomechanical forces in this disease is based on the simple geometric alterations that typically occur in AAAs. Thus, as the aorta gradually dilates during aneurysm formation, it also undergoes a progressive change in shape from a cylindrical structure to one more closely approximating a sphere. Mathematical calculations for a sphere indicate that this simple change in aortic geometry can reduce tensile wall stress to at least half of the values expected if based solely on the Law of Laplace (applicable to cylindrical geometry).[2]

A second role of geometric changes is in determining how biomechanical forces are distributed within the aortic wall. Computational studies based on finite element analysis have revealed that maximum diameter and aneurysm shape both have a substantial influence on the distribution of aortic wall stress. In some AAAs the maximum stress is located in areas other than the point of maximal diameter.[85–87] Indeed, in most AAAs the maximal tensile stress is located at geometric inflections and surface transitions, precisely the locations where aneurysm rupture most commonly occurs in patients. This information has recently been applied to effectively predict the risk of rupture beyond that projected from AAA size alone.[86] It appears quite likely that as tensile stress distribution measures become more widely available, they may supplement simple measurements of aortic diameter in clinical decision-making. Continued study of this issue may elucidate the mechanisms of aneurysm rupture, especially by delineating how regional differences in connective tissue structure or matrix metabolism might be associated with variations in cellular and molecular responses to tensile wall stress.

Finally, the presence of laminated mural thrombus, a recognized feature of AAAs, has been assumed not to contribute to the tensile strength of the aneurysmal aorta. Clinical observations, however, have suggested that either the thickness or circumferential extent of mural thrombus may be a predictor of rapid AAA expansion, with the thickness of mural thrombus within human AAAs being directly correlated with hypoxia in the underlying aortic wall.[88] Regions of the aortic wall subject to low oxygen conditions also exhibit decreased tensile strength as compared with thrombus-free areas of the aneurysm wall, providing one of the first direct links between the presence of mural thrombus and molecular mechanisms which might mediate its effects on the underlying tissue.[89,90]

PROSPECTS FOR MEDICAL MANAGEMENT

Currently, no therapeutic approaches are proven to reduce the rate of aneurysm expansion in patients. However, increasing basic knowledge and refined pathophysiologic concepts of aneurysmal disease have led to translational research efforts demonstrating that several different pharmacologic strategies can suppress aneurysmal degeneration in animal models. Early clinical studies also indicate that at least some of these approaches may be effective in patients, but further investigation is needed. Thus, in the near future, a major challenge will be to extend translational research efforts on the medical management of AAAs toward broader clinical evaluation and application.

General medical management

A key question is how general medical management might influence the natural history of aneurysmal disease. Based on the associations between AAAs and various risk factors in population-based studies, potential measures that would appear to have greatest promise include smoking cessation, blood pressure control, and cholesterol reduction. For example, Cronenwett and colleagues first demonstrated that COPD is associated with a greater rate of expansion and rupture in patients with small asymptomatic AAAs, a finding that has been repeatedly confirmed by others.[91] Moreover, patients who continue to smoke exhibit more rapid aneurysm expansion than non-smokers.[91,92] Therefore, smoking cessation is one of the most important medical measures that can be recommended for patients with AAAs. Hyperlipidemia is an important risk factor for atherosclerosis. There is now effective medical therapy, particularly in the form of hydroxymethyl coenzyme A reductase inhibitors (statins). The mechanisms by which these agents act to reduce clinical events associated with atherosclerosis may not be through direct reductions in plaque size or luminal obstruction, but rather through molecular mechanisms affecting inflammation and proteinase expression.[93–96] These findings suggest that statins may influence aneurysmal degeneration. However, this possibility has not yet been tested in animal models or clinical studies. Poorly controlled hypertension is another controllable risk factor associated with AAAs.[91] While the actual effects of antihypertensive therapy on aneurysm growth are still uncertain, blood pressure control is an important aspect of general medical care that reduces cardiovascular morbidity and mortality. In addition, recent studies using angiotensin-converting enzyme (ACE) inhibitors in animal models of AAAs have indicated that these agents may be of benefit beyond any effect on blood pressure alone.[97]

Propranolol

Early interest in modulating the growth of small AAAs focused on beta-blockers, particularly propranolol. These efforts were based on the use of beta-blockers to prevent aortic root dilatation in patients with Marfan syndrome,[98] a retrospective study suggesting a benefit of propranolol in patients with small AAAs,[99] and experimental work showing that propranolol specifically inhibits aortic dissections and aneurysms in small animal models.[100,101] To evaluate the effects of propranolol in patients with small asymptomatic AAAs (3.0–5.0cm diameter), a prospective, randomized, placebo-controlled, multicenter clinical trial was recently conducted in Canada.[102] Of greatest concern is that 42% of the 276 propranolol-treated patients initially enrolled in the trial were unable to continue the medication, primarily due to side effects associated with propranolol. Moreover, in the patients remaining for evaluation there was no detectable difference between treatment groups with respect to aneurysm growth rate, the need for AAA repair, or mortality. In a similarly designed but smaller clinical trial conducted in Denmark, Lindholt et al. found that 60% of patients randomized to propranolol experienced side effects severe enough to require dropping out of the trial (primarily dyspnea), and that the mortality rate in the propranolol group was significantly higher than in the placebo group (16.7% versus 4.2%).[103] This led the investigators to discontinue the study prematurely, after only 2 years of follow-up. Therefore, propranolol is not an effective or advisable strategy for the medical management of patients with AAAs. Despite their negative results, these efforts have nonetheless demonstrated that prospective randomized clinical trials of a given pharmacologic strategy can be safely and properly conducted in patients with small asymptomatic AAAs.

Non-steroidal anti-inflammatory drugs

Experimental studies have demonstrated that treatment with indomethacin inhibits elastase-induced AAAs in the rat, largely through inhibition of the inducible form of cyclo-oxygenase (COX-2) and a concomitant reduction in PGE_2, IL-6, and MMP-9.[54,55] Indomethacin also suppresses the secretion of inflammatory mediators from human AAA tissue in explant culture.[104] In an associated retrospective case-control study of 78 patients with small AAAs, Walton et al. also found a significantly lower rate of aneurysm expansion in the 15 who were treated with NSAIDs compared to the 63 controls (median 1.5mm versus 3.2mm per year).[104] While these findings clearly suggest that NSAIDs have the potential to reduce aneurysm growth in patients, larger prospective studies are needed to evaluate this possibility further.

Metalloproteinase inhibitors

Based on current knowledge of the role of MMPs in aneurysmal disease and the results of animal studies, MMP inhibition has been proposed as one therapeutic approach to slow aneurysm expansion. Tetracycline derivatives may be one of the most clinically applicable strategies to achieve this aim, since doxycycline has been uniformly successful in animal models of AAAs and because tetracyclines have already been used successfully as MMP inhibitors in patients with periodontitis, arthritis, and other conditions. Furthermore, exposure to tetracycline reduces the secretion of MMP-9 by cultured explants of human AAA tissue. In addition, intraoperative administration of tetracycline leads to rapid drug accumulation within aneurysm wall tissues.[105] In patients undergoing open repair of AAAs, preoperative treatment with oral doxycycline for 1 week resulted in a fivefold reduction in the amount of MMP-9 expressed within aneurysm wall tissue.[106] These observations have increased interest in evaluating MMP inhibition with doxycycline as a potential therapeutic strategy for small asymptomatic AAAs.

To examine the feasibility of this approach, Baxter and colleagues recently conducted a 6-month pilot study to evaluate compliance, side effects, and safety of prolonged treatment with doxycycline in a representative population of patients with small asymptomatic AAAs.[107] Of 36 patients enrolled into the study, 92% completed the full 6 months of treatment with doxycycline (100mg orally twice a day), with a high rate of compliance. Side effects of doxycycline were uncommon and easily managed; these included dermal photosensitivity reactions, reversible tooth discoloration, and non-specific gastrointestinal complaints. The mean plasma doxycycline level after 3 months was within the range required for MMP inhibition. There was no significant increase in mean AAA size over the 6-month period of study. Interestingly, the elevated plasma levels of MMP-9 observed in this population were reduced significantly after 6 months of treatment. Prolonged treatment with doxycycline is therefore considered safe and well tolerated by patients with small asymptomatic AAAs. However, further studies will need to evaluate the long-term effects of doxycycline on the rate and extent of aneurysm growth.

Morosin et al. recently reported the first prospective, double-blind, randomized, placebo-controlled study on the effects of doxycycline in patients with small asymptomatic AAAs.[108]

Thirty-two patients with small AAAs (3.0–5.5cm diameter) were randomly assigned to receive either doxycycline (150mg daily) or placebo during a 3-month period, followed by ultrasound surveillance over the next 18 months. The aneurysm expansion rate in the doxycycline group was significantly lower than in the placebo group during the 6- to 12-month and the 12- to 18-month periods. During the 18-month period of follow-up, 41% of patients in the placebo group experienced aneurysm expansion greater than 5mm as compared with only 7% of patients in the doxycycline group. Thus, despite the small size of the study and short period of drug treatment, these encouraging results strongly support further evaluation of doxycycline in the medical management of AAAs.

CONCLUSION

Basic research on aortic aneurysms is altering rapidly our concepts of this common and life-threatening disease. AAAs may eventually be amenable to remarkably different therapeutic strategies than those commonly in use today. Based on more fundamental understanding of the etiology and pathophysiology of aneurysmal degeneration, new therapeutic strategies to limit the growth of aortic aneurysms will be tested soon in clinical trials. These efforts may influence the overall clinical approach for aneurysmal disease. Eventually, there may be a shift in clinical management to include routine population screening and medical management (pharmacotherapy) for small asymptomatic AAAs. Randomized clinical trials to determine if medical treatment can reduce the rate or extent of expansion in patients with small asymptomatic AAAs, presently in development, can be expected to broaden our understanding of aneurysmal disease and its potential for pharmacologic management.

REFERENCES

1. Thompson RW, Geraghty PJ, Lee JK. Abdominal aortic aneurysms: basic mechanisms and clinical implications. Curr Probl Surg 2002; 39:93–232.
2. Dobrin PB. Elastin, collagen, and the pathophysiology of arterial aneurysms. In: Keen RR, Dobrin PB, eds. Development of aneurysms. Georgetown, TX:Landes Bioscience; 2000:43–73.
3. Dobrin PB, Baker WH, Gley WC. Elastolytic and collagenolytic studies of arteries: implications for the mechanical properties of aneurysms. Arch Surg 1984;119:405–9.
4. Dobrin PB, Mrkvicka R. Failure of elastin or collagen as possible critical connective tissue alterations underlying aneurysmal dilatation. Cardiovasc Surg 1994;2:484–8.
5. Alcorn HG, Wolfson SK Jr, Sutton-Tyrrell K, Kuller LH, O'Leary D. Risk factors for abdominal aortic aneurysms in older adults enrolled in The Cardiovascular Health Study. Arterioscler Thromb Vasc Biol 1996;16:963–70.
6. Lederle FA, Johnson GR, Wilson SE, et al. Prevalence and associations of abdominal aortic aneurysm detected through screening. Ann Intern Med 1997;126:441–9.
7. Kiechl S, Willeit J, Group BS. The natural course of atherosclerosis. Part II: Vascular remodeling. Arterioscler Thromb Vasc Biol 1999; 19:1491–8.
8. Clifton MA. Familial abdominal aortic aneurysms. Br J Surg 1977; 64:765–6.
9. Majumder PP, St Jean PL, Ferrell RE, Webster MW, Steed DL. On the inheritance of abdominal aortic aneurysm. Am J Hum Genet 1991;48:164–70.
10. Verloes A, Sakalihasan N, Koulischer L, Limet R. Aneurysms of the abdominal aorta: familial and genetic aspects in three hundred thirteen pedigrees. J Vasc Surg 1995;21:646–55.
11. Salo JA, Soisalon-Soininen S, Bondestam S, Mattila PS. Familial occurrence of abdominal aortic aneurysm. Ann Intern Med 1999; 130:637–42.
12. van Vlijmen-van Keulen CJ, Pals G, Rauwerda JA. Familial abdominal aortic aneurysm: a systematic review of a genetic background. Eur J Vasc Endovasc Surg 2002;24:105–16.
13. Rasmussen TE, Hallett JW Jr, Metzger RL, et al. Genetic risk factors in inflammatory abdominal aortic aneurysms: polymorphic residue 70 in the HLA-DR B1 gene as a key genetic element. J Vasc Surg 1997; 25:356–64.
14. Hirose H, Takagi M, Miyagawa N, et al. Genetic risk factor for abdominal aortic aneurysm: HLA-DR2(15), a Japanese study. J Vasc Surg 1998;27:500–3.
15. Gerdes LU, Lindholt JS, Vammen S, Henneberg EW, Fasting H. Apolipoprotein E genotype is associated with differential expansion rates of small abdominal aortic aneurysms. Br J Surg 2000;87:760–5.
16. Rossaak JI, van Rij AM, Jones GT, Harris EL. Association of the 4G/5G polymorphism in the promoter region of plasminogen activator inhibitor-1 with abdominal aortic aneurysms. J Vasc Surg 2000;31:1026–32.
17. Tung WS, Lee JK, Thompson RW. Simultaneous analysis of 1176 gene products in normal human aorta and abdominal aortic aneurysms using a membrane-based complementary DNA expression array. J Vasc Surg 2001;34:143–50.

18. Armstrong PJ, Johanning JM, Calton WC Jr, et al. Differential gene expression in human abdominal aorta: aneurysmal versus occlusive disease. J Vasc Surg 2002;35:346–55.

19. Schillinger M, Exner M, Mlekusch W, et al. Heme oxygenase-1 gene promoter polymorphism is associated with abdominal aortic aneurysm. Thromb Res 2002;106:131–6.

20. Wassef M, Baxter BT, Chisholm RL, et al. Pathogenesis of abdominal aortic aneurysms: a multidisciplinary research program supported by the National Heart, Lung, and Blood Institute. J Vasc Surg 2001;34:730–8.

21. Brophy CM, Reilly JM, Smith GJ, Tilson MD. The role of inflammation in nonspecific abdominal aortic aneurysm disease. Ann Vasc Surg 1991;5:229–33.

22. Curci JA, Liao S, Huffman MD, Shapiro SD, Thompson RW. Expression and localization of macrophage elastase (matrix metalloproteinase-12) in abdominal aortic aneurysms. J Clin Invest 1998;102:1900–10.

23. Koch AE, Haines GK, Rizzo RJ, et al. Human abdominal aortic aneurysms: immunophenotypic analysis suggesting an immune-mediated response. Am J Pathol 1990;137:1199–213.

24. Hance KA, Tataria M, Ziporin SJ, Lee JK, Thompson RW. Monocyte chemotactic activity in human abdominal aortic aneurysms: role of elastin degradation peptides and the 67-kD cell surface elastin receptor. J Vasc Surg 2002;35:254–61.

25. Anidjar S, Salzmann JL, Gentric D, Lagneau P, Camilleri JP, Michel JB. Elastase-induced experimental aneurysms in rats. Circulation 1990;82:973–81.

26. Koch A, Kunkel S, Pearce W, et al. Enhanced production of the chemotactic cytokines interleukin-8 and monocyte chemoattractant protein-1 in human abdominal aortic aneurysms. Am J Pathol 1993;142:1423–31.

27. Colonnello JS, Hance KA, Shames ML, et al. Transient exposure to elastase induces mouse aortic wall smooth muscle cell production of MCP-1 and RANTES during the development of experimental aortic aneurysm. J Vasc Surg 2003;38:138–46.

28. Pearce WH, Sweis I, Yao JS, McCarthy WJ, Koch AE. Interleukin-1 beta and tumor necrosis factor-alpha release in normal and diseased human infrarenal aortas. J Vasc Surg 1992;16:784–9.

29. Holmes DR, Wester W, Thompson RW, Reilly JM. Prostaglandin E2 synthesis and cyclooxygenase expression in abdominal aortic aneurysms. J Vasc Surg 1997;25:810–5.

30. Juvonen J, Surcel HM, Satta J, et al. Elevated circulating levels of inflammatory cytokines in patients with abdominal aortic aneurysm. Arterioscler Thromb Vasc Biol 1997;17:2843–7.

31. McMillan WD, Pearce WH. Inflammation and cytokine signaling in aneurysms. Ann Vasc Surg 1997;11:540–5.

32. Franklin IJ, Walton LJ, Greenhalgh RM, Powell JT. The influence of indomethacin on the metabolism and cytokine secretion of human aneurysmal aorta. Eur J Vasc Endovasc Surg 1999;18:35–42.

33. Miller FJ Jr, Sharp WJ, Fang X, Oberley LW, Oberley TD, Weintraub NL. Oxidative stress in human abdominal aortic aneurysms: a potential mediator of aneurysmal remodeling. Arterioscler Thromb Vasc Biol 2002;22:560–5.

34. Rajagopalan S, Meng XP, Ramasamy S, Harrison DG, Galis ZS. Reactive oxygen species produced by macrophage-derived foam cells regulate the activity of vascular matrix metalloproteinases in vitro: implications for atherosclerotic plaque stability. J Clin Invest 1996;98:2572–9.

35. Fu X, Kassim SY, Parks WC, Heinecke JW. Hypochlorous acid oxygenates the cysteine switch domain of pro-matrilysin (MMP-7). A mechanism for matrix metalloproteinase activation and atherosclerotic plaque rupture by myeloperoxidase. J Biol Chem 2001;276:41279–87.

36. Johanning JM, Franklin DP, Han DC, Carey DJ, Elmore JR. Inhibition of inducible nitric oxide synthase limits nitric oxide production and experimental aneurysm expansion. J Vasc Surg 2001;33:579–86.

37. Johanning JM, Armstrong PJ, Franklin DP, Han DC, Carey DJ, Elmore JR. Nitric oxide in experimental aneurysm formation: early events and consequences of nitric oxide inhibition. Ann Vasc Surg 2002;16:65–72.

38. Yajima N, Masuda M, Miyazaki M, Nakajima N, Chien S, Shyy JY. Oxidative stress is involved in the development of experimental abdominal aortic aneurysm: a study of the transcription profile with complementary DNA microarray. J Vasc Surg 2002;36:379–85.

39. Halme S, Juvonen T, Laurila A, et al. Chlamydia pneumoniae reactive T lymphocytes in the walls of abdominal aortic aneurysms. Eur J Clin Invest 1999;29:546–52.

40. Lindholt JS, Juul S, Vammen S, Lind I, Fasting H, Henneberg EW. Immunoglobulin A antibodies against Chlamydia pneumoniae are associated with expansion of abdominal aortic aneurysm. Br J Surg 1999;86:634–8.

41. Tambiah J, Franklin IJ, Trendell-Smith N, Peston D, Powell JT. Provocation of experimental aortic inflammation and dilatation by inflammatory mediators and Chlamydia pneumoniae. Br J Surg 2001;88:935–40.

42. Tambiah J, Powell JT. Chlamydia pneumoniae antigens facilitate experimental aortic dilatation: prevention with azithromycin. J Vasc Surg 2002;36:1011–7.

43. Kalayoglu MV, Libby P, Byrne GI. Chlamydia pneumoniae as an emerging risk factor in cardiovascular disease. JAMA 2002;288:2724–31.

44. Dal Canto AJ, Swanson PE, O'Guin AK, Speck SH, Virgin HW. IFN-gamma action in the media of the great elastic arteries, a novel immunoprivileged site. J Clin Invest 2001;107:R15–22.

45. Gregory AK, Yin NX, Capella J, Xia S, Newman KM, Tilson MD. Features of autoimmunity in the abdominal aortic aneurysm. Arch Surg 1996;131:85–8.

46. Davis VA, Persidskaia RN, Baca-Regen LM, Fiotti N, Halloran BG, Baxter BT. Cytokine pattern in aneurysmal and occlusive disease of the aorta. J Surg Res 2001;101:152–6.

47. Schonbeck U, Sukhova GK, Gerdes N, Libby P. TH2 predominant immune responses prevail in human abdominal aortic aneurysm. Am J Pathol 2002;161:499–506.

48. Lacraz S, Nicod L, Galve-de Rochemonteix B, Baumberger C, Dayer JM, Welgus HG. Suppression of metalloproteinase biosynthesis in human alveolar macrophages by interleukin-4. J Clin Invest 1992;90:382–8.

49. Lacraz S, Nicod LP, Chicheportiche R, Welgus HG, Dayer JM. IL-10 inhibits metalloproteinase and stimulates TIMP-1 production in human mononuclear phagocytes. J Clin Invest 1995;96:2304–10.

50. Anidjar S, Dobrin PB, Eichorst M, Graham GP, Chejfec G. Correlation of inflammatory infiltrate with the enlargement of experimental aortic aneurysm. J Vasc Surg 1992;16:139–47.

51. Dobrin PB, Baumgartner N, Anidjar S, Chejfec G, Mrkvicka R. Inflammatory aspects of experimental aneurysms: effect of methylprednisolone and cyclosporine. Ann N Y Acad Sci 1996;800:74–88.

52. Ricci MA, Strindberg G, Slaiby JM, et al. Anti-CD18 monoclonal antibody slows experimental aortic aneurysm expansion. J Vasc Surg 1996;23:301–7.

53. Hingorani A, Ascher E, Scheinman M, et al. The effect of tumor necrosis factor binding protein and interleukin-1 receptor antagonist on the development of abdominal aortic aneurysms in a rat model. J Vasc Surg 1998;28:522–6.

54. Holmes DR, Petrinec D, Wester W, Thompson RW, Reilly JM. Indomethacin prevents elastase-induced abdominal aortic aneurysms in the rat. J Surg Res 1996;63:305–9.

55. Miralles M, Wester W, Sicard GA, Thompson R, Reilly JM. Indomethacin inhibits expansion of experimental aortic aneurysms via inhibition of the cox2 isoform of cyclooxygenase. J Vasc Surg 1999;29:884–93.

56. Menashi S, Campa JS, Greenhalgh RM, Powell JT. Collagen in abdominal aortic aneurysm: typing, content, and degradation. J Vasc Surg 1987;6:578–82.

57. Minion DJ, Wang Y, Lynch TG, Fox IJ, Prorok GD, Baxter BT. Soluble factors modulate changes in collagen gene expression in abdominal aortic aneurysms. Surgery 1993;114:252–6.

58. Rizzo RJ, McCarthy WJ, Dixit SN, et al. Collagen types and matrix protein content in human abdominal aortic aneurysms. J Vasc Surg 1989;10:365–73.

59. Gargiulo M, Stella A, Spina M, et al. Content and turnover of extracellular matrix protein in human "nonspecific" and inflammatory abdominal aortic aneurysms. Eur J Vasc Surg 1993;7:546–53.
60. Sakalihasan N, Heyeres A, Nusgens BV, Limet R, Lapiere CM. Modifications of the extracellular matrix of aneurysmal abdominal aortas as a function of their size. Eur J Vasc Surg 1993;7:633–7.
61. Thompson RW, Parks WC. Role of matrix metalloproteinases in abdominal aortic aneurysms. Ann N Y Acad Sci 1996;800:157–74.
62. Thompson RW, Holmes DR, Mertens RA, et al. Production and localization of 92-kilodalton gelatinase in abdominal aortic aneurysms: an elastolytic metalloproteinase expressed by aneurysm-infiltrating macrophages. J Clin Invest 1995;96:318–26.
63. McMillan WD, Tamarina NA, Cipollone M, Johnson DA, Parker MA, Pearce WH. Size matters: the relationship between MMP-9 expression and aortic diameter. Circulation 1997;96:2228–32.
64. Hovsepian DM, Ziporin S J, Sakurai MK, Lee JK, Curci JA, Thompson RW. Elevated plasma levels of matrix metalloproteinase-9 (MMP-9) in patients with abdominal aortic aneurysms: a circulating marker of degenerative aneurysm disease. J Vasc Int Radiol 2000;11:1345–52.
65. Davis V, Persidskaia R, Baca-Regen L, et al. Matrix metalloproteinase-2 production and its binding to the matrix are increased in abdominal aortic aneurysms. Arterioscler Thromb Vasc Biol 1998;18:1625–33.
66. Dobrin PB. Animal models of aneurysms. Ann Vasc Surg 1999;13:641–8.
67. Carrell TW, Smith A, Burnand KG. Experimental techniques and models in the study of the development and treatment of abdominal aortic aneurysm. Br J Surg 1999;86:305–12.
68. Halpern VJ, Nackman GB, Gandhi RH, et al. The elastase infusion model of experimental aortic aneurysms: synchrony of induction of endogenous proteinases with matrix destruction and inflammatory cell response. J Vasc Surg 1994;20:51–60.
69. Chiou AC, Chiu B, Pearce WH. Murine aortic aneurysm produced by periarterial application of calcium chloride. J Surg Res 2001;99:371–6.
70. Allaire E, Forough R, Clowes M, Starcher B, Clowes AW. Local overexpression of TIMP-1 prevents aortic aneurysm degeneration and rupture in a rat model. J Clin Invest 1998;102:1413–20.
71. Petrinec D, Liao S, Holmes DR, Reilly JM, Parks WC, Thompson RW. Doxycycline inhibition of aneurysmal degeneration in an elastase-induced rat model of abdominal aortic aneurysm: preservation of aortic elastin associated with suppressed production of 92 kD gelatinase. J Vasc Surg 1996;23:336–46.
72. Curci JA, Petrinec D, Liao SX, Golub LM, Thompson RW. Pharmacologic suppression of experimental abdominal aortic aneurysms: a comparison of doxycycline and four chemically modified tetracyclines. J Vasc Surg 1998;28:1082–93.
73. Bigatel DA, Elmore JR, Carey DJ, Cizmeci-Smith G, Franklin DP, Youkey JR. The matrix metalloproteinase inhibitor BB-94 limits expansion of experimental abdominal aortic aneurysms. J Vasc Surg 1999;29:130–8.
74. Moore G, Liao S, Curci JA, et al. Suppression of experimental abdominal aortic aneurysms by systemic treatment with a hydroxamate-based matrix metalloproteinase inhibitor (RS 132908). J Vasc Surg 1999;29:522–32.
75. Pyo R, Lee JK, Shipley JM, et al. Targeted gene disruption of matrix metalloproteinase-9 (gelatinase B) suppresses development of experimental abdominal aortic aneurysms. J Clin Invest 2000;105:1641–9.
76. Longo GM, Xiong W, Greiner TC, Zhao Y, Fiotti N, Baxter BT. Matrix metalloproteinases 2 and 9 work in concert to produce aortic aneurysms. J Clin Invest 2002;110:625–32.
77. Tilson MD, Elefriades J, Brophy CM. Tensile strength and collagen in abdominal aortic aneurysm disease. In: Greenhalgh RM, Mannick JA, Powell JT, eds. The cause and management of aneurysms. London: WB Saunders; 1990:97–104.
78. Huffman MD, Curci JA, Moore G, Kerns DB, Starcher BC, Thompson RW. Functional importance of connective tissue repair during the development of experimental abdominal aortic aneurysms. Surgery 2000;128:429–38.
79. Satta J, Juvonen T, Haukipuro K, Juvonen M, Kairaluoma MI. Increased turnover of collagen in abdominal aortic aneurysms, demonstrated by measuring the concentration of the aminoterminal propeptide of type III procollagen in peripheral and aortal blood samples. J Vasc Surg 1995;22:155–60.
80. Satta J, Haukipuro K, Kairaluoma MI, Juvonen T. Aminoterminal propeptide of type III procollagen in the follow-up of patients with abdominal aortic aneurysms. J Vasc Surg 1997;25:909–15.
81. Lopez-Candales A, Holmes DR, Liao S, Scott MJ, Wickline SA, Thompson RW. Decreased vascular smooth muscle cell density in medial degeneration of human abdominal aortic aneurysms. Am J Pathol 1997;150:993–1007.
82. Henderson EL, Gang YJ, Sukhova GK, Whittemore AD, Knox J, Libby P. Death of smooth muscle cells and expression of mediators of apoptosis by T lymphocytes in human abdominal aortic aneurysms. Circulation 1999;99:96–104.
83. Liao S, Curci JA, Kelley B, Sicard GA, Thompson RW. Accelerated replicative senescence of medial smooth muscle cells derived from abdominal aortic aneurysms as compared to the adjacent inferior mesenteric artery. J Surg Res 2000;92:85–95.
84. Allaire E, Muscatelli-Groux B, Mandet C, et al. Paracrine effect of vascular smooth muscle cells in the prevention of aortic aneurysm formation. J Vasc Surg 2002;36:1018–26.
85. Vorp DA, Raghavan ML, Webster MW. Mechanical wall stress in abdominal aortic aneurysm: influence of diameter and asymmetry. J Vasc Surg 1998;27:632–9.
86. Fillinger MF, Raghavan ML, Marra SP, Cronenwett JL, Kennedy FE. In vivo analysis of mechanical wall stress and abdominal aortic aneurysm rupture risk. J Vasc Surg 2002;36:589–97.
87. Flora HS, Talei-Faz B, Ansdell L, et al. Aneurysm wall stress and tendency to rupture are features of physical wall properties: an experimental study. J Endovasc Ther 2002;9:665–75.
88. Vorp DA, Wang DH, Webster MW, Federspiel WJ. Effect of intraluminal thrombus thickness and bulge diameter on the oxygen diffusion in abdominal aortic aneurysm. J Biomech Eng 1998;120:579–83.
89. Vorp DA, Lee PC, Wang DH, et al. Association of intraluminal thrombus in abdominal aortic aneurysm with local hypoxia and wall weakening. J Vasc Surg 2001;34:291–9.
90. Fontaine V, Jacob MP, Houard X, et al. Involvement of the mural thrombus as a site of protease release and activation in human aortic aneurysms. Am J Pathol 2002;161:1701–10.
91. Cronenwett JL, Sargent SK, Wall MH, et al. Variables that affect the expansion rate and outcome of small abdominal aortic aneurysms. J Vasc Surg 1990;11:260–9.
92. MacSweeney ST, Ellis M, Worrell PC, Greenhaugh RM, Powell JT. Smoking and growth rate of small abdominal aortic aneurysms. Lancet 1994;344:651–2.
93. Vaughan CJ, Murphy MB, Buckley BM. Statins do more than just lower cholesterol. Lancet 1996;348:1079–82.
94. Bellosta S, Ferri N, Bernini F, Paoletti R, Corsini A. Non-lipid-related effects of statins. Ann Med 2000;32:164–76.
95. Maron DJ, Fazio S, Linton MF. Current perspectives on statins. Circulation 2000;101:207–13.
96. Liao JK. Isoprenoids as mediators of the biological effects of statins. J Clin Invest 2002;110:285–8.
97. Liao S, Miralles M, Kelley BJ, Curci JA, Borhani M, Thompson RW. Suppression of experimental abdominal aortic aneurysms in the rat by treatment with angiotensin-converting enzyme inhibitors. J Vasc Surg 2001;33:1057–64.
98. Shores J, Berger KR, Murphy EA, Pyeritz RE. Progression of aortic dilatation and the benefit of long-term beta-adrenergic blockade in Marfan's syndrome. N Engl J Med 1994;330:1335–41.
99. Leach SD, Toole AL, Stern H, DeNatale RW, Tilson MD. Effect of beta-adrenergic blockade on the growth rate of abdominal aortic aneurysms. Arch Surg 1988;123:606–9.
100. Brophy CM, Tilson JE, Tilson MD. Propranolol delays the formation of aneurysms in the male blotchy mouse. J Surg Res 1988;44:687–9.
101. Slaiby JM, Ricci MA, Gadowski GR, Hendley ED, Pilcher DB. Expansion of aortic aneurysms is reduced by propranolol in a hypertensive rat model. J Vasc Surg 1994;20:178–83.

102. Propranolol for small abdominal aortic aneurysms: results of a randomized trial. J Vasc Surg 2002;35:72–9.

103. Lindholt JS, Henneberg EW, Juul S, Fasting H. Impaired results of a randomised double blinded clinical trial of propranolol versus placebo on the expansion rate of small abdominal aortic aneurysms. Int Angiol 1999;18:52–7.

104. Walton LJ, Franklin IJ, Bayston T, et al. Inhibition of prostaglandin E2 synthesis in abdominal aortic aneurysms: implications for smooth muscle cell viability, inflammatory processes, and the expansion of abdominal aortic aneurysms. Circulation 1999;100:48–54.

105. Franklin IJ, Harley SL, Greenhalgh RM, Powell JT. Uptake of tetracycline by aortic aneurysm wall and its effect on inflammation and proteolysis. Br J Surg 1999;86:771–5.

106. Curci JA, Mao D, Bohner DG, et al. Preoperative treatment with doxycycline reduces aortic wall expression and activation of matrix metalloproteinases in patients with abdominal aortic aneurysms. J Vasc Surg 2000;31:325–42.

107. Baxter BT, Pearce WH, Waltke EA, et al. Prolonged administration of doxycycline in patients with small asymptomatic abdominal aortic aneurysms: report of a prospective (Phase II) multicenter study. J Vasc Surg 2002;36:1–12.

108. Mosorin M, Juvonen J, Biancari F, et al. Use of doxycycline to decrease the growth rate of abdominal aortic aneurysms: a randomized, double-blind, placebo-controlled pilot study. J Vasc Surg 2001;34:606–10.

CHAPTER
29

Abdominal Aortic Aneurysm Screening and Evaluation

Frank A Lederle

KEY POINTS

- Abdominal aortic aneurysms (AAAs) that rupture are often unknown to the patient until the day of the rupture.

- Consequently, earlier AAA detection by screening is reasonable in patients at risk for aneurysms.

- Three risk factors increase the likelihood of an AAA: male gender (>65 years old); history of smoking; and family history of AAA.

- The sensitivity of abdominal palpation to detect an AAA large enough to be considered for repair (≥ 5.0–5.5cm) is high, especially if the abdominal girth is less than 40in.

- Abdominal ultrasound is the initial diagnostic test of choice to confirm a clinical suspicion of AAA.

- The optimal age for initial ultrasound screening in patients at increased risk for AAA is 65 years.

- Two recent randomized clinical trials found no survival advantage of repair of AAAs smaller than 5.5cm. Periodic ultrasound suveillance with repair reserved for AAAs ≥ 5.5cm is less costly than repairing all AAAs ≥ 4.0cm.

- The first major randomized trial of screening in men has suggested it can reduce the aneurysm-related mortality by 42%. Governments will have to review the potential cost benefit advantages of screening to their populations.

BACKGROUND AND RATIONALE

Screening for abdominal aortic aneurysms (AAAs) was first reported 35 years ago by Schilling and colleagues.[1] Using physical examination and lateral abdominal radiography, they detected 26 AAAs ≥ 3.6cm in 873 men aged 55–64, a prevalence of 3.1%.[1,2] The study received little attention, but in 1983, Cabellon and colleagues reported using ultrasound and abdominal palpation to find AAAs in seven of 73 asymptomatic patients with vascular disease.[3] This study was followed by numerous similar studies and later by reports of larger, community-based programs. Since that time, screening for AAAs with ultrasound has been advocated by various authors and groups and debated extensively in the literature. As the large randomized trials currently underway are reported in the next few years, the place of AAA screening in the periodic health examination will soon be determined for the foreseeable future.

Early detection of disease through screening is an inherently appealing idea. However, screening must be undertaken with caution because the risks and costs apply to many whereas the benefits affect few, and in some instances may even be negligible compared with usual care. Cochrane and Holland[4] argued that when the practitioner initiates screening procedures, there is an ethical requirement for greater certainty regarding benefit than for routine health care, in which the patient asks the practitioner for help. In 1975, Frame and Carlson[5] proposed the following criteria for an acceptable screening program:

1. The disease must have a significant effect on the quality or quantity of life.
2. Acceptable methods of treatment must be available.
3. The disease must have an asymptomatic period during which detection and treatment significantly reduce morbidity and/or mortality.
4. Treatment in the asymptomatic phase must yield a therapeutic result superior to that obtained by delaying treatment until symptoms appear.
5. Tests must be available at reasonable cost to detect the condition in the asymptomatic period.
6. The incidence of the condition must be sufficient to justify the cost of screening.

Screening for AAA appears to meet these criteria. AAAs are common in older men, with AAAs ≥ 3.0cm occurring in 4–8%.[6,7] The prevalence of AAA, and hence the yield from screening, depends both on the population considered and on how AAA is defined. There is no widely accepted method of defining the cutoff point between AAA and normal. Most authors have used unadjusted aortic diameter (e.g. ≥ 3.0cm), which is known to be associated with the risk of rupture.[8] While such a 'one-size-fits-all' method could exaggerate the prevalence of AAA in larger people, we have found that age, gender, race, and body size have little influence on normal aortic diameter, suggesting that their use in defining AAA may not offer sufficient advantage to be warranted.[9] Small AAAs are much more common than large AAAs. Data from a large screening study conducted in older veterans show that with each 1cm decrease in AAA diameter, the number of AAAs of that diameter or larger more than doubles (**Table 29.1**). Aortic aneurysm is the 15th leading cause of death in the US,[10] and most of these deaths are due to rupture of AAAs.[11] Small AAAs enlarge at an average rate of 1cm every 3 years,[12,13] so there is usually a period of at least 5 years from the time that the abdominal aorta reaches 3cm in diameter (the most common definition of AAA) until symptoms of rupture develop, usually after the AAA is ≥ 6cm. During this period, AAAs are nearly always asymptomatic and elective repair can be carried out with relatively low operative mortality (2–5%) by experienced surgeons, whereas once rupture occurs, only a fifth of patients survive.[14] The screening tests that have been proposed (ultrasound or abdominal palpation with confirmatory ultrasound) are safe, inexpensive, and acceptable to patients.[15]

Prevalence of abdominal aortic aneurysms (AAAs) by diameter in male veterans aged 50–79 years.		
AAA diameter	No. of AAAs	%
≥3.0cm	5283	4.2
≥4.0cm	1644	1.3
≥5.0cm	571	0.45
≥5.5cm*	342	0.27
≥6.0cm	212	0.17
≥7.0cm	76	0.06
≥8.0cm	32	0.03
* Adapted from Lederle et al.[23]		

Table 29.1 Prevalence of abdominal aortic aneurysms (AAAs) by diameter in male veterans aged 50–79 years (n=126,196).

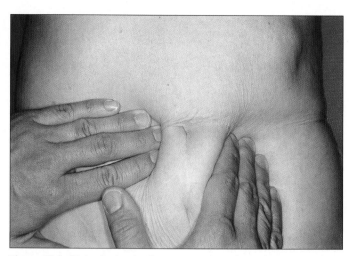

Figure 29.1 Abdominal palpation.

The great difficulty in justifying screening programs is in demonstrating that early detection improves outcome compared with usual care without screening. Because of the many possibilities for bias, randomized trials are usually necessary to make this determination. These are now becoming available for AAA screening and will be discussed below. The cost-effectiveness of AAA screening is also discussed below.

SCREENING MODALITIES

The diagnosis of asymptomatic AAA in the absence of screening must be incidental, as the result of a physical examination or imaging test done for reasons other than to detect AAA. The frequency of incidental diagnoses of AAA led to attempts to systematically apply tests to high-risk populations for the purpose of detecting asymptomatic AAA. Abdominal palpation is the oldest method of AAA detection. Few aneurysms will be found by 'routine' palpation of the abdomen,[16] but deliberate and careful evaluation of the aorta will detect most clinically important AAAs.[17] During the examination, the patient should be supine with the abdomen relaxed and the knees raised. The examiner places both hands palms down on the abdomen between the xyphoid process and the umbilicus and palpates deeply to detect the aorta pulsation between the two index fingers. Ample skin should be included between the two index fingers, and it is often helpful initially to probe for one side of the aorta at a time (**Fig. 29.1**).

It is the width, and not the intensity, of the aortic pulsation that determines the diagnosis; a normal aorta is often readily palpable in thin patients or those with loose abdominal muscles. The aorta is normally less than 1in (2.5cm) in diameter, and aortas larger than this (after allowing for skin thickness) warrant further investigation, usually with ultrasound. Findings of abdominal or femoral bruits or absent femoral pulses do not contribute to the diagnosis of asymptomatic AAA.[16] As Osler observed: 'No pulsation, however forcible, no thrill, however intense, no bruit, however loud – singly or together – justify the diagnosis of an aneurysm of the abdominal aorta, *only the presence of a palpable expansile tumour*'.[18]

The sensitivity of abdominal palpation for detecting AAA depends on the diameter of both aneurysm and patient. Three-quarters of AAAs ≥ 5.0cm in diameter are detectable by abdominal palpation, whereas less than one-quarter of AAAs 3.0–3.9cm are palpable.[17] The sensitivity of palpation is also much lower in patients with an abdominal girth of more than 100cm (a 40in waist) compared with thinner patients.[16,19] The sensitivity of palpation to detect AAAs large enough to be considered for repair (≥ 5cm) is quite high (100% in one small series of 12 cases[19]). Agreement between different examiners has been shown to be 'fair to good' (kappa = 0.53).[19] Only about one-third of elderly men suspected of having an enlarged aorta on abdominal palpation will be found to actually have AAA. This number (the positive predictive value) is much lower in women and young men,[17] but is not of great concern because ultrasound provides a safe and inexpensive confirmatory test. Thus, while abdominal palpation is not an ideal diagnostic test, many physicians consider it among the most worthwhile components of the physical examination, especially if the patient's health plan does not cover ultrasound screening for AAA.

A variety of abdominal imaging procedures will accurately diagnose AAA, but virtually all screening programs undertaken or considered to date have involved the use of ultrasound. Ultrasound is particularly useful because of its accuracy (**Fig. 29.2**), low cost, patient acceptance, lack of radiation exposure, and general availability. A variety of studies have shown the sensitivity and specificity of ultrasound for AAA to be nearly 100%.[16,20] Small portable ultrasonography equipment has increased the feasibility of mobile or temporary screening centers.

Plain radiography is a common means of incidental diagnosis of AAA and often provides early diagnostic clues to rupture, e.g. calcification, soft tissue mass, or loss of psoas or renal outlines.[21] However, plain radiography should not be used to confirm or exclude the diagnosis because many AAAs will be missed owing to insufficient calcification, resulting in sensitivities as low as 25%.[22] Computed tomography, angiography, magnetic resonance imaging, and their variants are all useful for detailed preoperative evaluation of AAA, but offer no advantage over ultrasound for initial diagnosis and are more expensive. Thus, for those practitioners interested in screening for AAA, two methods of screening can be recommended. Ultrasound is the preferred

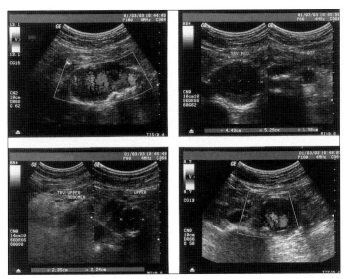

Figure 29.2 Ultrasound of abdominal aortic aneurysm.

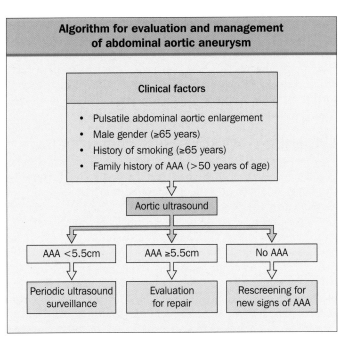

Figure 29.3 Algorithm for evaluation and management of abdominal aortic aneurysm.

method when feasible, but abdominal palpation with ultrasound confirmation of positive or suggestive examinations is a reasonable alternative.

PATIENT SELECTION

For screening to be efficient, it must target the population most likely to benefit. Published screening studies provide detailed information on factors associated with having an AAA detected at screening (**Fig. 29.3**). The factors that have been most important are gender and age. AAA is primarily a disease of men. Numerous studies have found that men are about four times as likely as women to have AAA.[6] Even after adjustment for other risk factors, men are still more than twice as likely to have AAA.[23] As a result, most published population screening programs and ongoing randomized trials of screening have not included women.[24] Age is an equally important consideration. Like most diseases, AAAs are more common in older people. Prevalence increases throughout life, but incidence may peak at age 65.[25] Very few people younger than 50 years of age have AAA, but the prevalence increases sharply afterwards (**Fig. 29.4**). Targeting young people will result in low yield, but targeting the very old is also of little value because many of those found to have AAA will not be candidates for repair or will not live long enough after repair to realize any benefit. AAA incidence and prevalence, death rates, and screening compliance rates from several population-based screening studies in England have led their directors to conclude that the preferred age for AAA screening is 65,[26,27] and none of the study groups have proposed screening those more than 80 years old.

In addition to gender and age, another potentially useful criteria for defining a target population for AAA screening is smoking history. Smoking is the strongest risk factor for AAA, with smokers having more than five times the risk of non-smokers.[23] The excess prevalence associated with smoking accounted for 75% of all the AAAs ≥ 4.0cm in a veteran population.[23] Several cross-sectional screening studies have demonstrated the strong association between smoking and AAA.[23,28] The effects of age and smoking on the prevalence of AAAs ≥ 4.0cm are shown in

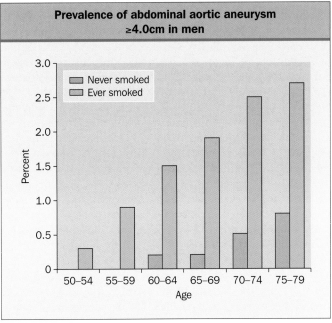

Figure 29.4 Prevalence of abdominal aortic aneurysms ≥4.0cm in men by age and smoking history. (Adapted from Lederle et al.[28] Redrawn with permission from Chesler E, ed. Clinical cardiology in the elderly, 2nd edn. Armonk, NY:Futura; 1999.)

Figure 29.4. Note that men who have never smoked have a prevalence of AAAs ≥ 4.0cm well below 1% regardless of age, whereas men in their 70s who had ever smoked had a prevalence greater than 2%. Limiting an AAA screening program to those who have ever smoked is therefore logical, but programs using this criterion have not been reported. Excluding non-smokers from screening would likely be unpopular, and would only reduce the number of persons screened by about 30%.[29] Limiting screening to current smokers cannot be recommended, as the majority of AAAs in the population would be missed using this requirement.[29]

Other moderately strong risk factors for AAA include white race, family history of AAA, coronary, cerebral or peripheral artery disease, and absence of diabetes.[23] However, efforts to further select a target population beyond that of men aged 65–80 years have not been found to be worthwhile.[29,30]

EVIDENCE THAT SCREENING IS BENEFICIAL

Assessment of the benefit of screening is difficult because of the large numbers of patients required and the difficulty of ascertaining AAA-related deaths, particularly in the unscreened group.[31] Nevertheless, useful data are rapidly becoming available. Two non-randomized community-based studies from England have reported beneficial results from AAA screening of older men.[32,33] One reported significant reductions in AAA-related deaths in men in the age group offered screening (65–73 years old) that was not seen in other men, based on a total of 83 AAA-related deaths.[32] The other reported a significant reduction in rupture rate in men after being invited for screening compared with before being invited.[33] Of concern, those considered unfit for surgery appear to have been included in the control group, the outcome did not include deaths from elective surgery, and there were only 62 ruptures in the study group.

In a randomized trial from Chichester, UK, that included 9342 women and 6433 men, no benefit was seen in women, but AAA screening and elective repair resulted in a 55% reduction in AAA ruptures in men.[34] The associated 41% reduction in AAA-related deaths (from 17 to ten) did not reach statistical significance, however. There were no operative deaths in 33 elective repairs in this study and repair was offered only for AAAs ≥ 6cm or rapid growth – two factors crucial to the success of the program but unlikely to be replicated in general practice. Recently, a second randomized trial of 12 658 men has been reported from Denmark.[35] AAA-related deaths were significantly reduced in the screening group, from 19 to six. These findings are highly suggestive of a benefit from screening, but the number of AAA-related deaths in the trials was very small. Several more randomized trials of AAA screening with ultrasound in older men are currently underway,[24] and their findings will be crucial to determining the effectiveness of screening for AAA.

The first randomized evaluation of population screening for AAA in men has recently been reported – The Multicentre Aneurysm Screening Study (MASS).[35a] Screening a population-based sample of 33,839 invited men reduced the risk of aneurysm-related mortality by 42% (53% of those actually screened). This trial has for the first time provided evidence for healthcare providers and governments to enable decisions about the costs and benefits of screening to be made in their populations.

RE-SCREENING

The studies discussed above describe the results of one-time screening programs. A related issue is whether re-screening at specified intervals would be worthwhile. Though no randomized trials have addressed this question, some information on the yield of re-screening is available. In a study by Lederle and colleagues, 2622 veterans who had aortic diameters <3.0cm by ultrasound at age 50–79 underwent repeat ultrasound after

4 years.[36] Fifty-eight (2.2%) had aortic diameters ≥ 3.0cm (meeting the usual definition of AAA), of which three were ≥ 4.0cm. Re-screening at 4 years was not considered worthwhile because of the low yield and small diameters of the AAAs detected. Crow et al.[27] described 223 men who had aortic diameters <2.6cm by ultrasound at age 65 and were then re-screened after 5 and 12 years. Six men had aortic diameters of 3.0–3.6cm (meeting the usual definition of AAA) at re-screening, but because of their age, none of these patients were considered likely to ever require elective repair. Based on these studies, it appears that screening, if implemented, need only be one-time. As noted previously, the ideal time for one-time screening appears to be at age 65.

COST-EFFECTIVENESS

Unlike many other screening programs, most of the cost of an ultrasound program of AAA screening results from treatment of detected AAA, with only about 15% coming from diagnosis.[37] Thus, the benefit of screening would appear to be closely linked to the benefit of treatment – that is to say, if repairing an AAA is worthwhile, then spending 15% more to detect it is probably also worthwhile.

At least six cost-effectiveness models of ultrasound screening for AAA have been published for men over age 60.[37,38] One concluded that screening did more harm than good; the others found screening to be beneficial at costs ranging from about $2000 to $41 550 per year of life saved. In addition, the previously mentioned Danish randomized trial[35] found that ultrasound screening prevented AAA-related deaths at a cost of only about $1000 per year of life saved. Cost-effectiveness ratios up to $40 000 per year of life saved are consistent with currently funded programs and those under $20 000 are considered to be 'very attractive', so screening for AAA looks very promising in this regard.[37] Screening with abdominal palpation and confirmatory ultrasound has been calculated to be more cost-effective than screening with ultrasound.[39]

Most of the cost-effectiveness studies based on models assumed that all AAAs ≥ 4.0cm would be repaired. However, two recent randomized trials[12,13] found no reduction in mortality from repair of asymptomatic AAAs smaller than 5.5cm, and the strategy of surveillance with repair reserved for AAAs ≥ 5.5cm is less costly than repairing all AAAs ≥ 4.0cm.[40] Revised cost-effectiveness models incorporating surveillance to 5.5cm would be expected to show improved cost-effectiveness.

MISCELLANEOUS CONCERNS REGARDING SCREENING

Screening identifies many small AAAs that are unlikely to rupture in the patient's lifetime. Adverse consequences for these patients include (a) needless worry and (b) risk from unnecessary procedures. Limited data are available on the possible adverse pyschological effects of screening in general, but false positive results have been associated with depression[41] and with increased anxiety that persists even after further testing rules out the disease.[42] Regarding AAA screening, a report of no difference in anxiety and depression scores between screened and unscreened subjects is encouraging,[43] but may not be reliable because the groups were small and dissimilar (the unscreened group had fewer married men). Another study reported that anxiety levels dropped after screening, regardless of whether AAA was detected.[44] Unfortunately, anxiety levels from before the screening invitation were not available for comparison.

More concerning for those with small AAAs detected at screening is the risk from unnecessary procedures. Despite publication of the two trials demonstrating that survival is not improved by elective repair of AAAs smaller than 5.5cm even in good operative candidates,[12,13] the inclination to repair smaller AAAs remains strong, at least in the US. Following publication of the first trial, several editorials endorsed elective repair of AAAs smaller than 5.5cm under various circumstances, contrary to the study's conclusions.[45,46] Patient anxiety regarding a condition that has been described as a 'U-boat in the belly'[47] also leads to repair of small AAAs. AAAs are most common in the oldest and sickest patients, who are least likely to benefit from repair even if their AAA is larger than 5.5cm. The operative mortality for elective AAA repair is higher in both the USA and the UK than it was in the randomized trials from those countries.[48,49]

The incentive to repair small AAAs may be increased by the advent of endovascular grafting. The effects of endograft manufacturers seeking return on their research and development investment, radiologists seeking to expand into the market of AAA repair, and vascular surgeons resisting that expansion, will all favor repair of smaller AAAs, since these make up the great majority of AAAs. Furthermore, the mortality of endovascular AAA repair has not yet proved to be less than that of open repair, and the long-term effectiveness of the procedure remains unknown. Currently, elective AAA repair causes about 2000 deaths per year in the US, compared with 9000 for AAA rupture.[11] If screening resulted in a large number of elective repair procedures in patients whose AAA would not have ruptured, overall mortality could potentially increase.

CURRENT RECOMMENDATIONS

The Vascular Surgical Society of Great Britain and Ireland has recommended a national ultrasound screening program for AAA,[50] and a review of the periodic physical examination found abdominal palpation for AAA to be one of the few maneuvers that could be recommended for older men.[51] The Canadian Task Force on the Periodic Health Examination[52] and the US Preventive Services Task Forces (USPSTF)[53] each gave AAA screening a 'C' rating (poor evidence to include or exclude from the periodic health examination) in recommendations issued before publication of the studies cited above under 'Evidence for screening'. The Canadian Task Force report noted that abdominal palpation of men over age 60 was 'prudent' and that ultrasound 'could be considered' in obese or high-risk patients. The USPSTF plans to reconsider the AAA recommendation in the near future, presumably after the remaining ongoing randomized trials report their findings (Russell Harris MD, 2001).

CURRENT PRACTICE

Screening for AAA remains uncommon in usual practice in the US, probably because of the lack of endorsement by the USPSTF. Merenstein et al.[54] interviewed medical directors of ten health plans and found that none covered routine ultrasound screening for AAA. Legs For Life®, a program developed by the Society of

Cardiovascular and Interventional Radiology and sponsored by several endovascular graft manufacturers, added AAA screening to its national screening week for peripheral vascular disease in 2001. Approximately 50 of the 400 Legs For Life® sites in the USA offered AAA screening with ultrasound to subjects over age 60 with two of the following three risk factors: male gender, history of smoking, and family history of AAA. The AAA screening program is expected to expand to nearly all Legs For Life® sites in the next few years.

The success of a screening program depends in part on the willingness of the target group to attend. Acceptance rates for AAA screening invitations have been reported for a number of investigational programs. Community screening programs using letters sent by the patients' general practitioner have reported acceptance rates of about 75%.[7,33,55] Acceptance rates are higher at age 65 than in more elderly patients.[33,55] A lower acceptance rate of 30% was observed when letters were sent to veterans from physicians whom they did not know.[28]

EVALUATION AND FOLLOW-UP

The success of a screening program depends to a large extent on how patients are managed after the screening test. For those who test negative, being actively informed of the negative results is more reassuring than telling the patient that 'no news is good news'.[41] For patients who screen positive for AAA by ultrasound, the first consideration is whether to recommend elective repair. As noted earlier, two randomized trials have demonstrated that survival is not improved by elective repair of AAAs <5.5cm, even in good operative candidates. Therefore, asymptomatic AAAs should be considered for repair when they are ≥ 5.5cm in good surgical candidates, and repair should be further deferred in patients with high operative risk until the risk of rupture outweighs that risk in the opinion of the attending vascular surgeon. For the majority of patients with AAA detected at screening, the management plan will be periodic imaging surveillance of the AAA until the AAA diameter crosses the threshold for elective repair in that patient. The patient and family must be educated that periodic follow-up is essential to the patient's safety. Patients with unrepaired AAAs who are potential operative candidates should have AAA measurement, usually with ultrasound, annually until the AAA is within 1cm of the threshold for repair, and then every 6 months afterwards until the AAA is repaired. Variations in AAA measurement of 0.5cm or more are not uncommon, and this should be taken into account in management decisions.[56]

The natural history of AAA is usually one of progressive slow growth with the risk of rupture increasing with the size of the aneurysm. AAAs of 4.0–5.5cm enlarge at a mean rate of 0.3cm per year, with less than 25% enlarging faster than 0.5cm per year.[12,13] Less than one-third of AAAs eventually rupture, and most patients with AAAs die of other causes, especially coronary artery disease.[57] Continued smoking is associated with increased AAA growth rate[58] and possibly with an increased likelihood of rupture.[59]

COMMENT

The continued high mortality from ruptured AAAs reflects the fact that many AAAs remain undetected during the years required to enlarge to the point of rupture. At the same time, many small AAAs that are detected incidentally and would not rupture are repaired, and operative mortality remains 2–8%. Both of these situations contribute to aortic aneurysms remaining the 15th leading cause of death in the US.[10] The public's health would clearly be better served by the policy employed in Chichester, UK, whereby men are screened once with ultrasound at age 65 and elective repair is undertaken when an AAA attains a diameter of 6.0cm or greater.[34] The Chichester policy is appealing, and now that the first randomized trial has reported

significant advantages, the completion of the other ongoing studies is awaited. If all the trials demonstrate a benefit from screening, recommendations from the influential Canadian and US Task Forces will likely soon follow, and themselves be followed by local health system guidelines and performance measures, at which point the era of widespread population screening for AAA will have begun. If screening is accompanied by prudent criteria for elective repair, the mortality associated with AAA may at last be reduced.

REFERENCES

1. Schilling FJ, Hempel HF, Becker WH, Christakis G. Asymptomatic aortic aneurysms detected on the abdominal roentgenogram. Circulation 1966;33(Suppl 3):209.

2. Schilling FJ, Christakis G, Hempel HH, Orbach A. The natural history of abdominal aortic and iliac atherosclerosis as detected by lateral abdominal roentgenograms in 2663 males. J Chronic Dis 1974;27:37–45.

3. Cabellon S, Moncrief CL, Pierre DR, Cavanaugh DG. Incidence of abdominal aortic aneurysms in patients with atheromatous arterial disease. Am J Surg 1983;146:575–6.

4. Cochrane AL, Holland WW. Validation of screening procedures. Br Med Bull 1971;27:3–8.

5. Frame PS, Carlson SJ. A critical review of periodic health screening using specific screening criteria. Part 1: Selected diseases of respiratory, cardiovascular, and central nervous systems. J Fam Pract 1975;2:29–36.

6. Lederle FA, Johnson GR, Wilson SE, for the Aneurysm Detection and Management Veterans Affairs Cooperative Study. Abdominal aortic aneurysm in women. J Vasc Surg 2001;34:122–6.

7. Boll AP, Verbeek AL, van de Lisdonk EH, van der Vliet JA. High prevalence of abdominal aortic aneurysm in a primary care screening programme. Br J Surg 1998;85:1090–4.

8. Nevitt MP, Ballard DJ, Hallett JW. Prognosis of abdominal aortic aneurysms: a population-based study. N Engl J Med 1989;321:1009–14.

9. Lederle FA, Johnson GR, Wilson SE, et al, and the ADAM VA Cooperative Study Investigators. Relationship of age, gender, race, and body size to infrarenal aortic diameter. J Vasc Surg 1997;26:595–601.

10. Hoyert DL, Arias E, Smith BL, Murphy SL, Kochanek KD. Deaths: final data for 1999. Natl Vital Stat Rep 2001;49:1–113.

11. Gillum RF. Epidemiology of aortic aneurysm in the United States. J Clin Epidemiol 1995;48:1289–98.

12. The UK Small Aneurysm Trial Participants. Mortality results for randomised controlled trial of early elective surgery or ultrasonographic surveillance for small abdominal aortic aneurysms. Lancet 1998;352:1649–55.

13. Lederle FA, Wilson SE, Johnson GR, et al, for the Aneurysm Detection and Management (ADAM) Veterans Affairs Cooperative Study Investigators. Immediate repair compared with surveillance of small abdominal aortic aneurysms. N Engl J Med 2002:346:1437–44.

14. Adam DJ, Mohan IV, Stuart WP, Bain M, Bradbury AW. Community and hospital outcome from ruptured abdominal aortic aneurysm within the catchment area of a regional vascular surgical service. J Vasc Surg 1999;30:922–8.

15. Lindholt JS, Juul S, Henneberg EW, Fasting H. Is screening for abdominal aortic aneurysm acceptable to the population? Selection and recruitment to hospital-based mass screening for abdominal aortic aneurysm. J Public Health Med 1998;20:211–7.

16. Lederle FA, Walker JM, Reinke DB. Selective screening for abdominal aortic aneurysms with physical examination and ultrasound. Arch Intern Med 1988;148:1753–6.

17. Lederle FA, Simel DL. The rational clinical examination. Does this patient have abdominal aortic aneurysm? JAMA 1999;281:77–82.

18. Osler W. Aneurysm of the abdominal aorta. Lancet 1905;2:1089–96.

19. Fink HA, Lederle FA, Roth CS, Bowles CA, Nelson DB, Haas MA. The accuracy of physical examination to detect abdominal aortic aneurysm. Arch Intern Med 2000;160:833–6.

20. Nusbaum JW, Freimanis AK, Thomford NR. Echography in the diagnosis of abdominal aortic aneurysm. Arch Surg 1971;102:385–8.

21. Loughran CF. A review of the plain abdominal radiograph in acute rupture of abdominal aortic aneurysms. Clin Radiol 1986;37:383–7.

22. Roberts A, Johnson N, Royle J, Buttery B, Buxton B. The diagnosis of abdominal aortic aneurysms. Aust N Z J Surg 1974;44:360–2.

23. Lederle FA, Johnson GR, Wilson SE, et al, and the ADAM VA Cooperative Study Investigators. The Aneurysm Detection and Management Study screening program: validation cohort and final results. Arch Intern Med 2000;160:1425–30.

24. Collaborative Aneurysm Screening Study Group (CASS Group). A comparative study of the prevalence of abdominal aortic aneurysms in the United Kingdom, Denmark, and Australia. J Med Screen 2001;8:46–50.

25. Vardulaki KA, Prevost TC, Walker NM, et al. Incidence among men of asymptomatic abdominal aortic aneurysms: estimates from 500 screen detected cases. J Med Screen 1999;6:50–4.

26. Scott RA, Vardulaki KA, Walker NM, Day NE, Duffy SW, Ashton HA. The long-term benefits of a single scan for abdominal aortic aneurysm (AAA) at age 65. Eur J Vasc Endovasc Surg 2001;21:535–40.

27. Crow P, Shaw E, Earnshaw JJ, Poskitt KR, Whyman MR, Heather BP. A single normal ultrasonographic scan at age 65 years rules out significant aneurysm disease for life in men. Br J Surg 2001;88:941–4.

28. Lederle FA, Johnson GR, Wilson SE, et al, for the Aneurysm Detection and Management (ADAM) Veterans Affairs Cooperative Study Group. Prevalence and associations of abdominal aortic aneurysm detected through screening. Ann Intern Med 1997;126:441–9.

29. Spencer CA, Jamrozik K, Norman PE, Lawrence-Brown MM. The potential for a selective screening strategy for abdominal aortic aneurysm. J Med Screen 2000;7:209–11.

30. Lindholt JS, Henneberg EW, Fasting H, Juul S. Mass or high-risk screening for abdominal aortic aneurysm. Br J Surg 1997;84:40–2.

31. Lederle FA. Screening for snipers: the burden of proof. J Clin Epidemiol 1990;43:101–4.

32. Heather BP, Poskitt KR, Earnshaw JJ, Whyman M, Shaw E. Population screening reduces mortality rate from aortic aneurysm in men. Br J Surg 2000;87:750–3.

33. Wilmink TB, Quick CR, Hubbard CS, Day NE. The influence of screening on the incidence of ruptured abdominal aortic aneurysms. J Vasc Surg 1999;30:203–8.

34. Scott RA, Wilson NM, Ashton HA, Kay DN. Influence of screening on the incidence of ruptured abdominal aortic aneurysm: 5-year results of a randomized controlled study. Br J Surg 1995;82:1066–70.

35. Lindholt JS, Juul S, Fasting H, Henneberg EW. Hospital costs and benefits of screening for abdominal aortic aneurysms. Results from a randomised population screening trial. Eur J Vasc Endovasc Surg 2002;23:55–60.

35a. The Multicentre Aneurysm Screening Study Group. The Multicentre Aneurysm Screening Study (MASS) into the effect of abdominal screening on mortality in men: a randomised controlled trial. Lancet 2002; 360:1531–9.

36. Lederle FA, Johnson GR, Wilson SE, et al, and the ADAM VA Cooperative Study Investigators. Yield of repeated screening for abdominal aortic aneurysm after a four-year interval. Arch Intern Med 2000;160:1117–21.

37. Lederle FA. Looking for asymptomatic abdominal aortic aneurysms. J Gen Intern Med 1996;11:774–5.

38. Pentikainen TJ, Sipila T, Rissanen P, Soisalon-Soininen S, Salo J. Cost-effectiveness of targeted screening for abdominal aortic aneurysm. Monte Carlo-based estimates. Int J Technol Assess Health Care 2000;16:22–34.

39. Frame PS, Fryback DG, Patterson C. Screening for abdominal aortic aneurysm in men ages 60 to 80 years: a cost-effectiveness analysis. Ann Intern Med 1993;119:411–6.

40. UK Small Aneurysm Trial Participants. Health service costs and quality of life for early elective surgery or ultrasonographic surveillance for small abdominal aortic aneurysms. Lancet 1998;352:1656–60.

41. Marteau TM. Psychological costs of screening. BMJ 1989;299:527.

42. Stewart-Brown S, Farmer A. Screening could seriously damage your health. BMJ 1997;314:533–4.

43. Khaira HS, Herbert LM, Crowson MC. Screening for abdominal aortic aneurysms does not increase psychological morbidity. Ann R Coll Surg Engl 1998;80:341–2.

44. Lucarotti ME, Heather BP, Shaw E, Poskitt KR. Psychological morbidity associated with abdominal aortic aneurysm screening. Eur J Vasc Endovasc Surg 1997;14:499–501.

45. Pretre R, Turina MI. Facts, at last, on management of small infrarenal aortic aneurysms. Lancet 1998;352:1642–3.

46. Cronenwett JL, Johnston KW. The United Kingdom Small Aneurysm Trial: implications for surgical treatment of abdominal aortic aneurysms. J Vasc Surg 1999;29:191–4.

47. Santiago F. Screening for abdominal aortic aneurysms: the U-boat in the belly. JAMA 1987;258:1732.

48. Bayly PJ, Matthews JN, Dobson PM, Price ML, Thomas DG. In-hospital mortality from abdominal aortic surgery in Great Britain and Ireland: Vascular Anaesthesia Society audit. Br J Surg 2001;88:687–92.

49. Lawrence PF, Gazak C, Bhirangi L, et al. The epidemiology of surgically repaired aneurysms in the United States. J Vasc Surg 1999;30:632–40.

50. Harris PL. Reducing the mortality from abdominal aortic aneurysms: need for a national screening programme. BMJ 1992;305:697–9.

51. Oboler SK, LaForce FM. The periodic physical examination in asymptomatic adults. Ann Intern Med 1989;110:214–26.

52. Canadian Task Force on the Periodic Health Examination. Periodic health examination, 1991 update: 5. Screening for abdominal aortic aneurysm. Can Med Assoc J 1991;145:783–9.

53. U.S. Preventive Services Task Force. Guide to clinical preventive services, 2nd edn. Baltimore:Williams & Wilkins; 1996:67–72.

54. Merenstein D, Rabinowitz H, Louis DZ. Health care plan decisions regarding preventive services. Arch Fam Med 1999;8:354–6.

55. Khoo DE, Ashton H, Scott RA. Is screening once at age 65 an effective method for detection of abdominal aortic aneurysms? J Med Screen 1994;1:223–5.

56. Lederle FA, Wilson SE, Johnson GR, et al, for the Abdominal Aortic Aneurysm Detection and Management Veterans Administration Cooperative Study Group. Variability in measurement of abdominal aortic aneurysms. J Vasc Surg 1995;21:945–52.

57. Darling RC, Messina CR, Brewster DC, Ottinger LW. Autopsy study of unoperated abdominal aortic aneurysms: the case for early resection. Circulation 1977;56(Suppl 2):161–4.

58. MacSweeney ST, Ellis M, Worrell PC, Greenhalgh RM, Powell JT. Smoking and growth rate of small abdominal aortic aneurysms. Lancet 1994;344:651–2.

59. Brown LC, Powell JT. Risk factors for aneurysm rupture in patients kept under ultrasound surveillance. UK Small Aneurysm Trial Participants. Ann Surg 1999;230:289–96.

CHAPTER
30
Abdominal Aneurysms – EVAR

Marc RHM van Sambeek, Lukas C van Dijk, and Johanna M Hendriks

KEY POINTS

- Endovascular aneurysm repair (EVAR) for abdominal aortic aneurysms offers an important new alternative to open surgical procedure.

- Compared with conventional open surgery, EVAR reduces operating time, blood transfusions, intensive care requirements, and length of hospital stay.

- Reported mortality rates after EVAR are between 0% and 5%.

- Long-term reports are not available, but mid-term follow-up of EVAR reveals an incidence of re-interventions between 10% and 20% and a rate of late rupture of between 0.5 and 1.5%/year.

- The perplexing problems of endoleaks and graft failure continue to be challenges which technological innovations must address.

- Until solutions for endoleaks and stent failure are found, EVAR remains an imperfect long-term treatment and requires regular life-long graft surveillance.

- Based on the available evidence, EVAR is an appropriate treatment for selected patients, especially those at high risk for open surgical repair.

INTRODUCTION

In recent years, the interest in minimally invasive surgery has grown and the same trend can be observed in vascular surgery and interventional radiology, leading to what is commonly referred to as 'endovascular surgery'. Although the 1990s represent a decade of technological revolution, it is a mistake to consider endovascular treatment as a recent development. In 1947, João Cid dos Santos described thromboendarterectomy;[1] this technique was modified by Vollmar in 1964, to a semi-closed endarterectomy using ringstrippers.[2] In the same year, other pioneers, including Dotter and Judkins, published preliminary results on what they called 'angioplasty' of the femoropopliteal artery using co-axial catheters.[3] This technique was later modified by Grüntzig in 1974, who replaced the co-axial catheters with dilatation balloons.[4] In the early 1990s, Volodos et al. and Parodi et al. introduced endovascular treatment of abdominal aortic aneurysm (AAA) with a device composed of a Dacron graft and a Palmaz stent.[5,6]

Since the first use of a stent-graft for the endovascular exclusion of an AAA, the use of endovascular treatment of AAA has greatly expanded, and more than 50 000 devices have now been implanted. This technique is currently being evaluated in several multicenter randomized trials in Europe and the USA. Endovascular repair may prove to be an effective alternative to open surgical repair if it can produce a substantial decrease in mortality and morbidity rates.

However, the current standard treatment for an AAA remains the transabdominal open surgical approach and replacement of the aneurysmal aorta by a prosthesis. Because the procedure may cause stress to both physical and mental health, there is a decreased quality of life for an extended period of time after the operation.

With endovascular treatment of AAA, a laparotomy is not required. The endovascular graft can be implanted from a remote access site in the groin with less anesthetic requirement. The endovascular graft is advanced over guidewires up the femoral and iliac arteries. Once in position, the graft is deployed immediately distal from the renal arteries. The aorta is not clamped, and the blood loss is less than with open surgery.

Many terms are used to describe the prostheses that are implanted during an endovascular procedure; these include: endovascular graft, stent-graft, grafted stent, endoprosthesis, transluminally placed endovascular graft (TPEG), endograft, and many others. The graft material creates a barrier that excludes the AAA, and the stent or metallic ultrastructures positions the graft precisely, without the need for a surgical anastomosis. At the same time, the stent provides a certain level of support. Most major companies that manufacture endovascular products are producing and distributing aortic stent-grafts. Some of the older models have already been removed from the market, and most have undergone one or more revisions.

PATIENT SELECTION AND PREOPERATIVE IMAGING

Not all patients with an AAA are suitable for endovascular repair. Pre-procedural assessment must reject unsuitable patients, identify potential difficulties, and allow selection of an appropriate stent-graft. The main criteria for patient selection apply to anatomic details of the vascular tree between the renal arteries and the external iliac artery. Endovascular repair of the aorta (EVAR) brings many new challenges for preoperative imaging. Unlike the case with conventional surgery, with endovascular repair the anatomic configuration of the infrarenal aorta must be known to a high degree of accuracy. Regardless of which kind of stent-graft is to be used, a similar series of measurements must be obtained for each patient. Every company, every study, and every registry has its own worksheet that can be filled out to record the most relevant details. One of the most commonly used is the worksheet from the Eurostar registry (**Fig. 30.1**).[7]

The most common reasons to reject a patient, based on anatomic configurations are listed below.

Visceral supply

Patency of the celiac axis and superior mesenteric artery should be assessed before a patent inferior mesenteric artery can be over-stented. Renal arteries and accessory renal arteries should be identified.

Diameter of proximal neck

Depending on the device used, an infrarenal neck with a diameter of more than 28–29mm is considered unsuitable. All stent-grafts need to achieve a seal between the device and the aortic wall. Usually, the stent-graft is oversized by 10–20% compared with the diameter of the proximal neck. The largest commercially available stent-grafts are 31mm in diameter.

Length of proximal neck

To achieve a good seal between the stent-graft and the aortic wall, a snug apposition over a length of 10–15mm is required.

Angulation of the proximal neck

Angulation of the proximal neck is not uncommon and is more often seen with larger aneurysms (>60mm). Aortic neck angulation appears to be an important determinant of outcome after EVAR. Mild angulation (<40°) is associated with favorable outcome, whereas those with moderate (40–59°) and severe (>60°) angulation have a higher risk of adverse events, especially type I endoleaks.[8]

Conical nature of the proximal neck

A contour change of the proximal neck of more than 10% is associated with a higher proximal endoleak rate, and therefore considered unfavorable (**Fig. 30.2**).[9]

Calcification and mural thrombus in proximal neck

Calcification and mural thrombus in the proximal neck are expressed in degrees of circumference. Mural thrombus in the neck over more than 90° is considered a risk factor for endoleak, whereas extended calcification will increase the probability of stent-graft migration.

Diameter of iliac artery

In general, the stent-graft will end in the common iliac artery. Therefore, there is a size limitation toward the diameter of the common iliac artery, depending on the device used. If the diameter of the common iliac artery is too large, the stent-graft can be extended to the external iliac artery. In such a case, it is advisable to coil-embolize the hypogastric artery, since retrograde flow from the hypogastric artery can cause an endoleak.

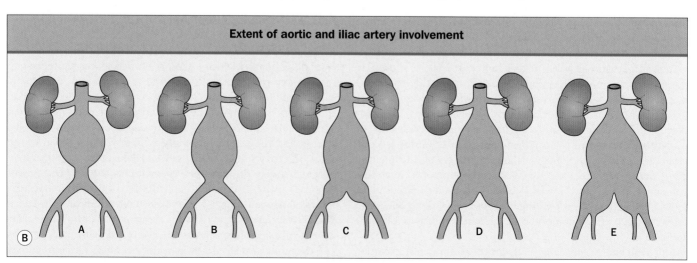

Figure 30.1 Endovascular repair of the aorta (A) Worksheet for documentation of diameters and length measurements for abdominal aortic aneurysms. (B) Worksheet for documentation of iliac artery involvement.

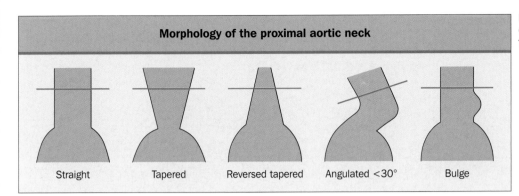

Figure 30.2 Worksheet for documentation of the morphology of the proximal aortic neck.

Morphology of the proximal aortic neck

Straight   Tapered   Reversed tapered   Angulated <30°   Bulge

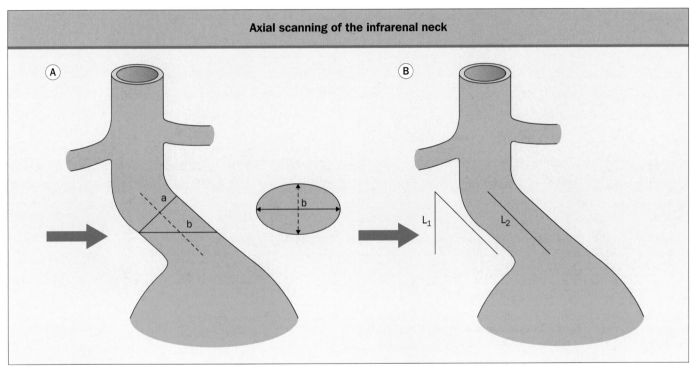

Axial scanning of the infrarenal neck

Figure 30.3 Axial scanning of the infrarenal neck. (A) With axial scanning of an angulated infrarenal neck, the neck may appear elliptical. Assessment of the largest diameter includes overestimation of the 'real' diameter. (B) With axial scanning the length of the infrarenal neck (L1) includes an underestimation of the 'real' length (L2).

Length of distal sealing zone

In a similar way to the proximal sealing zone, a snug apposition over a length of 10–15mm is required.

Tortuosity of iliac arteries

The introducer systems are large (16–28F in diameter) and relatively inflexible. If the iliac arteries are small, calcified, and tortuous, it will be difficult for the delivery system to pass without causing damage to the iliac tract. There are no strict criteria in this matter and a decision should be made based on diameter and flexibility of the delivery system and the surgeon's experience.

Almost all imaging modalities have been used in the diagnostic work-up of a patient. Ultrasound is most commonly used to establish the diagnosis of an AAA. Spiral computed tomography angiography (CTA) is used in most centers to categorize patients as suitable or unsuitable for EVAR and to assess the diameters at several levels. Longitudinal measurements of the aorta may be made from calibrated angiography.

Spiral CTA

High-quality contrast-enhanced CTA is essential and is currently the imaging technique of choice for EVAR. It provides detailed information on vascular anatomy and thus helps in selecting suitable patients and the right stent-graft. The patient should not have oral contrast as this may interfere with three-dimensional (3D) reconstructions. The scan must image from the celiac axis to the common femoral artery. CTA protocols vary considerably, but most require a large volume of iodinated contrast agent (100–150mL), narrow collimation (3–5mm) and reformatting of overlapping axial slices at short (2–4mm) intervals.

There is a potential pitfall when assessing axial scans. As the aorta expands, it can also lengthen. This can cause the aneurysm neck to deviate anteriorly and laterally. Axial scanning does not take this into account, and the neck or aneurysm may appear oval rather than round in cross-section. This can result in a tendency to overestimate the neck diameter and underestimate the neck length (**Fig. 30.3**). Mistakes in assessment can be overcome with image processing on a workstation. Curved linear

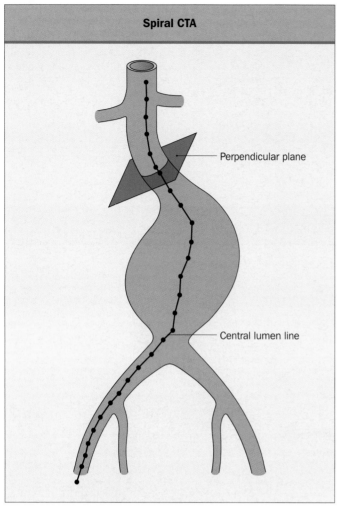

Spiral CTA

Perpendicular plane

Central lumen line

Figure 30.4 Spiral CTA. Curved linear reformats (created by imaging processing on a workstation) allow visualization in a plane perpendicular to the central lumen line. Oblique projections are avoided.

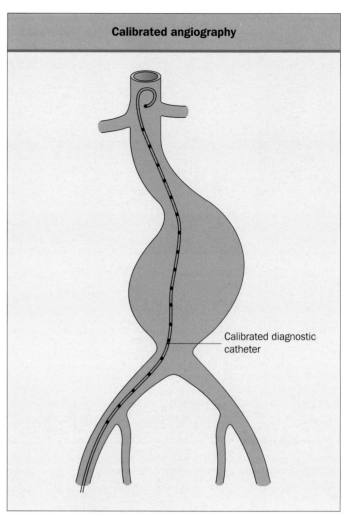

Calibrated angiography

Calibrated diagnostic catheter

Figure 30.5 Calibrated angiography.

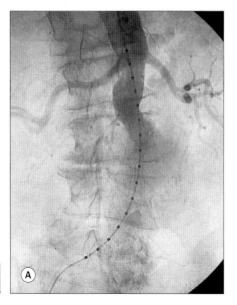

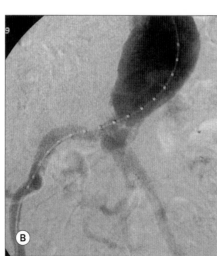

Figure 30.6 Calibrated angiography of a patient with abdominal aortic aneursym (AAA). A pigtail catheter with markers at 1cm intervals is positioned in the AAA. Because of the large volume of the AAA, assessment is performed in several runs.

reformats (CLR) can be used for accurate assessment of the diameters and length of the potential attachment zones in the aorta and iliac arteries. Unlike axial CT images, CLR allow visualization of the aortic and iliac lumen in a plane perpendicular to the central arterial axis. By avoiding oblique projection, the images represent the true cross-sectional shape of the aorta. CLRs perpendicular to the vessel axis can be acquired using central lumen lines, which can be created by positioning markers in the center of the aorta and iliac arteries at several levels (**Fig. 30.4**).[10]

Arterial angiography

Arterial angiography can provide additional information. It is superior to CTA in the assessment of the grade of stenosis of major branches of the aorta. By itself, it is insufficient for patient selection because thrombus in the aneurysm and arteriosclerotic disease of the arterial wall are not displayed.

A 5F pigtail catheter with markers at 1cm intervals is placed in the aneurysm and angiography performed by injecting 20mL contrast at 10mL/second, imaging at 2 frames/second (**Figs 30.5 & 30.6**). Anterior neck angulation causes considerable fore-shortening of the neck in the anteroposterior projection, and the markers will be aligned very close to each other. The catheter does not follow the center lumen line, and when assessing length measurements, this should be taken into account, especially in an angulated aneurysm.

If the arteries are very tortuous and not too calcified during the angiography, one can try to straighten the iliac artery by passing a super-stiff guidewire through the pigtail catheter. If the wire will not pass or the artery does not straighten, a stent-graft delivery is unlikely to succeed.

Magnetic resonance angiography

Like spiral CTA, magnetic resonance angiography (MRA) can produce multiplanar two-dimensional and 3D images. Although MRA is currently inferior to spiral CTA regarding spatial resolution, and is technically demanding and time-consuming, it certainly has advantages worthy of mention. For example, the patient is not exposed to ionizing radiation or nephrotoxic contrast. MRA cannot be used in all patients. Approximately 10–15% of patients are claustrophobic or have metal implants that make it impossible to use MRA.

SELECTION OF A STENT-GRAFT

The minimally invasive therapeutic option of treatment of an AAA is of great interest to various medical specialties, including cardiovascular surgery, interventional radiology, and interventional cardiology. Each year, approximately 50 000 patients undergo open repair for AAA in the USA alone. With such a large potential market, most of the important companies that manufacture endovascular products now produce and distribute stent-grafts.

Various materials have been tested, and all the major producers now use the two materials most frequently used in surgery, including polyester weaves and polytetrafluoroethylene (PTFE). Ideally, if stent-grafts are to provide the advantages they potentially offer over conventional surgery, they must have certain characteristics (**Table 30.1**).[11] Each device must have

Characteristics of the ideal stent-graft.	
Low overall cost	User-friendliness
Stent-graft size range	Column strength
Durability (metallic ultrastructure + graft material)	Sealing capacity
Biocompatibility	Radio-opacity
Sealing capacity	Low thrombogenicity
Lowest delivery device size	Lowest delivery device profile
Delivery device flexibility	Delivery device reliability
Radial force stability	Excellent apposition of graft
Customization	

Table 30.1 Characteristics of the ideal stent-graft.

as many of these characteristics as possible to warrant a safe implantation, high rates of immediate technical success, and excellent long-term clinical success.

Following the early use of improvised, non-commercial endovascular grafts for AAA, a number of commercially produced endovascular grafts are now available (**Table 30.2**).[12]

Components of endovascular devices
Delivery systems

Stent-grafts are delivered in the vascular tree using introducer sheaths, trocars, deployment capsules, and retractable covers. The profile of the introducer sheaths must be small enough to pass through the iliac tract, without causing vascular damage. However, the introducer sheaths must be wide enough for easy passage of the stent-graft, rigid enough to resist kinking, and flexible enough to follow the angulations in the iliac arteries. A hemostatic valve is mandatory.

Graft material

The graft material must be strong enough to resist late deterioration, damage due to friction with metallic parts of the stent, and yet thin enough to be compressed in a small delivery catheter. In most stent-grafts, conventional polyester has been preferred. Over time, companies have started using thinner polyester variations in order to downsize the profile of the delivery systems. PTFE is an alternative graft material that is currently used in the Excluder endograft and Powerlink endograft. Other materials such as polycarbonate, polyurethane, and other polymers are under investigation.

Graft attachment systems

Graft attachment systems can be divided into two groups, according to whether they are deployed by self-expandable or balloon expanding stents. Vascular stents can be constructed from stainless steel, elgiloy, tantalum, or nitinol. Friction with the vessel wall is the main mechanism of attachment, but hooks, anchors, and barbs are used in addition to secure a better fixation and seal inside the artery.

Name (Company)	Graft material	Stent material	Introducer size (OD)	Device composition	Expansion	Fixation
Ancure (Guidant)	Polyester	Elgiloy	22F	Unibody	Self-expanding	Hooks
AneuRx (Medtronic AVE)	Polyester	Nitinol	22F	Modular	Self-expanding	Friction
Talent (Medtronic AVE)	Polyester	Nitinol	18–22F	Modular	Self-expanding	Friction + juxta renal bare stent
Excluder (WL Gore)	PTFE	Nitinol	18F	Modular	Self-expanding	Friction + hooks
Zenith (Cook)	Polyester	Stainless steel	22F	Modular	Self-expanding	Hooks + juxta renal bare stent
LifePath (Edwards Lifesc.)	Polyester	Elgiloy	22F	Modular	Balloon-expandable	Friction + crimps
PowerLink (Endologix)	PTFE	Stainless steel	18–20F	Unibody	Self-expandable	Friction
Quantum LP (Cordis)	Polyester	Nitinol	22F	Modular	Self-expandable	Hooks + juxta renal bare stent

Available endovascular grafts.

Table 30.2 Available endovascular grafts. OD, outside diameter; PTFE, polytetrafluoroethylene.

Deployment accessories

Regular tools of interventional radiology are essential accessories for a successful stent-graft placement. Among these are floppy to super-stiff guidewires, angiographic and guiding catheters, dilatation balloons, snares, and power injectors.

Various structural differences between the different devices are potentially associated with both beneficial and deleterious effects. While most of these structural differences are considered to be important, until now there has been no evidence as to whether they are beneficial or not. Polyester weaves are claimed to be stronger materials than PTFE, especially in contact with the metallic skeleton. However, PTFE has a lower thrombogenicity, is thinner, and has a better graft apposition.[13] Another issue is the use of a metallic exo- or endoskeleton (stent frame at the outside or inside of the graft). Whereas an exoskeleton might be associated with better embedding into the vessel wall, with better fixation of the graft, an endoskeleton might have the advantage of better graft apposition to the wall and less potential turbulence. There is also an ongoing discussion concerning the unibody and modular design of stent-grafts. A unibody design may give rise to better overall stent-graft stability, with no risk of dislodgement of any components, and bearing a closer resemblance to surgical grafts. Modular designs have the advantage of increased size combinations and the possibility of 'tailoring' the stent-graft during the procedure. Suprarenal fixation will create a better fixation of the stent-graft and therefore decreases the risk of stent-graft migration. This technique could be particularly useful when the aortic neck is short, or has unfavorable features such as irregular shape, mural thrombus, or extensive calcification. Opponents of suprarenal fixation fear a more complicated procedure in case of a conversion.[14] To date, there is no evidence that suprarenal fixation is associated with a higher incidence of renal infarction.[15]

TECHNIQUE OF ENDOVASCULAR REPAIR

Endovascular repair of an AAA can be performed in the operating theater, radiologic angiosuite, or catheterization laboratory under general, regional, and even local anesthesia. The choice of one of these locations is subjective, and is influenced by the preference of the interventionist. If the procedure is not performed in an operating theater, it should meet the standards of hygiene and sterility associated with the latter.

Radiologic requirements

Minimum radiologic requirements for fluoroscopy are a mobile C-arm image intensifier with possibilities for cine loop angiography, digital subtraction, road-map, and frame-by-frame replay. Ceiling or floor mounted fluoroscopy equipment has several advantages over the portable image intensifier. Most important are better field size/spatial resolution ratio and a suitable radiolucent table that can be adjusted to the fluoroscopic field.

The typical aorta at the infrarenal level has a slight anterior angulation (10–15°) due to lordosis of the lumbar vertebrae. This angulation is more pronounced in the majority of patients with AAA (the angle can vary from 10° to 60°), because the aneurysm raises the aorta from the vertebral column. Fluoroscopy with the C-arm in the AP position produces projection errors and this may lead to less optimal or inaccurate placement of the stent-graft in the infrarenal aortic neck (**Fig. 30.7**).[16,17] In addition to an angulation of the C-arm, sometimes a rotation of the C-arm is required for optimal projection of the orifice of the renal arteries. It is essential to have aortic angulation and rotation data available preoperatively. Only lateral angiograms or CTA reconstructions can give an indication of neck angulation.

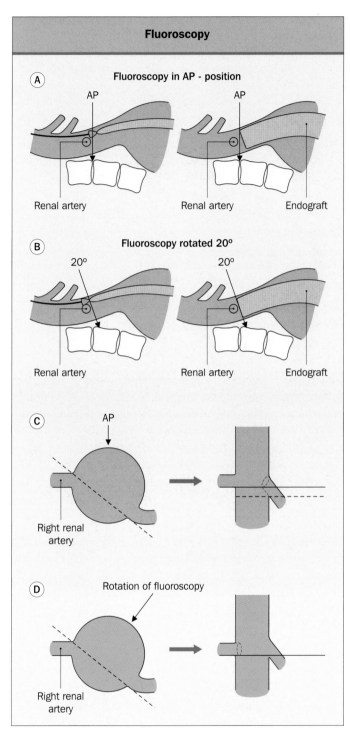

Fluoroscopy

A Fluoroscopy in AP - position

AP AP

Renal artery Renal artery Endograft

B Fluoroscopy rotated 20°

20° 20°

Renal artery Renal artery Endograft

C AP

Right renal artery

D Rotation of fluoroscopy

Right renal artery

Figure 30.7 Fluoroscopy. Fluoroscopy in the AP position produces projection errors which could lead to less accurate placement of the stent-graft in the infrarenal aortic neck (A & C). Angulation and rotation of the C-arm may be required for optimal projection (B & D) of the infrarenal neck and renal artery orifice.

Operating team

The patient should be positioned on a radiolucent operating table and draped for emergent open repair in the event of failed endovascular repair or occurrence of complications needing conversion.

The locations of the operating team and fluoroscopy equipment are illustrated in **Figure 30.8**. An endovascular procedure

should be performed by at least two interventionists and one scrub nurse/radiology technician. There should be two monitors, so that both interventionists have an unobstructed view of a monitor. Since the delivery devices are long (usually longer than 100cm), long guidewires are required. Therefore, it is advisable to extend the operating table with an extension table to enable safe manipulation of the devices.

Graft insertion

The common femoral artery in the ipsilateral groin is exposed through a surgical cut-down, and intravenous heparin is given to the patient. A 6–8F introducer sheath is inserted and a flexible guidewire is positioned in the suprarenal aorta. With the use of a (straight) diagnostic catheter, the flexible guidewire is exchanged for a super-stiff guidewire, which is positioned in the descending aorta. At the same time, another introducer sheath (6–8F) is inserted into the contralateral common femoral artery, either percutaneously or through a groin cut-down. With the use of a flexible guidewire, a pigtail catheter is positioned at the level of the renal arteries. The introducer sheath in the ipsilateral common femoral artery is removed and a transverse arteriotomy is performed in such a way that the super-stiff guidewire is situated within the arteriotomy. A large introducer sheath (depending on the device used) or the catheter and stent-graft within it are introduced under fluoroscopic control until the superior end of the prosthesis is at the assumed level of the renal arteries. If necessary, the image intensifier is angulated and rotated, and moved to place the superior end of the stent-graft in the center of the field, in order to eliminate errors caused by parallax. Magnification can be advantageous in identifying the superior end of the stent-graft in relation to the orifice of the renal arteries. At this time, the first aortogram is performed with the use of a power injector by injecting 20mL contrast at 10mL/second, imaging at two frames/second. Rotation of the stent-graft and repositioning can be performed. It is usually necessary to perform several aortograms in order to properly position the stent-graft.

Once it has been ascertained that the stent-graft is in the optimal position, immediately distal from the renal arteries, the pigtail catheter is pulled distally (**Fig. 30.9**). The trunk and ipsilateral limb of the stent-graft can be deployed under fluoroscopic control. If balloon dilatation of the proximal and distal attachment side is required, this will be performed at this time. After dilatation, a guidewire from the contralateral femoral artery is directed into the short contralateral stump of the stent-graft. This can usually be achieved with a 'free-style' catheterization using an angled guiding catheter. If difficulty is experienced, a guidewire can be passed from the ipsilateral side, through the ipsilateral limb of the stent-graft, and, with the aid of a 'cross-over' guiding catheter, over the bifurcation in the contralateral short limb into the aneurysm sac. With a snare catheter from the contralateral femoral artery, the guidewire can be retrieved. An approach from the brachial artery can also be used if the 'free-style' catheterization of the short contralateral stump fails. The brachial approach can also be used in the case of extreme tortuosity in the iliac tract. After retrieval of the brachial wire with the snare catheter, tension can be applied at the brachial and femoral ends. This technique of 'body-flossing' results in considerable straightening of the iliac arteries.

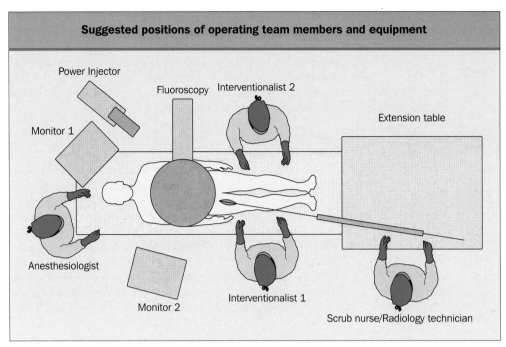

Figure 30.8 Suggested positions of operating team members and equipment.

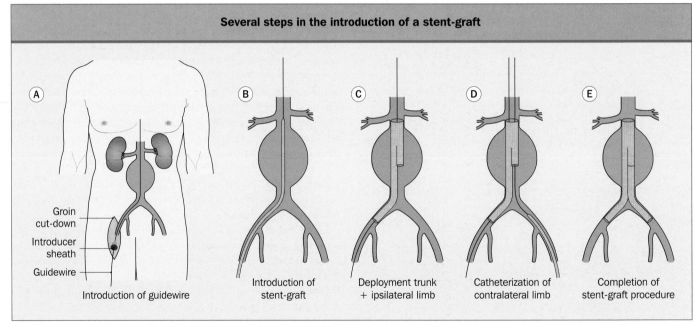

Figure 30.9 Several steps in the introduction of a stent-graft. (A) After a cut-down in the groin, a guidewire is introduced through an introducer sheath. (B) The delivery system is positioned under fluoroscopic control. (C) The trunk and ipsilateral limb is deployed. (D) Catheterization of the contralateral stump and introduction of the contralateral limb. (E) Deployment of contralateral limb and completion of stent-graft procedure.

After cannulation of the contralateral short stump, the guidewire is exchanged for a super-stiff guidewire. The 6–8F introducer sheath is exchanged for a larger sheath and the contralateral limb is directed under fluoroscopic control to a position within, and overlapping, the contralateral stump. The position of the hypogastric artery can be assessed by regular angiography or retrograde angiography through the introducer sheath. The contralateral limb is deployed under fluoroscopic control. The overlapping attachment site and distal attachment site can be dilated.

A pigtail catheter is reintroduced, and a post-intervention digital subtraction aortogram is performed several times for the detection of the presence of extravasation of contrast, which can indicate an endoleak. Stent-graft limbs and iliac arteries are examined for kinking or twisting.

The technique for introduction and deployment differs for every individual stent-graft, and discussion on these differences is beyond the scope of this chapter. For individual techniques of introduction and deployment, the reader is referred to the relevant specialized manuals.

PERIOPERATIVE COMPLICATIONS

Injuries to access arteries

Damage to the access vessels can easily occur due to the passage of large-bore catheters, containing stent-grafts. This may result in rupture, particularly in tortuous and diseased iliac arteries. One should be aware that the large catheter can have a tamponading effect, and the bleeding may only become apparent after removal of the catheter. Newer stent-grafts can be introduced through iliac arteries with a high degree of tortuosity and in the presence of extensive circumferential calcification. Visceral organs can be damaged by an uncontrolled introduction of (stiff) guidewires into the renal and suprarenal arteries. Therefore, it is mandatory that guidewires and catheters are only introduced under fluoroscopic control.

Embolization

Manipulation of endovascular devices within the aneurysm sac can result in microembolization and death from renal failure.[18] Every effort should be made to reduce catheter and balloon manipulations at the renal and suprarenal level, especially when mural thrombus is present at the renal and suprarenal level.

Distal embolization resulting in ischemia is also a recognized complication. Dislodgement of emboli from the mural thrombus in the aneurysm sac can be prevented by the use of stiff guidewires. Using the latter, the delivery device will follow the guidewires more easily, with a reduced risk of impinging on the mural thrombus.

Post-implant syndrome

Post-implant syndrome is characterized by febris eci (up to 40°C), general depression, and sometimes back pain. There is no leukocytosis or other signs of infection. Symptoms can last up to 10 days. The cause is unknown, and the incidence may be as high as 50%.[19] The post-implant syndrome is probably associated with thrombosis within the aneurysm sac. In general, it is considered benign: some consider it to be a favorable sign, signifying thrombosis of the aneurysm sac and complete exclusion of the aneurysm.

Groin and wound complications

Numerous groin and wound complications can occur and these complications are outlined in **Table 30.3**.

Post-operative mortality

It is generally accepted that EVAR represents a suitable treatment strategy for patients unfit for conventional open surgery. The option of having a less invasive treatment choice has been accepted favorably by the medical community and has been gaining consensus since its introduction. EVAR can be undertaken under local anesthesia; it can reduce operative risk and shorten recovery time. Mortality and morbidity increase in patients with significant co-morbidities and in the elderly population.

Comparative studies on mortality with EVAR and conventional open surgery have been carried out in single centers in the form of case control studies, and concurrent single or multicentric prospective non-randomized comparisons. The most published series report similar intraoperative mortality rates after EVAR and open repair (**Table 30.4**).[20–27]

Groin and wound complications.
(Post)operative bleeding
Access site hematoma
Access site false aneurysm
Access site lymphocele, lymphorrhea, lymphedema
Wound infection

Table 30.3 Groin and wound complications.

Comparative results after EVAR and conventional open repair.				
Author	Journal (year)	EVAR Mortality (%)	Open repair Mortality (%)	P
Brewster DC	J Vasc Surg (1998)	0	0	NS
Goldstone J	Proceedings (1998)	1.1	3.8	NS
May J	J Vasc Surg (1998)	5.6	5.6	NS
Zarins CK	J Vasc Surg (1999)	2.6	0	NS
De Virgilio C	Arch Surg (1999)	3.6	4.7	NS
Beebe HG	J Vasc Surg (2001)	1.5	3.1	NS
May J	J Vasc Surg (2001)	2.7	5.9	NS
Zarins CK	Proceedings (2001)	0.5	3.5	<0.05

Table 30.4 Comparative results after EVAR and conventional open repair. NS, not significant.

ENDOLEAK AND LATE COMPLICATIONS

Endoleak

Endoleak is a condition associated with endovascular stent-grafts, defined by persistent blood flow outside the lumen of the stent-graft but within the aneurysm sac or adjacent vascular segment being treated by the stent-graft.[28,29] An endoleak is evidence of incomplete exclusion of the aneurysm from the circulation. There is evidence that an endoleak may resolve spontaneously, but a proportion of those that do persist are associated with late aneurysm rupture.[30–32] Although intrasac pressure may approach systemic arterial pressure in the presence of an endoleak, some type II endoleaks have been associated with a decrease in aneurysm volume and intrasac pressures that are substantially less than systemic pressures.[33]

An endoleak can be classified according to the time of occurrence.[28] An endoleak first observed during the perioperative (<30 days) period is defined as a 'primary endoleak', and detection thereafter is termed a 'secondary endoleak'. Further categorization requires precise information regarding the course of the blood flow into the aneurysm sac (**Fig. 30.10**).[34]

A type I endoleak is indicative of a persistent perigraft channel of blood flow caused by inadequate seal at either the proximal (I-a) or distal (I-b) stent-graft end or attachment zones. In the case of an aorto-mono-iliac prosthesis, a type I endoleak may also refer to blood flow around an iliac occluder plug (I-c).

417

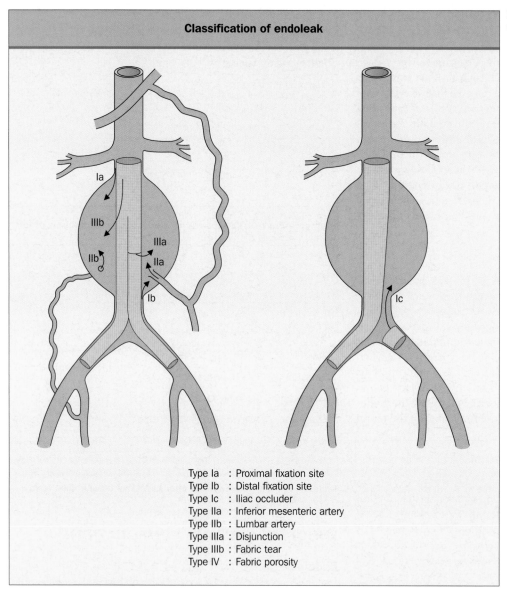

Classification of endoleak

Type Ia : Proximal fixation site
Type Ib : Distal fixation site
Type Ic : Iliac occluder
Type IIa : Inferior mesenteric artery
Type IIb : Lumbar artery
Type IIIa : Disjunction
Type IIIb : Fabric tear
Type IV : Fabric porosity

Figure 30.10 Classification of endoleak.

A *type II* endoleak is attributed to retrograde flow from the inferior mesenteric artery (II-a), lumbar arteries (II-b), or other collateral vessels. Origin and outflow sources of a type II endoleak should be specified, such as lumbar-lumbar, lumbar-inferior mesenteric artery (IMA), accessory renal-lumbar/IMA, hypogastric-lumbar/IMA, or undefined. It should be emphasized that any connection with a proximal or distal attachment zone will classify the endoleak as a type I endoleak.

A *type III* endoleak is caused by component disconnection (III-a) or fabric tear, fabric disruption, or graft disintegration (III-b). Type III-b endoleak can be further stratified as minor (<2mm) or major (>2mm).

A *type IV* endoleak is caused by blood flow through an intact but otherwise porous fabric, observed during the first 30 days after stent-graft implantation. This definition is not applicable to fabric-related endoleaks observed after the first 30-day period.

If an endoleak is visualized in imaging studies but the precise source cannot be determined, the endoleak is categorized as an endoleak of undefined origin.

It is recognized that an AAA can continue to enlarge after endovascular repair, even in the absence of a detectable endoleak, and that this enlargement may lead to aneurysm rupture. This phenomenon is currently defined as 'endotension'.[35,36] Explanations for persistent or recurrent pressurization of an aneurysm sac include blood flow that is below the sensitivity limits of detection with current imaging modalities or pressure transmission through thrombus or stent-graft material.[37–39]

The incidence of endoleak has been reported as between 10% and 44%.[40–42] If left untreated, an endoleak may seal spontaneously by thrombosis. This occurred in almost 50% of the cases reported by Moore, resulting in a permanent endoleak rate of approximately 20%.[40] Spontaneous sealing of an endoleak will result in a decrease in the size of the aneurysm sac. Conversely, the size of an AAA can increase when a secondary endoleak develops in a previously excluded AAA after endovascular repair. Type II endoleaks are more likely to seal than types I or III endoleaks. It has also been suggested that an AAA with a type II endoleak is less likely to rupture. This assumption is dangerous, since late ruptures of AAA treated with a stent-graft and with a type II endoleak have been reported. However, persistent types I and III endoleaks are more prone to cause a rupture following an endograft.[30]

Endoleaks may be managed by (1) observation, (2) a further endovascular procedure, (3) endoscopic treatment, and (4) conversion.

As some endoleaks seal spontaneously, the majority of interventionists are prepared to disregard endoleaks despite the knowledge that aneurysm rupture may occur. Although there is no proof that spontaneous sealing of an endoleak by thrombosis decreases pressure within the aneurysm sac, there is some evidence that this is the case, as a reduction in the diameter of treated aneurysms has been observed. The duration of the observation period varies according to the size of the aneurysm and the interventionist's personal experience and preference.

Type I endoleaks can be treated by secondary endoluminal interventions. A balloon dilatation, to compress the device against the vessel wall, is the most appropriate first step. If this fails, application of a 'giant' Palmaz stent is likely to be successful in resolving a proximal endoleak if the stent-graft has been positioned correctly. If migration of the proximal or distal attachment occurs, or when these fixations are in a less than optimal position, a secondary intervention to extend the stent-graft with an extension cuff is indicated. The same procedure can be performed in the case of type III endoleaks. Surgical band ligature has been used, and involves open exposure and placement of an external ligature around the proximal attachment site.[43] Although this technique necessitates a laparotomy or endoscopic approach, it is less disturbing hemodynamically than conversion in high-risk patients with a type I endoleak.

Type II endoleaks arising from the lumbar arteries or IMA may be treated by coil embolization with super-selective catheterization of the superior gluteal artery or superior mesenteric artery. The aneurysm can also be punctured by the translumbar or transperitoneal route. In this way, thrombogenic material can be injected directly into the aneurysm.

Retroperitoneal endoscopic ligation of the IMA and all lumbar arteries remains a popular alternative for the treatment of persistent type II endoleaks if the lesser invasive possibilities are not applicable or have failed.[44]

The perplexing problems of endoleaks will continue to be a challenge to the success of EVAR and will have to be addressed aggressively. Until solutions for endoleaks are found, EVAR will remain an imperfect long-term treatment and continued follow-up will be mandatory.[45]

Graft limb thrombosis

First-generation stent-grafts with unsupported fabric were prone to thrombosis of the limbs of the graft, due to kinking and twisting within the native arteries. This problem required primary stenting during the initial procedure or a secondary procedure to reopen or expand a limb in the iliac artery.[46] The problem can also occur in stent-grafts with full support of the limbs. Successful EVAR results in a reduction in the size of the AAA, both in length and in transverse diameter. The morphologic changes in the AAA may lead to kinking of the previously straight limbs, with possible progression to thrombosis. X-ray studies in AP and lateral planes are required at regular intervals to identify the problem of kinking in supported limbs and to prevent graft limb thrombosis. With unsupported limbs, a color flow duplex ultrasonography may be required to identify the problem.

Stent-graft infection

To date, there have been no published reports of infection of endovascular stent-grafts placed in the aorta. There has been one report of the development of an aortoenteric fistula after EVAR.[47] Anecdotal reports of a few infected endovascular stent-grafts have been made by oral communication. Over the last 6 years, stent-grafts have been used on a larger scale. The apparent low incidence of infection at this stage may suggest that the devices are more resistant to infection than conventional grafts placed by open surgery.

Device failure

One of the negative aspects of EVAR is the unknown long-term outcome. The durability of prostheses in the long term is, as yet, unknown. Despite extensive pre-marketing fatigue testing of stent-grafts, reports of structural failure throughout a wide range of device types continue to be noted with some frequency, including fractures of nitinol frames and elgiloy hooks, and disruption of stent-graft fabrics within 4 years of implantation (**Table 30.5**). Many patients who underwent EVAR with one of the first generation devices are currently encountering serious complications requiring surgical explantation.[48] Some of the first generation devices have in fact been taken off the market, and some of the encountered problems solved by using another choice of materials or a complete redesign of the stent-graft or delivery systems.

Device failure.		
Prosthesis (Manufacturer)	Device failure	Action or current status
EVT (Endovasc Techn)	Hook fractures	Problem solved
Stentor (Mintec)	Fabric defects Seam failures	Off the market
Vanguard (Boston Scientific)	Fabric defects Tie breaks Metal disintegration	Off the market Re-design
AneuRx (Medtronic AVE)	Microleaks Modular dislocation	Problem solved
LifePath (Baxter)	Wireform fractures	Problem solved
Talent (Medtronic AVE)	Wireform fractures	
Ancure (Guidant)	Delivery catheter	Problem solved
Excluder (WL Gore)	Wireform fractures in thoracic device	Re-design

Table 30.5 Device failure.

Dilatation of the proximal neck

Morphologic characteristics of the proximal neck influence the effectiveness of aneurysm exclusion and the durability of the stent-graft attachment. Gradual dilatation of the aorta at the level of the attachment systems may cause an endoleak and stent-graft migration. Studies in healthy people have shown that the infrarenal aortic diameter increases approximately 25% between the age of 25 and 70 years.[49] After conventional AAA repair, higher rates of increase have been described.[50-52]

Some studies have shown dilatation of the proximal neck following endovascular repair.[53-57] Two possible explanations can be given for the continued growth of the infrarenal neck after endovascular repair. It can be a continuation of the aneurysmal process or an effect of the outward force generated by the endovascular stent onto the aortic wall. If the outward force is the predominant cause of postoperative neck dilatation, the diameter will probably not stretch beyond the nominal stent size.

Late rupture

The most significant outcome measure of EVAR is the absence of abdominal aortic aneurysm rupture. Prevention of rupture is the reason for which EVAR is undertaken. A recently published large series of patients treated with EVAR reported late rupture rates up to 1.5% per year.[58-61] Multivariate analysis of risk factors for rupture has identified only three that are statistically significant: 1) the last diameter measurement of the aneurysm (relative risk: 1.057); 2) mid-graft endoleak (relative risk: 7.5); and 3) stent-graft migration (relative risk: 5.3).[59] Type I endoleak was a significant risk factor for late rupture on univariate analysis but dropped out on multivariate analysis, indicating that late type I endoleaks are usually secondary to migration.

A number of the reported late ruptures in all mentioned studies occurred in compassionate cases treated with first generation devices. On the basis of a decreasing trend, one can hypothesize that, with new generation devices and meticulous follow-up with 'state-of-art' imaging, concerns of rupture may lessen.

QUALITY OF LIFE

The long-term effects of EVAR on cognitive function and quality of life are not known. Patients treated with EVAR exhibit better physical and functional scores in the first weeks to months after intervention. They also return to baseline status significantly earlier than the conventional open surgery group.[62-64] The studies carried out document the temporary advantage of EVAR on quality of life.

ECONOMICS

EVAR is a less invasive method for the treatment of AAA compared to conventional open surgery. The potential benefits of EVAR include increased patient acceptance, less resource utilization, and, hopefully, cost saving. The cost-effectiveness of this technology is critically dependent on the potential to reduce morbidity and mortality rates, relative to conventional open surgery. EVAR is expensive due to the high cost of the devices and the need for close post-intervention surveillance and secondary interventions. The main possibility for cost savings is

Is EVAR cost-effective?		
Author	*Journal (year)*	
Holzenbein J	Eur J Vasc Endovasc Surg (1997)	Yes
Ceelen W	Acta Chir Belg (1999)	Equal
Patel SW	J Vasc Surg (1999)	Yes
Seiwert AJ	Am J Surg (1999)	Equal
Quinones WJ	J Vacs Surg (1999)	No
Sternbergh WC	J Vasc Surg (2000)	No
Clair DG	J Vasc Surg (2000)	No
Birch SE	Aus NZJ Surg (2000)	No
Turnipseed W	J Vasc Surg (2001)	No
Bosch JL	Radiology (2001)	No

Table 30.6 Is EVAR cost-effective?

reduced requirements for blood transfusion, shorter intensive care unit (ICU) and hospital stay, a lower 30-day mortality, and a lower systemic/remote complication rate.

Several studies have been carried out to evaluate the cost-effectiveness of EVAR compared to conventional open surgery (**Table 30.6**).[65-74] In most of these studies, only the hospital cost was included. So far, there is no convincing evidence that EVAR is cost-effective.

FOLLOW-UP

As the long-term outcome of endovascular repair is, as yet, unknown, careful and indefinite follow-up is required. Physical examination and CTA are recommended within 1 month of the procedure, at 6, 12, and 18 months after the intervention, and annually thereafter. CTA may fail to identify an endoleak if delayed images are not obtained after infusion of contrast.[75] Although conflicting studies exist, most investigations suggest that the sensitivity of CTA is superior to that of other non-invasive imaging techniques, such as duplex ultrasonography, for endoleak detection.[76,77] Color duplex ultrasonography is very operator dependent but does have the advantages of showing blood flow within the aneurysm sac, not requiring contrast, and being less costly.

Besides the search for endoleaks, changes in the dimension of the aneurysm sac may assist in defining the success or failure of aneurysm exclusion. Aneurysm growth after endovascular repair is an indicator of incomplete aneurysm exclusion and therefore a continued risk for late aneurysm rupture.[78] Aneurysm size should be expressed as either maximum diameter or volume. The maximum diameter should be measured perpendicular to the central lumen line of the vessel with 3D reconstructed CTA images. Because the aneurysm cross-section often appears elliptical on axial images, the minor axis of the ellipse (smallest diameter) is generally a closer assessment of the maximum aneurysm diameter.[79] Intraobserver and interobserver variability of diameter measurements obtained from CTA range between

2 and 5mm.[80] Therefore, only a diameter change of 5mm or more is considered significant.

Total aneurysm volume is comprised of luminal aneurysm volume and non-luminal aneurysm volume. An aneurysm can be considered completely excluded if the non-luminal aneurysm volume is less than 10% of the original non-luminal aneurysm volume noted after endograft implantation. The intraobserver and interobserver variability of volume measurements have ranged between 3% and 5%. Therefore, a volume change of 5% or more is considered significant.[81]

A plain abdominal X-ray in four planes should be obtained at regular intervals to assess kinking and migration of the stent-graft, and to assess the integrity of the support system. Structural failures have been reported in the majority of devices within 4 years from implantation. These structural failures include hook fractures, disintegration of the metal frame, wireform fractures, and lateral bar and proximal spring fractures.

CONVERSION

Conversions should be differentiated as primary conversions (at the original operation or within 30 days) or secondary conversions (at a later operation).

The current indications for primary conversion include vascular damage to the access vessels, iliac or aortic rupture, stent-graft migration with obstruction of renal or iliac arteries, and device-related problems (deployment failures, entrapment of the delivery catheter).

Secondary conversion might be indicated in persistent endoleak, growing aneurysm, graft thrombosis, graft infection, renal artery obstruction, and migration of the stent-graft.

The conversion rate in most series is 2–15%. In an analysis from the Eurostar registry, including 1871 patients, 2.6% of patients required conversion.[82] Nearly 80% of the conversions were performed in the first postoperative month (primary conversion). Primary conversion was mostly due to access problems and device migration. Secondary conversions were performed for rupture and for a persistent endoleak, with or without aneurysmal growth. Patients who required primary conversion had an 18% mortality rate. Secondary conversion was associated with a perioperative mortality of 27% and, when performed for rupture, a mortality of 50%.

At conversion, the aorta can be cross-clamped at a suprarenal or subdiaphragmal level. If it is impossible to cross-clamp the aorta, control can be obtained with an occluding balloon at the level of the visceral arteries. The aneurysm sac can be opened and the stent-graft removed by traction. After removal of the stent-graft, the clamp can be applied infrarenally and reconstruction can be continued. If the graft is incorporated in the aortic wall (e.g. suprarenal fixation) the stent-graft can be cut through the metal frame. The proximal part of the stent-graft remains *in situ* and a surgical anastomosis can be performed on the remaining stent-graft.

Due to extensive variations in stent-graft configurations, and the complications pending conversion, conversion needs a flexible intraoperative attitude towards clamping techniques and stent-graft extraction.

EVIDENCE

Evidence-based comparison between EVAR and open repair is not reliable at present. Prospective randomized trials are ongoing in The Netherlands (DREAM Trial), UK (EVAR Trial), France (ACE Trial) and the United States (OVER Trial). Comparative trials have been carried out in single centers in the form of case control studies, and concurrent single or multicentric prospective non-randomized studies. Recently, a meta-analysis was performed by Adriaensen et al.[83] In this meta-analysis, short-term results were defined as all measurable results within 30 days of the procedure, including: duration of procedure, blood loss during the procedure, number of days in the ICU, number of days in the hospital, and 30-day mortality and complication rates. The total complication rate was divided into a local/vascular and a systemic/remote complication rate. Nine studies were included, reporting 1318 procedures (687 EVAR and 631 conventional open surgery). To pool continuous variables, means weighted for sample size were calculated. A random-effects model was used to pool dichotomous data and to calculate pooled odds ratios (EVAR versus conventional open surgery). Mean blood loss was 456mL for EVAR and 1202mL for conventional open surgery (p=0.003). EVAR patients spent on average 0.5 days in the ICU and 3.9 days in the hospital, and conventional open surgery patients 2.2 days (p=0.04) and 10.3 days (p=0.02), respectively. The pooled 30-day mortality was 0.03 for EVAR (95% confidence interval: 0.02–0.04) and 0.04 for conventional open surgery (95% confidence interval: 0.00–0.07) (p=0.03); odds ratio 0.55 (95% confidence interval: 0.33–0.92). The pooled local/vascular complication rate was 0.16 for EVAR (95% confidence interval: 0.06–0.25) and 0.12 for conventional open surgery (95% confidence interval: 0.06–0.18) (p=0.46); the odds ratio was 0.97 (95% confidence interval: 0.62–1.54). The pooled systemic/remote complication rate was 0.17 for EVAR (95% confidence interval: 0.09–0.25) and 0.44 for conventional open surgery (95% confidence interval: 0.21–0.66) (p<0.001); odds ratio 0.22 (95% confidence interval: 0.11–0.45). From this meta-analysis, it was concluded that endovascular treatment of AAA compared to conventional open surgery resulted in less blood loss, shorter ICU and hospital stay, a lower 30-day mortality, and a lower systemic/remote complication rate. Endovascular repair will be a more effective alternative to open surgical repair if it can produce a substantial decrease in mortality and morbidity rates, which is most likely to occur in patients at high risk.

REFERENCES

1. Dos Santos JC. Sur la desobstruction des thrombose arterielle anciennes. Med Acad Chir 1947;409–11.

2. Vollmar J. Rekonstruktive chirurgie der arterien. Stuttgart 1967; 24–27:264–70.

3. Dotter CT, Judkins MP. Transluminal treatment of arteriosclerotic obstruction: description of a new technique and a preliminary report of its application. Circulation 1964;30:654–70.

4. Grüntzig A, Hophoff H. Perkutane rekanlisation chronischer arterieller Verschlüsse mit einem neuen Dilatationskatheter. Modification der Dotter-technik. Dtsch Med Wochenschr 1974;99:2502–5.

5. Volodos N, Karpovich I, Trojan V, et al. Clinical experience in the use of self-fixing synthetic prosthesis for remote endoprosthetics of the thoracic and abdominal aorta and iliac arteries through the femoral artery and as intraoperative endoprosthesis for aorta reconstruction. Vasa 1991;33:93–5.

6. Parodi JC, Palmaz J, Barone H. Transfemoral intraluminal graft implantation for abdominal aortic aneurysms. Ann Vasc Surg 1991;5:491–9.

7. Harris PL, Buth J, Miahle C, et al. The need for clinical trials of endovascular abdominal aortic repair. The EUROSTAR Project. EUROpean collaborators on Stent-graft techniques for abdominal aortic aneurysm repair. J Endovasc Surg 1997;1:72–7; discussion 78–9.

8. Sternbergh WC III, Carter G, York JW, et al. Aortic neck angulation predicts adverse outcome with endovascular abdominal aortic aneurysm repair. J Vasc Surg 2002;35:482–6.

9. Stanley BM, Semmens JB, Mai Q, et al. Evaluation of patient selection guidelines for endoluminal AAA repair with the Zenith stent-graft: the Australian experience. J Endovasc Ther 2001;8:457–64.

10. Broeders IAMJ, Balm R, Blankensteijn JD, et al. Preoperative sizing of grafts for transfemoral endovascular aneurysm management; a prospective comparative study of spiral CT angiography, arterial angiography and conventional CT imaging. J Endovasc Surg 1997;4:252–61.

11. Capasso P. Abdominal and thoracic aortic stent-grafts. Semin Interv Radiol 2001;18:299–319.

12. White G, May J. Endovascular grafts. In: Rutherford R, ed. Vascular surgery, 5th edn. Philadelphia:WB Saunders; 1999:584–618.

13. Palmaz JC. Biopolymers for endovascular use. Semin Interv Radiol 1998;15:13–9.

14. Malina M, Lindh M, Ivancev K, et al. The effect of endovascular aortic stents placed across the renal arteries. Eur J Vasc Endovasc Surg 1997; 13:207–13.

15. Kramer SC, Seifarth H, Pamler R, et al. Renal infarction following endovascular aortic aneurysm repair: incidence and clinical consequences. J Endovasc Ther 2002;9:98–102.

16. Beebe HG. Imaging modalities for aortic endografting. J Endovasc Surg 1997;4:111–23.

17. Broeders IAMJ, Blankensteijn JD. A simple technique to improve the accuracy of proximal AAA endograft deployment. J Endovasc Ther 2000;7:389–93.

18. Parodi JC. Endovascular repair of abdominal aortic aneurysms and other arterial lesions. J Vasc Surg 1995;21:549–55.

19. May J, White GH. Endovascular treatment of aortic aneurysms. In: Rutherford R, ed. Vascular surgery, 5th edn. Philadelphia:WB Saunders; 1999:1281–95.

20. Goldstone J, Brewster DC, Chaikoff EL, et al. Endoluminal repair versus standard open repair of abdominal aortic aneurysms: early results of a prospective clinical comparison trial. Proceedings of the 46th Scientific Meeting of the NA Chapter of the International Society for Cardiovascular Surgery. San Diego, CA; 1998.

21. Zarins CK, White RA, Schwarten D, et al. Investigators of the Medtronic AneuRx Multicenter Clinical Trial. AneuRx stent graft versus open surgical repair of abdominal aortic aneurysms: multicenter prospective clinical trial. J Vasc Surg 1999;29:292–308.

22. May J, White GH, Yu W, et al. Concurrent comparison of endoluminal versus open repair in the treatment of abdominal aortic aneurysms; analysis of 303 patients by life table method. J Vasc Surg 1998; 27:213–21.

23. Brewster DC, Geller CS, Kaufmann JA, et al. Initial experience with endovascular aneurysm repair: comparison of early results with outcome of conventional open repair. J Vasc Surg 1998;27:992–1003.

24. De Virgilio C, Bui H, Donayre C, et al. Endovascular vs open abdominal aortic aneurysm repair. Arch Surg 1999;134:947–51.

25. Beebe HG, Cronewett JL, Katzen BT, et al. Results of an aortic endograft trial: impact of device failure beyond 12 months. J Vasc Surg 2001;33:S55–63.

26. May J, White GH, Waugh R, et al. Improved survival after endoluminal repair with second generation prostheses compared with open repair in the treatment of abdominal aortic aneurysms: a 5-year concurrent comparison using life table method. J Vasc Surg 2001;33:S21–6.

27. Zarins CK, Arko FR, Lee WA, et al. Effectiveness of endovascular versus open repair in prevention of aneurysm related death. Proceedings of the 49th Scientific Meeting of the American Association for Vascular Surgery. Baltimore, MD; 2001.

28. White GH, Yu W, May J, et al. Endoleaks as a complication of endoluminal grafting of abdominal aortic aneurysms: classification, incidence, diagnosis and management. J Endovasc Surg 1997;4:152–68.

29. White GH, May J, Waugh R, et al. Type I and type II endoleak: a more useful classification for reporting results of endoluminal repair of AAA (Letter). J Endovasc Surg 1998;5:189–91.

30. Lumsden AB, Allen RC, Chaikof EL, et al. Delayed rupture of aortic aneurysms following endovascular stent grafting. Am J Surg 1995; 170:174–8

31. White GH, Yu W, May J, et al. Three-year experience with the White-Yu endovascular GAD graft for transluminal repair of aortic and iliac aneurysms. J Endovasc Surg 1997;4:124–36.

32. Torsello GB, Klenk E, Kasprzak B, et al. Rupture of abdominal aortic aneurysm previously treated by endovascular stentgraft. J Vasc Surg 1998;28:184–7.

33. Malina M, Ivancev K, Chuter TAM, et al. Changing aneurysmal morphology after endovascular grafting: relation to leakage or persistent perfusion. J Endovasc Surg 1997;4:23–30.

34. Chaikof EL, Blankensteijn JD, Harris PL, et al. Reporting standards for endovascular aneurysm repair. J Vasc Surg 2002;35:1048–60.

35. Gilling-Smith G, Brennan J, Harris PL, et al. Endotension after endovascular repair: definition, classification and implications for surveillance and intervention. J Endovasc Surg 1999;6:305–7.

36. White GH, May J, Petrasek P, et al. Endotension: an explanation for continued AAA growth after successful endoluminal repair. J Endovasc Surg 1999;6:308–15.

37. Schurink GW, Aarts N, Wilde J, et al. Endoleakage after stent-graft treatment of abdominal aneurysms: implications on pressure and imaging: an in-vitro study. J Vasc Surg 1998;28:234–41.

38. Faries PL, Sanchez LA, Marin ML, et al. An experimental model for the acute and chronic evaluation of intra-aneurysmal pressure. J Endovasc Surg 1997;4:290–7.

39. Schurink GW, van Baalen JM, Visser MJ, et al. Thrombus within an aortic aneurysm does not reduce pressure on the aneurysmal wall. J Vasc Surg 2000;31:501–6.

40. Moore WS, Rutherford RB, for the EVT Investigators. Transfemoral endovascular repair of abdominal aortic aneurysm: results of the North American EVT phase 1 trial. J Vasc Surg 1996;23:543–53.

41. Blum U, Voshage G, Lammer J, et al. Endoluminal stent-grafts for infrarenal abdominal aortic aneurysms. N Engl J Med 1997;336:13–20.

42. May J, White GH, Yu W, et al. Repair of abdominal aortic aneurysms by endoluminal method: outcome in the first 100 patients. Med J Aust 1996;165:549–51.

43. Yusuf SW, Whitaker SC, Chuter TA, et al. Early results of endovascular aortic aneurysm surgery with aortouniiliac graft, contralateral occlusion and femoro-femoral bypass. J Vasc Surg 1997;25:165–72.

44. Wisselink W, Cuesta MA, Berends PJ, et al. Retroperitoneal endoscopic ligation of lumbar and inferior mesenteric artery as a treatment of persistent endoleak after endovascular aortic aneurysm repair. J Vasc Surg 2000;31:1240–4.

45. Veith FJ, Baum RA, Ohki T, et al. Nature and significance of endoleaks and endotension: summary of opinions expressed at an international conference. J Vasc Surg 2002;35:1029–35.

46. Cuypers PW, Laheij RJ, Buth J. Which factors increase the risk of conversion to open surgery following endovascular abdominal aortic aneurysm repair? The EUROSTAR collaborators. Eur J Vasc Endovasc Surg 2000;20:183–9.

47. Norgren L, Jernby B, Engellau L. Aortoenteric fistula caused by a ruptured stent-graft: a case report. J Endovasc Surg 1998;5:269–72.

48. Schlensak C, Doenst T, Moreno JB, et al. Serious complications requiring surgical interventions after endoluminal stent graft placement for the treatment of infrarenal aortic aneurysms. J Vasc Surg 2001;34:198–20.3.

49. Sonesson B, Lanne T, Hansen F, et al. Infrarenal aortic diameter in the healthy person. Eur J Vasc Surg 1994;8:89–95.

50. Lipski DA, Ernst CB. Natural history of the residual infrarenal aorta after infrarenal abdominal aortic aneurysm repair. J Vasc Surg 1998; 27:805–11.

51. Sonesson B, Resch T, Lanne T, et al. The fate of the infrarenal aorta after open aneurysm surgery. J Vasc Surg 1998;28:889–94.

52. Illig KA, Green RM, Ouriel K, et al. Fate of the proximal aortic cuff: implications for endovascular aneurysm repair. J Vasc Surg 1997; 26:492–9.

53. Sonesson B, Malina M, Ivancev K, et al. Dilatation of the infrarenal aneurysm neck after endovascular exclusion of abdominal aortic aneurysm. J Endovasc Surg 1998;5:195–200.

54. Matsumura JS, Chaikof EL. Continued expansion of aortic necks after endovascular repair of abdominal aortic aneurysms. EVT Investigators. J Vasc Surg 1998;28:422–30.

55. May J, White GH, Yu W, et al. A prospective study of anatomico-pathological changes in abdominal aortic aneurysms following endoluminal repair: is the aneurysmal process reversed. Eur J Vasc Endovasc Surg 1996;12:11–7.

56. Wever JJ, de Nie AJ, Blankensteijn JD, et al. Dilatation of the proximal neck of infrarenal aortic aneurysms after endovascular AAA repair. Eur J Vasc Endovasc Surg 2000;19:197–201.

57. Prinssen M, Wever JJ, Mali WP, et al. Concerns for the durability of proximal AAA endograft fixation from a 2-year and 3-year longitudinal CT angiography study. J Vasc Surg 2001;33:64S.

58. Zarins CK, White RA, Moll FL, et al. Aneurysm rupture after endovascular repair using the AneuRx stent graft. J Vasc Surg 2000;31:960–70.

59. Harris PL, Vallabhaneni SR, Desgranges P, et al. Incidence and risk factors of late rupture, conversion, and death after endovascular repair of infrarenal aortic aneurysms: the EUROSTAR experience. J Vasc Surg 2000;32:739–49.

60. Zarins CK, White RA, Moll Fl, et al. The AneuRx stent graft: four-year results and worldwide experience 2000. J Vasc Surg 2001;33:S135–45.

61. Makaroun MS. The Ancure endografting system: an update. J Vasc Surg 2001;33:S129–34.

62. Lloyd AJ, Boyle J, Bell PR, et al. Comparison of cognitive function and quality of life after endovascular or conventional aortic aneurysm repair. Br J Surg 2000;87:443–7.

63. Malina M, Nilsson M, Brunkwall J, et al. Quality of life before and after endovascular and open repair of asymptomatic AAAs: a prospective study. J Endovasc Ther 2000;7:372–9.

64. Aquino RV, Jones MA, Zullo TG, et al. Quality of life assessment in patients undergoing endovascular or conventional AAA repair. J Endovasc Ther 2001;8:521–8.

65. Holzenbein J, Kretschmer G, Glanzl R, et al. Endovascular AAA treatment: expensive prestige or economic alternative? Eur J Vasc Endovasc Surg 1997;14:265–72.

66. Ceelen W, Sonneville T, Randon C, et al. Cost-benefit analysis of endovascular versus open abdominal aortic aneurysm treatment. Acta Chir Belg 1999;99:64–7.

67. Patel ST, Haser PB, Bush HL Jr, et al. The cost-effectiveness of endovascular repair versus open surgical repair of abdominal aortic aneurysms: a decision analysis model. J Vasc Surg 1999;29:958–72.

68. Seiwert AJ, Wolfe J, Whalen RC, et al. Cost comparison of aortic aneurysm endograft exclusion versus open surgical repair. Am J Surg 1999;178:117–20.

69. Quinones-Baldrich WJ. Achieving cost-effective endoluminal aneurysm repair. Semin Vasc Surg 1999;12:220–5.

70. Sternbergh WC III, Money SR. Hospital cost of endovascular versus open repair of abdominal aortic aneurysms: a multicenter study. J Vasc Surg 2000;31:237–44.

71. Clair DG, Gray B, O'Hara PJ, et al. An evaluation of the cost to health care institutions of endovascular aortic aneurysm repair. J Vasc Surg 2000;32:148–52.

72. Birch SE, Stary DR, Scott AR. Cost of endovascular versus open surgical repair of abdominal aortic aneurysms. Aust NZ J Surg 2000;70:660–6.

73. Turnipseed WD, Carr SC, Tefera G, et al. Minimal incision aortic surgery. J Vasc Surg 2001;34:47–53.

74. Bosch JL, Lester JS, McMahon PM, et al. Hospital costs for elective endovascular and surgical repairs of infrarenal abdominal aortic aneurysms. Radiology 2001;220:492–7.

75. Schurink GW, Aarts NJ, Wilde J, et al. Endoleakage after stent-graft treatment of abdominal aneurysm: implications on pressure and imaging: an in vitro study. J Vasc Surg 1998;28:234–41.

76. McWilliams RG, Martin J, White D, et al. Detection of endoleaks with enhanced ultrasound imaging: Comparison with biphasic computed tomography. J Endovasc Ther 2002;9:170–9.

77. Sato DT, Goff CD, Gregory RT, et al. Endoleak after aortic stent graft repair: diagnosis by color duplex ultrasound versus computed tomography. J Vasc Surg 1998;28:657–63.

78. Matsumura JS, Moore WS. Clinical consequences of periprosthetic leak after endovascular repair of abdominal aortic aneurysm. J Vasc Surg 1998;27:606–13.

79. Ouriel K, Green RM, Donayre C, et al. An evaluation of new methods of expressing aortic aneurysm size: relationship to rupture. J Vasc Surg 1992;15:12–20.

80. Aarts NJ, Schurink GW, Schultze Kool LJ, et al. Abdominal aortic aneurysm for endovascular repair: intra- and interobserver variability of CT measurements. Eur J Vasc Endovasc Surg 1999;18:475–80.

81. Singh-Ranger R, McArthur T, Corte MD, et al. The abdominal aortic aneurysm sac after endoluminal exclusion: a medium term morphologic follow-up based on volumetric technology. J Vasc Surg 2000; 31:490–500.

82. Cuypers PW, Laheij RJ, Buth J. Which factors increase the risk of conversion to open surgery following endovascular abdominal aortic aneurysm repair? The EUROSTAR collaborators. Eur J Vasc Endovasc Surg 2000;20:183–9.

83. Adriaensen ME, Bosch JL, Halpern EF, Myriam Hunink MG, Gazelle GS. Elective endovascular versus open surgical repair of abdominal aortic aneurysms: a systematic review of short term results. Radiology 2002; 224: 739–47.

CHAPTER
31

Abdominal Aneurysm – Open Repair

Patrick J O'Hara

KEY POINTS

- **Definition**: direct surgical replacement of an infrarenal abdominal aortic aneurysm utilizing transperitoneal or retroperitoneal incision.

- **Key features**:
  - Nearly universal applicability.
  - Low mortality and morbidity rates.
  - Exceptional durability.

- **Clinical considerations**:
  - Proximal and distal extent.
  - Patient selection and co-morbidities.
  - Preoperative strategy to treat all relevant aneurysmal/occlusive disease.
  - Tailor incision to suit anatomy.
  - Straightforward bifurcated graft preferred to difficult tube graft.
  - Proximal end-to-end anastomosis near renal arteries.
  - Preserve at least one hypogastric artery or implant inferior mesenteric.
  - Avoid embolization.
  - Assure distal perfusion adequate while in operating room.

INTRODUCTION

The first reported surgical repair of an infrarenal abdominal aortic aneurysm (AAA) took place 50 years ago and was performed using an arterial homograft to replace the aneurysmal infrarenal aorta.[1] Since that time, numerous advances in surgical and anesthetic techniques, graft materials, and perioperative management have led to dramatic improvements in the early mortality and morbidity rates associated with the procedure. As experience has accumulated, the durability of infrarenal aortic reconstruction has also been documented.[2,3] Until recently, the infrarenal abdominal aortic aneurysm repair has required direct surgical exposure of the abdominal aorta through a variety of incisions, but, with the first reported endovascular repair of an infrarenal abdominal aortic aneurysm just over 10 years ago, an additional method of aortic aneurysm repair, utilizing minimally invasive techniques, has become feasible in selected patients.[4] Open aneurysm repair refers to the direct surgical replacement of the infrarenal abdominal aortic aneurysm and the iliac arteries if indicated, utilizing direct exposure through a transperitoneal or retroperitoneal incision, by suturing a prosthetic graft to the uninvolved proximal and distal arteries.

The concept of endovascular aneurysm repair has much intuitive appeal, especially for patients who are clearly at high risk for traditional open repair, as its physiologic impact should be lower due to the smaller incisions needed and the elimination of the requirement for aortic cross-clamping. Multiple endovascular aortic stent graft devices are still in the developmental stages and the two that have been approved for clinical use in the USA (Medtronics Aneurx® and Guidant Ancure®) have been associated with low early mortality rates that are similar to, but not lower than, those observed for open aneurysm repair.[5–7] However, the technology is still new and is developing rapidly. Despite the encouraging early results, the long-term durability of endovascular stent-grafts has been called into question by reports of endoleaks leading to reintervention or sometimes explantation of the endoprosthesis.[8,9] Furthermore, although the influence of the presence of an endoleak is unclear, cumulative annual rupture rates of 1% have been reported for aortic aneurysms despite endovascular exclusion.[10,11] For these reasons, open aneurysm repair is still the standard of care for good risk patients with infrarenal abdominal aortic aneurysms requiring repair.[12] Until the long-term durability of endovascular aneurysm repair is known with assurance, the procedure should be reserved for patients who are clearly at high risk for open aneurysm repair.[13,14]

ANATOMIC DISTRIBUTION OF TRUE ANEURYSMS

The distribution of 2586 true aneurysms surgically treated at the Cleveland Clinic in the Department of Vascular Surgery from January 1, 1989 to December 31, 2001 is illustrated in **Figure 31.1** (departmental vascular registry, unpublished data). The most commonly encountered aneurysms involved the infrarenal aorto-iliac arteries, accounting for approximately 70% (1817/2586) of the total true aneurysms treated during the interval. Suprarenal (140) and thoracoabdominal (240) aortic aneurysms comprised 15% (380/2586) of true aneurysms, while femoral (5%; 130/2586) and popliteal (4%; 110/2586) aneurysms were less commonly encountered. One hundred forty-nine other true aneurysms (6%) encompassed a miscellaneous group consisting of brachio-cephalic or visceral aneurysms and other rare lesions. Although the precise distribution may vary among centers, the relative frequency of occurrence of aneurysmal disease in each arterial segment depicted in **Figure 31.1** is representative of the relative prevalence and recognition of each lesion.

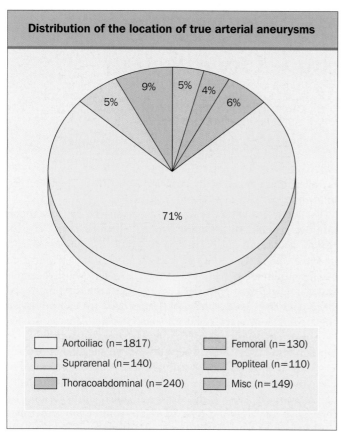

Distribution of the location of true arterial aneurysms

9% 5% 4%
5% 6%
71%

Aortoiliac (n=1817)   Femoral (n=130)
Suprarenal (n=140)   Popliteal (n=110)
Thoracoabdominal (n=240)   Misc (n=149)

Figure 31.1 The distribution of the location of true arterial aneurysms treated by surgical repair (n = 2586) at the Cleveland Clinic from January 1, 1989 through December 31, 2001 (unpublished data from the departmental vascular registry).

TECHNIQUE OF OPEN ANEURYSM REPAIR

Preoperatively, the surgeon should formulate a strategy for open repair of the abdominal aortic aneurysm with the goal, ideally, to treat all the aneurysmal and associated occlusive disease that is identified on preoperative imaging studies. Judgment, however, is required to modify the optimal plan according to the particular circumstances. Depending upon the clinical considerations, such as emergency or elective operation, and the associated co-morbidities, objectives must be prioritized and accomplished as time and circumstances permit.

Intraoperative autotransfusion for autologous blood salvage is routinely employed at the time of aortic aneurysm repair and has been shown to reduce the necessity for perioperative homologous blood transfusion, especially when combined with preoperative donation of autologous blood.[15–17] While preoperative autologous blood donation is not always feasible, it may often be utilized after the induction of anesthesia in association with intraoperative hemodilution and has the advantage of providing fresh coagulation factors when it is reinfused at the conclusion of the procedure.[18]

Important anesthetic considerations involve close monitoring of arterial pressure and intravascular volume status and are facilitated by the routine use of pulmonary artery pressure monitoring catheters, radial artery lines, and urinary catheters. The use of combined epidural and general anesthetic techniques

has permitted the safe management of patients with severe respiratory co-morbidities, formerly thought to represent prohibitive risks for open aneurysm repair, and has greatly facilitated the postoperative pain and respiratory management of these difficult patients.[19]

At the Cleveland Clinic, most aneurysms involving the aorto-iliac system are approached through the preferential use of a transperitoneal midline or, rarely, transverse incisions (**Fig. 31.2A**),[20] although some surgeons have advocated the routine use of a retroperitoneal approach through either a flank or low thoraco-abdominal incision, with similar excellent results (**Fig. 31.2B**).[21–24] The transperitoneal approach provides an opportunity for exploration of the intra-abdominal viscera and has the advantage of providing better exposure of the distal right common iliac system, when this is required, because of its involvement in aneurysmal or occlusive disease. The chief limitation of the transperitoneal approach, however, is difficulty with exposure of the proximal infrarenal or visceral aorta, especially in the obese patient. To solve this problem, some surgeons have advocated medial visceral rotation to allow proximal exposure of the visceral and proximal infrarenal aorta.[25] In contrast, the left retroperitoneal or low thoraco-retroperitoneal approach affords more flexibility when difficulty with proximal control is anticipated, because of juxtarenal or suprarenal extension of the aneurysm, the presence of a hostile abdomen from multiple prior intra-abdominal procedures, or the existence of morbid obesity. Furthermore, when the peritoneum is not opened with this approach, heat loss and resulting hypothermic complications are minimized. The left kidney may be either left in its bed or elevated if more proximal exposure of the visceral aortic segment is required. Since the choice of incision depends upon the anatomic features of the arterial disease, and also the associated co-morbidities that may be present, the versatile aortic surgeon should be comfortable with all available approaches to optimal aortic exposure.

Aneurysms involving the infrarenal aorto-iliac segment that are managed by open repair are replaced with a synthetic graft that is sutured to the uninvolved artery proximal and distal to the aneurysmal vessels. The dissection is performed with emphasis on minimal manipulation of the aneurysm, to minimize the risk of distal embolization, a feature that is especially important if the patient has had prior evidence of atheromatous embolization. Unless there are contraindications, systemic heparinization is routinely utilized and is usually supplemented with dilute regional heparinization infused into the distal iliac arteries. It is usually preferable to apply the outflow clamps before the inflow aortic clamp, if feasible, to minimize the risk of distal embolization. Following this, the aneurysm sac is incised along the right antero-lateral aspect to avoid the autonomic plexus, which usually lies along the left side of the aneurysm and typically crosses anterior to the left common iliac artery (**Fig. 31.3**). Preservation of this plexus is particularly important to male patients who are still sexually active, and its disturbance may lead to retrograde ejaculation.[26] Mural thrombus, if present, is carefully removed and special care is taken to avoid forcing particulate matter into the iliac arteries, since this material could be a source of embolization when flow is restored after graft placement. Expeditious control of retrograde bleeding from patent lumbar arteries may require local endarterectomy prior to suture ligation, especially if the posterior aortic wall is

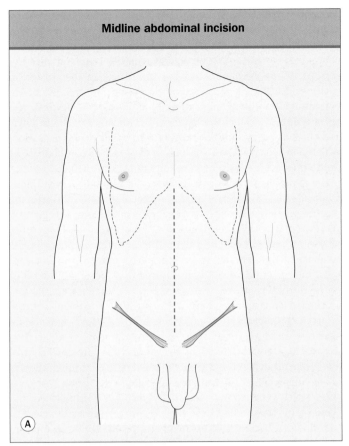

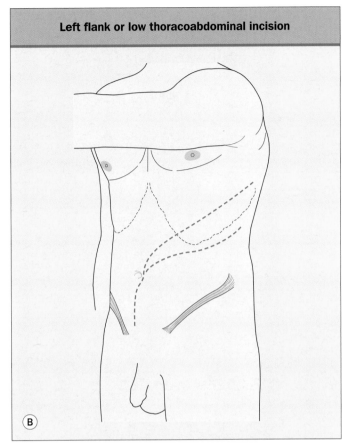

Figure 31.2 Abdominal aortic aneurysm repair. (A) The usual midline abdominal incision used for transperitoneal abdominal aortic aneurysm repair. (B) The left flank or low thoracoabdominal incision used for retroperitoneal abdominal aortic aneurysm repair (upper incision for juxtarenal or visceral aortic exposure).

heavily calcified. An appropriately sized synthetic graft, usually fabricated from collagen-coated knitted Dacron, is inserted by suturing it from within the aneurysm using the method described by Creech.[27] Alternatively, a woven Dacron or polytetra-fluoroethylene (PTFE) graft may be utilized with similar results. An end-to-end proximal anastomosis is required and should be placed immediately distal to the renal arteries to minimize the potential for late aneurysm formation in the aortic segment between the renal arteries and the proximal anastomosis (**Fig. 31.4**). The proximal anastomosis may often be carried out with a running monofilament permanent suture if the aorta is of good quality and has minimal calcification, but it may require buttressing with a Teflon® felt strip in the presence of friable or calcified aortic tissue (**Fig. 31.5A**).[28] Alternatively, the proximal anastomosis may be performed utilizing evenly spaced, interrupted, horizontal mattress sutures tied down over Teflon® felt pledgets, a technique particularly helpful when the aortic quality is poor or severely calcified (**Fig. 31.5B**). If the aneurysm ends sufficiently proximal to the aortic bifurcation, and the common iliac arteries are not significantly aneurysmal, an aortic interposition, or 'tube' graft may be an appropriate choice, especially if the distal aorta is not severely calcified. The distal anastomosis is carried out in an end-to-end fashion, similar to that used for the proximal anastomosis (**Fig. 31.6A**). Often, however, the distal aorta is aneurysmal or is calcified, especially in its posterior aspect. In this situation, it is usually more expeditious to perform a bifurcation graft, rather than to attempt a difficult interposition

graft. The waist of the bifurcation graft should be no more than 4–5cm in length, to minimize the tendency for the iliac limbs to kink, and the preferred configuration for the iliac anastomosis is end-to-end to the distal common iliac artery near its bifurcation, to eliminate as much common iliac artery as is feasible, especially if it is ectatic (**Fig. 31.6B**). In addition to preserving the autonomic plexus, an attempt is made to preserve perfusion to at least one, but ideally both, hypogastric arteries to diminish the likelihood of postoperative sexual dysfunction or colon ischemia.[26,29] This effort may require the performance of hypogastric endarterectomy if the artery is not aneurysmal (**Fig. 31.6C and D**). On occasion, implantation of the inferior mesenteric artery, which sometimes may require endarterectomy, is required if the colon circulation is compromised, especially if at least one of the hypogastric arteries cannot be revascularized.[29] The inferior mesenteric artery may be reimplanted into the body of the aortic graft or into the left iliac limb of the graft as a Carrel patch (**Fig. 31.7**). Care should be taken to keep the button as small as feasible to prevent late aneurysm formation of the patch. After perfusion to the lower extremities is confirmed to be adequate, and reclamping of the graft is no longer likely to be necessary, the remaining circulating heparin is neutralized with protamine sulfate and complete hemostasis is assured. The aneurysm sac is closed over the graft and the retroperitoneum is closed over the aneurysm sac to ensure separation of the synthetic graft from the abdominal viscera, thus minimizing the potential for graft enteric erosion leading to graft infection (**Fig. 31.8A**).

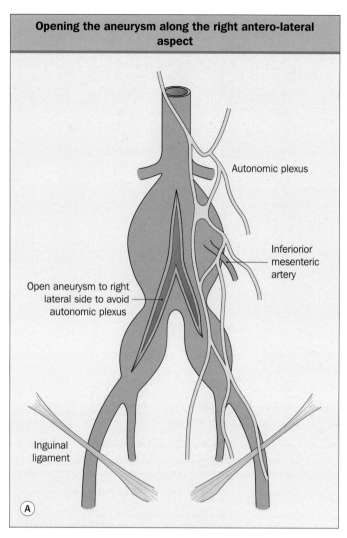

Opening the aneurysm along the right antero-lateral aspect

Autonomic plexus

Inferiorior mesenteric artery

Open aneurysm to right lateral side to avoid autonomic plexus

Inguinal ligament

(A)

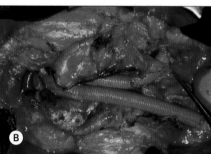

(B)

Figure 31.3 Open aneurysm repair.
(A) Representation of opening the aneurysm along the right antero-lateral aspect to preserve the autonomic plexus. (B) Intraoperative photo of autonomic plexus (indicated by forceps) during open aneurysm repair.

If the aneurysm sac or retroperitoneal tissue is inadequate to ensure coverage of the graft, a pedicle of omentum may be mobilized to place in the retroperitoneum for coverage (**Fig. 31.8B**). The incision is closed and the patient is transferred to the intensive care unit or recovery unit for close monitoring and support only after the surgeon is assured that distal perfusion is adequate.

Ruptured aneurysms

Rupture of an abdominal aortic aneurysm is an abdominal catastrophe. If the aneurysm freely ruptures anteriorly into peritoneal cavity, rapid exsanguination usually occurs and it is not possible to salvage the patient unless rapid control of the aorta proximal to the site of rupture is achieved in the operating room. If the aneurysm ruptures posteriorly into the retroperitoneal space, the resulting hemorrhage may be temporarily contained. Urgent operation is, nevertheless, required since the retroperitoneal hematoma usually ruptures into the peritoneal cavity, resulting in profound hypotension. In this situation, expeditious prepping and draping is undertaken while the anesthesia team establishes adequate volume replacement lines, and the surgeon should be prepared for rapid decompensation, which may occur with the induction of anesthesia and release of the tamponade effect when the abdomen is opened.

Rapid proximal control is most often facilitated by expeditious compression or clamping of the supraceliac aorta through the diaphragmatic crura, with subsequent replacement of the aortic clamp distal to the renal arteries following careful exposure of the infrarenal neck (**Fig. 31.9**). Control can sometimes be established by digital pressure from within aneurysm but care must be exercised with this maneuver to avoid embolization of mural thrombus into the visceral or lower extremity circulation. Occlusion of the supraceliac aorta utilizing a balloon catheter inserted through the femoral or left brachial artery may also be effective in some circumstances, but judgment is required to choose the method that will be likely to achieve proximal control most expeditiously. Distal control is established through the use of vascular clamps or intraluminal balloon occlusion catheters (**Fig. 31.9**). When hemodynamic stabilization is established, the aneurysm is repaired, as described for the elective procedure.

Following successful repair of ruptured abdominal aortic aneurysms, abdominal compartment syndromes may be a factor in the development of multisystem organ failure and may contribute to the increased early postoperative mortality and morbidity rates observed among such patients. Some have advocated delayed abdominal closure utilizing synthetic mesh in this situation, to minimize this problem.[30]

Associated considerations
Renal anomalies
Renal anomalies are among the most common vascular variations encountered by the vascular surgeon during open aneurysm repair, occurring in approximately one in 200 patients.[31] The variations in renal anatomy range in complexity from the presence of accessory renal arteries arising from the aneurysm to various forms of renal ectopia and fusion, usually associated with aberrant renal arteries and anomalies of the urinary collecting system. When these more complex variations are detected on preoperative computed tomography (CT) scanning, they are optimally managed by utilization of a left thoraco-retroperitoneal approach.[32–34] This approach allows the renal mass, as well as the collecting system, to be displaced anteriorly, thereby avoiding injury to these structures and the resulting risk of graft infection or renal ischemia. The retroperitoneal approach also greatly assists in the repair of anomalous renal arteries arising from the aneurysm by facilitating their reimplantation into the graft from within the aneurysm sac (**Fig. 31.10**).

Venous anomalies
Although abnormalities of the major intra-abdominal venous structures are relatively unusual, they are not rare.[35,36] Consequently, the vascular surgeon should also be familiar with the more frequent venous variations, since damage to these structures

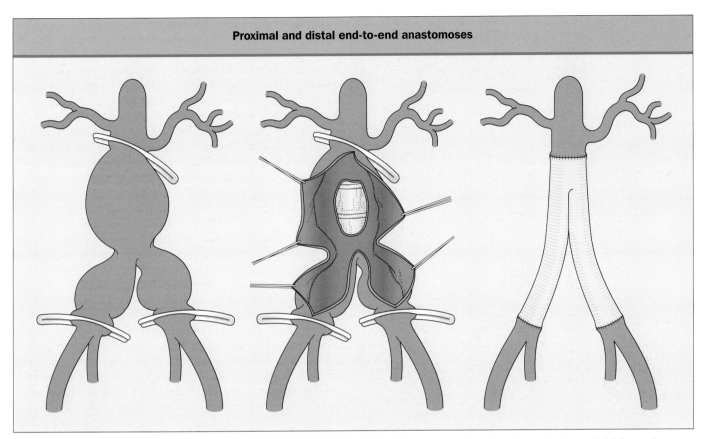

Proximal and distal end-to-end anastomoses

Figure 31.4 Diagrammatic representation of the proximal and distal end-to-end anastomoses preferred for the repair of a typical infrarenal abdominal aortic aneurysm. The proximal anastomosis is placed immediately distal to the renal arteries within the aneurysm sac. (Reprinted with the permission of The Cleveland Clinic Foundation.)

can lead to massive hemorrhage that may be difficult to control. Preoperative CT scanning can usually establish their presence and allows for the development of a preoperative strategy for their optimal management. The varieties of major venous anomalies most commonly encountered during open repair of abdominal aortic aneurysms are those involving the renal veins, with circumferential renal vein occurring in up to 6% of patients. If this anomaly is known to exist preoperatively, one of the divisions of the renal vein may be sacrificed, if necessary, for adequate exposure of the aortic neck. Adequate venous drainage from the left kidney may still take place through the remaining division. The retro-aortic renal vein is thought to be less common, occurring in 3.3% of patients with aortic aneurysms. It should be suspected if the renal arteries are encountered before the renal vein is exposed during dissection of the aneurysm neck through the anterior, transperitoneal approach (**Fig. 31.11**). This variation may be difficult to manage through the retroperitoneal approach, and may require the aortic graft to be tunneled under the renal vein, if space permits. Alternatively, an attempt to reconstruct the renal vein may be required if its division is essential to allow graft placement. The potential also exists for injury to the retro-aortic portion of this anomalous vein during placement of the aortic cross-clamp, and troublesome bleeding may be avoided by careful application of the clamp. Anomalies of the inferior vena cava are less common, occurring in 2.4% of patients, and usually consist of the left-sided or duplicated vena cava (**Fig. 31.12**). Division of the left renal vein may facilitate exposure of the aortic neck, if care is taken to preserve adequate venous decompression pathways through the gonadal or adrenal veins.[35–39]

Inflammatory aneurysms

At operation, inflammatory aneurysms are distinguished by their characteristic white appearance and the presence of a thickened aneurysm wall. They may be associated with a dense fibrotic response in the retroperitoneum (**Fig. 31.13**). While the etiology of these aneurysms is not known with certainty, they are usually not infected. Frequently, the fourth portion of the duodenum is densely adherent to the aneurysm, making exposure of the aneurysm neck problematic, especially from the anterior approach. Attempts to dissect the duodenum away from the aneurysm are likely to lead to duodenal injury, with contamination of the surgical field, and are best avoided. Once proximal control is obtained and the aneurysm sac is opened, the adherent duodenum and aneurysm sac can be retracted with impunity and the aneurysm can be repaired in the usual fashion. Temporary supraceliac aortic control may be required to facilitate exposure and the aortic clamp can subsequently be moved to the infrarenal location when the aneurysm has been opened and the duodenum is no longer under tension.[40–43]

Dissecting aneurysms

Dissecting aneurysms involving only the infrarenal aorta are unusual. The extent of proximal aortic involvement is usually apparent on the preoperative CT scan and angiography should

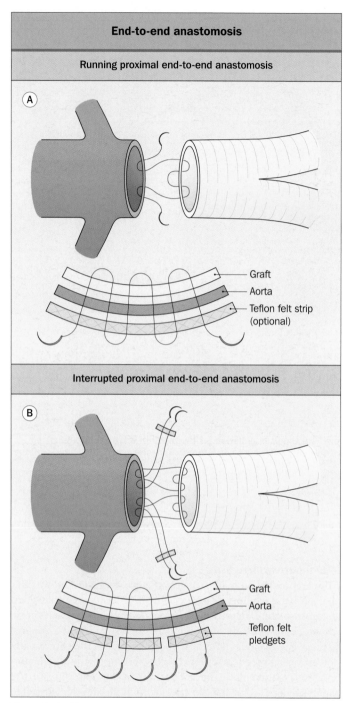

End-to-end anastomosis

Running proximal end-to-end anastomosis

(A)

— Graft
— Aorta
— Teflon felt strip
(optional)

Interrupted proximal end-to-end anastomosis

(B)

— Graft
— Aorta
— Teflon felt
pledgets

Figure 31.5 End-to-end anastomosis. (A) Diagrammatic representation of a running proximal end-to-end anastomosis used for the repair of an infrarenal abdominal aortic aneurysm. When required, a Teflon® felt strip may be used to buttress the suture line (insert). (B) Diagrammatic representation of an interrupted proximal end-to-end anastomosis used for the repair of an infrarenal abdominal aortic aneurysm. Teflon, felt pledgets may be used to buttress the suture line (insert).

be obtained, in this situation, to identify the source of perfusion of the visceral arterial branches. If the infrarenal portion of the abdominal dissection is large or enlarging, proximal fenestration and infrarenal graft replacement of the enlarging aneurysm may be required because obliteration of the false lumen may unfavorably alter the hemodynamics of proximal perfusion (**Fig. 31.14**).[44–47]

Associated non-vascular procedures

Occasionally, concomitant intra-abdominal pathology may be discovered either preoperatively or unexpectedly at the time of aneurysm repair, especially if a transperitoneal approach is employed. While the primary objective of abdominal aortic aneurysm repair is to prevent death from rupture of the aneurysm, an important long-term consideration is the prevention of synthetic graft infection, which is a catastrophic complication. By some estimates, up to 7% of patients with aneurysms may have coexistent cholelithiasis.[48] Although some surgeons have advocated the performance of cholecystectomy at the time of aneurysm repair, it has been reported that bile is colonized with bacteria in 13–46% of patients with cholelithiasis or choledocholithiasis.[49–51] Spillage of contaminated bile at the time of cholecystectomy has the potential to inoculate the synthetic graft with bacteria in this setting. Consequently, it seems unwise, without a compelling reason, to combine any procedure with aortic aneurysm repair that potentially might pose a risk for synthetic graft infection, a sentiment shared by others.[52] Concomitant colorectal malignancy and abdominal aortic aneurysm is unusual but may occur in as many as 0.5% of patients undergoing aortic aneurysm repair.[53] Furthermore, patients in that series who underwent treatment of the colon lesion first, had a tendency to die from the unresected aneurysm. The quandary posed by unanticipated discovery of simultaneous colon malignancy at the time of aortic aneurysm repair may be difficult to resolve with complete certainty,[54] but it seems most reasonable to treat each lesion at a separate procedure to minimize the risk of graft infection, and to treat the most threatening lesion first. Consequently, in the absence of bleeding or obstruction from the colon tumor, the aneurysm repair most often should precede colon resection, especially if the aneurysm is large (>6cm) or symptomatic.

Hostile abdomen

Patients who have had multiple prior abdominal operations or have a history of previous abdominal adhesions from sepsis or radiotherapy, and subsequently require abdominal aortic aneurysm repair, may be anticipated to be at increased risk for bowel or ureteral injury if the transperitoneal approach is utilized. In this circumstance, ureteral stents, placed cystoscopically prior to laparotomy, may assist in the identification of the ureters at the time of aneurysm dissection, and, consequently, aid in their protection in the presence of extensive retroperitoneal scarring. In this setting, the retroperitoneal approach can sometimes provide the considerable advantage of exposure for direct aneurysm replacement, with its demonstrated durability, while allowing the complete avoidance of the hostile intraperitoneal environment. This alternative, when feasible, is preferable to ligation of the aneurysm and extra-anatomic bypass, an approach that has been associated with late aneurysm rupture.[55–57] The mechanism of late aneurysm expansion and rupture following aneurysm ligation and extra-anatomic expansion bypass is related to continued pressurization of the sac from retrograde filling through patent inferior mesenteric or lumbar arteries, a mechanism strikingly similar to that causing aneurysm expansion observed in the presence of some persisting type II endoleaks following endovascular aortic aneurysm exclusion.

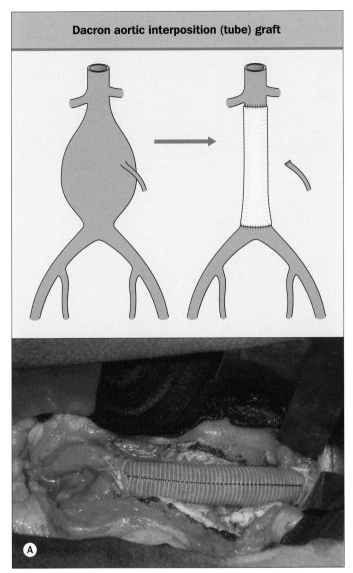

Dacron aortic interposition (tube) graft

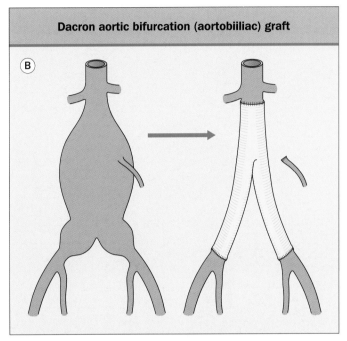

Dacron aortic bifurcation (aortobiiliac) graft

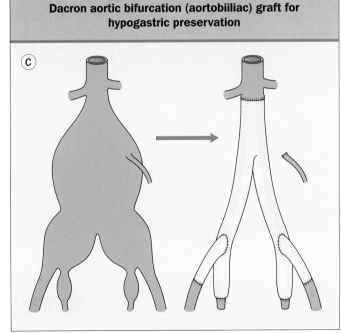

Dacron aortic bifurcation (aortobiiliac) graft for hypogastric preservation

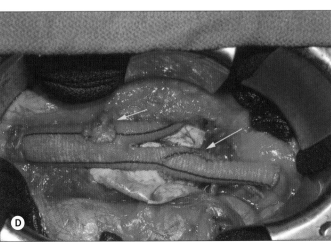

Figure 31.6 Abdominal aortic aneurysm repair. (A) Diagrammatic representation of a Dacron aortic interposition (tube) graft used for the repair of an infrarenal abdominal aortic aneurysm (with intraoperative photo). (B) Diagrammatic representation of a Dacron aortic bifurcation (aortobiiliac) graft used for the repair of an infrarenal abdominal aortic aneurysm. (C) Diagrammatic representation of a Dacron aortic bifurcation (aortobiiliac) graft used for hypogastric preservation during the repair of an infrarenal abdominal aortic aneurysm. The external iliac arteries are revascularized bilaterally by the use of interposition (jump) grafts. It is usually easier to perform the hypogastric anastomoses first since they are deeper in the pelvis from the anterior approach. (D) Intraoperative photograph of hypogastric graft with external iliac jump graft (arrow) and inferior mesenteric artery implantation into the body of the aortic graft (arrow).

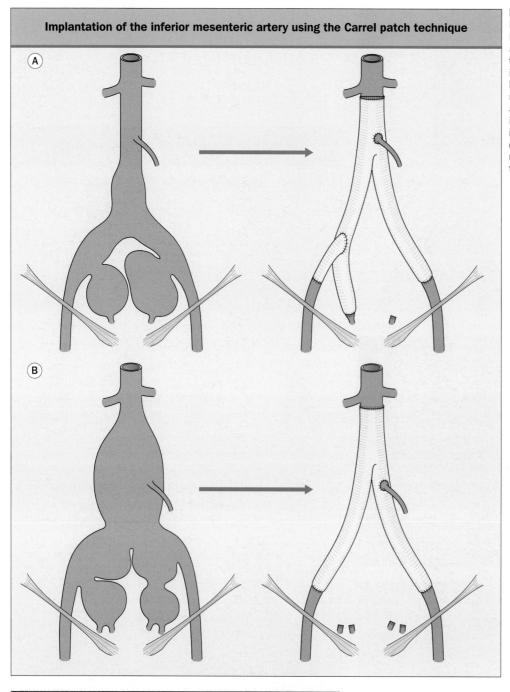

Implantation of the inferior mesenteric artery using the Carrel patch technique

(A)

(B)

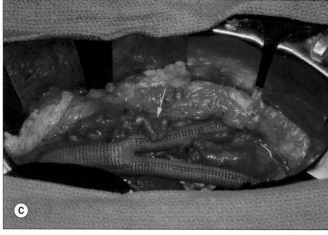

(C)

Figure 31.7 Carrel patch technique.
Diagrammatic representation of implantation of the inferior mesenteric artery, using the Carrel patch technique, into a Dacron aortic interposition graft (A), or into the left limb of a bifurcation graft (B) during the repair of an infrarenal abdominal aortic aneurysm. Endarterectomy of the inferior mesenteric artery may be required at the time of implantation. (C) Intraoperative photograph of inferior mesenteric artery (arrow) implanted into the left limb of aortic bifurcation graft.

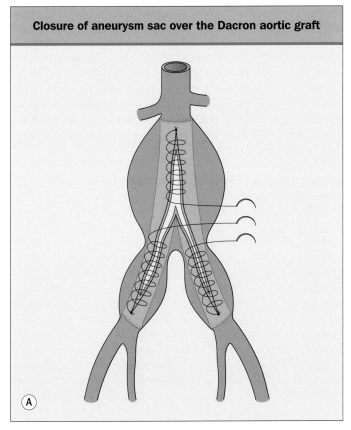

Closure of aneurysm sac over the Dacron aortic graft

(A)

SELECTION OF THERAPY

Co-morbidities and risk stratification

The presence of coronary artery disease, chronic obstructive pulmonary disease, impaired renal function, advanced hypertension, diabetes mellitus, and smoking are variables that have been consistently demonstrated to influence survival following open repair of abdominal aortic aneurysms.[58–61] The prevalence of concomitant severe, correctable coronary artery disease among patients presenting for repair of aortic aneurysms has been documented by coronary angiography, and its detection and treatment provides a unique opportunity to improve the outcome following aortic aneurysm repair.[62–64] In the classic study by Hertzer et al, 32% of 246 patients were found to have severe, correctable coronary artery disease prior to abdominal aortic aneurysm repair and 28% of these patients underwent myocardial revascularization prior to open aneurysm repair. Subsequent 5-year survival of those patients treated with preliminary myocardial revascularization was 75%, which was similar to that of patients without severe coronary artery disease and was significantly better than the 29% late survival rate observed for a subset of patients with severe, uncorrected coronary artery disease.[65–67] Consequently, at the Cleveland Clinic Foundation, cardiac risk stratification is currently pursued primarily utilizing non-invasive cardiac testing such as thallium stress or dobutamine stress echo

Figure 31.8 Closure of the aneurysm sac. Diagrammatic representation of the closure of the aneurysm sac over the Dacron aortic graft (A), or use of an omental pedicle flap (B) to separate the synthetic graft material from the gastrointestinal tract during closure following the repair of an infrarenal abdominal aortic aneurysm.

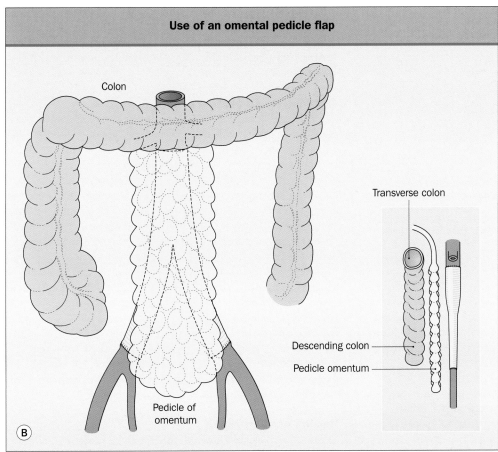

Use of an omental pedicle flap

Colon

Transverse colon

Descending colon

Pedicle omentum

Pedicle of omentum

(B)

433

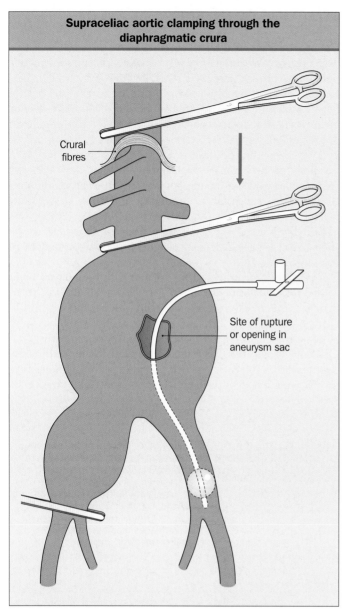

Supraceliac aortic clamping through the diaphragmatic crura

Crural fibres

Site of rupture or opening in aneurysm sac

Figure 31.9 Diagrammatic representation of supraceliac aortic clamping through the diaphragmatic crura during the repair of a ruptured abdominal aortic aneurysm. When control is established, the clamp is moved to the infrarenal location to allow visceral perfusion. Intraluminal balloon catheters may be useful for the control of back-bleeding from the iliac arteries.

examinations for patients who are under serious consideration for abdominal aortic aneurysm repair. If the stress test is abnormal, or if the patient initially presents with established indications of coronary artery disease, such as a prior history of myocardial infarction or angina, or electrocardiographic changes suggesting ischemia, coronary angiography and appropriate intervention are recommended prior to elective aneurysm repair.

Indications for open infrarenal aneurysm repair

Urgent operation is indicated for all ruptured or clearly symptomatic abdominal aortic aneurysms, irrespective of size, provided that the patient does not have an underlying pre-existing medical condition, such as widespread, untreatable, metastatic malignancy, that would already prevent meaningful survival. Asymptomatic

aneurysms should be repaired when the risk of aneurysm rupture exceeds the risk of operation. While the decision to operate must be individualized according to the rate of expansion of the aneurysm, the patient's age, and the presence of associated co-morbidities, the usual threshold for aneurysm repair is, currently, a diameter of 5.5cm or more. However, the observation that approximately 81% of abdominal aortic aneurysms reaching 5.0 to 5.4cm in diameter eventually require repair within 4 years of surveillance may justify repair at a lower threshold of 5cm in selected, good risk patients.[68–70]

Goals/therapeutic objectives of open infrarenal aneurysm repair

The primary risk of an abdominal aortic aneurysm is that of progressive expansion with eventual rupture leading to exsanguination and death. Less commonly, an abdominal aortic aneurysm can undergo thrombosis or become a source of distal embolization, which, in turn, can lead to critical limb ischemia. Consequently, the therapeutic objectives of open abdominal aortic aneurysm repair are primarily the prevention of death by rupture, and, secondarily, limb preservation by the maintenance of adequate arterial perfusion to the pelvis and lower extremities. Important related considerations include issues linked to the quality of life, such as minimizing associated gastrointestinal complications, maximizing the durability of the reconstruction, and the preservation of sexual function. As the economic impact of added costs involved with follow-up requirements, including the need for late imaging studies and subsequent maintenance procedures required with current endovascular methods, becomes more clear, it is likely that more attention will also be directed toward optimizing the overall cost of aortic aneurysm treatment, to increase the value obtained per unit of health care expenditure.

Alternatives to open repair

Since pharmacologic methods for definitive treatment of infrarenal aortic aneurysms are unavailable, once an aneurysm has enlarged sufficiently to pose a substantial risk of rupture, or has become symptomatic, there are currently no reasonable alternatives to surgical aneurysm repair. The forms of surgical therapy currently most widely available include open repair of the aneurysm with synthetic graft replacement, open ligation of the aneurysm with extra-anatomic bypass, and endovascular exclusion of the aneurysm utilizing an aortic stent graft. Attempts to repair aortic aneurysms utilizing laparoscopic techniques are currently investigational. With the current technology, the laparoscopic procedures are time consuming and have not yet achieved widespread applicability.[71–73] Some surgeons have advocated the performance of open aneurysm repair through a small abdominal incision, and believe that this relatively less invasive approach may lessen the length of hospitalization for selected patients.[74–76] Reports of late rupture of aneurysms treated by ligation and extra-anatomic bypass have lessened enthusiasm for this approach, except under unusual circumstances.[55–57]

Results of open repair

Several variables are known to influence the mortality and morbidity rates following open abdominal aortic aneurysm repair. The existence of several patient co-morbidities, especially untreated coronary artery disease, chronic obstructive pulmonary disease,

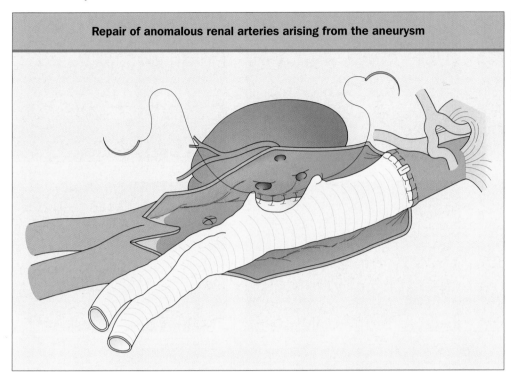

Repair of anomalous renal arteries arising from the aneurysm

Figure 31.10 Diagrammatic representation of the repair of anomalous renal arteries arising from the aneurysm facilitated by a retroperitoneal approach allowing their implantation into the graft. (Reprinted with the permission of The Cleveland Clinic Foundation.)

renal insufficiency, and advanced age, has each been shown to have a deleterious effect on both early and late results. Other factors, such as the necessity for emergency operation because of aneurysm rupture or the development of symptoms of aneurysm expansion or leak, as well as the experience of the surgical team, have also been demonstrated to influence the early postoperative mortality and morbidity rates.[77–79]

Early results
The operative mortality rates for open abdominal aortic aneurysm repair, based on a collected review of published series of patients who underwent infrarenal abdominal aortic aneurysm repair

from 1981–1991, are summarized in **Table 31.1**.[77] The early postoperative mortality rates following abdominal aortic aneurysm repair are considerably higher for emergency operations than for elective operations, a feature that justifies preventative repair of large aneurysms among patients likely to survive more than 1 to 2 years.[13,68–70,80–82] Representative early mortality rates for the emergency repair of symptomatic or ruptured abdominal aortic aneurysms range from 13% to 69% (**Table 31.1**).[80,83] Since patients who present with active intraperitoneal hemorrhage and profound hypotension are less likely to survive emergency operation than those who arrive in the operating room in a stable hemodynamic condition, the large disparity in reported early

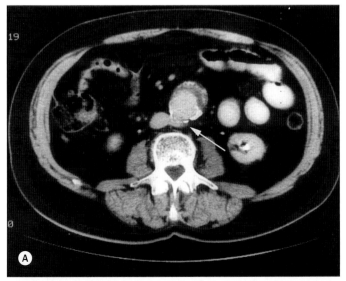
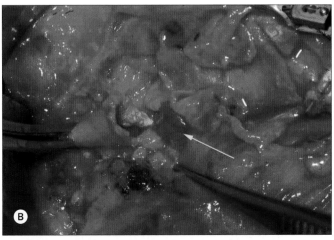

Figure 31.11 Retroaortic left renal vein. (A) Computed tomographic scan demonstrating retroaortic left renal vein (arrow). (B) Intraoperative photograph of retroaortic left renal vein (arrow). Note the absence of the renal vein in the usual position anterior to the aorta.

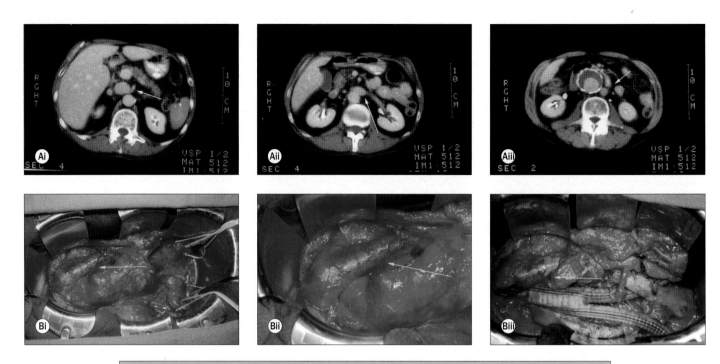

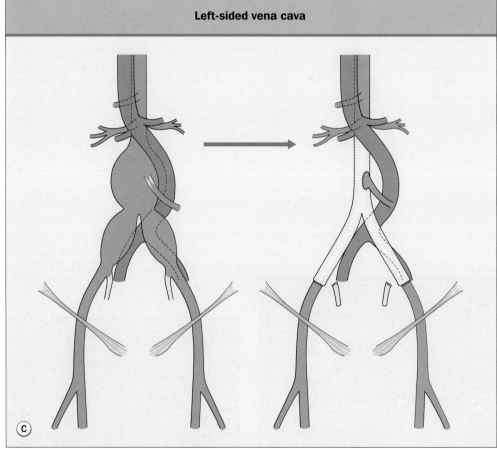

Figure 31.12 Left-sided vena cava. (A) Computed tomographic (CT) scans demonstrating left-sided vena cava (arrows, CT images i–iii). (B) Intraoperative photograph demonstrating left-sided vena cava (arrow, images i–iii). In this patient, the inferior mesenteric artery has been implanted into the left iliac limb of the synthetic graft. (C) Diagrammatic representation of left-sided vena cava.

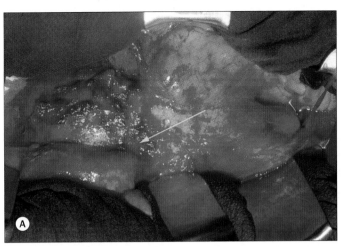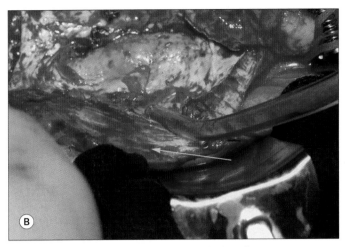

Figure 31.13 Inflammatory abdominal aortic aneurysm. (A) Intraoperative photographs of an intact, inflammatory abdominal aortic aneurysm upon initial exposure. Note the adherent duodenum (arrow). (B) Intraoperative photographs of an inflammatory abdominal aortic aneurysm after it has been opened. Note the thickness of the aneurysm wall (arrow).

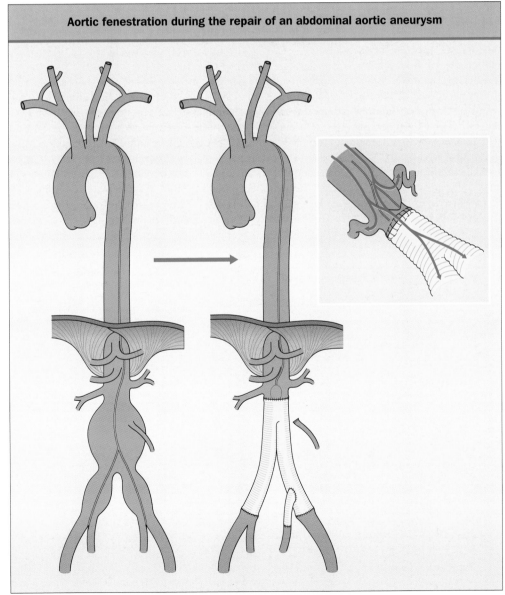

Aortic fenestration during the repair of an abdominal aortic aneurysm

Figure 31.14 Diagrammatic representation of aortic fenestration during the repair of an abdominal aortic aneurysm. (Reprinted with the permission of The Cleveland Clinic Foundation.)

Operative mortality for open abdominal aortic aneurysm repair			
Urgency of aneurysm repair	*n*	*Composite mortality rate (%)*	*Range (%)*
Ruptured	1040	48.4%	25.4–69.3
Urgent, non-ruptured	101	18.8%	13.3–27.3
Elective	3130	3.5%	0–5.1

Table 31.1 Operative mortality for open abdominal aortic aneurysm repair based on a collected review of published series of patients who underwent infrarenal abdominal aortic aneurysm repair from 1981–1991.[77]

Operative mortality for 1135 patients who underwent elective, open, infrarenal abdominal aortic aneurysm repair.			
30-day mortality (%)	*30-day complications (%)*	*5-year survival (%)*	*10-year survival (%)*
1.2	17	75	49

Table 31.2 Operative mortality for 1135 patients who underwent elective, open, infrarenal abdominal aortic aneurysm repair at the Cleveland Clinic Foundation from 1989–1998.[13]

mortality rates is probably greatly influenced by the condition of the patient at the time the emergency operation is undertaken. Representative early mortality rates reported for elective infrarenal aortic aneurysm repair, in contrast, typically range from 0% to 5.1% (**Table 31.1**).[13,80,83] More recently, the elective postoperative mortality rate for infrarenal abdominal aortic aneurysm repair has continued to improve, especially at experienced centers.[80] At the Cleveland Clinic Foundation, the mortality for 1135 elective infrarenal abdominal aortic aneurysms operated upon from January 1, 1989 through December 31, 1998 was 1.2% (**Table 31.2**). In this series, 21% (3/14) of the early postoperative deaths resulted from cardiac complications, 21% from pulmonary causes, 29% (4/14) from multisystem organ failure, and 29% (4/14) from miscellaneous causes.[13] These most recent results over the past decade represent a dramatic decline in the early postoperative mortality rate (9.6%) observed more than two decades ago at the same center from 1968 through 1973.

Late results

Late survival rates following successful open abdominal aortic aneurysm repair, based on a collected review of published series

Late survival following successful open abdominal aortic aneurysm repair.	
Interval after operation	*Range (%)*
1 year	90–95
5 years	60–84

Table 31.3 Late survival following successful open abdominal aortic aneurysm repair based on a collected review of published series of patients who underwent infrarenal abdominal aortic aneurysm repair from 1981–1991.[77]

of patients who underwent infrarenal abdominal aortic aneurysm repair from 1981–1991, are summarized in **Table 31.3**, and demonstrate 1-year cumulative survival rates ranging from 90% to 95% and typical 5-year survival rates of 60% to 84% at experienced centers.[77] At the Cleveland Clinic Foundation, the Kaplan-Meier estimates of late survival for 1135 elective infrarenal abdominal aortic aneurysms operated upon from January 1, 1989 through December 31, 1998 were 75% at 1 year and 49% at 10 years (**Fig. 31.15**).[13] Decreased postoperative survival was significantly associated with advancing age, the presence of coronary artery disease or congestive heart failure, and

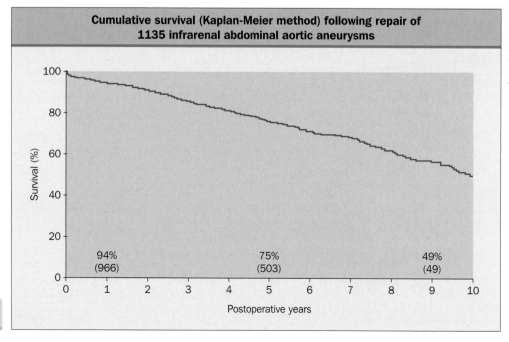

Figure 31.15 Cumulative survival (Kaplan–Meier method) following repair of 1135 infrarenal abdominal aortic aneurysms at the Cleveland Clinic Foundation from 1989 through 1998. (Reprinted with permission from the Journal of Vascular Surgery.[13])

Significant risk factors	Risk ratio	95% confidence intervals	p value
Age >75 years	2.2	1.7, 2.8	<0.001
Prior congestive heart failure	2.1	1.3, 3.4	0.004
Chronic obstructive pulmonary disease	1.5	1.2, 2.0	0.001
Creatinine >2mg/dL or prior dialysis	3.2	2.2, 4.6	<0.001

Multivariable analysis of risk factors associated with all deaths among 1135 patients who underwent elective infrarenal abdominal aortic aneurysm repair.

Table 31.4 Multivariable analysis of risk factors associated with all deaths among 1135 patients who underwent elective infrarenal abdominal aortic aneurysm repair at the Cleveland Clinic Foundation from 1989–1998.[13]

preoperative pulmonary or renal disease – associations reported by others (**Table 31.4**).[13,84,85]

The cumulative 6-year survival of patients who survive repair of ruptured abdominal aortic aneurysms (45%) is less than that of patients who undergo elective repair of their aneurysms (63%). Furthermore, cardiac complications were the leading cause, accounting for 29% of the late deaths.[85] These and other data emphasize that an aggressive approach to the detection and treatment of severe associated coronary artery disease is warranted to enhance late survival especially among non-diabetic men.[65–67]

Results in octogenarians

Although the severity of co-morbidities tends to increase with advancing age, we and others have concluded that repair of abdominal aortic aneurysms in properly selected octogenarians

is safe and durable. Consequently, when otherwise indicated, it should not be withheld on the basis of advanced age alone, even among the very elderly.

In our own experience with the management of infrarenal and juxtarenal abdominal aortic aneurysm repairs, performed in 114 consecutive octogenarians during a 10-year period from 1984 through 1993 at the Cleveland Clinic Foundation, the 30-day mortality rate for the entire series was 14%, but it declined from 23% during the first 5 years to 8% during the second 5 years of the study period (p=0.028). Fatal complications occurred in 9.6% of the patients with asymptomatic abdominal aortic aneurysms, and in 35% of those who had symptomatic abdominal aortic aneurysms (p=0.008). However, considering only patients with asymptomatic abdominal aortic aneurysms, the early mortality rate in the second 5 years (4%) improved significantly (p=0.038) in comparison to that for the first 5 years of the study period (17%).[86]

The cumulative 5-year survival rate for 97 available operative survivors was 48%, which was less than that for the normal male US population at the age of 80 years (59%; p<0.0001). However, the 5-year survival rate of 80% for 27 operative survivors who had received previous myocardial revascularization was significantly better compared to that for 70 others who did not (38%; p=0.0077), suggesting that prior treatment of severe coronary artery disease is associated with enhanced late survival, but patient selection probably is an important consideration in this respect (**Fig. 31.16**).[86]

Analysis of variables associated with postoperative survival among elderly patients at the Cleveland Clinic Foundation suggested that the presence of aneurysm symptoms or pre-existing renal disease was significantly associated with an adverse effect on the initial 30-day, but not the long-term, survival rate of operative survivors. Conversely, prior myocardial revascularization was not associated with an improved early postoperative survival rate, but it was associated with a more favorable late survival rate. Both early and late survival rates were reduced by high perioperative transfusion requirements.[86]

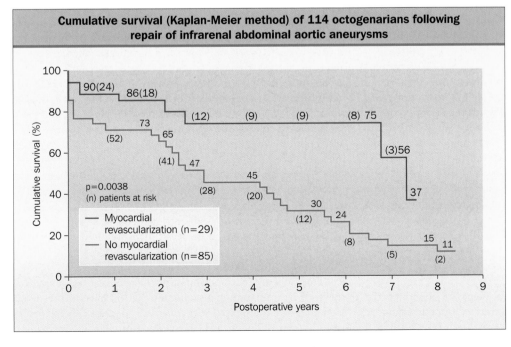

Figure 31.16 Cumulative survival (Kaplan–Meier method) of 114 octogenarians following repair of infrarenal abdominal aortic aneurysms at the Cleveland Clinic Foundation. Late survival was significantly better (p=0.0038) for those patients who underwent previous myocardial revascularization. (Reprinted with permission from the Journal of Vascular Surgery.[83])

Thirty-day complication rates among 1135 patients who underwent elective infrarenal abdominal aortic aneurysm repair.		
Complication	No.	%
Any complication		
None	939	83
Single	150	13
Multiple	46	4
Cardiac	64	5
Pulmonary	50	4
Renal	19	2
Miscellaneous	85	7
Wound	38	3
Intestinal obstruction	14	1
Intestinal ischemia	1	1
Sepsis	8	0.7
Retroperitoneal bleeding	5	0.4
Stroke	4	0.4
Deep venous thrombosis	4	0.4
Amputation	1	0.1

Table 31.5 Thirty-day complication rates among 1135 patients who underwent elective infrarenal abdominal aortic aneurysm repair at the Cleveland Clinic Foundation from 1989–1998.[13]

Multivariable analysis of risk factors associated with all 30-day complications among 1135 patients who underwent elective infrarenal abdominal aortic aneurysm repair.			
Significant risk factors	Risk ratio	95% confidence intervals	p value
Male gender	2.3	1.1, 5.2	0.035
Prior congestive heart failure	3.7	1.7, 7.8	0<.001
Chronic obstructive pulmonary disease	1.9	1.2, 2.9	0.004
Creatinine >2mg/dL or prior dialysis	2.5	1.3, 4.7	0.006

Table 31.6 Multivariable analysis of risk factors associated with all 30-day complications among 1135 patients who underwent elective infrarenal abdominal aortic aneurysm repair at the Cleveland Clinic Foundation from 1989–1998.[13]

Late complications 6–12 years following successful open abdominal aortic aneurysm repair.	
Late complication	Incidence (%)
Aorto-enteric fistula	0.9
Pseudoaneurysm	1.3
Graft infection	0.4
Bowel ischemia	0.3
Total	2.8

Table 31.7 Late complications 6–12 years following successful open abdominal aortic aneurysm repair based on a collected review of published series of patients who underwent infrarenal abdominal aortic aneurysm repair from 1981–1991.[77]

COMPLICATIONS

Early complication rates among 1135 patients who underwent elective infrarenal abdominal aortic aneurysm repair at the Cleveland Clinic Foundation from 1989–1998 are listed in **Table 31.5**. Eighty-three per cent of the patients had completely uncomplicated postoperative courses, whereas the remainder had at least one complication. Among this group of patients, multivariable analysis of risk factors associated with all 30-day complications yielded male gender, a history of congestive heart failure, or prior pulmonary or renal disease as variables significantly associated with an increased risk of the development of any postoperative complication (**Table 31.6**).[13]

Based on a collected review of published series of patients who underwent infrarenal abdominal aortic aneurysm repair from 1981–1991, late complications 6–12 years following successful open abdominal aortic aneurysm repair are distinctly unusual, with an overall incidence of 2.8% (**Table 31.7**).[77] In our own experience, only four late graft complications (0.4%) were identified among 1047 patients available for late follow-up. Two patients had graft infections, one had a graft limb occlusion, and one patient, who had undergone aortobifemoral graft placement at the time of aneurysm repair, developed a femoral pseudoaneurysm.[13]

SUMMARY

Key features

Open repair of an abdominal aortic aneurysm describes the direct surgical replacement of an infrarenal abdominal aortic aneurysm, utilizing either a transperitoneal or a retroperitoneal incision, and is currently the standard of treatment to which alternative treatment methods are compared. Due to the remarkable progress in preoperative imaging techniques, the recognition and management of patient co-morbidities, surgical and anesthetic techniques, and postoperative management, this approach has nearly universal applicability for the treatment of even extensive aneurysmal and associated occlusive disease. Multiple, first-rate, reproducible studies have firmly established that low mortality and morbidity rates are consistently achievable with this approach in experienced centers. Perhaps the most noteworthy feature of open aneurysm repair is its exceptional durability. Numerous well-documented reports have demonstrated that, once the aneurysm is repaired with an open procedure, it is distinctly unusual for a patient to develop a subsequent related problem with the reconstruction, even at very late follow-up intervals.

Future developments

It seems unlikely that open aneurysm repair will be completely replaced by interventional techniques in the near future. Consequently, it is important for vascular surgeons not only to acquire endovascular skills, but also to maintain proficiency in standard open vascular procedures. Not all patients with aneurysms have anatomy that is optimal, or even suitable, for stent-grafting utilizing currently available technology. It is also unlikely that any single device or refinement will eliminate the need for all the other tools we have available in vascular surgery.[14] With current technology, open operations are frequently required to supplement endovascular procedures as attempts are made to broaden the applicability of these new devices.[87,88]

Techniques for open aneurysm repair employing minimal incisions have been proposed and appear to have application in selected patients. These procedures, which do not require expensive imaging equipment, may prove to be cost effective alternatives or supplements to endovascular repair if the anatomy is favorable.[74–76]

Innovative techniques, involving laparoscopic assisted aneurysm repair, are in the preliminary stages of development. These methods will require careful evaluation of the risks and benefits associated with this approach before they are practical for widespread application.[71–73,89,90] It seems most likely that a combination of various approaches will evolve.

REFERENCES

1. Dubost C, Allary M, Oeconomos N. Resection of an aneurysm of the abdominal aorta: reestablishment of the continuity by a preserved human arterial graft, with result after five months. Arch Surg 1952;64:405–8.
2. Plate G, Hollier LA, O'Brien P, Pairolero PC, Cherry KJ, Kazmier FJ. Recurrent aneurysms and late vascular complications following repair of abdominal aortic aneurysms. Arch Surg 1985;120:590–4.
3. Hallett JW Jr, Marshall DM, Petterson TM, et al. Graft-related complications after abdominal aortic aneurysm repair: reassurance from a 36-year population-based experience. J Vasc Surg 1997;25:277–84.
4. Parodi JC, Palmaz JC, Barone HD. Transfemoral intraluminal graft implantation for abdominal aortic aneurysms. Ann Vasc Surg 1991; 5:491–9.
5. Zarins CK, White RA, Schwarten D, et al. AneuRx stent graft versus open surgical repair of abdominal aortic aneurysms: multicenter prospective clinical trial. J Vasc Surg 1999;29:292–305.
6. Zarins CK, White RA, Moll FL, et al. The AneuRx stent graft: four-year results and worldwide experience 2000. J Vasc Surg 2001; 33(2 Suppl): S135–45.
7. Makaroun MS. The Ancure endografting system: an update. J Vasc Surg 2001;33(2 Suppl):S129–34.
8. Buth J, Laheij RJ. Early complications and endoleaks after endovascular abdominal aortic aneurysm repair: report of a multicenter study. J Vasc Surg 2000; 31:134–46.
9. Wolf YG, Hill BB, Rubin GD, Fogarty TJ, Zarins CK. Rate of change in abdominal aortic aneurysm diameter after endovascular repair. J Vasc Surg 2000;32:108–15.
10. Zarins CK, White RA, Hodgson KJ, Schwarten D, Fogarty TJ. Endoleak as a predictor of outcome after endovascular aneurysm repair: AneuRx multicenter clinical trial. J Vasc Surg 2000; 32:90–107.
11. Harris PL, Vallabhaneni SR, Desgranges P, Becquemin JP, van Marrewijk C, Laheij RJ. Incidence and risk factors of late rupture, conversion, and death after endovascular repair of infrarenal aortic aneurysms: the EUROSTAR experience. European Collaborators on Stent/graft techniques for aortic aneurysm repair. J Vasc Surg 2000;32:739–49.
12. Zarins CK, Harris EJ Jr. Operative repair for aortic aneurysms: the gold standard. J Endovasc Surg 1997;4:232–41.
13. Hertzer NR, Mascha EJ, Karafa MT, O'Hara PJ, Krajewski LP, Beven EG. Open infrarenal abdominal aortic aneurysm repair: the Cleveland Clinic experience from 1989 to 1998. J Vasc Surg 2002; 35:1145–54.
14. O'Hara PJ. Gentlemen, this is no humbug: The role of natural selection in vascular surgery. J Vasc Surg 2002; 35:841–6.
15. O'Hara PJ, Hertzer NR, Krajewski LP, Cox GS, Beven EG. Reduction in the homologous blood requirement for abdominal aortic aneurysm repair by the use of preadmission autologous blood donation. Surgery 1994;115:69–76.
16. Cali RF, O'Hara PJ, Hertzer NR, Diehl JT, Beven EG. The influence of autotransfusion on homologous blood requirements during aortic reconstruction. Cleve Clin Q 1984;51:143–8.
17. O'Hara PJ, Hertzer NR, Santilli PH, Beven EG. Intraoperative autotransfusion during abdominal aortic reconstruction. Am J Surg 1983; 145:215–20.
18. Kramer AH, Hertzer NR, Beven EG. Intraoperative hemodilution during elective vascular reconstruction. Surg Gynecol Obstet 1979;149:831–6.
19. Gottlieb A. Aortic reconstructive surgery: Anesthetic considerations. Curr Opin Anesthesiol 1992;6:35.
20. Lord RS, Crozier JA, Snell J, Meek AC. Transverse abdominal incisions compared with midline incisions for elective infrarenal aortic reconstruction: predisposition to incisional hernia in patients with increased intraoperative blood loss. J Vasc Surg 1994;20:27–33.
21. Sicard GA, Reilly JM, Rubin BG, et al. Transabdominal versus retroperitoneal incision for abdominal aortic surgery: report of a prospective randomized trial. J Vasc Surg 1995; 21:174–81.
22. Cambria RP, Brewster DC, Abbott WM, et al. Transperitoneal versus retroperitoneal approach for aortic reconstruction: a randomized prospective study. J Vasc Surg 1990;11:314–24.
23. Leather RP. Comparative analysis of retroperitoneal and transperitoneal aortic replacement for aneurysm. Surg Gynecol Obstet 1989;168:387.
24. Darling RC, Leather RP, Paty PS, Chang BB, Shah DM. Flank vs. abdominal approach for abdominal aortic surgery: the flank approach. Adv Surg 1997;31:237–52.
25. Reilly LM, Ramos TK, Murray SP, Cheng SW, Stoney RJ. Optimal exposure of the proximal abdominal aorta: a critical appraisal of transabdominal medial visceral rotation. J Vasc Surg 1994;19:375–89.
26. O'Hara PJ. Aortoiliac revascularization. In: Montague DK, ed. Disorders of male sexual function. Chicago:Year Book Medical Publishers Inc; 1987.
27. Creech O Jr. Endo-aneurysmorrhaphy and treatment of aortic aneurysm. Ann Surg 1966;164:935–46.
28. Hertzer NR. Teflon reinforcement of an uninterrupted aortic anastomosis. Surg Gynecol Obstet 1983;157:480–1.
29. Brewster DC, Franklin DP, Cambria RP, et al. Intestinal ischemia complicating abdominal aortic surgery. Surgery 1991;109:447–54.
30. Rasmussen TR, Hallett JW Jr, Noel AA, et al. Early abdominal closure with mesh reduces multiple organ failure after ruptured abdominal aortic aneurysm repair: guidelines from a 10-year case-control study. J Vasc Surg 2002;35:246–53.
31. Hallett JW Jr. Management of aneurysms. In: Strandness JE, van Breda A, eds. Vascular diseases. New York:Churchill Livingstone; 1994:605–12.
32. O'Hara PJ, Hakaim AG, Hertzer NR, Krajewski LP, Cox GS, Beven EG. Surgical management of aortic aneurysm and coexistent horseshoe kidney: review of a 31-year experience. J Vasc Surg 1993;17:940–7.
33. Crawford ES, Coselli JS, Safi HJ, Martin TD, Pool JL. The impact of renal fusion and ectopia on aortic surgery. J Vasc Surg 1988;8:375–83.
34. Hollis HW Jr, Rutherford RB, Crawford GJ, Cleland BP, Marx WH, Clark JR. Abdominal aortic aneurysm repair in patients with pelvic kidney. Technical considerations and literature review. J Vasc Surg 1989;9:404–9.
35. Aljabri B, MacDonald PS, Satin R, Stein LS, Obrand DI, Steinmetz OK. Incidence of major venous and renal anomalies relevant to aortoiliac surgery as demonstrated by computed tomography. Ann Vasc Surg 2001;15:615–8.
36. Brener BJ, Darling RC, Frederick PL, Linton RL. Major venous anomalies complicating abdominal aortic surgery. Arch Surg 1974;108:159–65.
37. Bartle EJ, Pearce WH, Sun JH, Rutherford RB. Infrarenal venous anomalies and aortic surgery: avoiding vascular injury. J Vasc Surg 1987;6:590–3.

38. Ruemenapf G, Rupprecht H, Schweiger H. Preaortic iliac confluence: a rare anomaly of the inferior vena cava. J Vasc Surg 1998;27:767–71.

39. Giordano JM, Trout HH III. Anomalies of the inferior vena cava. J Vasc Surg 1986;3:924–8.

40. Crawford JL, Stowe CL, Safi HJ, Hallman CH, Crawford ES. Inflammatory aneurysms of the aorta. J Vasc Surg 1985;2:113–24.

41. Nitecki SS, Hallett JW Jr, Stanson AW, et al. Inflammatory abdominal aortic aneurysms: a case-control study. J Vasc Surg 1996; 23:860–8.

42. Sterpetti AV, Hunter WJ, Feldhaus RJ, et al. Inflammatory aneurysms of the abdominal aorta: incidence, pathologic, and etiologic considerations. J Vasc Surg 1989;9:643–9.

43. Green RM, Ricotta JJ, Ouriel K, DeWeese JA. Results of supraceliac aortic clamping in the difficult elective resection of infrarenal abdominal aortic aneurysm. J Vasc Surg 1989;9:124–34.

44. Panneton JM, Teh SH, Cherry KJ Jr, et al. Aortic fenestration for acute or chronic aortic dissection: an uncommon but effective procedure. J Vasc Surg 2000; 32:711–21.

45. Becquemin JP, Deleuze P, Watelet J, Testard J, Melliere D. Acute and chronic dissections of the abdominal aorta: clinical features and treatment. J Vasc Surg 1990; 11:397–402.

46. Cambria RP, Morse S, August D, Gusberg R. Acute dissection originating in the abdominal aorta. J Vasc Surg 1987;5:495–7.

47. Graham D, Alexander JJ, Franceschi D, Rashad F. The management of localized abdominal aortic dissections. J Vasc Surg 1988;8:582–91.

48. Thomas JH. Abdominal aortic aneurysmorrhaphy combined with biliary or gastrointestinal surgery. Surg Clin North Am 1989;69:807–15.

49. Csendes A, Burdiles P, Maluenda F, Diaz JC, Csendes P, Mitru N. Simultaneous bacteriologic assessment of bile from gallbladder and common bile duct in control subjects and patients with gallstones and common duct stones. Arch Surg 1996;131:389–94.

50. Kaufman HS, Magnuson TH, Lillemoe KD, Frasca P, Pitt HA. The role of bacteria in gallbladder and common duct stone formation. Ann Surg 1989;209:584–91.

51. Delikaris PG, Michail PO, Klonis GD, Haritopoulos NC, Golematis BC, Dreiling DA. Biliary bacteriology based on intraoperative bile cultures. Am J Gastroenterol 1977;68:51–5.

52. Hugh TB, Masson J, Graham AR, Tracy GD. Combined gastrointestinal and abdominal aortic aneurysm operations. Aust NZ J Surg 1988; 58:805–10.

53. Nora JD, Pairolero PC, Nivatvongs S, Cherry KJ, Hallett JW, Gloviczki P. Concomitant abdominal aortic aneurysm and colorectal carcinoma: priority of resection. J Vasc Surg 1989;9:630–5.

54. Morris HL, da Silva AF. Co-existing abdominal aortic aneurysm and intra-abdominal malignancy: reflections on the order of treatment. Br J Surg 1998;85:1185–90.

55. Darling RC III, Ozsvath K, Chang BB, et al. The incidence, natural history, and outcome of secondary intervention for persistent collateral flow in the excluded abdominal aortic aneurysm. J Vasc Surg 1999; 30:968–76.

56. Paty PS, Darling RC III, Chang BB, Shah DM, Leather RP. A prospective randomized study comparing exclusion technique and endoaneurysmorrhaphy for treatment of infrarenal aortic aneurysm. J Vasc Surg 1997;25:442–5.

57. Resnikoff M, Darling RC III, Chang BB, et al. Fate of the excluded abdominal aortic aneurysm sac: long-term follow-up of 831 patients. J Vasc Surg 1996;24:851–5.

58. Hertzer NR. Fatal myocardial infarction following abdominal aortic aneurysm resection. Three hundred forty-three patients followed 6–11 years postoperatively. Ann Surg 1980;192:667–73.

59. Johnston KW. Multicenter prospective study of nonruptured abdominal aortic aneurysm. Part II. Variables predicting morbidity and mortality. J Vasc Surg 1989;9:437–47.

60. Crawford ES, Saleh SA, Babb JW III, Glaeser DH, Vaccaro PS, Silvers A. Infrarenal abdominal aortic aneurysm: factors influencing survival after operation performed over a 25-year period. Ann Surg 1981;193:699–709.

61. Diehl JT, Cali RF, Hertzer NR, Beven EG. Complications of abdominal aortic reconstruction. An analysis of perioperative risk factors in 557 patients. Ann Surg 1983;197:49–56.

62. Hertzer NR, Young JR, Kramer JR, et al. Routine coronary angiography prior to elective aortic reconstruction: results of selective myocardial revascularization in patients with peripheral vascular disease. Arch Surg 1979;114:1336–44.

63. Hertzer NR, Beven EG, Young JR, et al. Coronary artery disease in peripheral vascular patients: a classification of 1000 coronary angiograms and results of surgical management. Ann Surg 1984;199:223–33.

64. Young JR, Hertzer NR, Beven EG, et al. Coronary artery disease in patients with aortic aneurysm: a classification of 302 coronary angiograms and results of surgical management. Ann Vasc Surg 1986;1:36–42.

65. Hertzer NR, Young JR, Beven EG et al. Late results of coronary bypass in patients with peripheral vascular disease. I. Five-year survival according to age and clinical cardiac status. Cleve Clin Q 1986;53:133–43.

66. Hertzer NR, Young JR, Beven EG, et al. Late results of coronary bypass in patients with peripheral vascular disease. II. Five-year survival according to sex, hypertension, and diabetes. Cleve Clin J Med 1987;54:15–23.

67. Hertzer NR, Young JR, Beven EG, et al. Late results of coronary bypass in patients with infrarenal aortic aneurysms. The Cleveland Clinic Study. Ann Surg 1987;205:360–7.

68. Brewster DC, Cronenwett JL, Hallett JW, et al. Guidelines for the treatment of abdominal aortic aneurysms: Report of a subcommittee of the Joint Council of the American Association for Vascular Surgery and the Society for Vascular Surgery. J Vasc Surg 2003;37:1106–17.

69. The UK Small Aneurysm Trial Participants. Mortality results for randomized controlled trial of early elective surgery or ultrasonographic surveillance for small aortic aneurysms. Lancet 1998;353:1649–55.

70. Lederle FA, Wilson SE, Johnson GR, et al. Immediate repair compared with surveillance of small aortic aneurysms. N Engl J Med 2002; 346:1437–44.

71. Alimi YS, Hartung O, Valerio N, Juhan C. Laparoscopic aortoiliac surgery for aneurysm and occlusive disease: when should a minilaparotomy be performed? J Vasc Surg 2001;33:469–75.

72. Bruns C, Wolfgarten B, Walter M, Pichlmaier H, Koebke J. Gasless videoendoscopic implantation of an aortobifemoral vascular prosthesis via a transperitoneal versus extraperitoneal approach: an experimental study. J Endovasc Surg 1996;3:290–6.

73. Fogarty TJ. Minimally invasive vascular surgery: laparoscopic as well as endovascular. J Endovasc Surg 1996;3:297–8.

74. Turnipseed WD, Carr SC, Tefera G, Acher CW, Hoch JR. Minimal incision aortic surgery. J Vasc Surg 2001;34:47–53.

75. Turnipseed WD. A less-invasive minilaparotomy technique for repair of aortic aneurysm and occlusive disease. J Vasc Surg 2001;33:431–4.

76. Cerveira JJ, Halpern VJ, Faust G, Cohen JR. Minimal incision abdominal aortic aneurysm repair. J Vasc Surg 1999;30:977–84.

77. Hollier LH, Taylor LM, Ochsner J. Recommended indications for operative treatment of abdominal aortic aneurysms. Report of a subcommittee of the Joint Council of the Society for Vascular Surgery and the North American Chapter of the International Society for Cardiovascular Surgery. J Vasc Surg 1992;15:1046–56.

78. Huber TS, Wang JG, Derrow AE, et al. Experience in the United States with intact abdominal aortic aneurysm repair. J Vasc Surg 2001; 33:304–10.

79. Huber TS, Harward TR, Flynn TC, Albright JL, Seeger JM. Operative mortality rates after elective infrarenal aortic reconstructions. J Vasc Surg 1995;22:287–93.

80. Katz DJ, Stanley JC, Zelenock GB. Operative mortality rates for intact and ruptured abdominal aortic aneurysms in Michigan: an eleven-year statewide experience. J Vasc Surg 1994;19:804–15.

81. Dardik A, Burleyson GP, Bowman H, et al. Surgical repair of ruptured abdominal aortic aneurysms in the state of Maryland: factors influencing outcome among 527 recent cases. J Vasc Surg 1998;28:413–20.

82. Noel AA, Gloviczki P, Cherry KJ Jr, et al. Ruptured abdominal aortic aneurysms: the excessive mortality rate of conventional repair. J Vasc Surg 2001;34:41–6.

83. Taylor LM Jr, Porter JM. Basic data related to clinical decision-making in abdominal aortic aneurysms. Ann Vasc Surg 1987;1:502–4.

84. Johnston KW. Nonruptured abdominal aortic aneurysm: six-year follow-up results from the multicenter prospective Canadian aneurysm study. Canadian Society for Vascular Surgery Aneurysm Study Group. J Vasc Surg 1994;20:163–70.

85. Johnston KW. Ruptured abdominal aortic aneurysm: six-year follow-up results of a multicenter prospective study. Canadian Society for Vascular Surgery Aneurysm Study Group. J Vasc Surg 1994;19:888–900.

86. O'Hara PJ, Hertzer NR, Krajewski LP, Tan M, Xiong X, Beven EG. Ten-year experience with abdominal aortic aneurysm repair in octogenarians: early results and late outcome. J Vasc Surg 1995;21:830–8.

87. Chang DW, Chan A, Forse RA, Abbott WM. Enabling sutureless vascular bypass grafting with the exovascular sleeve anastomosis. J Vasc Surg 2000;32:524–30.

88. Quinones-Baldrich WJ, Panetta TF, Vescera CL, Kashyap VS. Repair of type IV thoracoabdominal aneurysm with a combined endovascular and surgical approach. J Vasc Surg 1999;30:555–60.

89. Cerveira JJ, Cohen JR. Laparoscopically assisted abdominal aortic aneurysm repair. Semin Laparosc Surg 1999;6:144–52.

90. Kline RG, D'Angelo AJ, Chen MH, Halpern VJ, Cohen JR. Laparoscopically assisted abdominal aortic aneurysm repair: first 20 cases. J Vasc Surg 1998;27:81–7.

CHAPTER

32

Complex Aortic Aneurysm: Pararenal, Suprarenal, and Thoracoabdominal

W Darrin Clouse and Richard P Cambria

KEY POINTS

- Complex aortic aneurysms represent a continuum of disease involving multiple aortic segments.

- Patient-specific variables that may enhance rupture risk include: chronic obstructive pulmonary disease, renal insufficiency, smoking, hypertension, prior stroke, Marfan's syndrome, pain/symptoms attributable to the aneurysm, and female gender.

- Aneurysm-specific variables that enhance rupture risk include: aneurysm size, dissection, extent of disease, and expansion rate.

- The decision to undertake operative reconstruction in patients with complex aortic aneurysms is made weighing the above characteristics with the patient's overall medical condition.

- Refinements in computed tomography and helical reconstruction have made this the imaging modality of choice and frequently the only study required for evaluating complex aneurysmal disease.

- Results of open reconstruction have improved due to the multiplicity of operative strategies and adjuncts applied attempting to minimize the principal complications.

- Emerging technology is proving endovascular repair of complex aortic aneurysm feasible and may become part of management strategies in the near future.

INTRODUCTION

While the majority of degenerative aortic aneurysms are isolated infrarenal lesions, some 7–15% involve segments at or above the renal arteries. These lesions represent varying points on an anatomic continuum of aneurysmal disease, and multiple aortic segments are commonly affected. For example, most studies examining natural history data for thoracic aortic aneurysms indicate that between 20% and 30% of these patients will also be found to have aneurysms of the abdominal aorta (AAA).[1–3] Our experience indicates that roughly 20% of patients undergoing thoracoabdominal aneurysm (TAA) repair will proceed to have expansion of remaining aortic segments.[4] In a large Mayo Clinic series encompassing nearly 6000 aortic resections for aneurysmal disease, 2% of patients undergoing AAA repair and 18% of patients with TAA underwent multiple aneurysm repairs.[5] Crawford and Cohen noted in a series of 1500 patients treated for AAA that some 12.5% harbored aneurysms in other aortic segments.[6]

Aside from the obvious more proximal extent of aorta involved, TAA can also be distinguished from the more routine AAA because of differing etiologies and shifts in patient demographic profiles. While a majority are degenerative in nature and occur in association with hypertension, smoking, and frequently with evidence of vascular disease in other territories, up to 20% of TAAs in most series result from chronic aortic dissection.[7–11] Furthermore, the male:female sex ratio of TAA is 1:1, whereas AAA patients have a 5:1 male:female ratio. Others have noted the tendency for aneurysmal disease in females to involve proximal aortic segments more frequently, and women appear to be at increased risk of rupture.[12–14]

Successful operation on an abdominal aneurysm involving the visceral aortic segment was first reported by Etheredge et al. in 1955.[15] Thereafter, DeBakey and colleagues reported Dacron graft aortic replacement with multiple sidearms for visceral vessel reconstruction.[16] The modern era of successful surgical management of TAA began with the pioneering work of E Stanley Crawford, whose technical modifications laid the foundation for the widespread successful management of TAA. Crawford described a simplified operative approach to these lesions using the inclusion technique wherein visceral and intercostal vessels were reconstructed from within the aneurysm by directly anastomosing openings in the main Dacron graft to the aortic origin of these vessels.[17,18] Despite various surgical and adjunctive strategies applied in different centers to minimize overall operative morbidity, the state of the art in contemporary management still entails a 5–10% risk of perioperative mortality and/or morbidity in the form of renal, respiratory, and spinal cord ischemic complications.[7–10,19,20] Given this fact, and while acknowledging conventional surgical repair remains the only treatment option in most environments, endovascular stent-graft repair providing for side-branch flow may in the near future alter the treatment of pararenal aneurysms and TAA.[21,22]

Aneurysm extent

While a degree of confusion exists regarding the terms juxta- and pararenal aneurysm, the Ad Hoc Committee on Reporting Standards of the Society for Vascular Surgery and the American Association for Vascular Surgery has identified *pararenal* as synonymous with *juxtarenal* (**Fig. 32.1**).[23] *Juxtarenal* and *pararenal* aneurysms are those that extend cephalad sufficiently close to the renal arteries (less than a 1 cm neck) to require suprarenal, or higher, aortic cross-clamping. The term *suprarenal* aneurysm implies that at least one renal artery arises from the aneurysm, yet it does not extend proximally to involve the superior mesenteric artery (SMA). Further extension cephalad to involve the visceral vessels is considered a total abdominal aneurysm or, synonymously, a type IV TAA, as described below. Thus, lesions

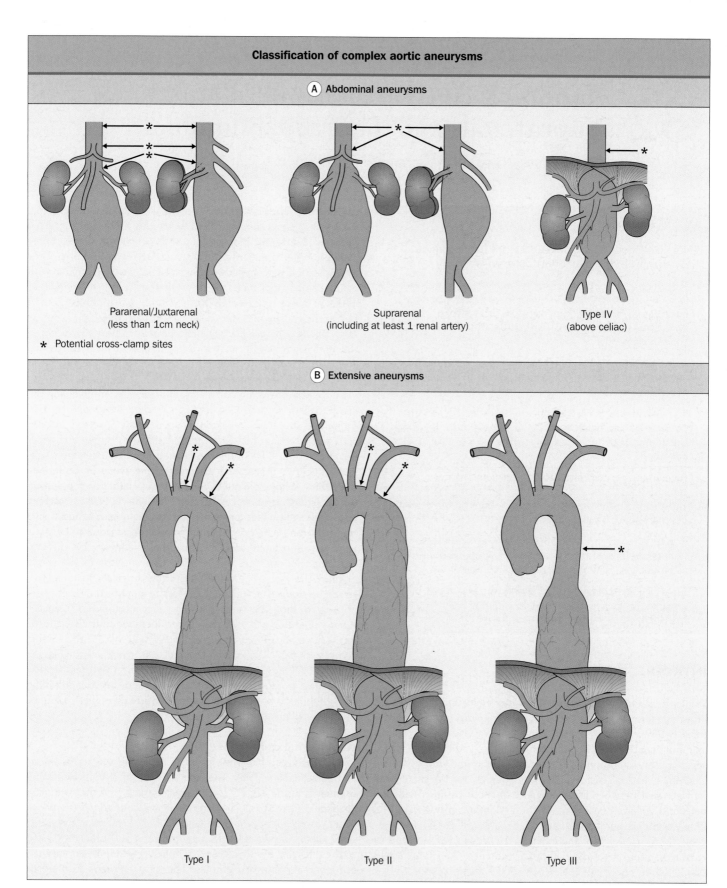

Figure 32.1 Classification of complex aortic aneurysms. (A) Abdominal aneurysms: *pararenal* with infrarenal neck of less than 1cm; *suprarenal* with at least one renal artery involved in aneurysm; total abdominal or *type IV* thoracoabdominal aneurysm (TAA) when it is necessary to carry graft above celiac axis. (B) Extensive TAA: *types I–III*. Notice potential aortic cross-clamp sites for each extent.

simultaneously involving the thoracic and abdominal aorta as well as those which include the visceral aortic segment are termed *thoracoabdominal* aneurysms.

Thoracoabdominal aneurysms are classified according to the scheme originally devised by Crawford, which, in the most basic terms, considers whether the lesion is primarily a caudal extension of a descending thoracic aneurysm, or a cephalad extension of a total abdominal aneurysm (**Fig. 32.1**).[18] This classification is clinically useful since it has direct implications for both the technical conduct of operation, and the incidence of operative complications, in particular, ischemic spinal cord injury. There is considerable variation in the spectrum and overall scope of operation required to deal with aneurysms within the classification of TAA. For example, in contemporary practice, management of the type IV aneurysm should be accomplished with an overall morbidity and mortality not significantly different from the management of routine AAA.[24] In fact, delineating between a suprarenal aneurysm and a type IV TAA amounts to no more than a few centimeters of the visceral aortic segment. We define *type IV* repair as one in which it is necessary to extend the graft proximal to the celiac axis.

Type I and *type II* lesions are more extensive and require resection of the entire descending thoracic aorta. Repair of these aneurysms typically requires a clamp placed at or even proximal to the left subclavian artery. We reserve the designation type II aneurysm for those patients where the *entire* descending thoracic and abdominal aorta is involved. *Type III* aneurysms involve variable lengths of the descending aorta and abdominal aorta. Furthermore, the aneurysm should be classified according to the extent of aorta resected during a single procedure. For example, it is commonplace to resect a type I aneurysm into a prior infrarenal aneurysm repair. Such lesions should be classified as a type I rather than a type II aneurysm.

There is considerable variation reported in the literature with respect to the distribution of TAA. While this reflects, to a degree, referral biases, the issue of precision in aneurysm classification, as discussed above, likely also accounts for some of the variability. Displayed in **Table 32.1** are data from representative contemporary series regarding the relative distribution of TAA

extent. Virtually all major clinical series of TAA reconstruction emphasize a significant incidence of prior aortic resections, and in our experience this is seen in nearly one-third of patients presenting for TAA resection.[25] The most common pattern is the patient who has undergone a prior infrarenal AAA repair (60% of total prior resections). However, virtually every pattern can be seen, including prior proximal thoracic aortic grafts and/or prior TAA resections where part of the visceral aortic segment was encompassed in the original operation.[26,27]

The classification scheme outlined in **Figure 32.1** does not consider the patient with concomitant discontinuous aneurysm of parts or all of the ascending aorta and aortic arch. While synchronous proximal aneurysm is noted in 6–13% of TAA patients, contiguous arch aneurysm is rare, typically occurring only in patients with a prior DeBakey type I aortic dissection, especially those with Marfan's syndrome.[28] Patients with incontinuity arch/thoracoabdominal aortic aneurysm usually require complex, staged procedures.[29,30] Since patients with degenerative TAA or prior distal dissections most often have an aneurysm 'neck' in the region of the aortic isthmus, TAA resection is usually, and more safely, performed staged after surgical correction of ascending/arch aneurysms when both require resection.[30]

Etiology

The majority of pararenal and thoracoabdominal aortic aneurysms are degenerative in nature and most authorities agree the terms *atherosclerotic* and *degenerative* may be used interchangeably. With the exception of the rare primary abdominal aortic dissection or infected aneurysm, abdominal aneurysm etiology is limited to degenerative disease and para-anastomotic pseudoaneurysm. In contrast, some 20% of TAAs are the sequelae of chronic aortic dissection.[7–11] Of patients experiencing acute aortic dissection, 25–40% will progress to have aneurysmal dilation of the dissected aorta.[31–35] DeBakey et al.[36] found this phenomenon occurred in 30% of over 500 aortic dissection patients treated surgically. Recently, Marui et al.[37] reported that 43% of patients initially treated medically during the acute phase of type III

Aneurysm extent (Crawford classification) among major series of patients undergoing thoracoabdominal aneurysm repair.						
Reference	*Year*	*Number of repairs*	*Type I* No. (%)	*Type II* No. (%)	*Type III* No. (%)	*Type IV* No. (%)
Svensson et al.[11]	1993	1509	378 (25)	442 (29)	343 (23)	346 (23)
Schepens et al.[64]	1996	172	33 (19)	53 (31)	55 (32)	31 (18)
Grabitz et al.[150]	1996	260	68 (26.2)	81 (31.2)	87 (33.5)	24 (9.2)
Acher et al.[7]	1998	176	35 (19.9)	66 (37.5)	29 (16.5)	46 (26.1)
Hamilton et al.[198]	1998	265	40 (15.1)	74 (27.9)	78 (29.4)	73 (27.5)
Coselli et al.[61]	2000	1220	423 (34.7)	371 (30.4)	201 (16.5)	225 (18.4)
Estrera et al.[89]	2001	508	164 (25.1)	165 (25.2)	84 (12.8)	95 (14.5)
Cambria et al.[25]	2002	337	92 (27)	59 (17)	120 (36)	66 (20)
Total		**4447**	**1233 (28)**	**1311 (30)**	**997 (22)**	**906 (20)**

Table 32.1 Aneurysm extent (Crawford classification) among major series of patients undergoing thoracoabdominal aneurysm repair.

dissection progressed to have aortic enlargement. Moreover, dilation to 6cm or greater occurred in nearly 30%. Factors that appear to have a significant impact on chronic aneurysm development after dissection include poorly controlled hypertension, maximal aortic diameter of at least 4cm in the acute phase, and continued patency of the false lumen.[37–40] Furthermore, some 10–20% of those with dissection will subsequently experience rupture.[31,38] Confounding this issue is the fact some patients with degenerative lesions will go on to develop dissection within the pre-existing aneurysm, an inherently unstable condition.[14,41] Aneurysms that are the sequelae of chronic dissection tend to be more extensive and occur in younger patients compared with degenerative aneurysms. Patients with true cystic medial necrosis, such as those with Marfan's syndrome, have an increased risk of aneurysm and dissection formation. Marfan's syndrome is an autosomal dominant, inherited mutation of the fibrillin-1 gene leading to disarrayed microfibrillar connective tissue formation and subsequent aortic degeneration. In addition to disorders of other connective tissue, cystic medial degeneration of the aorta, perhaps caused by smooth muscle cell apoptosis mediated by angiotensin II receptors, leads to a spectrum of aortic pathology including root and sinotubular aneurysm, annuloaortic ectasia, and acute and chronic dissection.[42] While aortic disease has traditionally led to early death in patients with Marfan's syndrome, the surgical and diagnostic advances in aortic disease during the last three decades have allowed their life-expectancy to approach that of the population at large.[43,44] Frequently these patients have either total aortic ectasia or multiple aneurysms. Ascending aortic and aortic valve disease is the most common lesion addressed, with 90% of initial operations occurring in this segment. However, 40% proceed to a second aortic procedure, which typically involves the thoracoabdominal aorta.[45] Aggressive beta-blockade has been shown to retard the growth of the aortic root and may have a similar effect on the thoracoabdominal aorta.[46]

Aortitis leading to aneurysm development is rare. Lesions secondary to the sequelae of giant cell arteritis are typically seen in women. Aneurysms can result from either Takayasu's disease or giant cell aortitis. Evans et al.[47] found that patients with giant cell arteritis were 17.3 and 2.4 times more likely to develop thoracic and abdominal aneurysms, respectively, when compared with the general population. There may be no known prior diagnosis of aortitis or other associated collagen vascular disease. Such aneurysms can be either focal or diffuse along the thoracoabdominal aorta, and are frequently associated with other known sequelae of inflammatory aortitis, namely, visceral and renal artery occlusive disease. TAAs secondary to infectious processes present challenging management issues because the dual goals of eradication of sepsis and arterial reconstruction typically demand an in-situ type of reconstruction (i.e. placement of a prosthetic graft in a contaminated field). The term *mycotic* aneurysm continues to be applied to these lesions, although, as originally described by Osler,[48] this term more precisely relates to aneurysms secondary to embolization from an infected cardiac vegetation. A more proper term is *infected* aneurysm. In contemporary practice, the pathogenesis of these lesions is usually hematogenous seeding of atherosclerotic plaque, the development of focal aortitis with dissolution of the aortic wall, and the formation of a false aneurysm. All such aneurysms are, in fact, contained ruptures of false aneurysms.

In summary, the distribution of TAA etiology is approximately 80% degenerative, 15–20% secondary to chronic dissection (including those with familial connective tissue diseases), 2% infectious, and 1–2% resulting from aortitis.[8,25,28]

Natural history

Natural history data aid in balancing aneurysm rupture risk with surgical morbidity. The expected natural history of pararenal aneurysms and TAA is progressive enlargement and eventual rupture regardless of etiology. Since these aneurysms are uncommon compared with AAA, fewer natural history studies are available. Furthermore, natural history studies of degenerative TAA are confused by inclusion of patients with acute aortic dissection, many of whom succumb in the acute phase of the disease.[1,12] Size criteria for operation in TAA are not as clearly defined compared with AAA. Since rupture risk and factors associated with rupture of pararenal aneurysms are similar to those for AAA described elsewhere in this text, we herein concentrate on natural history studies of TAA.

Population-based studies, since they are exempt from the inherent bias of referral center series, offer the best insight. Two studies performed 20 years ago form the foundation of thoracic aneurysm epidemiology. Bickerstaff and colleagues from the Mayo Clinic reported an incidence of 5.9 thoracic aortic aneurysms per 100 000 person-years over a 30-year period (1951–1980) in Rochester, Minnesota.[1] They found that rupture occurred in 74% of their patients and was nearly always fatal. Actuarial 5-year survival was a mere 13%. If patients with aortic dissection were eliminated, the prognosis of degenerative thoracic aortic aneurysm in the first 3 years after diagnosis was considerably worse when compared with a prior Mayo Clinic study of unoperated AAA.[49] Similar data with respect to the incidence of concomitant AAA (25%), the higher risk of rupture with aortic dissection, and a substantial rupture risk for thoracic aneurysm were reported by McNamara and Pressler.[2] The latter study is valuable since no patients were operated upon and the 3-year survival of patients with degenerative thoracic aortic aneurysm was only 35%. Almost half of the deaths were related to aneurysm rupture.

Recently, Clouse and associates re-evaluated the prognosis of degenerative thoracic aortic aneurysms found in Olmsted County, Minnesota, between 1980 and 1994[14] and compared this experience to Bickerstaff's prior communication.[1] The descending aorta was the principal segment affected in 60% of patients. The incidence of degenerative aneurysm had nearly tripled and the 5-year survival had improved to 56% in the 15 years of study. This was attributed to the development of computed tomography (CT) and echocardiography, with earlier diagnosis, and potentially improved surgical techniques. Notably, the overall 5-year rupture risk was 20%. Nearly 80% of ruptures occurred in women, and female gender was independently associated with rupture risk (relative risk, 6.8; 95% confidence interval [CI], 2.3–19.9; p=0.01). Aneurysm-specific variables also strongly correlated with rupture and included symptoms attributable to the aneurysm and dissection developing within the degenerative aneurysm, further establishing their importance in surgical decision-making.[41,50] Increasing aneurysm size led to higher rupture risk (**Fig. 32.2**). Rupture accounted for 30% of all deaths and occurred with an incidence of 3.5 per 100 000 patient-years.[51] The 30-day mortality for

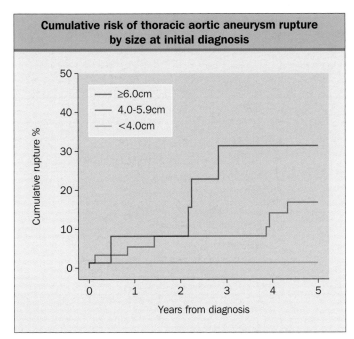

Figure 32.2 Cumulative risk of thoracic aortic aneurysm rupture by size at initial diagnosis. Five-year rupture risk for aneurysms 6.0cm or larger, 31%; for 4–5.9cm, 16%; and for those <4cm, 0%. (Adapted from Clouse et al.[14] ©2004 American Medical Association.)

elective repair was 8%, versus 54% for emergent cases. The authors suggested 6cm as the size criterion for intervention in appropriate-risk, asymptomatic patients. Johansson et al.[12] also reported the incidence of ruptured thoracic aortic aneurysm in two separate time intervals (1989 and 1980). The incidence of presentation for treatment of ruptured thoracic aortic aneurysm was 5 per 100 000 patient-years. The incidence was stable over the decade examined and rupture was usually fatal. Interestingly, these investigators found an equal sex distribution among patients with ruptured thoracic aortic aneurysm.

Although natural history data from referral center populations are biased, such studies remain valuable since issues surrounding the selection of patients for operative therapy are considered. Crawford and colleagues reported on nearly 100 patients referred for, but subsequently denied, surgical treatment for TAA, usually related to advanced age or associated co-morbid conditions. Survival at 2 years was only 24%, and half of all deaths were related to aneurysm rupture. Interestingly, chronic obstructive pulmonary disease (COPD) was noted in 80% of patients denied reconstruction because of associated co-morbid conditions. Not surprisingly, the 2-year survival in these authors' comparative series of surgically treated patients (70%) was far superior to the observed survival in the non-operated cohort.[52] Size criteria for recommending operation were initially inferred from another report from Crawford's group. In a series of 117 patients treated for ruptured thoracic or thoracoabdominal aortic aneurysm, they found 80% of all ruptures occurred in aneurysms less than 10cm, dispelling the previously held myth that only exceedingly large thoracic aneurysms rupture. Rupture occurred in smaller aneurysms when acute dissection was the pathology. Rupture occurred with equal frequency in the chest and abdominal cavities, and 60% of all TAA ruptures occurred in cases where the abdominal component was less than 8cm in

diameter. Since rupture was observed in some 10% of patients with aneurysms less than 6cm in diameter, the authors recommended elective operation for TAA when a 5cm-diameter threshold was exceeded.[53]

Recent referral center reports give further insight into the expected natural history and rupture risk in patients considered for TAA resection. These valuable data have delineated both patient-specific and aneurysm-specific factors that are important elements in aneurysm prognosis (**Table 32.2**). TAAs appear to expand at more rapid rates as they become larger, and several investigators have correlated increased expansion rates with rupture.[54–56] Furthermore, these studies indicate that TAA rupture risk is negligible in aneurysms less than 5cm, is equivalent to the risk of surgical morbidity in the 5–6cm range, and increases substantially at aneurysm diameters above 6cm and growth rates of ≥ 10mm/year.

SELECTION FOR OPERATION

These natural history observations have led us to use 6cm as a generally appropriate size threshold to recommend surgical intervention for extent I–III TAA. In view of recent Society for Vascular Surgery guidelines for AAA treatment, 5.5cm is used for abdominal lesions.[57] Increasing expansion rate is used as an indicator of heightened rupture risk and consideration is given to earlier operation, while in chronic dissection and patients with Marfan's syndrome, a 5cm size threshold is maintained due to rupture tendency at smaller sizes.[38,58,59]

Asymptomatic presentation with radiographic detection is common, yet symptoms due to aneurysm expansion, rupture, and local compression are seen and should be quickly evaluated in view of enhanced rupture potential. Juvonen et al.[50] noted even the presence of atypical symptoms was an independent rupture correlate. The usual dismissal of such complaints, if they are chronic, is inappropriate in patients with known TAA. Frequent symptoms reported include back pain localized to the left lower hemithorax, or, when the aortic hiatus is significantly involved, a typical mid-back and/or epigastric pain. When the aneurysm erodes into the thoracolumbar spine or chest wall, complaints of chest and back pain can be both prominent and present for weeks to months, as they nearly always represent contained rupture. Depending on the topography of the aneurysm, other symptoms may be referable to a variety of compression and/or erosion phenomena. New onset of hoarseness related to left recurrent laryngeal nerve palsy, compression or erosion of the tracheobronchial tree or pulmonary parenchyma producing cough, hemoptysis or dyspnea, and dysphagia are all possible but uncommon symptomatic manifestations of TAA.[60] Similar to AAA, distal embolization of atheromatous debris can be observed, but has constituted a rare indication, in and of itself, for operation in our experience. Perhaps related to reluctance to recommend operation because of the threat of surgical morbidity, between 40% and 70% of TAA patients will present with symptoms.[8,11,25,61] This explains the higher proportion of patients treated for rupture when compared with AAA operations. Approximately 25% of patients will be treated in urgent or emergent circumstances with half presenting with frank rupture.[7,8,11,25,61,62]

Co-morbid conditions associated with diffuse atherosclerosis and global vascular disease are commonplace in patients with

	Referral center reports describing thoracic/thoracoabdominal aortic aneurysm prognosis.	
Reference	*Prognostic factors (end-point)* *Aneurysm-specific*	*Patient-specific*
Cambria et al.[192]	Size ≥5cm (rupture)	COPD (expansion; rupture trend) Chronic renal failure (rupture trend)
Dapunt et al.[193]	Size ≥5cm (expansion, survival)	Smoking (expansion)
Perko et al.[13]	Dissection (rupture) Size ≥6cm (rupture, survival)	Hypertension (survival) Respiratory insufficiency (survival) Renal failure (rupture, survival)
Masuda et al.[54]	Size (expansion) Abdominal aneurysmal disease (expansion)	Diastolic hypertension (expansion) Renal failure (expansion)
Griepp et al.[59]	Dissection (rupture, survival) Smaller max size (dissection rupture) Increasing extent (rupture)	Age (rupture) Hypertension (dissection rupture) COPD (rupture) Pain – even atypical (rupture)
Coady et al.[58,194]	Size ≥6cm (rupture or dissection)	
Bonser et al.[195]	Intraluminal thrombus (expansion) Mid descending aorta (expansion)	Smoking (expansion) Prior stroke (expansion) Peripheral vascular disease (expansion)
Juvonen et al.[38,50]	Size ≥5cm (smaller max for dissection rupture)	Age (rupture) COPD (rupture) Pain – even atypical (rupture) Hypertension (dissection rupture)
Lobato et al.[55]	Size ≥5cm (rupture) Expansion (rupture)	
Davies et al.[196]	Size ≥5cm (rupture) Size ≥6cm rupture or acute dissection) Descending aorta (survival) Elective repair (survival) Expansion (rupture trend)	Female gender (rupture or acute dissection) Prior stroke (rupture or acute dissection) Marfan's syndrome (rupture or acute dissection)

Table 32.2 Referral center reports describing thoracic/thoracoabdominal aortic aneurysm prognosis. COPD, chronic obstructive pulmonary disease.

TAA. A familial aneurysm history is present in about 10% of patients. Prior aortic grafting for aneurysmal disease is seen in nearly one-third of patients with TAA. The most common scenario is a previous infrarenal aneurysm repair. Coselli et al. detailed experience in 123 patients undergoing TAA resection after prior infrarenal AAA repair. These patients presented for TAA repair a mean of 8 years after the initial AAA operation.[26] While many of these represent de-novo development of a second aneurysm, it is also clear that an inadequate initial infrarenal operation will create the necessity for a second, more definitive procedure. The presence of a previous infrarenal or more proximal thoracic aortic graft does not unduly complicate the subsequent TAA repair. Coselli and colleagues have indicated that TAA operation after a prior aortic graft produces results similar to those seen with de-novo TAA resection, although a prior proximal graft appears to increase the risk of spinal cord ischemia.[27]

Patients treated for degenerative aneurysm generally have advanced diffuse atherosclerosis, with an average age of 70 years. Hypertension is nearly universal. Cerebrovascular disease, prior stroke, and lower extremity arterial occlusive disease occur in 20–25% of patients. Associated renovisceral occlusive disease occurs in 30–40% of patients, with nearly 35% requiring

endarterectomy or bypass of these vessels.[25] About 15% of patients will have significant renal insufficiency (serum creatinine ≥1.8mg/dL).[8,25] Renal dysfunction accompanied by renal artery occlusive disease has important implications for both accurate assessment of perioperative risk and long-term preservation of renal function. Some of these patients will have the potential for retrieval or salvage of renal function with renal artery reconstruction. However, the presence of an abnormal preoperative serum creatinine is at least a univariate correlate of perioperative mortality.[7,8,11,19,25,63–65] As a result, assessment of renal function and associated renovascular disease becomes an important component of preoperative patient evaluation and surgical decision-making. Preoperative azotemia (serum creatinine >2.5mg/dL) constitutes a relative contraindication to elective operation unless preoperative studies indicate renal artery reconstruction may possibly salvage or recover renal function.

An accurate assessment of cardiopulmonary function and associated co-morbid conditions is mandatory to guide appropriate decision-making with respect to recommending operation. Cigarette smoking and/or significant COPD are frequently encountered. Pulmonary function tests are recommended in all such patients. Approximately one-third of patients have moderately compromised pulmonary function, with 15% having severe

COPD manifested by an FEV1 of less than 50% predicted. In patients with clinically evident heart disease, some type of non-invasive cardiac testing is appropriate. In addition, patients with a history or symptoms suggestive of heart failure should have an assessment of left ventricular function. Advanced age must be considered if it is accompanied by overall fragility and impaired functional status. Accordingly, advanced age in itself is not an absolute reason to deny operation.[66]

Preoperative hydration is critical, especially in patients with impaired renal function. In the past, preoperative dopamine infusion was used in patients with renal insufficiency; however, preliminary results with intravenous infusion of the D_1-selective dopamine agonist, fenoldopam, suggest a salutary effect on post-repair renal function, and some now use this adjunct when any degree of renal impairment is present. Patients may undergo mechanical and antibiotic bowel preparation, based on evidence indicating that bacterial translocation during supraceliac clamping may contribute to disorders of blood coagulation.[67,68]

Non-operative therapy may be selected initially in very frail patients, those with modest-size aneurysms, and those for whom associated co-morbid conditions make the short-term risk of surgery prohibitive and/or life expectancy limited to a degree that surgical treatment is not rational. Patients selected for non-operative therapy should be treated aggressively with beta-blockade, hypertension control, and cessation of cigarette smoking.[69]

Imaging

Accurate and complete radiographic evaluation is mandatory. Based on review of preoperative studies, there should be no equivocation in the surgeon's mind as to the proximal and distal extent of resection. In contemporary practice, a dynamic, fine-cut, contrast-enhanced CT scan with or without helical reconstruction provides the surgeon with:

- the location of proximal aortic cross-clamping and anastomosis;
- a qualitative assessment of the aorta in the region of the proximal cross-clamp;
- the assessment of patency and orificial stenosis of the visceral vessels;
- the topography of the renal artery origins in relation to aneurysm contour, in addition to kidney size and adequacy of perfusion; and
- the distal extent of the resection including major aneurysmal disease of the iliac vessels.

Traditionally, complete contrast arteriography has also been used to evaluate patients treated in elective settings to assist in examination of the aortic arch and renovisceral vessels. Further, surgeons who utilize retrograde transfemoral aortic perfusion have routinely used pelvic arteriography to exclude significant iliac occlusive disease. However, in conjunction with its ability to provide the best topographic information, refinements in helical CT reconstruction have made renovisceral and iliac evaluation by this means more than adequate (**Fig. 32.3**). Magnetic resonance angiography (MRA) may also be used for renovisceral evaluation.[70] Contrast arteriography remains beneficial in selected situations. Chronic dissection generally requires complete arteriography. It is critical to understand preoperatively exactly how each renovisceral and iliac orifice is related to the true and false lumens. When distal aortic reconstruction is required in patients with previous colon resection, arteriography

may also provide useful information about the remaining collateral colonic blood supply. Patients with rare anatomic variants such as horseshoe kidneys and anomalous arterial anatomy generally require arteriography. Further, arteriography may be useful in providing some assessment of the number and location of patent intercostal vessels. While decisions about intercostal vessels are ultimately made intraoperatively, knowledge of multiple patent arteries in the critical aortic segment (T_8 to L_1) can prepare the surgeon for their reconstruction and potentially save operative and clamp time and lessen neurologic morbidity. Kieffer et al.[71] have recently commented on spinal cord arteriography safety and efficacy in 480 patients. They reported complications in six (1.2%) patients with only two (0.4%) being spinal cord related. Adamkiewicz's artery was identified in 86% of cases and the anterior spinal artery was able to be completely or partially visualized in 89%. MRA technology is another advancing imaging option to identify intercostal vessels.[72]

Contrast studies should be minimized in patients with any degree of renal insufficiency; likewise, catheter manipulation in patients with excessive atherosclerotic debris in the visceral aortic segment. All elective iodinated contrast diagnostic studies should be performed well in advance of surgery. Serum creatinine should be rechecked after contrast-related imaging and operative repair delayed until renal function is stable.

OPERATIVE MANAGEMENT

Standard central venous access including a pulmonary artery catheter and arterial lines appropriate for the site of anticipated cross-clamping are essential. Fluid warming and passive external warming devices should be standard, to avoid systemic hypo-thermia. An epidural catheter is recommended for intraoperative anesthesia and postoperative analgesia. When epidural cooling or spinal drainage is used, a lower thoracic epidural catheter is necessary, and a cerebrospinal fluid (CSF) drainage catheter should be placed in the lower lumbar area and connected to a pressure transducer.

Packed red blood cells (RBC) and fresh frozen plasma are started early as the primary fluid replacement; platelets are administered when the visceral or distal aortic anastomoses are completed. Autotransfusion is routinely used to retrieve shed blood and generally accounts for half the RBC volume returned to the patient. In preparation for aortic cross-clamping, 12.5–25g of mannitol and/or furosemide is administered to promote diuresis. Patients with renal insufficiency are maintained on dopamine or fenoldopam infusions. When CSF drainage and/or epidural cooling are in place, 20mL of CSF are removed prior to clamping. Operative cases involving a very difficult proximal aortic reconstruction or significant renal dysfunction preoperatively may benefit from partial left heart bypass and distal aortic perfusion.

Aortic cross-clamping proceeds slowly and the epidural anesthetic is often reinforced to aid in lowering the blood pressure prior to aortic clamping. Sequential clamping of the left iliac and visceral vessels prior to proximal aortic clamping facilitates a more controlled blood pressure manipulation with vasodilator agents. With more proximal TAA, lower blood pressures are required during the cross-clamp time. While some controversy exists regarding the spinal cord blood flow effects of vasodilators, particularly sodium nitroprusside, for control of

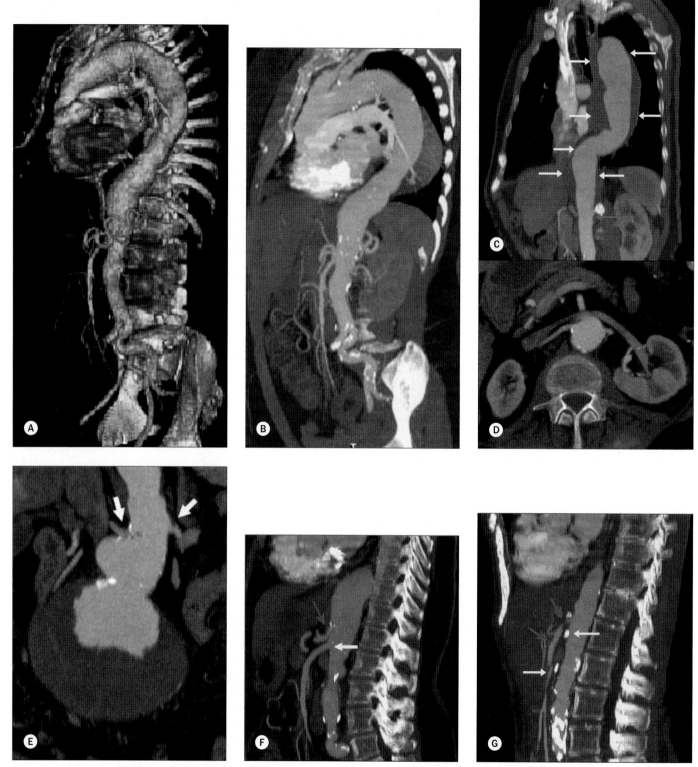

Figure 32.3 Computed tomography reformat. (A) & (B) Computed tomography (CT) reformat and 3D reconstruction of type I thoracoabdominal aneurysm (TAA) showing aneurysm extent. Note clear visualization of aortic bifurcation and iliac arteries without significant disease. (C) CT reformat revealing type I TAA aneurysm extent (white arrows) and where the aorta returns to normal caliber at the visceral aortic segment (red arrow). (D) & (E) Axial cut and CT reformat of pararenal aortic aneurysm, allowing evaluation of the proximal neck. Note less than 1cm neck below the renal arteries (white arrows). (F) CT reformat of the celiac (red arrow) and superior mesenteric artery (SMA) (white arrow) in a type I TAA, delineating no significant occlusive disease. In (G) note severe celiac stenosis (red arrows) and occlusion of the SMA at its calcific origin with distal reconstitution (white arrows).

proximal hypertension during aortic cross-clamping, we continue to use nitroprusside as the principal afterload reducing agent.[73-75] It provides rapid and easily reversible manipulation of arterial pressure. CSF is removed to maintain pre-clamp baseline CSF pressures. Aortic unclamping is associated with significant hemodynamic alterations during two stages – visceral reperfusion and distal reperfusion. Sodium bicarbonate is given prior to visceral vessel unclamping unless an in-line mesenteric shunt (see Fig. 32.11) has been used, and may be needed with distal unclamping. The temporary use of vasopressors may also be required during these times. Repeat administration of mannitol is given and renal-dose dopamine or fenoldopam is continued. Further dosing through the epidural catheter may be discontinued so that a lower extremity neurologic examination can be done at the procedure's end. Emergence from anesthesia usually requires therapy for hypertension. In the intensive care unit, the blood pressure should be maintained in the upper levels of normal, and hypotension should be aggressively treated. When used, CSF catheters must be transduced and pressures maintained at less than 12mmHg for 24–48 hours after operation.

Abdominal aneurysms (pararenal, suprarenal and type IV TAA)

Operative decision-making includes the aortic clamp site in relation to the renal and visceral vessels, necessary renovisceral reconstructions, and the proper proximal and distal graft configurations. Complete resection of the aneurysm is the objective. Too often, resection is confined to the infrarenal aorta, placing suture lines in diseased, aneurysmal aorta, creating the milieu for eventual graft failure and reintervention. Adequate operative exposure is the sine qua non of a complete and safe reconstruction. Adjuncts for spinal cord and visceral protection are not routinely used in repair of these lesions. Proximal clamp times for re-establishing visceral flow can be 20–30min with type IV TAA. Additionally, most pararenal lesions allow positioning the proximal aortic clamp to provide flow in at least one mesenteric artery and occasionally one renal artery. Similar to more extensive aneurysmal disease, a cross-clamp time over 30min has been associated with postoperative renal dysfunction.[76] Mannitol and, if necessary, furosemide should be used to maintain diuresis intraoperatively. Dopamine and fenoldopam infusion may benefit those with renal insufficiency. Further, cold renal perfusion is recommended when access to the renal ostia is safe.

Several options exist for exposure of abdominal aneurysms. They can be divided into anterior and lateral approaches.

Anterior approaches
Transperitoneal approach with supraceliac clamping
The traditional midline transperitoneal approach supplemented by supraceliac aortic clamping is adequate for some juxtarenal aneurysms (**Fig. 32.4**). Adequate exposure starts with extending the midline incision onto the xiphoid process. Inferior traction on the stomach with division of the lesser omentum and mobilization with rightward retraction of the left lateral liver segment provide access to the aorta at the hiatus. Nasogastric intubation assists in esophageal identification. A clamp may be placed with the tips against the vertebral column posteriorly, or circumferential control with a tape may facilitate improved aortic clamping. The clear disadvantage of this approach is dis-

continuous exposure of the visceral segment with repositioning of the retractors and transverse colon. Thus, it is only useful for juxtarenal aneurysms where exposure and treatment of visceral occlusive disease is not necessary. The left renal vein may hinder adequate aneurysm exposure. However, mobilization and retraction of this vein is possible in most cases (**Fig. 32.5**). We eschew division of the vein.

Transperitoneal approach with medial visceral rotation
Medial visceral rotation from the left, introduced by Stoney, provides exposure of the entire abdominal aorta without the theoretic morbidity of a combined thoracoabdominal approach.[77] A full-length laparotomy is made. The small bowel is wrapped and retracted superiorly and to the right, as with all transperitoneal approaches. The left colon is mobilized along the line of Toldt. Cephalad, the phrenocolic and splenorenal ligaments are divided. A plane may be developed anterior to the kidney, ureter, and adrenal gland while rotating the stomach, colon, spleen, and pancreas medially (**Fig. 32.6**). Control and mobilization of the left renal vein may be enhanced with this exposure specifically by ligating the adrenal, gonadal, and renal-lumbar branches (**Fig. 32.5**). Alternatively, the plane may be developed posterior to the left kidney, thus rotating venous structures to the midline and allowing unimpeded access to the suprarenal aorta (**Fig. 32.6**). Splenic and/or pancreatic injury is a potential complication of this technique.[78] During medial visceral rotation from the right, the small bowel mesentery is mobilized from its retroperitoneal attachments. This is extended to include right colon medialization in continuity with the duodenum and pancreatic head. Dissection along the posterior pancreatic border with superior displacement of the viscera reveals the SMA origin 90 degrees to the anterior surface of the aorta (**Fig. 32.7**). Division of the autonomic tissue surrounding the SMA and division of the left diaphragmatic crus allow clamping above the renal arteries or above the SMA (**Fig. 32.7**). The right-sided rotation provides excellent visualization for pararenal aneurysm repair with particular advantages when full right renal artery or right iliac artery visualization is essential. When continuous exposure of the visceral aortic segment is required, however, we opt for the lateral approaches.

Lateral approaches
Retroperitoneal/thoracoabdominal approach
We reserve the term *retroperitoneal* for those incisions no higher than the 11th rib where the peritoneum is not entered, and consider incisions higher than the 10th interspace *thoracoabdominal* irrespective of peritoneal entry (**Fig. 32.8**). In our view, it is now obsolete to debate the merits of lateral versus anterior approaches. Both randomized and uncontrolled studies delineate the merits of both.[79-81] Certain technical and anatomic circumstances dictate the use of lateral approaches. For patients with significant visceral segment disease and true type IV lesions where distal thoracic control is required, it is the method of choice. It is clearly advantageous in obese patients or those with multiple prior abdominal procedures and adhesive obliteration of the peritoneal space. The main disadvantage is poor access to right-sided aortic branches.

The main considerations when using this type of exposure is the level of the flank incision necessary and whether the left kidney and ureter are to be left in anatomic position or swept

Maneuver of supraceliac clamping for aortic control from the anterior transperitoneal approach

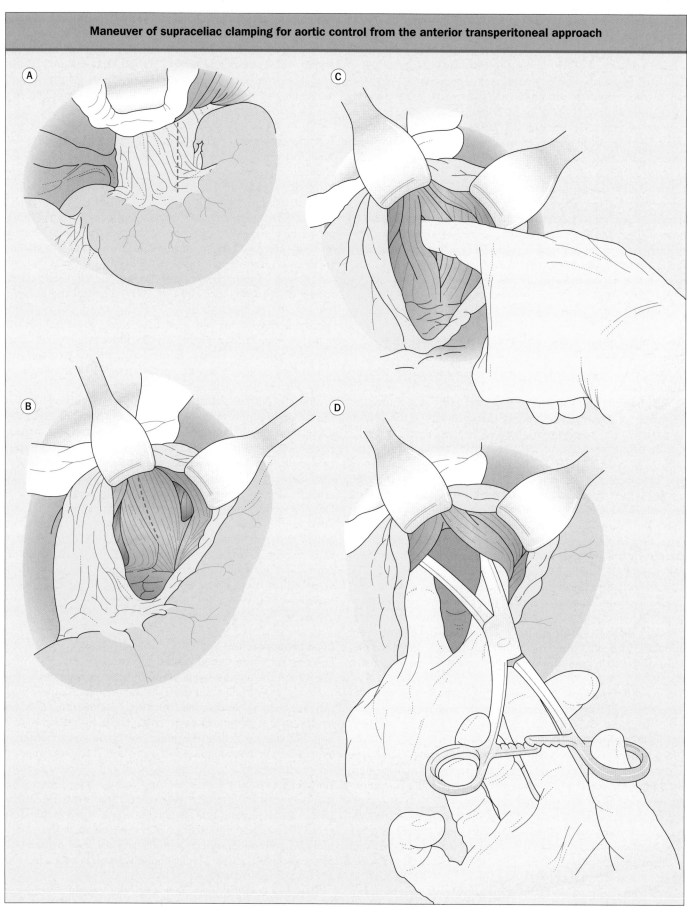

Figure 32.4 Maneuver of supraceliac clamping for aortic control from the anterior transperitoneal approach. The lesser omentum is opened and the crus divided. The periaortic tissue is cleared with a finger and the aortic clamp placed with tips against the vertebral bodies.

Mobilization of the left renal vein

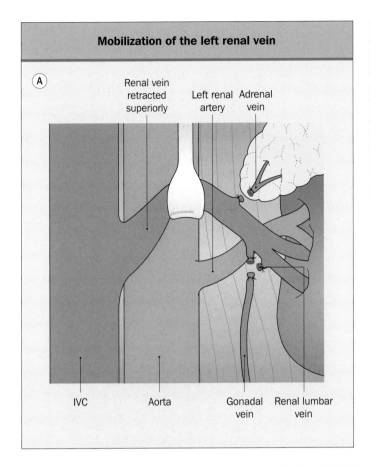

(A) Renal vein retracted superiorly · Left renal artery · Adrenal vein · IVC · Aorta · Gonadal vein · Renal lumbar vein

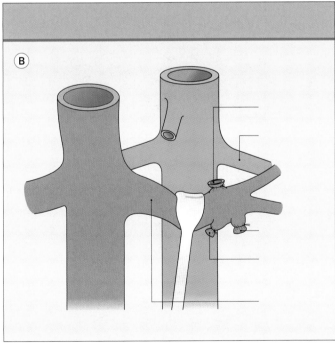

(B)

Figure 32.5 Mobilization of the left renal vein. (A) Ligation of the adrenal, gonadal, and renal-lumbar veins. (B) The left renal artery usually courses behind the vein.

Left medial visceral rotation

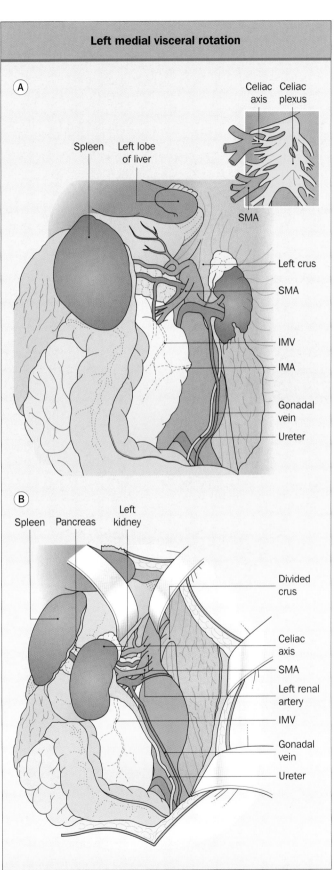

(A) Celiac axis · Celiac plexus · Spleen · Left lobe of liver · SMA · Left crus · SMA · IMV · IMA · Gonadal vein · Ureter

(B) Spleen · Pancreas · Left kidney · Divided crus · Celiac axis · SMA · Left renal artery · IMV · Gonadal vein · Ureter

Figure 32.6 Left medial visceral rotation. (A) Approach with left kidney remaining in retroperitoneum. (B) Approach with kidney mobilized and rotated anteriorly with other viscera. Note renal-lumbar vein courses across the aorta near the left renal artery.

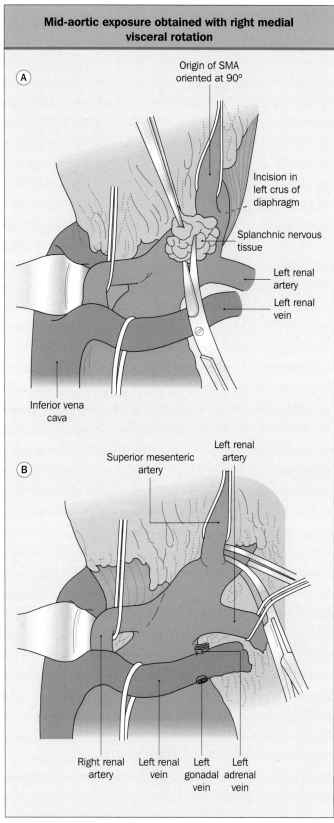

Mid-aortic exposure obtained with right medial visceral rotation

(A)

Origin of SMA oriented at 90°

Incision in left crus of diaphragm

Splanchnic nervous tissue

Left renal artery

Left renal vein

Inferior vena cava

(B)

Superior mesenteric artery

Left renal artery

Right renal artery

Left renal vein

Left gonadal vein

Left adrenal vein

Figure 32.7 Mid-aortic exposure obtained with right medial visceral rotation. (A) Note superior mesenteric artery elevated to 90° angle with aorta. (B) After left renal vein mobilization, excellent access to the pararenal aorta is obtained.

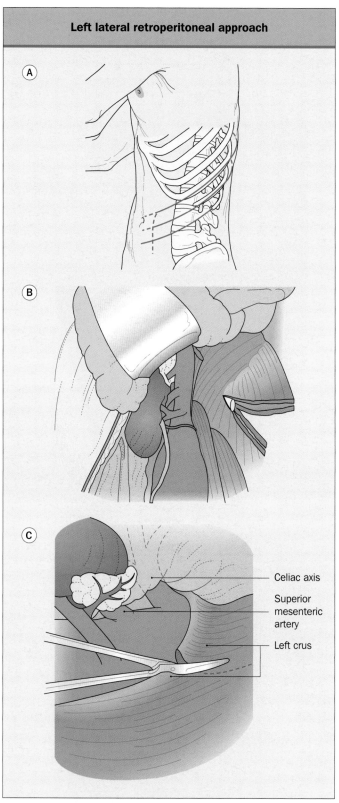

Left lateral retroperitoneal approach

(A)

(B)

(C)

Celiac axis

Superior mesenteric artery

Left crus

Figure 32.8 Left lateral retroperitoneal approach. (A) Various levels of incision depend upon extent of aneurysmal disease. The abdominal portion is not carried to midline so as to keep the viscera intraperitoneal, to decrease evaporative and heat losses. (B) Excellent contiguous exposure to the visceral aortic segment is obtained. Again note the renal-lumbar vein at the level of the left renal artery. (C) Division of the left crus at the aortic hiatus facilitates supraceliac aortic exposure.

medially with the peritoneum and its contents. For pararenal aneurysms, the incision is somewhat higher than for infrarenal repairs. If full supraceliac exposure is required, then extension into the 9th or even 8th interspace is used. The left pleural space is usually entered on these approaches, and the diaphragm may need to be partially divided. For type IV TAA, extension into the 8th interspace with costal margin division and a phrenic-sparing incision provides excellent visualization. The patient is placed on an air-vacuum styrofoam beanbag in a right lateral decubitus position with the torso at a 65–70° rotation, with the hips and lower extremities rotated back as close as possible to horizontal. The table is jackknifed to open the left flank. The incision is carried through the abdominal wall musculature and transversalis fascia until the pre-peritoneal space is entered laterally. The peritoneal sac is swept anteromedially, defining the retroperitoneal space (**Fig. 32.8**). This is continued until the peritoneal envelope is dissected over the aneurysmal segments. Ligation of the inferior mesenteric artery facilitates full inferior exposure. As with left medial visceral rotation, a plane anterior or posterior to the kidney may be developed. For most aneurysm surgery, a retrorenal plane is preferred with the exception of a retroaortic left renal vein. The left diaphragmatic crus is divided, completing exposure of the entire suprarenal aorta (**Fig. 32.8**). The retroperitoneal approach with renal elevation is preferable for pararenal aneurysm repair as it facilitates dissection, aortic control, and reconstruction. For type IV lesions or those where any significant visceral segment work must be accomplished, thoracoabdominal exposure with peritoneal entry for visceral inspection and distal vessel palpation is ideal.

Aortic clamping

Clamping above the renal arteries and below the SMA is possible in many pararenal aneurysms. However, this may not be ideal in some patients due to associated side-branch occlusive disease, aortic calcification, and differences in anatomic spacing of the branch vessels. When clamping between the renal and superior mesenteric arteries is feasible, construction of the proximal anastomosis can be accomplished with less involved proximal dissection and potentially less cardiac strain and hemodynamic compromise, as visceral flow remains open. It may also decrease coagulation disturbances, as supraceliac clamping with hepatic and bowel ischemia with bacterial translocation have been implicated in this process.[65,66,82,83] The advantages of clamping below the celiac have been challenged by Green and co-workers. They found less renal dysfunction with supraceliac clamping in their aneurysm experience.[84] Renal dysfunction may be related to atheromatous embolization during clamping or surgical dissection of diseased aortic segments, as the supraceliac aorta is usually less involved by atherosclerotic disease. Also, mechanical or hemodynamic factors related to clamping near the renal orifices are potential factors. These considerations must be weighed when evaluating preoperative imaging studies. Helical CT with and without contrast allows for critical evaluation of aortic calcification and mural thrombus, aiding in choosing the most appropriate clamp location. However, clamp sites may not be selected until intraoperatively or may change during the conduct of operation. The vascular surgeon dealing with complex abdominal aneurysms should be familiar with all exposures and clamping maneuvers. The Henry Ford Hospital pararenal aneurysm experience revealed that 7% of clamps were between the celiac and SMA, 17% were between the two renal arteries, 36% between the renal arteries and the SMA, and 40% at the supraceliac level.[85] Constructs for the configuration of the proximal anastomosis vary according to the extent of proximal aneurysmal disease (**Figs 32.9 & 32.10**).

Extensive TAA (type I–III)

There is consensus that the inclusion technique, refined by Crawford, is the preferred operative method for replacement of

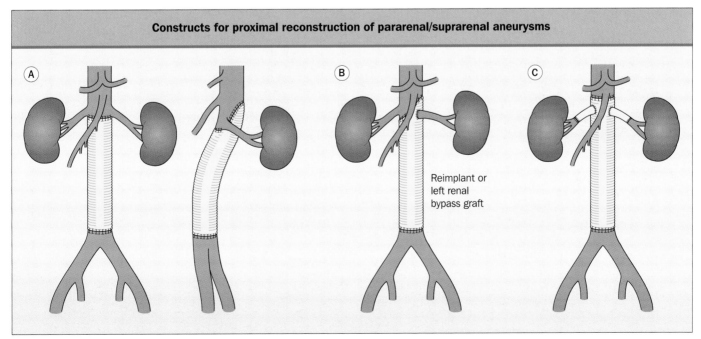

Figure 32.9 Constructs for proximal reconstruction of pararenal/suprarenal aneurysms. (A) Posterior bevel. (B) Left lateral bevel with left renal reconstruction. (C) Suprarenal flush graft with bilateral renal artery reconstruction.

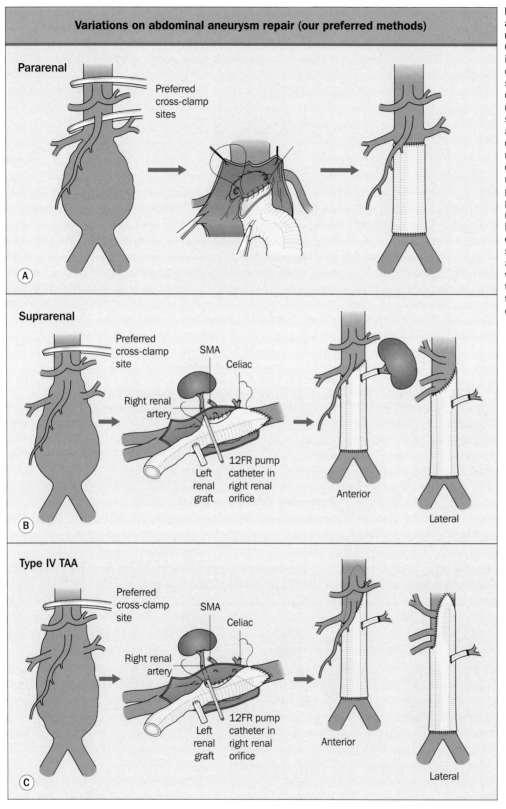

Variations on abdominal aneurysm repair (our preferred methods)

Pararenal

Preferred cross-clamp sites

(A)

Suprarenal

Preferred cross-clamp site

SMA

Celiac

Right renal artery

Left renal graft

12FR pump catheter in right renal orifice

Anterior

Lateral

(B)

Type IV TAA

Preferred cross-clamp site

SMA

Celiac

Right renal artery

Left renal graft

12FR pump catheter in right renal orifice

Anterior

Lateral

(C)

Figure 32.10 Variations on abdominal aneurysm repair (our preferred methods). (A) *Pararenal aneurysm.* Cross-clamp: supraceliac or suprarenal inframesenteric depending upon aortic disease and renovisceral artery spacing. Inset: sewing proximally to the cuff of aorta at the renal artery orifices. (B) *Suprarenal aneurysm.* Cross-clamp: supraceliac. Inset: beveled proximal anastomosis with 12F perfusion catheter as stent-of-sorts in the right renal artery to inhibit orificial compromise. Left renal artery reconstruction with 6mm polytetrafluoroethylene (PTFE) pre-attached to aortic prosthesis. (C) *Type IV.* Cross-clamp: thoracic aorta. Inset: beveled proximal anastomosis encompassing the entire visceral segment and pre-attached left renal artery PTFE graft. When sewing to the visceral aortic segment, care must be taken to place the suture line as close to the visceral vessels as possible, to exclude diseased aorta.

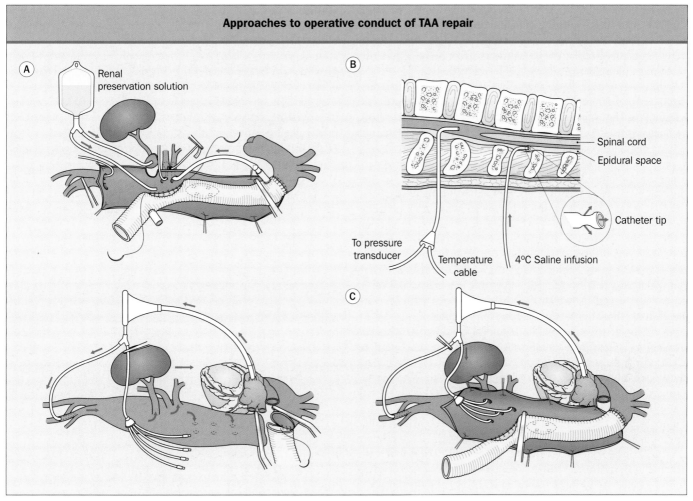

Approaches to operative conduct of TAA repair

Figure 32.11 Approaches to operative conduct of thoracoabdominal aneurysm repair. (A) Our modified clamp-and-sew technique with in-line mesenteric shunting after proximal anastomosis completion, providing pulsatile arterial flow that can be inserted into either the celiac axis (as depicted) or the superior mesenteric artery (SMA), and cold renal perfusion into both kidneys. Critical intercostal reconstruction and single inclusion button anastomosis of the celiac axis, SMA, and right renal artery with 6mm polytetrafluoroethylene sidearm graft for the left renal reconstruction. (B) Epidural cooling for regional spinal cord hypothermia is accomplished with 4°C saline infusion via an epidural catheter, achieving 25°C prior to clamping. CSF temperature and pressure are monitored simultaneously with a separate intrathecal catheter. (C) Repair with atriofemoral bypass and sequential aortic clamping. Two clamps are placed proximally to initially allow proximal anastomosis completion with retrograde, transfemoral aortovisceral perfusion. Subsequently, the distal clamp is moved caudad to allow critical intercostal reconstruction while renovisceral perfusion is provided by 'octopus' catheters.

extensive TAA (**Fig. 32.11**).[17,18] Crawford also emphasized operative expediency and simplicity without the use of external shunts or bypasses, minimal cross-clamp times, minimal dissection on the anterior aspects of the aorta, and avoidance of systemic anticoagulation because of its potential contribution to intraoperative bleeding complications.[86]

These general principles of operation are recommended with certain modifications. The two general approaches involve (1) a clamp-and-sew technique versus (2) the use of distal aortic perfusion combined with a sequential clamping technique (**Fig. 32.11**). The rationale for distal aortic perfusion is the reduction of ischemic times to the spinal cord and viscera since their vascular beds are perfused during creation of the proximal anastomosis. Some surgeons use an initial right axillary to femoral bypass graft to provide passive distal aortic perfusion.[87] However, most authors who prefer distal aortic perfusion use active distal perfusion with atrial-femoral bypass utilizing the

Bio-Medicus pump. This centripetal, motorized pump is used with heparin-impregnated tubing and can be placed without systemic heparin.[88] However, the majority of surgeons prefer systemic heparin if using atrial-femoral bypass. Partial left heart bypass using a femoral vein to femoral artery technique becomes more complicated because of the necessity to add an in-line oxygenator and higher doses of heparin. Although recent reports continue to suggest potential benefit,[10,89–91] the atrial-femoral bypass technique with sequential clamping only saves the cross-clamp time required to complete the proximal aortic anastomosis, which is a minimum of the overall clamp time. After constructing the proximal aortic anastomosis, reconstruction of critical intercostal vessels and visceral aortic segment must then proceed, with distal perfusion providing only retrograde pelvic perfusion and some additional spinal cord circulation via the lateral sacral branches of the hypogastric vessels. However, visceral perfusion by various catheter arrangements may be used (**Fig. 32.11**).

459

These have the disadvantage of multiple catheters interfering with surgical exposure. The pressure/flow relationships of multiple small catheters may be problematic. At least two studies demonstrated a paradoxical detrimental effect on renal function using multiple selective visceral perfusion catheters.[92,61]

While some have been aggressive about the application of distal perfusion methods for all TAA,[89,91,93] others advocate their use only in the more extensive type I and type II aneurysms. Others utilize atrial-femoral bypass and distal aortic perfusion selectively in accordance with individual patient anatomy.[9,90] Currently, we favor the selective use of atrial-femoral bypass. Since its principal advantage is visceral/spinal cord protection during the performance of the proximal aortic reconstruction, distal aortic perfusion is most beneficial when the proximal reconstruction is likely to be complex, for example in patients with chronic dissection. Clearly, comparable results have been achieved in contemporary practice using both clamp/sew and distal perfusion techniques.[7,8,25,61,89,91,94,95] In addition, atrial-femoral bypass will provide easily titratable mechanical unloading of the left ventricle, which may be desirable in patients with significant valvular or left ventricular dysfunction.

Our general approach to the technical conduct of operation involves a clamp/sew technique with specific adjuncts for spinal cord, visceral, and renal protection (**Fig. 32.11**). We have developed a technique to provide for regional hypothermic protection to that segment of the spinal cord typically at risk for ischemic injury during TAA repair.[96–98] As schematized in **Figure 32.11**, this epidural cooling system uses an iced saline epidural infusion which provides moderate (25–27°C) hypothermia to the spinal cord during the critical period when the aorta is cross-clamped. Direct installation of renal preservation fluid (4°C lactated Ringer's solution with 25g/L of mannitol and 1g/L of methylprednisolone) into the renal artery ostia is performed after the aorta is opened. Initially, 250cc of this solution is instilled into each renal artery ostium and a continuous drip of the same begun through perfusion balloon-tipped catheters. Experience has shown that such an infusion will result in a rapid decline of renal parenchymal temperature to 15°C after the bolus infusion and it remains at roughly 25°C during the continuous infusion.

The final adjunct in our overall approach involves in-line mesenteric shunting. As displayed in **Figure 32.11**, a 10mm Dacron sidearm graft is sewn to the main aortic graft so as to be located just beyond the region of the proximal anastomosis. A 20F to 24F arterial perfusion cannula is attached to the sidearm graft and immediately after completion of the proximal anastomosis, prograde pulsatile perfusion can be established into either the celiac axis or SMA to minimize visceral ischemic time. In our experience, pulsatile arterial perfusion can thus be re-established to the mesenteric circulation within 25min of initial aortic cross-clamp placement.[99] This system can be modified by using a bifurcated graft and placing a separate cannula into the left renal artery origin in patients at particular risk for perioperative renal failure.

The concept of hypothermic protection for spinal cord and visceral organs can be extended to the extreme by the use of complete cardiopulmonary bypass, profound hypothermia, and circulatory arrest. Although this method has been utilized as a routine operative approach for patients with extensive TAA in at least one center,[100–102] the majority of surgeons specifically

avoid this technique because of the potential for bleeding and pulmonary complications. While this technique is essential for the repair of complex lesions of the ascending aorta or aortic arch, in patients with TAA, its use is only recommended when proximal control and clamping of the aorta is either hazardous or not technically possible.[103]

Regardless of individual preferences concerning the conduct of operation, broad continuous exposure of the entire left posterolateral aspect of the aorta is key to technical success (**Fig. 32.12**). The posterior portion of a standard posterolateral thoracotomy is only necessary for type I and type II aneurysms. We keep the thoracic portion of the incision low and have found the 5th or 6th interspace with posterior division of the 6th and 7th ribs provides adequate exposure in the majority of even

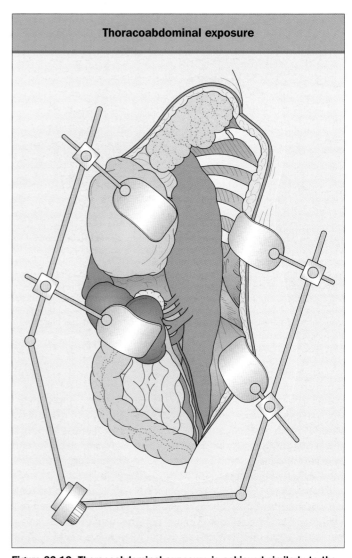

Thoracoabdominal exposure

Figure 32.12 Thoracoabdominal exposure is achieved similarly to the retroperitoneal abdominal approach, with extension of a posterolateral thoracotomy into the 6th or even 7th interspace for extensive aneurysms. The Omnitract self-retaining retractor is placed opposite the patient's back to allow unimpeded access to the field. Again, the abdominal portion is not extended to midline so as to keep the peritoneal contents intra-abdominal; however, the peritoneum is opened to provide an avenue to assess visceral perfusion and arterial flow.

proximal aneurysms. A self-retaining retractor system is essential to have continuous exposure of the entire operative field (**Fig. 32.12**). We prefer to keep the abdominal portion of the incision well lateral on the abdominal wall rather than extending to the midline. This allows the visceral contents to lay within the abdominal cavity and decreases evaporative fluid and heat losses. The abdominal portion of the incision is transperitoneal to allow direct inspection and assessment of the visceral circulation at the conclusion of operation. Exposure of the abdominal aorta is obtained by entering the plane posterior to the spleen, left kidney, and left colon. Located topographically close to the renal-lumbar vein as it courses across the aorta is the left renal artery (**Fig. 32.5**). A key point in the dissection is identifying the renal artery and dissecting it back to its aortic origin. This is a convenient starting point for cephalad and caudad division of the retroperitoneal tissues over the aorta inferiorly and division of the median arcuate ligament and diaphragmatic crura superiorly.

The incision in the diaphragm can be by one of several methods. Direct radial division of the diaphragm to the aortic hiatus is the quickest, simplest, and affords excellent exposure. However, such radial division of the diaphragm will irrevocably paralyze the left hemidiaphragm and contributes to postoperative respiratory compromise. Some surgeons prefer a circumferential division of the diaphragm through its muscular portion, leaving a few centimeters attached laterally to the chest wall. Engle et al.[104] have emphasized the benefit of preserving the phrenic innervation to the left hemidiaphragm by dividing only a portion lateral to the phrenic nerve insertion and then taking down the muscular fibers of the aortic hiatus. A large Penrose drain can be passed around the diaphragm pedicle for retracting superiorly and inferiorly during different stages of the subsequent reconstruction (**Fig. 32.13**). We have applied this method liberally, particularly in patients with evidence of preoperative pulmonary compromise. Following deflation of the left lung, the thoracic component of the dissection is usually straightforward. The mediastinal pleura over the aneurysm and proximal aorta are divided. Additional mobility on the vagus nerve can be obtained by dividing it distal to the origin of the left recurrent nerve. Should more proximal control be necessary, the ligamentum arteriosum is divided on the aorta, and in this region, care is taken to keep dissection directly on the underside of the aortic arch to avoid injury to the left pulmonary artery. In patients with degenerative aneurysm, dissection in this area is generally straightforward. When chronic dissection is the pathology, the prior inflammation from the dissecting process makes dissection more difficult. The aorta is surrounded with a vessel tape on either side of the left subclavian artery depending on the proximal extent of the aneurysm. Sufficient normal aorta should be cleared with blunt dissection on the posterior aspect of the aorta to allow room for clamp placement and an accurate proximal aortic anastomosis. External control of the left subclavian artery is not necessary as intraluminal balloon control can be obtained if the cross-clamp needs to be placed proximal to the left subclavian artery.

The aneurysm is opened initially in the abdomen, atherothrombotic debris is evacuated, and backbleeding from the right iliac or distal aorta is controlled with balloon catheters. In cases where the entire descending thoracic aorta is resected, proximal intercostal vessel orifices between T_4 and T_8 are typically

vigorously backbleeding and are rapidly oversewn. Intercostal arteries in the critical T_8 to L_1 aortic segment are evaluated for potential reimplantation into the graft and these vessels are balloon occluded to prevent both backbleeding and the negative 'sump' effect on net spinal cord perfusion that can result from these orifices being exposed to atmospheric pressure.[105] The proximal aortic neck is prepared for reconstruction, and circumferential division of the aorta is mandatory if chronic dissection is present at the site of proximal anastomosis. If the anastomosis is carried out in the distal arch, division of the aneurysm neck is helpful in preventing late suture line-esophageal erosion.

Reconstruction of intercostal vessels in the T_8–L_1 segment is usually the next step in the operation. The most common technique utilized is an inclusion button anastomosis. Intercostal vessels in the region of a proximal or distal aortic anastomosis can be reconstructed by use of a long beveled suture line (**Fig. 32.14**). Depending on the topography of intercostal vessel origins, it may be possible to defer intercostal vessel reconstruction until after completion of the visceral vessel anastomosis by utilizing partial occluding clamps on the main aortic graft. Since we have the protective effect of regional spinal cord hypothermia until all aspects of the reconstruction have been completed, there is no urgency to re-establish intercostal blood flow. The important intercostal vessels are those in the T_8–L_1 segment; therefore, it is common for the intercostal inclusion button to nearly overlap (on the opposite side of the aorta) the visceral segment inclusion button.

Visceral and renal artery reconstruction is carried out next. Significant occlusive lesions of the right renal and mesenteric arteries should be treated with orificial or visceral segment endarterectomy (**Fig. 32.15**). This method involves incising the diseased intima and media and entering the correct endarterectomy plane typically evidenced by the pinkish color of the inner adventitia. Sufficient length of the superior mesenteric and celiac arteries should be dissected out to facilitate countertraction from the external side of the vessel, although this is not possible with the right renal artery. Should the calcified end of the obstructing lesion not break off easily, sharp division under direct vision is the preferred method. The most common method of visceral/renal artery reconstruction, which has been applied in the overwhelming majority of our cases, is a single inclusion button to encompass the origins of the celiac, superior mesenteric, and right renal arteries (**Fig. 32.15**). If the aneurysm is excessively large in the visceral aortic segment, wide separation of the visceral/renal ostia may necessitate individual inclusion button anastomoses or grafts. Suture bites should be close to the visceral vessel origins to avoid leaving too much aneurysmal aortic wall. As the posterior aspect of this suture line continues around the inferior border of the right renal artery, we exchange the 6F perfusion catheter for a 12F perfusion catheter to serve as a stent of sorts in the right renal artery origin. This catheter is gently agitated up and down as the suture line moves around the renal artery, to ensure that the latter is not compromised by the suture bites. The topography and course of the right renal artery should be interrogated with this indwelling catheter because in circumstances where the right renal artery drapes over a large infrarenal component of the aneurysm, occlusion of the right renal artery is a definite technical complication of operation (**Fig. 32.15**). Just prior to completion of this suture line, backbleeding and patency of the celiac,

Diaphragm management during extensive TAA repair

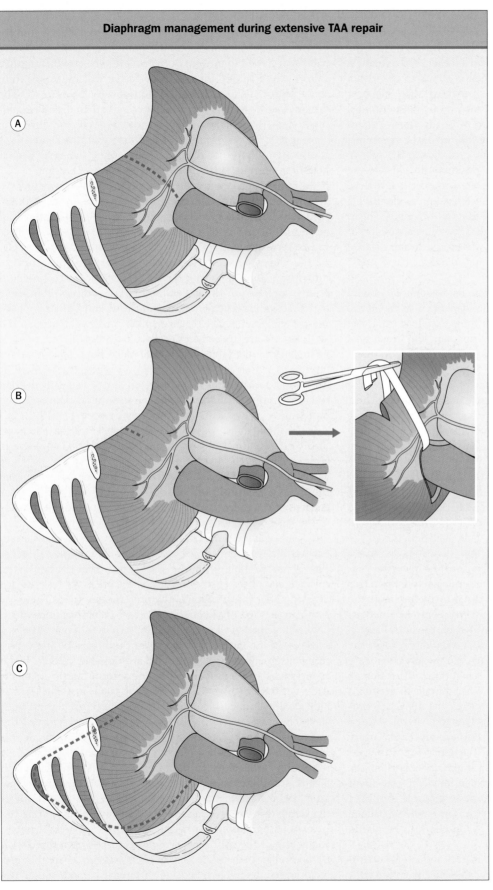

Figure 32.13 Diaphragm management during extensive thoracoabdominal repair. (A) Radial division provides rapid, direct, and uncompromised aortic exposure but causes left hemidiaphragm paralysis. (B) Partial division under the costal margin and dissection of the aortic hiatus preserves the phrenic nerve, and the diaphragmatic pedicle can be mobilized with a large Penrose drain. (C) Circumferential division of the muscular diaphragm is time-consuming and less hemostatic but spares the phrenic nerve.

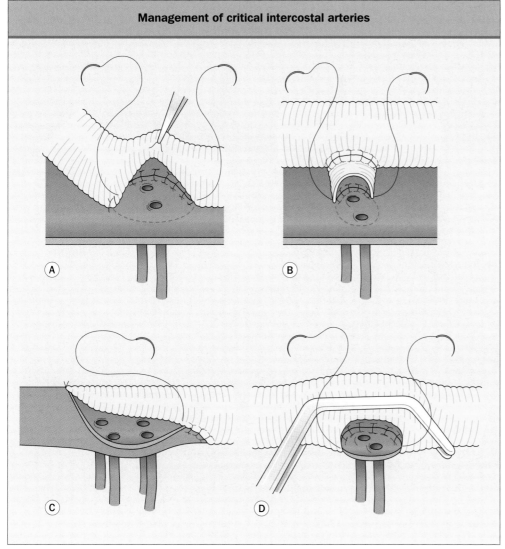

Management of critical intercostal arteries

A

B

C

D

Figure 32.14 Methods of management of critical intercostal arteries.
(A) Inclusion button anastomosis.
(B) Separate sidearm graft.
(C) Beveled anastomosis preservation when possible. (D) Carrell patch mobilization and direct reimplantation into the graft.

superior mesenteric, and right renal arteries are verified and the in-line mesenteric shunt is clamped and removed.

Reconstruction of the left renal artery is now accomplished with a separate sidearm graft of 6mm polytetrafluoroethylene (PTFE). This allows a direct, deliberate anastomosis in end-to-end fashion and permits flexibility in dealing with the spectrum of occlusive lesions, multiple renal arteries, and so forth that may be encountered. As noted in **Figure 32.15**, care must be taken to place this sidearm graft in an orientation where it will not kink when returned to its anatomic position. Some surgeons prefer to use a single inclusion button to encompass both renal arteries along with the visceral vessels, but in our experience, this will include too great an area of aneurysmal aorta unless the aneurysm is exceedingly small in the visceral aortic segment. When a single, pristine left renal artery and orifice are encountered, direct reimplantation may be entertained. The clamp is then moved again to a position inferior to the origin of the left renal artery graft and the distal aortic anastomosis is carried out. We make every effort to perform tube reconstructions to the aortic bifurcation unless there is gross aneurysmal disease of the proximal common iliac arteries. After re-

establishment of flow to the lower extremities and verification of adequate perfusion by intraoperative pulse volume recordings, Doppler signals in the left renal, celiac, and superior mesenteric vessels are checked in addition to palpation of the SMA pulse in the root of the mesentery. Hemostasis will usually be adequate at this point, but infusions of platelets and fresh frozen plasma are typically increased now, when a final check for hemostasis is made. Careful inspection of the inferior aspect of the aneurysm sac in both the chest and abdomen is necessary to detect backbleeding of lumbar and/or intercostal vessels, which can be an important source of postoperative hemorrhage. The redundant aneurysm sac is then sutured securely over the aortic prosthesis in the abdomen and the chest. Occasionally, in patients with modest-size aneurysms, chronic dissections, or prior proximal thoracic aortic grafts, there will be insufficient aneurysm wall to totally cover the proximal suture line and aortic graft. In selected cases, we have used a PTFE patch to exclude the aortic prosthesis from the left lung. The left kidney is returned to its bed and perinephric fat usually suffices to provide adequate coverage of the aortic graft in the region of the visceral aortic segment. During closure, renal artery reconstructions are

Aortic and visceral orifice endarterectomy

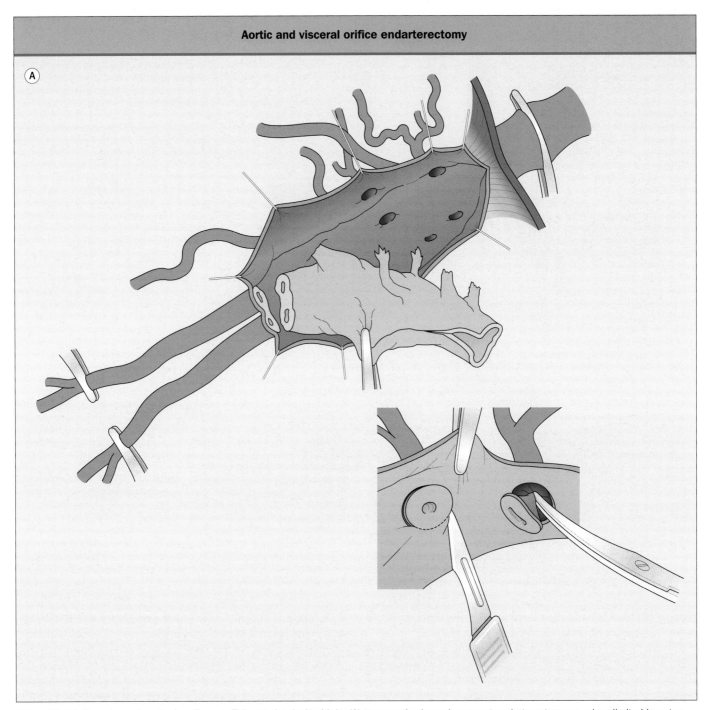

Figure 32.15 Renovisceral occlusive disease. This may be dealt with by (A) transaortic visceral segment endarterectomy or, when limited in nature, by orificial endarterectomy.

interrogated one final time. As displayed in **Table 32.3**, clamp times, blood turnover, and blood component replacement will vary as a function of aneurysm extent, but overall operative time can be kept in the 5–6 hour range for most patients.

Endovascular reconstruction

Initial success with endoluminal treatment for isolated infrarenal aortic aneurysms was described by Parodi et al. in Argentina.[106] The feasibility of isolated thoracic aortic stent-grafting was introduced 3 years later, in 1994, by Dake et al.[107] Information

supporting the safety and efficacy of transrenal fixation for proximal seating of endovascular aortic grafts in pararenal aneurysms with short neck lengths now exists and most authorities consider this acceptable.[108,109] However, endografting of the aortic visceral segment is the final technical barrier to total contiguous endovascular repair of the thoracic and abdominal aorta.

Proprietary development of thoracic aortic devices has lagged behind those for infrarenal AAA and reports of this technology are largely those of custom-made grafts. Our initial experience with 28 patients undergoing thoracic aortic stent-grafting was

Standard visceral button and left renal bypass graft

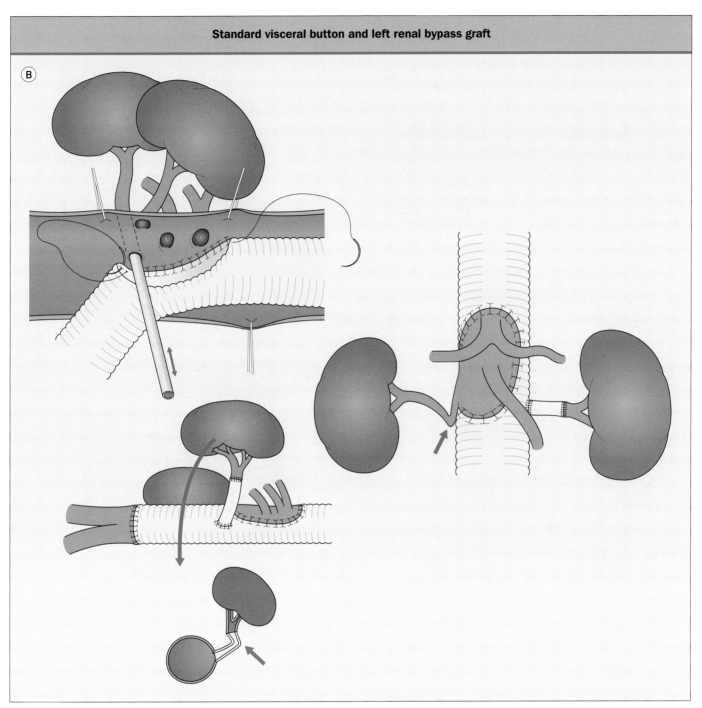

Figure 32.15 Renovisceral occlusive disease (*cont'd*) (B) Creation of a standard visceral button inclusion anastomosis of the celiac axis, SMA, and right renal artery and 6mm polytetrafluoroethylene sidearm bypass for left renal artery reconstruction. When performing this, we use a 12F perfusion catheter as a stent-of-sorts in the right renal artery to prevent compromise of its orifice as the anastomosis is carried around these arterial origins. Care must be taken with both renal reconstructions. If the infrarenal portion of the aneurysm is large and the right renal artery drapes over this portion, once reconstructed the right renal may kink against the aortic graft. Also, when the left kidney is returned to the retroperitoneum, unless the sidearm graft has been trimmed to the precise length, it may also kink.

recently reported and there was a 3.5% peri-procedural mortality.[110] While this figure lies in the lower end of reported rates for thoracic endografts, which have been up to 20%,[111,112] it is twice that of our updated experience with 362 infrarenal AAA endovascular repairs (1.6%)[113] and slightly higher than the 30-day mortality evidenced in the EUROSTAR trial (2.9%).[114] This must be tempered by the fact that most thoracic stent-graft studies consist of small cohort numbers and many of these

patients have been treated in desperate anatomic or co-morbid circumstances where conventional open repair was not a realistic option.

Further confounding endografting in the thoracic position are the larger relative proportion of female patients afflicted with thoracic aortic disease and the unique difficulties in proximal deployment. Females tend to have smaller access vessels, which limit large profile systems. Not unlike other reports, 20% of our patients required arterial access at sites other than the femoral arteries, with 21% experiencing an access site complication.[110] Available reviews suggest that 8–43% of landing sites in descending aortic aneurysms will not allow an appropriate 2cm length for secure proximal fixation.[111,112,115] Pre-procedural subclavian

artery transposition has been necessary in 21% of our early patients.[110] Although an early concern with first-generation devices, the 'windsock' effect of ventricular ejection, leading to inaccurate proximal deployment (particularly when performed near the arch), has now been overcome by superior design attributes. Construct-related issues have also contributed to mortality. Graft migration with aneurysm rupture, stroke, mesenteric ischemia, and massive embolization have all been described as sequelae of thoracic aortic endografting.[111,112,115,116]

Spinal cord ischemia has been reported in 0–12% of patients after thoracic endografting. However, it does appear to occur less frequently than with open reconstruction, as most series report rates of roughly 5%.[111,112,115,117] Gravereaux et al. recently noted three of their 53 (5.7%) thoracic aortic aneurysm endograft patients suffered cord ischemia,[118] and we have observed two such cases now in 50 endografts. Factors implicated as relevant to development of cord ischemia after thoracic endografting are the extent of descending aorta excluded as well as previous or concomitant AAA repair.[111,112,118] In the latter, it is unclear if infrarenal clamping or lumbar sacrifice contribute to ischemic injury, and, while combined repair is an attractive option in 'dumbell' aneurysms, this risk must be considered.[111,119] It has been suggested that patients with these risk factors be managed with protective adjuncts (i.e. CSF drainage) similar to

Operative characteristics in 337 thoracoabdominal aneurysm repairs.

Intraoperative data	Type I and 2 (n=151)	Type III and IV (n=186)	p
OR time (min)	329±95	298±93	0.0025
Visceral XC time (min)	52.5±16.8	42.7±11.4	<0.0001
Total XC time (min)	72.7±28.8	76.1±23.7	0.22
Total transfusion (cm³)	3341±2035	2301±1755	<0.0001
FFP (units)	6.4±4.2	4.4±3.8	<0.0001
Platelets (units)	10.1±5.9	5.6±5.5	<0.0001

Table 32.3 Operative characteristics in 337 thoracoabdominal aneurysm repairs.[25] FFP, fresh frozen plasma; OR, operating room; XC, cross-clamping.

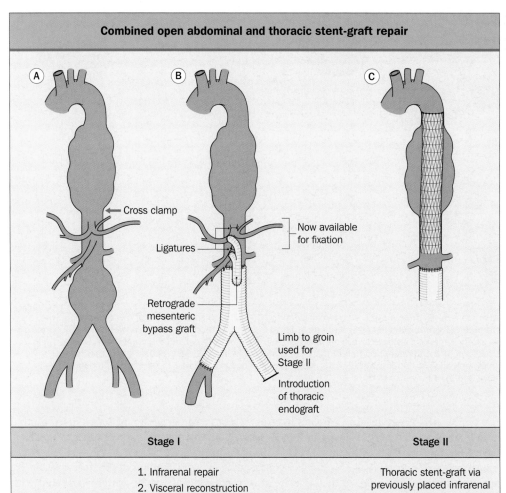

Combined open abdominal and thoracic stent-graft repair

(A)

(B)

(C)

← Cross clamp

Ligatures

Now available for fixation

Retrograde mesenteric bypass graft

Limb to groin used for Stage II

Introduction of thoracic endograft

Stage I

1. Infrarenal repair
2. Visceral reconstruction
3. Celiac/SMA ligation

Stage II

Thoracic stent-graft via previously placed infrarenal graft limb

Figure 32.16 Combined open abdominal and thoracic stent-graft repair. (A) Thoracoabdominal aneurysm with sparing of the visceral segment or the so-called 'dumbbell' aneurysm. (B) Initial standard open repair of the infrarenal abdominal portion is performed using a bifurcated prosthesis accompanied by retrograde mesenteric reconstruction using a bifurcated graft to the celiac and superior mesenteric artery, followed by ligation of these vessels. Now the visceral aortic segment may be used as the distal fixation site for the thoracic endograft. (C) This is performed in a staged fashion, allowing spinal cord perfusion to accommodate, using one limb of the prior placed infrarenal graft for adequate access.

open repair.[118] The benefit of such adjuncts remains unproven. We have had success with our early experience combining open abdominal repair with thoracic endografting (**Fig. 32.16**). Initially, the infrarenal portion of the aneurysm is repaired with a bifurcated graft. Prior to celiac and superior mesenteric ligation, retrograde reconstruction of these vessels from the infrarenal graft is performed with a bifurcated Dacron prosthesis. This permits use of the visceral segment for distal fixation of the thoracic endograft. Because of the current data on cord ischemia, the thoracic endograft is performed in a staged manner with one infrarenal graft limb used for endoluminal access and re-anastomosed at the appropriate level once endografting is complete.

To date, two methods for incorporation of the renoviseral vessels in endograft repair have been developed: graft fenestration and side-branch extension grafts. The construct, feasibility, and implantation technique of one fenestrated visceral segment endograft has been developed by Anderson et al.[21] Based on preoperative 1mm-interval CT scanning with reconstruction each endograft is custom-made with fenestrations placed at specific, measured locations for the renoviseral ostia (**Fig. 32.17**). These fenestrations are radiopaquely marked. The device itself is based on the Zenith system. It is modular (unilimbed and a contra-limb extension) with an uncovered Gianturco Z-stent (William Cook, Europe; Bjaeverskov, Denmark) for proximal fixation. No stent wiring crosses the fenestrations, and radiopaque markers are placed on the posterior and anterior graft surface for proper axial placement. Apposition of the renal fenestrations to the ostia is provided by modified Palmaz P204 stents (Cordis Endo-vascular, Warren, NJ, USA). These stents are placed with a small portion in the endograft lumen. The modification consists of laser cutting to facilitate flaring to 90° in one end of the stent. This provides for graft-wall approximation and the ability to endoluminally access the renal arteries in the future. The graft is loaded with the prongs of the proximal stent separately capped and deployable to allow manipulation and positioning of the graft in the neck. In a series of 13 patients, Anderson's group has communicated feasibility and technical success in 100% of 19 renal arteries, five accessory renal arteries, and nine superior mesenteric arteries targeted for fenestration. Two type II endo-leaks occurred.[21]

A second method to permit even more proximal endograft placement using multiple side-branch grafts has been reported by Chuter et al.[22] Using this system, they have recently grafted a type III TAA; however, the patient suffered delayed para-plegia, again reinforcing the continued potential of ischemic cord injury with endovascular technology.[120] The device is modular and consists of a proximal attachment portion anastomosed to a graft segment incorporating stumps for renoviseral vessel extensions and a 20mm distal aortic stump in which a modified

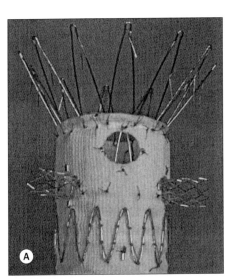
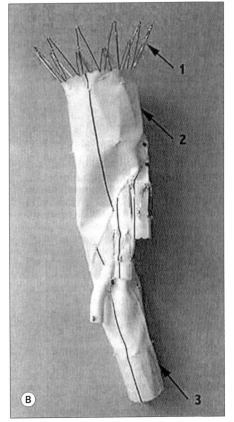
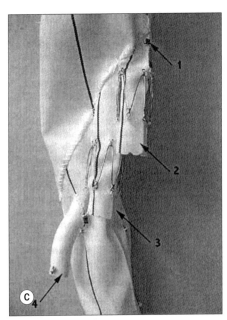

Figure 32.17 Endovascular constructs currently used for repair of aneurysms involving the visceral aortic segment. (A) Custom fenestrated device used by Anderson et al.[21] Based upon preoperative imaging, the fenestrations are made and surrounded by radiopaque markers. The renal fenestrations are supported by modified Palmaz-204 stents that flare and approximate the graft to the renal orifices. (B) Side-branch extension type graft developed by Chuter et al.[22] Note the proximal fixation stent (1) and the distal segment (3) in which a standard AAA endovascular graft is placed for completion of distal reconstruction. (C) Visceral segment portion of graft showing radiopaque markers (1) and closer view of celiac artery (2), superior mesenteric artery (3), and right renal artery (4) stumps. Reprinted with permission from J Endovasc Ther.

standard infrarenal AAA device is inserted to complete distal reconstruction. Stumps for the celiac and SMA are 2.5cm long and 8mm in diameter and are surrounded by a 12mm stent to mark the stump. Radiopaque rings mark the unsupported renal artery stumps. The inventors prefer a SMART stent (non-covered) with both luminal and external stents for the renovisceral extension grafts, which provide for high-friction graft-to-graft apposition. Although progress in technology has rendered endovascular complex aneurysm repair possible, such work has, to date, been preliminary and at the province of a few acknowledged innovators in stent-graft technology.

SURGICAL RESULTS AND COMPLICATIONS

Operative mortality

Pararenal aneurysmorraphy operative mortality approaches 5%, while in large clinical series of TAA repair it averages roughly 10% (**Table 32.4**). However, other reports detail considerably higher perioperative mortality in TAA.[19,63] Several preoperative patient characteristics may influence the patient's ultimate outcome regardless of operative conduct. The circumstances of clinical presentation are a dominant factor associated with operative mortality in pararenal/suprarenal aneurysms and TAA. In the recent update of our experience, operative mortality was 6.7% for elective TAA operations, while it increased to 13.4% in non-elective situations (p=0.06). Similar data have been reported by others, regardless of aneurysm extent.[7,9,63,89,121,122] Although not universal, some contemporary series have demonstrated an increased operative mortality in elderly patients undergoing either complex abdominal or extensive TAA repair.[7,9,11,61,122] The presence of increasing numbers of co-morbid conditions can naturally be expected to increase overall operative risk. Individual series variously demonstrate increased operative risks with patients with coronary artery disease, COPD, and renal insufficiency.[7,8,11,19,25,61,63,64,95,122] Dysfunction in these respective organ systems increases the risks of organ-specific complications after operation and patients who sustain major neurologic deficits, postoperative renal failure, and cardiopulmonary complications have a significantly increased risk of operative mortality.[7-9,10,11,25] Previously, we reported the risk of operative mortality with TAA repair was increased more than sixfold in patients with postoperative renal failure and increased by a factor of 16 in those with paraplegia,[8,25] findings similar to those of Svensson et al.[11] Visceral ischemic time during repair has been shown to enhance plasma concentrations of proinflammatory mediators and thus predispose to multiple system organ failure (MSOF).[123] Fifty percent of in-hospital deaths after TAA repair were associated with MSOF.[25,64] These data emphasize the importance of minimizing such complications.

Operative series of complex aortic aneurysm: morbidity and mortality.					
Reference	No. of patients	Aneurysm extent	Early mortality No. (%)	Paraplegia/paraparesis No. (%)	Renal failure No. (%)
Qvarfordt et al.[132]	77	Pararenal	1 (1.3)	0	2 (2.5)*
Crawford et al.[189]	101	Pararenal	8 (7)	†	7 (7)
Poulias et al.[76]	38	Pararenal	2 (5.2)	0	5 (13)*
Nypaver et al.[85]	53	Pararenal	2 (3.5)	0	3 (5.6)*
Allen et al.[197]	65	Para/suprarenal	1 (1.5)	1 (1.5)	2 (3)*
Faggioli et al.[122]	50	Pararenal	6 (12)	0	1 (2)
Martin et al.[121]	57	Suprarenal	1 (1.8)	0	1 (2; elective only)*
Svensson et al.[11]	1509	TAA	155 (10)	234 (16)	269 (18)
Coselli et al.[61]	1220	TAA	89 (7.3)	56 (4.6)	133 (11.1)
Schepens et al.[64]	172	TAA	18 (10.5)	24 (14.7)	18 (10.4)*
Hamilton et al.[198]	265	TAA	21 (7.9)	12 (4.5)	† (†9)
Grabitz et al.[151]	260	TAA	37 (14.2)	39 (15)	27 (10.4)*
Acher et al.[7]	217§	TAA	21 (9.7)	17 (7.8)	4 (3.8)*
Estrera et al.[89]	654§	TAA	106 (16)	33 (5)	† (†¶29%)
Cambria et al.[25]	337	TAA	28 (8.3)	38 (11)	45 (13)

*Only those requiring hemodialysis.
†Not reported.
‡From prior report from group.
§Includes descending thoracic aneurysms.
¶Strict criteria; increase in serum creatinine of 1 mg/dl for two consecutive days.

Table 32.4 Operative series of complex aortic aneurysm: morbidity and mortality. TAA, thoracoabdominal aneurysm.

Perioperative hemorrhage

Intraoperative bleeding complications can occur from technical mishaps and/or from dilutional coagulopathy caused by excessive blood turnover, and previously were an important source of early mortality. Blood turnover in extensive aneurysm cases is, of necessity, significant, since large type II aneurysms, for example, can contain up to several liters of blood in the aneurysm sac alone. This is routinely returned to the patient in the form of autotransfused blood. Approximately half the blood turnover during TAA resection is returned to the patient by autotransfusion methods. Total blood transfusion for resection of the more extensive type I and type II aneurysms averages >3L, and this figure varies with the extent of aortic replacement (**Table 32.3**). An expected correlation exists between blood turnover, aneurysm extent, and perioperative mortality. In our updated TAA experience, operative transfusion requirement was an independent correlate of perioperative mortality (odds ratio [OR], 1.4; 95% CI, 1.1–1.7; p=0.0015). Coselli et al.[9] documented that blood and plasma transfusions increased with use of partial cardiopulmonary bypass.

Prior to restoration of visceral and lower extremity perfusion, blood component replacement with fresh frozen plasma and platelet transfusions alleviates coagulopathic bleeding. Minimizing systemic heparin and careful hemostasis throughout the course of operation also reduce coagulopathic bleeding. Hepatic and mesenteric ischemia contribute to intraoperative coagulopathic bleeding.[67,68,93,124–126] Significant depletion of coagulation factors occurs during supraceliac aortic clamping. These changes are quantitatively more severe when compared with an infrarenal aortic cross-clamp.[82,127] Regardless of whether the mechanism of coagulopathic bleeding is hepatic ischemia or bacterial translocation in ischemic gut, experimental data and clinical observations suggest that minimizing mesenteric ischemia is critical in avoiding coagulopathic bleeding.[125,127] Minimizing the supraceliac cross-clamp duration along with the use of adjuncts to achieve mesenteric blood flow during repair (see Operative Management) is also an important component of operative success (**Fig. 32.11**).[99,128]

Re-exploration for bleeding complications has a highly significant impact on overall operative mortality.[11] Currently, bleeding complications occur in roughly 2–5% of TAA patients and should be less with pararenal aneurysmorrhaphy.[8,9,25,121] Postoperative splenic bleeding and undetected backbleeding from intercostal or lumbar vessels have been the principal sources of postoperative hemorrhage. A careful search of the entire aneurysm sac, after all suture lines have been completed, for backbleeding lumbar and intercostal vessels, and an aggressive posture towards splenectomy for even apparently trivial splenic tears should prevent these complications.

Respiratory insufficiency

Despite emphasis on spinal cord ischemic complications and renal failure in the majority of clinical series, postoperative respiratory failure is the single most common complication after TAA resection, occurring in 25–45% of patients.[8,11,20,25,61,64] While the incidence may be somewhat less after pararenal and suprarenal aneurysm repair, it remains one of the most frequently encountered postoperative problems.[85] A slow wean from ventilatory support, often planned to proceed over several days, is appropriate management in patients with baseline pulmonary insufficiency. Despite varying definitions, postoperative respiratory insufficiency occurs commonly and the variables predictive of this complication include active cigarette smoking, baseline COPD, and cardiac, renal, or bleeding complications.[8,25,64,104,129,130] Prior to elective operation, the patient should discontinue tobacco use for a minimum of a month. Preoperative consultation with a pulmonologist for optimization of bronchodilator therapy and pulmonary toilet is an important component in the management of patients with significant COPD. It is intuitive that paralysis of the left diaphragm by its radial division to the aortic hiatus will significantly contribute to postoperative respiratory failure. Accordingly, a diaphragm-sparing technique should be applied and has been reported to ameliorate pulmonary compromise after repair (**Fig. 32.13**).[104]

Perioperative renal insufficiency

Various criteria have been used to define postoperative renal failure. Doubling of the baseline serum creatinine level or an absolute postoperative creatinine level of >3.0mg/dL is a definition applied in most major clinical series. Etiologic factors important in the development of postoperative renal failure include the duration of renal ischemia, baseline renal dysfunction, cholesterol embolization from surgical manipulation of the aneurysm in the region of the renal artery orifices, and failure of renal artery reconstruction. Transient and modest decreases in overall excretory function are the inevitable consequence of some obligatory period of renal ischemia. In the great majority of patients, postoperative renal insufficiency is both non-oliguric and also reversible with maintenance of intravascular volume (**Table 32.5**). Preoperative renal insufficiency is the most powerful predictor of postoperative renal failure. Both an abnormal preoperative serum creatinine and a prolonged aortic cross-clamp time increase the risk of postoperative renal failure by a factor of four.[7,11,61,92,131]

The risk of postoperative renal insufficiency is higher for reconstructions involving pararenal aneurysms compared with infrarenal lesions.[76,85,132] As aortic aneurysmal extent increases, so does the risk of renal complications (**Table 32.4**).[25,95] In Crawford's experience, significant postoperative renal failure occurred in about 20% of patients, with dialysis being required in half. The risk of operative mortality increased fivefold in patients sustaining postoperative renal failure.[11] We previously reviewed over 180 TAA operations and found that in the 8% of

Stratification, by postoperative renal function, of patients undergoing 334 thoracoabdominal aneurysm repairs.	
	No. (%)
0–50% elevation in baseline creatinine	195 (58.4)
50–100% elevation in baseline creatinine	77 (23)
>100% elevation in baseline creatinine	19 (5.7)
Doubling and creatinine rising to >3.0mg/dL	27 (8)
Dialysis	16 (4.8)

Table 32.5 Stratification, by postoperative renal function, of patients undergoing 334 thoracoabdominal aneurysm repairs.[25]

patients who sustained significant postoperative renal failure, the risk of mortality was increased almost tenfold (OR, 9.1; 95% CI, 2.5–33; p<0.005).[131] About one-third of patients who develop significant postoperative renal dysfunction die perioperatively.[25]

The most important maneuver to minimize the risk of postoperative renal failure is minimizing renal ischemic time. Some authors prefer the use of distal aortic perfusion and a sequential clamping technique so that the renal arteries can be perfused during construction of the proximal aortic anastomosis. The addition of individual visceral/renal perfusion catheters from the atrial femoral bypass circuit, at least in theory, provides for continuous renal artery perfusion during all phases of the operation (**Fig. 32.11**). However, the size of such catheters may not permit adequate perfusion pressure or flow to the renal vessels, and at least two reports of this method suggest an apparent paradoxical detrimental effect on overall renal function with this technique.[61,92] The other frequently applied intraoperative adjunct, and the one preferred on our service, is selective hypothermic renal artery perfusion (**Fig. 32.11**). While such regional renal hypothermia is likely unnecessary in patients with normal renal function and with renal ischemic times less than 1 hour, it can provide a margin of safety in circumstances of either technical difficulty or prolongation of renal ischemia. An additional intraoperative adjunct employed to minimize the risk of postoperative renal failure is correction of renal artery occlusive lesions.[61,133] Perioperative continuous infusions of dopamine or fenoldopam may benefit patients with renal insufficiency.[65,134]

Management of perioperative renal failure is usually conservative if the patient remains non-oliguric. Patients taking diuretic medications preoperatively will generally require some in the postoperative period, and renal-dose dopamine or fenoldopam infusions may also help to maintain an appropriate diuresis. We prefer to avoid the use of hemodialysis therapy unless clear-cut indications exist on either a metabolic or blood volume basis. Conventional hemodialysis is accompanied by a substantial risk of hemodynamic instability after TAA resection, and we have observed such hypotension precipitating spinal cord ischemic events even weeks after surgery. Continuous venovenous hemodialysis may provide a smoother hemodynamic course than conventional hemodialysis. Currently, some 2–5% of patients will require hemodialysis for renal failure postoperatively.[25,61,131]

Spinal cord ischemic complications

Two morphologic factors referable to human spinal cord circulation explain ischemic risk to the spinal cord during TAA.[135,136] The first is the anatomic vagaries of the anterior spinal artery, which is variable both in caliber and continuity. Angiographic studies have shown that the anterior spinal artery may be discontinuous, with the typical pattern being extreme narrowing cephalad to its joining the greater radicular artery. The second factor is that the radiculomedullary arterial supply to the human spinal cord is inconsistent. Although radicular arteries are contributed at each segmental level, only a few actually go on to contribute medullary (i.e. actually reaching the cord) components. The cervical thoracic territory is richly supplied with radiculomedullary arteries, but the middle thoracic segment has but one or two such arteries. However, the anterior spinal artery in this region remains well developed. The thoracolumbar watershed region is at highest risk for ischemic injury because this region is typically supplied by a single radiculo-

medullary artery, the artery of Adamkiewicz or the greater radicular artery. This artery enters the vertebral canal between the 9th to 12th thoracic vertebral segments in 75–80% of individuals and arises between T_8 and L_1 in 86%. Angiographic studies confirm that one or more intercostal arteries can contribute to it and, in some three-quarters of patients, it arises from the left side.[71,137]

In the presence of an aneurysm, additional anatomic variability may be added by mural thrombus obliterating many or all of the intercostal vessels. Such gradual obliteration of intercostal vessels in a chronic degenerative aneurysm serves to establish antecedent collateral circulation prior to surgical correction. Most authors agree that the risk of cord injury is considerably less in patients where intercostal vessels in the critical T_8–L_1 zone have been obliterated by mural thrombus.[62,138,139] In aneurysms caused by chronic dissection, the typical pattern is aneurysmal dilatation of the false lumen and a narrow, compressed true lumen giving rise to multiple patent intercostals. Furthermore, obliteration of intercostals in a chronic degenerative aneurysm is virtually never accompanied by spontaneous cord injury, while sudden obliteration of multiple intercostal vessels, as might be seen in acute aortic dissection, can cause acute paraplegia.[140] This difference in intercostal patency between degenerative and dissecting aneurysms accounts for the increased risk of cord ischemia when dissection is the etiology.

Despite improvements in surgical and adjunctive techniques, spinal cord ischemia remains an unsolved problem and is the most feared and devastating non-fatal complication of TAA reconstruction. The pathogenesis of spinal cord injury after aortic replacement is likely multifactorial, but ultimately results from ischemic insult caused by temporary or permanent interruption of spinal cord blood supply. Debate continues about the relative importance of the initial ischemic insult versus reperfusion injury. Spinal cord ischemic complications manifest along a clinical spectrum from complete flaccid paraplegia to varying degrees of temporary or permanent paraparesis. The clinical observation of delayed deficits has led some to speculate that swelling in the rigid bony spinal canal, accompanied by relative increases in CSF pressure, are the pathogenesis of such delayed deficits.[141,142] Others have speculated that the initial ischemic insult in the operating room creates the milieu for programmed neuronal cell death as an inevitable consequence.[101] We and others have noted the striking correlation between perioperative hypotension and delayed-onset neurologic deficit, suggesting that the principal and collateral circulation to the cord may be in a delicate balance for some time after operation.[8,25,138] Indeed, delayed deficits occur just as frequently as those evident on emergence from anesthesia.[89,97,138] Careful attention to maintain adequate perfusion pressure in the days following TAA resection is important in limiting the occurrence of delayed deficit, but other mechanisms such as thrombosis of reconstructed vessels and microembolization may contribute to subsequent delayed deficits. Efforts to minimize spinal cord ischemia have been the principal driving force in the development and application of the variety of operative approaches. Svensson et al.,[11] in reviewing Crawford's experience, reported a 16% incidence of lower extremity neurologic deficits. As detailed in **Table 32.4**, contemporary results from centers of excellence find a rough halving of the overall incidence of spinal cord ischemia compared with Crawford's summary report. While good functional outcome after delayed deficit is commonly possible, some 30–60% of patients experiencing spinal cord ischemia suffer total paraplegia without any hope of meaningful recovery.[11,25,61,89,97,143,144]

The main difficulty in interpreting literature regarding spinal cord ischemic complications revolves around differing study populations based upon operative urgency, aneurysm extent, and etiology, as well as individual operative approaches using multiple adjuncts. There is general consensus that the clinical variables of aortic cross-clamp duration, aneurysm extent, emergency operations, and dissection increase spinal cord injury risk, although the latter has recently been disputed.[7–9,89,93] In our series of 337 reconstructions,[25] as well as Coselli's series of 1220 repairs[61] and Estrera's recent report in 654 operations,[89] dissection did not augment the risk of spinal cord ischemia. Crawford initially demonstrated that with increasing TAA extent, risk of cord injury increased with longer aortic cross-clamp duration.[11] We reported that a visceral cross-clamp time longer than 60min was significantly associated with ischemic cord injury.[96] In our latest analysis, total aortic and visceral clamp times increased ischemic cord injury risk. Total clamp time was an independent predictor for spinal cord ischemia.[25] Clinically significant spinal cord ischemia with pararenal/suprarenal aneurysm repair is rare. However, the incidence clearly increases in treatment for more extensive aneurysms. Svensson and colleagues noted a 24% incidence of cord injury in treatment of type I and type II TAA, as opposed to a 5.5% incidence for types III and IV TAA.[11] While absolute rates were improved in Coselli's contemporary communication, increasing aneurysm extent still correlated with cord ischemia, as 8.2% of type II patients and 1.3% of type IV patients suffered paraplegia/paraparesis.[61] Similar results have been conveyed by Estrera et al. of Safi's group.[89] We also have detected substantial ischemic risk in reconstructions for type I and type II TAA (12%) compared with those for less extensive aneurysms (6.5%).[25,97]

The circumstances of clinical presentation will have great bearing on cord injury risk. In Crawford's experience, cord injury rates doubled in treatment for ruptured versus intact aneurysms.[11] In our earlier data, operation for acute presentation (half for frank rupture and/or dissection) was independently associated with postoperative lower extremity neurologic deficit (RR, 7.7; 95% CI, 1.7–37.7; p=0.009).[8] Rupture itself has been proven an independent predictor of spinal cord ischemia.[25] Also, most authors contend that sacrifice of critical intercostal arteries and/or the inability to reperfuse these arteries in a timely fashion are important factors in the pathogenesis of ischemic cord injury. Griepp et al.[145] noted that cord ischemia increased dramatically when ten or more intercostal pairs were sacrificed (i.e. resection of the entire descending thoracic aorta). Our group and others have demonstrated that the sacrifice of intercostal vessels in the critical T_8–L_1 zone correlates with postoperative cord injury.[8,9,25,62,96,138] In fact, in our experience, sacrifice of patent intercostal arteries in the critical zone is an independent correlate with cord ischemia.[25]

A variety of clinical strategies and adjuncts have been applied in an effort to prevent ischemic spinal cord injury.[135,136] These methods can be divided into two general categories. The first of these are surgical or adjunctive methods designed to preserve relative spinal cord perfusion pressure. Localization techniques (preoperative angiography and intraoperative evoked potential or polargraphic) act as guides for the surgeon to preserve or

reconstruct critical intercostal arteries. Preoperative spinal arteriography can demonstrate the location and intercostal feeder vessels to the greater radicular artery in 65–85% of TAA patients studied.[71,137] However, except for predicting the risk of cord injury when the resection needs to encompass the critical aortic segment, clinical benefit of preoperative spinal arteriography has been debatable.[137,146–148] The hydrogen ion polargraphic technique, described by Svensson, has been elegantly documented with postoperative angiographic studies and has significant research promise, but has not been applied clinically in other centers.[149] Evoked potential monitoring evaluates the ability of the long tracks of the spinal cord to conduct an impulse during the cross-clamp period. Variations in the latency and amplitude of recorded potentials imply ischemia of the cord. Somatosensory evoked potentials (SSEP) was the original technique used, but this method has been plagued by lack of sensitivity and specificity, likely related to the fact that the peripheral nerve recording electrode is located distal to the cross-clamp.[150] Newer techniques used for evoked potential monitoring such as epidural electrode spinal cord stimulation (scSSEP) and motor evoked potentials (MEP) have shown promise in both correlation between cord deficits and intraoperative evoked potential abnormalities and as a guide for application of intraoperative adjuncts when detected with initial cross-clamping.[151–156]

Intercostal vessel reanastomosis is the most commonly applied surgical maneuver used to preserve spinal cord perfusion. When excessive atheroma or acute dissection surrounds intercostal vessel origins, this may be technically challenging. Further, the critical intercostal zone is in topographic proximity to the visceral aortic segment, and separate reconstruction to minimize intercostal clamp time may be impossible. Also, the surgeon typically faces the intraoperative dilemma of expending total aortic cross-clamp time to reattach intercostal vessels. Some authors have suggested expending aortic clamp time for this is a worthless maneuver, and routinely oversew or occlude all intercostal vessels, often using other adjuncts directed against spinal cord ischemia.[7,145] As described, we rapidly oversew the backbleeding intercostals in the T_4–T_8 region and balloon occlude those intercostals selected for reconstruction in the critical T_8–L_1 zone. Svensson's and Safi's groups have previously detailed specifics of intercostal management during operation.[62,138] It must be acknowledged, however, that intercostal reattachment is a 'blind' maneuver unless some reliable method of preoperative or intraoperative critical vessel localization is applied.[156] Documentation detailing the merit of directed intercostal vessel reattachment was provided by Grabitz et al. using scSSEP. These investigators reported more neurologic deficits when rapid loss of scSSEPs occurred after aortic cross-clamping. Furthermore, neurologic outcome for each group of SSEP responses correlated with achieving rapid evoked potential return by early intercostal reimplantation.[151] Jacobs and co-workers, using MEP to guide intercostal reconstruction or sacrifice, demonstrated this modality can provide rapid detection of intraoperative spinal cord ischemia and its reversal by either hemodynamic manipulations or intercostal reconstruction.[152,157] These authors have recently obtained a very impressive 2.7% neurologic deficit rate using this strategy in 184 patients with type I–III TAA.[156] The supposition that MEP may be more useful than SSEP in guiding intraoperative preventive strategies

471

has also recently been supported by van Dongen and associates.[155] However, restoring intercostal perfusion may be inadequate as a stand-alone adjunct simply because it cannot be performed rapidly enough.

The rationale for CSF pressure monitoring and drainage relates to the concept of spinal cord perfusion pressure as the difference between distal arterial pressure below the clamp and CSF pressure.[158] Thoracic aortic clamping results in an abrupt increase in intracerebral blood flow, which is likely the principal mechanism leading to increases in CSF pressure that may accompany clamping. However, the absolute degree of this rise is typically modest,[159,160] and Kazama et al. found CSF drainage favorably influenced spinal cord blood flow only when CSF pressure was experimentally elevated to four times baseline values.[161] Thus, assumptions on which the theoretic benefit of CSF drainage are based may not be valid. In fact, several studies have failed to demonstrate benefit for CSF drainage.[162,163] However, elevated CSF pressure has correlated with delayed-onset deficit in particular, and many authors continue to use CSF drainage either alone or more typically in combination with other strategies[7,89,93,164,165] since it is simple, safe, and it has shown promise in experimental studies.[166,167] Furthermore, reversal of delayed deficits by CSF drainage has been reported and chances of delayed deficit reversal appear greater than those of reversing immediate deficits.[141–143,168] Coselli's group recently reported a prospective, randomized trial of CSF drainage in type I and II repairs. Thirteen percent of those without drainage experienced clinically significant spinal cord ischemia while this occurred in significantly fewer (only 2.6%) drained patients.[169–171]

The second preventive method, neuroprotective adjuncts, are intended to increase spinal cord tolerance to ischemia. Two general categories of such adjuncts exist: systemic or regional hypothermia and pharmacologic agents. The latter can be classified according to intended mechanisms of actions:

- non-specific neuroprotective agents (e.g. steroids, prostaglandins, magnesium, and barbiturates);[20,172–176] and
- excitatory neurotransmitter inhibitors such as naloxone,[164,165,177] calcium channel blockers,[178] and oxygen free radical scavengers.[179]

Determining benefits of these agents in the clinical setting is difficult because they are typically used in combination with other strategies. The pre-eminent clinical experience involving this general strategy has been reported by Acher et al., applying endorphin receptor blockade with naloxone in combination with CSF drainage and routine intercostal ligation. Utilizing this technique in patients with thoracic aneurysms and TAA, these authors have reported overall spinal cord ischemic injury rates of 3.5%.[7]

Oxygen requirements of spinal cord tissue decrease 6–7% for each degree Celsius reduction in cord temperature. Hypothermia for cord protection during TAA surgery can be either regional (i.e. confined to the spinal cord itself) or systemic. The protective effect of hypothermia is presumed due to decreased tissue metabolism. However, the mechanism may be more complex, involving membrane stabilization and attenuation of excitatory neurotransmitter release.[180] Hypothermic spinal cord protection may ablate the hyperemic phase of cord reperfusion, resulting in less edema after circulation is restored.[181,182] The specifics of applying hypothermic protection range from modest systemic hypothermia simply achieved by passively cooling the

operating room and allowing evaporative and respiratory heat losses, to profound hypothermia (15° to 18°C) with complete cardiopulmonary bypass and temporary circulatory arrest. Lesser degrees can be achieved actively by adding a heat exchanger to a partial cardiopulmonary bypass circuit. This technique provides for active systemic hypothermia, the degree of which is limited by cardiac arrhythmias.[183] Regional hypothermia has the distinct advantage of avoiding systemic hypothermia, a concept we believe critical to the operative management of TAA patients. Systemic hypothermia has been independently associated with the development of complications after elective abdominal aortic surgery.[184] Regional hypothermia can be indirectly administered via the doubly clamped thoracic aorta,[185] or directly onto the spinal cord.[98] Our experience with the rate and volume of cooled epidural perfusate necessary to achieve moderate regional cord hypothermia indicates that effective cooling through intercostal vessels alone is likely not feasible. Application of regional hypothermic techniques is based on convincing experimental data revealing near complete protection against cord injury.[182,186] Marsala and colleagues established a clinically applicable closed epidural infusion system that achieved moderate (26° to 28°C) cord hypothermia and was 100% effective against spinal cord ischemia induced by double thoracic aortic clamping in a dog model.[187] Moreover, newer experimental evidence indicates moderate regional cord hypothermia is compatible with MEP monitoring and does not lessen its ability to detect cord ischemia in pigs.[188]

Stimulated by these data and the potential to fit regional hypothermia into our operative strategy, we developed a clinically applicable epidural cooling system and have utilized it since 1993. The mechanics of this clinically applicable system as displayed in **Figure 32.11** are straightforward, with an epidural catheter used for infusion of 4°C saline and a separate intrathecal catheter used to measure CSF temperature and pressure. It is necessary to maintain a continuous infusion to achieve moderate (approximately 25°C) levels of cord hypothermia, and the infusion must be initiated some 45 min prior to the anticipated application of the cross-clamp. Technically, the principal limitation of the system is pressure increases during epidural infusion – averaging twice baseline in our patients – and is a significant concern relative to spinal cord perfusion above the cooling level. It therefore is necessary to maintain an arbitrary 30–40mmHg between mean arterial pressure and mean CSF pressure by either decreasing the epidural infusion rate or increasing systemic arterial pressure. Neurologic outcomes in our first 70 patients using this method were significantly improved compared with institutional controls. Those without regional cord hypothermia experienced nearly a tenfold increase in ischemic cord injury.[96] This effect remained verified in our latest evaluation of the technique. Devastating neurologic deficits after 170 thoracic aneurysm or extensive TAA (types I, II, and III) resections were reduced to the 2–3% range with use of epidural cooling.[97] In recent examination of our overall experience with TAA repair, use of epidural cooling produced a significant reduction in cord ischemia in types I–III aneurysms.[25] Using our modified clamp-and-sew technique, patients with extensive aneurysms unable to have epidural cooling as part of their operative strategy suffered a 20% rate of cord ischemic injury of any degree while this was reduced to 8.6% in those undergoing reconstruction with epidural cooling.

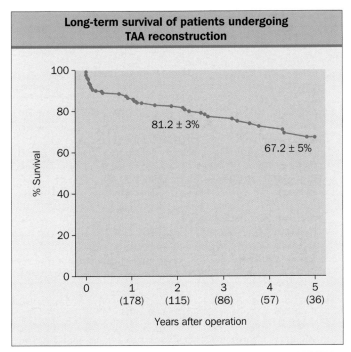

Figure 32.18 Long-term survival of 333 patients undergoing 337 TAA reconstructions at the Massachusetts General Hospital. Two-year and 5-year survival are 81.2±3% and 67.2±5%, respectively.

Long-term survival in series of repaired aortic aneurysm of various extent.			
Reference	*Year*	*Aneurysm extent*	*5-Year survival*
Svensson et al.[11]	1993	TAA	61%
Schepens et al.[64]	1996	TAA	53%
Schwartz et al.[24]	1996	Type IV	50%
Hallett et al.[190]	1997	AAA	67%
Faggioli et al.[122]	1998	Pararenal	40%
Martin et al.[121]	2000	Suprarenal/ Type III or IV	50%
Coselli et al.[61]	2001	TAA	72%
Biancari et al.[191]	2002	AAA	66.8%
Cambria et al.[25]	2002	TAA	67.2%

Table 32.6 Long-term survival in series of repaired aortic aneurysm of various extent. AAA, abdominal aortic aneurysm; TAA, thoracoabdominal aneurysm.

Late survival

Late survival in patients after complex AAA repair has been reported to be 40–75% at 5 years.[121,122,189] Svensson et al. indicated survival projections in the 60% range at 5 years after TAA operation.[11] Displayed in **Figure 32.18** are our late survival data in 333 patients undergoing 337 TAA repairs, with a 5-year survival of 67.2% (95% CI, 59–77%).[25] Long-term actuarial survival in a variety of clinical series are displayed in **Table 32.6.** Results are comparable regardless of aneurysm extent.[11,24,25,61,64,121,122,190,191] These data indicate that the substantial resource investment required to support TAA patients through successful operation and recovery is an appropriate expenditure of such resources.

The majority of operative survivors return to their preoperative independent living status.[19,64] Cardiac events are the most common source of late mortality.[11,64,121] Further, the negative impact of postoperative lower extremity neurologic deficit and dialysis dependence on perioperative survival remains significant as these patients also have distinctly inferior late survival.[11] Some 10% of patients will go on to have another aortic event, whether it be remote aneurysm or graft-related, and rupture of another aneurysm has accounted for approximately 10% of late deaths.[4,11,64] In determining long-term aortic outcome in our patients, we have found 10.5% of patients went on to have a second aortic event at an average of just over 2 years after repair.[4] Interestingly, aortic disease-related events occurred in 7% of patients and accounted for 71% of late events with the great majority being repair of another aneurysm (n=20; 87%). Graft-related complications occurred in only 3% of repairs and accounted for the remaining 29% of late aortic events. Clinically

evident renovisceral occlusion was the most common graft-related event (n=5; 56%). Inclusion anastomosis pseudo-aneurysm, graft infection, and graft-esophageal fistula were rare, occurring in less than 1% of patients. One-year and 5-year freedom from another aortic event was 96% and 71%, respectively. Independent predictors of late aortic events were female gender, initial aneurysm rupture, partial aneurysmal disease resection, and expansion of remaining aortic segments on imaging surveillance. This evaluation suggests TAA repair is durable with few long-term sequelae related to grafting. However, these patients are at risk for further aortic problems and aortic surveillance after successful TAA reconstruction is important in those with the above risk factors.

SUMMARY

There has been substantial progress in the overall results of operative treatment of pararenal and suprarenal aortic aneurysms as well as TAA. Given the unfavorable natural history of these lesions, an aggressive posture towards graft replacement is clearly justified in environments with demonstrated surgical expertise. The multiplicity of surgical strategies and adjuncts applied in efforts to minimize the principal complications of operation for complex aortic aneurysms indicate that the evolution of surgical sophistication is, as yet, incomplete. Similar to the evolution of surgical treatment of standard infrarenal AAA, an increase in the percentage of patients treated in elective circumstances will improve overall results in the future. It appears that endovascular strategies or combination open/endovascular approaches will be imminently feasible for select patients.

REFERENCES

1. Bickerstaff LK, Pairolero PC, Hollier LH, et al. Thoracic aortic aneurysms: a population-based study. Surgery 1982;92:1103–8.
2. McNamara JJ, Pressler VM. Natural history of arteriosclerotic thoracic aortic aneurysms. Ann Thorac Surg 1978;26:468–73.
3. Svensjö S, Bengtsson H, Bergqvist D. Thoracic and thoracoabdominal aortic aneurysm and dissection: an investigation based on autopsy. Br J Surg 1996;83:68–71.
4. Clouse WD, Marone LK, Davison JK, et al. Late aortic and graft-related events after thoracoabdominal aneurysm repair. J Vasc Surg 2003;37:254–61.
5. Gloviczki P, Pairolero P, Welch T, et al. Multiple aortic aneurysms: the results of surgical management. J Vasc Surg 1990;11:19–28.
6. Crawford ES, Cohen ES. Aortic aneurysm: a multifocal disease. Arch Surg 1982;117:1393–400.
7. Acher CW, Wynn MM, Hoch JR, Kranner PW. Cardiac function is a risk factor for paralysis in thoracoabdominal aortic replacement. J Vasc Surg 1998;27:821–30.
8. Cambria R, Davison JK, Zannetti S, et al. Thoracoabdominal aneurysm repair: perspectives over a decade with the clamp-and-sew technique. Ann Surg 1997;226:294–305.
9. Coselli JS, LeMaitre SA, Poli de Figueiredo L, et al. Paraplegia after thoracoabdominal aortic aneurysm repair: is dissection a risk factor? Ann Thorac Surg 1997;63:28–36.
10. Safi HJ, Campbell MP, Muller CC, et al. Cerebral spinal fluid drainage and distal aortic perfusion decrease the incidence of neurological deficit: the results of 343 descending and thoracoabdominal aortic aneurysm repairs. Eur J Vasc Endovasc Surg 1997;14:118–24.
11. Svensson LG, Crawford ES, Hess KR, et al. Experience with 1509 patients undergoing thoracoabdominal aortic operations. J Vasc Surg 1993;17:357–70.
12. Johansson G, Markstrom U, Swedenborg J. Ruptured thoracic aortic aneurysms: a study of incidence and mortality rates. J Vasc Surg 1995;21:985–8.
13. Perko MJ, Norgaard M, Herzog TM, et al. Unoperated aortic aneurysm: a survey of 170 patients. Ann Thorac Surg 1995;59:1204–9.
14. Clouse WD, Hallett JW, Schaff HV, et al. Improved prognosis of thoracic aortic aneurysms. JAMA 1998;280:1926–9.
15. Etheredge SN, Yee J, Smith JV, et al. Successful resection of large aneurysm of the upper abdominal aorta and replacement with homograft. Surgery 1955;38:1071–81.
16. DeBakey ME, Creech O Jr, Morris CG. Aneurysms of the thoracoabdominal aorta involving the celiac, superior mesenteric, and renal arteries: report of four cases treated by resection and homograft replacement. Ann Surg 1956;44:549–73.
17. Crawford ES. Thoracoabdominal and abdominal aortic aneurysm involving renal, superior mesenteric and celiac arteries. Ann Surg 1974;179:763–72.
18. Crawford ES, Crawford JL, Safi H, et al. Thoracoabdominal aortic aneurysms: preoperative and intraoperative factors determining immediate and long term results of operation in 605 patients. J Vasc Surg 1986;3:389–404.
19. Gilling-Smith GL, Worswick OL, Knight PF, et al. Surgical repair of thoracoabdominal aortic aneurysm: 10 years experience. Br J Surg 1995;82:624–9.
20. Hollier L, Money SR, Naslund TC, et al. Risk of spinal cord dysfunction in patients undergoing thoracoabdominal aortic replacement. Am J Surg 1992;164:210–3.
21. Anderson JL, Berce M, Hartley DE. Endoluminal aortic grafting with renal and superior mesenteric artery incorporation by graft fenestration. J Endovasc Ther 2001;8:3–8.
22. Chuter TAM, Gordon RL, Reilly LM, et al. An endovascular system for thoracoabdominal aortic aneurysm repair. J Endovasc Ther 2001;8:25–33.
23. Johnston KW, Rutherford RB, Tilson MD, et al. Ad Hoc Committee on reporting standards, SVS/NAISCVS. Suggested standards for reporting on arterial aneurysms. J Vasc Surg 1991;13:452–8.
24. Schwartz LB, Belkin M, Donaldson M, et al. Improvements in results of repair of Type IV thoracoabdominal aortic aneurysms. J Vasc Surg 1996;24:74–81.
25. Cambria RP, Clouse WD, Dorer DJ, et al. Thoracoabdominal aortic aneurysm repair: results with 337 operations performed over a 15-year interval. Ann Surg 2002;216:471–9.
26. Coselli JS, LeMaire SC, Buket S, et al. Subsequent proximal aortic operations in 123 patients with previous infrarenal abdominal aortic aneurysm surgery. J Vasc Surg 1995;22:59–67.
27. Coselli JS, Poli de Figuerrado LF, LeMaire SA. Impact of previous thoracic aneurysm repair on thoracoabdominal aortic aneurysm management. Ann Thorac Surg 1997;64:639–50.
28. Panneton JM, Hollier LM. Basic data underlying clinical decision making: non-dissecting thoracoabdominal aortic aneurysms: Part I. Ann Vasc Surg 1995;9:503–14.
29. Heineman MK, Buehner B, Jurmann MJ, et al. Use of 'elephant trunk technique' in aortic surgery. Ann Thorac Surg 1995;60:2–7.
30. Safi HJ, Miller CC 3rd, Estrera A, et al. Staged repair of extensive aortic aneurysms: morbidity and mortality in the elephant trunk technique. Circulation 2001;104:2938–42.
31. Neya K, Omoto R, Kyo S. Outcome of Stanford Type B acute aortic dissection. Circulation 1992;86(Suppl 5):II1–7.
32. Schor JS, Yerlioghu ME, Galla JD, et al. Selective management of acute Type B aortic dissection: long-term follow-up. Ann Thorac Surg 1996;61:1339–41.
33. Fattori R, Bacchi-Reggiani L, Bertaccini P, et al. Evolution of aortic dissection after repair. Am J Cardiol 2000;86:868–72.
34. Iguchi A, Tabayashi K. Outcome of medically treated Stanford Type B aortic dissection. Jpn Circ J 1998;62:102–5.
35. Kato M, Bai H, Sato K, et al. Determining surgical indications for acute type B dissection based on enlargement of aortic diameter during the chronic phase. Circulation 1995;92(Suppl 2):II107–12.
36. DeBakey ME, McCollum CH, Crawford ES, et al. Dissection and dissecting aneurysms of the aorta. Twenty-year follow-up of five hundred twenty-seven patients treated surgically. Surgery 1982;92:1118–34.
37. Marui A, Mochizuki T, Mitsui N, et al. Toward the best treatment for uncomplicated patients with type B acute aortic dissection: a consideration for sound surgical indication. Circulation 1999;100(Suppl 2):275–80.
38. Juvonen T, Ergin MA, Galla JD, et al. Risk factors for rupture of chronic type B dissections. J Thorac Cardiovasc Surg 1999;117:776–86.
39. Bernard Y, Zimmermann H, Chocron S, et al. False lumen patency as a predictor of late outcome in aortic dissection. Am J Cardiol 2001;87:1378–82.
40. Kozai Y, Watanabe S, Yonezawa M, et al. Long-term prognosis of acute aortic dissection with medical treatment: a survey of 263 unoperated patients. Jpn Circ J 2001;65:359–63.
41. Cambria RP, Brewster DC, Moncure AC, et al. Spontaneous aortic dissection in the presence of coexistent or previously repaired atherosclerotic aortic aneurysm. Ann Surg 1988;208:619–24.
42. Nagashima H, Sakomura Y, Aoka Y, et al. Angiotensin II type 2 receptor mediates vascular smooth muscle cell apoptosis in cystic medial degeneration associated with Marfan's syndrome. Circulation 2001;104(Suppl 1):I282–7.
43. Murdoch JL, Walker BA, Halpern BL, et al. Life expectancy and causes of death in the Marfan syndrome. N Engl J Med 1972;286:804–8.
44. Silverman DI, Burton KJ, Gray J, et al. Life expectancy in the Marfan syndrome. Am J Cardiol 1995;75:157–60.
45. Finkbohner R, Johnston D, Crawford ES, et al. Marfan syndrome: long-term survival and complications after aortic aneurysm repair. Circulation 1995;91:728–33.
46. Shores J, Berger KR, Murphy EA, et al. Progression of aortic dilatation and the benefit of long-term beta-adrenergic blockade in Marfan's syndrome. N Engl J Med 1994;330:1335–41.
47. Evans JM, O'Fallon WM, Hunder GG. Increased incidence of aortic aneurysms and dissection in giant cell (temporal) arteritis. Ann Intern Med 1995;122:502–7.

48. Osler W. The Gulstonian lectures on malignant endocarditis. BMJ 1885;1:467.

49. Estes JE Jr. Abdominal aortic aneurysm: a study of one hundred and two cases. Circulation 1950;2:2582–64.

50. Juvonen T, Ergin MA, Galla JD, et al. Prospective study of the natural history of thoracic aortic aneurysms. Ann Thorac Surg 1997; 63:1533–45.

51. Clouse WD, Hallett JW, Schaff HV, et al. Acute aortic dissection; the most common aortic catastrophe? (in press)

52. Crawford ES, DeNatale RW. Thoracoabdominal aortic aneurysm: observations regarding the natural course of the disease. J Vasc Surg 1986;3:578–82.

53. Crawford ES, Hess KR, Cohen JS, et al. Ruptured aneurysm of the descending thoracic and thoracoabdominal aorta. Ann Surg 1991; 213:417–26.

54. Masuda Y, Takanashi K, Takasu J, et al. Expansion rate of thoracic aortic aneurysms and influencing factors. Chest 1992;102:461–6.

55. Lobato AC, Puech-Leao P. Predictive factors for rupture of thoraco-abdominal aortic aneurysm. J Vasc Surg 1998;27:446–53.

56. Galla JD, Ergin MA, Lansman SL, et al. Identification of risk factors in patients undergoing thoracoabdominal aneurysm repair. J Card Surg 1997;12:292–9.

57. Brewster DC, Cronenwett JL, Hallett JW, et al. Guidelines for the treatment of abdominal aortic aneurysms. J Vasc Surg 2003; 37:1106–17.

58. Coady MA, Rizzo JA, Hammond GL, et al. Surgical intervention criteria for thoracic aortic aneurysms: a study of growth rates and complications. Ann Thorac Surg 1999;67:1922–6.

59. Griepp RB, Ergin MA, Galla JD, et al. Natural history of descending thoracic and thoracoabdominal aneurysms. Ann Thorac Surg 1999; 67:1927–30.

60. Cooke J, Cambria RP. Simultaneous tracheobronchial and esophageal obstruction secondary to thoracoabdominal aneurysm. J Vasc Surg 1993;18:90–4.

61. Coselli JS, LeMaire SA, Miller CC 3rd, et al. Mortality and paraplegia after thoracoabdominal aortic aneurysm repair: a risk factor analysis. Ann Thorac Surg 2000;69:409–14.

62. Safi HJ, Miller CC 3rd, Carr C, et al. Importance of intercostal artery reattachment during thoracoabdominal aortic aneurysm repair. J Vasc Surg 1998;27:58–68.

63. Cox GS, O'Hara PJ, Hertzer N, et al. Thoracoabdominal aneurysm repair: a representative experience. J Vasc Surg 1992;15:780–8.

64. Schepens MA, Dekkar E, Hanerlijnck RP, et al. Survival and aortic events after graft replacement for thoracoabdominal aortic aneurysm. Cardiovasc Surg 1996;4:713–9.

65. Safi HJ. Fenoldopam improves renal function following thoraco-abdominal aortic aneurysm surgery. 27th Global: Vascular and Endovascular Issues, Techniques and Horizons. (abstract)

66. Huynh TT, Miller CC, Estrera AL, et al. Thoracoabdominal and descending thoracic aortic aneurysm surgery in patients aged 79 years and older. J Vasc Surg 2002;36:469–75.

67. Cohen JR, Angus L, Asher A, et al. Disseminated intravascular coagulation as a result of supraceliac clamping: implications for thoraco-abdominal aneurysm repair. Ann Vasc Surg 1987;1:552–7.

68. Cohen JR, Sardari F, Paul J, et al. Increased intestinal permeability: implications for thoracoabdominal aneurysm repair. Ann Vasc Surg 1991;6:433–7.

69. Gadowski GR, Pilcher DB, Ricci MA. Abdominal aortic aneurysm expansion rate: effects of size and beta-adrenergic blockade. J Vasc Surg 1994;19:727–31.

70. Rieumont MJ, Kaufman JA, Geller SC, et al. Evaluation of renal artery stenosis with dynamic gadolinium-enhanced magnetic resonance angiography. Am J Radiol 1997;169:39–44.

71. Kieffer E, Fukui S, Chiras J, et al. Spinal cord arteriography: a safe adjunct before descending thoracic or thoracoabdominal aortic aneurysmectomy. J Vasc Surg 2002;35:262–8.

72. Yamada N, Takamiya M, Kuribayashi M, et al. MRA of the Adamkiewicz artery: a preoperative study for thoracic aortic aneurysm. J Comput Assist Tomogr 2000;24:362–8.

73. Cernaianu A, Olah A, Cilley JJ, et al. Effect of sodium nitroprusside on paraplegia during cross-clamping of the thoracic aorta. Ann Thorac Surg 1993;56:1035–8.

74. Shine T, Nugent M. Sodium nitroprusside decreases spinal cord perfusion pressure during descending thoracic aortic cross-clamping in the dog. J Cardiothorac Anesth 1990;4:185–93.

75. Simpson J, Eide T, Schiff G, et al. Isoflurane versus sodium nitroprusside for the control of proximal hypertension during thoracic aortic cross-clamping: effects on spinal cord ischemia. J Cardiothorac Vasc Anesth 1995;9:491–6.

76. Poulias GE, Doundalikis N, Skoutas B, et al. Juxtarenal abdominal aneurysmectomy. J Cardiovasc Surg 1992;127:520–4.

77. Sauer L, Stoney RJ. Transabdominal exposure of the pararenal and suprarenal aorta by medial visceral rotation. Semin Vasc Surg 1989; 2:209–13.

78. Goldstone J. Aneurysms of the aorta and iliac arteries. In: Moore WS, ed. Vascular surgery: a comprehensive review, 6th edn. Philadelphia: WB Saunders; 2001:457–80.

79. Cambria RP, Brewster DC, Abbott WM, et al. Transperitoneal versus retroperitoneal approach for aortic reconstruction. A randomized prospective study. J Vasc Surg 1990;11:314–25.

80. Kirby LB, Rosenthal D, Atkins CP, et al. Comparison between the transabdominal and retroperitoneal approaches for aortic reconstruction in patients at high risk. J Vasc Surg 1999;30:400–6.

81. Sicard GA. Surgical techniques for repair of abdominal aortic aneurysms. In: Gewertz BL, Schwartz LB, eds. Surgery of the aorta and its branches. Philadelphia:WB Saunders; 2000:124–75.

82. Gertler JP, Cambria RP, Laposata M, et al. Coagulation changes during thoracoabdominal aneurysm repair. J Vasc Surg 1996;24:936–45.

83. Illig KA, Green RM, Ouriel K, et al. Primary fibrinolysis during supraceliac aortic clamping. J Vasc Surg 1997;25:244–54.

84. Green RM. Supraceliac aortic clamping for infrarenal aortic surgery: value and technical precautions. In: Veith FJ, ed. Current critical problems in vascular surgery, vol. 4. St. Louis:Quality Medical; 1992:211–6.

85. Nypaver TJ, Shepard AD, Reddy DJ, et al. Repair of pararenal abdominal aortic aneurysms: an analysis of operative management. Arch Surg 1993;128:803–13.

86. Crawford ES, Mizrahi EM, Hess KR, et al. The impact of distal per-fusion and somatosensory evoked potential monitoring on prevention of paraplegia after aortic aneurysm operation. J Thorac Cardiovasc Surg 1988;95:357–66.

87. Comerota AJ, White JV. Reducing morbidity of thoracoabdominal aneurysm repair by preliminary axillofemoral bypass. Am J Surg 1995;170:218–22.

88. Connolly J, Wakabayashi A, German J, et al. Clinical experience with pulsatile left heart bypass without anticoagulation for thoracic anerysms. J Thorac Cardiovasc Surg 1971;62:568–76.

89. Estrera AL, Miller CC 3rd, Huynh TTT. Neurologic outcome after thoracic and thoracoabdominal aortic aneurysm repair. Ann Thorac Surg 2001;72:1225–31.

90. Coselli JS, LeMaire SA. Left heart bypass reduces paraplegia rates after thoracoabdominal aortic aneurysm repair. Ann Thorac Surg 1999;67:1931–4.

91. Schepens MAA, Vermeulen FEE, Morshuis WJ. Impact of left heart bypass on the results of thoracoabdominal aortic aneurysm repair. Ann Thorac Surg 1999;67:1963–7.

92. Safi HJ, Harlin SA, Miller CC 3rd. Predictive factors for acute renal failure in thoracic and thoracoabdominal aortic aneurysm surgery. J Vasc Surg 1996;24:338–45.

93. Safi H, Hess KR, Randel M, et al. Cerebrospinal fluid drainage and distal aortic perfusion: reducing neurologic complications in repair of thoracoabdominal aortic aneurysms, Type I and Type II. J Vasc Surg 1996;23:223–8.

94. Mauney M, Tribble C, Cope J, et al. Is clamp and sew still viable for thoracic aortic resection? Ann Surg 1996;223:534–43.

95. LeMaire SA, Miller CC 3rd, Conklin LD, et al. A new predictive model for adverse outcomes after elective thoracoabdominal aortic aneurysm repair. Ann Thorac Surg 2001;71:1233–8.

96. Cambria RP, Davison JK, Zannetti S, et al. Clinical experience with epidural cooling for spinal cord protection during thoracic and thoracoabdominal aneurysm repair. J Vasc Surg 1997;25:234–43.

97. Cambria RP, Davison JK, Carter C, et al. Epidural cooling for spinal cord protection during thoracoabdominal aneurysm repair: a five-year experience. J Vasc Surg 2000;31:1093–102.

98. Davison J, Cambria R, Vierra D, et al. Epidural cooling for regional spinal cord hypothermia during thoracoabdominal aneurysm repair. J Vasc Surg 1994;20:304–10.

99. Cambria RP, Davison JK, Giglia JS, et al. Mesenteric shunting decreases visceral ischemic time during thoracoabdominal aneurysm repair. J Vasc Surg 1998;27:745–9.

100. Kouchoukos N, Daily BB, Rokkas CK, et al. Hypothermic bypass and circulatory arrest for operations on the descending thoracic and thoracoabdominal aorta. Ann Thorac Surg 1995;60:67–77.

101. Rokkas CK, Kouchoukos NT. Profound hypothermia for spinal cord protection in operations on the descending and thoracoabdominal aorta. Semin Thorac Cardiovasc Surg 1998;10:57–60.

102. Kouchoukos NT, Masetti P, Rokkas CK, et al. Safety and efficacy of hypothermic cardiopulmonary bypass and circulatory arrest for operations on the descending thoracic and thoracoabdominal aorta. Ann Thorac Surg 2001;72:699–708.

103. Safi HJ, Muller CC, Subramanian MH, et al. Thoracic and thoraco-abdominal aortic aneurysm repair using cardiopulmonary bypass, profound hypothermia and circulatory arrest via left side of the chest incision. J Vasc Surg 1998;28:591–8.

104. Engle J, Safi HJ, Miller CC 3rd, et al. The impact of diaphragm management on prolonged ventilator support following thoracoabdominal aortic repair. J Vasc Surg 1999;29:150–6.

105. Wadouh F, Arndt C, Oppermann E, et al. The mechanism of spinal cord injury after simple and double aortic cross-clamping. J Thorac Cardiovasc Surg 1986;92:121–7.

106. Parodi JC, Palmaz JC, Barone HD. Transfemoral intraluminal graft implantation for abdominal aortic aneurysms. Ann Vasc Surg 1991; 5:491–9.

107. Dake MD, Miller DC, Semba CP, et al. Transluminal placement of endovascular stent-grafts for the treatment of descending thoracic aortic aneurysms. N Engl J Med 1994;331:1729–34.

108. Marin ML, Parsons RE, Hollier LH, et al. Impact of transrenal aortic endograft placement on endovascular graft repair of abdominal aortic aneurysms. J Vasc Surg 1998;28:638–46.

109. Greenberg RK, Lawrence-Brown M, Bhandari G, et al. An update of the Zenith endovascular graft for abdominal aortic aneurysms: initial implantation and mid-term follow-up data. J Vasc Surg 2001; 33:S157–64.

110. Cambria RP, Brewster DC, Lauterbach SR, et al. Evolving experience with thoracic aortic stent-graft repair. J Vasc Surg 2002;35:1129–36.

111. Mitchell RS, Miller DC, Dake MD, et al. Thoracic aortic aneurysm repair with an endovascular stent graft: the 'first generation'. Ann Thorac Surg 1999;67:1971–4.

112. Greenberg MD, Resch T, Nyman U, et al. Endovascular repair of descending thoracic aortic aneurysms: an early experience with intermediate-term follow up. J Vasc Surg 2000;31:147–56.

113. Dattilo JB, Brewster DC, Fan C, et al. Clinical failures of endovascular AAA repair: incidence, causes, and management. J Vasc Surg 2002; 35:1137–44.

114. van Marrewijk C, Buth J, Harris P, et al. Significance of endoleaks after endovascular repair of abdominal aortic aneurysms: the Eurostar experience. J Vasc Surg 2002;35:461–73.

115. Grabenwoger M, Hutschala D, Ehrlich MP, et al. Thoracic aortic aneurysm: treatment with endovascular self-expandable stent grafts. Ann Thorac Surg 2000;69:441–5.

116. White R, Donayre CE, Walot I, et al. Endovascular exclusion of descending thoracic aortic aneurysm and chronic dissections: initial clinical results with the AneuRx device. J Vasc Surg 2001;33:927–34.

117. Kasirajan K, Dolmatch B, Ouriel K, et al. Delayed onset of ascending paralysis after thoracic aortic stent graft deployment. J Vasc Surg 2000;31:196–9.

118. Gravereaux EC, Faries PF, Burks JA, et al. Risk of spinal cord ischemia

after endograft repair of thoracic aortic aneurysms. J Vasc Surg 2001; 34:997–1003.

119. Moon MR, Mitchell RS, Dake MD, et al. Simultaneous abdominal aortic replacement and thoracic stent-graft placement for multilevel aortic disease. J Vasc Surg 1997;25:332–40.

120. Chuter TAM, Gordon RL, Reilly LM, et al. Multi-branched stent-graft for Type III thoracoabdominal aortic aneurysm. J Vasc Interv Radiol 2001;12:391–2.

121. Martin GH, O'Hara PJ, Hertzer NR, et al. Surgical repair of aneurysms involving the suprarenal, visceral, and lower thoracic aortic segments: early results and late outcome. J Vasc Surg 2000;31:851–62.

122. Faggioli G, Stella A, Freyrie A, et al. Early and long-term results in the surgical treatment of juxtarenal and pararenal aortic aneurysms. Eur J Vasc Endovasc Surg 1998;15:205–11.

123. Welborn MB, Oldenburg SA, Hess PJ, et al. The relationship between visceral ischemia proinflammatory cytokines, and organ injury in patients undergoing thoracoabdominal aneurysm repair. Crit Care Med 2000;28:3191–7.

124. Cambria R, Brewster D, Moncure A, et al. Recent experience with thoracoabdominal aneurysm repair. Arch Surg 1989;124:620–4.

125. Cohen JR, Schroder W, Leal J, et al. Mesenteric shunting during thoracoabdominal aortic clamping to prevent disseminated intra-vascular coagulation in dogs. Ann Vasc Surg 1988;2:261–7.

126. Safi HJ, Miller CC 3rd, Yawn DH, et al. Impact of distal aortic and visceral perfusion on liver function during thoracoabdominal and descending thoracic aortic repair. J Vasc Surg 1998;27:145–53.

127. Anagnostopoulos PV, Shepard AD, Pipinos II, et al. Hemostatic alterations associated with supraceliac aortic cross-clamping. J Vasc Surg 2002;35:100–8.

128. Gertler JP, Cambria RP, Makary MA, et al. Correction of coagulation defect in thoracoabdominal aneurysm repair by mesenteric shunting. 24th meeting of the New England Society for Vascular Surgery,1997 (abstract).

129. Money SR, Rice K, Crockett D, et al. Risk of respiratory failure after repair of thoracoabdominal aortic aneurysms. Am J Surg 1994; 168:152–5.

130. Svensson LG, Hess KR, Coselli JS, et al. A prospective study of respiratory failure after high-risk surgery on the thoracoabdominal aorta. J Vasc Surg 1991;14:271–82.

131. Kashyap VS, Cambria RP, Davison JK, et al. Renal failure after thoracoabdominal aortic surgery. J Vasc Surg 1997;26:949–57.

132. Qvarfordt PG, Stoney RJ, Reilly LM, et al. Management of pararenal aneurysms of the abdominal aorta. J Vasc Surg 1986;3:84–93.

133. Svensson LG, Crawford ES, Hess KR, et al. Thoracoabdominal aortic aneurysms associated with celiac, superior mesenteric and renal artery occlusive disease. Methods and analysis of results in 271 patients. J Vasc Surg 1992;16:378–90.

134. DeLasson L, Hanson HE, Juhl B, et al. A randomized, clinical study on the effect of low-dose dopamine on central and renal hemodynamics in infrarenal aortic surgery. Eur J Vasc Endovasc Surg 1995;10:82–90.

135. Cambria RP, Giglia J. Prevention of spinal cord ischemic complications after thoracoabdominal aortic surgery. Eur J Vasc Endovasc Surg 1998;15:96–109.

136. Cambria RP, Davison JK. Spinal cord ischemic complications after thoracoabdominal aortic surgery. In: Gewertz BL, Schwartz LB, eds. Surgery of the aorta and its branches. Philadelphia:WB Saunders; 2000:212–30.

137. Savader SJ, Williams GM, Trerotola SO, et al. Preoperative spinal artery localization and its relationship to postoperative neurologic complications. Radiology 1993;189:165–71.

138. Svensson LG, Hess KR, Coselli JS, et al. Influence of segmental arteries, extent and atriofemoral bypass on postoperative paraplegia after thoracoabdominal aortic operations. J Vasc Surg 1994;20:255–62.

139. Svensson LG, Rickards E, Coull A, et al. Relationship of spinal cord blood flow to vascular anatomy during thoracic aortic cross-clamping and shunting. J Thorac Cardiovasc Surg 1986;91:71–8.

140. Lauterbach SR, Cambria RP, Brewster DC, et al. Contemporary management of aortic branch compromise resulting from acute aortic dissection. J Vasc Surg 2001;33:1185–92.

141. Safi HJ, Miller CC 3rd, Arizzadeh A, et al. Observations on delayed neurologic deficit after thoracoabdominal aneurysm repair. J Vasc Surg 1997;26:616–22.

142. Azizzadeh A, Huynh TTT, Miller CC 3rd, et al. Reversal of twice-delayed neurologic deficits with cerebrospinal fluid drainage after thoracoabdominal aneurysm repair: a case report and plea for a national database collection. J Vasc Surg 2000;31:592–8.

143. McGarvey M, Hogan MS, Cheung AT, et al. Interventions for reversing delayed-onset postoperative paraplegia after thoracic aortic reconstruction. Program of the 38th annual meeting of the Society of Thoracic Surgeons 2002; 202 (abstract).

144. Maniar HS, Pradad SM, Chu CM, et al. Delayed paraplegia after thoracoabdominal aneurysm repair. Program of the 38th annual meeting of the Society of Thoracic Surgeons 2002; 200 (abstract).

145. Griepp RB, Ergen MA, Galla JD, et al. Looking for the artery of Adamkiewicz: a quest to minimize paraplegia after operations for aneurysm of the descending thoracic and thoracoabdominal aorta. J Thorac Cardiovasc Surg 1996;112:1202–15.

146. Kieffer E, Richard T, Chiras J, et al. Preoperative spinal cord arteriography in aneurysmal disease of the descending thoracic and thoracoabdominal aorta: preliminary results in 45 patients. Ann Vasc Surg 1989;3:34–46.

147. Williams GM, Perler BA, Burdick JF, et al. Angiographic localization of spinal cord blood supply and its relationship to postoperative paraplegia. J Vasc Surg 1991;13:23–35.

148. Heinemann MK, Brassel F, Herzog T, et al. The role of spinal angiography in operations on the thoracic aorta: myth or reality? Ann Thorac Surg 1998;65:346–51.

149. Svensson LG, Patel V, Robinson MF, et al. Influence of preservation or perfusion of intraoperatively identified spinal cord blood supply on spinal motor evoked potentials and paraplegia after aortic surgery. J Vasc Surg 1991;13:355–65.

150. Cunningham JJ, Laschinger JC, Spencer FC. Monitoring of somatosensory evoked potentials during surgical procedures on the thoracoabdominal aorta. IV. Clinical observations and results. J Thorac Cardiovasc Surg 1987;94:275–85.

151. Grabitz K, Sandmann W, Stuhmeirer K, et al. The risk of ischemic spinal cord injury in patients undergoing graft replacement for thoracoabdominal aortic aneurysms. J Vasc Surg 1996;23:230–40.

152. deHaan P, Kalkman CJ, De Mol BA, et al. Efficacy of transcranial motor-evoked myogenic potentials to detect spinal cord ischemia during operations for thoracoabdominal aneurysms. J Thorac Cardiovasc Surg 1997;113:87–101.

153. Laschinger J, Owen J, Rosenbloom M, et al. Direct noninvasive monitoring of spinal cord motor function during thoracic aortic occlusion: use of motor evoked potentials. J Vasc Surg 1988;7:161–71.

154. Matsui Y, Goh K, Shiiya N, et al. Clinical application of evoked spinal cord potentials elicited by direct stimulation of the cord during temporary occlusion of the thoracic aorta. J Thorac Cardiovasc Surg 1994;107:1519–27.

155. van Dongen EP, Schepens MA, Morshuis WJ, et al. Thoracic and thoracoabdominal aortic aneurysm repair: use of evoked potential monitoring in 118 patients. J Vasc Surg 2001;34:1035–40.

156. Jacobs MJ, de Mol BA, Elenbaas T, et al. Spinal cord blood supply in patients with thoracoabdominal aortic aneurysms. J Vasc Surg 2002;35:30–7.

157. Jacobs M, Meylaerts S, de Haan P, et al. Strategies to prevent neurologic deficit based on motor-evoked potentials in types I and II thoracoabdominal aortic aneurysm repair. J Vasc Surg 1999;29:48–59.

158. Grubbs PJ, Marini C, Toporoff B, et al. Somatosensory evoked potentials and spinal cord perfusion pressure are significant predictors of postoperative neurologic dysfunction. Surgery 1988;104:216–23.

159. Svensson LG, Grum DF, Bednarski M, et al. Appraisal of cerebrospinal fluid alterations during aortic surgery with intrathecal papaverine administration and cerebrospinal fluid drainage. J Vasc Surg 1990; 11:423–9.

160. Berendes J, Bredee J, Schipperheyn J, et al. Mechanism of spinal cord injury after cross-clamping of the descending thoracic aorta. Circulation 1982;66(Suppl 1):112–6.

161. Kazama S, Masaki Y, Maruyama S, et al. Effect of altering cerebrospinal fluid pressure on spinal cord blood flow. Ann Thorac Surg 1994; 58:112–5.

162. Crawford ES, Svensson LG, Hess KR, et al. A prospective randomized study of cerebrospinal fluid drainage to prevent paraplegia after high risk surgery on the thoracoabdominal aorta. J Vasc Surg 1991;13:36–46.

163. Murray MJ, Bower TC, Oliver WCJ, et al. Effects of cerebrospinal fluid drainage in patients undergoing thoracic and thoracoabdominal aortic surgery. J Cardiothorac Vasc Anesth 1993;7:266–72.

164. Acher CW, Wynn MM, Hoch JR, et al. Combined use of cerebral spinal fluid drainage and naloxone reduces the risk of paraplegia in thoracoabdominal aneurysm repair. J Vasc Surg 1994;19:236–48.

165. Acher CW, Wynn MM, Archibald J. Naloxone and spinal fluid drainage as adjuncts in the surgical treatment of thoracoabdominal and thoracic aneurysms. Surgery 1990;108:755–62.

166. McCullough J, Hollier L, Nugent M. Paraplegia after thoracic aortic occlusion: influence of cerebrospinal fluid drainage. J Vasc Surg 1988; 7:153–60.

167. Bower TC, Murray MJ, Gloviczki P, Yaksh TL, Hollier LH, Pairolero PC. Effects of thoracic aortic occlusion and cerebrospinal fluid drainage on regional spinal cord blood flow in dogs: correlation with neurologic outcome. J Vasc Surg 1989;9:135–44.

168. Hill A, Kalman P, Johnston K, et al. Reversal of delayed-onset paraplegia after thoracic aortic surgery with cerebrospinal fluid drainage. J Vasc Surg 1994;20:315–7.

169. LeMarire SA, Köksoy C, Schmittling ZC, et al. Cerebrospinal fluid drainage during thoracoabdominal aortic aneurysm repair prevents spinal cord ischemia. Ann Thorac Surg 2000;70:1790 (abstract).

170. Coselli JS, LeMaire SA, Schmittling ZC, et al. Cerebrospinal fluid drainage in thoracoabdominal aortic surgery. Semin Vasc Surg 2000; 13:308–14.

171. Coselli JS, LeMaire SA, Köksoy C, et al. Cerebrospinal fluid drainage reduces paraplegia after thoracoabdominal aortic aneurysm repair: Results of a randomized clinical trial. J Vasc Surg 2002;35:631–9.

172. Fowl R, Patterson R, Gewirtz R, et al. Protection against postischemic spinal cord injury using a new 21-aminosteroid. J Surg Res 1990; 48:597–600.

173. Francel P, Long B, Malik J, et al. Limiting ischemic spinal cord injury using a free radical scavenger 21-aminosteroid and/or cerebrospinal fluid drainage. J Neurosurg 1993;79:742–51.

174. Laschinger J, Cunningham JJ, Cooper MM, et al. Prevention of ischemic spinal cord injury following aortic cross-clamping: use of corticosteroids. Ann Thorac Surg 1984;38:500–7.

175. Nylander W, Plunkett RJ, Hammon JW Jr, et al. Thiopental modification of ischemic spinal cord injury in the dog. Ann Thorac Surg 1982;33:64–8.

176. Simpson I, Eide T, Schiff G, et al. Intrathecal magnesium sulfate protects the spinal cord from ischemic injury during thoracic aortic cross-clamping. Anesthesiology 1994;81:1493–9.

177. Follis F, Miller K, Scremin O, et al. NMDA receptor blockade and spinal cord ischemia due to aortic crossclamping in the rat model. Can J Neurol Sci 1994;21:227–32.

178. Gelbfish J, Phillips T, Rose D, et al. Acute spinal cord ischemia: prevention of paraplegia with verapamil. Circulation 1986;74:I5–10.

179. Agee JM, Flanagan T, Blackbourne LH, et al. Reducing postischemic paraplegia using conjugated superoxide dismutase. Ann Thorac Surg 1991;51:911–5.

180. Rokkas C, Cronin C, Nitta T, et al. Profound systemic hypothermia inhibits the release of neurotransmitter amino acids in spinal cord ischemia. J Thorac Cardiovasc Surg 1995;110:27–35.

181. Allen BT, Davis C, Osborne D, et al. Spinal cord ischemia and reperfusion metabolism: the effect of hypothermia. J Vasc Surg 1994; 19:332–40.

182. Rokkas C, Sundaresan S, Shuman TA, et al. Profound systemic hypothermia protects the spinal cord in a primate model of spinal cord ischemia. J Thorac Cardiovasc Surg 1993;106:1024–35.

183. Svensson LG, Hess KR, D'Agostino RS, et al. Reduction of neurologic injury after high-risk thoracoabdominal aortic surgery. Ann Thorac Surg 1998;66:132–8.

184. Bush HJ, Hydo LJ, Fischer E, et al. Hypothermia during elective abdominal aortic aneurysm repair: the high risk of avoidable morbidity. J Vasc Surg 1995;21:392–400.

185. Fehrenbacher J, McCready R, Hormuth D, et al. One-stage segmental resection of extensive thoracoabdominal aneurysms with left-sided heart bypass. J Vasc Surg 1993;18:366–71.

186. Wisselink W, Becker M, Nguyen J, et al. Protecting the ischemic spinal cord during aortic clamping: the influence of selective hypothermia and spinal cord perfusion pressure. J Vasc Surg 1994;19:788–96.

187. Marsala M, Vanicky I, Galik J, et al. Panmyelic epidural cooling protects against ischemic spinal cord damage. J Surg Res 1993;55:21–31.

188. Meylaerts SA, de Haan P, Kalkman CJ, et al. The influence of regional spinal cord hypothermia on transcranial myogenic motor-evoked potential monitoring and the efficacy of spinal cord ischemia detection. J Thorac Cardiovasc Surg 1999;118:1038–45.

189. Crawford ES, Beckett WC, Greer MS. Juxtarenal infrarenal aortic aneurysm: special diagnostic and therapeutic considerations. Ann Surg 1986;203:661–70.

190. Hallett JW, Marshall DM, Petterson TM, et al. Graft-related complications after abdominal aortic aneurysm repair: reassurance from a 36-year population-based experience. J Vasc Surg 1997;25:277–86.

191. Biancari F, Ylönen K, Anttila V, et al. Durability of open repair of infrarenal abdominal aortic aneurysm: a 15-year follow-up study. J Vasc Surg 2002;35:87–93.

192. Cambria RA, Gloviczki P, Stanson A, et al. Outcome and expansion rate of 57 thoracoabdominal aortic aneurysms managed nonoperatively. Am J Surg 1995;170:213–7.

193. Dapunt OE, Galla JD, Sadeghi AM, et al. The natural history of thoracic aortic aneurysms. J Thorac Cardiovasc Surg 1994; 107:1323–33.

194. Coady MA, Rizzo JA, Hammond GL, et al. What is the appropriate size criterion for resection of thoracic aortic aneurysms? J Thorac Cardiovasc Surg 1997;113:476–91.

195. Bonser RS, Pagano D, Lewis ME, et al. Clinical and patho-anatomical factors affecting expansion of thoracic aortic aneurysms. Heart 2000; 84:277–83.

196. Davies RR, Goldstein LJ, Coady MA, et al. Yearly rupture or dissection rates for thoracic aortic aneurysms: simple prediction based on size. Ann Thorac Surg 2002;73:17–28.

197. Allen BT, Anderson CB, Rubin BG, et al. Preservation of renal function in juxtarenal and suprarenal abdominal aortic aneurysm repair. J Vasc Surg 1993;17:948–59.

198. Hamilton IN Jr, Hollier LH. Adjunctive therapy for spinal cord protection during thoracoabdominal aortic aneurysm repair. Semin Thorac Cardiovasc Surg 1998;10:35–9.

CHAPTER

33

Peripheral Aneurysms

Matthew T Menard and Michael Belkin

KEY POINTS

- An **aneurysm** is a permanent localized (i.e. focal) dilation of an artery, having at least a 50% increase in diameter compared with the expected normal diameter of the artery in question.

- **Arteriomegaly** is diffuse enlargement involving several arterial segments (i.e non-focal), with an increase in diameter of greater than 50% compared with the expected normal diameter.

- **Ectasia** is characterized by dilation with an increase in diameter of less than 50% of the normal arterial diameter.

- Popliteal artery aneurysms are the most frequent of peripheral aneurysms, exhibit a strong male predominance, and are commonly associated with aneurysms at other sites.

- Diagnosis is made by physical examination or ultrasound, while angiography is useful for operative planning.

- Given the high rate of complications, early operative intervention with autologous saphenous vein is recommended whenever possible.

- Femoral artery aneurysms, like popliteal aneurysms, are usually atherosclerotic in origin.

- Upper extremity aneurysms are infrequently encountered, with subclavian-axillary artery aneurysms arising from compression against a congenital bony abnormality being the most common.

- Evidence of emboli to the hand should trigger a search for a causative aneurysm more proximally.

- Careful monitoring of all patients with peripheral aneurysms is indicated given the high prevalence of additional aneurysms.

LOWER EXTREMITY ANEURYSMS

Popliteal aneurysms
History
Since popliteal aneurysms were first described in early Greek manuscripts, a colorful literature has documented their evolving management over the centuries. Antyllus's initial report in 200 BC described ligation and open packing of the aneurysm sac. Philagrius' 18th century proposals for aneurysm excision led to Pott's recommendation of above-the-knee amputation in 1779. This gave way to compression therapy, including Parker's deployment in the 19th century of teams of medical students applying pressure continuously over a period of days.[1] Linton popularized

sequential lumbar sympathectomy and extirpation of the aneurysm, and from Edwards' recommendations in 1969 onwards, popliteal artery exclusion accompanied by surgical bypass with saphenous vein has remained the mainstay of operative repair. More recent proposals have included applying percutaneous endoluminal technology to popliteal artery aneurysm treatment. In general, the incidence of lower extremity aneurysms appears to be increasing, perhaps due to better surveillance of the aging population, as does the ratio of aneurysms in the periphery to that of the abominal aorta.[2–4]

Although much less frequently encountered than aortic aneurysms, popliteal aneurysms are the most common of peripheral aneurysms, representing nearly 80% of cases. There is a strong male predominance, with an average male:female ratio of 30:1. They typically occur in men in their fifth and sixth decades, while women with popliteal aneurysms are usually in their eighth decade. They are associated with aortic aneurysms 40% of the time, and are bilateral in 50% to 70% of cases. Patients with bilateral aneurysms have a 70% chance of having a concomitant abdominal aortic aneurysm and the overall rate of second aneurysms in patients with popliteal aneurysms is nearly 80%.[4] Popliteal aneurysms are almost exclusively atherosclerotic in etiology. Trauma, cystic degeneration of the adventitia, entrapment, and infection are additional less common causes. There is a high rate of associated atherosclerotic disorders in this population, with myocardial dysfunction present in up to 40%, hypertension in up to two-thirds, smoking in 50–75%, and diabetes mellitus in 15% of patients.[5,6]

Signs and symptoms
Peripheral aneurysms can be asymptomatic or can present with significant complications. The most common clinical presentation of popliteal aneurysms is one of thrombosis and/or embolism with resultant acute limb ischemia. Early symptoms may be limited to petechial hemorrhage or localized digital gangrenous changes secondary to microemboli. Claudication as a first symptom has typically been found in 30–45% of patients in case series of popliteal aneurysms, although Bouhoutsos et al.[7] reported 73% of 116 patients had initial claudication. With aneurysmal growth in the absence of developed collaterals, acute dissection of mural thrombus or propagation of clot can precipitate severe, often irreversible ischemia. Left untreated, the incidence of future thromboembolic events in initially asymptomatic aneurysms is high; in one series of popliteal aneurysms managed conservatively, only 32% of patients were without complication at 5 years.[3] Similarly, in a study of 26 asymptomatic aneurysms followed for an average of 3 years, 31% developed limb-threatening complications, with two requiring amputation and two developing rest pain.[5] More rarely, the initial symptoms are secondary to

popliteal nerve compression from the growing aneurysm, leading to paresthesias, neuropraxia, and muscular dysfunction. Popliteal vein compression by the aneurysm can lead to thrombosis, manifest by leg swelling, superficial varicosities, or phlebitis. In the unlikely event of popliteal artery rupture, ischemia from arterial compression by the contained hematoma is more typical than exsanguination. Isolated case reports have also described arteriovenous fistula formation following aneurysm rupture into the popliteal vein.[8]

Diagnosis

Although smaller aneurysms or those protected by the supra- or infrageniculate muscles may not be readily detectable on palpation, a careful physical examination will lead to the diagnosis in the majority of cases of popliteal aneurysms. A prominent pulsatile mass will typically be identified with the knee in a slightly flexed position. They are most often located at or just above the level of the knee joint and less often below the joint. In the event of thrombosis, the mass may be firm and non-pulsatile. Widened pulses detected in the contralateral leg or elsewhere on examination are additional clues to the presence of a popliteal aneurysm. Cutaneous stigmata of distal embolism or the presence of more severe lower extremity ischemia from an acute thromboembolic event in this setting should always raise the suspicion for a newly symptomatic popliteal aneurysm.

When the physical examination is not definitive, ultrasound can often confirm the presence or absence of a popliteal aneurysm. Scanning of the contralateral leg as well as other sites of possible concomitant aneurysmal change should always be performed given the high likelihood of detecting extra-popliteal or bilateral aneurysms. When the aneurysm walls are calcified, plain radiographs of the knee may suggest the diagnosis. Computed tomography and magnetic resonance imaging are both highly accurate in establishing the diagnosis of popliteal aneurysms. These modalities are particularly helpful in distinguishing aneurysms from other entities (e.g. Baker's cysts) in the differential diagnosis of popliteal fossa masses. Angiography done during the process of a workup for extremity ischemia can uncover previously unsuspected aneurysms, but in the presence of occlusion or extensive laminated intramural thrombus, it can also be misleading in underestimating the size or even presence of a popliteal aneurysm. Its principal role in the management of popliteal aneurysms is that of operative planning. Specifically, it can frequently delineate both the status of the inflow and outflow vasculature and the full axial extent of the aneurysm.

Management

Given that even small aneuryms can give rise to serious complications, the presence of a popliteal aneurysm is usually sufficient indication for treatment. It is generally agreed upon that all symptomatic aneurysms should undergo operative repair, given the high rate of limb loss with conservative management. The true natural history of untreated asymptomatic popliteal aneurysms is poorly defined, however, and the indications for surgical repair of a small, incidentally noted, asymptomatic popliteal aneurysm are somewhat controversial. Lowell and colleagues[9] reported on a subset of 94 asymptomatic aneurysms followed for nearly 7 years; 18% of the limbs eventually developed symptoms (25% acute, 75% chronic) and three (4%) required amputation after attempted repair. Aneurysm size >2cm, the presence of

thrombus and poor distal runoff were significant predictors of the development of symptoms in this study. In a review of the available literature between 1980 and 1994, involving 1673 patients with 2445 popliteal aneurysms, Dawson and co-workers[10] found that on average 35% of patients treated non-operatively ultimately developed ischemic complications, and of those in whom surgical repair was later attempted, 25% went on to require amputation. In another single-institution report of a cohort of popliteal aneurysm patients followed expectantly, 100% developed symptoms of ischemia over time and required surgery, half within 2 years of initial presentation.[11] When statistical modeling was applied to determine outcomes in operatively versus non-operatively managed patients, intermediate-term results clearly favored surgical treatment.[12]

In view of these collective results, and the generally unfavorable long-term limb salvage rate following conservative treatment, most authors recommend surgical repair of asymptomatic popliteal aneurysms in all but certain high-risk patients. Some surgeons have modified these recommendations when autogenous vein is unavailable for use as a bypass conduit, given the poor results with prosthetic reconstruction in the distal popliteal and tibial position, or in the rare cases when suitable runoff targets are lacking. Similarly, given the overall limited life-expectancy of patients with multiple aneurysms (16% 10-year survival compared with 66% for those with a single aneurysm at initial presentation), other authors support conservative management in this subset of patients.[13]

Surgical therapy of popliteal aneurysms is principally directed at excluding the aneurysm from the circulation, thereby eliminating the potential development of limb-threatening ischemia, and providing adequate distal arterial flow. For typical aneurysms of small or modest size in which compression is not part of the presenting symptom profile, the aneurysm need not be opened or excised. In fact, it is often advantageous to avoid direct dissection of the aneurysm sac, to avert injury to the nerves and veins that may be densely adherent from associated chronic inflammation. The aneurysm is usually ligated both proximally and distally, and a bypass graft fashioned from autogenous greater saphenous vein. In cases in which there is significant atherosclerotic or aneurysmal disease of the superficial femoral or common femoral arteries, the proximal anastomosis should originate at the level of the common femoral artery. If the aneurysm is limited to the popliteal segment, the bypass graft may originate from the above-knee popliteal artery or, more typically, from the distal superficial femoral artery just proximal to the adductor canal. The placement of the distal anastomosis will be guided by the presence or degree of propagated thrombus in the below-knee popliteal segment, using the tibial or peroneal vessels as targets as dictated by the angiographic findings (**Fig. 33.1**). The aneurysm will usually thrombose to the level of the geniculate arteries or the point of proximal ligation. While most surgeons advocate ligation of the distal superficial femoral artery or suprageniculate popliteal artery just proximal to the aneurysmal segment, some defer this step in hopes of preserving presumed valuable collateral flow through these superior geniculate branches. This maneuver may be associated with a slight risk of continued perfusion and pressurization of the bypassed aneurysm, with the attendant possibility of late expansion and rupture.

In cases when the popliteal aneurysm is large enough to result in compression of the adjacent nerve and vein, it is advisable to

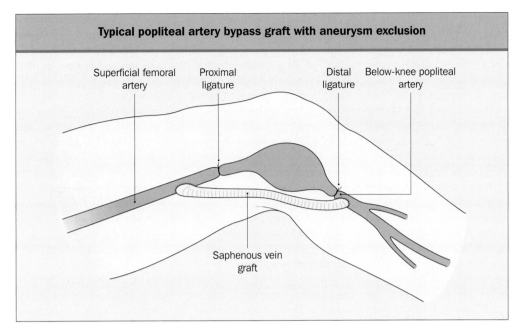

Typical popliteal artery bypass graft with aneurysm exclusion

Superficial femoral artery

Proximal ligature

Distal ligature

Below-knee popliteal artery

Saphenous vein graft

Figure 33.1 Typical popliteal artery bypass graft with aneurysm exclusion. Typical popliteal artery aneurysm bypass graft, extending from the distal superficial femoral artery to the below-knee popliteal artery, with suture ligation proximal and distal to the aneurysm.

expose and open the sac and perform an endoaneurysmorrhaphy similar to that of abdominal aortic aneurysm repair. Thrombus is removed and all encountered bleeding geniculate branches are ligated from within the sac while excision of the sac is avoided. Although feasible through a medial approach, a posterior approach with the patient in a prone position affords optimal exposure for this procedure, particularly when the aneurysm is limited to the popliteal fossa. Harvesting of the lesser saphenous vein if of adequate size avoids the need for an additional incision when using this technique. Finally, the sequence of repair in instances of multiple aneurysms is dictated by the severity of symptoms. In the absence of limb-threatening complications from a popliteal aneurysm, the repair of a concomitant abdominal aortic aneurysm would generally take preference.

Intra-arterial thrombolytic therapy has become an important adjunct in the management of acute ischemia resulting from popliteal aneurysms. Patients presenting with thromboembolic complications may have obliteration of their popliteal artery outflow tract, with potential involvement of all three tibial vessels and the more distal microcirculation. Attempts at intraoperative thromboembolectomy may be insufficient to clear the clot burden and obtain vessel patency, severely limiting the surgical options. In such cases, preoperative or intraoperative use of thrombolytics may successfully restore a suitable runoff vessel and enhance distal outflow, thereby improving the success of subsequent bypass surgery.[14] Several reports have documented lower amputation rates and reduced occlusive complications employing a strategy of combined thrombolysis and surgery compared with surgery alone.[15] While it has recently been argued that one should proceed directly to amputation in the event of failed thrombolyis for acute thrombosis of popliteal aneurysms,[16] this is not a commonly practiced strategy.

More recently, attempts at treating popliteal aneurysms with endoluminal stent grafting have been reported.[17] Self-expanding or balloon-expandable covered stents delivered via a percutaneous or open femoral route under fluoroscopic guidance have been used to exclude the aneurysm sac. However, the results of this minimally invasive therapy have not equaled that of surgical bypass, and the approach should be considered experimental at present.

Outcome

The results of operative repair of popliteal aneurysms vary considerably depending on the preoperative status of the patient and the type of conduit employed. For asymptomatic aneurysms with good outflow, the long-term patency rate is excellent. In one recent study, 5-year primary patency rates for saphenous grafts were 92%, compared with 66% for a matched cohort with occlusive disease.[18] Ten-year patency is approximately 80% and limb salvage rates are higher still, surpassing 95% at 10 years.[11,19] Urgent surgical intervention, in contrast, is associated with a less favorable outcome. In the setting of a thrombosed aneurysm or an extremity with severely attenuated outflow, 5- and 10-year patency rates of 60% and 48% and limb salvage rates of 60% and 80%, respectively, have been reported.[11,19] Highlighting the importance of the status of the tibial runoff vessels on patency rates, Lilly et al.[20] observed 5-year patency rates of 91% for asymptomatic lesions compared with 54% for symptomatic lesions, with a direct correlation of outcome to the quality of the distal outflow.

Long-term patency rates of saphenous vein grafts are nearly four times that of non-vein alternatives. In one representative study, seven of 31 popliteal aneurysmorrhaphies using prosthetic grafts resulted in limb loss compared with only one of 42 done with saphenous vein reconstruction.[9] Results from other reported series of non-autologous reconstructions of popliteal aneurysms are equally as poor, with 5-year primary patency rates ranging from 29% to 40%.[5,13,21] Of note, saphenous vein grafts performed in patients with popliteal aneurysms have been found to uniformly dilate over time, in distinction to those performed for occlusive disease, which trend toward a normalized diameter.[18] The perioperative mortality associated with popliteal aneurysm repair is generally low; in a multicenter study conducted in the UK, a rate of <2.0% was reported, with outcome influenced by the initial presentation.[22]

Femoral aneurysms
History

Femoral artery aneurysms are the second most prevalent peripheral artery aneurysm, following those of the popliteal artery. They are relatively uncommon clinical entities, with a combined incidence of both femoral and popliteal aneurysms in the USA population of 7.39 per 100 000 hospitalized men and 1.00 per 100 000 hospitalized women.[23] True aneurysms are primarily atherosclerotic in nature and are most often located in the common femoral artery. The femoral artery is also the most common site of pseudoaneurysms, including those of mycotic and anastomotic etiology as well as those secondary to trauma and percutaneous cannulation. As with peripheral aneurysms elsewhere, there is a frequent association of femoral aneurysms with both abdominal aortic aneurysms and extremity aneurysms at other sites. In their landmark review of patients with multiple aneurysms, Dent at al.[4] found that of those with a common femoral aneurysm, 95% had a second aneurysm, 92% had an aortoiliac aneurysm and nearly 60% had bilateral femoral aneurysms. Conversely, the incidence of femoral and popliteal aneurysms in patients with abdominal aortic aneurysms has ranged from 3.1% to 14% in the literature.[4,24] Notably, in the report by Diwan and colleagues[24] on abdominal aortic aneurysm patients with lower extremity aneurysms, all patients were men and only one had a family history of aneurysmal disease. The presence of peripheral artery occlusive disease was the only detectable differentiating factor of these men when compared with those with abdominal aortic aneurysms but no additional aneurysms.[24] Other investigators have confirmed this clear predilection for men to develop lower extremity aneurysms compared with women. Graham et al.[25] reported a male:female ratio of 15:1 for femoral artery aneurysms, clearly increased from that typically seen with abdominal aortic aneurysms. Different biologic and genetic processes than those present in abdominal aortic aneurysm patients are presumably responsible for this strong gender disparity. Experiments using a mouse strain with known X-chromosome mutations and abnormal elastin function have shown these animals to have a marked tendency toward aneurysm development, but as of yet no predisposition for peripheral aneurysms over those of the aorta.[26]

The factors leading to the development of typical femoral artery aneurysms are not clearly delineated. It has been postulated that constriction at the level of the inguinal ligament leads to relative turbulence in the post-stenotic common femoral artery. Consistent with this idea is the fact that femoral artery aneurysms rarely extend proximally to involve the external iliac artery and most commonly involve the common femoral artery in a segmental fashion. Repetitive hip flexion with resultant shear stress and vessel distortion proximal to a major branch point has also been postulated as a contributing component. Others have focused on the role of inflammatory cells or a more systemic defect in the vessel architecture to explain why peripheral aneurysms are so frequently multiple. There is a high incidence of coexistent cardiovascular disease in patients with femoral aneurysms, particularly hypertension and coronary artery disease, as well as a history of cigarette smoking. Interestingly, some authors have noted a particularly low incidence of lower extremity aneurysms in patients with diabetes mellitus,[27] perhaps due to the counterbalancing effect of vessel wall calcification seen with this disease.

Recognizing the more technically challenging nature when the deep arterial system is involved, femoral aneurysms have been classified as either Type I, limited to the common femoral artery, or Type II, extending to the profunda femoral artery. In their initial series describing 55 common femoral aneurysms, Cutler and Darling[27] found a distribution of 44% Type I and 56% Type II aneurysms. Isolated profunda artery aneurysms are uncommon, comprising only 2% of all femoral aneurysms. Similarly, aneurysms limited to the superficial femoral artery are unusual, with most being mycotic or traumatic in etiology. Aneurysms in this location tend to present at a later mean age compared with other femoral and popliteal aneurysms and are more typically seen in patients with generalized degenerative enlargement of the entire superficial femoral artery, a situation known as arteriomegaly.[28]

Signs and symptoms

Asymptomatic femoral artery aneurysms, representing 30–40% of cases in reported series, are often incidentally noted during routine physical examination. Palpation of a smooth, pulsatile, fusiform and non-tender groin mass is sufficiently diagnostic in the majority of cases. Local pain, swelling, and tenderness are typical features when femoral artery aneurysms become symptomatic. Pain as the sole symptom of the aneurysm is present in 20% of cases[25] and is characterized by mild and focal groin or anterior thigh pain secondary to chronic compression of the femoral nerve. Compression of the femoral vein by a slowly expanding aneurysm can lead to lower extremity edema, phlebitis, and venous stasis changes.

Complications of femoral artery aneurysms include embolization, thrombosis, and rupture. In one series of 45 patients with 63 aneurysms, nearly one-half (47%) of patients had suffered a major complication by the time of first presentation.[27] Thirty-two percent of these were thromboses, while another 10% were ruptures. The incidence of embolic complications in patients with femoral aneurysms is typically reported to be between 5% and 10%.[25,27,29] Acute thrombosis can result in a critically threatened limb with sensorimotor deficits or frank gangrene, particularly if the deep arterial system is involved. Patients with subacute or chronic thrombosis and who have had intervening collateral recruitment, on the other hand, more typically present with ischemic rest pain or claudication. Investigation has failed to correlate thrombosis of femoral artery aneurysms with prolonged postural changes, exercise, or other identifiable precipitants.

Emboli from femoral artery aneurysms can be either clinically silent or, in the absence of significant occlusive disease, manifest by foot or calf pain or distal cutaneous stigmata. If the embolic shower is mild, it may be limited to petechial hemorrhage evident on the distal aspect of the toes or a transient skin pattern of livedo reticularis. More severe or recurrent episodes of embolism can result in greater degrees of ischemia, ranging from end-digit gangrene seen with 'blue toe syndrome' to limb-threatening ischemia necessitating emergency surgery. As the fibrous femoral sheath serves to confine the femoral artery, rupture of femoral aneurysms is a relatively rare event, and exsanguination following rupture even more so. When rupture does occur, however, it is heralded by groin ecchymosis and local pain, and pressure effects of the vessels within the space-limited sheath may lead to severe distal ischemia. All told, 40% of patients with femoral artery aneurysms have some manifestation of either acute or chronic ischemia. Of note, it can at times be difficult to determine to what degree concomitant arterial occlusive disease or an associated popliteal or aortic aneurysm is responsible for the symptoms present.

Diagnosis

In instances in which the diagnosis is not made by physical examination, ultrasonography is a reliable means of documenting both the presence and size of femoral artery aneurysms. It also serves to reliably screen for associated popliteal or aortoiliac aneurysms and, combined with duplex scanning, can provide useful information on sac morphology. Computed tomography and magnetic resonance imaging are additional highly accurate diagnostic modalities available that can help define the status of the proximal and distal vasculature. Once the diagnosis is secure, however, angiography remains the imaging technique of choice. It can most accurately delineate the extent of thromboembolic disease and optimize preoperative planning by detailing the patency of the inflow as well as the lower extremity outflow tract. If prolonged ischemia time renders formal preoperative arteriography inadvisable, an intraoperative angiogram is indicated.

Management

There is little disagreement that patients presenting with a symptomatic femoral artery aneurysm should undergo operative repair. Certainly, any aneurysm presenting with ischemic complications of rest pain or tissue loss is best served by operative treatment. Claudication resulting from thromboembolic sequelae of a femoral aneurysm and not from associated occlusive disease also warrants intervention, given the risk of recurrent events and progression of ischemia. Similarly, those presenting with pain from local expansion or evidence of venous compromise should be offered surgery if they are otherwise medically appropriate. Finally, aneurysms that serial monitoring suggests are enlarging should undergo prophylactic surgical treatment.

As with peripheral aneurysms elsewhere, to what extent an aggressive management strategy should be employed for asymptomatic femoral aneurysms remains an area of active controversy. Some conservative authors argue that the risk of thromboembolic complications is reduced compared with that of popliteal aneurysms. Further, they note that little evidence exists correlating the size of a femoral artery aneurysm to the rate of ischemic complications. Others, conversely, cite the potential for dire outcomes in patients who have been followed nonoperatively and the unacceptably high rate of limb loss in these patients to support a more aggressive operative policy. The literature in general would support the latter position. In one study of 12 patients with femoral aneurysms followed conservatively over a 10-year period, five (43%) thrombosed and all required amputation.[30] Similarly, in a series of 44 patients from the Mayo Clinic treated non-operatively, there was a 16% rate of amputation secondary to complications of the femoral aneurysm.[31] In practice, most surgeons consider any femoral aneurysm reaching a size of 2.5–3.0cm appropriate for repair. Further, small asymptomatic aneurysms in the presence of a popliteal aneurysm or distal occlusive disease warranting repair should also be simultaneously addressed.

The most common surgical treatment of femoral aneurysms is that of aneurysmorrhaphy with short interposition graft placement. Other than rare cases where resection of the aneurysm is

indicated (e.g. with mycotic aneurysms), the sac is usually opened and debrided of its thrombus but left *in situ*. Following reconstruction, the sac walls can then be closed over the interposition graft. The specific configuration of the replacement graft is determined by the anatomic extent of the aneurysm. The proximal anastomosis is typically at the level of the distal external iliac artery or proximal common femoral artery. Occasionally it will be necessary to obtain proximal control of the iliac artery via a retroperitoneal flank incision. Extension of the aneurysm into both the profunda and superficial arteries requires either reimplantation of the more distal, non-aneurysmal profunda into a common-to-superficial femoral artery interposition graft or utilization of a sidearm graft to the profunda (**Fig. 33.2**). Alternatively, the interposition graft can be sewn directly into a reconstructed bifurcation fashioned by suturing a new common wall between the profunda and superficial femoral artery orifices, a technique known as 'syndactilization'.

If the entire superficial femoral artery is arteriomegalic or frankly aneurysmal, or in the event of a concomitant popliteal artery aneurysm or significant femoral artery occlusive disease, the distal anastomosis will of necessity be at the level of the popliteal or tibial vessels. In these cases, it is often advisable to fashion a separate common femoral artery interposition graft from which the proximal anastomosis of the planned outflow graft can be based. The choice of conduit for femoral artery aneurysm reconstructions is one of surgeon preference. For reconstructions limited to the common femoral artery, size considerations may confer some benefit to synthetic grafts. For more distal artery involvement, however, both synthetic and saphenous vein grafts have been used with equal efficacy.

Outcome

In general, the results of operative repair of femoral artery aneurysms are excellent. There is minimal perioperative mortality in published series and the long-term patency rates in asymptomatic patients have been in the 80–95% range.[25,27] When preoperative claudication, rest pain, or gangrene was present, however, the clinical outcome was satisfactory in only 70% of cases at a mean follow-up of 2 years.[25]

Profunda femoral artery aneurysms

As mentioned above, isolated profunda artery aneurysms are rare, and usually arise secondary to penetrating trauma or iatrogenic groin cannulation. Based largely on isolated case reports, they have a reputation for relatively rapid enlargement and rupture compared with other femoral and popliteal aneurysms. It is unclear whether this reputation is deserved given the possibility that many profunda aneurysms may go undetected. Although in one review of 20 patients 50% of isolated profunda femoral artery aneurysms were treated with ligation and resection alone with reported success, the long-term outcome of these patients was poorly documented.[32] In general, resection or ligation with reconstruction is the recommended treatment strategy for aneurysms in this location.

Infrapopliteal aneurysms

Aneurysms of the tibial and pedal arteries are also uncommon. Although a percentage are degenerative in etiology, most are pseudoaneurysms that arise following trauma or infection or as a delayed complication of balloon catheter embolectomy.[33–35]

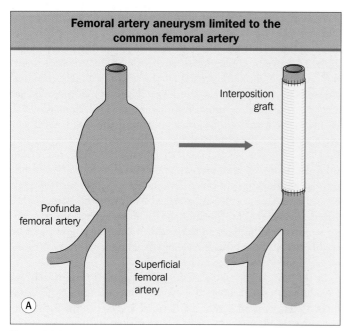

Femoral artery aneurysm limited to the common femoral artery

Interposition graft

Profunda femoral artery

Superficial femoral artery

A

Figure 33.2 Femoral artery aneursym. (A) Femoral artery aneurysm limited to the common femoral artery. Typical operative reconstruction with end-to-end interposition graft. (B) Femoral artery aneurysm with extension to superficial and profunda femoral arteries. Reconstructive options include interposition grafting to the superficial femoral artery with reimplantation of non-aneurysmal profunda or utilization of a sidearm graft to the profunda.

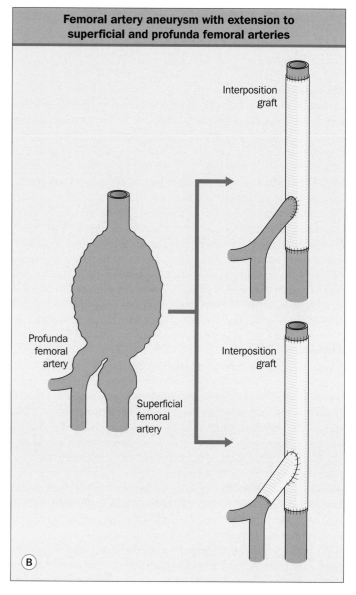

Femoral artery aneurysm with extension to superficial and profunda femoral arteries

Interposition graft

Profunda femoral artery

Interposition graft

Superficial femoral artery

B

Isolated case reviews of tibial artery aneurysms in association with polyarteritis nodosa have also been reported.[36] These aneurysms are often asymptomatic and are discovered during routine arteriography undertaken for other reasons. Alternatively, they may present as a painful mass or with digital or calf ischemia secondary to thromboembolism. Small, asymptomatic aneurysms may be safely observed, while symptomatic lesions should be surgically addressed. If the remaining vessels are healthy, ligation of the aneurysm is acceptable. In the presence of diabetes or concomitant atherosclerosis in the remaining infrageniculate vessels, ligation or excision with saphenous vein bypass is the recommended treatment.

Femoral pseudoaneurysms

Femoral pseudoaneurysms, encompassing those of iatrogenic, anastomotic, traumatic, and mycotic origin, are the most frequently encountered subset of femoral artery aneurysms. Their increasing incidence is largely due to the expanding use of catheter-based interventions in the treatment of cardiovascular

disease; pseudoaneurysms are reported to occur in 0.2% of all femoral arterial access procedures.[37] Longer procedure time, larger-bore catheters, thrombolytic or antiocoagulation therapy, and use of multiple catheters are risk factors for pseudoaneurysm development.[38] Drug abuse and more frequent use of arterial closure devices following needle cannulation are in turn responsible for an increasing incidence of infected femoral false aneurysms. Femoral suture line pseudoaneurysms occur in 3% of all femoral anastomoses and 6–8% of aortofemoral anastomoses,[39] presenting an average of 6 years following graft placement. They have been found to be six times more likely to occur with prosthetic grafts than with vein grafts.[40]

Often detected as a pulsatile groin mass following percutaneous intervention, femoral pseudoaneurysms may be asymptomatic or associated with neuropathic pain secondary to femoral nerve compression from rapid expansion. Mycotic aneurysms typically appear as a tender, erythematous groin swelling, with or without associated purulent or sanguinous discharge. Ultrasonography is the preferred diagnostic modality, although computed tomography is helpful to determine the presence or extent of infection in the case of anastomotic and mycotic pseudoaneurysms. For uncomplicated traumatic pseudoaneurysms, surgical repair is the traditional therapy; local or regional anesthesia is appropriate if co-morbid disease renders general anesthesia inadvisable. Of note, ultrasound-guided thrombin ablation is increasingly being employed as an easier, less invasive, and more cost-effective treatment option for routine iatrogenic pseudoaneurysms.[41] Operative treatment of the technically more challenging mycotic and suture-line pseudoaneurysms usually entails reconstruction with an interposition vein or prosthetic graft, respectively. Proximal and distal control may be simplified by using balloon catheters, but ensuring patency of the relevant outflow vessels is imperative.

UPPER EXTREMITY ANEURYSMS

History
Aneurysms of the upper extremity are relatively uncommon. In their review of nearly 1500 patients documenting the incidence of multiple aneurysms, Dent et al.[4] observed a 3.5% incidence of peripheral aneurysms but only two cases of subclavian artery aneurysm and one case of brachial artery aneurysm. Reviewing the reported world literature, Hobson et al.[42] discovered only 195 cases of subclavian and axillary aneurysms, representing approximately 1% of all peripheral aneurysms. Eighty-eight percent of these were located in the subclavian artery. Subclavian artery aneurysms can be divided into atherosclerotic-related aneurysms of the proximal vessel, subclavian–axillary artery aneurysms typically associated with post-stenotic enlargement from thoracic outlet syndrome and those associated with aberrant anatomy. The first report of a subclavian aneurysm in proximity to a first rib exostosis and resultant thoracic outlet syndrome was by Mayo in 1813, and Coote first performed a cervical rib resection to decompress the subclavian artery as early as 1861. Based on experimental dog models, Halsted in 1916 first postulated a connection between post-stenotic dilatation and the development of aneurysms. Proximal upper extremity aneurysms can have a variety of clinical sequelae, ranging from exsanguinating rupture to compressive neuropathy to thromboembolism-induced ischemia. While antegrade clot propagation with distal ischemia is far more common, the risk of cerebral ischemia from retrograde propagation has been recognized since Symonds' initial description in 1927. Aneurysms located more distally in the upper extremity are primarily complicated by thromboembolism. As with lower extremity aneurysms, intervention prior to the development of limb-threatening complications is generally recommended given the potential long-term morbidity associated with symptom development.

Proximal subclavian artery aneurysms
Aneurysms of the proximal subclavian artery represent less than 25% of all subclavian aneurysms. While cystic medial necrosis, trauma, infection from syphilis or tuberculosis, and congenital factors are all well-documented causes, the majority of aneurysms in this location are atherosclerotic in origin. They typically occur in patients over 60 years of age and are slightly more common in men. Diagnostic and management features are included in the discussion below on subclavian–axillary aneurysms.

Subclavian–axillary artery aneurysms
Aneurysms of the distal subclavian artery often extend into the axillary artery and are typically classified as subclavian–axillary artery aneurysms. They are the most common subset of subclavian artery aneurysms, representing 75% of all cases. They usually occur in younger patients; in one series of 31 patients from the Mayo Clinic, the mean age was 47.[43] Other institutional reviews of aneurysms in this location consistently demonstrate a slight female predominance and a slight predilection for the right side. The former phenomenon may be because cervical ribs are more frequently found in women, while the latter finding may be explained by a higher incidence of right-handedness and resultant increased right-sided thoracic outlet muscle use, with subsequent impingement of the adjacent vessel. Between 33% and 45% of patients with subclavian–axillary aneurysms will have a second aneurysm, usually in the abdominal aorta.[43,44]

Subclavian–axillary artery aneurysms are nearly always secondary to long-standing compression of the vessel against a congenital bony abnormality. Cervical ribs – present in 0.6% of the population, and bilateral up to 80% of the time – are the predominant anatomic element responsible for compression (**Fig. 33.3**). Abnormal first ribs, congenital bands, and malalignment following clavicular fracture are less common causes of arterial thoracic outlet syndrome. Vascular complications of thoracic outlet

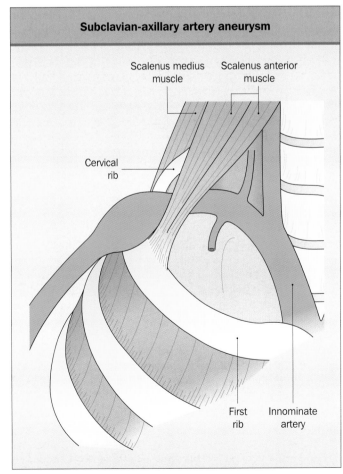

Figure 33.3 Subclavian–axillary artery aneurysm. Compression of the subclavian artery from an abnormal cervical rib can lead to formation of a subclavian–axillary artery aneurysm.

syndrome are infrequent and are estimated to occur in less than 5% of cases. Of note, in a large review by Halsted[45] of 716 patients with cervical ribs, only 4% had associated subclavian–axillary artery aneurysms. Complete cervical ribs articulate with a tubercle on the superior aspect of the first rib, behind the distal insertion point of the anterior scalene muscle. Long-standing compression where the artery crosses the first rib results in a localized stenosis as well as angulation of the distal subclavian artery. Repeated mechanical trauma with shoulder movement leads to inflammation and fibrotic scarring of the vessel wall. Ultimately, post-stenotic turbulence develops as a consequence of both the angulation and the intrinsic luminal narrowing, and the resultant alterations in wall shear stress give rise to post-stenotic dilation and aneurysm formation. Rarely, localized jet flow from very tight lesions can produce saccular aneurysms.

Signs and symptoms

It is sometimes possible to diagnose subclavian–axillary aneurysms prior to symptom development by detection of a pulsatile palpable mass in the supraclavicular fossa or axilla. In the absence of complete thrombosis, an associated loud bruit and thrill are usually present. Isolated neurologic symptoms stemming from compression of the brachial plexus by a cervical rib or other bony abnormality may also prompt a radiographic workup revealing an asymptomatic concomitant aneurysm. Most often, however, the presence of a subclavian–axillary aneurysm, as with peripheral aneurysms elsewhere, is heralded by thromboembolic complications. Up to 90% of patients in reported series are symptomatic at the time of presentation.[42] Digital ischemia from embolization of laminated thrombus from either the atheroma-rich stenotic segment or the aneurysm, reported to occur in 70% of symptomatic cases,[42] is the most frequently seen symptom. It typically manifests as small, punctate, cyanotic lesions focused in the fingers and palm. Trafficking of emboli down the relatively more straightforward course of the radial artery results in a preponderance of thumb and index finger involvement. Platelet aggregates at the site of an intimal disruption or at the point of impact of a post-stenotic jet are believed to be another source of microemboli contributing to Raynaud's syndrome, which is not uncommonly seen in subclavian-axillary aneurysms. Episodic pallor and cyanosis, pain, and marked cold sensitivity are hallmarks of this component of the disease, the arterial ischemic implications of which are important to realize. More severe degrees of ischemia may result from repeated embolic events and progressive obliteration of the distal arterial bed. This may lead to loss of distal radial and ulnar pulses and the development of upper extremity claudication, digital ulceration, or limb-threatening tissue loss, the latter of which is seen in 10% of cases.[42]

An enlarging subclavian–axillary aneurysm may stretch the fibers of the brachial plexus or adjoining soft tissues, producing persistent shoulder pain or distal neurologic sequelae. The reported incidence of pain is between 20% and 40%,[42,43] while brachial plexus palsy is seen 10% of the time. If the recurrent laryngeal nerve is stretched by a right-sided aneurysm, hoarseness may result. Thrombosis of a subclavian–axillary aneurysm is relatively rare and often without serious symptomatic consequence in the presence of good collateral flow. Rupture of subclavian–axillary aneurysms is also an uncommon occurrence, but can result in fatal exsanguination.

Diagnosis

Occasionally, plain film radiography has been used to identify proximal subclavian aneurysms, seen as an upper mediastinal or apical mass. If the diagnosis of a subclavian–axillary aneurysm is suspected based on the history and physical examination, ultrasonography has been used to confirm the presence of arterial compression and post-stenotic dilatation, as well as to detail the presence of mural thrombus, thrombosis, or collateral development. Computed tomography has also served to diagnose bony abnormalities and associated aneurysmal change in this region. For both diagnosis and preoperative planning, however, the imaging modality of choice for subclavian-level aneurysms remains arteriography. It is usually performed through a femoral approach, and at times requires additional maneuvers such as dynamic imaging to fully demonstrate subtle degrees of stenosis or a thrombus-lined aneurysm in the presence of thoracic outlet syndrome. Vasodilator administration is often necessary to elucidate the full extent of collateral flow as well as digital artery embolic disease, especially in the presence of Raynaud's syndrome.

Management

In general, the presence of a subclavian aneurysm is sufficient indication to proceed to operative repair. In the setting of either acute or chronic ischemia of the upper extremity stemming from thromboembolic sequelae of the aneurysm, there is little disagreement that surgery is warranted. Although several approaches have been described, including transaxillary and transclavicular, the supraclavicular approach is optimal in most cases. When thoracic outlet syndrome is present, this incision allows full decompression of the arterial channel through resection of the involved cervical and/or first rib, anterior scalenectomy, and lysis of any constricting fibrous bands. Most authors feel that concomitant clavicular resection is unnecessary and can lead to disabling shoulder instability. If the aneurysm is localized to the proximal subclavian artery, a median sternotomy for right-sided lesions or a left thoracotomy for left-sided lesions affords optimal exposure. Occasionally, additional access to the axillary artery will be necessary through a separate transaxillary or deltopectoral incision.

After mobilization and resection of the subclavian–axillary aneurysm, a primary reconstruction of the artery is carried out if possible. If an interposition graft is necessary, which is often the case, both autogenous saphenous vein and synthetic (Dacron or polytetrafluoroethylene) grafts have been successfully used. Generally, a prosthetic graft is preferred for subclavian artery reconstruction, while autogenous conduit is thought more appropriate for replacement of the smaller axillary artery.

A different, more limited, approach to the treatment of aneurysms of this location, favored by some surgeons, is that of distal ligation with axilloaxillary bypass. This option is particularly well suited for high-risk patients or those with technically challenging proximal subclavian aneurysms. If the aneurysm is large or adherent, the sac may alternatively be opened and left in place and the aneurysm repaired via an inclusion technique. Proximal and distal ligation alone without reconstruction has also been described, but in one report resulted in claudication in 25% of cases.[43]

The optimal management of small, asymptomatic aneurysms with mild post-stenotic dilatation but without clinical or radiographic evidence of mural thrombus remains debatable.[43,46]

Blank and Connar[47] have suggested that thoracic outlet decompression alone may suffice and result in return of the artery to a normal caliber. Others favor operative repair given that the risk of subsequent aneurysm enlargement or serious embolic complications with conservative management is not insignificant and that few cases of actual regression have been documented.[46,48] Still others believe that at the very least, such situations merit exploration of the vessel to rule out subtle intimal disease or mural thrombus, reserving the possibility of resection and reconstruction if appropriate.

If a subclavian–axillary aneurysm is complicated by occlusive embolic disease with significant ischemia, intraoperative thromboembolectomy should be performed as an initial step. This will usually entail separate access at the level of the brachial artery bifurcation or wrist. Preoperative thrombolysis, although less well supported in the literature, is another, often effective way to optimize brachial and forearm outflow. If clearance of subacute or chronic thrombus proves impossible, an upper extremity bypass procedure will often be required at the same time as definitive treatment of the aneurysm. Autogenous vein, preferably the distal saphenous vein, is the conduit of choice,[49] and in such cases the aneurysm can be simply resected or ligated. Given the documented risk of retrograde embolization, proximal as well as distal ligation should be performed. Analogous to the situation in the lower extremity, when the proximal superficial outflow is compromised, revascularizing the deep brachial artery will often suffice to adequately perfuse the hand provided collateral flow through the elbow joint is intact. If bypass is necessary to the level of the forearm vessels and the radial or ulnar arteries are unsuitable, the interosseus artery is often an acceptable outflow target. When restoration of adequate flow to the distal extremity is not possible, especially in the setting of vasospasm or distal tissue loss, a cervicodorsal sympathectomy may be indicated. In general, however, the once prominent role of this modality has diminished as the efficacy of more definitive revascularization has become clear.

Outcome

Although few modern series are available, the published results of operative treatment of subclavian aneurysms are favorable, particularly in the absence of distal extremity occlusion. In one study of 18 patients undergoing aneurysm resection and reconstruction without distal extremity bypass, graft or arterial patency was 100% at an average 9-year follow-up.[43] There was no operative mortality and no evidence of recurrent aneurysmal development amongst those repaired primarily. In another review of 33 bypass grafts for upper extremity ischemia, of which only six were for complications of thoracic outlet syndrome, patency of the entire cohort was 73% at 2 years and 67% at 3 years. Of somewhat limited value given the mixed nature of the study population, 2-year patency was 83% for grafts at or above the brachial artery and only 53% for grafts distal to the brachial bifurcation.[49] Limb loss is rare in the reported literature and usually follows multiple unsuccessful attempts to revascularize the upper extremity in the face of an obliterated outflow tract. A single forearm amputation was required in the 31 patients reported by Pairolero et al.[43]

Aberrant subclavian artery aneurysms

An aberrant subclavian artery arising from the proximal descending thoracic aorta is the most frequently encountered

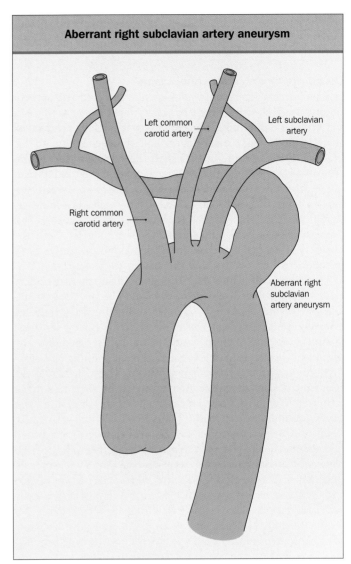

Aberrant right subclavian artery aneurysm

Left common carotid artery

Left subclavian artery

Right common carotid artery

Aberrant right subclavian artery aneurysm

Figure 33.4 Aberrant right subclavian artery aneurysm. An aberrant right subclavian artery typically arises from the proximal descending thoraric aorta. When it is aneurysmal, it is known as a Kommerell's diverticulum.

anomaly of the aortic arch, present in 0.5% of normal adults. It is rarely associated with aneurysmal change at the vessel origin, a phenomenom referred to as Kommerell's diverticulum since the original description in 1936 (**Fig. 33.4**). Although predominantly asymptomatic and detected on routine chest radiography as an incidental mediastinal mass, such aneurysms are a well-recognized cause of esophageal compression, a condition known as dysphagia lusoria. Other presenting symptoms include dyspnea or coughing from tracheal compression, chest pain from aneurysmal expansion, and right upper extremity ischemia from thromboembolic complications. Given the risk of potentially fatal rupture or associated complications, surgical repair is recommended. Several techniques have been described, including resection of the aneurysm via either a right or left thoracotomy or median sternotomy and reconstruction of the subclavian artery from either the ascending aortic arch or via an end-to-side anastomosis off the right common carotid artery. A separate supraclavicular incision becomes necessary for this latter step when a left thoracotomy approach is utilized. Highlighting the increased technical challenge these cases represent, Kieffer et al.[50] reported a 30% operative mortality in the largest series to date of patients with Kommerell's diverticulum.

Distal upper extremity aneurysms

Isolated axillary artery aneurysms are rare and predominantly of traumatic origin. Crutch-induced aneurysmal dilation of the axillary artery is a well-recognized entity, and is typically heralded by acute ischemia from aneurysm thrombosis or embolism to the brachial artery or more distal vessels. Pseudoaneurysms in this area usually follow penetrating trauma or are distant sequelae of humeral fractures or shoulder dislocations. Undetected aneurysm-related hemorrhage into the axillary sheath can lead to compression of the brachial plexus and significant neurologic impairment. Surgical excision with vein interposition grafting has been the mainstay of treatment of these aneurysms, although more recently endolumenal stent grafts have been successfully employed.[51]

The hypothenar hammer syndrome, or dilatation of the ulnar artery following repeated use of the hand in a pushing, pounding, or twisting motion, is another well-described syndrome affecting the upper extremity. Typically occurring in male laborers, repetitive damage leads to medial degeneration and aneurysm formation. Subsequent thrombosis and/or embolism produces varying degrees of digital ischemia. The pathophysiology results from the unique anatomic course of the distal ulnar artery, in that the aneurysmal changes invariably arise at a point beyond where the artery leaves the protection of the volar carpal ligament, known as Guyon's canal, and lies relatively unprotected just anterior to the hook of the hamate bone (**Fig. 33.5**). It is a frequently overlooked cause of secondary Raynaud's phenomenon, differing slightly in that the thumb is characteristically spared and the classic triphasic color changes are usually absent. Resection with microsurgical reconstruction offers the best chance for optimal digital perfusion, and removes the often painful source of ulnar nerve compression.[52] Cervicodorsal sympathectomy and thrombolytic therapy are adjunctive maneuvers that have been used in select cases to further improve outcome.[53,54]

Isolated aneurysms of the brachial, radial, and more proximal ulnar artery, as well as aneurysms of the palmar arch, are rare and often the focus of individual case reports. Most stem from recre-

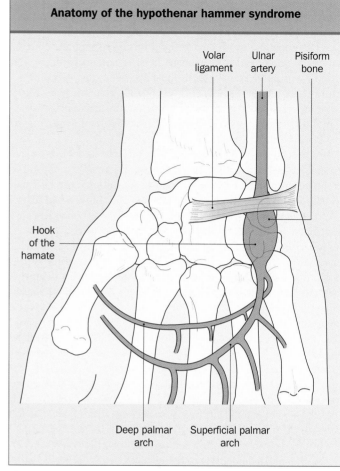

Anatomy of the hypothenar hammer syndrome

Figure 33.5 Anatomy of the hypothenar hammer syndrome. Distal to the volar ligament, the ulnar artery lies relatively unprotected and vulnerable to trauma in a position anterior to the hook of the hamate.

ational or occupational trauma, although some are of mycotic origin. Unless small and asymptomatic, they are usually best treated with resection followed by revascularization with vein conduit.[53,55]

REFERENCES

1. Hardy JD, Tompkins WC, Hatten LE, et al. Aneurysms of the popliteal artery. Surg Gynecol Obstet 1975;140:401–4.
2. Ramesh S, Michaels JA, Galland RB. Popliteal aneurysm: morphology and management. Br J Surg 1993;80:1531–3.
3. Szilagyi DE, Schwartz RL, Reddy DJ. Popliteal arterial aneurysms. Their natural history and management. Arch Surg 1981;116:724–8.
4. Dent TL, Lindenauer MS, Ernst CB, et al. Multiple arteriosclerotic arterial aneurysms. Arch Surg 1972;105:338–44.
5. Vermilion BD, Kimmins SA, Pace WG, et al. A review of one hundred forty-seven popliteal aneurysms with long-term follow-up. Surgery 1981; 90:1009–14.
6. Reilly MK, Abbott WM, Darling RC. Aggressive surgical management of popliteal artery aneurysms. Am J Surg 1983;145:498–502.
7. Bouhoutsos J, Martin P. Popliteal aneurysm: a review of 116 cases. Br J Surg 1974;61:469–75.
8. Reed MK, Smith BM. Popliteal aneurysm with spontaneous arteriovenous fistula. J Cardiovasc Surg 1991;32:482–4.
9. Lowell RC, Gloviczki P, Hallett JW, et al. Popliteal artery aneurysms: the risk of nonoperative management. Ann Vasc Surg 1994;8:14–23.
10. Dawson I, Sie RB, Van Bockel JH. Atherosclerotic popliteal aneurysm. Br J Surg1997;84:293–9.
11. Roggo A, Brunner U, Ottinger LW, et al. The continuing challenge of aneurysms of the popliteal artery. Surg Gynecol Obstet 1993;177:565–72.
12. Michaels JA, Galland RB. Management of asymptomatic popliteal aneurysms: the use of a Markov decision tree to determine the criteria for a conservative approach. Eur J Vasc Surg 1993;7:136–43.
13. Dawson I, Van Bockel JH, Brand R, et al. Popliteal artery aneurysms: long-term follow-up of aneurysmal disease and results of surgical treatment. J Vasc Surg 1991;13:398–407.
14. Wyffels PL, DeBord JR, Marshall JS, et al. Increased limb salvage with intraoperative and postoperative ankle level urokinase infusion in acute lower extremity ischemia. J Vasc Surg 1992;15:771–9.
15. Hoelting T, Paetz B, Richter GM, et al. The value of preoperative lytic therapy in limb-threatening acute ischemia from popliteal artery aneurysm. Am J Surg 1994;168:227–31.
16. Marty B, Wicky S, Ris HB, et al. Success of thrombolysis as a predictor of outcome in acute thrombosis of popliteal aneurysms. J Vasc Surg 2002;35:487–93.

17. Henry M, Amor M, Henry I, et al. Percutaneous endoluminal treatment of peripheral aneurysms: a single center experience with a series of 35 aneurysms. J Vasc Interv Radiol 1998;9(Suppl 1):183–4.
18. Upchurch GR, Gerhard-Herman MD, Sebastian MW, et al. Improved graft patency and altered remodeling in infrainguinal vein graft reconstruction for aneurysmal versus occlusive disease. J Vasc Surg 1999;29:1022–30.
19. Anton GE, Hertzer NR, Beven EG, et al. Surgical management of popliteal aneurysms: trends in presentation, treatment, and results from 1952 to 1984. J Vasc Surg 1986;3:125–34.
20. Lilly MP, Flinn WR, McCarthy WJ, et al. The effect of distal arterial anatomy on the success of popliteal aneurysm repair. J Vasc Surg 1988;7:653–60.
21. Hagino RT, Fujitani RM, Dawson DL, et al. Does infrapopliteal arterial runoff predict success for popliteal artery aneurysmorrhaphy? Am J Surg 1994;168:652–8.
22. Varga ZA, Locke-Edmunds JC, Baird RN. A multicenter study of popliteal aneurysms. J Vasc Surg 1994;20:171–7.
23. Lawrence PF, Lorenzo-Rivero S, Lyon JL. The incidence of iliac, femoral, and popliteal artery aneurysms in hospitalized patients. J Vasc Surg 1995;22:409–16.
24. Diwan A, Sarkar R, Stanley JC, et al. Incidence of femoral and popliteal artery aneurysms in patients with abdominal aortic aneurysms. J Vasc Surg 2000;31:863–9.
25. Graham LM, Zelenock GB, Whitehouse WM, et al. Clinical significance of arteriosclerotic femoral artery aneurysms. Arch Surg 1980;115:502–7.
26. Brophy CM, Tilson JE, Braverman IM, et al. Age of onset, pattern of distribution, and histology of aneurysm development in a genetically predisposed mouse model. J Vasc Surg 1988;8:45–8.
27. Cutler BS, Darling RC. Surgical management of arteriosclerotic femoral aneurysms. Surgery 1977;74:764–73.
28. Rigdon EE, Monajjem N. Aneurysms of the superficial femoral artery: a report of two cases and review of the literature. J Vasc Surg 1992;16:790–3.
29. Baird RJ, Gurry JF, Kellam J, et al. Arteriosclerotic femoral artery aneurysms. Can Med Assoc J 1977;117:1306–7.
30. Tolstedt GE, Radhe HM, Bell JW. Late sequelae of arteriosclerotic femoral aneurysms. Angiology 1961;12:601–2.
31. Pappas G, Janes JM, Bernatz PE, et al. Femoral aneurysms. JAMA 1964;190:489–93.
32. Tait WF, Vohra RK, Carr HMH, et al. True profunda femoris aneurysms: are they more dangerous than other atherosclerotic aneurysms of the femoropopliteal segment? Ann Vasc Surg 1991;5:92–5.
33. Cronenwett JL, Walsh DB, Garret HE. Tibial artery pseudoaneurysms: delayed complication of balloon catheter embolectomy. J Vasc Surg 1988;8:483–8.
34. Monig SP, Walter M, Sorgatz S, et al. True infrapopliteal artery aneurysms: report of two cases and literature review. J Vasc Surg 1996;24:276–8.
35. McKee TI, Fisher JB. Dorsalis pedis artery aneurysm: case report and literature review. J Vasc Surg 2000;31:589–91.
36. Borozan PG, Walker HSJ, Peterson GJ. True tibial artery aneurysms: case report and literature review. J Vasc Surg 1989;10:457–9.
37. Messina LM, Brothers TE, Wakefield TW, et al. Clinical characteristics and surgical management of vascular complications in patients undergoing cardiac catheterization: interventional versus diagnostic procedures. J Vasc Surg 1991;13:593–600.
38. Skillman JJ, Ducksoo K, Baim DS. Vascular complications of percutaneous femoral cardiac interventions: incidence and operative repair. Arch Surg 1988;123:1207–12.
39. Biancari F, Ylonen K, Anttila V, et al. Durability of open repair of infrarenal abdominal aortic aneurysm: a 15-year follow-up study. J Vasc Surg 2002;35:87–93.
40. Szilagyi DE, Smith RF, Elliott JP, et al. Anastomotic aneurysms after vascular reconstruction: problems of incidence, etiology, and treatment. Surgery 1975;78:800–16.
41. Kang SS, Labropoulos N, Mansour A, et al. Expanded indications for ultrasound-guided thrombin injection of pseudoaneurysms. J Vasc Surg 2000;31:289–98.
42. Hobson RW II, Israel MR, Lynch TG. Axillosubclavian arterial aneurysms. In: Bergan JJ, Yao JST, eds. Aneurysms: diagnosis and treatment. New York:Grune & Stratton; 1982:435–47.
43. Pairolero PC, Walls JT, Payne S, et al. Subclavian-axillary artery aneurysms. Surgery 1981;90:757–63.
44. McCollum CH, Da Gama AD, Noon GP, et al. Aneurysm of the subclavian artery. J Cardiovasc Surg 1979;20:159–64.
45. Halsted WS. An experimental study of circumscribed dilation of an artery immediately distal to a partially occluding band, and its bearing on the dilation of the subclavian artery observed in certain cases of cervical rib. J Exp Med 1916;24:271.
46. Scher LA, Veith FJ, Samson RH, et al. Vascular complications of thoracic outlet syndrome. J Vasc Surg 1986;3:565–8.
47. Blank RH, Connar RG. Arterial complications associated with thoracic outlet syndrome. Ann Thor Surg 1974;17:315–24.
48. Banis JC, Rich N, Whelan TJ Jr. Ischemia of the upper extremity due to noncardiac emboli. Am J Surg 1977;134:131–9.
49. McCarthy WJ, Flinn WR, Yao JST, et al. Result of bypass grafting for upper limb ischemia. J Vasc Surg 1986;3:741–6.
50. Kieffer E, Bahnini A, Koskas F. Aberrant subclavian artery: surgical treatment in thirty-three adult patients. J Vasc Surg 1994;19:100–11.
51. Sullivan TM, Bacharach JM, Perl J, et al. Endovascular management of unusual aneurysms of the axillary and subclavian arteries. J Endovasc Surg 1996;3:389–95.
52. Kalisman M, Laborde K, Wolff TW. Ulnar nerve compression secondary to ulnar artery false aneurysm at the Guyon's canal. J Hand Surg 1982;7:137–9.
53. Clark ET, Mass DP, Bassiouny HS, et al. True aneurysmal disease in the hand and upper extremity. Ann Vasc Surg 1991;5:276–81.
54. Lawhorne TW Jr, Sanders RA. Ulnar artery aneurysm complicated by distal embolization: management with regional thrombolysis and resection. J Vasc Surg 1986;3:663–5.
55. Nehler MR, Dalman RL, Harris EJ, et al. Upper extremity arterial bypass distal to the wrist. J Vasc Surg 1992;16:633–42.

CHAPTER
34

Aortic Arch Branch Disease

Jeffrey M Rhodes and Kenneth J Cherry Jr

KEY POINTS

- Aortic arch branch disease is defined as disease of the innominate, subclavian, or common carotid arteries resulting in flow-limiting stenosis or embolization to the brain and/or upper extremities.

- Etiology of these lesions is most frequently atherosclerotic. However, large vessel arteritis must also be considered in the differential diagnosis.

- Short-segment extra-anatomic reconstructions (subclavian-to-carotid grafting) are safe and durable reconstructions for isolated proximal lesions.

- Direct trans-sternal reconstructions are necessary when multiple vessels are involved, and are superior to extra-anatomic bypasses in this situation.

- Endovascular reconstructions, when technically feasible, have a low morbidity and very good mid-term patency rates.

INTRODUCTION

While carotid bifurcation disease is frequently encountered by the vascular surgeon, the need to treat the more proximal disease of the great vessels is uncommon in practice. Despite this, the vascular specialist must always consider the possibility of proximal disease when approaching patients with neurologic or upper extremity symptoms.

Throughout the 1960s, reports emerged regarding the treatment of occlusive lesions of the great vessels. Crawford at al.[1] reported their experience with both extra-anatomic and direct trans-sternal repairs. Although they demonstrated the technical feasibility of both approaches, they also demonstrated a significant difference in mortality between the two. As their experience increased, they shifted from 100% trans-sternal repairs to approximately 20% by the end of the decade. Their preferred alternative became short-segment extra-anatomic reconstructions such as carotid–subclavian bypasses, but they still advocated direct repairs for multiple lesions and when adequate inflow was a concern. In attempts to find a revascularization option with less morbidity than trans-sternal repairs, some investigators pursued remote extra-anatomic repairs such as axilloaxillary[2] or femoral-to-axillary bypasses. Contemporary surgical series have demonstrated decreased morbidity and mortality for each type of revascularization, with excellent long-term patency for both direct trans-sternal repairs and short-segment extra-anatomic bypasses.[3,4] Even remote extra-anatomic reconstructions can

produce excellent long-term results.[5] However, some authors have reported a significantly decreased mid-term patency, making extra-anatomic reconstructions more controversial.[6] When considering open surgical approaches only, short-segment extra-anatomic bypasses are the preferred reconstruction. However, if multiple vessels are involved, a direct trans-sternal repair is best, saving the remote extra-anatomic bypasses for those patients who are prohibitive operative risks.

With the emergence of endovascular therapies, the debate now centers less on the ideal surgical approach but instead on whether endovascular or 'conventional' surgical approaches should be used as primary therapy for great vessel occlusive disease.[7] While endovascular therapy does not have the four decades of experience of surgical revascularization, promising mid-term data are emerging which support strong consideration of this approach when technically feasible. Similar to treating lower extremity occlusive disease, a combination of endovascular correction of the inflow lesion and either subsequent or simultaneous repair of the 'outflow' lesion may be warranted. The goal of this chapter will be to discuss the etiology and clinical presentation of aortic arch branch vessel disease, the indications for therapy, and the outcomes of various surgical and endovascular approaches.

ANATOMY AND PATHOLOGY

Occlusive lesions of the great vessels are predominately atherosclerotic in nature. In surgical series of direct trans-sternal revascularization, the incidence of atherosclerotic lesions has been reported to be 69–100%.[4,8] Takayasu's arteritis is the next most common in the US, with the Mayo Clinic series reporting a 22% incidence in patients requiring surgery.[4] Secondary arteritis from radiation is also seen occasionally and can represent a formidable clinical challenge.

Since the pathologic features of atherosclerotic vascular disease have been discussed in a previous chapter (see Chapter 2), we will focus on those vasculitic changes specific to the great vessels. The etiology of Takayasu's arteritis remains unclear but is likely multifactorial. The arterial inflammation is an immune-mediated response with a genetic predisposition. Infectious agents have been implicated by some as the triggering event, but these findings are inconsistent.[9] Initial histopathologic changes consist of plasma cells and lymphocytes within the adventitia and media. Giant cells can form within the media, and elastic fibers can be identified within these lesions. After degradation of the media elastic fibers, it becomes fibrotic. It is this fibrosis that results in the long tapered stenosis of the affected vessels. The intimal injury and subsequent proliferation/thickening are secondary

Anatomic distribution of disease in Takayasu's arteritis.		
	Degree of stenosis	
	≥50% No. (%)	100% No. (%)
Innominate artery	10 (77)	5 (38)
Right common carotid artery	9 (69)	4 (31)
Left common carotid artery	8 (62)	4 (31)
Right subclavian artery	8 (62)	5 (38)
Left subclavian artery	12 (92)	10 (77)

Table 34.1 Anatomic distribution of disease in Takayasu's arteritis. Distribution of hemodynamically significant (>50%) stenoses and complete (100%) occlusions in 13 patients with symptomatic great vessel disease from Takayasu's arteritis.

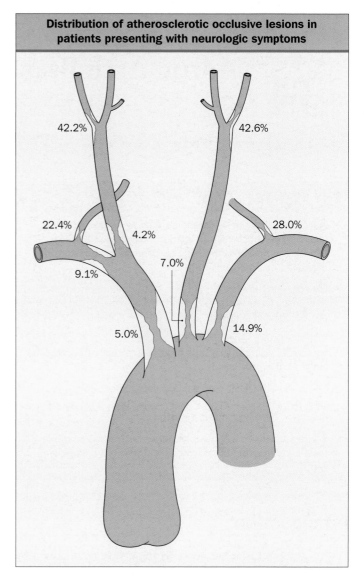

Distribution of atherosclerotic occlusive lesions in patients presenting with neurologic symptoms

42.2%   42.6%
22.4%   4.2%   28.0%
7.0%
9.1%
5.0%   14.9%

Figure 34.1 Distribution of atherosclerotic occlusive lesions in patients presenting with neurologic symptoms. (Adapted from Hass et al.[12])

results from damage in the vaso vasorum. This intimal damage contributes to development of atherosclerosis that can later cause significant stenoses and occlusions years after quiescence of the inflammatory stage.[9]

The anatomic distribution of disease in Takayasu's arteritis varies depending on ethnicity and/or location of the study population. Japanese populations have a higher incidence of isolated supra-aortic and aortic arch involvement. The distribution of disease in the US is not well defined. **Table 34.1** demonstrates the frequency with which each vessel may be involved, highlighting the diffuse nature of this disease.

Atherosclerosis often affects multiple arteries. Contemporary surgical series of trans-sternal repairs have documented multiple great vessel involvement in 70–80% of patients.[4,8,10] When considering all reconstructions of the innominate, common carotid, or subclavian arteries, Crawford and colleagues reported only a 24% incidence of multiple vessel involvement.[1] The discrepancy may be due to the inclusion of isolated subclavian lesions that underwent carotid–subclavian bypass. Perhaps the more important question is what is the likely distribution of disease in a patient who presents with neurologic symptoms? DeBakey et al.[11] reported on 942 consecutive patients with neurologic symptoms, all of whom underwent arteriography. Extracranial stenoses were identified in 41% of patients. Not surprisingly, the most common location of occlusive disease in this symptomatic population was the carotid bifurcation (64% of lesions), although 67% of patients were noted to have multiple vessels involved. The vertebral arteries accounted for 19% of lesions; the subclavians, 8%; and both the common carotids and innominate arteries accounted for 3.6% each.

Hass et al.[12] reported the anatomic results of the Joint Study of Extracranial Arterial Occlusion. Nearly 5000 patients were included in this prospective registry of patients presenting with neurologic symptoms. **Figure 34.1** summarizes the frequency with which a given artery was involved, including both stenosis and occlusions, on a per patient basis. Strikingly similar to DeBakey's series, 67.3% of patients had multiple vessels involved. No identifiable lesion was seen in 19% of patients and surgically inaccessible lesions alone were seen in 6%. Again, despite the carotid bifurcation being the most common lesion, proximal great vessel disease must be considered in every patient.

PATHOPHYSIOLOGY

Like for occlusive lesions at the carotid bifurcation, the morbidity from great vessel occlusive disease can result from thromboembolic events to either the brain or upper extremity. In addition, given the frequency of multiple vessel involvement, low-flow states resulting in global ischemic symptoms or vertebrobasilar insufficiency play a significant role in the pathophysiology. This is particularly true for patients with Takayasu's arteritis. Such patients in the Mayo Clinic series had a 70% incidence of global ischemic symptoms due to flow-limiting lesions.[4] Fifty-four percent also had upper extremity claudication from innominate or subclavian stenoses. Despite the smooth tapering lesions seen with Takayasu's, embolic events do also occur. Thirty-one percent of these patients had neurologic events due to emboli, half of whom also had microemboli to the digits.

The pathophysiology of atherosclerotic lesions is different given the potentially irregular nature of the luminal surface. For those lesions requiring surgical intervention, it is twice as likely that an embolic event will be the cause of the presenting symptom. In the atherosclerotic (atherosclerosis obliterans, ASO) patients from the same Mayo Clinic series,[4] 63% had embolic events; 53% causing neurologic symptoms and 10% causing pure upper extremity symptoms, with 5% of patients having both territories affected.

CLINICAL PRESENTATION

The clinical scenario of a patient presenting with symptomatic great vessel disease varies based on the type of lesion, the location and extent of those lesions, and, most importantly, on the underlying pathology, which will affect not only the presentation but also the long-term outcome.

The typical patient with Takayasu's arteritis is female. Initial presentation is before the age of 40.[9] However, the age that the patient seeks intervention for vascular complaints has been reported in two series to range from 18 to 58 years.[4,13] During the early phases of the disease, complaints can be non-specific, including fever, malaise, and myalgia. Some patients will complain of limb claudication or pain overlying an involved artery. Hypertension and its sequelae represent the most frequent presentation.[9] Hypertension can be from renal artery stenosis, aortic coarctation, or carotid involvement with alteration in the usual baroreflex. Neurologic symptoms related to the hypertension can include headache, visual changes, stroke, or even encephalopathy. As the disease advances and the subclavian, innominate, and carotid arteries develop progressive diameter reduction, low-flow symptoms can emerge. Lightheadedness, dizziness, photophobia, visual disturbances, and clinical subclavian steal syndrome can all occur. Upper extremity claudication without clinical steal remains more common than true symptomatic steal.

Most patients with Takayasu's arteritis will have signs of significant vascular involvement on initial presentation. The classic description is of pulselessness of one or both upper extremities. Early in the course of disease, there may only be discrepancies in blood pressures between the arms or between the arms and the lower extremities. Subclavian or carotid bruits can often be heard, as well as intra-abdominal bruits. Carotid pulses may also be blunted or absent. In the presence of significant subclavian disease, the hands can be pale with sluggish capillary refill. In the case of embolic lesions, splinter hemorrhages may occur. Rarely, embolization may even occur to the lateral chest wall, causing ulceration. These physical examination findings are not specific for Takayasu's and apply to atherosclerotic patients as well.

Some of the differences between ASO patients and those with Takayasu's arteritis were discussed in the pathophysiology section. Specifically, ASO patients are more likely to have lesions that result in embolic events. The typical neurologic symptoms that result from emboli include hemispheric events referable most frequently to the anterior circulation and amaurosis fugax. The other major area of difference is the demographics and associated co-morbidities. Comparing the risk factors of the ASO and Takayasu's patients from the Mayo Clinic series,[4] the mean age was significantly older for the ASO group (59±10 years versus 40±11 years, p<0.001), and all Takayasu's patients were female compared with 66% in the ASO group (p<0.05). When comparing other variables including history of previous transient ischemic attack/cerebrovascular accident (TIA/CVA), diabetes, hypertension, tobacco use, hyperlipidemia, known coronary artery disease, renal insufficiency, or previous symptomatic lower extremity peripheral vascular disease, the only significant difference was history of tobacco use. Tobacco abuse was almost uniform in the ASO patients, with 95% reporting a significant or ongoing use of tobacco. The Takayasu's group still had a high rate of tobacco use (69%), but this was significantly less than for ASO patients (p=0.02). The risk factors are almost identical to those of Berguer and colleagues,[10] including age, female predominance, and tobacco use.[10]

Patients with radiation-induced stenosis of the carotid arteries and great vessels can present with both embolic and low-flow signs and symptoms. The duration from therapeutic irradiation to development of symptomatic arterial disease is usually a decade, but this is variable and may be within years to several decades later.[14,15] The radiation injury predisposes to atherosclerotic changes in the vessels, often in locations not typical of uncomplicated atherosclerosis. Despite the relatively frequent use of radiation therapy in the treatment of malignancy, it is relatively infrequent that these patients develop significant lesions that require revascularization. The presenting symptoms are often global ischemia from a low-flow state since multiple vessels are frequently involved. Vertebrobasilar and upper extremity symptoms have also been reported.[14]

Regardless of the etiology of occlusive disease, an often talked about phenomenon is the subclavian steal syndrome. True subclavian steal syndrome occurs when a proximal subclavian stenosis/occlusion is present. During upper extremity activity, blood flows retrograde down the vertebral to supply the arm and results in compromised cerebral perfusion. Although the radiographic finding of subclavian steal is common, the clinical syndrome is rare.[16] Of 168 patients identified with true radiographic subclavian steal in the Joint Study of Extracranial Arterial Occlusion, none was reported to have worsening symptoms with arm use, and 80% had significant lesions in other vessels which likely contributed to the vertebrobasilar/low-flow state symptoms.[17] The radiographic finding is more important as a marker for proximal disease rather than for its clinical relevance.

Taking into consideration that it is rare for patients to present to the vascular specialist's office with a pathologic and anatomic diagnosis in hand, the questions when seeing these patients are:

1. What is the lesion responsible for the symptom?
2. What is the cause of that lesion?
3. What are the risks of correcting that lesion?

One must always be aware of the possibility that the cause of the presenting neurologic symptom may not be the carotid bifurcation lesion seen on duplex ultrasound. This is especially true if the severity of that lesion does not correspond to the given symptom. Based on history and physical examination findings, one must consider further imaging/investigation. A female patient with a history of heavy tobacco use who presents at a relatively young age (fifth or sixth decade of life) constitutes a subgroup that has an increased risk of proximal great vessel disease. This is true regardless of the etiology of the lesion. While not an indication in itself to image the great vessels, a low threshold should exist in this population. Physical examination findings of a proximal bruit or discrepancies in blood pressures also warrant further investigation of the great vessels.

DIAGNOSTIC TECHNIQUES

Although the proximal extent of the carotid and subclavian arteries can not be directly visualized using duplex ultrasound, significant information can be gained from this imaging modality. On rare occasions, the origin of the right common carotid artery and even a portion of the innominate artery can be seen directly in slender individuals. Usually, the presence of proximal carotid or innominate disease is inferred from the Doppler waveform characteristics in the common carotid artery. The normal waveform has a sharp systolic upstroke, is triphasic, and has a clear spectral window. In the presence of hemodynamically significant proximal disease, the waveform may be blunted, monophasic, and have spectral broadening consistent with turbulent flow (**Fig. 34.2**). Other findings on duplex scan indicating more proximal disease include abnormal subclavian flow similar to the changes mentioned for the common carotid, retrograde vertebral flow indicating a flow-limiting proximal subclavian stenosis, or a discrepancy of 10mmHg or greater in upper extremity blood pressure measurements.

Although it is now common practice to intervene on carotid bifurcation disease based on duplex ultrasound findings alone, initial criticism of this approach was that significant proximal disease would be missed. Akers et al.[18] examined 1000 consecutive arch angiograms to determine if this added to patient management over non-invasive testing alone. These studies were not compared directly with duplex ultrasound studies, and it appears that asymptomatic patients were included. There was a 10.5% incidence of proximal disease, but the majority was vertebral artery occlusive disease. When excluding the vertebral arteries, 1.8% of patients had significant proximal lesions. The authors concluded that routine arteriography is not necessary except when there is a significant discrepancy in upper extremity blood pressures or if non-invasive testing does not find a lesion that adequately accounts for the patient's symptoms. To better define the role of duplex ultrasound for the diagnosis of aortic arch branch vessel disease, McLaren et al.[19] examined a series of 650 consecutive carotid duplex scans that all underwent confirmatory arteriography. Using the criteria mentioned above, they accurately predicted the presence of 27 proximal lesions (4%). Only one lesion was missed by duplex. This yielded a sensitivity and specificity of 96% and 100%, respectively. More importantly, the positive and negative predictive values were 100% and 99%, respectively. The authors stressed that 50% of the proximal lesions identified did require surgical intervention, highlighting the importance of recognizing these lesions. These findings were confirmed in a prospective manner by Kadwa and colleagues,[20] who examined 129 patients undergoing carotid endarterectomy.

They found a 14.5% incidence of proximal disease, half involving either the innominate or common carotid artery and half involving the subclavians. All proximal lesions could be predicted by a combination of pulse and blood pressure abnormalities, presence of bruits, and/or duplex findings. Thirty-seven percent of these patients required surgical correction of these additional lesions.

The gold-standard examination to delineate the extent and location of great vessel pathology remains arch aortography with four-vessel runoff. With present digital subtraction techniques, the contrast load has decreased, as has the time to complete the study. A typical study can now be performed with 100ml or less of contrast. **Figure 34.3** demonstrates a standard arch aortogram in a patient with atherosclerotic occlusive disease (**Fig. 34.3A**) and in a patient with Takayasu's arteritis (**Fig. 34.3B**). The criticisms of intra-arterial contrast studies have been their invasive nature, the risk of stroke from catheter manipulations, nephrotoxicity of the contrast agents, and the possibility of missing irregular lesions due to inability to visualize them through the column of contrast. Although gadolinium can be used as an alternative agent to decrease renal toxicity, the image quality may be suboptimal. The ACAS study identified the risk of stroke in asymptomatic patients undergoing angiography to be 1.2%.[21] A contemporary series by Johnston and associates compared the risk of neurologic complications in patients undergoing cerebral angiography – 50% of whom were symptomatic – at a university medical center versus a community hospital practice.[22] They found no difference in cerebrovascular risk between the two settings. The overall risk of stroke and TIA was 0.5% and 0.4%, respectively.

Although conventional arteriography is associated with a low risk, it is certainly not risk-free. The desire of both the patient and physician to find a safer and less invasive means of imaging the aortic arch and its branches has led to further developments in both computed tomography (CT) angiography and magnetic resonance angiography (MRA) (**Fig. 34.3C**). Much of the data published on MRA centers around cervical carotid disease. The American Heart Association published a summary on use of MRA imaging, and, for carotid artery disease, stated that it should be used in conjunction with duplex ultrasound, reserving conventional angiography for discrepant results.[23] In a review of 11 studies comparing MRA with conventional angiography in a total of nearly 700 patients, the median sensitivity was 93% (range, 86–100%) and the median specificity was 88% (range, 75–98%), making it a reasonable adjunct to duplex ultrasound for cervical carotid artery disease.[23]

The criticism that duplex ultrasound first received – the possibility of missing more proximal lesions – is now directed towards MRA. Carpenter et al.[24] prospectively studied MRA for

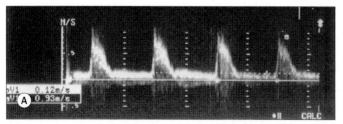
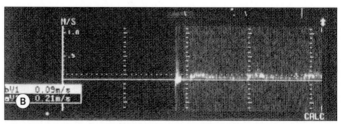

Figure 34.2 Spectral analysis of the left (A) and right (B) common carotid arteries. The left has mild diffuse stenotic (16–49%) disease. The right spectral waveform is altered by a significant (>50%) stenosis of the innominate artery that can not be directly visualized in this patient.

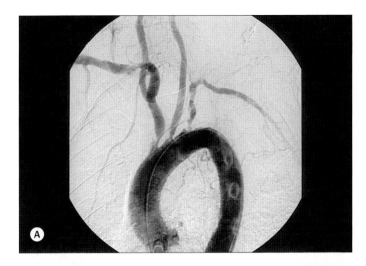

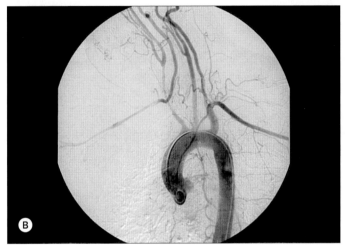

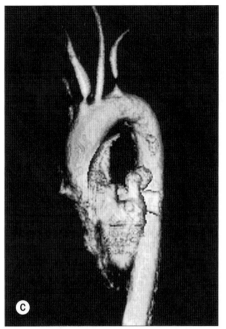

Figure 34.3 Standard arch aortogram in a patient with atherosclerotic occlusive disease (A) and in a patient with Takayasu's arteritis (B). MRA of atherosclerotic disease involving innominate and left common carotid arteries (C).

aortic arch occlusive disease, all patients having both MRAs and conventional angiograms performed. The sensitivity of MRA was only 73% (specificity, 89–98%), leading the authors to conclude that, although a normal study excludes significant disease, the technology was not yet to the point that MRA could replace conventional angiography. Prince et al.[25] summarized their experience with thoracic aortic MRA for various aortic and non-aortic pathologies. A subset of 19 patients was analyzed who had occlusive disease of major aortic branches. This included not only great vessel disease (excluding vertebrals) but also mesenteric and renal disease. Despite these limitations, the sensitivity and specificity at detecting a hemodynamically significant stenosis was promising, at 90% and 96%, respectively. As the technology and techniques for both obtaining and analyzing data are improved, MRA is likely to become accurate enough to replace conventional arteriography of the aortic arch and its branches.

Proponents of MRA also point out that, in regards to plaque morphology and ulceration, MRA may be more sensitive than conventional angiography, which can obscure the details of a lesion by the column of contrast.[23] Randoux et al.[26] confirmed this finding for carotid bifurcation lesions, but no data exist for aortic branch vessel pathology. The other aspect of their study was the validation of CT angiography in the evaluation of the cervical carotid artery. This technique can also be used to image the aortic arch and branch vessels, but data are limited.

In summary, the radiographic evaluation of a patient suspected of having symptomatic carotid bifurcation or great vessel occlusive disease should begin with duplex ultrasonogaphy. If the study does not demonstrate a lesion that is clearly responsible for the symptom or is suggestive of a proximal stenosis, further imaging of the aorta arch and great vessels should be performed. If there is a low clinical suspicion for significant proximal disease, a magnetic resonance angiogram beginning at the level of the aorta should be obtained. A normal study will exclude significant pathology. If there is a high suspicion of a lesion that will require intervention, a conventional intra-arterial angiogram is recommended, especially if a percutaneous intervention at the time of angiography is being considered. In patients with significant renal insufficiency, MRA is preferred even if a percutanous intervention is being entertained, in order to direct that intervention and limit the subsequent contrast load.

MANAGEMENT AND PROGNOSIS

Direct trans-sternal reconstruction for aortic branch vessel occlusive disease remains the gold standard for patients with disease affecting multiple vessels. For isolated disease of the common carotid or subclavian arteries, short-segment extra-anatomic bypasses (subclavian–carotid bypass) is the surgical treatment of choice. When comparing the results of either remote extra-anatomic bypasses or endovascular approaches, it

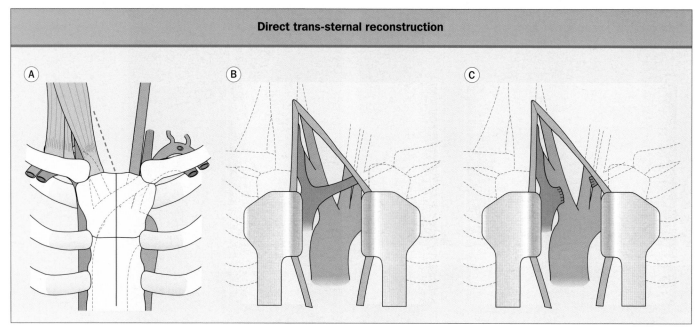

Direct trans-sternal reconstruction

Ⓐ   Ⓑ   Ⓒ

Figure 34.4 Direct trans-sternal reconstruction. Initial exposure of the ascending aorta and its branches by a trans-sternal approach (A,B). The left brachiocephalic vein can be divided and oversewn to facilitate exposure (C).

is important to compare treatments of similar lesions to understand which therapy is best. In this section, we will discuss both the technical aspects of each of the therapies and data regarding both complications and long-term success.

Direct trans-sternal repair is performed through a median sternotomy with extension of the incision to the right neck if needed (**Figs 34.4A&B**). Alternatively, a mini-sternotomy to the third intercostal space can be performed with transection of the sternum at that level.[27] The left brachiocephalic vein is fully mobilized, and, if necessary, this can be divided and oversewn to facilitate exposure and allow proper lie of the graft without significant long-term sequelae to the left upper extremity (**Fig. 34.4C**).[4] Separate cervical incisions are made if the target vessels are the carotid bifurcations. Extending the sternal incision into the right neck can facilitate exposure of the innominate and proximal right subclavian and common carotid arteries (**Fig. 34.5**). The proximal anastomosis is placed as far lateral on the ascending aorta as possible (**Fig. 34.6**). This allows for a smooth lie of the graft and keeps the bulk in the anterior mediastinum to a minimum, preventing encroachment onto the graft after closure of the chest. We prefer the use of knitted 7, 8, or 10 mm polyester grafts with additional sidearms placed as needed (**Figs 34.6B & 34.7**). Some authors prefer the use of bifurcated grafts (**Fig. 34.6D**) but, again, care must be taken to avoid excessive mediastinal contents that could kink or impinge on the graft. Resection of the diseased innominate artery is one way to provide additional space for a graft.

When planning revascularization, arteries that have complete proximal occlusions are grafted first, in order to maximize cerebral blood flow during each stage of the procedure. If available, electroencephalographic (EEG) monitoring can be helpful, but the need for shunt placement is uncommon (<10%) and often the decision to place a shunt is based on the preoperative clinical scenario (**Fig. 34.8**).[4] Although the Texas Heart Group has favored reconstructing all occluded vessels, we have found

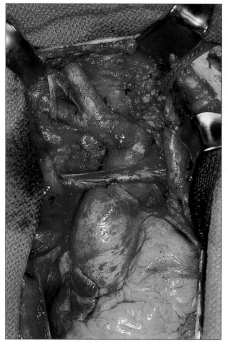

Figure 34.5 Intraoperative photograph of the trans-sternal approach to the ascending aorta and innominate bifurcation. The brachiocephalic vein was left intact.

that the left subclavian can be dealt with in a staged fashion if necessary (**Fig. 34.9**). In our recent series, none of the 16 patients who had left subclavian artery occlusions required a subsequent bypass.

The other procedural aspect of aortic branch vessel occlusive disease is the utility of innominate artery endarterectomy. This is technically more demanding than bypass grafting, and patients must have proper anatomy to allow its use. Specifically, the aorta at the innominate origin must not have significant calcification. Also, there needs to be approximately one centimeter between the innominate origin and the left carotid origin, to allow proper

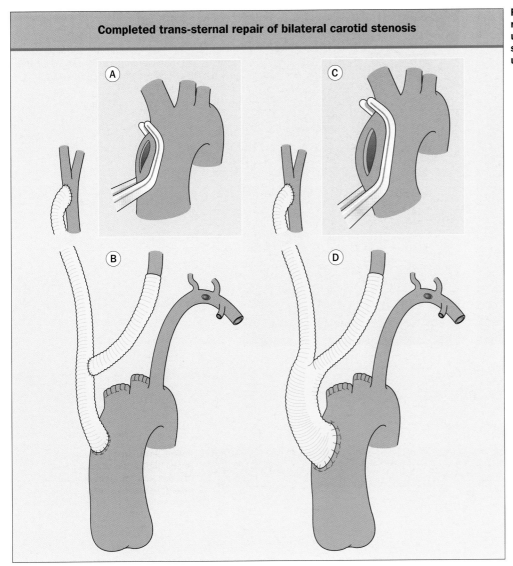

Completed trans-sternal repair of bilateral carotid stenosis

Figure 34.6 Completed trans-sternal repair of bilateral carotid stenosis using an 8mm polyester graft with a sidearm that was added (A,B), or using a bifurcated graft (C,D).

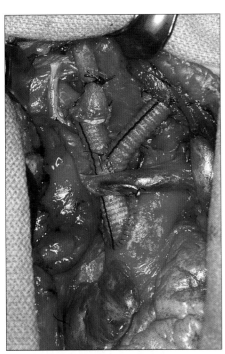

Figure 34.7 Intraoperative photograph of a completed aorto-innominate and left common carotid bypass using an 8mm polyester graft to the innominate bifurcation with a single sidearm added that goes to the left common carotid artery (not pictured) in a patient with Takayasu's arteritis.

clamping without compromising perfusion to both hemispheres (**Fig. 34.10**). Extensive experience with this technique by the group at the University of California at San Francisco demonstrated its utility, with patency rates equal to or better than those achieved with bypass grafting.[28] It is particularly useful when simultaneous coronary artery bypass grafting will be necessary, since the ascending aorta can be left free for the proximal vein grafts.

When feasible, short-segment cervical reconstructions (subclavian–carotid bypasses) are performed for disease isolated to a single vessel. Synthetic conduits, 8mm knitted polyester, are preferred over vein grafts in this location. Remote, non-anatomic bypass grafts can also be performed in patients who are at a prohibitive risk for trans-sternal repairs and are not candidates for short-segment cervical bypasses owing to involvement of the usual inflow vessel. These reconstructions include axilloaxillary bypasses, carotid–carotid bypasses (with either pre-tracheal or retroesophageal tunneling), and femoral–axillary bypasses (**Fig. 34.11**). Synthetic materials, often externally supported, are used for these reconstructions.

Endovascular therapy for aortic branch vessel occlusive disease has been reported for atherosclerotic lesions, radiation-

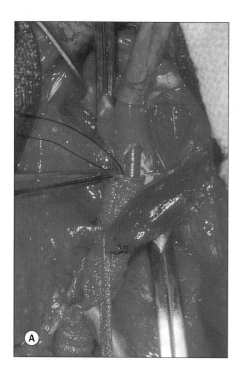

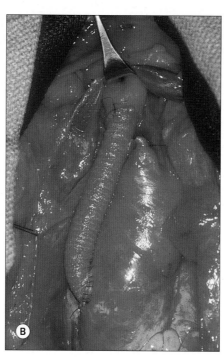

Figure 34.8 Shunt placement. (A) Intraoperative photograph of an aorto-innominate bypass utilizing a shunt for cerebral protection. Note that this is secured into the graft and common carotid arteries with Rummel tourniquets, and the right subclavian artery is clamped. (B) Completed repair after shunt removal.

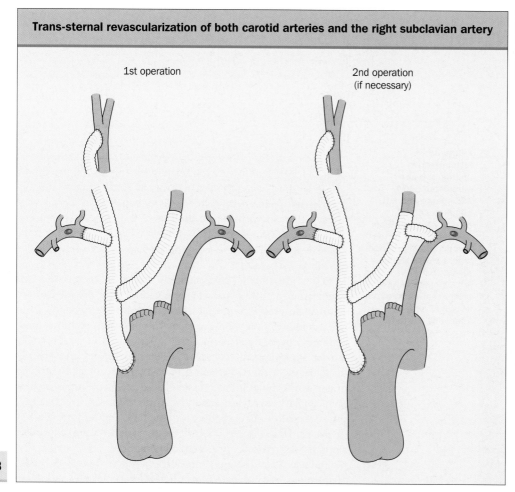

Trans-sternal revascularization of both carotid arteries and the right subclavian artery

1st operation

2nd operation
(if necessary)

Figure 34.9 Trans-sternal revascularization of both carotid arteries and the right subclavian artery. Revascularization of the left subclavian artery can be performed at a later date, but is rarely necessary.

Arteriotomy during an innominate endarterectomy

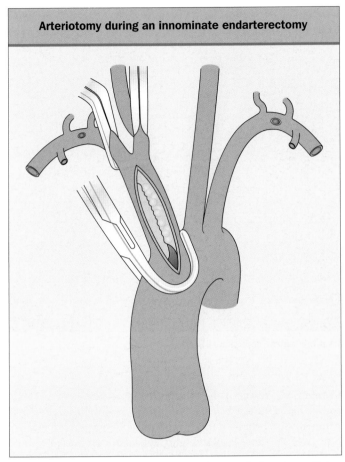

Figure 34.10 **Arteriotomy during an innominate endarterectomy.** Note that the arteriotomy is carried onto the aorta as needed and that the proximal clamp is placed such as to allow adequate flow to the left common carotid artery.

Possible extra-anatomic options for surgical revascularization

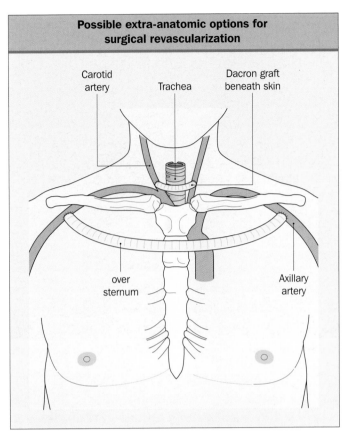

Figure 34.11 **Possible extra-anatomic options for surgical revascularization.** Both an axillo–axillary artery bypass and a carotid–carotid bypass are depicted. The retroesophageal tunnel for the carotid–carotid bypass is an alternative option (not pictured).

induced stenoses, and Takayasu's arteritis.[29] Percutaneous approach can be from the ipsilateral brachial/axillary artery or from either femoral approach. Both 0.035in and 0.018in systems are available. Although the use of cerebral protection devices has not been reported for common carotid origin or innominate lesions, they may be beneficial for symptomatic embolic lesions. Intraoperative angioplasty and stenting may also allow for correction of a proximal inflow lesion via a retrograde approach during operative correction of a carotid bifurcation lesion, with the benefit of distal carotid control to prevent embolization (**Fig. 34.12**). Although it is technically feasible to recanalize a completely occluded segment using angioplasty and stent placement, there is a higher rate of both technical failure and restenosis/occlusion.[30]

When trying to decide which revascularization option is best for a given patient, one must consider the risk of the given procedure and the long-term benefits of that procedure. When comparing various approaches, it is also important to compare treatment of similar lesions, similar extent of disease and similar pathologies. These comparisons also need to be among contemporary series when available. There is no prospective comparison between the various surgical approaches, nor are there any data regarding direct, prospective comparisons of open versus endovascular options. Farina et al.[31] assessed carotid–subclavian bypass versus percutaneous transluminal angioplasty (PTA) without

stenting for proximal stenoses of <4cm length in a retrospective cohort fashion. Patients with innominate or common carotid disease were excluded, as were those with complete occlusions. In this group of 36 patients, there was no difference in the incidence of immediate complications between the two procedures; however, 5-year primary patency data favored surgical reconstruction (87% versus 54%). The authors concluded that PTA should be reserved for elderly patients or those who have prohibitive medical co-morbidities for surgery. Whether the addition of stents to the PTA arm would have improved patency is unclear.

The remainder of the data on revascularization of aortic branch vessel disease comes from individual series. **Tables 34.2 & 34.3** summarize available contemporary data over the past decade for surgical and endovascular repairs. Although direct comparisons can be made for the initial outcomes and complications, it is more difficult to compare long-term outcomes since those data are incomplete for endovascular therapies. Very little life-table data exist for endovascular repairs, and the use of 'long-term' often applies to follow-up periods of less than 2 years.

Direct, trans-sternal repair carries with it the highest morbidity and mortality of all the approaches discussed, owing to the scope of the operative procedure and the extent of disease. The overall neurologic event rate is 7%, with a perioperative death rate of 5% (**Table 34.2, upper panel**). Risk factors identified for

499

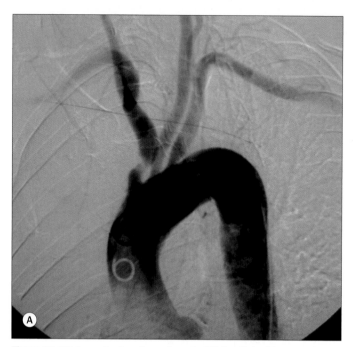
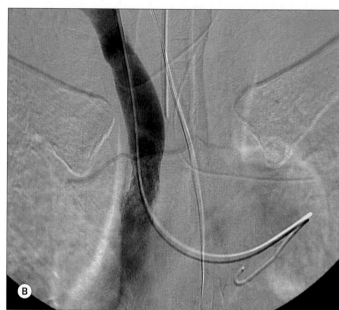

Figure 34.12 Innominate artery stenosis (A) treated with stent placement from the carotid approach (B).

poor early outcomes have included the presence of a hyper-coaguable state (or thrombophilia) and renal insufficiency.[4] Although identifying hypercoaguable patients preoperatively would likely improve these results, screening of all patients undergoing great vessel repair would not be cost-effective. We advocate screening only those patients who have a history of multiple graft thromboses, regardless of the location of those grafts. This approach is relevant whether considering a direct, extra-anatomic or endovascular repair. In addition, any patient who experiences an acute graft, endarterectomy, or PTA site/stent thrombosis should be evaluated. Renal insufficiency should be considered a significant risk factor for poor initial outcome, and these patients may benefit from minimizing the complexity/invasiveness of the procedure. Unfortunately, the extent of disease is more likely to be the determinant of which approach is necessary. The etiology of disease (ASO, Takayasu's or radiation-induced arteritis) is not a predictor of initial outcomes.

It was the higher rate of perioperative complications that influenced Crawford and DeBakey to shift from a universal trans-sternal approach for all patients to short extra-anatomic bypasses in 80%.[1] The contemporary perioperative neurologic event rate for short-segment extra-anatomic (subclavian–carotid and carotid–subclavian) bypass grafting is 1%, with a death rate of 0.6% (**Table 34.2, middle panel**). It is also a durable repair, with 5-year patency rates in the high-80s to mid-90 percent range and excellent stroke-free survival rates. This is the open revascularization approach of choice when the anatomy is suitable.

Some authors have advocated remote extra-anatomic approaches, such as axilloaxillary bypass, when a suitable ipsilateral inflow vessel is not available. Although the recent reported series often included significant numbers of patients with pure upper extremity symptoms, the axilloaxillary bypass has low stroke and death rates of 0% and 1.4%, respectively

(**Table 34.2, lower panel**). Patency has also been acceptable, from 87% to 90% at 5 years. However, not all series share these patency rates. Schanzer et al.[37] reported a 5-year primary patency rate of 72%, and Brewster and colleagues[6] reported a 50% occlusion rate. The other theoretic disadvantage of this approach is the course of the graft, which traverses the sternum, making future procedures through a median sternotomy potentially problematic. Despite these concerns, axilloaxillary bypass grafting is a reasonable option for the patient who is a prohibitive operative risk for a trans-sternal repair, is not a candidate for subclavian–carotid grafting owing to anatomic considerations, and for whom an endovascular solution is not possible.

Much of the available data on endovascular therapy for aortic branch vessel occlusive disease is from individual series with follow-up data expressed as patency during a mean follow-up period rather than by life-table analysis. This makes direct comparisons with the contemporary surgical literature problematic. In addition, the claim of having long-term follow-up data when the mean follow-up period is often less than 2 years is inadequate. Acknowledging these limitations, meaningful comparisons can be made on complication rates, and trends for patency can be noted. An example of how patency data can be misleading is seen in Farina's study,[31] where they did report 5-year life-table patency rates. The raw value for patency of subclavian PTA was 78% at a mean of 40 months; however, the 5-year patency by life-table analysis was only 54%.

The technical success and complication data for endovascular therapy versus open surgical techniques are directly comparable. For isolated subclavian lesions, technical success was achieved in 93% of cases (**Table 34.3, upper panel**). Those series with a higher rate of total occlusions tended to have a lower technical success rate. This was often due to an inability to cross the lesion. Data regarding the routine use of stents are not clear. Presently, there are no definitive data to support one approach over the other. Significant complications with endovascular therapy were

Trans-sternal surgical repairs

Author	No.	CVA/TIA No. (%)	Death No. (%)	Primary patency (5 year)	Secondary patency (5 year)	Stroke-free survival (5 year)	Survival (5 year)
Kieffer[8]	148	8 (5)	8 (5)	98%	99%	89%	78%
Berguer[10]	100	10 (10)	8 (8)	94%	97%	87%	73%
Rhodes[4]	58	4 (7)	2 (3)	80%	91%	86%	88%
Azakie[28]	94	6 (6)	3 (3)	–	–	–	85%
Total	**400**	**28 (7)**	**21 (5)**	**n/a**	**n/a**	**n/a**	**n/a**

Short-segment extra-anatomic bypass

Author	No.	CVA/TIA No. (%)	Death No. (%)	Primary patency (5 year)	Secondary patency (5 year)	Stroke-free survival (5 year)	Survival (5 year)
Law[3]	60	2 (3.3)	1 (1.7)	88%	–	86%	84%
AbuRahma[32]	51	0	0	96%	98%	82%	86%
Perler[33]	31	1 (3.2)	0	92%	–	71%	88%
Synn[34]	32	0	0	77%	–	74% (87% CVA-free)	–
Vitti[35]	124	0	1 (0.8)	94%	–	90%	83%
Farina[31]	15	0	0	87%	100%	100%	–
Total	**313**	**3 (1.0)**	**2 (0.6)**	**n/a**	**n/a**	**n/a**	**n/a**

Axilloaxillary bypass

Author	No.	CVA/TIA No. (%)	Death No. (%)	Primary patency (5 year)	Secondary patency (5 year)	Stroke-free survival (5 year)	Survival (5 year)
Mingoli[5]	61	0	1 (1.6)	87%	88%	98%	93%
Rosenthal[36]	32	0	0	90%	–	–	92%
Schanzer[37]	33	0	1 (3.0)	72%	–	–	–
Weiner[38]	19	0	0	89%	–	–	–
Total	**145**	**0**	**2 (1.4)**	**n/a**	**n/a**	**n/a**	**n/a**

Table 34.2 Results of contemporary surgical series for repair of aortic arch branch lesions by direct trans-sternal repair, short-segment extra-anatomic bypass grafting (subclavian–carotid and carotid–subclavian bypass), and remote extra-anatomic bypass (axilloaxillary bypass). CVA, cerebrovascular accident; n/a, not applicable; TIA, transient ischemic attack.

rare or non-existent. When they occurred, they were most often related to the access site. The mortality rate was 0.7%, comparable to that seen with carotid–subclavian bypass grafting (0.6%, **Table 34.2, middle panel**). There were no neurologic events reported, thus comparing favorably with carotid–subclavian grafting, which had a 1.0% stroke rate.

The durability of endovascular repair of proximal subclavian lesions remains less clear. In distinction to Farina's series,[31] Selby et al.[39] reported a 97% 5-year life-table patency in 32 non-occluded lesions treated with PTA alone. The remaining available data do not give life-table information. Realizing the limitation of comparing raw data with life-table data, the aggregate patency of subclavian PTA with or without stenting at a mean of 27

months was 84%. While the 5-year life-table patency is less, endovascular therapy is a reasonable first choice for isolated proximal stenotic lesions. The treatment of total occlusions remains controversial.

When examining the results of endovascular treatment of the innominate and common carotid arteries, it is not surprising that the complication rates increase. In the 43 reported cases, all underwent stent placement (**Table 34.3, lower panel**). The neurologic event rate in this group was 4.7%, with a mortality of 2.3%. These events occurred during simultaneous surgical treatment of concomitant carotid bifurcation lesions, however. The patency at a mean follow-up of 23 months was 95%. These numbers are promising, but more data are needed before wide-

Endovascular treatment of subclavian artery stenoses							
Author	No.	Death No. (%)	Occlusion No. (%)	Stents No. (%)	Technical success No. (%)	Primary patency*	Follow-up (months)
Duber[30]	8	0	8 (100)	0	7 (88)	38%	17
Selby[39]	29	0	0	0	32 (100)[†]	97%	36
Marques[40]	31	1 (3)	6 (19)	4 (13)	31 (100)	97%	37
Sullivan[41]	66	–	10 (15)	62 (100)[†]	62 (94)	89%	13
Queral[42]	12	0	5 (42)	10 (100)[‡]	10 (83)	66%	27
Hebrang[43]	52	0	9 (17)	0	45 (87)	79%	29
Farina[31]	21	0	0	0	21 (91)[¶]	78%	40
Total	**219**	**1 (0.7)**	**38 (17)**	**76 (35)**	**208 (93)**	**84%**	**27**

*Based on intent to treat.
[†]32 lesions treated in 29 patients.
[‡]All lesions able to be crossed were stented.
[¶]23 lesions in 21 patients.

Endovascular treatment of innominate and common carotid stenoses							
Author	No.	CVA/TIA No. (%)	Death No. (%)	Occlusion No. (%)	Stents No. (%)	Technical success No. (%)	Primary patency	Follow-up (months)
Ruebben[44]	8	0	0	0	8 (100)	8 (100)	100%	17
Sullivan[42]	21	2 (9.5)	1 (4.8)	0	21 (100)	20 (95)	–	–
Queral[43]	14	0	0	3 (21)	14 (100)	14 (100)	93%	27
Total	**43**	**2 (4.7)**	**1 (2.3)**	**3 (7.0)**	**43 (100)**	**42 (98)**	**95%**	**23**

Table 34.3 Results of endovascular therapy for subclavian stenoses and for innominate and common carotid lesions.

spread use is considered. Again, in a patient who is at increased surgical risk due to medical co-morbidities, endovascular therapy should be strongly considered based on the limited data available.

There have been numerous reports of endovascular treatment for Takayasu's arteritis involving the aortic branch vessels. Tyagi et al.[45] directly compared the results of PTA alone for symptomatic subclavian artery stenosis in patients with either Takayasu's arteritis or ASO. The lesions included were stenoses <6cm in length and occlusions <2cm. Although there was a trend toward worse outcomes in patients with Takayasu's arteritis (19% restenosis versus 5% in ASO, at a mean of 43 months), it did not reach statistical significance. All lesions were amenable to repeat angioplasty and one required an additional dilatation. Other workers have reported the use of stents for patients with Takayasu's disease, but no data exist other than short-term follow-up, to determine if this is superior to PTA alone.[13,29]

Use of PTA with or without stenting has appeal in those patients who have post-irradiation stenosis, given the risk of graft infection and wound healing difficulties encountered with direct repairs.[4] The data on endovascular repair of these lesions are very limited. Melliere et al.[46] reported a group of six patients who had angioplasty of carotid, subclavian, iliac, or femoral vessels. Four of six were successful, but data were lacking on follow-up. Given the poor results with surgical therapy in this

population, despite minimal available data, PTA with or without stenting should be considered where feasible.

SUMMARY

Aortic arch branch disease is a relatively uncommon cause of significant neurovascular symptoms in the general population. Although the true incidence is unknown, duplex ultrasound and angiographic studies suggest the incidence of significant proximal lesions to be about 2–4% in a symptomatic population.[18,19] Symptoms can be related to emboli from these lesions or from low-flow states when multiple vessels are involved. Low-flow symptoms include pre-syncope and other vertebrobasilar complaints. In addition, 50% of patients will have isolated or concomitant upper extremity symptoms.[4]

The etiology of occlusive disease of the great vessels is most often atherosclerosis, with Takayasu's arteritis accounting for one-fifth of patients in contemporary surgical series.[4] Radiation arteritis is an infrequent cause but often difficult to deal with due to high delayed wound healing and infection rates. Diagnostic imaging should include a duplex ultrasound, and any suggestion of a more proximal lesion on this or by physical examination (i.e. proximal non-cardiac bruit or blood pressure discrepancy) will warrant further imaging. Intra-arterial angiography remains the gold standard for definitive imaging but MRA is an acceptable alternative, especially if the suspicion for proximal disease is low.

Surgical options to treat these lesions include direct trans-sternal repairs including endarterectomy or bypass grafting originating from the ascending aorta. Isolated stenoses of the subclavian or carotid origins can be treated with short-segment extra-anatomic bypasses (subclavian–carotid bypass). Remote extra-anatomic bypasses (axilloaxillary bypass) are reserved for those patients who represent a high surgical risk. PTA and stenting is gaining popularity as first-line therapy for proximal lesions because of

its low morbidity and rare mortality, both of which compare favorably with surgical therapies. The long-term patency of these endovascular approaches remains unclear; mid-term results are promising, however, although appear somewhat inferior to those achieved with surgical repairs. If restenosis occurs, these lesions can often be retreated by endovascular means with good assisted primary patency. As stent technology evolves and both drug-eluting stents and cerebral protection devices become available, the already promising results of endovascular therapy are likely to improve further.

REFERENCES

1. Crawford ES, DeBakey ME, Morris GC, Howell JF. Surgical treatment of occlusion of the innominate, common carotid, and subclavian arteries: a 10 year experience. Surgery 1969;65:17–31.
2. Myers WO, Lawton BR, Sautter RD. Axillo-axillary bypass graft. JAMA 1971;217:826.
3. Law MM, Colburn MD, Moore WS, et al. Carotid-subclavian bypass for brachiocephalic occlusive disease: choice of conduit and long-term follow-up. Stroke 1995;26:1565–71.
4. Rhodes JM, Cherry KJ, Clark RC, et al. Aortic-origin reconstruction of the great vessels: risk factors for early and late complications. J Vasc Surg 2000;31:260–9.
5. Mingoli A, Sapienza P, Feldhaus RJ, et al. Long-term results and outcomes of crossover axilloaxillary bypass grafting: a 24-year experience. J Vasc Surg 1999;29:894–901.
6. Brewster DC, Moncure AC, Darling C, et al. Innominate artery lesions: problems encountered and lessons learned. J Vasc Surg 1985;2:99–112.
7. Hadjipetrou P, Cox S, Piemonte T, Eisenhauer A. Percutaneous revascularization of atherosclerotic obstruction of aortic arch vessels. J Am Coll Cardiol 1999;33:1238–45.
8. Kieffer E, Sabatier J, Koskas F, Bahnini A. Atherosclerotic innominate artery occlusive disease: early and long-term results of surgical reconstruction. J Vasc Surg 1995;21:326–37.
9. Sharma BK, Jain S. Takayasu's arteritis. In: Ball GV, Bridges SL, eds. Vasculitis. New York:Oxford University Press; 2002:278–89.
10. Berguer R, Morasch MD, Kline RA. Transthoracic repair of innominate and common carotid artery disease: immediate and long-term outcome for 100 consecutive surgical reconstructions. J Vasc Surg 1998;27:34–42.
11. DeBakey ME, Crawford ES, Morris GC, Cooley DA. Surgical consideration of occlusive disease of the innominate, carotid, subclavian, and vertebral arteries. Ann Surg 1961;154:698–725.
12. Hass WK, Fields WS, North RR, et al. Joint Study of Extracranial Arterial Occlusions: II. Arteriography, techniques, sites, and complications. JAMA 1968;203:159–66.
13. Bali HK, Jain S, Jain A, Sharma BK. Stent supported angioplasty in Takayasu arteritis. Int J Cardiol 1998;66S:S213–7.
14. Andros G, Schneider PA, Harris RW, et al. Management of arterial occlusive disease following radiation therapy. Cardiovasc Surg 1996;4:135–42.
15. Phillips GR, Peer RM, Upson JF, et al. Late complications of revascularization for radiation-induced arterial disease. J Vasc Surg 1992;16:921–5.
16. Gosselin C, Walker PM. Subclavian steal syndrome: existence, clinical features, diagnosis and management. Semin Vasc Surg 1996;9:93–7.
17. Fields WS, Lemak NA. Joint Study of Extracranial Arterial Occlusion: VII. Subclavian steal – a review of 168 cases. JAMA 1972;222:1139–43.
18. Akers DL, Markowitz IA, Kerstein MD. The value of aortic arch study in the evaluation of cerebrovascular insufficiency. Am J Surg 1987;154:230–2.
19. McLaren JT, Donaghue CC, Drenzer AD. Accuracy of carotid duplex examination to predict proximal and intrathoracic lesions. Am J Surg 1996;172:149–50.
20. Kadwa AM, Robbs JV, Abdool-Carrim AT. Aortic arch angiography prior to carotid endarterectomy. Is its continued use justified? Eur J Vasc Endovasc Surg 1997;13:527–30.
21. Executive Committee for ACAS. Endarterectomy for asymptomatic carotid artery stenosis. JAMA 1995;273:1421–8.
22. Johnston DCC, Chapman K, Goldstein LB. Low rate of complications of cerebral angiography in routine clinical practice. Neurology 2001;57:2012–4.
23. Yucel EK, Anderson CM, Edelman RR, et al. Magnetic resonance angiography: update on applications for extracranial arteries. Circulation 1999;100:2284–301.
24. Carpenter JP, Holland GA, Golden MA, et al. Magnetic resonance angiography of the aortic arch. J Vasc Surg 1997;25:145–51.
25. Prince MR, Narasimham DL, Jacoby WT, et al. Three-dimensional gadolinium-enhanced MR angiography of the thoracic aorta. AJR Am J Roentgenol 1996;166:1387–97.
26. Randoux B, Marro B, Koskas F, et al. Carotid artery stenosis: prospective comparison of CT, three-dimensional gadolinium enhanced MR, and conventional angiography. Radiology 2001;220:179–85.
27. Sakopoulos AG, Ballard JL, Gundry SR. Minimally invasive approach for aortic arch branch vessel reconstruction. J Vasc Surg 2000;31:200–2.
28. Azakie A, McElhinney DB, Hagashima R, et al. Innominate artery reconstruction: over 3 decades of experience. Ann Vasc Surg 1998;228:402–10.
29. Sharma BK, Jain S, Bali HK, et al. A follow-up study of balloon angioplasty and de-novo stenting in Takayasu's arteritis. Int J Cardiol 2000;75:S147–52.
30. Duber C, Klose KJ, Kopp H, Schmiedt W. Percutaneous transluminal angioplasty for occlusion of the subclavian artery: short and long-term results. Cardiovasc Intervent Radiol 1992;15:205–10.
31. Farina C, Mingoli A, Schultz RD, et al. Percutaneous transluminal angioplasty versus surgery for subclavian artery occlusive disease. Am J Surg 1989;158:511–4.
32. AbuRahma AF, Robinson PA, Jennings TG. Carotid-subclavian bypass grafting with polytetrafluoroethylene grafts for symptomatic subclavian artery stenosis or occlusion: a 20-year experience. J Vasc Surg 2000;32:411–9.
33. Perler BA, Williams GM. Carotid-subclavian bypass – a decade of experience. J Vasc Surg 1990;12:716–23.
34. Synn AY, Chalmers RTA, Sharp WJ, et al. Is there a conduit of preference for a bypass between the carotid and subclavian arteries? Am J Surg 1993;166:157–62.
35. Vitti MJ, Thompson BW, Read RC, et al. Carotid-subclavian bypass: a twenty-two year experience. J Vasc Surg 1994;20:411–8.
36. Rosenthal D, Ellison RG, Clark MD, et al. Axilloaxillary bypass: is it worthwhile? J Cardiovasc Surg 1988;29:191–5.
37. Schanzer H, Chung-Loy H, Kotok M, et al. Evaluation of axillo-axillary artery bypass for the treatment of subclavian or innominate artery occlusive disease. J Cardiovasc Surg 1987;28:258–61.
38. Weiner RI, Deterling RA, Sentissi J, O'Donnell TF. Subclavian artery insufficiency: treatment with axilloaxillary bypass. Arch Surg 1987;876–80.
39. Selby JB, Matsumoto AH, Tegtmeyer CJ, et al. Balloon angioplasty above the aortic arch: immediate and long-term results. AJR Am J Roentgenol 1993;160:631–5.

40. Marques KMJ, Ernst SMPG, Mast EG, et al. Percutaneous transluminal angioplasty of the left subclavian artery to prevent or treat the coronary-subclavian steal syndrome. Am J Cardiol 1996;78:687–90.

41. Sullivan TM, Gray BH, Bacharach JM, et al. Angioplasty and primary stenting of the subclavian, innominate, and common carotid arteries in 83 patients. J Vasc Surg 1998;28:1059–65.

42. Queral LA, Criado FJ. The treatment of focal aortic arch branch lesions with Palmaz stents. J Vasc Surg 1996;23:368–75.

43. Hebrang A, Maskovic J, Tomac B. Percutaneous transluminal angioplasty of the subclavian arteries: long-term results in 52 patients. AJR Am J Roentgenol 1991;156:1091–4.

44. Ruebben A, Tettoni S, Muratore P, et al. Feasibility of intraoperative balloon angioplasty and additional stent placement of isolated stenosis of the brachiocephalic trunk. J Thorac Cardiovasc Surg 1998;115:1316–20.

45. Tyagi S, Verma PK, Gambhir DS, et al. Early and long-term results of subclavian angioplasty in aortitis (Takayasu disease): comparison with atherosclerosis. Cardiovasc Intervent Radiol 1998;21:218–24.

46. Melliere D, Becquemin JP, Berrahal D, et al. Management of radiation-induced occlusive arterial disease: a reassessment. J Cardiovasc Surg 1997;38:261–9.

CHAPTER
35

Surgery for Vertebrobasilar Insufficiency

Edouard Kieffer

KEY POINTS

- Anatomic variations of the vertebral artery (VA) are common and most of them are clinically relevant.

- Atherosclerotic lesions of the VA are often bilateral and may be associated with lesions of the carotid bifurcations or intrathoracic great vessels which significantly affect the pathophysiology of symptoms and the surgical choices.

- Extrinsic compressions of the VA are anatomically frequent, although they do not always have a clinical expression.

- Studies using strict criteria for vertebrobasilar transient ischemic attack (TIA) have shown a 5-year stroke rate of 22–35%, very similar to that of carotid TIA.

- Hemodynamic compromise of the posterior circulation is the primary cause of vertebrobasilar insufficiency (VBI).

- The hindbrain is particularly susceptible to ischemia.

- Reconstruction of the VA may be indicated in three circumstances, of decreasing clinical importance: VBI, concomitant carotid artery disease, and anatomic indications.

- Surgery for thromboembolic VBI should be considered only in patients with TIAs or a small residual deficit.

- The indications for surgery in hemodynamic VBI are quite different: (1) in the presence of significant carotid artery disease, (2) if medical treatment of incapacitating VBI has been unsuccessful.

- The relationship between clinical symptoms and certain positions of the head and neck should lead to the performance of positional arteriograms.

- Reconstruction of the VA is now possible at the level of any of its four segments.

- The technique of choice for proximal VA reconstruction is transposition of the VA into the common carotid artery.

- Clinical and anatomic results of VA reconstructions have been very satisfactory in the most recently reported series.

Although more than 40 years have elapsed since the first surgical repairs of proximal vertebral artery (VA) disease,[1,2] VA surgery has not been widely accepted, neither among neurologists nor by many vascular surgeons. However, renewed interest has recently arisen among several groups of workers, who have reported series of operated patients with logical indications and good results.[3–23]

Several reasons may explain these difficulties:

- there has been a lot of controversy about the definition of and criteria for 'vertebrobasilar insufficiency' (VBI), some neurologists still questioning its individuality as a syndrome;

- investigators have noticed in some patients an apparent lack of correlation between clinical manifestations and arterial lesions seen at angiography;

- although occipital, cerebellar, or brainstem infarcts due to vertebral and basilar artery disease have been described precisely for several decades, the prognosis of vertebrobasilar transient ischemic attacks (TIAs) has long been wrongly considered of a benign nature, especially in comparison with those occurring in the carotid territory;

- angiography of the VA has long suffered a bad reputation due to complications related to the nature of contrast media and direct injections into the VA; and

- besides being limited to the first segment of the artery, VA surgery was deemed difficult and was complicated by a significant number of failures caused by postoperative occlusions.

This chapter will attempt to discuss each of the above-mentioned points and present a logical, comprehensive approach to the problems of VA lesions, VBI, and VA reconstruction. It will emphasize the wide spectrum of anatomic lesions, the pathophysiology of symptoms, the rationale for surgical indications, as well as the feasibility and safety of VA reconstruction at all levels of the cervical and intracranial courses of the artery.

SURGICAL ANATOMY

The rather complicated anatomic course of the VA may be conveniently divided into four consecutive segments (**Fig. 35.1**).[24,25] The first segment (V1) is in the medial part of the supra-clavicular fossa from the subclavian artery to the bony canal of the transverse process of C6. The second segment (V2) runs vertically on the lateral side of the cervical spine, passing through the bony canals from C6 to C2. The third segment (V3) curves laterally and then medially around C1 into the atlanto-occipital membrane. The fourth segment (V4) has a short intracranial course towards the opposite VA, forming the basilar artery on the anterior aspect of the brainstem.

Cervical branches of the VA arise exclusively from the V2 and V3 segments. Besides small muscular, osteoarticular, and meningeal branches, radicular arteries follow each of the cervical nerve roots. Some of them – the radiculospinal arteries – may participate in the arterial supply to the spinal cord together with branches originating from other collaterals of the subclavian artery. Intracranial branches, arising from the V4 segment, include the spinal arteries (anterior and posterior) and the posteroinferior

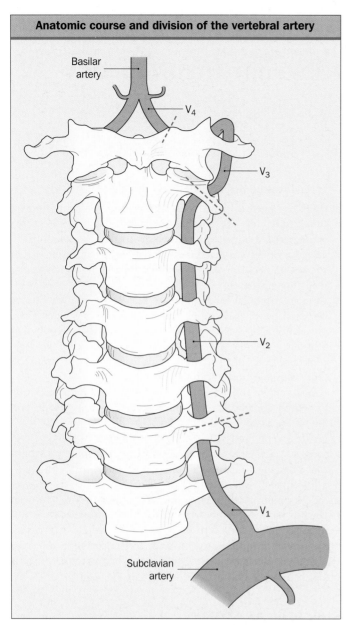

Anatomic course and division of the vertebral artery

Basilar artery

V4

V3

V2

V1

Subclavian artery

Figure 35.1 Anatomic course and division into four consecutive segments of the vertebral artery running from the subclavian artery (SCA) to the basilar artery (BA).

cerebellar artery (PICA), which is the largest collateral branch of the VA.

Anatomic variations of the VA are common and most of them are clinically relevant. The left VA originates from the aortic arch in 6–10% of individuals. In the majority of cases (around 60%), the VAs are not symmetrical ('equivalent'), with one large ('dominant') artery, usually the left, and a small ('minor') contralateral artery. While penetration into the bony canal occurs in C6 in 90% of cases, it is either lower (C7) or higher (C5 to C3) in the remaining 10%. The basilar artery may originate only from the dominant VA, while the minor one ends into the ipsilateral PICA. In such cases, the ipsilateral posterior cerebral artery usually originates from the internal carotid artery. Finally, embryological carotid-basilar anastomoses may persist in a small number of individuals.[26] The most common are the trigeminal

and hypoglossal arteries. These abnormal anastomoses are usually associated with small VA and hypoplasia or atresia of one or both posterior communicating arteries.

ANATOMIC LESIONS

Each of the four segments of the VA may be affected by a variety of diseases. Intrinsic, parietal, diseases do not differ in nature from those observed in other parts of the body. Extrinsic compressions by bony, muscular, or fibrous elements are more specific of the VA pathology and will therefore be studied in some detail.

Intrinsic disease
Atherosclerotic disease
Atherosclerotic lesions are commonly located at the origin of the VA. They are usually in continuity with lesions of the subclavian artery and remain limited to the first centimeter of the artery, except in a few hypertensive, diabetic, or elderly patients. A post-stenotic dilatation may be present in cases with tight stenosis. In contradistinction to the usual carotid plaques, intimal ulceration, with or without mural thrombosis, is rarely present. Most plaques of the VA, whether fibrous or calcified, have a smooth surface without intimal damage.[27]

Atherosclerotic disease of the intracranial (V4) segment is second in frequency. It may be associated with lesions of the basilar artery and its branches, emphasizing the need for complete angiographic visualization of both extracranial and intracranial vessels.

The V2 segment is rarely affected by atherosclerotic disease, except in patients with cervical irradiation. Of utmost surgical importance is the fact that the V3 segment is usually spared from atherosclerosis.[28–30]

Atherosclerotic lesions of the VA are often bilateral and may be associated with lesions of the carotid bifurcations or intrathoracic great vessels which significantly affect the pathophysiology of symptoms and the surgical choices.

Fibromuscular disease
Fibromuscular disease is much less common than atherosclerotic disease. It usually affects the V2 and/or V3 segments.[31,32] The most common aspect is that of 'strings of beads' with or without an excess in length resulting in buckling or kinking of the artery. Dysplastic aneurysms are much rarer. Fibromuscular disease of the VA may be complicated by dissection, arteriovenous (AV) fistula, or thromboembolic manifestations. Associated disease of the internal carotid artery is nearly constant. Intracranial berry aneurysms are found in a small number of patients. Renal and visceral arteries, as visualized by panarteriography, may also be affected.

Arteritis
Takayasu's disease is a non-specific aortoarteritis that affects mainly the intrathoracic great vessels and subclavian-axillary arteries.[33] Except for its origin from the subclavian artery, the VA is usually spared by arteritis. It may in fact enlarge considerably in cases with bilateral lesions of the carotid arteries and thus become the main arterial supply to the brain. Extensive occlusions of the VA in Takayasu's disease are usually due to secondary thrombosis and not to the disease itself.

Giant cell (temporal) arteritis may affect the vertebral artery in a small number of cases.[34]

Trauma

Although routine arteriography for stable patients with penetrating neck trauma may disclose more lesions of the VA than are usually acknowledged, penetrating trauma to the VA remains a rarity.[35–39] Its initial consequences are usually minimal and patients may remain clinically silent. A self-containing cervical hematoma may compress and occlude the VA or lead to a false aneurysm.[40] AV fistulas are frequent due to the close relationship between the VA and its surrounding venous plexus.

Blunt trauma to the VA may affect the V2 segment in conjunction with fractures or dislocations of the spine.[41,42] More often the V3 segment will be the site of traumatic lesions secondary to hyperextension and rotation of the cervical spine resulting from accidental trauma or cervical manipulation with forceful stretching of the VA.[43] Complete or subadventitial rupture occurs rarely. The usual lesion is purely intimal and may lead to thromboembolic complications with or without a traumatic dissection of the VA.

Iatrogenic trauma usually complicates direct puncture following attempts at carotid arteriography or catheterization of the internal jugular vein.[44] An AV fistula is the usual consequence of such trauma. Trauma to the VA has also been reported following surgery of the cervical spine.[45]

Spontaneous aneurysms, dissections, and AV fistulas

Spontaneous aneurysms[46–50] and dissections[51–57] are rare lesions that usually affect the V3 segment. Most of them are dysplastic in origin and complicate fibromuscular disease, Ehlers–Danlos syndrome, or neurofibromatosis.

Spontaneous AV fistulas are at least as common as traumatic AV fistulas.[58,59] They are usually located in the V2–V3 segments. Although they may complicate fibromuscular disease, spontaneous AV fistulas, whether single or multiple, are usually congenital in nature. AV malformations are complex lesions that develop in the cervical soft tissues and muscles. In addition to arterial supply from the VA, they are usually fed by other cervical arteries originating from the subclavian and external carotid arteries.

Extrinsic disease (compressions)

Close relations of the VA with the cervical spine and fibromuscular elements account for the possibility of extrinsic compressions that are specific of VA disease and which may affect any of the different segments of the artery.[60–64]

The normal VA is tightly attached to several anatomic elements:

- the sympathetic chain with the stellate ganglion completely surrounding the proximal VA in the supraclavicular fossa;
- in the V2–V3 segments, the VA is fixed by its adventitia to the periosteum of each transverse foramen and, at the top of the spine, to the upper aspect of the atlas; and
- finally, the VA is tightly fixed to the atlanto-occipital membrane as it crosses this structure to enter the dura mater.

The normal VA thus has a certain mobility between these points of fixation:

- in the V1 segment, on each side of the stellate ganglion; and
- in the V2–V3 segments, between each vertebra.

In the V2 segment, the corresponding cervical spine allows only for limited flexion, extension, rotation, and lateral inclination. In sharp contrast, the VA around C1 and C2 is a very mobile segment, with an excess in arterial length that has been described as a 'safety buckle', allowing for an adaptation of the VA to the considerable amplitude of motion in this area, especially during rotation of the neck.

Extrinsic compressions of the VA are anatomically frequent, although they do not always have a clinical expression. They may appear late in life due to progressive degenerative disc disease, elevation of the aortic arch and lengthening of the subclavian artery due to age or hypertension. While some of these compressions may be permanent, most appear or worsen during extreme positions of the neck (rotation, lateral inclination, flexion, and extension).[65,66] The arterial consequences of such compressions vary according to the nature, length, and degree of compression. Although the VA may remain normal for years, tight and long-standing compressions may lead to intimal damage with an attending risk of thromboembolic complications.[67–69]

A list of the most significant elements of compression with their topography according to each segment of the VA and their trigger position is indicated in **Table 35.1**. Although there are many causes of extrinsic compression of the VA,[16,18,60,61,63,67,69–79] two of them deserve special emphasis because of their frequency and clinical importance.

Cervical spondylosis is a classic and frequent cause of VA compression in the bony canal of the transverse processes.[60,67,69,72,79] Compression is usually limited to one or two of the lower cervical vertebrae (C4 to C6). The two main factors that contribute to disturbances in VA flow are:

- osteolytic proliferation of the uncinate processes, which pushes the VA towards the back and the outside of its normal pathway; and
- shortening of the cervical spine due to degenerative disc disease, which produces an excess in length between each transverse process.

The VA compression is progressive and leads to gentle curving of the artery, provided the neck remains in a neutral position. When the neck rotates ipsilaterally, the vertebral interspace tends to become shorter, and tight stenosis or even complete occlusion of the VA may appear (**Fig. 35.2**).

Compression of the VA at the normal V1–V2 junction in C6 has been described for a long time.[74] The VA may be compressed at the cross insertion of hypertrophic or laterally displaced muscular or tendinous fibers of the longus colli and anterior scalene muscles that insert on the transverse process of the C6 vertebra.[71,73] The compression is usually intermittent and triggered by rotation of the neck. When the V1–V2 junction is at an abnormally located level, extrinsic muscular compressions are more frequent and may be permanent (**Fig. 35.3**) or intermittent.[63] The usual trigger position is hyperextension of the neck because of the abnormal arterial pathway: perpendicular or hairpin turn in abnormally low (C7) penetration; tight and S-shaped in abnormally high (C5 to C3) penetration.

PATHOPHYSIOLOGY OF VERTEBROBASILAR INSUFFICIENCY

Postmortem studies and clinical evaluation of patients with VBI have identified two different pathologic mechanisms: thromboembolism and hemodynamic compromise.[63,80–83] Although these

Elements compressing vertebral artery in the neck.		
Segment	*Elements of compression*	*Trigger position*
V1	Stellate ganglion Fibrous band Anterior scalene muscle (with or without thoracic outlet syndrome)	Ipsilateral rotation and lateral inclination of the neck Same as above and lateral inclination of the neck Hyperabduction of the arm
V1–V2 junction	Insertion of longus colli and anterior scalene muscle on C6 Abnormal entrance into the bony canal: – high (C5–C3) – low (C7)	Rotation of the neck Hyperextension of the neck Same as above and hyperflexion of neck
V2	Cervical spondylosis Cervical spine trauma Neural or bony tumor	Ipsilateral rotation of the neck
V3	Extraosseous course of the VA Anterior branch of C2 nerve Hypermotility of C1–C2 joint Bony canal of the upper aspect of C1	Contralateral rotation of the neck Same as above Same as above Hyperextension of the neck
V3–V4	Foramen of the atlanto-occipital membrane Bony abnormalities of the atlanto-occipital joint	Hyperextension or hyperflexion of the neck Same as above

Table 35.1 Elements compressing vertebral artery in the neck.

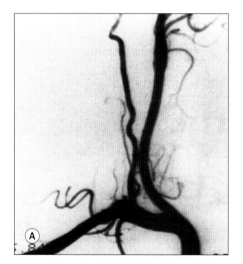

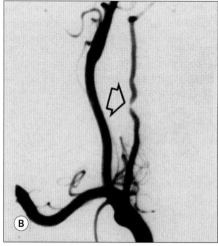

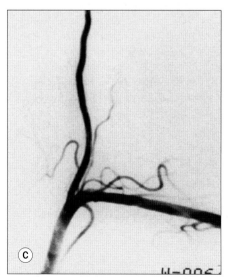

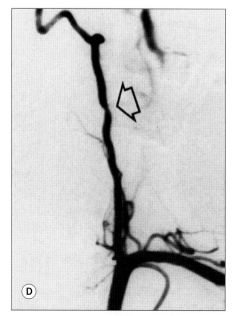

Figure 35.2 Bilateral compression of equivalent vertebral arteries due to spondylosis. While the vertebral arteries are widely patent in neutral positions of the neck (A, C), tight stenosis is apparent on both sides (open arrows) during ipsilateral rotations of the neck (B, D).

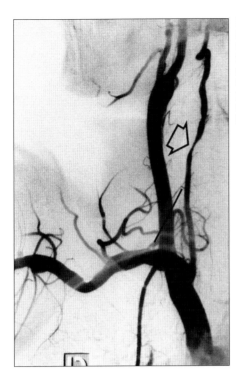

Figure 35.3 Abnormally high penetration of the vertebral artery into the transverse foramen of C4 with tight stenosis due to permanent compression (open arrow).

two mechanisms may combine in a few patients, they are usually caused by different anatomic lesions, account for different clinical manifestations, and have different prognostic implications.

Thromboembolic VBI

Although it is the least frequently involved, thromboembolism may occur in the vertebrobasilar territory much in the same way as it occurs in the carotid territory.[84]

Atherosclerosis does not play a major role in this mechanism because of the usually smooth nature of the atherosclerotic plaques of the VA. Non-atherosclerotic lesions, especially traumatic or spontaneous aneurysms or dissections, are the most frequent etiologies, due to the frequency of intimal disease and the possibility of mural thrombus formation in such lesions.[67,69]

Because of the anatomy of the basilar artery and its branches, most large emboli stop at the top of the basilar artery or in one or both of the posterior cerebral arteries (**Fig. 35.4**). They produce severe and different neurologic complications that have been described under the term 'top of the basilar syndrome'.[82] The smallest emboli may produce TIAs that usually last several hours or RINDs in which neurologic symptoms may take several days to a few weeks to disappear.

The distal end of the occlusions may reach different levels depending on anatomic, hemodynamic, and rheologic factors. Four types of VA occlusion may be distinguished. Segmental VA occlusions with revascularization at the C1–C2 level through the 'occipital connection'[28,29,63,83] are the most favorable (**Fig. 35.5**). They are usually well compensated by collateral circulation and thus remain accessible to surgical reconstruction by means of a distal bypass. Occlusions may also extend intracranially up to the origin of the PICA, which remains patent through the opposite VA. Such segmental VA occlusions are compatible with absent or minimal neurologic complications.[85,86] In more extensive occlusions that involve the origin of the PICA or the basilar artery itself, neurologic complications are usually severe, ranging from

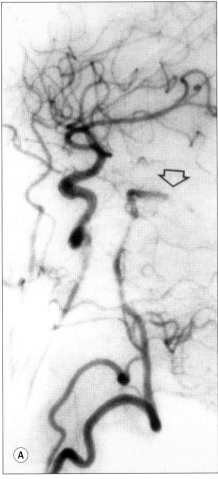

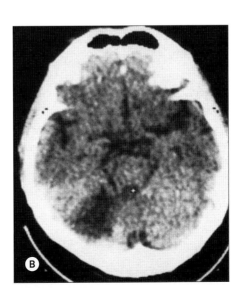

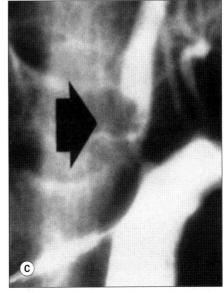

Figure 35.4 Embolic occlusion of the posterior cerebral artery (A) **(open arrow) causing large infarction of the occipital lobe** (B) **in a patient with tight stenosis and mural thrombus of the proximal vertebral artery** (C) **(black arrow).**

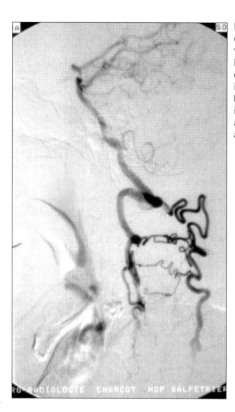

Figure 35.5 Segmental occlusion of the vertebral artery. Patency of the distal cervical vertebral artery is maintained through branches of the ipsilateral subclavian and external carotid arteries.

variety of factors that may be classified into four main categories (**Table 35.2**).

Anatomic factors

The posterior circulation has two anatomic peculiarities that must be considered in the discussion of hemodynamic VBI. First, the basilar artery is normally formed by the union of the two VAs. The direct consequence of this fact is that, provided it is of sufficient diameter, one patent VA is usually enough to ensure satisfactory blood flow to the basilar artery.[3,5,63] The anatomic requisites for hemodynamic VBI are thus either bilateral VA disease or unilateral VA disease with contralateral absent or hypoplastic VA or a small contralateral VA ending in the PICA without participating in the formation of the basilar artery (**Fig. 35.6**). These anatomic situations logically constitute the only justified indications for VA reconstruction in hemodynamic VBI.

The second factor to be considered is the continuity of the normal basilar artery with the anterior circulation through the posterior elements of the circle of Willis, namely both posterior communicating arteries. The two anatomic factors that may therefore increase potential for VBI are:

- associated carotid artery disease, a finding that is particularly frequent in atherosclerotic patients; and
- congenital absence or hypoplasia of the posterior communicating artery on one or both sides, a finding that is present in approximately 30% of normal individuals (**Fig. 35.7**).

However, these factors are not constantly present in the most severe and indisputable hemodynamic VBI, owing to the combined influence of other factors that are discussed below. They will therefore not be considered as being indispensable to a justified surgical indication for hemodynamic VBI.

Susceptibility of the hindbrain to ischemia

The hindbrain is particularly susceptible to ischemia.[98] There are three main reasons for this. The first is a competition between flow coming from the vertebrobasilar system and that coming from the carotid system through the posterior communicating arteries.[8] This 'dead point' located somewhere in the middle part of the basilar artery varies according to local factors affecting vertebrobasilar flow (such as extrinsic compression) and this may be responsible for rapid variations in brainstem perfusion.[96] This accounts for the apparently paradoxical fact that patency of

limited latero-medullary or cerebellar infarcts to massive infarction of the brainstem. The clinical picture of these vertebrobasilar infarctions has been fully and precisely described for several decades in the classic neurologic literature.[87–89]

Although complete or near complete clinical recovery occurs in about 50% of patients with vertebrobasilar strokes, the early mortality remains as high as 20% to 30%,[90–92] which is significantly more than for carotid strokes. The prognosis for thromboembolic TIA is probably not as good as is usually believed. Studies using strict criteria for vertebrobasilar TIA have shown a 22% to 35% 5-year stroke rate, very similar to that of carotid TIA.[93–95]

Hemodynamic VBI

Hemodynamic compromise of the posterior circulation is the primary cause of VBI.[8,63,82–84,96–98] It is usually explained by a

Factors compromising vertebral artery flow.		
	Contributing factors	*Management*
Watershed ischemia	Hindbrain	Carotid reconstruction
Autoregulation disturbances	Alpha-blocking medication	Stop drug
Obstruction (permanent or transient)	Vertebral arteries	VA reconstruction
Anemia, hypoxemia, thrombocytosis, polycythemia	Blood	Medical treatment
Orthostatic hypotension	Systemic pressure	Medical treatment
Cardiac failure, rhythm disturbances, AV conduction defects	Heart	Medical treatment, pacemaker implantation

Table 35.2 Factors compromising vertebral artery flow.

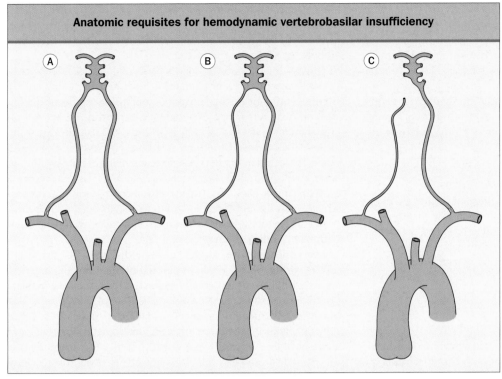

Anatomic requisites for hemodynamic vertebrobasilar insufficiency

Figure 35.6 Anatomic requisites for hemodynamic vertebrobasilar insufficiency: (A) bilateral vertebral artery disease; (B) unilateral vertebral artery disease with a contralateral absent or hypoplastic vertebral artery; or (C) a small contralateral vertebral artery ending in the posteroinferior cerebellar artery without participating in the formation of the basilar artery.

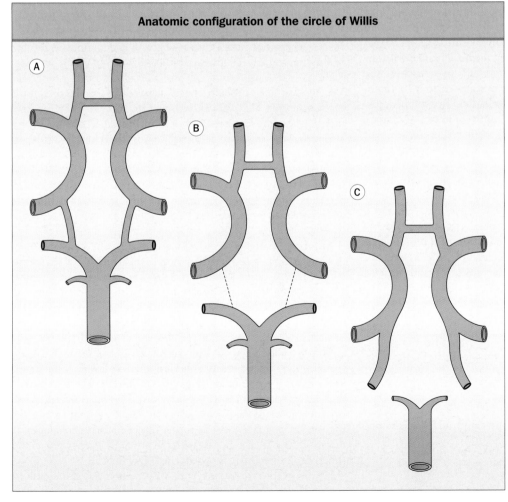

Anatomic configuration of the circle of Willis

Figure 35.7 Anatomic configuration of the circle of Willis. A normal configuration (A) is present in only half of the general population. The most common variations include absence or hypoplasia of one or both of the posterior communicating arteries (B) and origin of one or both of the posterior cerebral arteries from the carotid arteries (C).

both posterior communicating arteries is not a protection against VBI. Second, the branches of the basilar artery that perfuse the brainstem are small, terminal arteries, a situation that favors the appearance of watershed ischemia. This also explains why the vestibular nucleus, which is fed by very long, small, and terminal arteries, is one of the most frequently ischemic structures in patients with hemodynamic VBI. And third, elderly people, especially if hypertensive or diabetic, tend to have poor cerebral autoregulation,[96] a fact that often accounts for the failure of local compensatory mechanisms.

Cardiac and peripheral hemodynamic factors

Cardiac function is obviously an important factor in hemo-dynamic VBI. Low cardiac output due to cardiac insufficiency, rhythm disturbances, or atrioventricular conduction defects may lower total cerebral blood flow. Similarly, patients with postural (orthostatic) hypotension, either spontaneous or due to medication, also have a tendency to decrease vertebrobasilar blood flow.

Rheologic factors

Anemia, hypoxemia, thrombocytosis, polycythemia, and hyper-lipemia are also well known contributors to tissue ischemia and may aggravate hemodynamic VBI. Although one of these five factors may largely predominate in an individual patient, they usually combine in different manners to cause hemodynamic VBI.[80] In these cases, symptoms are of short duration and repetitive. They affect mainly the territories that are fed by long terminal arteries. This fact accounts for the nearly constant vestibular symptoms in hemodynamic VBI, due to the fact that vestibulo-labyrinthine arteries are long, terminal branches arising in the mid-portion of the basilar artery in the vicinity of the hemodynamic dead point. Other symptoms related to brain-stem or cerebellar ischemia are due similarly to hypoperfusion in watershed areas of the cerebellum, brainstem nuclei, reticulate substance, long motor or sensory tracts of the brainstem, or upper part of the medulla. Ischemia of the occipital lobe is frequent when posterior cerebral arteries act as terminal arteries, i.e. in the absence of functioning posterior communicating arteries.

The prognosis of hemodynamic VBI seems to be relatively good. Although the daily repetition of TIAs may become a functional and social handicap, vertebrobasilar strokes are rather rare in this setting. However, the repetition of TIAs and the presence of symptoms related to ischemia of the long tracts of the brainstem should be considered as ominous manifestations and harbingers of vertebrobasilar strokes.

In our opinion, the clinical and prognostic differences between thromboembolic and hemodynamic vertebrobasilar TIAs are of utmost importance and have not been clearly appreciated in the literature.

SURGICAL INDICATIONS

Reconstruction of the VA may be indicated in three circum-stances of decreasing clinical importance:[62,63,99]

- VBI;
- concomitant carotid artery disease; and
- anatomic indications.

Vertebrobasilar insufficiency

VBI is by far the most common indication for reconstruction of the VA. The rationale for operation is different in thrombo-embolic as opposed to hemodynamic VBI.

Surgery for thromboembolic VBI should be considered only in patients with TIAs or a small residual deficit. It is aimed at the prevention of further thromboembolic events. Even though the contralateral VA may be widely patent, the presence of an embolic source is a logical indication for surgical treatment using either a direct reconstruction or a distal bypass excluding the lesion.[63] Occlusion of the VA is an indication for surgery only in cases with limited distal extension, leaving the V3 segment accessible for bypass.[28] In patients with more extensive occlusions, surgery may be indicated in order to reconstruct a large con-tralateral stenotic VA and therefore to avoid bilateral occlusion with its attending risk of stroke.

The indications for surgery in hemodynamic VBI are quite different (**Fig. 35.8**). We have developed the following practical approach.[63] The patient is fully evaluated for associated medical problems and the presence of significant carotid artery disease. Maximal treatment of medical problems is undertaken and a specific medical treatment of VBI, including antiplatelet and alpha-blocking drugs, is prescribed. Medical management is successful in a good number of patients. Four-vessel arteriography is indicated only in suitable surgical candidates:

- in the presence of significant carotid artery disease, with or without symptoms; or
- if medical treatment of incapacitating VBI has been unsuc-cessful in a patient without significant carotid artery disease.

Four situations may arise according to the degree of VA disease, the association of carotid artery disease, and the possibility for reconstruction of the diseased carotid and vertebral arteries. Patients with significant, reconstructible carotid artery and VA disease have usually been treated by isolated carotid reconstruction.[100–103] VA reconstruction was performed a few months later if symptoms of VBI persisted. Although many attempts have been made at predicting the clinical results of isolated carotid operations, this usually has not been possible. Failure to cure the symptoms of VBI has been noted in 30–50% of patients. Associated carotid and vertebral reconstructions in the same operative session solve the problem with a minimal added operative risk and therefore should be performed more widely.[104,105]

Secondly, patients with VBI and significant carotid artery disease and non-significant or non-reconstructible VA disease should have a carotid reconstruction whether or not they have carotid symptoms. This situation may arise in the rare patient with diffuse non-reconstructible VA occlusions or more fre-quently in patients with bilateral, small hypoplastic VA, charac-teristic of hypoplasia of the vertebrobasilar arterial system.

Thirdly, patients with VBI, significant VA lesions, and non-significant or non-reconstructible carotid artery lesions should have isolated VA reconstruction (**Figs 35.9 & 35.10**). The presence of non-reconstructible carotid artery disease (such as extensive common and internal carotid artery occlusion or tight stenosis of the carotid siphon) may lead to the use of unusual techniques of reconstruction such as bypass with the proximal anastomosis in the subclavian or external carotid arteries (**Fig. 35.11**).

Finally, in the rare patients with VBI and non-significant or non-reconstructible lesions of both the vertebral and carotid arteries,

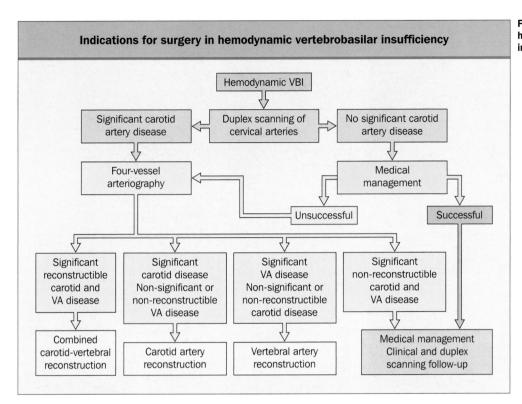

Figure 35.8 Indications for surgery in hemodynamic vertebrobasilar insufficiency (VBI). VA, vertebral artery.

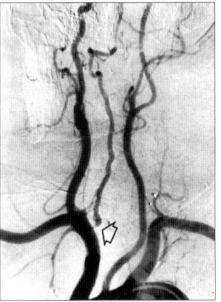

Figure 35.9 Isolated vertebral artery reconstruction. Indication for a vertebral artery reconstruction is logical in this patient with hemodynamic vertebrobasilar insufficiency, absence of the left vertebral artery, tight stenosis of the right proximal vertebral artery (open arrow), and non-significant carotid artery disease.

maximal medical management is the only available therapeutic modality.

In each of these cases with hemodynamic VBI, VA reconstruction should be limited to the large 'dominant' VA; very few patients, if any, need bilateral reconstructions. It should, however, be recognized that one or both of the VA occlusive lesions may not be evident on standard arteriograms because of its positional nature. The relationship between clinical symptoms and certain positions of the head and neck should lead to the performance of positional arteriograms under local anesthesia with the patient in the sitting position.

Carotid artery disease without VBI

In the absence of VBI, VA lesions combined with carotid artery disease may become an indication for VA reconstruction in two circumstances. Both of these indications have solely hemodynamic justification and apply only to large, dominant VA.

VA reconstruction may be combined with carotid endarterectomy during the same operation.[4,62] This may be performed with a minimal added morbidity and has the same rationale as simultaneous reconstruction of significant though asymptomatic lesions of the renal or visceral arteries in the course of aortoiliac reconstructions.

More importantly, patients with non-reconstructible carotid artery lesions such as extensive internal carotid artery occlusions without a stenosis of the external carotid artery may be benefitted by the reconstruction of a large diseased VA.[106,107] This may dramatically increase hemispheric cerebral blood flow to a much greater extent than extracranial-intracranial anastomoses do, and possibly prevent the appearance or recurrence of hemispheric TIAs or strokes.

Anatomic indications

Finally, VA reconstruction may be indicated in a few asymptomatic patients with isolated VA disease:

- to prevent thromboembolic complications in patients with severe bilateral VA disease;
- to treat AV fistulas or malformations – often in conjunction with interventional radiologic procedures;[59] or
- to allow the removal of bony or nervous tumors in proximity to the VA.[62,63,108,109]

In the majority of these patients, a distal bypass to the V3 segment, excluding the proximal part of the VA, allows surgical management or embolization of the proximal lesion.[39]

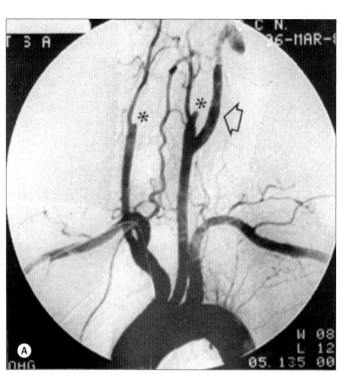

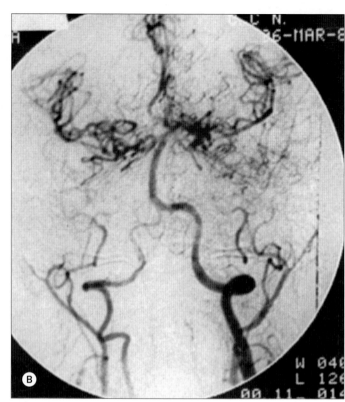

Figure 35.10 Distal vertebral artery reconstruction (open arrow) in a patient with bilateral internal carotid occlusion. Both hemispheres are supplied by the vertebral bypass through the basilar artery and both posterior communicating arteries.

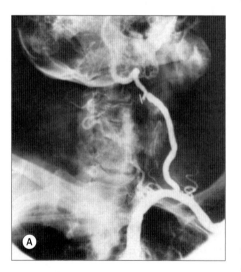

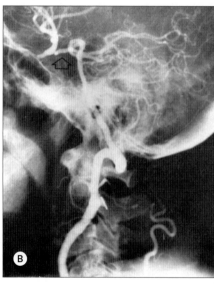

Figure 35.11 Subclavian artery to distal vertebral artery bypass using autogenous saphenous vein graft in a patient with occlusion of the ipsilateral common and internal carotid arteries. The basilar artery supplies the ipsilateral carotid territory through the posterior communicating artery (open arrow).

RECONSTRUCTIVE TECHNIQUES

Reconstruction of the VA is now possible at the level of any of its four segments. The techniques have been described extensively in the literature[18,62,99,110,111] and thus will be only briefly discussed here.

Surgery of the V1 segment

Approach is either through a transverse supraclavicular incision with dissociation of both heads of the sternomastoid muscle or through a low pre-sternomastoid incision. The VA is approached between the common carotid artery and the internal jugular vein, with the vagus nerve being left adjacent to the vein. Lymphatic elements, including the thoracic duct on the left side, and the vertebral vein are carefully divided and cut in order to avoid a postoperative lymphatic drainage. The VA is then exposed along with the sympathetic chain and the stellate ganglion, which should be preserved in order to avoid a postoperative Horner's syndrome.

Atherosclerotic lesions at the origin of the VA have been treated using closed (trans-subclavian) or open endarterectomy with good results.[22] We seldom use this technique because:

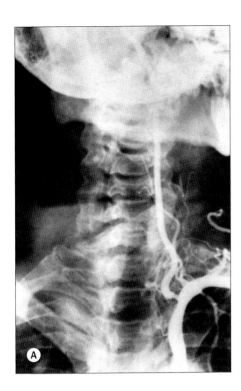
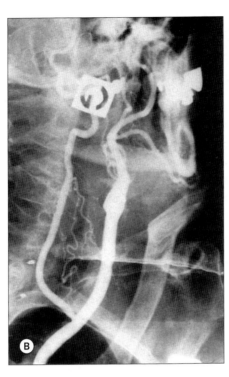

Figure 35.12 Tight stenosis of the proximal vertebral artery (A) treated by transposition into the common carotid artery (B). While neglecting moderate subclavian artery disease, this procedure is facilitated by an excessive length of the first segment of the vertebral artery.

- it needs complete exposure of the proximal subclavian and its branches;
- it may lead to an extensive endarterectomy of the subclavian artery, which may necessitate distal tacking sutures;
- it does not take into account the frequent excess in length of the V1 segment, which may lead to postoperative kinking of the VA; and
- it entails the risk of a distal intimal flap in the VA, which may be the cause of postoperative stenosis or occlusion.

Similarly, transposition into, or venous bypass from, the distal subclavian artery[3] are rather complicated procedures since they necessitate complete dissection of the subclavian artery. Moreover, their late results may be compromised by progression of atherosclerotic disease in the subclavian artery itself. In our opinion, these two techniques should be considered only when the ipsilateral common carotid artery is not usable because of occlusion or advanced mural atherosclerosis, severe siphon stenosis, or advanced contralateral carotid occlusive disease, making clamping impossible or potentially dangerous.

The technique of choice for proximal VA reconstruction is transposition of the VA into the common carotid artery (**Fig. 35.12**).[9–11,15,62,99,110–112] It is a simple procedure that necessitates only limited exposure of the proximal VA and adjacent common carotid artery. It has the advantage of completely neglecting the lesions of the subclavian artery. It allows for simultaneous management of excessive length of the VA. Lastly, progression of atherosclerotic disease is seldom encountered in the common carotid artery on late follow-up. Requirements for this technique are a normal common carotid and intracranial internal carotid arteries. Atherosclerotic lesions of the carotid bifurcation should be treated simultaneously using the same pre-sternomastoid incision.[7,104,105,110,111] Clamping of the normal common carotid artery does not entail an added risk of cerebral ischemia because antegrade perfusion of the internal carotid artery is maintained during clamping through the ipsilateral external carotid artery.

Surgery of the V2 segment

Although tedious and potentially difficult, a direct approach to the VA in the V2 segment is feasible by unroofing the VA in the bony canal of the transverse processes.[113] In this segment, the VA is surrounded by venous plexus, which has to be coagulated and transsected and may constitute an operative difficulty.

While this approach has been used extensively for direct decompression of the VA in patients with cervical spondylosis, a much simpler distal bypass from the carotid or subclavian to the V3 segment is usually preferred. In our opinion, the only remaining indications for a direct approach of the V2 segment is penetrating trauma to the VA[38] or combined neurologic and arterial decompression in patients with cervical spondylosis[72] or tumors.[62,108,109]

Surgery of the V3 segment

The introduction of a direct approach to the distal cervical VA has been a major advance in the management of VA disease.[6,8,17,28,29,62] The VA is usually approached in the C1–C2 interspace using a high pre-sternomastoid incision (**Fig. 35.13**). The internal jugular vein is left in the anterior part of the surgical field. The spinal accessory nerve is identified and preserved. The C1 transverse process leads to the underlying C1–C2 interspace, which is opened by resecting the muscles inserting in the lower aspect of C1. The VA is then dissected from the anterior branch of the C2 nerve and freed from the surrounding venous plexus. Two to three centimeters of healthy VA are available for the distal implantation of a saphenous bypass originating from the common carotid artery (**Fig. 35.10**) or, much less frequently, from the external carotid, internal carotid, or subclavian arteries (**Fig. 35.11**).

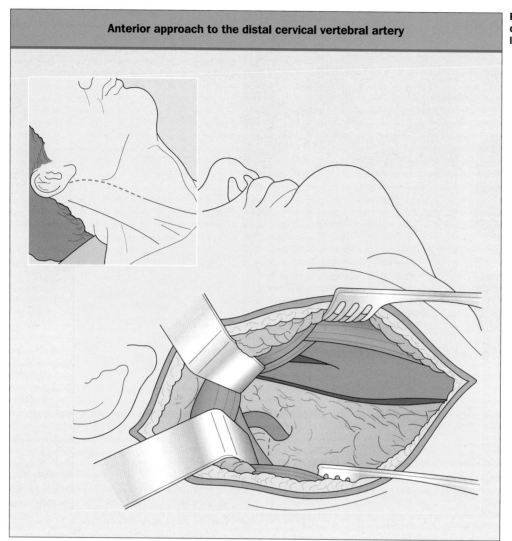

Anterior approach to the distal cervical vertebral artery

Figure 35.13 Anterior approach to the distal cervical vertebral artery at the level of the C1–C2 interspace.

Alternative techniques include transposition of the distal VA into the internal carotid artery,[114] transposition of the occipital artery into the VA,[6] or the use of arterial autograft obtained from the proximal V1 segment or from an endarterectomized internal carotid artery.[29] These techniques have the advantage of bypassing all the lesions of the V2 segment, with a distal anastomosis or implantation in a usually healthy portion of the VA.

Rarely, a more distal (above C1) approach to the VA is needed (**Fig. 35.14**).[115] It may be obtained through a posterior extension of the previous incision or through a posterior midline incision with a lateral extension. In both cases, resection of the posterior arch of C1 allows a relatively easy approach to the VA, which can be dissected up to the atlanto-occipital membrane.

Surgery of the V4 segment

Direct approach to the V4 segment in the posterior fossa is feasible. Successful segmental endarterectomy of the intracranial VA has been reported.[116] However, the usual technique has been extra-intracranial revascularization using occipital artery to PICA anastomosis[117] or venous graft from the external carotid artery to the posterior cerebral artery.[118]

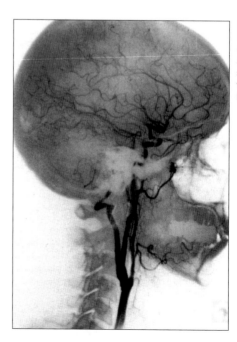

Figure 35.14 Reconstruction of the distal vertebral artery at the C1 level using a saphenous vein graft from the carotid bifurcation.

CONCLUSION

Although it is not yet widely accepted by the medical community, the concept of hemodynamic VBI appears to be valid. Management of the patients should be performed by a multidisciplinary team including neurologists, neuroradiologists, otolaryngologists, vascular surgeons, neurosurgeons, and other specialists if indicated. Using modern diagnostic tools and logical criteria for diagnosis and indications, as well as precise techniques for surgery, clinical

and anatomic results of VA reconstructions have been very satisfactory in the most recently reported series.[119] Our own experience now numbers more than 900 VA reconstructions. Mortality for isolated VA procedures has been less than 1%. Early occlusion rate has dropped to less than 4%, with very few late occlusions. Cure or maximal improvement of clinical symptoms has been obtained in more than 90% of the patients with hemodynamic VBI.

REFERENCES

1. Cate WR, Scott HW Jr. Cerebral ischemia of central origin: relief by subclavian-vertebral artery thromboendarterectomy. Surgery 1959; 45:19–31.
2. Crawford ES, De Bakey ME, Fields WS. Roentgenographic diagnosis and surgical treatment of basilar artery insufficiency. JAMA 1958; 168:509–14.
3. Berguer R, Bauer RB. Vertebral artery reconstruction: a successful technique in selected patients. Ann Surg 1981;193:441–7.
4. Berguer R, Feldman AJ. Surgical reconstruction of the vertebral artery. Surgery 1983;93:670–5.
5. Berguer R, Flynn LM, Kline RA, Caplan L. Surgical reconstruction of the extracranial vertebral artery: management and outcome. J Vasc Surg 2000;31: 9–18.
6. Berguer R, Morasch MD, Kline RA. A review of 100 consecutive reconstructions of the distal vertebral artery for embolic and hemodynamic disease. J Vasc Surg 1998;27:852–9.
7. Branchereau A, Magnan PE. Results of vertebral artery reconstruction. J Cardiovasc Surg 1990;31:320–6.
8. Carney AL. Vertebral artery surgery: historical development, basic concepts of brain hemodynamics, and clinical experience of 102 cases. Adv Neurol 1981;30:249–82.
9. Cormier JM, Ricco JB, Franceschi C. 82 cas de réimplantation de la sous-clavière ou de la vertébrale dans la carotide primitive. Chirurgie 1979;105:592–6.
10. Deriu GP, Ballotta E, Franceschi L, et al. Surgical management of extracranial vertebral artery occlusive disease. J Cardiovasc Surg 1991; 32:413–9.
11. Diaz FG, Ausman JI, de los Reyes RA, et al. Surgical reconstruction of the proximal vertebral artery. J Neurosurg 1984;61:874–81.
12. Edwards WH, Mulherin JL. The surgical approach to significant stenosis of vertebral and subclavian arteries. Surgery 1980;87:20–8.
13. Edwards WH, Mulherin JL Jr. The surgical reconstruction of the proximal subclavian and vertebral artery. J Vasc Surg 1985;2:634–42.
14. Giangola G, Imparato AM, Riles TS, Lamparello PJ. Vertebral artery angioplasty in patients younger than 55 years: long-term follow-up. Ann Vasc Surg 1991;5:121–4.
15. Habozit B. Vertebral artery reconstruction: results in 106 patients. Ann Vasc Surg 1991;5:61–5.
16. Imparato AM. Vertebral arterial reconstruction: a nineteen-year experience. J Vasc Surg 1985;2:626–34.
17. Kieffer E, Praquin B, Chiche L, et al. Distal vertebral artery reconstruction: long-term outcome. J Vasc Surg 2002;36:549–54.
18. Pauliukas PA, Barkauskas EM, Shifrin EG, Portnoi IM. Experience with reconstruction of vertebral arteries. In: Caplan LR, Shifrin EG, Nicolaides AN, Moore WS, eds. Cerebrovascular ischemia: investigation and management. London:Med-Orion; 1996:577–601.
19. Reul GJ, Cooley DA, Olson SK, et al. Long-term results of direct vertebral artery operations. Surgery 1984;96:854–62.
20. Roon AJ, Ehrenfeld WK, Cooke PB, Wylie EJ. Vertebral artery reconstruction. Am J Surg 1979;138:29–36.
21. Rosset E, Ayari R, Magnan PE, et al. Long-term results of reconstructions of the vertebral artery. In: Branchereau A, Jacobs M, eds. Long-term results of arterial interventions. Armonk:Futura; 1997:67–79.
22. Thevenet A, Ruotolo C. Surgical repair of vertebral artery stenoses. J Cardiovasc Surg 1984;25:101–10.
23. Van Schil PE, Ackerstaff RG, Vermeulen FE, et al. Long-term clinical and duplex follow-up after proximal vertebral artery reconstruction. Angiology 1992;43:961–8.
24. Argenson C, Francke JP, Sylla S, et al. Les artères vertébrales (segments V1 et V2). Anatomia Clinica 1979;2:29–41.
25. Francke JP, Di Marino V, Pannier M, et al. Les artères vertébrales: segments atlanto-axoïdien V3 et intracrânien V4, collatérales. Anatomia Clinica 1980;2:229–42.
26. Ouriel K, Green RM, DeWeese JA. Anomalous carotid-basilar anastomoses in cerebrovascular surgery. J Vasc Surg 1988;7:774–7.
27. Fisher CM, Gore I, Okabe N, White PD. Atherosclerosis of the carotid and vertebral arteries extracranial and intracranial. J Neuropathol Exp Neurol 1965;24:455–76.
28. Berguer R. Distal vertebral artery bypass: technique, the "occipital connection", and potential uses. J Vasc Surg 1985;2:621–6.
29. Kieffer E, Rancurel G, Richard T. Reconstruction of the distal cervical vertebral artery. In: Berguer R, Bauer RB, eds. Vertebrobasilar arterial occlusive disease. New York:Raven Press; 1984:265–90.
30. Laurian C, Georges B, Houdart R, Cormier JM. Revascularisation de l'artère vertébrale distale (3°segment): indications dans le traitement de l'insuffisance vertébro-basilaire. Sem Hop Paris 1984;16:547–52.
31. Chiche L, Bahnini A, Koskas F, Kieffer E. Occlusive fibromuscular disease of arteries supplying the brain: results of surgical treatment. Ann Vasc Surg 1997;11:496–504.
32. Stanley JC, Fry WJ, Seeger JF, et al. Extracranial internal carotid and vertebral artery fibrodysplasia. Arch Surg 1974;109:215–22.
33. Kieffer E, Natali J. Supraaortic trunk lesions in Takayasu's arteritis. In: Bergan JJ, Yao JST, eds. Cerebrovascular insufficiency. New York: Grune & Stratton; 1983:395–415.
34. Thielen KR, Wijdicks EFM, Nichols DA. Giant cell temporal arteritis: involvement of the vertebral and carotid arteries. Mayo Clinic Proc 1998;73:444–6.
35. Blickenstaff KL, Weaver FA, Yellin AE, et al. Trends in the management of traumatic vertebral artery injuries. Am J Surg 1989;158:101–6.
36. Demetriades D, Theodorou D, Asensio J, et al. Management options in vertebral artery injuries. Br J Surg 1996;83:83–6.
37. Golueke P, Sclafani S, Phillips T, et al. Vertebral artery injury: diagnosis and management. J Trauma 1987;27:856–65.
38. Meier DE, Brink BE, Fry WJ. Vertebral artery trauma: acute recognition and treatment. Arch Surg 1981;116:236–9.
39. Reid JDS, Weigelt JA. Forty-three cases of vertebral artery trauma. J Trauma 1988;28:1007–12.
40. Jean WC, Barrett MD, Rockswold G, Bergman TA. Gunshot wound to the head resulting in a vertebral artery pseudoaneurysm at the base of the skull. J Trauma 2001;50:126–8.
41. Biffl WL, Moore EE, Elliott JP, et al. The devastating potential of blunt vertebral arterial injuries. Ann Surg 2000;231:672–81.
42. Hayes P, Gerlock AJ, Cobb CA. Cervical spine trauma: a cause of vertebral artery injury. J Trauma 1980;20:904–5.
43. Sherman DG, Hart RG, Easton JD. Abrupt change in head position and cerebral infarction. Stroke 1981;12:2–6.

44. Van Tets WF, Van Drullemen HM, Tjan GT, Van Berge Henegouwen D. Vertebral arteriovenous fistula caused by puncture of the internal jugular vein. Eur J Surg 1992;158:627–8.

45. Smith MD, Emery SE, Dudley A, et al. Vertebral artery injury during anterior decompression of the cervical spine: a retrospective review of ten patients. J Bone Joint Surg 1993;75:410–5.

46. Buerger T, Lippert H, Meyer F, Halloul Z. Aneurysm of the vertebral artery near the atlas arch. J Cardiovasc Surg 1999;40:387–9.

47. Catala M, Rancurel G, Koskas F, et al. Ischemic stroke due to spontaneous extracranial vertebral giant aneurysm. Cerebrovasc Dis 1993; 3:322–6.

48. Hoffman K, Hosten N, Liebig T, et al. Giant aneurysm of the vertebral artery in neurofibromatosis type I: report of a case and review of literature. Neuroradiology 1998;40:245–8.

49. Rifkinson-Mann S, Laub J, Haimov M. Atraumatic extracranial vertebral artery aneurysm: case report and review of the literature. J Vasc Surg 1986;4:288–93.

50. Thompson JE, Eilber F, Baker JD. Vertebral artery aneurysm: case report and review of the literature. Surgery 1979;85:583–5.

51. Caplan LR, Zarins CK, Hemmati M. Spontaneous dissection of the extracranial vertebral arteries. Stroke 1985;16:1030–8.

52. Chiche L, Praquin B, Koskas F, Kieffer E. Spontaneous dissection of the extracranial vertebral artery: indications and long-term outcome of surgical treatment. Ann Vasc Surg (accepted for publication).

53. Chiras J, Marciano S, Vega Molina J, et al. Spontaneous dissecting aneurysm of the extracranial vertebral artery. Neuroradiology 1985; 27:327–33.

54. Mas JL, Bousser MG, Hasboun D, Laplane D. Extracranial vertebral artery dissections: a review of 13 cases. Stroke 1987;18:1037–47.

55. Mokri B, Houser OW, Sandok BA, Piepgras DG. Spontaneous dissections of the vertebral arteries. Neurology 1988;38:880–5.

56. Schievink WI. Spontaneous dissection of the carotid and vertebral arteries. N Engl J Med 2001;344:898–906.

57. Touzé E, Randoux B, Méary E, et al. Aneurysmal forms of cervical artery dissection: associated factors and outcome. Stroke 2001;32:418–23.

58. Cluzel P, Pierot L, Leung A, et al. Vertebral arteriovenous fistulae in neurofibromatosis: report of two cases and review of the literature. Neuroradiology 1994;36:321–5.

59. Vinchon M, Laurian C, George B, et al. Vertebral arteriovenous fistulas: a study of 49 cases and review of the literature. Cardiovasc Surg 1994; 2:359–69.

60. Bauer RB. Mechanical compression of the vertebral arteries. In: Berguer R, Bauer RB, eds. Vertebrobasilar arterial occlusive disease. New York:Raven Press; 1984:45–71.

61. George B, Laurian C. Impairment of vertebral artery flow caused by extrinsic lesions. Neurosurgery 1989;24:206–14.

62. George B, Laurian C. The vertebral artery: pathology and surgery. Vienna:Springer Verlag; 1987:183–230.

63. Kieffer E, Rancurel G, Branchereau A. Insuffisance vertébrobasilaire par lésion de l'artère vertébrale. J Mal Vasc 1985;10(Suppl C):253–313.

64. Toole JF. Positional effects of head and neck on vertebral artery blood flow. In: Berguer R, Caplan LR, eds. Vertebrobasilar arterial disease. St Louis:Quality Medical Publishing; 1992:11–4.

65. Hedera P, Bujdakova J, Traubner P. Blood flow velocities in basilar artery during rotation of the head. Acta Neurol Scand 1993;88:229–33.

66. Koskas F, Comizzoli I, Gobin P, et al. Effects of spinal mechanics on the vertebral artery: anatomic basis of positional postural compression of the cervical vertebral artery. In: Berguer R, Caplan LR, eds. Vertebrobasilar arterial disease. St Louis:Quality Medical Publishing; 1992:15–28.

67. Alexandrov AV, Norris JW. Recurrent stroke caused by spondylotic compression of the vertebral artery. Ann Neurol 1994;35:126–8.

68. Matskevichus ZK, Pauliukas PA. Morphologic changes of the arterial wall at the site of the loops and kinks of the carotid and vertebral arteries. Arch Pathol 1990;52:53–8.

69. Sullivan HG, Harbison JW, Vines FS, Becker D. Embolic posterior cerebral artery occlusion secondary to spondylitic vertebral artery compression. J Neurosurg 1975;43:618–22.

70. Barton JW, Margolis MT. Rotational obstructions of the vertebral artery at the atlantoaxial joint. Neuroradiology 1975;9:117–20.

71. Dadsetan MR, Skerhut HE. Rotational vertebrobasilar insufficiency secondary to vertebral artery occlusion from fibrous band of the longus coli muscle. Neuroradiology 1990;32:514–5.

72. Hardin CA. Vertebral artery insufficiency produced by cervical osteoarthritic spurs. Arch Surg 1965;90:629–33.

73. Hurvitz SA, Bonecutter GE. Surgical decompression of the first part of vertebral artery for ischemic brainstem dysfunction. J Cardiovasc Surg 1999;40:395–400.

74. Husni EA, Bell HS, Storer J. Mechanical occlusion of the vertebral artery: a new clinical concept. JAMA 1966;196:474–8.

75. Kojima N, Tamaki N, Fujita K, Matsumoto S. Vertebral artery occlusion at the narrowed "scalenovertebral angle": mechanical vertebral occlusion in the distal first portion. Neurosurgery 1985;16:672–4.

76. Lang J, Kessler B. About the suboccipital part of the vertebral artery and the neighboring bone-joint and nerve relationships. Skull Base Surg 1991;1:64–72.

77. Mapstone T, Spetzler RF. Vertebrobasilar insufficiency secondary to vertebral artery occlusion from a fibrous band. J Neurosurg 1982; 56:581–3.

78. Radojevic S, Negovanovic B. La gouttière et les anneaux osseux de l'artère vertébrale de l'atlas (étude anatomique et radiologique). Acta Anat 1963;55:186–94.

79. Sheehan S, Bauer RB, Meyer JS. Vertebral artery compression in cervical spondylosis: arteriographic demonstration during life of vertebral artery insufficiency due to rotation and extension of the neck. Neurology 1960;10:968–86.

80. Buge A, Rancurel G, Kieffer E, Denvil D. L'insuffisance vertébrobasilaire: revue des critères sémiologiques cérébro-vasculaires et des indications chirurgicales. Concours Med 1980;41:102–41.

81. Caplan LR. Vertebrobasilar disease: time for a new strategy. Stroke 1981;12:111–4.

82. Caplan LR. Vertebrobasilar occlusive disease. In: Barnett HJM, Stein BM, Mohr JP, Yatsu FM, eds. Stroke: overview, pathophysiology, diagnostis and management. Philadelphia:Churchill Livingstone; 1986:549–619.

83. George B, Laurian C. Vertebro-basilar ischaemia: its relation to stenosis and occlusion of the vertebral artery. Acta Neurochir Wien 1982; 62:287–95.

84. Caplan LR, Amarenco P, Rosengart A, et al. Embolism from vertebral artery origin occlusive disease. Neurology 1992;42:1505–12.

85. Caplan LR. Occlusion of the vertebral or basilar artery: follow-up analysis of some patients with benign outcome. Stroke 1979;10:277–82.

86. Fisher CM. Occlusion of the vertebral arteries causing transient basilar symptoms. Arch Neurol 1970;22:13–9.

87. Caplan LR. Patterns of posterior circulation infarctions: correlation with vascular pathology. In: Berguer R, Bauer RB, eds. Vertebrobasilar arterial occlusive disease. New York:Raven Press; 1984:15–25.

88. Castaigne P, Lhermitte F, Gautier J, et al. Arterial occlusion in the vertebrobasilar system: a study of 44 patients with post-mortem data. Brain 1973;96:133–54.

89. Hauw J-J, Amarenco P, Duyckaerts C, et al. Neuropathologie de l'ischémie vertébro-basilaire. Sem Hop Paris 1986;62:2757–61.

90. Jones HR Jr, Millikan CH, Sandok BA. Temporal profile (clinical course) of acute vertebrobasilar system cerebral infarctions. Stroke 1980; 11:173–7.

91. McDowell FH, Potes J, Groch S. The natural history of internal carotid and vertebral-basilar artery occlusion. Neurology 1961;1:153–7.

92. Patrick BK, Ramirez-Lassepas M, Snyder BD. Temporal profile of vertebrobasilar territory infarction: prognostic implications. Stroke 1980;11:643–8.

93. Cartlidge NEF, Whisnant JP, Elveback LR. Carotid and vertebral-basilar transient cerebral ischemic attacks: a community study, Rochester, Minnesota. Mayo Clin Proc 1977;52:117–20.

94. Heyman A, Wilkinson WE, Hurwitz BJ, et al. Clinical and epidemiologic aspects of vertebrobasilar and nonfocal cerebral ischemia. In: Berguer R, Bauer RB, eds. Vertebrobasilar arterial occlusive disease. New York: Raven Press; 1984:27–36.

95. Whisnant JP, Cartlidge NEF, Elveback LR. Carotid and vertebral-basilar transient ischemic attacks: effects of anticoagulants, hypertension and

cardiac disorders on survival and stroke occurrence: a population study. Ann Neurol 1978;3:107–15.

96. Naritomi H, Sakai F, Meyer JS. Pathogenesis of transient ischemic attacks within the vertebrobasilar arterial system. Arch Neurol 1979; 36:121–8.

97. Rosset E, Magnan PE, Branchereau A, et al. Hemodynamic vertebrobasilar insufficiency caused by multiple arterial lesions: results of surgical treatment. Ann Vasc Surg 1993;7:243–8.

98. Valerio N, Rosset E, Ede B, et al. Compromised hemodynamics associated with multipedicular lesions of cerebral arteries. Ann Vasc Surg 2001;15:219–26.

99. Kieffer E. Chirurgie de l'artère vertébrale. Encycl Med Chir (Techniques chirurgicales) Paris, 1984.

100. Branchereau A, Ede B, Magnan PE, et al. Surgery for asymptomatic carotid stenosis: a study of three patient subgroups. Ann Vasc Surg 1998; 12:572–8.

101. Cardon A, Kerdiles Y, Lucas A, et al. Results of isolated carotid surgery in patients with vertebrobasilar insufficiency. Ann Vasc Surg 1998; 12:579–82.

102. Humphries AW, Young JR, Beven EG, et al. Relief of vertebrobasilar symptoms by carotid endarterectomy. Surgery 1965;57:48–52.

103. Ouriel K, May AG, Ricotta JJ, et al. Carotid endarterectomy for non-hemispheric symptoms: predictors of success. J Vasc Surg 1984; 1:339–45.

104. Kieffer E, Rancurel G. Surgical management of combined carotid and vertebral disease. In: Berguer R, Bauer RB, eds. Vertebrobasilar arterial occlusive disease. New York:Raven Press; 1984:305–11.

105. Malone JM, Moore W, Hamilton R, Smith M. Combined carotid-vertebral vascular disease: a new surgical approach. Arch Surg 1980; 115:783–5.

106. Archie JP. Improved carotid hemodynamics with vertebral reconstruction. Ann Vasc Surg 1992;6:138–41.

107. Berguer R, McCaffrey JF, Bauer RB. Bilateral internal carotid artery occlusion: its surgical management. Arch Surg 1980;115:840–3.

108. Merland JJ, Riche MC, George B, et al. Current trends in the combined radiological and surgical management of vascular malformations, tumors and dysplasia involving the vertebral artery. J Neuroradiol 1979; 6:269–86.

109. Sen C, Eisenberg M, Casden AM, et al. Management of the vertebral artery in excision of extradural tumors of the cervical spine. Neurosurgery 1995;36:106–16.

110. Berguer R, Kieffer E. Surgery of the arteries to the head. New York: Springer Verlag; 1992.

111. Edwards WH Sr. Vertebral artery reconstruction: indications and techniques. Semin Vasc Surg 1996;9:105–10.

112. Spetzler RF, Hadley MN, Martin NA, et al. Vertebrobasilar insufficiency. Part 1: Microsurgical treatment of extracranial vertebrobasilar disease. J Neurosurg 1987;66:648–61.

113. Brink B. Approach to the second segment of the vertebral arteries. In: Berguer R, Bauer RB, eds. Vertebrobasilar arterial occlusive disease. New York:Raven Press; 1984:257–64.

114. Koskas F, Kieffer E, Rancurel G, et al. Direct transposition of the distal cervical vertebral artery into the internal carotid artery. Ann Vasc Surg 1995;9:515–24.

115. Berguer R. Suboccipital approach to the distal vertebral artery. J Vasc Surg 1999;30:344–9.

116. Allen GS, Cohen RJ, Preziosi TJ. Microsurgical endarterectomy of the intracranial vertebral artery for vertebro-basilar transient ischemic attacks. Neurosurgery 1981;8:56–9.

117. Sundt TM Jr, Piedgras DG. Occipital to posterior inferior cerebellar artery bypass surgery. J Neurosurg 1978;48:916–28.

118. Sundt TM Jr, Piepgras DG, Houser OW, Campbell JK. Interposition saphenous vein grafts for advanced occlusive disease and large aneurysms in the posterior circulation. J Neurosurg 1982;56:205–15.

119. Kline RA, Berguer R. Vertebral artery reconstruction. Ann Vasc Surg 1993;7:497–501.

CHAPTER

36

Carotid Artery Disease: Natural History and Diagnosis

William C Mackey and A Ross Naylor

KEY POINTS

Natural history:

- Carotid plaque progression and degeneration determine the clinical natural history.

- The clinical natural history is well described for patients with transient ischemic attacks or stroke related to carotid disease.

- The clinical natural history for asymptomatic patients is less well understood.

- Improved understanding of the clinical natural history in asymptomatic patients awaits improved understanding of plaque evolution and degeneration.

- Treatment with aspirin or other antiplatelet agents and, in selected patients, carotid endarterectomy, improves the clinical outcome in patients with carotid disease.

Diagnosis:

- Duplex ultrasound imaging is the best overall study currently available for the diagnosis of carotid disease.

- Magnetic resonance angiography and standard contrast angiography have a role in selected patients.

- Brain imaging is not routinely required as a part of the diagnostic evaluation but has an important role in selected patients.

INTRODUCTION

While there has been substantial progress in understanding the evolution of atherosclerotic plaques at the carotid bifurcation, the pathophysiologic events that result in plaque instability, rupture, embolization, or arterial occlusion and that lead to transient cerebral ischemia or stroke are not fully understood. Until a more complete understanding of the events that trigger plaque instability are elucidated, the understanding of the natural history of carotid disease will depend on clinical studies of patients with carotid disease subjected to a variety of treatments. Over the past 12 years, many scientifically valid clinical studies have been carried out that have improved knowledge of the clinical course of both symptomatic and asymptomatic carotid lesions dramatically. Until the basic mechanisms underlying carotid plaque evolution and degeneration are understood, however, this knowledge will be incomplete and any management protocols imperfect.

Diagnostic imaging for carotid disease has changed significantly over the past decade. Conventional contrast arteriograms – once the gold standard in the diagnostic evaluation of patients with carotid disease – are now required in fewer than 10% of all patients being evaluated for carotid endarterectomy. Duplex ultrasonography provides a reliable non-invasive assessment of the degree of carotid stenosis in virtually all patients, and can usually assess plaque characteristics. Magnetic resonance angiography (MRA) provides a more comprehensive flow map of the carotid circulation, including the aortic arch, proximal common carotid, and intracranial arteries. When coupled with magnetic resonance imaging (MRI) of the brain, detailed images of the cerebral circulation, plus cerebral anatomy and pathology, are obtained. Computed tomography (CT) techniques are available to provide cross-sectional and reconstructed three-dimensional imaging regarding plaque burden, plaque anatomy, and detailed anatomic assessment of non-atherosclerotic lesions of the carotid artery, as well as the brain. Conventional contrast arteriography, now with digitized images, allows anatomic assessment of the entire cerebral circulation, though because of its associated risks and costs, it is appropriate only in patients undergoing endovascular treatment of their carotid lesion or in the rare patient for whom the other less invasive and less costly techniques provide insufficient data for diagnosis and/or surgical planning.

CLINICAL SYNDROMES ASSOCIATED WITH CAROTID ARTERY DISEASE

Patients with carotid disease may be asymptomatic or may present with a wide variety of symptoms. The detection of a cervical bruit may lead to duplex ultrasound imaging that reveals severe but asymptomatic disease, prompting referral for surgical evaluation. Furthermore, non-invasive screening of high-risk populations may result in the detection of significant asymptomatic lesions. The natural history associated with asymptomatic carotid lesions is discussed below.

Events related to carotid artery lesions are usually classified as either transient ischemic attacks (TIAs) or strokes. TIAs are defined as neurologic events that are sudden in onset without preceding aura, last for less than 24 hours, resolve completely to leave the patient at neurological baseline, and are referable to a definable vascular distribution of the central nervous system. TIAs may be related either to hypoperfusion (related to vascular stenoses or occlusions) or to embolization. Strokes are infarctions of central nervous system tissue related to hypoperfusion, embolization, or intracranial hemorrhage. Reversible ischemic neurologic deficit (RIND) is a term used to describe a focal neurologic event that lasts longer than 24 hours but resolves completely within 1 week. The duration of symptoms in patients with RIND suggests that some degree of structural damage to the brain must have occurred, though it may be very limited and undetectable by clinical imaging studies.

Stroke, TIA, and RIND are descriptions of clinical events. The correlation of these events with findings on brain imaging studies is imprecise. Approximately 24% of patients with clinical events consistent with TIA will be found to have infarction in an anatomic distribution consistent with the transient neurologic event on brain imaging.[1]

Sometimes, the differentiation between TIA and stroke can be less than clear-cut. Patients who present with frequent severe TIAs (crescendo TIAs) can be difficult to distinguish from patients with acute or evolving stroke. Early in the course of these events, brain imaging studies may not be helpful, since the anatomically detectable lesions evolve after the clinical events. Magnetic resonance brain imaging has improved the ability to detect very early brain infarction and may allow a more precise differentiation of these clinical syndromes.

Carotid territory TIAs can involve the eye only (transient monocular blindness or transient monocular field cuts, termed amaurosis fugax). More insidious chronic monocular visual deterioration can be associated with critical stenosis or occlusion of the ipsilateral internal carotid artery (ICA; chronic ocular ischemic syndrome). Carotid TIAs may also result in speech deficits (dysarthria, dysphasia, or aphasia). Motor manifestations range from mild clumsiness of a single limb to hemiplegia of the side opposite the carotid lesion. Sensory manifestations may include numbness or paresthesias on the side opposite the carotid lesion. Headache, mild confusion, and lightheadedness may accompany the above symptoms, but these non-specific and non-localizing symptoms are not symptoms of carotid TIA when they occur alone.

Stroke deficits related to carotid disease are similar to the temporary deficits seen with TIA. Permanent monocular blindness, aphasia, mono- or hemiparesis or hemiplegia, and hemisensory deficits are the most common manifestations of carotid-disease-related stroke.

Of equal importance to the recognition of symptoms likely to be related to carotid disease is the recognition of symptoms unlikely to be carotid-related. Common symptoms not likely to be related to carotid territory TIA or stroke are shown in **Table 36.1**.[2]

On occasion, carotid disease can present with symptoms consistent with more global cerebral hypoperfusion. Patients with critical stenosis or occlusion of several extracranial vessels can present with decreased mental acuity, orthostatic presyncope, or even vertebrobasilar-like symptoms. In the context of severe hemodynamic compromise related to multiple vascular lesions, these global symptoms may be properly attributed to carotid disease. With more localized vascular disease or with carotid lesions such as ulcers that might produce emboli, these symptoms are not usually related.

THE NATURAL HISTORY OF ASYMPTOMATIC CAROTID DISEASE

The presence of carotid artery atherosclerosis predisposes patients to TIAs and strokes, and the risk of these events is roughly correlated with the severity of the carotid disease. Chambers and Norris[3] followed 500 patients with neck bruits and varying

Signs and symptoms unlikely to be related to carotid disease.
Unconsciousness (including syncope)
Tonic/clonic activity
March of sensory deficit
Vertigo alone
Dysphagia alone
Dysarthria alone
Bowel or bladder incontinence
Visual loss with alteration of consciousness
Focal symptoms with migraine
Scintillating scotmata
Confusion alone
Amnesia alone

Table 36.1 Signs and symptoms unlikely to be related to carotid disease.[2] Most of these symptoms are more likely to be a manifestation of cardiac arrhythmias, seizures, migraine, or other non-vascular-related conditions.

degrees of carotid disease confirmed and graded by Doppler ultrasound. At 1 year, TIA or stroke had occurred in five of 239 patients (2.1%) with 0–29% stenosis, in nine of 157 (5.7%) with 30–74% stenosis, and in 22 of 113 (19.5%) with 75–100% stenosis. The authors further noted that the incidence of cardiac ischemic events also correlated with the severity of carotid stenosis in this cohort.

O'Holleran et al.[4] also noted that TIA and stroke risk were related to the degree of carotid stenosis. In this study, 60% of 121 patients with >75% stenosis by B-mode ultrasound had a stroke or TIA during 5-year follow-up. Only 13% of patients with <75% stenosis suffered a neurologic event during follow-up. These authors further correlated clinical outcome with the echogenicity of the carotid lesions. Calcified plaques were much less likely to be associated with symptoms than soft, primarily echolucent plaques. The findings of this study are summarized in **Table 36.2**. From these data it is apparent that both degree of stenosis and plaque density, as determined by duplex echo characteristics, are correlated with clinical outcome.

Risk of neurologic event and carotid plaque characteristics.				
Duplex characteristics	Stenosis	n	TIA	Stroke
Calcified	>75%	37	4 (11%)	1 (3%)
	<75%	53	0	0
Dense	>75%	42	23 (55%)	4 (10%)
	<75%	76	7 (9%)	1 (1%)
Soft	>75%	42	32 (76%)	9 (21%)
	<75%	46	10 (21%)	4 (9%)

Table 36.2 Risk of neurologic event and carotid plaque characteristics. TIA, transient ischemic attack. (Modified with permission from O'Holleran et al.[4])

Plaque progression has also been noted to correlate with outcome. Roederer et al.[5] found that in asymptomatic patients who initially presented with <80% stenosis, progression to >80% was associated with a high incidence of stroke, TIA, or progression to carotid occlusion. These authors noted a 35% risk of ischemic symptoms or carotid occlusion within 6 months of disease progression and a 46% incidence within 12 months. Conversely, only 1.5% of patients whose plaques remained stable developed symptoms over 12-month follow-up.

Further natural history data are available from the control, non-surgical groups in the more recent randomized trials of asymptomatic carotid atherosclerosis. These data do not really reflect the natural history of carotid disease, but rather the outcome associated with 'best medical management' of asymptomatic carotid disease. In the Veterans Administration Cooperative Trial,[6] medical management of asymptomatic carotid lesions (≥ 50% stenosis) resulted in a 20.6% incidence of ipsilateral TIA or stroke with 4 years of follow-up. In the Asymptomatic Carotid Atherosclerosis Study (ACAS),[7] medical management of ≥60% carotid stenosis was associated with a 19.2% estimated risk of TIA, stroke, or death over a 5-year follow-up.

Carotid plaques clearly place asymptomatic patients at risk for TIA and stroke. Degree of stenosis, plaque density, and plaque progression are correlates of the relative risk related to carotid artery atherosclerotic lesions. Patients at highest risk for TIA or stroke are those with >80% stenosis caused by a soft, echolucent plaque, or those whose plaque progresses from <80% to >80% stenosis during follow-up. These clinical findings are consistent with the current understanding of plaque evolution and degeneration. Benign fatty streaks progress to fibrous plaques. Continued lipid infiltration into the arterial wall leads to macrophage infiltration and chronic inflammation, with slow increase in plaque mass. Macrophage lysis with release of proteolytic enzymes, coupled with further lipid infiltration, results in a complex plaque with areas of lipid accumulation, ongoing chronic inflammation, and calcification. Neovascularity within the arterial wall and overlying plaque results from this cycle of ongoing inflammation and healing. Intraplaque hemorrhage resulting from neovascularity in the unstable plaque environment can result in sudden plaque expansion with thrombosis and arterial occlusion or in rupture of the fibrous cap overlying the lipid pool or area of intraplaque hemorrhage, with resultant embolization (**Fig. 36.1**). Given the current understanding of the pathogenesis of cerebrovascular events based on this scenario, it is understandable that low-density plaques (more lipid pool or intraplaque hemorrhage), plaques causing severe stenosis, or plaques that progress, would be associated with a greater risk of cerebrovascular events.

Medical therapy can favorably alter the natural history of asymptomatic carotid disease. Reductase inhibitors may slow the progression of carotid plaques and decrease the incidence of TIA and stroke, even in patients with normal cholesterol levels.[8] The role of aspirin or other antiplatelet agents in patients with asymptomatic carotid lesions has been established on the basis of several large-scale trials demonstrating benefit in the prevention of several cardiovascular endpoints (cardiac death, stroke death, stroke, and non-fatal myocardial infarction) in patients with known atherosclerosis and in patients at risk for atherosclerosis.

In addition, medical management of asymptomatic carotid disease has been compared with medical management plus

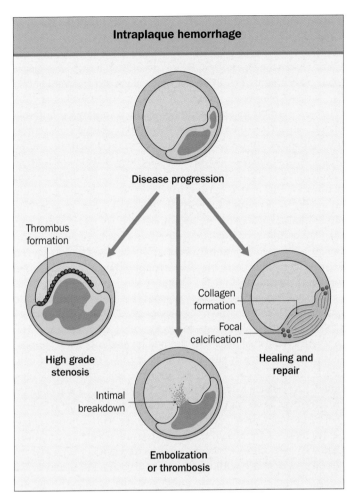

Intraplaque hemorrhage

Disease progression

Thrombus formation

High grade stenosis

Intimal breakdown

Embolization or thrombosis

Collagen formation

Focal calcification

Healing and repair

Figure 36.1 Intraplaque hemorrhage. Intraplaque hemorrhage may result in acute progression to high-grade carotid stenosis or occlusion, to fibrous cap rupture with embolization and ulceration, or to healing and repair with fibrosis and focal calcification. The events leading up to intraplaque hemorrhage and the determinants of which chain of events will follow such are at present poorly understood. (From Bergan & Yao, eds. Cerebrovascular insufficiency. New York: Grune & Stratton; 1983:51.)

carotid endarterectomy in several large-scale randomized trials. In ACAS,[7] surgery was marginally, but statistically significantly, beneficial for patients with ≥ 60% carotid stenosis. The 5-year ipsilateral stroke risk in the surgically treated group was 5.1%, including perioperative stroke or death. In the medically treated cohort, the 5-year stroke risk was 11% (p=0.004). While this result suggests a benefit for surgery, the benefit is indeed meager. One hundred carotid endarterectomies would have to be performed in this group of patients in order to prevent six strokes over 5 years. Subgroup analysis of the ACAS patients did not reveal greater benefit in patients with greater stenosis. The relative stroke risk reductions attributable to surgery were 45%, 67%, and 45% in the subgroups with 60–69%, 70–79%, and 80–89% stenosis, respectively.[7] Attempts to define groups more likely to benefit from surgery are currently underway.[9] It is clear that the identification of asymptomatic patients who will derive greater benefit from endarterectomy awaits a more sophisticated understanding of the natural history of atherosclerotic plaques. The key question that remains to be answered is: 'What are the markers that differentiate a potentially unstable plaque from a benign stable plaque?'

THE NATURAL HISTORY OF SYMPTOMATIC CAROTID ARTERY DISEASE

Once the pathophysiologic events described above have taken place, resulting in TIA or stroke, patients are at continuing risk for further neurologic events. A patient with stroke or TIA related to carotid disease could be assumed to have an unstable plaque, and it would seem logical that this plaque will remain unstable. Most studies of symptomatic carotid disease use stroke and death as endpoints. In fact, the real natural history of symptomatic carotid disease cannot be discerned from recent studies for the simple reason that TIA and stroke are generally accepted to represent compelling indications for intervention, either medical or surgical. A randomized study of the management of TIA or stroke patients including a placebo control group would never be allowed by modern human investigation review committees. The basis for the certainty that TIA and stroke demand treatment lies in several older studies. First, The Canadian Cooperative Study[10] showed that in 139 symptomatic patients, placebo treatment was associated with a 22% risk of stroke or death over a mean follow-up of 26 months. Similarly, in an American trial of aspirin therapy for patients with symptomatic cerebrovascular disease, Fields et al.[11] found a stroke or death risk of 21% at 2 years for patients treated with placebo. Finally, in a French trial,[12] placebo treatment of symptomatic patients was associated with a 3-year stroke/mortality risk of 19%. In each of these trials, medical therapy with aspirin significantly reduced the risk of stroke. These studies clearly establish that TIA and minor stroke are associated with a high risk of stroke and/or death within a few years after the index event. No sophisticated brain or carotid imaging studies were performed in these trials, hence they may have included some strokes and TIAs unrelated to carotid disease.

Because the placebo-controlled trials clearly demonstrated the high risk of subsequent stroke and death associated with untreated TIA or minor stroke events, and because aspirin and more recently clopidogrel have been shown to reduce this risk, all modern trials are conducted without placebo control. Current studies compare the 'natural' histories of medically treated carotid lesions with those treated medically plus surgically. Future studies will compare outcomes of medical and surgical management with endovascular management.

The North American Symptomatic Carotid Endarterectomy Trial (NASCET) has provided a remarkable amount of information about the risk of stroke associated with symptomatic carotid atherosclerosis.[13] The stroke risk in NASCET-eligible patients randomized to medical therapy (aspirin plus risk factor management using lipid-lowering agents, antihypertensives, etc.) was correlated with the presence of risk factors identified at the time of study entry (**Table 36.3**).

For patients with symptomatic severe carotid disease managed medically, the risk of stroke is high and predictable, based on well-established risk factors and on the severity of carotid stenosis. More recently, the NASCET collaborators have better defined the outcome of moderate and mild carotid disease. Patients managed medically with 50–69% and <50% stenosis had 5-year ipsilateral stroke rates of 22.2% and 18.7%, respectively.[14]

Similar results were noted in the European Carotid Surgery Trial (ECST),[15] which, like NASCET, compared outcomes in symptomatic carotid artery disease treated with medical manage-

Risk factors for stroke in symptomatic patients managed medically.	
Risk factors:	
Age >70 years	
Systolic BP >160 mmHg	
Diastolic BP >90 mmHg	
Recent stroke	
Stenosis >80%	
Ulcerated plaque	
History of tobacco use	
Diabetes	
Claudication	
Hyperlipidemia	
Stroke risk at 2 years:	
Low risk (0–5 factors)	17%
Moderate risk (6 factors)	23%
High risk (>6 factors)	39%
Stroke risk at 2 years based on severity of carotid stenosis:	
70–79%	12%
80–89%	18%
90–99%	26%

Table 36.3 Risk factors for stroke in symptomatic patients managed medically. (Data from NASCET)[14]

Three-year stroke risk in patients managed medically in the European Carotid Surgery Trial (ECST).				
	Annual risk of stroke (%)			
Stenosis	Year 1	Year 2	Year 3	Cumulative 3-year risk
70–79%	6%	6%	5%	17%
80–89%	11%	6%	3%	20%
90–99%	18%	14%	3%	35%

Table 36.4 Three-year stroke risk in patients managed medically in the European Carotid Surgery Trial (ECST).[15] As in the North American Symptomatic Carotid Endarterectomy Trial (NASCET), the rate of stroke was high and correlated with the degree of carotid stenosis.

ment alone versus medical management plus surgery. The results of NASCET and ECST are not directly comparable because the method of defining the degree of carotid stenosis in the two trials was quite different, such that 80% and 90% stenoses in the ECST were approximately equivalent to 61% and 80% stenoses, respectively, in NASCET. Even with this difference, the outcome in medically managed patients in ECST was similar to those in NASCET (**Table 36.4**).

In addition, the stroke rate was greatest in the first year following presentation and declined over time. The finding that stroke risk after TIA or minor stroke is highest in the early aftermath of the herald event is common to several studies, including the earliest trials of aspirin therapy. In the aspirin trial conducted by Fields et al.,[11] the placebo group had a 17.3% risk of cerebral or retinal infarction in the first year following randomization, but only a 5% risk in the second year. In NASCET,[13] the ipsilateral stroke rate in the cohort managed medically was approximately 18% in the first year and 8% in the second.

From all current randomized studies that compare medical management alone versus medical management plus carotid endarterectomy for symptomatic, severe carotid disease, it is clear that surgery favorably alters the natural history of medically treated carotid artery disease. In NASCET, the 2-year risk of ipsilateral stroke in patients with 70–99% stenosis who were managed medically was 26%, whereas carotid endarterectomy plus medical management was associated with a 2-year stroke risk of 9% (including perioperative risk of 5.5%).[13] The difference between outcomes in the two groups was highly statistically significant (p<0.001). In ECST, ipsilateral stroke was noted in 20.6% of patients with 80–99% stenosis managed medically, as compared with 6.8% of those undergoing surgery (p<0.0001).[16] There was smaller benefit from surgery in NASCET patients with less severe stenosis: for those with 50–69% stenosis, the 5-year ipsilateral stroke rate was 15.7% and 22.2% in the surgically and medically treated groups, respectively (p=0.045), while for those with <50% stenosis, surgery had no beneficial effect on stroke risk.[14] In ECST patients, carotid endarterectomy had no beneficial effect on stroke rate in patients with <70% stenosis and offered only marginal benefit for those with 70–80% stenosis.[16]

In summary, in asymptomatic patients, stroke risk is determined by degree of stenosis, plaque density, and plaque progression. The natural history of asymptomatic carotid lesions can be influenced favorably by medical therapies (reductase inhibitors and antiplatelet agents). Selected patients with asymptomatic carotid disease derive additional benefit from carotid endarterectomy, although at present the identification of asymptomatic patients likely to benefit from endarterectomy is imprecise and less than optimal. More precise patient selection awaits a better understanding of the factors that create carotid plaque instability. In symptomatic patients, the natural history of carotid atherosclerosis is well defined. Both medical and surgical management offer significant benefit. In symptomatic cases with ≥ 70% stenosis (NASCET criteria) or ≥ 80% stenosis (ECST) criteria, carotid endarterectomy offers significant benefit when compared with medical management alone. In patients with 50–70% stenosis (NASCET criteria), surgery provides modest benefit. Surgery offers no additional benefit for patients with <50% carotid stenosis. Of course, the potential benefits offered by surgery in reducing the stroke risk associated with both asymptomatic and symptomatic carotid disease are contingent on the safety of the surgical procedure itself. Excessive stroke morbidity could potentially offset any potential benefit in stroke risk reduction from surgery.

THE DIAGNOSIS AND EVALUATION OF CAROTID DISEASE

The diagnosis of carotid disease is usually made from the history and physical examination. Asymptomatic patients are most frequently found to have carotid disease after a bruit is detected on routine physical examination. While the presence of a bruit is neither sensitive nor specific for carotid disease, it is a reliable marker for the presence of atherosclerosis and its related risks.[17] Detection of a bruit usually prompts non-invasive evaluation of the carotids. Symptomatic patients present with carotid territory TIAs or strokes, or occasionally with less specific symptoms suggesting global cerebral hypoperfusion. Such symptoms should automatically prompt a search for the source of the symptoms. Once carotid disease is suspected on the basis of history and/or physical examination, detailed assessment can be carried out using a variety of imaging and hemodynamic studies: duplex ultrasound, transcranial Doppler, MRA, CT angiography, and traditional contrast angiography. The brain parenchyma can be imaged reliably with either CT scanning or MRI.

The goals of the evaluation of patients with carotid atherosclerosis are:

- to ascertain whether or not carotid disease is present;
- to assess the severity of carotid disease;
- to determine whether or not the carotid lesion is responsible for the patient's symptoms;
- to assess the potential operability of the carotid lesion; and
- to assess any unusual features of the carotid disease.

These goals must be achieved while subjecting the patient to minimal risk, and, in the current climate, while minimizing cost. No single carotid evaluation protocol is appropriate for all patients. MRI or CT imaging of the brain is required only in selected patients. Contrast angiography is now rarely indicated unless carotid angioplasty and stenting are being considered.

Duplex ultrasound imaging

Duplex ultrasound imaging is the most appropriate initial investigation because it is non-invasive, free of risk, relatively inexpensive, and accurate in determining degree of stenosis, in assessing plaque density, and in detecting plaque progression. It is also the most appropriate method for following patients with carotid atherosclerosis. Degree of stenosis is assessed accurately by Doppler-derived velocity data, while density and other morphologic characteristics are assessed with high-resolution ultrasound imaging. **Figures 36.2–36.5** show duplex data from representative studies. In **Figures 36.4 & 36.5**, color-flow duplex images are shown. In color-flow duplex, velocity data are color coded and superimposed over the ultrasound image to create a flow map.

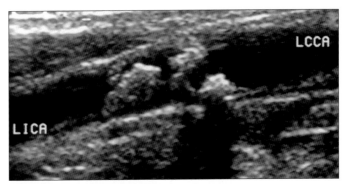

Figure 36.2 Duplex imaging. Duplex image of a highly irregular and ulcerated plaque in a patient with repeated episodes of transient monocular blindness. Peak systolic velocity equals 204cm/s, consistent with 50–79% stenosis.

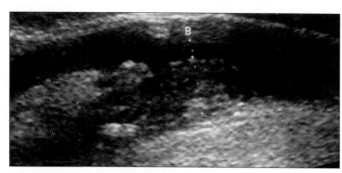

Figure 36.3 Duplex imaging. Duplex image of a soft, smooth, echolucent plaque at the carotid bifurcation. Peak systolic velocity equals 275cm/s, indicative of 50–79% stenosis.

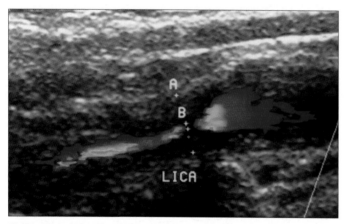

Figure 36.4 Color-flow duplex imaging. Color-flow duplex image of an apparent high-grade stenosis of the left internal carotid origin in a patient with a minor hemispheric stroke. Peak systolic velocity equals 500cm/s and end-diastolic velocity equals 153 cm/s, indicative of 80–99% stenosis.

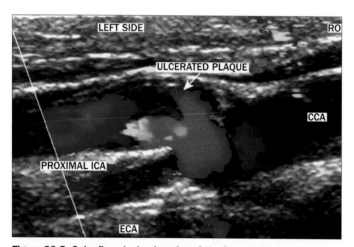

Figure 36.5 Color-flow duplex imaging. Color-flow duplex image of an ulcerated plaque at the left internal carotid origin. Note flow into ulcer cavity (arrow). Peak systolic velocity equals 589cm/s and end-diastolic velocity equals 173cm/s, indicative of 80–99% stenosis. The patient had multiple episodes of right-arm weakness.

Duplex velocity and Doppler waveform criteria for determination of carotid stenosis.			
Stenosis	*PSV (cm/s)*	*EDV (cm/s)*	*Spectral broadening*
<30%	<120	Any	Minimal
30–49%	<120	Any	Present
50–79%	>120	<140	Present
80–99%	>120	>140	Present

Table 36.5 Duplex velocity and Doppler waveform criteria for determination of carotid stenosis. EDV, end-diastolic velocity; PSV, peak systolic velocity.

angiographic or operative findings.[5,18,19] These criteria are shown in **Table 36.5**.

While these velocity criteria are accurate, they are not completely helpful in selecting patients for surgery based on the NASCET or ACAS criteria. Moneta et al.[20] found that an internal carotid to common carotid peak systolic velocity ratio of 4.0 detected a 70–99% stenosis by NASCET criteria with 91% sensitivity, 87% specificity, 76% positive predictive value, 96% negative predictive value, and 88% overall accuracy. The velocity ratio of 4.0 provided the best overall accuracy in the detection of ≥ 70% carotid stenosis by NASCET criteria.

Similarly, for asymptomatic patients, these same authors have evaluated the ≥60% ICA stenosis threshold used to determine ACAS eligibility. They found that the combination of a peak systolic velocity of ≥ 290cm/s and an end-diastolic velocity (EDV) of ≥ 80cm/s predicted ≥ 60% stenosis with a sensitivity of 78%, specificity of 96%, positive predictive value of 95%, negative predictive value of 84%, and overall accuracy of 88%.[21] While this finding is of interest, most carotid surgeons still select only patients with more critical (≥ 80%) stenosis for consideration for endarterectomy for asymptomatic disease. At the New England Medical Center, the criterion for patient selection for endarterectomy for asymptomatic stenosis is most frequently EDV ≥ 140cm/s, the University of Washington criterion for ≥ 80% stenosis.

Duplex imaging is also useful in evaluating plaque density and surface morphology. Plaque density and surface morphology data are not currently quantified for routine clinical use in carotid assessment. Nicolaides' group[22] have attempted to use the Gray-Scale Median as a means of quantifying plaque density. While they have shown that, in general, less dense plaques (higher lipid content or higher incidence of intraplaque hemorrhage) with Gray Scale Medians of 32 or less are more often associated with stroke than are more dense plaques (calcified), their correlation is imprecise. At present, the clinical use of density and morphology data is limited to a qualitative appreciation of their relevance in determining clinical outcome. More precise assessment of their significance awaits a practical, precise, and clinically relevant means for quantifying these plaque attributes.

Figures 36.2, 36.3 & 36.5 illustrate the capability of duplex to assess plaque morphology. **Figure 36.2** shows an example of a heterogeneous (mixed calcific and soft) plaque with a highly irregular surface. **Figure 36.3** illustrates a soft plaque of very low echogenicity. **Figure 36.5** shows a large ulcerated plaque.

Duplex ultrasound velocity data are reliable in the assessment of carotid stenosis. There are, however, a number of different criteria that may be used to define the severity of carotid stenosis. In our laboratory, velocity criteria modified from the University of Washington studies have provided the best correlation with

Carotid duplex imaging is also useful in detecting carotid occlusion and, therefore, in disqualifying selected patients from further consideration for surgical intervention. Sensitivity and specificity of 97% for the detection of internal carotid occlusion were reported even in early experience with duplex technology.[18] Criteria for diagnosis of occlusion include absence of flow in the ICA, blunted diastolic flow (EDV = 0) in the common carotid artery, and accelerated flow in the external carotid artery. Transcranial Doppler assessment of the ophthalmic artery for detection of reversal of flow provides additional evidence of internal carotid occlusion.

Duplex ultrasound suffers from two major shortcomings. First, the quality of duplex data is dependent on the ultrasound technologist's experience and diligence and the technique of measurement used. It remains an important part of quality control for each vascular laboratory, that results from individual technologists are audited against measured carotid stenosis. Second, duplex has no capability to image the arch, great vessel origins, distal ICA, or intracranial vasculature. Information regarding the intracranial circulation can be obtained non-invasively using transcranial Doppler (TCD), although anatomic variability in the cranial acoustic windows and other technical limitations often result in a less than complete survey of the intracranial circulation. TCD can provide useful data confirming the hemodynamic significance of intracranial lesions detected by MRA or other modalities. TCD is most useful as a means of detecting embolic events in the intracranial vessels.

Magnetic resonance angiography

Because of the shortcomings of duplex ultrasound imaging, and despite its proven accuracy in grading stenosis, many clinicians hesitate to base decisions on ultrasound data alone. Through the 1980s, duplex was used primarily as a screening tool and was followed by contrast angiography where surgical intervention was contemplated. Because of the risk, invasiveness, and cost associated with contrast angiography, a non-invasive study complementary to duplex was sought. MRA can complement duplex by providing images of the arch, great vessel origins, distal ICA, and intracranial circulation. While MRA, like duplex, is a flow map rather than an image of the arterial wall, MRA data can be rendered into images that closely mimic the anatomic data familiar from traditional contrast angiography. Furthermore, MRA data can be acquired along with MRI brain imaging data, allowing detailed assessment of the brain parenchyma along with assessment of the cerebral circulation.

As MRA technology advances, the data become more reliable and more useful for making clinical decisions. MRA depends on the detection of the differences in energy emitted from moving versus stationary protons after application of radiofrequency energy pulses within a magnetic field. This technique for differentiating energy released from stationary versus moving protons is called 'time of flight' technology. In two-dimensional time of flight (2D TOF) MRA, images are acquired in thin 2–3mm cross-sections and reassembled to give an image of the flowing blood. In three-dimensional time of flight (3D TOF) MRA, an entire vessel segment is subjected to the energy pulses at once and then partitioned for later reconstruction. The differences in these two data acquisition modes result in different image characteristics. The use of 2D and 3D modes in a complementary manner enhances the reliability of MRA data, and

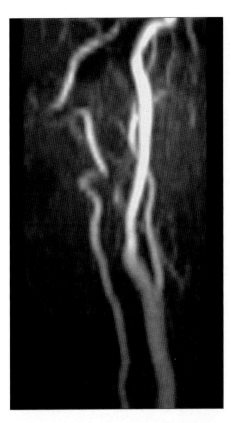

Figure 36.6 Two-dimensional time of flight magnetic resonance angiography (2D TOF MRA). 2D TOF MRA of near-normal carotid artery and small tortuous vertebral artery.

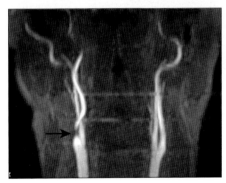

Figure 36.7 Magnetic resonance angiography (MRA). MRA showing both carotid arteries. The left is normal and the right has moderate-to-severe stenosis at the internal carotid origin (arrow).

most current MRA studies utilize both modalities to insure optimal images. In general, 2D TOF MRA allows for imaging of longer arterial segments and, therefore, is preferred for imaging the proximal common carotid and distal internal carotid arteries. Motion-related image degradation is less of a problem with 2D TOF because the images are acquired in thin slices and reconstructed later. Also, because each cross-sectional segment is energized individually, signal loss is minimized and very sluggish flow can be differentiated from no flow. This may make the 2D mode more sensitive than 3D in differentiating occlusive from preocclusive lesions. In 3D mode, the reconstructed cross-sectional segments are thinner, yielding better spatial resolution and allowing a more accurate assessment of degree of stenosis. Furthermore, because in 3D mode the volume to be imaged is energized simultaneously and not in sequenced perpendicular slices, tortuous vessels and areas of flow turbulence are better imaged. Representative MRA images are shown in **Figures 36.6–36.9**. These figures illustrate the potential for MRA to image the most proximal portions of the common carotid arteries (**Fig. 36.8**), the

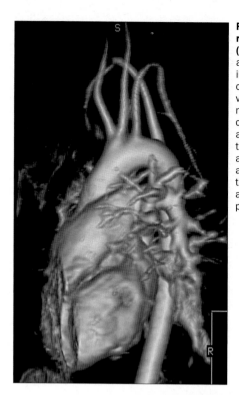

Figure 36.8 Magnetic resonance angiography (MRA). MRA of heart and great vessels, illustrating the capability of MRA to visualize proximal to most portions of the common carotid arteries. In this case, the common carotids are normal, but there is an aberrant origin of the right subclavian artery, explaining this patient's dysphagia.

Sensitivity and specificity of magnetic resonance angiography in detection of carotid stenosis and occlusion.				
Reference	Stenosis	Sensitivity	Specificity	Method
Young et al.[23]	70–99%	86%	93%	2D + 3D
Patel et al.[24]	70–99%	84%	75%	2D
Patel et al.[24]	70–99%	94%	85%	3D
Turnipseed et al.[25]	70–99%	100%	93%	2D
Mittl et al.[26]	70–99%	92%	75%	2D
Patel et al.[24]	Occlusion	100%	100%	2D + 3D
Young et al.[23]	Occlusion	80%	99%	2D + 3D

Table 36.6 Sensitivity and specificity of magnetic resonance angiography in detection of carotid stenosis (70–99%) and occlusion. (Contrast angiography as standard for comparison). 2D, two-dimensional; 3D, three-dimensional.

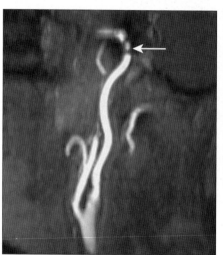

Figure 36.9 Magnetic resonance angiography (MRA). MRA done to evaluate a right hemispheric stroke in a patient with minimal disease at the carotid bifurcations by duplex imaging. Study shows a significant lesion in the right carotid siphon region (arrow). MRA is useful in diagnosing intracranial vascular disease.

cervical carotid arteries (**Figs 36.6 & 36.7**), and the intracranial carotid (**Fig. 36.9**). The accuracy of MRA technology depends on familiarity and expertise with computer software, and should be validated within each X-ray department.

The sensitivity and specificity of MRA in the detection of carotid stenoses and occlusions have been reported by several radiologists (**Table 36.6**). In these studies, duplex imaging was also assessed for sensitivity and specificity versus the 'gold standard' of contrast angiography. In most studies, the sensitivity and specificity for duplex were very similar to those of MRA.

In current practice, MRA is sensitive in the detection of carotid stenosis. A normal or near normal MRA virtually eliminates the possibility of a hemodynamically significant lesion. On the other hand, the specificity of MRA has been somewhat inconsistent. Turbulence related to moderate stenosis may result in more random motion of blood such that the axis of flow is inconsistent

and no longer perpendicular to the imaging plane. Signal dropout may occur as a result of turbulence, resulting in a flow void (see **Fig. 36.3**). In 2D TOF mode, a flow void may represent anything from 30% to 99% stenosis. Riles et al.[27] observed that using 2D TOF the sensitivity and specificity for detecting 50–99% stenosis were 100% and 60%, respectively. An MRA that revealed minimal disease was virtually certain to be accurate, but an MRA that predicted 50–99% stenosis was accurate only 60% of the time. This tendency to over-read the degree of stenosis because of the flow void phenomenon limits the utility of 2D TOF MRA in making surgical decisions, because it does not allow accurate discrimination between minimal (30–49%), moderate (50–69%), and critical (70–99%) stenoses. Improved sensitivity has been achieved using 3D TOF, although specificity for the diagnosis of 70–99% stenosis in some series employing this mode has been as low as 78–85%.[24,28]

The lack of specificity in the diagnosis of critical carotid stenosis remains a shortcoming for MRA and limits its value, especially as a screening tool. Duplex remains the preferred method, and most clinicians who use MRA for making clinical decisions use it in conjunction with duplex imaging. Patel et al.[24] found that the diagnostic accuracy of MRA and duplex for determining a stenosis of 70–99% were 86% and 88%, respectively; however, when the two studies were concordant, the diagnostic accuracy increased to 94%.

Computed tomography

Rapid-acquisition spiral CT scanning allows image acquisition to be timed with contrast administration, and enhanced computer image reconstruction gives CT angiograms nearly the same anatomic detail and resolution as standard contrast angiography. Furthermore, the cross-sectional source images give added information on plaque morphology not available with standard arteriograms. Because CT angiography requires a significant contrast load and is less readily available than standard contrast angiography, it is not used widely. Data supporting its routine application before carotid surgery are lacking. As more is learned about the influence of plaque morphology on natural history and as plaque morphology comes to play a greater role in patient selection for carotid endarterectomy, CT angiography will likely become a routine part of patient assessment.

Contrast angiography

Contrast angiography remains for many the standard against which all other diagnostic studies are measured. Newer digital imaging systems have further enhanced image quality, allowing multiplanar high-resolution images of the arch, carotids, vertebrals, and intracranial vessels. Examples of digital angiographic images of the carotid circulation are shown in **Figures 36.10–36.12**. Despite the traditional acceptance of contrast angiography as

the 'gold standard', this technique remains subject to significant inter-observer variability in interpretation. The discrepancy between the NASCET and ECST methods for determining carotid stenosis highlights the potential for significant variability in image interpretation. In NASCET, the stenosis was calculated as the ratio of the diameter at the narrowest point to the diameter at the point at which the ICA walls again become parallel, beyond the area of post-stenotic dilatation. In ECST, the stenosis was calculated as the ratio of the diameter at the narrowest point to the carotid bulb diameter reconstructed as if there were no disease. This variation has led to significant differences in angiographic interpretation such that a 60% stenosis in ECST is only an 18% stenosis in NASCET, a 70% stenosis in ECST is a 40% stenosis in NASCET, an 80% stenosis in ECST is a 61% stenosis in NASCET, and a 90% stenosis in ECST is an 80% stenosis in NASCET. Radiologists and surgeons looking at exactly the same film can arrive at significantly different interpretations of the degree of carotid stenosis. Even if the method of stenosis calculation is agreed, the inter-observer variability for contrast angiography can be significant and nearly as great as that for MRA.[23] While no one questions the ease with which contrast angiograms can be reviewed and their reliable depiction of carotid anatomy, contrast angiography should not be accepted uncritically in the assessment of carotid disease.

In addition to inter-observer variability, potential morbidity and cost limit the applicability of contrast angiography. Contrast allergy and nephrotoxicity remain significant issues despite newer contrast agents and improved protocols for prevention of anaphylaxis and renal failure. Arterial puncture can be associated with significant morbidity from hemorrhage, pseudoaneurysm formation, and arterial thrombosis. Selective carotid studies are associated with stroke risk. In ACAS, the risk of stroke from angiography was 1.2%.[7] Contrast angiography is more expensive than the less invasive diagnostic studies. At the New England Medical Center, the charge for diagnostic cerebral angiography averages approximately $2500, while for duplex ultrasonography and MRA, the charges average approximately $420 and $1100,

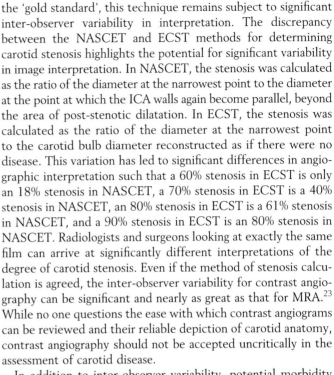

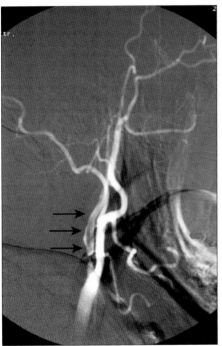

Figure 36.10 Contrast angiography. Critical internal carotid stenosis with a tail of thrombus extending into the more distal internal carotid artery (arrows). The patient had an evolving stroke. Duplex imaging suggested critical stenosis but the velocities were damped (peak systolic velocity = 55; end-diastolic velocity = 17), and no patent distal vessel could be identified. Endarterectomy was carried out uneventfully with an excellent neurologic recovery.

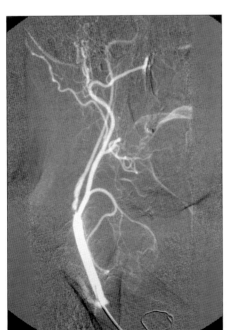

Figure 36.11 Contrast angiography. Carotid angiogram showing critical carotid stenosis with a small underperfused distal internal carotid artery (string sign). Duplex had been unable to rule out internal carotid artery occlusion.

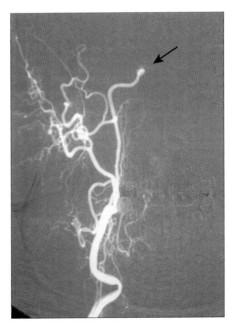

Figure 36.12 Contrast angiography. Carotid angiogram revealing moderate bifurcation disease, a small internal carotid artery (ICA), and occlusion of the intracranial ICA (arrow) in a patient with a middle cerebral artery stroke. Duplex had shown moderate ICA stenosis by image but very sluggish ICA velocities (peak systolic velocity = 25, end-diastolic velocity = 6).

respectively. Because of improvements in duplex and MRA and because of the morbidity and cost associated with contrast angiography, most centers performing a high volume of carotid surgery use contrast angiography in only occasional patients not adequately evaluated by duplex or MRA. **Figures 36.10–36.12** illustrate clinical scenarios in which contrast angiography was deemed necessary.

Investigation before carotid intervention

Neither CT scan nor MRI is indicated routinely in patients being evaluated for carotid endarterectomy. While CT and MRI evidence for stroke may be detected in up to 16% of asymptomatic patients and 35% of patients who had a TIA, it is not clear that these findings alter surgical outcomes or should have any influence on surgical decisions.[29] Some authors have reported increased neurologic morbidity associated with the presence of silent infarcts found on CT or MRI.[30,31] Others have found that incidentally discovered infarcts have no prognostic significance.[32,33] Martin et al.[32] performed routine CT scans on 469 patients being considered for carotid endarterectomy. Scans were abnormal in 62% of patients with a history consistent with stroke and in only 14% of patients with no history of stroke. There were no incidental tumors, arteriovenous malformations, intracranial aneurysms, or other significant brain lesions identified. The CT scans did not alter clinical judgement with respect to treatment selection in any patient. The perioperative stroke rate for the 230 endarterectomies performed in these patients was 1.3%. Given these results, it is hard to argue that routine brain imaging with CT or MRI is likely to have a beneficial impact on surgical outcome.

Brain imaging studies are clearly indicated in selected patients. Acute or evolving stroke, atypical neurological signs or symptoms, and a prior history of significant head injury or intracranial lesions are all legitimate indications for preoperative brain imaging. A remote history of stroke may be an indication for preoperative imaging, especially in the presence of residual neurological deficits. Of course, in patients undergoing MRA for evaluation of the cervical and intracranial vasculature, MRI can be performed with no added morbidity or patient inconvenience, and with little additional cost. In this case, it is hard to argue against brain imaging, though the anticipated influence of the MRI on surgical decisions should be minimal.

The preoperative imaging studies should be tailored to the needs of each individual patient. Selected patients may have sur-

Use of carotid and brain imaging at the New England Medical Center.	
Study	*Indication*
Duplex alone	1,2
Duplex + MRA	3–8
Contrast angiography	9–12
CT angiography	13
Brain imaging	14–16

1. >80% asymptomatic stenosis (EDV>140cm/s)
2. >70% stenosis with TMB, carotid TIA, or stroke with minimal residual signs
3. 1 or 2 above with suboptimal duplex, borderline velocities, or discrepant velocity and image data
4. 50–70% stenosis with TMB, carotid TIA, or stroke with minimal residual signs
5. Prior stroke with residual signs
6. Possible occlusion by duplex with ongoing symptoms
7. Decreased carotid pulses, suspected vertebrobasilar or severe intracranial disease
8. Sluggish velocities by duplex with high grade stenosis by duplex image
9. 3–8 with contraindication to MRA
10. Inability to differentiate high-grade stenosis and occlusion by duplex/MRA
11. Cannot determine distal extent of plaque by duplex
12. Plans for carotid stenting
13. Carotid territory symptoms with mild to moderate disease by duplex/MRA and no other source for symptoms
14. Acute stroke/evolving stroke
15. Atypical symptoms
16. Prior intracranial pathology/surgery

Table 36.7. Use of carotid and brain imaging at the New England Medical Center. CT, computed tomography; EDV, end-diastolic volume; MRA, magnetic resonance angiography; TIA, transient ischemic attack; TMB, transient monocular blindness.

gery with duplex data alone, while other patients will require more extensive evaluation including contrast angiography and brain imaging. **Table 36.7** outlines the New England Medical Center protocol for carotid and brain imaging studies in the commonly encountered clinical scenarios.

REFERENCES

1. Murros KE, Evans GW, Toole JF, et al. Cerebral infarction in patients with transient ischemic attacks. J Neurol 1989;236:182–6.
2. Toole JF, Dibert SW, Harpold GJ. Transient ischemic attacks and stroke in the distribution of the carotid artery: clinical manifestations. In: Moore, ed. Surgery for cerebrovascular disease, 2nd edn. Philadelphia:WB Saunders; 1996: 73.
3. Chambers BR. Norris JW. Outcome in patients with asymptomatic neck bruits. N Engl J Med 1986;315:860–5.
4. O'Holleran LW, Kennelly MM, McClurken M, Johnson JM. Natural history of asymptomatic carotid plaque. Five year follow-up study. Am J Surg 1987;154:659–62.
5. Roederer GO, Langlois YE, Jager KA, et al. The natural history of carotid arterial disease in asymptomatic patients with cervical bruits. Stroke 1984; 15:605–13.
6. Hobson RW, Weiss DG, Fields WS, et al. Efficacy of carotid endarterectomy for asymptomatic carotid stenosis. N Engl J Med 1993;328:221–7.
7. Executive Committee for Asymptomatic Carotid Atherosclerosis Study. Endarterectomy for asymptomatic carotid artery stenosis. JAMA 1995; 273:1421–8.
8. Crouse JR, Byington RP, Hoen HM, Furberg CD. Reductase inhibitor monotherapy and stroke prevention. Arch Intern Med 1997; 157:1305–10.
9. Nicolaides AN. Asymptomatic carotid stenosis and risk of stroke: identification of a high-risk group. Int Angiol 1995;14:21–8.
10. Canadian Cooperative Study Group. A randomized trial of aspirin and sulfinpyrazone in threatened stroke. N Engl J Med 1978;299:53–9.
11. Fields WS, Lemak NA, Frankowski RF, Hardy RJ. Controlled trial of aspirin in cerebral ischemia. Stroke 1977;8:301–15.

12. Bousser MG, Eschwege E, Haguenau M, et al. 'AICLA' controlled trial of aspirin and dipyridamole in secondary prevention of athero-thrombotic cerebral ischemia. Stroke 1983;14:5–14.

13. North American Symptomatic Carotid Endarterectomy Trial Collaborators. Beneficial effect of carotid endarterectomy in symptomatic patients with high-grade carotid stenosis. N Engl J Med 1991;325:445–53.

14. Barnett HJM, Taylor DW, Eliaziw M, et al. Benefit of carotid endarterectomy in patients with symptomatic moderate or severe stenosis. N Engl J Med 1998;339:1415–25.

15. European Carotid Surgery Trialists' Collaborative Group. MRC European Carotid Surgery Trial: interim results for patients with severe (70–99%) or mild (0–29%) carotid stenosis. Lancet 1991;337:1235–43.

16. European Carotid Surgery Trialists' Collaborative Group. Randomised trial of endarterectomy for recently symptomatic carotid stenosis: final results of the MRC European Carotid Surgery Trial (ECST). Lancet 1998;351:1379–87.

17. Wolf PA, Kannel WB, Sorlie P, McNamara P. Asymptomatic carotid bruit and risk of stroke: the Framingham Study. JAMA 1981;245:1442–5.

18. Roederer GO, Langlois YE, Chan ATW, et al. Ultrasonic duplex scanning of the extracranial carotid arteries: improved accuracy using new features of the common carotid artery. J Cardiovasc Ultrasonography 1982; 1:373–80.

19. Moneta GL, Taylor DC, Nicholls SC, et al. Operative versus nonoperative management of asymptomatic high-grade internal carotid artery stenosis: improved results with endarterectomy. Stroke 1987;18:1005–10.

20. Moneta GL, Edwards JM, Chitwood RW, et al. Correlation of North American Symptomatic Carotid Endarterectomy Trial (NASCET) angiographic definition of 70–99% internal carotid artery stenosis with duplex scanning. J Vasc Surg 1993;17:152–9.

21. Moneta GL, Edwards JM, Papanicolaou G, et al. Screening for asymptomatic internal carotid artery stenosis: duplex criteria for discriminating 60–99% stenosis. J Vasc Surg 1995;21:989–94.

22. El-Barghouty N, Geroulakos G, Nicolaides A, et al. Computer assisted carotid plaque characterization. Eur J Vasc Endovasc Surg 1995;9:389–93.

23. Young GR, Humphrey PRD, Nixon TE, et al. Variability in measurement of extracranial internal carotid artery stenosis as displayed by both digital subtraction and magnetic resonance angiography: an assessment of three caliper techniques and visual impression of stenosis. Stroke 1996; 27:467–73.

24. Patel MR, Kuntz KM, Klufas RA, et al. Pre-operative assessment of the carotid bifurcation: can magnetic resonance angiography and duplex ultrasonography replace contrast angiography? Stroke 1995;26:1753–8.

25. Turnipseed WD, Kennell TW, Turski PA, et al. Magnetic resonance angiography and duplex scanning: non-invasive tests for selecting symptomatic carotid endarterectomy candidates. Surgery 1993;114:643–8.

26. Mittl RL, Broderick M, Carpenter JP, et al. Blinded reader comparison of magnetic resonance angiography and duplex ultrasonography for carotid bifurcation stenosis. Stroke 1994;25:4–10.

27. Riles TS, Eidelman EM, Litt AW, et al. Comparison of magnetic resonance angiography, conventional angiography, and duplex scanning. Stroke 1992; 23:341–6.

28. Anderson CM, Lee RE, Levin DL, et al. Measurement of internal carotid artery stenosis from source MR angiograms. Radiology 1994;193:219–26.

29. Street D, O'Brien M, Ricotta J, et al. Observations on cerebral computed tomography in patients having carotid endarterectomy. J Vasc Surg 1988; 7:798–801.

30. Graber J, Vollman R, Levine H, et al. Stroke following carotid endarterectomy: risk predicted by preoperative CT scan. Am J Surg 1984; 147:492–7.

31. Vollman R, Eldrup-Jorgensen J, Hoffman M. The role of computed tomography in carotid surgery. Surg Clin North Am 1986;66:255–68.

32. Martin J, Valentine R, Myers S, et al. Is routine CT scanning necessary in the preoperative evaluation of patients undergoing carotid endarterectomy? J Vasc Surg 1991;14:267–70.

33. Ricotta J, Ouriel K, Green R, DeWeese J. Use of computerized cerebral tomography in selection of patients for elective and urgent carotid endarterectomy. Ann Surg 1985;202:783–7.

CHAPTER
37
Endovascular Treatment of Carotid Disease

Jean-Pierre Becquemin

KEY POINTS

- The optimal management of symptomatic carotid stenosis remains highly controversial.

- The first large randomized comparison of carotid endarterectomy with angioplasty demonstrated equivalent results.

- Cerebral protection devices may make angioplasty with stenting the safest option.

- Definitive randomized trials are awaited.

- Carotid stenting is technically difficult and requires considerable radiologic expertise; consequently, there is a significant learning curve.

INTRODUCTION

Endovascular treatment of carotid disease is a highly controversial new treatment for patients with severe carotid stenosis. Proponents, mostly in the rank of cardiologists, believe that 'carotid angioplasty is another nail in the coffin of carotid surgery'.[1] Opponents, most of them surgeons, reply by quoting George Bernard Shaw: 'when you have a new hammer, everything looks like a nail.' The debate will probably continue for some time, since firm evidence is lacking concerning the immediate and long-term benefits of stenting over carotid endarterectomy. However, encouraging results from clinical series indicate that carotid stenting may become the preferred option for a significant subset of patients with carotid disease.[2-4]

The basis of the controversy is no longer the feasibility, which is well demonstrated, but the risk of stroke, which remains the most dramatic complication of all carotid interventions. Most strokes are caused by dislodgment of atherosclerotic debris, which may occur at any time during arterial navigation, crossing the lesion with a guidewire, or stent deployment. Transcranial Doppler monitoring has shown that carotid stenting produces more microemboli than carotid surgery.[5] Also, acute stent occlusion has been reported even after apparently uneventful procedures.[6,7] Crushing of fresh thrombus in the plaque or mistakes in adjuvant medication may be explanatory.

To prevent these adverse effects and their consequences on neurologic outcome, there have recently been substantial technical improvements. Current refinements include new thin caliber catheters, low-profile balloons, specifically designed stents, monorail systems, and cerebral protection devices. Furthermore, derived from the coronary trials, there is a better understanding of adjuvant drug regimens that help to avoid acute stent occlusion.[8]

Finally, after the pioneers' learning curve, the technique itself is becoming routine and reproducible.

Carotid angioplasty remains, nevertheless, a relatively sophisticated procedure which needs great care in patient selection, a good knowledge of the available devices, good imaging facilities, and excellent skill in endovascular navigation.

MATERIALS, DEVICES, AND TECHNIQUES

This section describes the materials and the techniques used currently by the author. It is recognized that other excellent products are available on the market.

Materials and devices
Guidewires and catheters
Three types of guidewire are required:

- an angled, 0.035in, 1.5m long, soft hydrophilic guidewire (Terumo);
- an angled, 0.035in, 2.6m long, stiff hydrophilic (Terumo) guidewire; and
- a 0.014in soft hydrophilic wire.

The latter may not be necessary if a cerebral protection device is used.

The introducer sheath is 7F, 10cm long, with a valve and a lateral channel. Different types of catheters should be available: a vertebral catheter (from Terumo) or a JB-2 (from Cook) are adequate in 70% of the procedures. For difficult angulated arteries and/or the left common carotid artery, a glide vertebral catheter and/or a Simmons or a Mani catheter are more appropriate (**Fig. 37.1**). To get the required shape, the Simmons

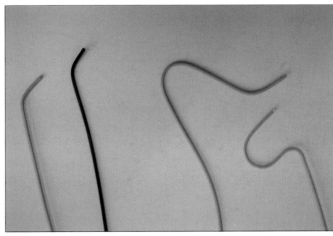

Figure 37.1 Catheters for carotid angioplasty/stenting.

catheter is shaped either in the iliac artery opposite from the introducer site, or in the renal, superior mesenteric, left sub-clavian artery, or against the aortic valve. The size of the Simmons or Mani catheter (there are three sizes) must be chosen to fit the size and shape of the aorta at the level of the arch. Finally, a 7F, 90cm long Arrow delivery catheter is used routinely at our institution.

Balloons

The author uses monorail balloons (**Fig. 37.2**), usually 2 or 3mm in diameter and 2 to 3cm in length. Crossail 0.014in monorail from Guidant for predilatation or the coronary Speedy or Gazel monorail from Boston Scientific are appropriate. Larger balloons (5 to 6mm) are also necessary to model the stent after deployment.

Stents

Most early carotid stenting was carried out using stainless steel balloon expandable stents such as the Palmaz stent (Cordis, Johnson and Johnson). Balloon expandable stents have two main advantages:

- the stent placement and the crushing of the plaque is a one-shot procedure, which avoids material manipulation; and
- the radial force of the stent is among the strongest available.

However, they have several drawbacks:

- the diameter of the balloon with the stent is relatively large, which can be an issue when trying to cross a tight stenosis safely;
- they are rigid and the stent is not protected by an outer sheath, thereby increasing the risk of plaque dislodgment, stent escape or blockage; and,
- any subsequent external compression may deform the stent.

Most currently available stents are self-expanding. They are made of stainless steel, such as the Carotid Wallstent (**Fig. 37.3A&B**), or of nitinol, such as the Herculink, AVE (Medtronic), or the Smart-stent (Cordis). These stents have good flexibility, are able to cross a tortuous artery, can match the size discrepancy between the common and internal carotid arteries. Moreover, the radial forces with these stents are acceptable. Of note is that the carotid Wallstent is more radio-opaque than the nitinol stents; this may be of importance when dealing with difficult lesions. Some of the stents shorten during their release, a phenomenon that must be anticipated to allow careful positioning.

Cerebral protection devices

There are two types of cerebral protection devices. One is based on carotid internal occlusion with a balloon, the other relies on a filter technique.

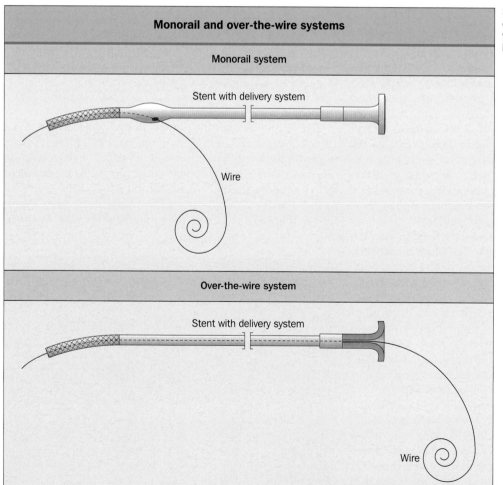

Monorail and over-the-wire systems

Monorail system

Stent with delivery system

Wire

Over-the-wire system

Stent with delivery system

Wire

Figure 37.2 Artist's impression of conception of monorail and over-the-wire systems for balloon catheter insertion.

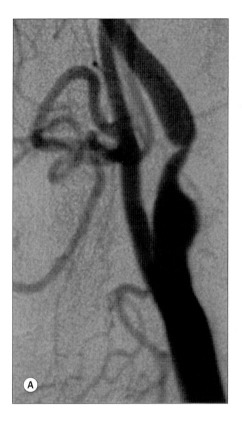

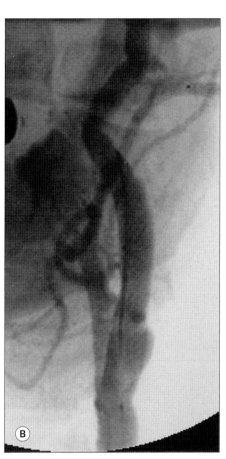

Figure 37.3 Severe carotid stenosis before (A) and after (B) implantation of a Wallstent.

The Percusurge GuardWire system (Medtronic)

This system includes a hollow Teflon-coated microcatheter available in 0.014in and 0.018in sizes with the balloon close to its distal tip. A disposable sealing system enables the balloon to be inflated and also deflated. The balloon diameter can be varied from 3.5 to 6mm. The very distal tip of the wire is floppy and radio-opaque; radio-opaque markers close to the balloon allow its accurate placement above the carotid stenosis (**Fig. 37.4**). The wire permits exchange of interventional devices, balloons, and stents, and the placement of an aspiration catheter. Before deflation of the balloon, by decompression with a syringe and slowly removing the aspiration catheter, debris is removed from the carotid artery. The system handles excellently, with good torque and forward movement. Very tight, eccentric, and irregular stenoses can be crossed relatively easily. However, the preparation of the system, notably the sealing system and the aspiration catheter, is relatively sophisticated.

The Arteria system

This is based on the principle of reverse flow. A guiding catheter with a large balloon is placed in the common carotid artery, proximal to the carotid bifurcation. A lateral channel on the guiding catheter allows, when necessary, a second balloon to be inflated in the external carotid artery (**Fig. 37.5**). The whole system is linked to a line, which is placed into one of the femoral veins. When the two balloons are inflated, the carotid inflow is stopped and the back flow from the internal carotid is diverted into the venous system. A filter between the arterial and venous

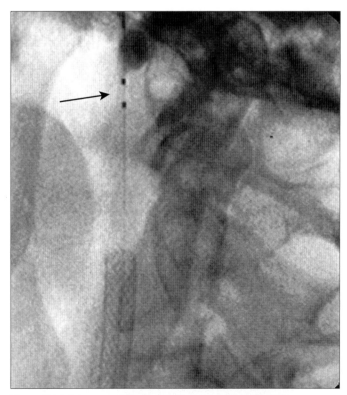

Figure 37.4 Intraoperative view of the Percusurge GuardWire protection device showing the radio-opaque markers above the carotid stenosis (arrow).

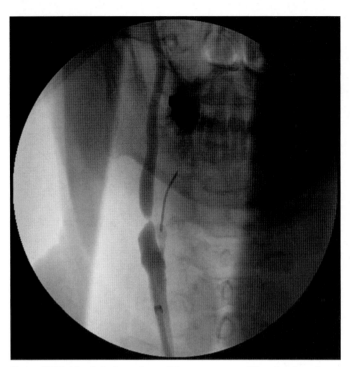

Figure 37.7 Angioguard carotid filter system in position.

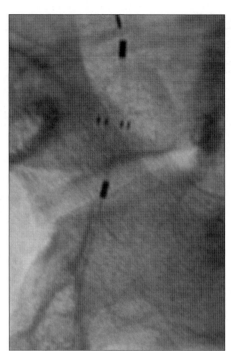

Figure 37.5 The Arteria system with common carotid and external carotid occlusion balloons.

side traps any debris. Since the flow in the internal carotid is reversed continuously, there is no risk of brain embolization during carotid stenting. However, the system requires a 10F introducer sheath and is relatively cumbersome and complex.

The EPI system (Boston Scientific)
This consists of a basket-like, porous membrane at the tip of a 0.014in guidewire (**Fig. 37.6**). An outer sheath protects the

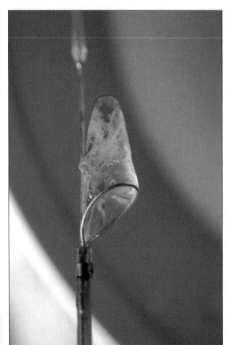

Figure 37.6 EPI carotid filter.

filter, which is released when the sheath is displaced caudally. The filter has to be deployed about 2cm above the stenosis in a relatively straight arterial segment. The filter, and particularly its base, should be applied carefully against the arterial wall in order to offer maximum efficacy. After carotid stent deployment, the filter containing trapped debris is retrieved by pulling it partially within the outer sheath.

The Angioguard system (Cordis)
This is also a basket-like filter fixed by longitudinal metallic wires. The filter presents micropores, 0.5mm in diameter. The basket is deployed and captured by pushing or pulling the outer sheath (**Fig. 37.7**).

The Neuroshield system
The principles of this system are similar to the two previously described filters.

The main advantage of filters is their simplicity, and the fact that they do not stop carotid blood flow during the procedure. The drawbacks are the relative instability of the devices, which may move during the different maneuvers of carotid stenting. Additionally, there is uncertainty concerning the full apposition of the filter on the arterial wall. Occasionally, when a large amount of fresh thrombus is trapped in the filter, carotid occlusion may occur.

Techniques of ICA angioplasty/stenting
Operating room installation
A well-appointed operating room is essential for a successful procedure. The operating table must be radiolucent. Before starting the endovascular maneuver, a clinician must check that no radio-opaque bars or wires cross the operating field, including the

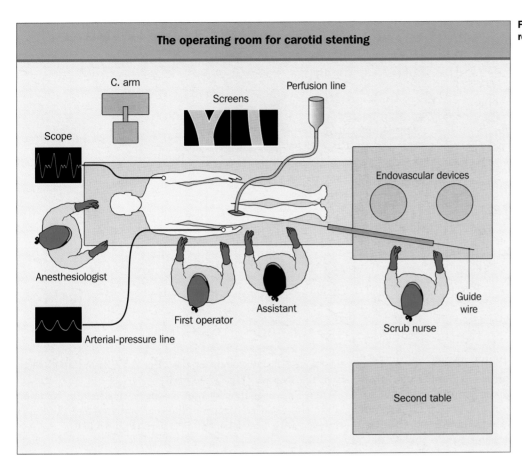

The operating room for carotid stenting

C. arm

Screens

Perfusion line

Scope

Endovascular devices

Anesthesiologist

Assistant

First operator

Guide wire

Scrub nurse

Arterial-pressure line

Second table

Figure 37.8 Diagram of the operating room for carotid stenting.

groin, the whole aorta, the neck, and the skull. Antero-posterior and lateral views must be easily and rapidly obtained and it must be possible to rotate the C-arm freely around the neck of the patient. The operating team, including the surgeon, the assistant, and the scrub nurse stand to the right of the patient. A disposable table is placed at the patient's feet (**Fig. 37.8**). This allows positioning of the endovascular devices 'in line', limiting the risk of dropping any wires or catheters, and septic contamination. The C-arm faces the operating team, with the screen opposite the main operator. The patient is draped in one large sterile sheet with two openings in the groin. The groin should have been shaved and washed with antiseptic solution. A variety of endovascular materials (guidewire, catheters, and stents, all of different sizes and length) should be stored in the vicinity of the operating theatre and be easily and rapidly accessible.

Anesthesia, monitoring, and medication

Except for combined procedures, patients have carotid procedures under local anesthesia. Since severe bradycardia may occur, continuous cardiac monitoring and intra-arterial pressure measurement is essential. Conscious level and motor functions should be surveyed regularly. Transcranial Doppler imaging of the middle cerebral artery may be useful, although not mandatory. Anesthesiologists should be available in the hospital for the rare occasions when general anesthesia is required urgently.

Patients are given 75mg aspirin and 75mg clopidogrel on the day prior to surgery. At the start of the guidewire manipulation, 1mg/kg of heparin should be given intravenously. Heparin is not reversed at the end of the procedure, and low molecular weight

heparin is started 6 hours afterwards and continued daily for 48 hours. Clopidogrel is given for 1 month and aspirin indefinitely. In order to prevent severe bradycardia and arterial spasm, 1mg of atropine may be given before angioplasty, or on demand.

Approaches to the carotid artery

There are three basic approaches.

1. Direct percutaneous carotid puncture was employed in the first attempts at carotid angioplasty. Very few indications remain, since it is relatively difficult to perform and may be hazardous. Arterial dissection, blind crossing of the carotid stenosis, and postoperative cervical hematoma have led progressively to its abandonment. However, following surgical exposure of the common carotid artery, direct puncture may occasionally be used. The main indication is the presence of tandem lesions, involving the common carotid and the carotid bifurcation.

2. The brachial approach through the axillary artery may be useful when the femoral approach is not adequate, but has risks of neurologic damage.

3. The femoral approach is used routinely. A 5F introducer sheath is placed into the femoral artery. A soft Terumo guidewire is then pushed into the aorta, up to the aortic arch.

Common carotid catheterization

The vertebral catheter is pushed up the guidewire. Once the catheter is in the arch, the wire is pulled out and the catheter gently pulled back while exercising clockwise rotation. Generally, the innominate artery trunk is easily catheterized. A small

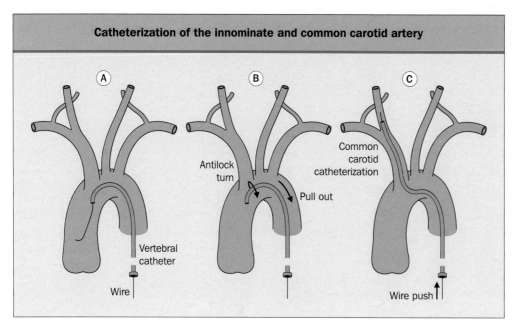

Figure 37.9 Catheterization of the innominate and common carotid artery.

amount of contrast medium is used to check that the positioning is correct (**Fig. 37.9**). For the left common carotid artery, the catheter is pulled back again for a few centimeters. In favorable cases, it jumps into the common carotid ostium. If not, a Simmons or Mani catheter should be used (**Fig. 37.10**). Once in the ostium, the wire and then the catheter (while holding the wire) are advanced into the common carotid artery. It is of prime importance to verify that the distal tip of the wire remains proximal to the carotid bifurcation and does not cross the carotid stenosis blindly.

External carotid catheterization
The C-arm is placed at the level of the neck to obtain lateral views. The guidewire is pulled out and contrast medium injected to help to locate the carotid bifurcation. The distal tip of the catheter is placed close to the external carotid ostium and the wire is pushed into the external carotid artery. Once in place, the vertebral catheter is advanced into the external carotid artery. The soft wire is then exchanged for a stiff guidewire, which is blocked into a tributary, the lingual or occipital artery.

Delivery catheter placement
The vertebral catheter is retrieved and replaced by the 7F Arrow catheter. The radio-opaque distal tip is placed in the common carotid artery. Then dilatator and wire are pulled out. An angiogram is performed through the Arrow catheter. Images are generally then of excellent quality. With the Arteria system, the Arrow catheter is not necessary.

Cerebral protection devices placement
With the filter devices or the distal protection balloon system, the distal flexible tip of the device is placed proximal to the carotid bifurcation through the Arrow catheter. Then, using road-mapping, the internal carotid artery is catheterized and the stenosis is crossed. This maneuver is generally easy to perform. In the case of an angulated internal carotid artery, the distal tip of the wire must be pre-shaped. Only a very gentle push is employed, to avoid plaque injury. Once the lesion has been

crossed, the distal balloon or the filter is deployed about 2cm above the stenosis (**Fig. 37.11A&B**).

When a reverse flow system has been chosen, the common carotid and external carotid balloons are inflated and the lesion is crossed with a 0.014in standard wire (**Fig. 37.11C**).

Predilatation
Predilatation is necessary only for a very tight carotid stenosis (>95%); this avoids any friction during the crossing by the stent and also makes the intra-stent balloon angioplasty easier to perform. Without this procedure, it may be impossible to cross the stenosis with the stent or to place the balloon after the release of the stent.

Stenting and angioplasty
This step is similar to angioplasty and stenting in peripheral arteries. The authors use a relatively long stent (3 or 4cm), to avoid it slipping off the lesion. For lesions located distal to the bifurcation, 5 to 6mm stents are used. For lesions located close to the bifurcation, 7 to 8mm stents are used. Whatever the location, adequate sizing must be assessed from the angiogram. The stent is released by pulling back the outer sheath, while holding the inner component of the delivery system. This step is crucial and must be followed carefully on both the road map and plain screens. The smaller field of the C-arm is used for this step (22cm). When correctly placed, the stent shows a typical hourglass shape. The delivery system is removed, while holding the wire of the protection device. A balloon, 2 to 3cm long and 5 to 6mm in diameter, is placed within the stent and inflated. When radio-opaque, the stent is well shown by plain X-ray. For less visible stents, a further angiogram checks opening and position. With distal balloon protection devices this step cannot be performed at this time, since the flow is still blocked.

Debris is removed with the aspiration catheter of the distal balloon protection device or by repositioning the filter in the outer sheath.

A final angiogram is performed with anteroposterior and lateral views of the neck, and of the intracerebral circulation.

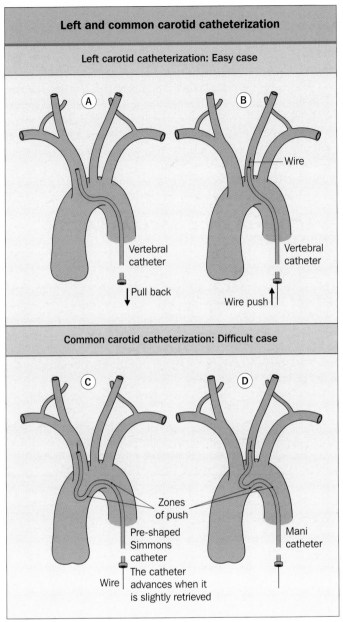

Figure 37.10 Left and common carotid catheterization.
(A&B) Catheterization of the left common carotid artery with a vertebral catheter. (C&D) Catheterization of the left common carotid artery with a Simmons and a Mani catheter.

At the end of the procedure, all material is removed and the groin is compressed manually for half an hour. Alternatively, a Perclose or Angioseal system can be used.

Techniques of common carotid artery angioplasty/stenting

For isolated common carotid lesions, the technique is similar to the one described previously; however, guidewire exchange and cerebral protection device placement is more risky, since the stenosis is proximal to the external carotid.

For tandem lesions of the common and internal carotid arteries, the internal carotid is treated in the conventional way; before closing the arteriotomy, the common carotid is punctured with a 5F introducer sheath. Guidewire, balloon, and stent are placed in the proximal common carotid lesion. It is useful to place a

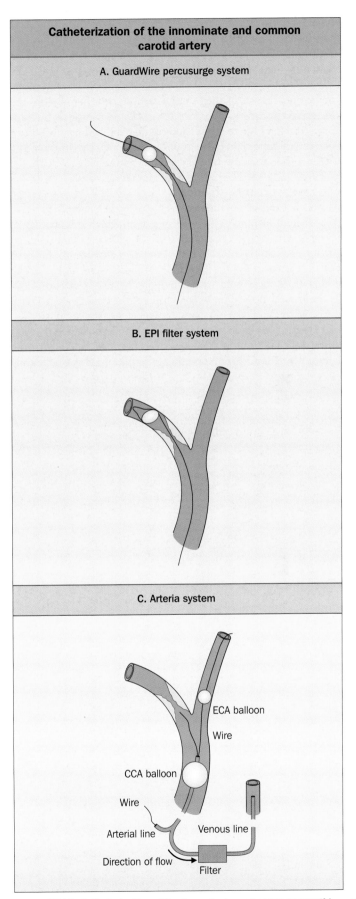

Figure 37.11 Catheterization of the innominate and common carotid artery. (A) Percusurge GuardWire cerebral protection device placement. (B) Filter placement. (C) Arteria system placement.

pigtail catheter in the aortic arch coming from the groin. It is then easy to survey the correct position of the stent.

Alternatively, the proximal common carotid stenosis can be treated by angioplasty and the internal carotid stenosis by conventional surgical repair. The authors prefer to start with the conventional repair of the internal carotid, and then, before the closure of the artery, puncture the common carotid in a retrograde fashion. Once the endovascular procedure has been completed, debris and clots are flushed through the arteriotomy, which is then repaired by conventional suture (**Fig. 37.12**).

The case for routine stenting

Although the current consensus for carotid angioplasty is to place a stent routinely, the evidence upon which this attitude is based is slim. In the Carotid and Vertebral Artery Transluminal Angioplasty Study (CAVATAS), the percentages of transient ischemic attack (TIA)/stroke and restenosis were similar in the group of patients who had undergone a stent procedure and in the group who had undergone balloon angioplasty alone. With transcranial Doppler assessment, however, Orlandi et al. showed that there were fewer microemboli in the middle cerebral artery in patients in whom a stent was placed compared to those in whom it was not.[9] From a pathologic point of view, this finding

appears logical. Balloon angioplasty widens the arterial lumen by fracturing the plaque. Thus, atherosclerotic debris and clots contained in the plaque may migrate in the bloodstream. Stents, by permanently crushing the plaque, prevent early recoil. The atherosclerotic material is trapped between the metallic frame and the arterial wall, which may limit migration. The disadvantage of routine stenting is its propensity to develop intimal hyperplasia and excess tissue growth within the struts of the stent, although so far, this problem does not seem to be relevant clinically. It may arise from the relatively short length of stent in a relatively high-flow situation. Nevertheless, longer term follow-up is required before any firm conclusions can be drawn on whether there is any place for balloon angioplasty alone.

SELECTION OF ENDOVASCULAR CAROTID TREATMENT

Patient selection

The current selection criteria used by the author are summarized in **Table 37.1**. However, there is no evidence, nor consensus, on patient selection for carotid angioplasty. Before choosing between carotid stenting or surgery, the balance of risks should be examined carefully; this includes general, local, and neurologic risk. Also, the risk of technical failure due to anatomic peculiarities must be taken into account.

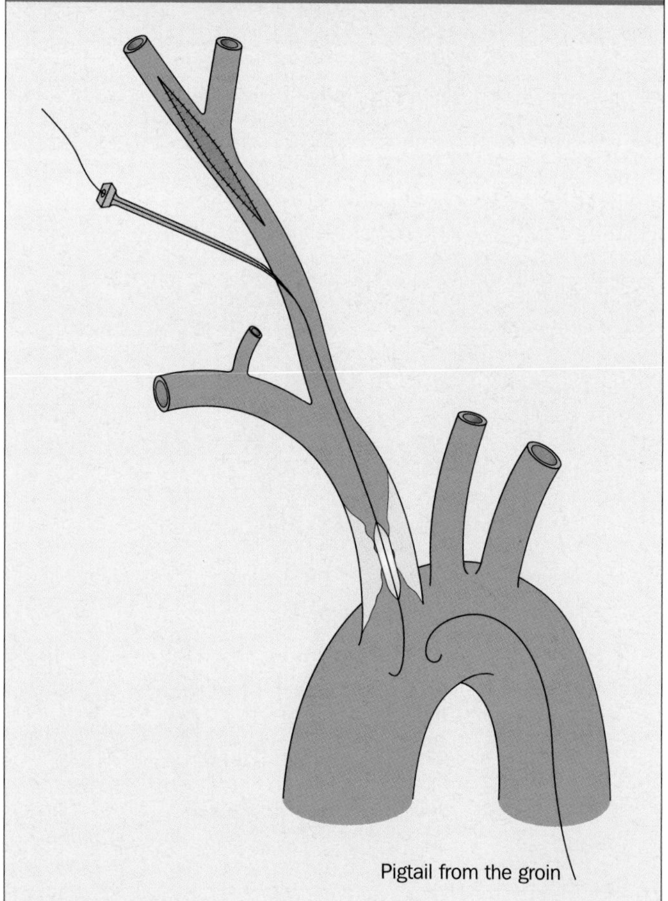

Figure 37.12 **Combined treatment of innominate and internal carotid artery stenosis.**

Comparison of current selection criteria for angioplasty/stenting or surgery for carotid stenosis.		
	Angioplasty/stenting	*Surgery*
Severe coronary disease	?	?
Calcified aortic valve	+/−	+++
Renal insufficiency	+	++
Pulmonary disease	+++	+/−
Age >80 years	−	+++
Aortic arch disease	−	+++
Severe angulations	+	+++
Severe tortuosity	+	+++
Aorto-iliac disease	+	+++
Hemorrhagic risk	+++	−
Unstable plaque	+	+++
Echolucent plaque	−	+++
Circular calcification	−	+++
Floating thrombus	−	+++
Restenosis	+++	+
Post-radiation stenosis	+++	+
Inflammatory arteritis	+	++
Atherosclerotic plaque	+++	+++

Table 37.1 **Comparison of current selection criteria for angioplasty/stenting or surgery for carotid stenosis.**

The general risk

Since surgery is associated with a very low mortality (particularly under local anesthetic), it is not easy to predict which patients may benefit from carotid angioplasty rather than surgery. It has been shown that patients with severe coronary, pulmonary, or renal disease have a higher risk of neurologic and general complications.[10,11] Unfortunately, it has still not been established whether angioplasty/stenting is less risky in these patients. Patients with severe respiratory disorders are probably the least disputable indication, since groin anesthesia is obviously a better option than general or cervical block anesthesia. In a cardiac patient, angioplasty may be hazardous, since hemodynamic instability is not well tolerated in those with severe coronary disease or with calcified aortic cardiac valve disease. Finally, patients with renal insufficiency are also not the best candidates for angioplasty, due to the need of contrast injection and the risk of contrast nephropathy. In addition, these patients often have unfavorable anatomic lesions.

The local risk

The risk of cervical nerve injury after surgery is in the range of 7%, although this is usually only temporary.[12] This rate is increased to 17% in patients who have had a previous neck operation[13] or neck irradiation. The risk of infection is quite low, except in those patients with a tracheostomy.

Thus, although still challenged by some authors,[14] there is a consensus to consider patients with restenosis following a previous carotid endarterectomy, or patients with radiation-induced stenosis (especially those with a tracheostomy), as an accepted indication for carotid stenting (**Fig. 37.13**).[15] Unfortunately, the durability of stenting for this indication is questioned, since severe intra-stent restenosis has been reported.[16]

The neurologic risk

Plaques which are ulcerated, unstable, or full of fresh thrombotic material and floating thrombus are clearly at risk from an endovascular procedure and are probably best treated by open surgery (**Fig. 37.14**). Conversely, fibrotic soft plaque gives rise to less risk. Duplex imaging may help to select these patients, although the criteria for plaque classification are still controversial.[17]

Contralateral occlusion of the internal carotid artery gives rise to a risk of intolerance to clamping, and a shunt is frequently required during carotid surgery. These patients may be considered for angioplasty instead.

The status of the aortic arch is also an important issue. It has been shown by transesophagal duplex imaging that the aortic arch is often the origin of spontaneous cerebral emboli,[18] and that the frequency of thrombus and significant unstable aortic plaque increase with age.[19] In these patients, endovascular treatment, at least from the groin, is not the best option.

The risk of technical failure

Angioplasty may fail because of navigation problems or failure of stent deployment. Failure must be anticipated in order to avoid serious clinical complications.

Iliac stenosis or occlusion is an annoying cause of failure that should be avoidable by preoperative duplex imaging. Sharp angulation of the aortic arch and common carotid arteries also risks failure of catheterization. The threshold is difficult to define, however, since skilled interventionalists may succeed where

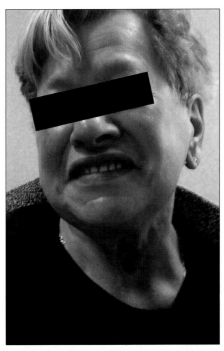

**Figure 37.13
A 67-year-old female with a symptomatic left carotid stenosis.** She had previously been treated by surgery and radiotherapy for head and neck cancer. This is an excellent indication for carotid stenting.

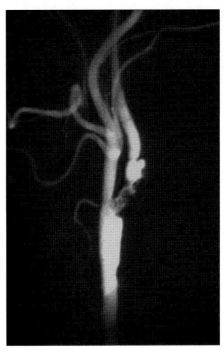

**Figure 37.14
Angiography of a carotid bifurcation showing unstable plaque and thrombus.** This is a contraindication to carotid stenting.

the less experienced fail. Severe common carotid tortuosity may preclude the delivery of the stent. Internal carotid artery tortuosity may also be difficult to deal with, since a kink may occur at the distal end of the stent.

Finally, heavy circular calcified plaque or very dense fibrotic plaque may be impossible to crush. In this case, if predilatation has not previously been attempted, the stent may remain blocked or partially deployed in the carotid artery.

Goals of therapy

The first goal of carotid endovascular therapy is to prevent stroke. Thus, only patients at significant risk of stroke should be treated.

Patients with asymptomatic <80% stenosis do not require treatment, nor do those with symptomatic <60% stenosis, since the natural history of these lesions is benign.

Cost-effectiveness

Carotid endarterectomy is a proven procedure with a very low mortality/neurologic complication rate and durable results.[20,21] The challenge for carotid angioplasty is at least to equal the results of surgery, even in high-risk patients.

The cost of the materials, including stents, cerebral protection devices, and the ancillary materials, is high. In Europe, it can be estimated to be in the range of 2500 euros. When all costs are taken together (materials, operating theater, physicians' and nurses' time and fees, intensive care unit, and total hospitalization time), the estimated cost in a US institution was $30 140 for angioplasty/stenting and $21 670 for surgery.[22] When complex patients were excluded, the cost was $24 848 for stenting and $19 480 for surgery. However, the calculation of costs may vary from one institution or one country to the other. Brooks et al. showed that, for a community hospital, charges were only slightly higher for stent.[23] Gray et al. found that the costs were higher with surgery ($5409) than with stenting ($3417).[24]

In the near future, it is expected that the cost of the devices will probably decline if the market increases and if there is competition between firms selling the devices.

The evidence for surgery or angioplasty/stenting

There are two current questions regarding carotid stenting that require scientific evidence. Is endovascular treatment at least equivalent to surgery? Are cerebral protection devices useful?

Is endovascular treatment at least equivalent to surgery?
Comparative cohort studies

To date, four published randomized trials are available. Two of these showed inferior results with carotid stenting and two showed similar results (**Table 37.2**).

Naylor et al. reported a single center study that was stopped prematurely after 23 procedures due to an unacceptably high complication rate in the endovascular group.[25] This study was criticized because the complication rate in the endovascular group was 75% – much higher than in all other series of carotid stenting. Patient selection (all comers were included) and the technique of angioplasty were the main issues questioned. This

study served to draw the attention of the medical community to the hazards of the endovascular approach.

The Wallstent study (unpublished) compared carotid stenting endarterectomy and included 219 out of a total of 700 planned patients. The trial was terminated prematurely because the total stroke and death rate was 12.1% at 1 year in the stented group and 3.6% in the surgical group.

Brooks et al. reported a series of 104 patients randomly allocated to carotid angioplasty and stenting or surgery for symptomatic carotid stenosis >70%.[23] One death occurred in the surgical group (1/51) and one TIA in the stent group (1/53); no individual sustained a stroke. The perception of procedure-related pain/discomfort was similar. Hospital stay was similar, although the stent group tended to be discharged earlier (mean 1.8 days versus 2.7 days). Return to full activity was achieved within 1 week by 80% of the stent group and 67% of the patients who had undergone carotid surgery.

CAVATAS is the largest multicenter study published to date.[12]. Some 504 patients with carotid stenosis were randomly assigned to endovascular treatment (n=251) or carotid endarterectomy (n=253). For endovascular patients, stents were used in 55 (26%) and balloon angioplasty alone in 158 (74%). Independent neurologists followed up the patients. In an intention-to-treat analysis, the rates of major outcome events within 30 days did not differ significantly between endovascular treatment and surgery (6.4% versus 5.9%, respectively, for disabling stroke or death; 10.0% versus 9.9% for any stroke lasting more than 7 days, or death). Cranial nerve injury was reported in 22 (8.7%) operated patients, but none after endovascular treatment (p<0.0001). Major groin or neck hematoma occurred less often after endovascular treatment than after surgery (three cases [1.2%] versus 17 [6.7%], p<0.0015). At 1 year after treatment, severe (70–99%) ipsilateral carotid stenosis was more common after endovascular treatment (25 [14%] versus seven [4%], p<0.001). However, no substantial difference in the rate of ipsilateral stroke was noted with survival analysis up to 3 years after randomization.

The high rate of major complications (10%) in the surgical group was criticized by some vascular surgeons. Also, the angioplasty group included outdated techniques (percutaneous transluminal angioplasty alone, no cerebral protection devices) and the complication rate was greater than in previously published series (between 3% and 6%).

		Summary of evidence comparing angioplasty/stenting and surgery for carotid stenosis.		
Authors	N° patients	Grade of evidence	Clinical outcome	Restenosis rate
Naylor[25]	23	Randomized	Surgery>Angioplasty	
Brooks[23]	104	Randomized	Surgery=Angioplasty	
CAVATAS[12]	504	Randomized	Surgery=Angioplasty	Surgery>Angioplasty
Aburahma[13]	83	Non-randomized	Surgery=Angioplasty	Surgery>Angioplasty
Jordan[26]	377	Non-randomized	Surgery>Angioplasty	
Golledge[27]	33 studies	Systematic review	Surgery>Angioplasty	

Table 37.2 Summary of evidence comparing angioplasty/stenting and surgery for carotid stenosis.

Several non-randomized comparative cohort studies have been published so far (level B). In two of these, the authors concluded that the risk of stroke was significantly greater with angioplasty than with carotid endarterectomy.

Jordan et al. reported a retrospective analysis of 377 patients who underwent 414 procedures.[26] The total stroke and death rates were 9.7% in the carotid stenting group and 0.9% in the surgical group (p=0.0015). There were more cardiopulmonary complications in the stented group (32.8%) than in the surgical group (17.4%) (p=0.002).

Golledge et al. reported a meta-analysis of 33 open studies (13 angioplasty and 20 carotid endarterectomy).[27] Carotid stents were deployed in 44% of angioplasty procedures. Mortality within 30 days of angioplasty was 0.8%, compared with 1.2% after endarterectomy (p=0.6). The stroke rate was 7.1% for angioplasty and 3.3% for endarterectomy (p<0.001), while the risk of fatal or disabling stroke was 3.2% and 1.6%, respectively (p<0.01). The risk of stroke or death was 7.8% for angioplasty and 4% for endarterectomy (p<0.001), while that for disabling stroke or death was 3.9% after angioplasty and 2.2% after endarterectomy (p<0.01).

Non-comparative cohort studies

These studies have focused on different aspects of carotid angioplasty and stenting. Safety and efficacy of these procedures have been evaluated by large, single center and multicenter studies, all of which favored carotid stenting.

Roubin et al. reported 528 consecutive patients (604 hemispheres/arteries) undergoing carotid stenting.[2] There was a 0.6% (n=3) fatal stroke rate and 1% (n=5) non-stroke death rate at 30 days. The major stroke rate was 1% (n=6) and the minor stroke rate was 4.8% (n=29). The overall 30-day stroke and death rate was 7.4% (n=43). After 30 days, the incidence of fatal and non-fatal stroke was 3.2% (n=31). On Kaplan–Meier analysis, the 3-year freedom from ipsilateral or fatal stroke was 92±1%.

Bergeron et al. reported a multicenter trial of carotid stenting performed by vascular surgeons in 99 patients.[28] Postoperatively, there was a 1% minor stroke rate and 4% had a TIA. No neurologic event was observed in the 1- to 24-month follow-up (mean 13 months). Stent patency was 98% at 1 year.

Wholey et al. reported the results of a survey of carotid stenting performed in 36 centers around the world.[29] In 5210 procedures involving 4757 patients, the technical success rate was 98.4%, the TIA rate 2.82%, the minor stroke rate 2.72%, the major stroke rate 1.49%, and death within 30 days was reported as 0.86%. The combined minor and major strokes and procedure-related death rate was 5.07%.

Ahmadi et al. reported a series of 303 patients in whom a significant reduction in the frequency of neurologic complications was seen after the initial 80 interventions (p=0.03).[30] Roubin et al. reported that over a 5-year study interval, the 30-day minor stroke rate improved from 7.1% (n=7) for the first year, to 3.1% (n=5) for the fifth year (p<0.05 for trend).[2]

Risk factors

Age
Gupta et al. reported excellent results in a group of patients over 65 years of age considered to be inoperable.[31] In contrast, Marthur et al.,[32] Chastain et al.,[19] and Roubin et al.[2] gave strong

indications that advanced age (>80 years) was an independent predictor of procedural strokes after angioplasty/stenting.

Cardiopathy
Waigand et al.[33] and Al Mubarak et al.[34] reported a series of patients with severe coronary artery disease, and/or mitral incompetence, aortic stenosis, rhythm disorders, or generalized arteriosclerosis treated by carotid stenting. In both series, the mortality rate was zero and the stroke rate minimal. These encouraging results need confirmation by larger prospective series.

Other risk factors
Shawl et al. evaluated the safety and efficacy of carotid artery stenting in 170 consecutive high-risk patients, defined as those with unstable angina, previous ipsilateral carotid endarterectomy, contralateral carotid artery occlusion, and other severe co-morbid illnesses.[35] Postoperatively, the total 30-day stroke rate was 2.9%, and there were no myocardial infarctions or deaths. Again, these results were favorable, but the series included patients with different levels of risk.

Role of degree of stenosis and plaque aspects
In two series,[32,36] the degree of stenosis (as defined by North American Symptomatic Carotid Endarterectomy Trial [NASCET] criteria) did not correlate with peri-procedural neurologic deficits. However, long and/or multiple lesions were shown to be independent variables of new, or worsening, transient or permanent neurologic deficits following carotid stenting.[32,36]

Echolucent stenosis on duplex scan may be a detrimental factor. A multicenter study showed that very soft echolucent plaques were associated with 81% of neurologic complications after stenting, compared to 4.7% in echogenic plaque.[17]

Nature of the stenosis
Stenting for restenosis following a previous endarterectomy offers excellent immediate and mid-term clinical outcome. New et al. reported a multicenter series of 338 patients (358 arteries).[15] The overall 30-day stroke and death rate was 3.7%. The minor stroke rate was 1.7%, the major non-fatal stroke rate was 0.8%, the fatal stroke rate was 0.3%, and the non-stroke-related death rate was 0.9%. The overall 3-year rate of freedom from all fatal and non-fatal strokes was 96%±1% (±SE).

However, these lesions may be prone to intra-stent restenosis. Aburahma et al. reported a comparative series of 83 carotid redo procedures, with 56% restenosis in the stented group versus 0% in the surgical group (p<0.0001).[13] The rate of restenosis was even higher in the small series from Leger et al., where 75% of patients developed a severe recurrent stenosis.[16]

Post-radiation angioplasty is also an accepted indication for carotid stenting. Unfortunately, only anecdotal cases are available. Seemingly favorable results are presented but short-term follow-up does not permit firm conclusions to be reached.[37–39]

Are cerebral protection devices useful?
There are no randomized studies to date comparing protected and unprotected carotid angioplasty, but the use of cerebral protection seems appropriate.

The risk of emboli during carotid angioplasty has been proved by in-vitro testing, intraoperative transcranial Doppler scanning, and debris examination of aspiration and filters.[6,40–43] However, clinical consequences are less obvious, and neurologic outcome probably depends upon particle size. Small particles have no apparent clinical adverse effects, in contrast to medium-sized particles, which may result in TIA or minor stroke. Large particles may provoke a major stroke.

Henry et al. in a historical series of 315 carotid angioplasty procedures, reported fewer clinical neurological events when a protection device was used than when it was not.[44]

Anecdotal reports with filters have also shown a good efficacy both *in vitro*[45] and in clinical series.[46–48] The Arteria system has also been tested *in vitro* with a good efficacy.[49]

Unfortunately, cerebral protection devices may fail. With the Percusurge GuardWire device, large particles were associated with a persistent risk of neurologic events.[50] Using pre- and post-procedure magnetic resonance angiography, Crawley et al. showed new infarcts in 15% of patients, despite the use of a protection device.[51]

In the light of these fragmentary, and still controversial, results, should a cerebral protection device be used in every case or selectively? Despite the lack of proof, common sense suggests that the best chance for the patient is to avoid any risk of cerebral emboli. Therefore, even if the systems are still not ideal, and perhaps not always useful, the author prefers to use one routinely.

Complications associated with carotid angioplasty and stenting: the ways to prevent and to manage them.		
Complications	*Prevention*	*Treatment*
Access:		
Iliac blockage	Pre-op duplex	Try contralateral side
Iliac dissection	Gentle manipulation	Try contralateral side
Groin hematoma	Compression, Perclose, Angioseal	Surgery if major bleeding
Difficulty with common carotid catheterization due to angles due to proximal stenosis	Patient selection	Appropriate catheter; if still unsuccessful, surgical conversion
Difficulty crossing internal carotid artery	Patient selection	Try 0.014in wire; if still unsuccessful, surgical conversion
Internal carotid artery stenting:		
Stent blockage	Choose a stent long enough; use self-expandable stent; drug regimen, avoid fresh hemorrhagic plaque	Surgical conversion
Stent gliding		Put in a second stent
Stent crushing		New dilatation
Stent thrombosis		Thrombolysis/ ReoPro
Internal carotid artery angioplasty:		
Cardiac arrest	Smooth inflation	Rapid balloon deflation, atropine
Severe bradycardia	Atropine, temporary pacemaker	
Plaque resistance to crushing	Patient selection	Highly resistant balloon
Post-stent complications:		
Spasm	Avoid over dilatation	Wait a few minutes, then intravenous atropine
Carotid dissection	Non-traumatic maneuvers	Coronary stenting
Syphon and middle cerebral embolism, thrombosis	Adequate drug regimen	Thrombolysis/ReoPro
Balloon problems:		
Burst	Control pressures	
Blockage at the stent extremities	Use low-profile balloon	Try to modify the position of the wire with a vertebral catheter
Cerebral protection problems:		
Balloon burst	Choose appropriate size	
Deflation impossible	Check the system before use	Cut the wire
Poor apposition of the filter	Check positioning	Turn the wire
Filter thrombosis	Rapid procedure, adequate drug regimen	Retrieve the filter without closing it
Intolerance to clamping	Use filter	Deflate the balloon, change for filter
Neurologic outcome:		
Ischemic events		
TIA	Patient selection	Wait and see
Stroke	Good technique	Urgent treatment according to mechanism
Hemorrhagic events	Blood pressure control	Blood pressure control; stop anticoagulants

Table 37.3 Complications associated with carotid angioplasty and stenting: the ways to prevent and to manage them.

Which is the best cerebral protection system?

To date, there is no answer to this question. The technology is too recent and also too rapidly evolving, the number of treated patients is too few, and the evaluation not yet complete. However, different situations seem to be logical indications for the mechanism of protection. Filters may be the option selected for use when the patient has poorly developed collateral vessels or previous brain tissue damage. The Percusurge GuardWire system, which has a remarkably good forward positioning and low-profile design, could be chosen when a very severe stenosis needs to be crossed. Unstable plaques may be best treated with the Arteria system.

COMPLICATIONS

Many complications interfere with the course of carotid angioplasty (**Table 37.3**). However, most can be prevented by adequate patient selection and technique. **Table 37.3** includes possible solutions to difficult situations.

SUMMARY

Carotid stenting is a sophisticated procedure whose efficacy is challenged by the excellent results of surgery. Evidence is still lacking concerning the overall benefit in reduction of stroke and death. There is also concern about the long-term value, since several studies have shown a higher rate of intimal hyperplasia in patients treated with a stent than in patients treated surgically. The only obvious and demonstrated advantages are the reduction of cervical nerve injuries and the possibility of treating lesions which are difficult to treat surgically.

However, major improvements have recently been made which make carotid stenting safer. The rate of postoperative complications is clearly reduced by technical expertise, better devices, and proper patient selection. It is not known at present whether carotid stenting will become the routine procedure in the foreseeable future. Further improvements to devices, notably toward simplicity of use, better protection devices, and prevention of intra-stent hyperplasia[52] may increase the number of patients eligible for this technique. Moreover, the results of major ongoing randomized trials and cohort studies, from both sides of the Atlantic, are awaited with interest. The battle between vascular surgeons, who understandably prefer to stick to open surgery, and cardiologists, who are looking for a new market, is not over. The author may risk a prediction, however, that, similar to other arterial territories, surgery and endovascular techniques will be complementary, rather than competitive, for the best care of vascular patients.

Recent evidence has emerged from two randomized studies designed to compare carotid stenting versus carotid endarterectomy. 1) The SAPPHIRE trial, whose latest analysis was presented at the June 2003 SVS/AAVS meeting, investigated patients at high risk for endarterectomy based on medical or anatomic factors. Composite endpoint including death stroke and myocardial infarction was significantly in favour of stent (5.8% versus 12.6% p=0.05). 2) A subgroup analysis of patients enrolled in the French EVA 3S trial (Endarterectomy versus Angioplasty in Severe Symptomatic Stenosis) showed that stenting without cerebral protection devices increased the absolute risk of post-stenting stroke by 3 fold (in submission). As a consequence, the safety committee of the study made mandatory the use of cerebral protection devices in patients allocated to carotid stenting.

REFERENCES

1. White CJ. Another nail in the coffin of carotid endarterectomy. J Am Coll Cardiol 2001;38:1596–7.
2. Roubin GS, New G, Iyer SS, et al. Immediate and late clinical outcomes of carotid artery stenting in patients with symptomatic and asymptomatic carotid artery stenosis: a 5-year prospective analysis. Circulation 2001; 103:532–7.
3. Veith FJ, Amor M, Ohki T, et al. Current status of carotid bifurcation angioplasty and stenting based on a consensus of opinion leaders. J Vasc Surg 2001;33(2 Suppl):S111–6.
4. Diethrich EB. Carotid angioplasty and stenting. Will they match the gold standard? Tex Heart Inst J 1998;25:1–9.
5. Jordan WD Jr, Voellinger DC, Doblar DD, Plyushcheva NP, Fisher WS, McDowell HA. Microemboli detected by transcranial Doppler monitoring in patients during carotid angioplasty versus carotid endarterectomy. Cardiovasc Surg 1999;7:33–8.
6. Chaturvedi S, Sohrab S, Tselis A. Carotid stent thrombosis: report of 2 fatal cases. Stroke 2001;32:2700–2.
7. D'Audiffret A, Desgranges P, Kobeiter H, Becquemin JP. Technical aspects and current results of carotid stenting. J Vasc Surg 2001; 33:1001–7.
8. Bhatt DL, Kapadia SR, Bajzer CT, et al. Dual antiplatelet therapy with clopidogrel and aspirin after carotid artery stenting. J Invasive Cardiol 2001;13:767–71.
9. Orlandi G, Fanucchi S, Fioretti C, et al. The case for routine stenting. Arch Neurol 2001;58:1410–3.
10. Ouriel K, Hertzer NR, Beven EG, et al. Preprocedural risk stratification: identifying an appropriate population for carotid stenting. J Vasc Surg 2001;33:728–32.
11. Jordan WD Jr, Alcocer F, Wirthlin DJ, et al. High-risk carotid endarterectomy: challenges for carotid stent protocols. J Vasc Surg 2002; 35:16–22.
12. Endovascular versus surgical treatment in patients with carotid stenosis in the Carotid and Vertebral Artery Transluminal Angioplasty Study (CAVATAS): a randomised trial. Lancet 2001;357:1729–37.
13. Aburahma AF, Bates MC, Stone PA, Wulu JT. Comparative study of operative treatment and percutaneous transluminal angioplasty/stenting for recurrent carotid disease. J Vasc Surg 2001;34:831–8.
14. Hill BB, Olcott C, Dalman RL, Harris EJ, Zarins CK. Reoperation for carotid stenosis is as safe as primary carotid endarterectomy. J Vasc Surg 1999;30:26–35.
15. New G, Roubin GS, Iyer SS, et al. Safety, efficacy, and durability of carotid artery stenting for restenosis following carotid endarterectomy: a multicenter study. J Endovasc Ther 2000;7:345–52.
16. Leger AR, Neale M, Harris JP. Poor durability of carotid angioplasty and stenting for treatment of recurrent artery stenosis after carotid endarterectomy: an institutional experience. J Vasc Surg 2001;33:1008–14.
17. Biasi GM. Is it time to reconsider the selection criteria for conventional or endovascular repair of carotid artery stenosis in the prevention of cerebral ischemia? J Endovasc Ther 2001;8:339–40.
18. Cohen A, Tzourio C, Bertrand B, Chauvel C, Bousser MG, Amarenco P. Aortic plaque morphology and vascular events: a follow-up study in patients with ischemic stroke. FAPS Investigators. French Study of Aortic Plaques in Stroke. Circulation 1997;96:3838–41.
19. Chastain HD, Gomez CR, Iyer S, et al. Influence of age upon complications of carotid artery stenting. UAB Neurovascular Angioplasty Team. J Endovasc Surg 1999;6:217–22.

20. Beneficial effect of carotid endarterectomy in symptomatic patients with high-grade carotid stenosis. North American Symptomatic Carotid Endarterectomy Trial Collaborators. N Engl J Med 1991;325:445–53.

21. Randomised trial of endarterectomy for recently symptomatic carotid stenosis: final results of the MRC European Carotid Surgery Trial (ECST). Lancet 1998;351:1379–87.

22. Jordan WD Jr, Roye GD, Fisher WS III, Redden D, McDowell HA. A cost comparison of balloon angioplasty and stenting versus endarterectomy for the treatment of carotid artery stenosis. J Vasc Surg 1998;27:16–22.

23. Brooks WH, McClure RR, Jones MR, Coleman TC, Breathitt L. Carotid angioplasty and stenting versus carotid endarterectomy: randomized trial in a community hospital. J Am Coll Cardiol 2001;38:1589–95.

24. Gray WA, White HJ Jr, Barrett DM, Chandran G, Turner R, Reisman M. Carotid stenting and endarterectomy: a clinical and cost comparison of revascularization strategies. Stroke 2002;33:1063–70.

25. Naylor AR, Bolia A, Abbott RJ, et al. Randomized study of carotid angioplasty and stenting versus carotid endarterectomy: a stopped trial. J Vasc Surg 1998;28:326–34.

26. Jordan WD Jr, Schroeder PT, Fisher WS, McDowell HA. A comparison of angioplasty with stenting versus endarterectomy for the treatment of carotid artery stenosis. Ann Vasc Surg 1997;11:2–8.

27. Golledge J, Mitchell A, Greenhalgh RM, Davies AH. Systematic comparison of the early outcome of angioplasty and endarterectomy for symptomatic carotid artery disease. Stroke 2000;31:1439–43.

28. Bergeron P, Becquemin JP, Jausseran JM, et al. Percutaneous stenting of the internal carotid artery: the European CAST I Study. Carotid Artery Stent Trial. J Endovasc Surg 1999;6:155–9.

29. Wholey MH, Wholey M, Mathias K, et al. Global experience in cervical carotid artery stent placement. Catheter Cardiovasc Interv 2000;50:160–7.

30. Ahmadi R, Wilifort A, Lang W, et al. Carotid artery stenting: effect of learning curve and intermediate-term morphological outcome. J Endovasc Ther 2001;8:539–46.

31. Gupta A, Bhatia A, Ahuja A, Shalev Y, Bajwa T. Carotid stenting in patients older than 65 years with inoperable carotid artery disease: a single-center experience. Catheter Cardiovasc Interv 2000;50:1–8.

32. Mathur A, Roubin GS, Iyer SS, et al. Predictors of stroke complicating carotid artery stenting. Circulation 1998;97:1239–45.

33. Waigand J, Gross CM, Uhlich F, et al. Elective stenting of carotid artery stenosis in patients with severe coronary artery disease. Eur Heart J 1998;19:1365–70.

34. Al Mubarak N, Roubin GS, Liu MW, et al. Early results of percutaneous intervention for severe coexisting carotid and coronary artery disease. Am J Cardiol 1999;84:600–2.

35. Shawl F, Kadro W, Domanski MJ, et al. Safety and efficacy of elective carotid artery stenting in high-risk patients. J Am Coll Cardiol 2000;35:1721–8.

36. Qureshi AI, Luft AR, Janardhan V, et al. Identification of patients at risk for periprocedural neurological deficits associated with carotid angioplasty and stenting. Stroke 2000;31:376–82.

37. Hernandez-Vila E, Strickman NE, Skolkin M, Toombs BD, Krajcer Z. Carotid stenting for post-endarterectomy restenosis and radiation-induced occlusive disease. Tex Heart Inst J 2000;27:159–65.

38. Houdart E, Mounayer C, Chapot R, Saint-Maurice JP, Merland JJ. Carotid stenting for radiation-induced stenoses: a report of 7 cases. Stroke 2001;32:118–21.

39. Sharma BK, Jain S, Bali HK, Jain A, Kumari S. A follow-up study of balloon angioplasty and de-novo stenting in Takayasu arteritis. Int J Cardiol 2000;75(Suppl 1):S147–52.

40. Al Mubarak N, Roubin GS, Vitek JJ, Iyer SS, New G, Leon MB. Effect of the distal-balloon protection system on microembolization during carotid stenting. Circulation 2001;104:1999–2002.

41. Angelini A, Reimers B, Della BM, et al. Cerebral protection during carotid artery stenting: collection and histopathologic analysis of embolized debris. Stroke 2002;33:456–61.

42. Martin JB, Murphy KJ, Gailloud P, et al. In vitro evaluation of the effectiveness of distal protection in the prevention of cerebral thromboembolism during carotid stent placement. Acad Radiol 2001;8:623–8.

43. Williams DO. Carotid filters: new additions to the interventionist's toolbox. Circulation 2001;104:2–3.

44. Henry M, Amor M, Henry I et al. Carotid stenting with cerebral protection: first clinical experience using the PercuSurge GuardWire system. J Endovasc Surg 1999;6:321–31.

45. Ohki T, Roubin GS, Veith FJ, Iyer SS, Brady E. Efficacy of a filter device in the prevention of embolic events during carotid angioplasty and stenting: an ex vivo analysis. J Vasc Surg 1999;30:1034–44.

46. Parodi JC, La Mura R, Ferreira LM, et al. Initial evaluation of carotid angioplasty and stenting with three different cerebral protection devices. J Vasc Surg 2000;32:1127–36.

47. Reimers B, Corvaja N, Moshiri S, et al. Cerebral protection with filter devices during carotid artery stenting. Circulation 2001;104:12–5.

48. Al Mubarak N, Colombo A, Gaines PA, et al. Multicenter evaluation of carotid artery stenting with a filter protection system. J Am Coll Cardiol 2002;39:841–6.

49. Ohki T, Parodi J, Veith FJ, et al. Efficacy of a proximal occlusion catheter with reversal of flow in the prevention of embolic events during carotid artery stenting: an experimental analysis. J Vasc Surg 2001;33:504–9.

50. Tubler T, Schluter M, Dirsch O, et al. Balloon-protected carotid artery stenting: relationship of periprocedural neurological complications with the size of particulate debris. Circulation 2001;104:2791–6.

51. Crawley F, Stygall J, Lunn S, Harrison M, Brown MM, Newman S. Comparison of microembolism detected by transcranial Doppler and neuropsychological sequelae of carotid surgery and percutaneous transluminal angioplasty. Stroke 2000;31:1329–34.

52. Hong MK, Kornowski R, Bramwell O, Ragheb AO, Leon MB. Paclitaxel-coated Gianturco-Roubin II (GR II) stents reduce neointimal hyperplasia in a porcine coronary in-stent restenosis model. Coron Artery Dis 2001;12:513–5.

CHAPTER 38

The Surgical Treatment of Carotid Disease

A Ross Naylor and William C Mackey

KEY POINTS

- A number of major randomized clinical trials have informed vascular surgeons that carotid endarterectomy is an operation justified by a firm evidence base.

- Carotid endarterectomy has the potential to reduce the risk of stroke, particularly in selected high-risk patients with neurologic symptoms and a tight internal carotid artery stenosis.

- Careful patient selection and obsessive attention to operative detail improves the results from surgery and enhances the benefit of carotid endarterectomy to the population.

- Areas of controversy remain, such as the exact role of carotid endarterectomy in asymptomatic patients and in patients undergoing coronary artery bypass.

- Carotid surgeons should be familiar with a number of rare syndromes and conditions that they may occasionally be called on to manage.

ATHEROSCLEROTIC CAROTID DISEASE

Atherosclerosis at the origin of the internal carotid artery (ICA) accounts for up to 50% of ischemic carotid territory strokes. This chapter summarizes the principles of treatment with emphasis on the selection for, technique, and outcomes of carotid endarterectomy (CEA).

Guidelines for CEA have largely evolved from three studies.[1-5] For symptomatic patients, these are the European Carotid Surgery Trial (ECST) and the North American Symptomatic Carotid Endarterectomy Trial (NASCET). The Asymptomatic Carotid Atherosclerosis Study (ACAS) has been the most important trial to evaluate the role of CEA in asymptomatic patients. However, the rationale underlying individual management decisions will inevitably reflect local, national, international, and cost-based factors. Where possible, discrepancies in practice will be discussed.

The international trials

No operation has been subjected to such intense scientific scrutiny as CEA. The results have provided level I evidence to guide overall practice and have been the foundation for almost every guideline for local practice. However, surgeons have occasionally tended to generalize the results of these trials uncritically into clinical practice. Surgeons must remember that the trial results were attributable specifically to those clinicians, surgeons, and centers that randomized patients. It has become customary to assume that all surgeons perform CEA with similar outcomes, that all patients receive optimal medical therapy, and that the trial cohorts still represent the current population of patients at risk. None of these assumptions is entirely valid.

Provision of 'best medical therapy' has improved greatly since 1991. Moreover, fewer than 0.5% of CEAs performed in North America between 1988 and 1989 were randomized within NASCET[6] and 94% of CEAs in the US are now performed in non-NASCET centers who report a significantly higher mortality rate than NASCET centers.[7] Community-based and other randomized trials in the US and Europe also suggest that the operative risk is generally worse than in ECST and NASCET.[7-10] Accordingly, interpretation of the data, grading of evidence, and recommendations for practice must take into account the additional effect of the individual surgeon's operative risk.

ECST and NASCET

ECST and NASCET included 6462 patients with carotid symptoms in the preceding 6 months.[11] All underwent angiography, computed tomography (CT), and neurologic assessment. Randomization was stratified for degree of stenosis, but the measurement method differed (Fig. 38.1). Both trials measured the luminal diameter (the numerator). The ECST denominator was the estimated diameter of the carotid bulb. In NASCET, this was the diameter of disease-free ICA above the stenosis. In practice, a 60% NASCET stenosis approximates to an 80% ECST stenosis.

Table 38.1 presents the principal findings from ECST and NASCET. NASCET found no evidence that CEA benefitted patients with a stenosis <50%. Patients with 50–69% stenoses gained a small, but significant, benefit. Stroke-free survival was maximal in patients with 70–99% stenoses. ECST observed that CEA only benefitted patients with 70–99% carotid stenoses.

In order to participate in the trials, each surgeon had to submit a 'track record'. Only those with low complication rates were included. However, evidence suggests that the operative risk in current clinical practice may be significantly higher[7-10] and could even nullify any long-term benefit. Table 38.2 therefore reanalyzes the data for NASCET 50–69%, ECST 80–99%, and NASCET 70–99% stenoses relative to varying operative risks. Not surprisingly, the higher the 30-day death/stroke rate, the lower the benefit. For example, if a surgeon chooses to operate on symptomatic patients with 50–69% NASCET stenoses and has an operative risk of 8%, the absolute risk reduction (ARR) falls to 5% at 3 years and 20 CEAs must be performed to prevent one stroke (i.e. questionable benefit). However, if the same surgeon were only to operate on patients with NASCET 70–99% disease with the same 8% operative risk, the ARR would be 17.2% and only six CEAs are needed to prevent one stroke at 3 years.

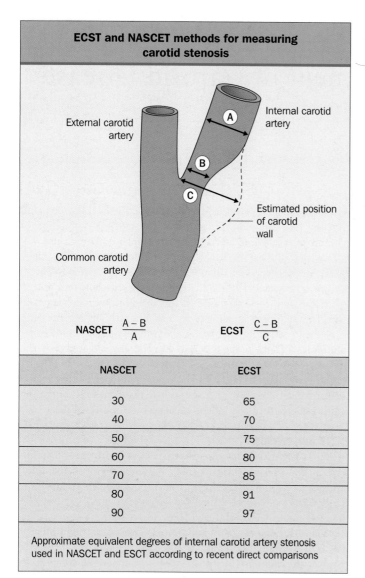

ECST and NASCET methods for measuring carotid stenosis

$$\text{NASCET} \quad \frac{A-B}{A} \qquad \text{ECST} \quad \frac{C-B}{C}$$

NASCET	ECST
30	65
40	70
50	75
60	80
70	85
80	91
90	97

Approximate equivalent degrees of internal carotid artery stenosis used in NASCET and ESCT according to recent direct comparisons

Figure 38.1 ECST and NASCET methods for measuring carotid stenosis. The table indicates how the two methods compare. (Adapted from Donnan et al.[80])

Surgeons cannot just implement the trial results without at least considering the impact of their own operative risk on the overall clinical effectiveness of the procedure.

ACAS

In ACAS,[5] 1662 patients with asymptomatic 60–99% stenosis were randomized to CEA plus best medical therapy (BMT) or BMT alone (**Table 38.1**). CEA conferred a statistically significant benefit with an ARR of 5.9% at 5 years (53% relative risk reduction). The operative risk (2.3%) was extremely low and 1.2% (50%) of the risk was from angiography. **Table 38.2** illustrates how the surgeon's operative risk alters the long-term reduction in stroke. If it were to exceed 4%, there would be no long-term benefit.[12]

EC–IC study

The Extracranial–Intracranial (EC–IC) bypass study[13] included 1377 patients with ICA occlusion randomized to BMT or EC–IC bypass (revascularization of the ipsilateral middle cerebral artery with inflow from the superficial temporal artery). The rationale

was that this might prevent stroke ipsilateral to the occluded carotid artery. This study found that surgery conferred no early or late benefit. The trial methodology aroused much debate[14] and there are renewed calls for a better designed study. It is hypothesized that if the new trial only included patients with ICA occlusion and exhausted hemodynamic reserve, surgery might confer significant benefit.[15] Until then, patients should not undergo EC–IC bypass routinely.

SELECTION OF PATIENTS FOR CAROTID SURGERY

Asymptomatic patients

The management of asymptomatic disease continues to arouse much debate. Following publication of ACAS,[5] it was recommended that provided a patient was anticipated to remain in good health and the surgeon had a low operative risk (<3%), it was appropriate to recommend CEA.

In response to the findings from ACAS, there has been a significant increase (perhaps as much as tenfold) in the number of CEAs performed in the US and mainland Europe. Indiscriminate application of the basic recommendations has, however, generated worldwide concerns,[12] particularly in units where the results of surgery may not be comparable to ACAS. The concerns relate to the following observations:

- ACAS showed no apparent benefit in women (17% relative risk reduction versus 66% for men)
- ACAS showed no evidence that CEA reduced the risk of disabling stroke
- ACAS found no correlation between stenosis severity and late stroke (in fact it was an inverse relationship)
- ACAS did not show whether patients with bilateral disease had a worse outcome
- although the relative risk reduction was 53%, this equated to an actual annual risk reduction of only 1% in stroke
- the patient should be expected to survive 5 years to gain maximum benefit, yet in some states, the largest single increase in the number of CEAs was in the very elderly[16]
- the cost per stroke prevented is extremely high.[17]

Surgeons in mainland Europe and the US have adopted the ACAS recommendations more liberally than colleagues in the UK and Scandinavia. In the latter, few asymptomatic patients undergo CEA outside the (ongoing) Asymptomatic Carotid Surgery Trial (ACST). Canadian neurologists have also advised against indiscriminate implementation of the ACAS guidelines.[18]

There is no doubt that CEA confers benefit in selected patients. However, even the most ardent carotid enthusiast must also concede that even if they could operate on every patient with an asymptomatic 60–99% stenosis with an operative risk equivalent to ACAS, only 3% of *all* strokes destined to occur in their community would be prevented.[17] In practice, therefore, each surgeon must interpret the ACAS data in the context of their operative risk and hospital priorities. For some, this will mean operating upon patients within the ACST, or not at all. Others (especially those with a low operative risk) can adopt a more liberal interpretation and offer CEA to patients who fit the ACAS criteria. However, if the operative risk were to exceed 4%, the surgeon should not recommend CEA in any patient with asymptomatic disease. Surgeons seeking a more pragmatic

Long-term risk of ipsilateral stroke (including perioperative stroke or death).

Stenosis (%)	Surgical risk (%)	Medical risk (%)	ARR (%)	RRR (%)	NNT	Strokes prevented per 1000 CEAs
ECST						
<30	9.8 at 5 years	3.9 at 5 years	−5.9	n/a	n/a	n/a
30–49	10.2 at 5 years	8.2 at 5 years	−2.0	n/a	n/a	n/a
50–69	15.0 at 5 years	12.1 at 5 years	−2.9	n/a	n/a	n/a
70–99	10.5 at 5 years	19.0 at 5 years	+8.5	45	12	83 at 5 years
NASCET						
30–49	14.9 at 5 years	18.7 at 5 years	+3.8	20	26	38 at 5 years
50–69	15.7 at 3 years	22.2 at 3 years	+6.5	29	15	67 at 3 years
70–99	8.9 at 3 years	28.3 at 3 years	+19.4	69	5	200 at 3 years
ACAS						
60–99	5.1 at 5 years	11.0 at 5 years	+5.9	53	17	59 at 5 years

Table 38.1 Long-term risk of ipsilateral stroke (including perioperative stroke or death). ARR, absolute risk reduction; CEAs, carotid endarterectomies; n/a, not applicable; NNT, number of CEAs to prevent one ipsilateral stroke; RRR, relative risk reduction.

Effect of operative risk on stroke prevention based on ACAS, ECST, and NASCET data.

Operative risk (%)	ACAS 60–99%		NASCET 50–69%		ECST 80–99%		NASCET 70–99%	
	ARR at 5 years	NNT at 5 years	ARR at 3 years	NNT at 3 years	ARR at 3 years	NNT at 3 years	ARR at 3 years	NNT at 3 years
0	8.2%	12	13%	8	18.8%	5	25.2%	4
2	6.2%	16	11%	9	16.8%	6	23.2%	4
4	4.2%	24	9%	11	14.8%	7	21.2%	5
6	2.2%	45	7%	14	12.8%	8	19.2%	5
8	0.2%	500	5%	20	10.8%	9	17.2%	6
10	n/a	n/a	3%	33	8.8%	11	15.2%	7
Trial risk	2.3%	6.5%	4.8%	5.8%				

Table 38.2 Effect of operative risk on stroke prevention based on ACAS, ECST, and NASCET data. The shaded boxes indicate the statistics that most closely apply to the results actually observed in the quoted trial. ARR, actual risk reduction; n/a, not applicable; NNT, number of carotid endarterectomies (CEAs) that must be performed to prevent one stroke at the specified time interval. Thus, for a surgeon with an operative risk of 4%, 24 asymptomatic patients with a 60–99% stenosis would have to undergo CEA to prevent one stroke at 5 years.

approach might only operate on 'higher'-risk patients. To date, no randomized trial has identified these reliably, but, intuitively, they are likely to include men with bilateral severe (>75%) stenoses or contralateral occlusion and irregular or ulcerated lesions. It is hoped that the combined ACST and ACAS databases will enable more discriminating guidelines to be developed in future.

Symptomatic patients
What degree of stenosis?
Using the NASCET criteria, there is no evidence that symptomatic patients with a stenosis <50% benefit from CEA. The equivalent threshold is <70% for centers using the ECST

measurement method. The only exception might be the rare patient with repeated TIAs despite optimal medical therapy. In this situation (not least for medicolegal reasons), the surgeon should seek the input of a neurologist or stroke physician. Patients with NASCET 50–69% (70–79% ECST) gain a small, but significant, benefit from CEA. However, this benefit is inextricably linked to the operative risk. Surgeons with a 30-day death/stroke rate >7.0% should consider whether BMT is the better option in these patients, especially if they are women or have suffered a single ocular event.

There is unequivocal evidence that patients with NASCET 70–99% stenoses (ECST 80–99%) benefit from CEA. Although the actual benefit varies according to the patient and other surgical factors, any patient with carotid symptoms and a severe ipsilateral stenosis should at least be considered for surgery. Exceptions include those with life-threatening co-morbidity or senility, but all will benefit from assessment and optimization of risk factor management.

There have been concerns that patients aged >75 years may not benefit from CEA because it is perceived that their increased operative risk outweighs any long-term benefit. In fact, secondary analyses from NASCET[19] suggest that patients over 75 years gain the most benefit, especially those with the most severe disease (ARR = 29% at 2 years, number of CEAs to prevent one stroke = 3). Accordingly, CEA should not be denied on the basis of chronological age; general fitness and biological age should always be the principal determinants.

Management of patients with a 'string sign' or near occlusion

Patients with subocclusion (string sign) have previously been considered to be at high risk of stroke, and suspicion of sub-occlusion on duplex imaging has prompted magnetic resonance angiography (MRA) or urgent contrast angiography (with its risks). Patients are usually heparinized and submitted to urgent CEA. Secondary analyses of ECST and NASCET data suggest that a reappraisal of practice may be required in some of these patients.

Table 38.3 presents the 30-day and 1-year risk of ipsilateral stroke in patients from NASCET related to the severity of carotid disease.[20] A string sign is defined as a critical stenosis with underfilling/collapse of the distal ICA (**Fig. 38.2**). Near occlusion with no string sign implies that the ICA opens into a normal caliber vessel. CEA conferred the lowest ARR (4.4%) in patients with a string sign. Corroborative data come from the ECST.[21] Of most practical importance, NASCET showed that emergency CEA was not necessary. No medically treated patient with a string sign suffered a stroke within 30 days.

Accordingly, evidence suggests that CEA confers an incrementally significant benefit in patients with increasingly severe carotid disease and a normal-caliber distal vessel. However, the long-term benefit is significantly reduced in patients with a string sign/hypoplastic distal ICA. In Leicester, UK, these patients are usually anticoagulated unless they are having ongoing cerebral events. This is because it is believed the embolic risk is low. Moreover, because NASCET data suggest that two-thirds of patients with a string sign have already recruited intracranial collateral pathways,[22] the risk of hemodynamic stroke must also be low.

Timing of CEA after the most recent cerebral event

As NASCET and ECST included patients within 6 months of the last neurologic event, this threshold has been retained for selecting patients for CEA. Clearly, if a more liberal approach towards treating asymptomatic disease is adopted, then the debate over thresholds becomes moot. For those whose practice comprises predominantly symptomatic patients, secondary analyses from ECST and NASCET suggest that the threshold may be extended beyond the traditional 6 months in selected patients. ECST has shown that the 1- and 2-year stroke risk for patients with 90–99% stenoses was 18% and 14%, respectively.[23] NASCET patients with 80–89% stenoses had a 19% 1-year risk, increasing to 35% for those with 90–94% stenoses.[4]

It would therefore seem appropriate to extend the threshold for surgery to 12 months after the last neurologic event in patients with 80–99% carotid stenoses. There might even be an argument for extending this to 18 months in those with 90–95% stenoses, particularly if they are men and have a contralateral occlusion. Conversely, the 6-month threshold should still be retained for patients with 70–79% stenoses.

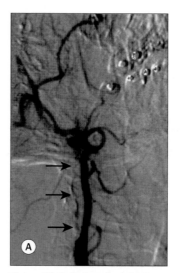 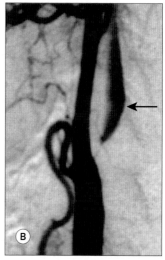

Figure 38.2 String sign. (A) Near occlusion with a string sign is defined as a 95–99% stenosis with underfilling/non-visualization or collapse of the distal internal carotid artery (arrows). (B) Near occlusion with no string sign. Here, the distal internal carotid artery opens into a normal-caliber vessel (arrow).

Thirty-day and 1-year risk of ipsilateral stroke relative to degree of stenosis and presence of string sign.								
Degree of stenosis (+/– string)	Surgical risk (%) 30 days	12 months	Medical risk (%) 30 days	12 months	ARR 12 month (%)	RRR 12 month (%)	NNT 12 month	Strokes prevented per 1000 CEAs
70–79%	3.9	4.6	1.4	12.8	+8.2	64	12	83
80–89%	6.3	8.7	6.4	18.5	+9.8	53	10	100
90–94%	8.7	8.7	4.6	35.1	+26.4	75	4	250
95–99% + no string	6.1	9.1	2.3	18.3	+9.2	50	11	91
95–99% + string sign	6.7	6.7	0.0	11.1	+4.4	40	23	43

Table 38.3 Thirty-day and 1-year risk of ipsilateral stroke relative to degree of stenosis and presence of string sign. ARR, absolute risk reduction; RRR, relative risk reduction; NNT, number of carotid endarterectomies (CEAs) to prevent one ipsilateral stroke. (Adapted from Morgenstern et al.[20])

Fast-track referral

An overview of the secondary analyses from NASCET and ECST have been helpful in predicting which patients have the greatest risk of stroke.[11] **Table 38.4** presents a 'league table' of ARR conferred by CEA, together with the number of CEAs required to prevent one stroke. CEA confers the maximum benefit in a patient with a 95% stenosis plus plaque ulceration, or a 70–99% stenosis with contralateral occlusion (ARR 47–54%). Only two operations are required to prevent one stroke at 2 years. The least benefit (ten times less) is obtained by operating on patients with a string sign (ARR = 4%, number needed to treat = 23).

Relative scale of benefit for carotid endarterectomy over best medical therapy in symptomatic patients from NASCET.		
Stenosis	*ARR*	*NNT*
String sign	4% at 1 year	23
50–69% (all patients)	7% at 3 years	15
70–79% (all patients)	8% at 1 year	12
50–99% + lacunar stroke	9% at 3 years	11
95–99% + no string	9% at 1 year	11
70–99% + patients aged <65	10% at 2 years	10
80–89% (all patients)	10% at 1 year	10
70–99% + symptom onset <6 months	11% at 2 years	9
75% + no plaque ulceration	11% at 2 years	9
85% + no plaque ulceration	11% at 2 years	9
95% + no plaque ulceration	11% at 2 years	9
50–99% + cortical stroke	15% at 3 years	7
70–99% + aged 65–74	15% at 3 years	7
75% + plaque ulceration	20% at 2 years	5
70–99% (all patients)	20% at 3 years	5
70–99% + contralateral 70–99% stenosis	20% at 2 years	5
70–84% + intracranial disease	23% at 3 years	4
90–94% (all patients)	26% at 1 year	4
70–99% + patients aged >75	28% at 2 years	3
70–99% + >7 concurrent risk factors	30% at 2 years	3
70–99% + recurrent events >6 months	30% at 2 years	3
85–99% + no intracranial collaterals	31% at 2 years	3
85% + plaque ulceration	32% at 2 years	3
85–99% + intracranial disease	37% at 3 years	3
70–99% + contralateral occlusion	47% at 2 years	2
95% + plaque ulceration	54% at 2 years	2

Table 38.4 Relative scale of benefit for carotid endarterectomy (CEA) over best medical therapy in symptomatic patients from NASCET. ARR, actual risk reduction; NNT, number of CEAs required to prevent one stroke at specified time period.

Clinicians can now identify patients for fast-track investigation and expedited referral for CEA. Factors suggesting increased early risk include male sex, age >75 years, cortical stroke presentation, and recurrent symptoms for over 6 months. Angiographic factors (and by analogy duplex/MRA) include plaque irregularity/ulceration and contralateral occlusion. Intracranial markers of increased risk (in medically treated patients only) include intracranial disease or failure to recruit collaterals.

Expedited or emergency carotid endarterectomy

In the 1960s, there was a vogue for emergency CEA in patients with acute stroke secondary to carotid occlusion. This practice was associated with hemorrhagic transformation of the infarct in up to 60% of patients.[24] Since then, emergency CEA has largely been abandoned. The only exceptions (apart from in a trial) would be the immediate treatment of acute thrombotic stroke after CEA or carotid angioplasty.

In contrast to emergency CEA, urgent CEA (within 24 hours) should be considered in patients with crescendo TIAs or stroke in evolution. The former implies that the patient is suffering repeated TIAs, with full neurologic recovery between each event. Stroke in evolution suggests that there is partial recovery of the deficit followed by repeated deterioration but never complete recovery. It is assumed that both syndromes follow repeated embolization from an unstable plaque (**Fig. 38.3**).

Following recognition that emergency CEA conferred no benefit after acute thrombotic stroke, it became customary to defer CEA for up to 8 weeks in all patients who had a stroke. NASCET has now corroborated a number of studies[25] which have shown that expedited CEA (within 4 weeks of completed stroke) in selected patients is not associated with an increased operative risk.[26] Patients undergoing CEA within 30 days of stroke in NASCET had a 4.8% operative risk compared with 5.2% when surgery was deferred for >30 days. Not all stroke patients will be suitable for early CEA. Surgery should be reserved for patients with small cortical infarcts who make a rapid neurologic recovery.

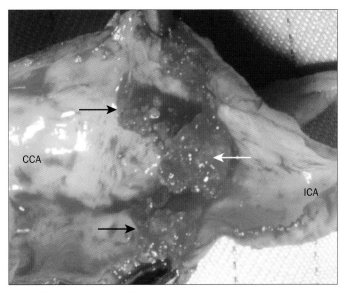

Figure 38.3 Opened carotid endarterectomy specimen in a patient presenting with crescendo transient ischemic attacks. The transected stenosis (black arrows) contains loose debris. Immediately distal to the stenosis is adherent fresh thrombus (white arrow).

Staged or synchronous CEA in patients with severe cardiac disease?

This is an enduring controversy with insufficient 'quality' data to answer the debate. With increasing awareness that aortic arch disease is an important cause of stroke after coronary artery bypass grafting (CABG), there has been renewed debate as to the value of staged or synchronous CEA. In a recent systematic review,[27] it was observed that 2% of patients suffered a stroke after CABG. Factors predictive of an increased risk of operative stroke (predominantly with asymptomatic carotid stenoses) included:

- carotid bruit (hazard ratio 3.6)
- a history of prior stroke/TIA (hazard ratio 3.6)
- carotid stenosis >50% or occlusion (hazard ratio 4.3).

However, the review also observed that 50% of those who had a stroke did not have any carotid disease, while 60% had territorial infarctions on CT/autopsy that were incompatible with their underlying carotid disease. The review did indicate that the risk of stroke increased with the degree of carotid stenosis but was maximal (7–11%) in those with carotid occlusion. The stroke risk for patients who had a CABG with asymptomatic bilateral 50–99% stenoses was only about 5%.

Patients usually fall into two categories: (i) patients undergoing CABG with asymptomatic carotid disease; and (ii) symptomatic carotid patients with severe ischemic heart disease. In these situations, management strategies should be based on the available evidence and clinical reason for doing the operation. The majority of patients awaiting CEA do not need coronary revascularization. Symptomatic patients with severe cardiac disease are, however, at increased risk of perioperative myocardial events. The first-line strategy should always be optimization of medical management. For those in whom medical management is considered maximal, the second-line approach is to see whether the coronary lesions are amenable to angioplasty, thereby enabling the surgeon to proceed with discrete CEA. If angioplasty is not possible, the surgeon has to decide between CEA under locoregional anesthesia, staged CEA then CABG, or synchronous CEA–CABG. Synchronous procedures are currently preferred in Boston and Leicester, but there is no randomized trial evidence to support this strategy.

The main controversy relates to the treatment of patients booked for CABG with asymptomatic carotid disease. Meta-analyses suggest that staged (CEA–CABG), reverse staged (CABG–CEA), and synchronous CEA+CABG carry similar overall risk, but the morbidity varies according to which procedure is done first.[28] Reverse-staged procedures incur a higher risk of stroke, whereas staged operations have a higher incidence of cardiac events. Results for synchronous operations lie midway between. The American Heart Association[29] sanctions CEA (staged or synchronous) in asymptomatic patients provided that the surgeon has an operative risk <5% for discrete CEA in asymptomatic patients. Each surgeon must therefore review their outcomes regularly and management decisions must be made individually.

MANAGEMENT OF CAROTID DISEASE

Best medical management

All patients benefit from optimization of risk factors and anti-platelet therapy. This should not be delegated to the most junior member of the firm. There is more to this aspect of patient care than simply advising patients to stop smoking and take aspirin.

Ischemic heart disease was the main cause of death in ECST and NASCET. Accordingly, the cardiac status should be evaluated and therapy for angina optimized. There is controversy as to whether routine preoperative cardiologic assessment is necessary. This is more commonly practised in North America. In the UK, cardiac referral is normally reserved for patients with cardiac failure and poor functional capacity, recent myocardial infarction (within 8 weeks), severe or unstable angina, severe valvular disease, symptomatic arrhythmias, or recurrence of symptoms after cardiac surgery or angioplasty.[30]

Treatment of hypertension remains the cornerstone of stroke prevention. Thresholds vary between countries and by age. In practice, patients less than 60 years old with a blood pressure (BP) >140/90mmHg require treatment. As the patient ages, slight relaxation in thresholds is permissible. Meta-analyses suggest that for every 5mmHg reduction in diastolic BP there is a 15% relative reduction in stroke.[31,32] No patient should undergo CEA with a systolic BP >180mmHg as this is an independent risk factor for operative stroke.[33]

Wherever possible, patients should be on antiplatelet therapy. Aspirin (cyclo-oxygenase pathway inhibitor) will confer a 15% reduction in late stroke in patients presenting with TIA or stroke.[34] The optimal dose of aspirin is controversial. NASCET suggested that higher doses (600–1200mg) were associated with a lower risk of operative events.[2] However, a large randomized trial has now clearly shown the converse to be true.[35] Although clopidogrel (ADP inhibitor) confers a small but significant reduction in any vascular event, there is no evidence that it specifically reduces the risk of stroke.[36] It does, however, significantly increase the bleeding time.[37] This should be borne in mind in patients scheduled for surgery. Meta-analyses suggest that the combination of aspirin plus dipyridamole reduces the risk of stroke by 23%. Unfortunately, up to 25% of patients will have to stop treatment because of adverse side effects.[38] Thus, for all practical purposes, the evidence suggests that all patients should be on 75–300mg aspirin and that this should not be stopped prior to surgery. Clopidogrel is probably the second-line drug in those unable to take aspirin. Some surgeons stop clopidogrel treatment several days before CEA, particularly in patients taking the combination of clopidogrel and aspirin.

Careful control of blood glucose in diabetic patients is essential for the avoidance of diabetic complications. However, there is no evidence[39] that tight glycemic control actually reduces the risk of stroke. The UK Prospective Diabetes Study Group[40] has reported that type 2 diabetic patients require extremely tight control of BP [mean <144/82mmHg]. Evidence suggests that this reduces the risk of late stroke by up to 44%.

Treatment of hyperlipidemia is controversial and again varies geographically. Previous meta-analyses[41] have suggested that low levels of cholesterol increase the risk of hemorrhagic stroke, while high levels increase the risk of ischemic stroke. Sticking to evidence-based principles alone,[42] existing guidelines suggest that lipid-lowering therapy should only be offered to patients who have a TIA/stroke and have a history of ischemic heart disease. In North America,[43] therapy would also be given to patients with other vascular risk factors. More recently, the Medical Research Council/British Heart Foundation (MRC/BHF) Heart Protection Study (over 20 000 randomized patients) showed that 40mg simvastatin daily conferred a 12% reduction in total mortality, a 17% reduction in vascular mortality, a 24% reduction in coronary events, and a 27% reduction in stroke.[44] This trial will almost certainly alter the advice given in the UK regarding the treatment of hyperlipidemia,[44] which will be more along the North American guidelines. Of great importance was the observation that there appeared to be no cholesterol threshold below which statin therapy was not associated with long-term cardiovascular benefit. There is some evidence that statin therapy stabilizes carotid plaque, as well as reducing lipid levels.

In the past, there have been concerns that patients with multiple co-morbidity gain less benefit from CEA, either because of an increased operative risk or because the patient is unlikely to live long enough to gain clinical benefit. NASCET has now shown that the presence of increasing co-morbidity does not influence the long-term risk of stroke after CEA. Conversely, multiple risk factors significantly increased the risk of stroke in medically treated patients with severe carotid disease.[2]

PRINCIPLES OF SURGICAL MANAGEMENT

Preoperative checklist

Before submitting a patient to surgery, it is important that the surgeon completes a 'checklist' to minimize morbidity and mortality and potential exposure to medicolegal investigation (**Table 38.5**). In particular, reasons for doing the operation should be documented clearly in the case notes, together with a review of the procedural risks (stroke, death, cranial nerve injury).

The surgeon must also ensure that the patient is receiving optimal medical therapy. No patient should undergo CEA with uncontrolled hypertension (systolic BP >180mmHg) or unstable cardiac symptoms. Uncontrolled hypertension is an independent risk factor for operative stroke,[33] and increases the risk of cardiac events, hyperperfusion syndrome, and intracranial hemorrhage.

The status of the cranial nerves should be reviewed at this stage. Any patient who has previously undergone thyroid, radical neck surgery or contralateral CEA should have undergone indirect laryngoscopy and evaluation of hypoglossal and glossopharyngeal nerve function. Bilateral recurrent laryngeal or hypoglossal nerve injuries can be fatal. If there is any evidence of injury, the surgeon must review the indication for surgery. It might, for example, be

appropriate to abandon CEA in an asymptomatic patient with laryngoscopic evidence of contralateral vocal cord palsy. Alternatively, carotid angioplasty might be more appropriate. If surgery is still deemed necessary, the patient must be warned of the potential for emergency (even permanent) tracheostomy.

In the UK and many parts of Europe, it is considered ideal to repeat the duplex examination immediately before operation. In North America, this is less commonly performed, largely because the majority of patients have undergone imaging within the preceding 7–14 days. Repeat duplex imaging enables the level of the bifurcation to be marked and ensures that the ICA has not occluded while awaiting surgery (thereby avoiding an unnecessary procedure). It also serves as a validatory study against which the original MRA/duplex/angiogram or resected plaque can be compared and enables a regular review of duplex technologist practice (internal validation and quality control). Finally, it provides the surgeon with a chance to exclude unexpected inflow and outflow disease or unrecognized distal disease extension. It is essential to anticipate high carotid disease. Temporomandibular subluxation cannot readily be performed once the operation is underway.

TECHNIQUE OF CAROTID ENDARTERECTOMY

Position

The operation side is marked preoperatively. The patient lies supine with the head extended and rotated away from the operation side. A sandbag beneath the shoulders and head ring facilitates this. To reduce venous congestion, the head of the table is raised (**Fig. 38.4**). A urethral catheter minimizes discomfort from a full bladder, which can aggravate postoperative hypertension. The patient should receive the first of three doses of intravenous antibiotics (cephalosporin +/– metronidazole).

Choice of anesthesia

Carotid surgery has traditionally been performed under general anesthesia (GA), largely because the surgeon finds it less stressful, the operation does not need to be rushed (especially when supervising trainees), patient movement is avoided, and there are theoretical benefits regarding reduced cerebral metabolic requirements. More recently, there has been a vogue towards CEA under either local anesthesia or regional anesthesia – hereafter to be described as locoregional anesthesia (LRA) – because it is the optimal method for neurologic monitoring and selective shunting. Anesthesia is produced by varying combinations of local infiltration and/or deep and superficial cervical plexus blockade with 0.5% bupivacaine. Light intravenous sedation may also be employed if a patient is agitated or anxious.

The evidence regarding LRA versus GA is conflicting. Few randomized trials have been performed and none has shown that LRA reduces the overall stroke or cardiovascular risk.[45] However, a meta-analysis of non-randomized studies suggested that LRA may be associated with a reduction in the rate of perioperative stroke, myocardial infarction, and pulmonary complications.[45] In the UK, the GALA trial is currently randomizing patients to CEA under GA or LRA.

Is distal disease extension a possibility?

The possibility that the disease process might extend distally must be anticipated in advance, not least because the operative

Preoperative surgical checklist.
Is the reason for surgery clearly documented?
Are there any atypical symptoms warranting further investigation?
Is the degree of stenosis appropriate for surgery?
Have the perioperative risks been documented in the notes?
Is the patient on optimal medical therapy?
Consider rescanning the carotid arteries prior to surgery
Is high carotid disease anticipated?
Assess cranial nerve status in all patients with previous neck surgery
Mark the operation side with an indelible marker

Table 38.5 Preoperative surgical checklist.

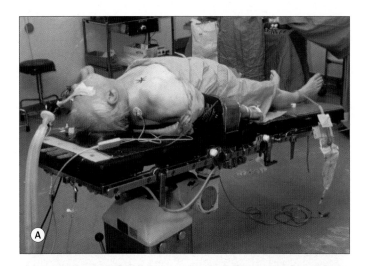

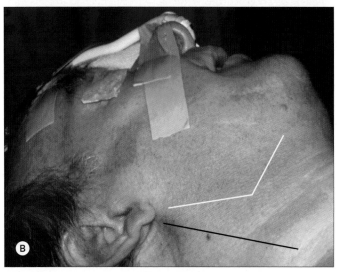

Figure 38.4 Technique of carotid endarterectomy. (A) The side of the operation should be clearly marked. The patient is positioned head up to reduce venous congestion and the table slightly rotated away from the operative side. (B) Patients with a 'short neck' or suspected high disease extension benefit from nasolaryngeal intubation. This opens up the angle of access between mastoid process/sternomastoid (black line) and the mandible (white line).

risks increase. It is difficult (if not impossible) to perform temporomandibular subluxation during CEA. The strict definition of high disease is when the plaque extends above a line drawn between the ramus of the mandible and the mastoid process. In practical terms, this generally means above the digastric muscle. For those reliant on duplex imaging, high disease must be suspected when the technologist cannot visualize the ICA above the stenosis clearly.

Simple measures to facilitate distal access include nasolaryngeal intubation (**Fig. 38.4B**), which opens the angle between the mandible and mastoid process. Temporomandibular dislocation has largely been replaced by subluxation. With dislocation, the mandibular condyle is pulled anteriorly over the articular eminence into the infratemporal fossa and is associated with an increased risk of joint dysfunction. The alternative is subluxation.[46] Here, the condyle is pulled anteriorly to rest under the articular eminence and stabilized by intraoral fixation wires, which are removed at the end of the procedure. Mandibular subluxation is

associated with few complications and surprisingly little post-operative and long-term discomfort.

Exposure of the carotid bifurcation

The skin incision is made over the anterior border of sternomastoid, preserving the great auricular nerve superiorly. Skin edge bleeding is minimized by infiltrating the skin and subcutaneous tissues with 0.5% bupivacaine with adrenaline. Dissection continues anterior to sternomastoid. The common facial vein traverses the operative field and overlies the carotid bifurcation. This is divided and dissection continues in a plane immediately medial to the internal jugular vein.

In individuals with a fat neck, there is often a large pad of fat and lymph nodes overlying the bifurcation. The fat pad should be mobilized towards the operating surgeon. This minimizes troublesome bleeding and exposes a relatively avascular triangle bounded superiorly by digastric muscle. The bifurcation can also become slightly rotated and branches may appear to emerge at unusual angles. This can be corrected by remembering to mobilize all external carotid artery (ECA) branches towards the first assistant.

Access to the ICA distal to the bifurcation is facilitated by: (i) division of the digastric muscle (**Fig. 38.5A**); (ii) division of the sternomastoid branch of the ECA (plus vein) which tethers the hypoglossal nerve (**Fig. 38.5B**); and (iii) careful retraction of the hypoglossal nerve. This is aided by dividing the ansa cervicalis. A suture tie on the divided ansa acts as a useful retractor/elevator of the hypoglossal nerve and avoids the damage associated with a sling (**Fig. 38.5C**). Finally, more distal branches of the ECA may have to be divided (**Fig. 38.5D**) to mobilize the hypoglossal nerve and expose the diseased segment of the ICA completely.

Dissection continues until the ICA, common carotid artery (CCA), and ECA are mobilized above and below the disease (**Fig. 38.6**). The bifurcation should not be 'skeletonized' as this predisposes to functional elongation and kinking and increases the risk of embolization during the dissection phase. The patient is given 5000 units of heparin intravenously. Few centers measure the coagulation profiles as there is no evidence that modifying the heparin dose alters outcome.

Minimizing cranial nerve injury

The keys towards minimizing cranial nerve injury are: (i) knowledge of the anatomy; (ii) care not to divide any neural tissue traversing the bifurcation (**Fig. 38.7**) apart from the ansa (**Figs 38.5B and 38.5C**); (iii) avoiding inclusion of the vagus nerve in the carotid clamps; (iv) avoiding diathermy in the vicinity of the cranial nerves; and (v) minimizing division of the tissue immediately anterior to the ICA when dissecting above digastric. This tissue contains small pharyngeal branches from the vagus and glossopharyngeal nerves.

Whether to shunt

Insertion of a plastic shunt between the CCA and ICA during endarterectomy can maintain cerebral flood flow. Surgeons tend to be routine, selective, or never shunters. An overview of the randomized trials by the Cochrane Collaboration[47] has failed to show that any one strategy is better than another. There is, however, a consensus that routine/selective shunting is preferable to never shunting. Surgeons who shunt routinely argue that CEA

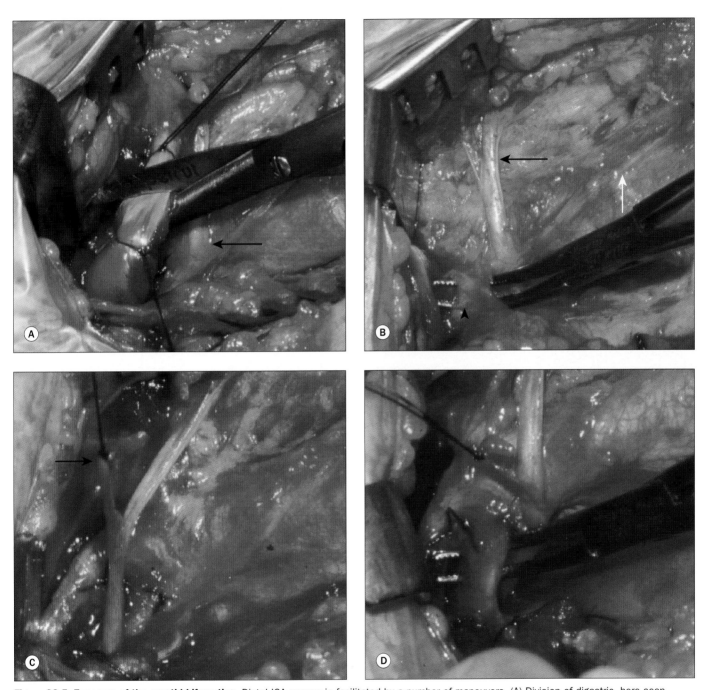

Figure 38.5 Exposure of the carotid bifurcation. Distal ICA access is facilitated by a number of maneuvers. (A) Division of digastric, here seen overlying the hypoglossal nerve (arrow). (B) Division of sternomastoid artery/vein (arrowhead) which tethers the hypoglossal nerve (black arrow). The ansa cervicalis (white arrow) has not yet been divided. (C) Division of the ansa cervicalis. A suture tie (arrow) allows the hypoglossal nerve to be retracted without traumatizing the nerve. (D) Further access is facilitated by progressively dividing higher external carotid artery branches.

need not be hurried, trainees are supervised in a less stressful environment, while familiarity with shunt insertion means that it is generally easier to operate around the shunt (**Fig. 38.6B**), especially during high exploration. Selective users argue that shunts are only necessary in 10–15% of patients,[48] they can cause intimal damage and secondary thromboembolism, and that they get in the way!

It is important to remember that having a shunt in place does not mean it is working. About 3% of shunts malfunction, usually due to impaction on distal ICA coils or kinks.[49] Unless some form of monitoring is available, this will be missed. Selective

users must accept that awake testing under LRA is the only infallible method for determining who needs a shunt. Other methods (stump pressure, back flow, electroencephalography [EEG], somatosensory-evoked potential [SEP], transcranial Doppler [TCD], near infra-red spectometry [NIRS]) are not completely reliable. However, selective users must accept that hemodynamic failure accounts for only 20% of intraoperative strokes. The remainder (due to thromboembolism) may still occur unless some other form of monitoring is employed.[50]

The most commonly used shunts are the Javid and Pruitt–Inahara. The Javid is tapered and held in place with

555

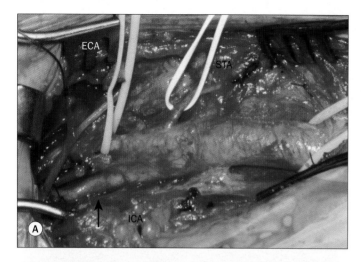

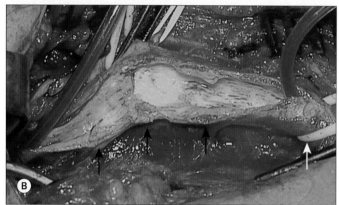

Figure 38.6 Exposure of the carotid bifurcation. The common carotid artery (CCA), internal carotid artery (ICA), external carotid artery (ECA), and superficial temporal artery (STA) are mobilized but not 'skeletonized'. The aim is to ensure that access is cleared well above and below the stenosis (A) so that it is possible to insert a shunt easily and atraumatically (B). Note the three individual stenoses in this patient (black arrows). The sling around the CCA (white arrow) is secured around the hub of a West retractor to prevent accidental dislodgment of the proximal balloon of the Pruitt–Inahara shunt.

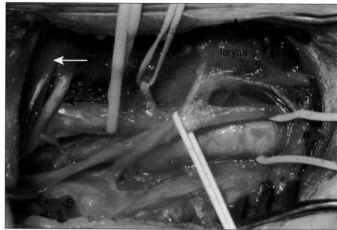

Figure 38.7 Aberrant cranial nerve anatomy. The hypoglossal nerve (black arrow) is immediately inferior to digastric (white arrow). The sling encircles a complex series of aberrant neural structures traversing the bifurcation. These should not be divided.

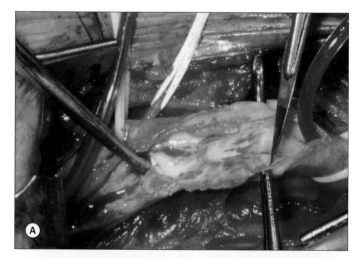

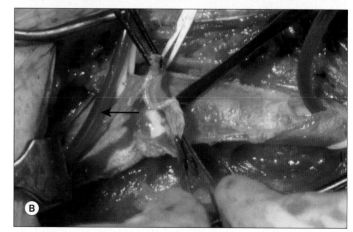

Figure 38.8 Traditional endarterectomy starts with a Watson–Cheyne retractor insinuated between the plaque and media in the distal common carotid artery. The plaque is divided over the retractor (A). The plaque is then removed by cephalad endarterectomy (arrow).

proximal and distal retaining clamps. It has higher flow rates than the Pruitt. Its main limitation is the need for more distal dissection to position the clamp. The Pruitt has balloons that hold the shunt in position (**Fig. 38.6B**) and facilitate access to the distal ICA. The Pruitt has lower flow rates; however, 90% of patients have flows within 10% of their preclamp value[51] and there is no systematic evidence that shunt type alters outcome.

Traditional or eversion endarterectomy

In a traditional endarterectomy, a Watson–Cheyne dissector is insinuated between the plaque and the media (**Fig. 38.8**). The plaque is divided proximally and the dissection plane extended distally up the ICA until it either feathers or is transected. The ECA plaque is everted. There is no evidence that tacking sutures alter outcome. In NASCET, tacking sutures were associated with an increased operative risk. However, this could simply mean that a smooth intimal step was more difficult to achieve because of technical problems (high disease, posterior tongue of plaque, excessively thinned wall). Following plaque removal, loose intimal flaps are removed from the endarterectomy zone

(**Fig. 38.9**). The arteriotomy is then closed primarily, or with a patch (see below).

Eversion CEA requires transection of the ICA at its origin (**Fig. 38.10**). The ICA is then 'everted' and the tube of atheroma expelled. Once the distal limit is exposed, the lesion is excised. The ICA is then shortened, as appropriate, and reanastomosed to the bifurcation after endarterectomy of the CCA. Advantages of eversion CEA include no lengthening/kinking of the ICA and no patching. Clamp time is generally shorter. However, it is not usually possible to insert a shunt until after the endarterectomy has been completed and there is always the worry that a distal intimal flap may go unnoticed. Few randomized trials have been performed. However, a systematic review of the available data[52] has shown no evidence that either eversion or traditional endarterectomy is safer or preferable.

Whether to patch

An overview of the randomized trials by the Cochrane Group (**Table 38.6**) showed that a policy of routine patching (**Fig. 38.11**) was preferable to routine primary closure and conferred a threefold reduction in the rate of perioperative stroke and thrombosis.[53] Late stroke and restenosis was also reduced. No randomized trials have compared routine with selective patching. For those surgeons who prefer a policy of selective patching, criteria usually include: female patients; ICA diameter <5mm; and an ICA arteriotomy >2cm. There is no evidence that patch

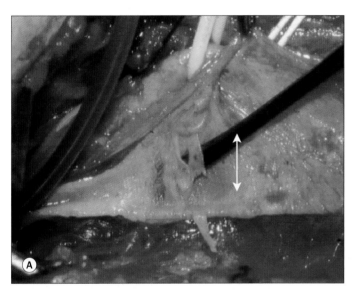
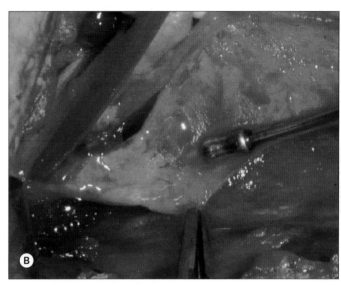

Figure 38.9 Traditional endarterectomy. (A) The distal intimal step is defined, intimal flaps are removed in a radial direction (arrow). Axial (longitudinal) removal of intimal flaps causes a deepening of the endarterectomy plane and may damage the integrity of the arterial wall. (B) Here, the distal intimal step has been tacked down and is being irrigated with heparinized saline to identify undiagnosed flaps.

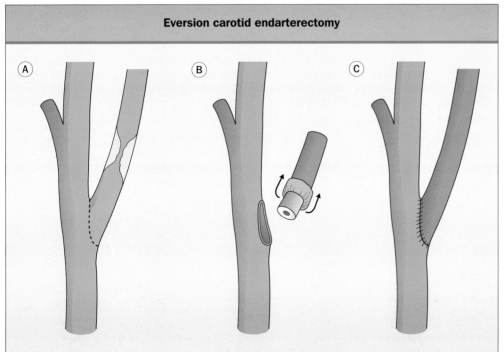

Eversion carotid endarterectomy

Figure 38.10 Eversion carotid endarterectomy. The internal carotid artery (ICA) is detached from the bifurcation along the dotted line (A). The adventitia/residual media is everted and the core of atheroma expelled (B). The ICA can be shortened as appropriate and reanastomosed to the bifurcation after distal common carotid artery (CCA) endarterectomy (C).

Cochrane Collaboration meta-analysis of the randomized trials of routine patching versus primary closure after carotid endarterectomy.			
	Routine patching	Primary closure	Odds ratio of increased risk with primary closure
30-day outcomes			
Ipsilateral stroke	1.3%	3.9%	2.9 (95% CI 1.3–6.7)
All strokes	1.6%	4.2%	2.6 (95% CI 1.1–6.7)
Carotid thrombosis	0.3%	3.9%	5.9 (95% CI 2.2–17)
Long-term outcomes			
Ipsilateral stroke	1.6%	4.4%	2.6 (95% CI 1.1–6.3)
All strokes	2.2%	5.9%	2.6 (95% CI 1.2–5.9)
50–100% restenosis	4.5%	13%	3.1 (95% CI 1.9–5.3)

Table 38.6 Cochrane Collaboration meta-analysis of the randomized trials of routine patching versus primary closure after carotid endarterectomy. (Adapted from Counsell et al.[53])

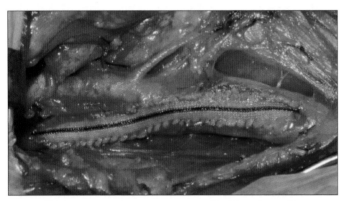

Figure 38.11 Completed endarterectomy with thin-walled collagen-impregnated Dacron patch.

type (prosthetic or vein) alters outcome. Vein patches are susceptible to central rupture (overall incidence 1%). The risk is increased in women with hypertension, but most particularly in those in whom the vein is harvested from the ankle. Advocates of vein patching should harvest the groin saphenous vein. Alternatives include the jugular vein. Prosthetic patches are vulnerable to a 1% incidence of infection (see later).

Monitoring and quality control assessment

Despite awareness that the majority of strokes after CEA follow inadvertent technical error,[54] few surgeons incorporate completion quality control assessment and there is no consensus on the role of monitoring during carotid surgery. Reasons include: (i) the absence of any randomized trials; (ii) the lack of accurate audits of the actual causes of perioperative stroke; (iii) a tendency to overinterpret 'single issues' such as the role of the shunt or patch; (iv) logistical issues relating to access to equipment and personnel; (v) the mistaken view that one monitoring method is infallible; and, most importantly, (vi) a failure to ask the right questions.[55]

Each unit must audit their own practice. The first question is whether the majority of strokes are intraoperative (apparent upon recovery from anesthesia) and therefore attributable to an adverse event during the operation. Postoperative strokes occur after normal recovery from anesthesia. Intraoperative strokes (historically the commonest) are thromboembolic (the majority) or hemodynamic. Thus, when trying to develop a monitoring protocol, methods must be used that will answer the question posed. **Table 38.7** presents the chronological sequence from embolus through hemodynamic failure to the onset of a neurologic deficit and indicates which monitoring technique will detect the underlying problem. For example, neither awake testing nor EEG can be blamed for failing to warn a surgeon that embolization is occurring. Both document that something is wrong, but not why. Only TCD warns the surgeon of an unstable plaque during dissection, or of embolization preceding on-table thrombosis. Similarly, for 'selective shunters' the only infallible way of identifying hemodynamic failure is to perform CEA under LRA. Awake testing, however, will not prevent intraoperative embolic stroke.

A similar approach should apply when evaluating methods for assessing the technical performance of CEA. **Table 38.8** lists the principal technical errors and those methods best able to identify them. The choice of technique will inevitably reflect each center's access to resources and personnel. What is appropriate for one unit may not be effective in another. Surgeons with an operative risk under 3% will feel that change is unnecessary. Others may apply one or more monitoring modalities once a review has been made of when the majority of complications occur. It is not acceptable for surgeons with poor outcomes simply to dismiss the concept of monitoring and quality control assessment just because others can achieve complication rates under 2% without them.[56]

In Leicester, a combination of monitoring methods is used (intraoperative TCD, completion angioscopy, and 3 hours of

The role of monitoring techniques during carotid surgery.			
Detection of embolism $\longrightarrow$	Detection of reduced perfusion $\longrightarrow$	Detection of loss of electrical activity $\longrightarrow$	Detection of neuronal injury
TCD	Reduced stump pressure Reduced ICA back flow Near infra-red spectroscopy Jugular venous O_2 saturation Xenon–CBF measurement TCD	EEG SSEP	Awake testing

Table 38.7 The role of monitoring techniques during carotid surgery. CBF, cerebral blood flow; EEG, electroencephalography; ICA, internal carotid artery; SSEP, somatosensory evoked potential; TCD, transcranial Doppler. (Adapted from Naylor & Mackey.[56])

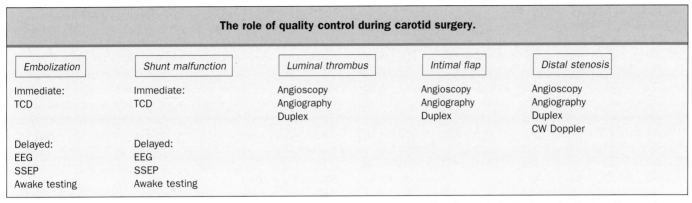

The role of quality control during carotid surgery.				
Embolization	**Shunt malfunction**	**Luminal thrombus**	**Intimal flap**	**Distal stenosis**
Immediate: TCD	Immediate: TCD	Angioscopy Angiography Duplex	Angioscopy Angiography Duplex	Angioscopy Angiography Duplex CW Doppler
Delayed: EEG SSEP Awake testing	Delayed: EEG SSEP Awake testing			

Table 38.8 The role of quality control during carotid surgery. CW Doppler, continuous wave Doppler analysis; Duplex, color Duplex ultrasound; EEG, electroencephalography; SSEP, somatosensory evoked potential; TCD, transcranial Doppler (Adapted from Naylor & Mackey.[56])

postoperative TCD monitoring). Each has specific questions to answer based on a series of prospective audit studies in 1200 patients.[57] Intraoperative TCD:

- enables warning of embolization from unstable plaques during carotid dissection and allows the surgeon to modify operative technique
- ensures optimal shunt function by immediately identifying kinking, impaction of the distal shunt lumen against a distal ICA coil, and ensuring mean middle cerebral artery (MCA) velocity is above 15cm/s
- enables rapid identification of the very rare patient who is at risk of developing on-table thrombosis.[57]

Completion angioscopy enables the lumen of the endarterectomy zone to be inspected before flow is restored (**Fig. 38.12**). This

is important as the commonest cause of intraoperative stroke is embolization of luminal thrombus following clamp release. The thrombus is derived from bleeding from the vasa vasorum onto the endarterectomized surface (**Fig. 38.12**). Angiography and duplex may identify luminal irregularities but only after flow has been restored. Finally, all patients are monitored for 3hours postoperatively with TCD. This is because early postoperative thrombosis is preceded by 1–2hours of increasing embolization, which can be arrested by incremental infusions of Dextran-40.[57] Since implementing this protocol, the rate of intraoperative stroke has fallen from 4% to 0.3% in the last 1200 patients and no patient has suffered a stroke due to postoperative carotid thrombosis. Implementation of this monitoring program has been associated with a 60% reduction in the overall operative risk.[57]

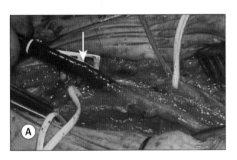

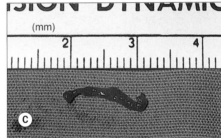

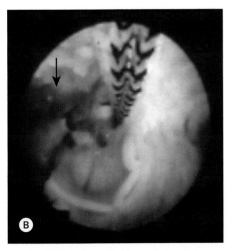

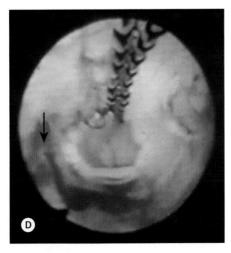

Figure 38.12 Completion angioscopy. (A) The angioscope (this is a hysteroscope) is inserted into the endarterectomy zone prior to patch closure (arrow). (B) Thrombus adherent to the proximal common carotid artery (arrow) despite prior irrigation with heparinized saline. (C) Size of thrombus retrieved from (B). (D) Bleeding from the vasa vasorum (arrow) is the source of these luminal thrombi. (Figures 38.12B & C reproduced with permission from Lennard et al.[81])

Technical operative problems

Occasionally, a surgeon will encounter unexpectedly high carotid disease. If the risk–benefit analysis compels the surgeon to continue, distal access is facilitated by division of digastric muscle, mobilization of the hypoglossal nerve, division of the styloid musculature (styloglossus, stylopharyngeus), and, finally, styloid process fracture. It is not usually possible to undertake temporomandibular subluxation intraoperatively.

Redundant endarterectomy zones predispose to kinking and thrombosis. Eversion plication or shortening can correct this (see below). Excessive thinning, tearing of the thinned endarterectomy zone, or marked coiling of the ICA can be treated by reversed vein bypass (see below).

Occasionally, a surgeon will encounter a hypoplastic carotid artery. As discussed earlier, this pattern of disease is associated with a very low incidence of late stroke. Accordingly, if this is suspected before opening the vessel, an on-table angiogram should be performed. If confirmed, it is probably best to abandon the procedure and anticoagulate the patient. The rationale is to minimize the risks of thrombus propagation across the circle of Willis in the event of ICA thrombosis. If the artery has been opened, ligation of the hypoplastic ICA and anticoagulation is appropriate.

One other rare phenomenon – the thrombosed carotid artery – may confront the surgeon. This manifests itself in two forms. First, the acutely thrombosed artery, which will be avoided if the ICA is rescanned prior to surgery. If encountered, the artery should be left and the procedure abandoned. In practice, the patient will have occluded asymptomatically and attempts to restore flow could lead to a severe thromboembolic stroke. The second presentation is the partially recanalized ICA. Here, a string of thrombus is adherent to the ICA wall up to the skull base. TCD should show if MCA flow is dependent upon the ipsilateral ICA (MCAV <15cm/s). If so, strenuous attempts should be made to reconstruct the vessel (probably with a vein bypass). If not, the artery should be ligated and the patient anticoagulated.

Shortening the redundant endarterectomy zone

Occasionally, the endarterectomy zone may be too redundant after CEA and attempts to close the artery will predispose to corrugation of the intima or kinking of the bifurcation. There are two methods for treating this. The first is to transect the intima and remove a segment of redundant wall. Continuity is restored by a continuous 6:0 Prolene (Ethicon Ltd) anastomosis. One of the problems with this method is that in a very thin-walled vessel after endarterectomy (especially elderly women), the sutures can tear out.

Eversion plication

Here, the redundant endarterectomy zone is shortened by everting a segment of wall (**Fig. 38.13**). The first step is to place two stay sutures on either side of the vessel wall, incorporating the redundant segment of artery. The sutures are tied and pulled apart, which causes the eversion to occur. A continuous 6:0 Prolene suture completes the anastomosis. The principal advantages are that the distal intimal step can be incorporated into the eversion, and the strength and integrity of the arterial wall are maintained.

Carotid bypass

Occasionally it is necessary to perform a carotid bypass. Both prosthetic material and saphenous vein may be used and there is no randomized trial evidence that either is preferable. We prefer to use reversed saphenous vein harvested from the groin. If a shunt has been deployed, this will have to be removed temporarily. If no shunt has been used, now is the time to get one ready. The flexibility of the Pruitt–Inahara shunt, together with the absence of any need for retaining clamps, makes this an excellent stent for anastomosis and maintenance of distal perfusion. The reversed vein is placed over the distal limb of the shunt, which is reinserted into the distal ICA (**Fig. 38.14**). The opposing vein and ICA are then spatulated and anastomosed.

There are several ways of completing the anastomosis. One is to perform a continuous suture to the posterior wall with interrupted sutures anteriorly. Our preference is to complete the

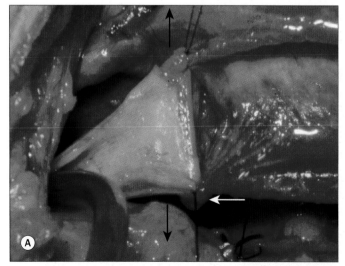
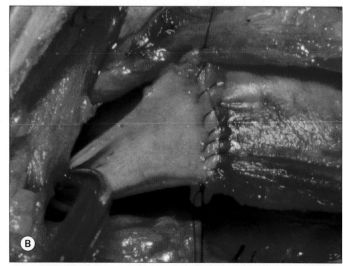

Figure 38.13 Eversion plication of redundant endarterectomy zone. (A) Two stay sutures are placed at opposing sides of the wall incorporating the excess redundancy. The sutures are tied and pulled apart (black arrows), thereby causing eversion of the redundant wall posteriorly (white arrow). The adjacent segments of intima/endarterectomized artery are then reanastomosed to restore arterial continuity (B).

anastomosis with interrupted 6:0 Prolene sutures. Stay sutures are positioned at 12 and 6 o'clock and tied. The anastomosis can then be rotated so that either the medial or lateral wall is accessible. The anastomosis is facilitated by placing a further (untied) suture midway between the stay sutures (**Fig. 38.14B**). This allows the vessel walls to be eased away from the shunt and facilitates accurate suture apposition. Once completed, it is helpful at this stage to deflate the distal Pruitt balloon and retract the shunt to see if there are any obvious bleeding points. Once the shunt has been removed, further suture insertion may lead to unwanted stenosis formation at the anastomosis.

The next step is reconstruction of the carotid bifurcation. Alternatives include end-to-end anastomosis with the CCA or oversewing of the distal ICA and reimplantation end-to-side onto the CCA. The bifurcation should be reconstructed where possible. The first step is to open the back wall of the vein with fine scissors to a point where it is felt that the heel of the anastomosis will lie comfortably against the distal apex of the origin of the ECA (**Fig. 38.14C**). Care should be taken to avoid graft redundancy as this will lead to kinking when flow is restored. A 6:0 Prolene suture anastomoses the heel of the graft to the ICA–ECA origin and down onto the distal CCA.

Any patient who has had a carotid vein bypass must undergo regular duplex ultrasound surveillance. Evidence suggests that up to 20% will develop a severe recurrent stenosis within 12 months,[58] significantly higher than observed after standard endarterectomy. Vein bypass stenosis may be treated by angioplasty. About one-third will require repeated angioplasty to maintain graft patency.

COMPLICATIONS OF CAROTID SURGERY

Operative stroke/death

The operative risk is defined as the rate of death and/or *any* stroke within the first 30 days after CEA. In NASCET and ECST, the operative mortality rate was 0.6–1.0%, the death/disabling stroke rate was 2–4%, while the death/any stroke rate was 5–7%.[1-4] Surgeons participating in ECST and NASCET had to submit their recent 'track record' for scrutiny. Accordingly, some have criticized ECST and NASCET as not being representative of true clinical practice. Operative mortality and stroke rates are significantly higher in community studies and more recent randomized trials.[7-10] This is important to resolve as only 6% of CEAs in the US are currently performed in a NASCET hospital.[7]

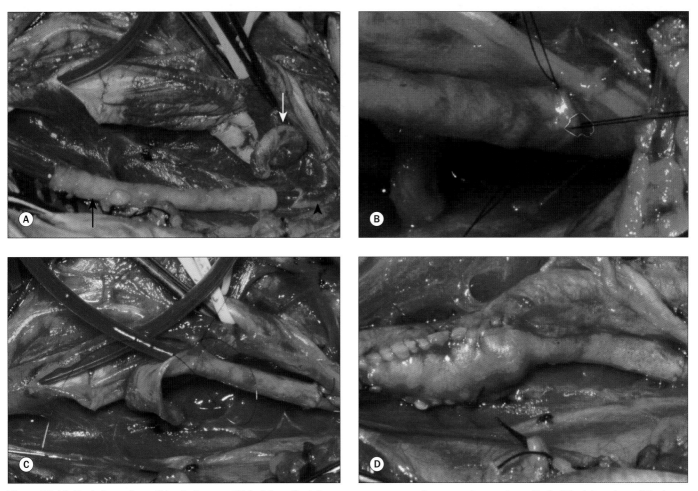

Figure 38.14 Technique of carotid vein bypass. (A) In this patient, bypass was necessary because of excessive coiling of the internal carotid artery (ICA) distal to the endarterectomy zone (white arrow). The saphenous vein has been harvested from the groin, reversed, and placed over the distal limb of a Pruitt–Inahara shunt (black arrow). The shunt is reinserted into the distal ICA (arrowhead) and flow restored. **(B)** The distal anastomosis starts with interrupted stay sutures at 6 and 12 o'clock, facilitated by a further suture placed midway to enable accurate positioning of each suture (left). **(C)** The vein graft is shortened as necessary and an end-to-end anastomosis to the external carotid artery (ECA) origin, proximal ECA, and distal common carotid artery reconstructs the bifurcation. The shunt does not need to be removed until the last minute. **(D)** Completed saphenous vein bypass.

ECST[33] identified three factors on multivariate analysis that were predictive of increased operative risk: female sex (odds ratio [OR] 2.1); peripheral vascular disease (OR 2.5); and a systolic blood pressure >180mmHg (OR 2.2). Similar factors from NASCET[59] included: hemispheric as opposed to ocular events (OR 2.3); left versus right CEA (OR 2.3); contralateral occlusion (OR 2.2); ipsilateral infarct on CT or MRI (OR 1.8); and irregular as opposed to smooth plaque (OR 1.5). Neither in NASCET nor ECST was there any association between age and operative risk.

In NASCET it was observed that patients taking aspirin <650mg daily were more likely to suffer an operative stroke.[2] A randomized trial has shown the converse to be true.[35] Randomized evidence suggests that low-dose aspirin (75–300mg) significantly reduces perioperative cardiovascular morbidity/mortality, while avoiding the side effects associated with higher-dose therapy.

The incidence of intracranial hemorrhage/hyperperfusion stroke is about 1%. Both have similar predisposing factors, including severe bilateral extracranial disease, a history of hypertension, poor intracranial collateralization, and impaired autoregulation. Current thinking is that the two may be part of a common phenomenon where impaired autoregulation takes some time to reset after CEA, during which time the brain is exposed to increased blood flow. The patient can therefore present with several symptoms, including headache, irritability, drowsiness, seizure, and ultimately stroke, which may be either ischemic or hemorrhagic.

Management of operation-related stroke
Intraoperative stroke
It has become conventional to assume that any patient who recovers from anesthesia with a new neurologic deficit must have suffered a stroke due to endarterectomy site thromboembolism. Accordingly, these patients should be re-explored immediately. Delay beyond 1 hour reduces the chances of success.[60] In Leicester, the patient would receive the first of three 8mg doses of intravenous dexamethasone, although there is no randomized trial evidence to support this strategy. Care should be taken to avoid unnecessary neck movement, which may precipitate embolization. If the artery was closed primarily, a patch should now be inserted at re-exploration following thrombectomy. Completion angiography should be performed to exclude persisting technical error or distal mural thrombus. If the thrombus does not clear, extreme care should be employed when passing a number 2/3 Fogarty catheter into the distal reaches of the ICA to minimize the risk of causing a carotid–cavernous sinus fistula. Anecdotal case reports have indicated that there might be a role for catheter-guided thrombolysis in the future.[61]

Postoperative stroke
Any stroke that occurs in the first 24 hours should be assumed to be embolic, especially the initial 12 hours. A CT scan is unlikely to alter decision-making and this should not delay the patient being returned to theater. Although the stroke may have been due to focal embolism, as opposed to carotid thrombosis, the surgeon has no way of knowing if there is an underlying technical error or mural endarterectomy zone thrombus with the potential for further embolization.

Any patient who has a stroke after 24 hours has elapsed should undergo emergency CT scan to exclude intracranial hemorrhage.

Patients with intracranial hemorrhage require careful BP control so as to avoid the extremes of rising intracranial pressure or hypoperfusion.

Patients who report severe headache and/or seizure in the early postoperative phase require urgent hospitalization. Almost invariably they will have grossly elevated BP and are at some danger of intracranial hemorrhage. The mainstay of treatment is rapid control of seizures (titrated intravenous diazepam initially), followed by attempts to reduce the BP (titrated intravenous labetolol).

Prevention of operative stroke
Although the introduction of a program of monitoring and quality control has virtually abolished intraoperative stroke, it had no effect on the 2.7% rate of stroke secondary to postoperative carotid thrombosis.[57]

The rare patient destined to suffer postoperative carotid thrombosis often has 1–2 hours of increasing embolization before the onset of any neurologic deficit.[62,63] This observation has been corroborated worldwide.[64–67] This high rate of embolization can be arrested by incremental infusion of Dextran-40, which prevents progression to thrombosis.[57] Carotid thrombosis can occur in the absence of any technical error[63] and may be mediated by factors that enhance platelet function in individual patients, rather than by the actual surgical technique.

Evidence supporting the latter observation comes from research which shows that: postoperative embolization is unrelated to patch type[68]; patients undergoing staged bilateral CEAs have similar degrees of embolization after each procedure[69]; and embolization is unrelated to aspirin therapy but the platelets of patients with high-rate embolization are significantly more sensitive to ADP stimulation.[70] More recently, a randomized trial has shown that 75mg clopidogrel (ADP inhibitor) administered the night before surgery confers a significant reduction in the rate of postoperative embolization.[71]

Medical complications
A secondary analysis from NASCET indicated that 10% of patients suffered a medical complication in the perioperative period after CEA.[72] The commonest were cardiovascular (8%) or respiratory (0.8%). None, however, suffered a pulmonary embolus. Overall, 70% of medical morbidity after CEA was classed as mild and 27% were considered moderately severe. Only five patients (0.3%) suffered a major medical complication (all myocardial infarction).

Hypertension is a common clinical problem after CEA that was not specifically addressed in either ECST or NASCET. Depending on the threshold applied, up to 40% of patients may require antihypertensive therapy in the early postoperative phase. Preliminary evidence suggests that the incidence may be reduced significantly in patients who have CEA under LRA.[45] The majority settle within 12 hours. Persisting hypertension beyond this merits review by a cardiovascular specialist so as to minimize both the cardiac risk and the potential for progressing on to the hyperperfusion syndrome and intracranial hemorrhage.

Cranial nerve injury
Cranial nerve injuries were documented in 8.6% of patients in NASCET.[59] Almost all were classified as mild and all recovered within 30 days. None suffered a major cranial nerve injury. The

commonest nerves to be injured were the hypoglossal (3.7%), vagus (2.5%), and mandibular branch of the facial nerve (2.2%). No patient in NASCET suffered glossopharyngeal nerve palsy, reflecting the exclusion of patients with high carotid disease from the trial.

A recent review of the literature by Forsell[73] identified 13 series (2911 patients). Here, the overall prevalence of cranial nerve injury was 15%. The mandibular branch of the facial nerve was injured in about 4%, the glossopharyngeal nerve in 0.5%, the recurrent laryngeal nerve was traumatized in 5%, and the hypoglossal in 7%.

Most surgeons have placed relatively little importance on discussing the potential for cranial nerve injury with patients before carotid surgery. The NASCET and Forsell series indicate that this stance is no longer acceptable. The majority will undoubtedly be transient, but the risks and implications of permanent nerve injury must be accepted by the patient as they consent to surgery.

Patch infection

Prosthetic patch infection complicates about 1% of CEAs. In a recent review (43 patients), 37% occurred within 2 months of surgery, while 56% occurred after 6 months had elapsed.[74] Early postoperative cases usually present with deep wound infection or false aneurysm formation and the majority usually report an early wound complication (hematoma, infection). Published cases of prosthetic patch rupture are extremely rare (four to date) and can occur at any time following operation. Late infections (over 6 months) tend to present with chronic sinus discharge or false aneurysm formation. The vast majority of organisms responsible for prosthetic patch infection (90%) are either staphylococci or streptococci.[74]

Management depends on the mode and urgency of presentation. Preoperative investigation is unnecessary in patients with massive hemorrhage. Less urgent cases benefit from duplex/angiographic assessment. Radioisotope-labeled white cell scans can be unreliable and there is no evidence that CT results alter outcome. The golden rule is that an abscess overlying a carotid incision must never be incised unless a vascular colleague is present.

Surgical options for patch infection include:

- patch removal and autologous venous reconstruction with either patch or bypass
- patch removal followed by ligation of the CCA, ICA, and ECA
- debridement and cover with a muscle flap.

Ligation should be considered only in patients with a chronically occluded ICA or in the rare patient in whom catastrophic hemorrhage cannot be controlled. Up to 50% of patients who have ligation will suffer a stroke. Evidence suggests that the optimal treatment is patch removal with autologous reconstruction (90% alive, stroke-free and infection-free at 2 years). Reconstruction using prosthetic material has a very poor outcome and is not recommended.[74]

Postoperative surveillance

With the exception of the management of asymptomatic disease and postoperative surveillance, there is remarkable similarity in transatlantic attitudes towards the surgical treatment of atherosclerotic carotid artery disease. In the UK and Scandinavia, few patients undergo serial clinical or ultrasound surveillance

outwith clinical trials. This is based on evidence that the risk of ipsilateral stroke in patients with a recurrent stenosis greater than 50% is only about 6% at 3 years as compared with 3% in patients with normal carotid arteries or a stenosis less than 50%.[75] Only one ACAS patient (0.12%) underwent reoperation for a symptomatic severe recurrent stenosis and there was no association between late stroke and recurrent stenosis.[76] In the US and mainland Europe, serial ultrasound surveillance receives greater emphasis, partly because surgeons in these countries adopt a more active stance in the treatment of asymptomatic carotid disease.

NON-ATHEROMATOUS CAROTID DISEASE

Arteritis
Takayasu's arteritis
Takayasu's arteritis (TA) is an extremely rare, chronic inflammatory arteritis of unknown etiology. Because of its rarity, few clinicians (especially in the Western world) have acquired substantial experience in its management. TA is predominantly a disease of the aorta and its principal branches (**Table 38.9**) and comprises varying combinations of occlusion, stenosis, and dilatation. Extracranial carotid involvement can occur on its own (type I) or in combination with multiple disease locations (types IIa, IIb, V). Accordingly, the patient can present with a variety of symptoms and signs (cerebral, coronary, mesenteric, renovascular hypertension, etc.).

The strategy of investigation must, therefore, take account of the fact that multiple sites of disease may be present. From the surgical point of view, baseline investigations should include full blood count (looking for anemia, thrombocytosis, and leukocytosis), urea and electrolytes (looking for evidence of end-organ damage to the kidneys), and simple markers of systemic illness (elevated plasma viscosity [PV], erythrocyte sedimentation rate [ESR], C-reactive protein [CRP]). If the clinical history or duplex findings (**Fig. 38.15**) suggest a diagnosis of TA, digital subtraction thoracic and abdominal aortograms (including the principal branches) should be performed.

The first-line treatment is prednisolone therapy (40–60mg daily). If this fails to control the symptoms or active phase of the disease (which can be monitored using duplex measurement of

Classification of Takayasu's arteritis.	
Type I	Branches of the aortic arch (subclavian, carotid, vertebral)
Type IIa	Ascending aorta Aortic arch + branches
Type IIb	Ascending aorta, aortic arch Aortic arch branches Descending thoracic aorta
Type III	Descending thoracic aorta Abdominal aorta +/– renal arteries
Type IV	Abdominal aorta +/– renal arteries
Type V	Combination of Types IIb and IV

Table 38.9 Classification of Takayasu's arteritis.

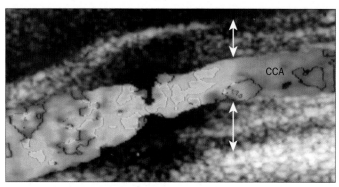

Figure 38.15 Takayasu's disease. Color duplex ultrasound image showing Takayasu's disease at the distal common carotid artery in a 20-year-old woman who presented with amaurosis fugax and hemispheric transient ischemic attacks. Note the gross thickening of the vessel wall (arrows). This extended down to the aortic arch on magnetic resonance angiography. Severe stenotic/occlusive disease was also present in the contralateral carotid artery, both subclavians, and one vertebral.

arterial wall thickness or by serial ESR, CRP, or PV), immunosuppression may be added to the regimen (methotrexate, cyclophosphamide). In the past, angioplasty has generally been considered contraindicated in TA because of the long lengths of disease involvement. There have, however, been anecdotal reports of its application in patients with short segment disease or carotid involvement, particularly following the introduction of synchronous stenting. Surgical intervention should be reserved, where possible, for patients over the active phase of the disease. This is indicated by no evidence of worsening constitutional symptoms or end-organ symptoms; reducing ESR, CRP, or PV; and no deterioration in duplex or angiographic occlusions or stenoses. Care should be taken to avoid any anastomosis in arteries involved with TA. Accordingly, carotid bypass should generally derive inflow from the aortic arch as opposed to the subclavian arteries.

Giant cell arteritis

Giant cell arteritis (GCA) is another chronic inflammatory disorder of arteries. Most clinicians are aware of the involvement of branches of the ECA, but GCA can also affect the thoracic and abdominal aorta, carotid and subclavian arteries, as well as the femoropopliteal vessels. The symptoms may be very similar to those in patients with atherosclerosis (especially as the disease tends to start in patients aged over 50 years), but prodromal non-specific symptoms, jaw claudication, and tenderness over the temporal artery should raise suspicions.

Surgery has little role in the management of cerebral GCA apart from rare occlusive complications presenting with end-organ injury. Stroke/TIA can follow carotid or vertebral artery involvement but is rare. The principal fear is unilateral or bilateral blindness, which can occur rapidly following occlusion of the posterior ciliary arteries. Any patient in whom there is reasonable suspicion of GCA should have a temporal artery biopsy as soon as possible. If there is to be any significant delay, oral steroid therapy (20–60mg prednisolone daily) should be started empirically. Patients with acute blindness should be admitted immediately and receive intravenous corticosteroid therapy. There is limited evidence that immunosuppression improves the outcome in steroid-resistant patients.

Radiation arteritis

Exposure to radiation predisposes to an increased risk of carotid stenosis. In the first 3–5 years after radiotherapy, the primary injury leads to intimal hyperplasia. These lesions can be quite extensive within segments of the common and internal carotid arteries but tend to be smooth. Thereafter, evidence suggests that radiotherapy can predispose towards accelerated atherogenesis.

In clinical practice, the incidence of symptomatic lesions requiring intervention is extremely small. There is no consensus regarding the management of asymptomatic lesions. In the UK, these patients would probably be treated conservatively unless there is a contralateral occlusion. In North America, surveillance and interventional strategies are less conservative. It would not, however, be appropriate simply to apply the ACAS findings to asymptomatic postradiation stenoses that were non-atherosclerotic. The risks of surgery are inevitably higher. This is because:

- carotid dissection is made more difficult by the scarring associated with the radiotherapy and any previous radical neck surgery
- the normal planes of dissection between intima and media disappear because of radiation-induced fibrosis
- the segments of diseased artery can be long and extensive
- the risks of secondary infection (primary arterial, patch) increase because of poor wound healing, especially in the presence of an adjacent tracheostomy.

Surgical options previously included endarterectomy, patching the stenosis, or formal carotid vein bypass. Surgery has, however, largely been superseded by angioplasty with stenting,[77] which is now the first-line treatment.

Carotid aneurysm

As with aneurysms anywhere else in the body, carotid aneurysms (CA) can be true or false. Causes of true CA include atherosclerosis, fibromuscular dysplasia, TA, or GCA. False CA can follow iatrogenic dissection (postangioplasty, post-CEA), spontaneous dissection, infected carotid vein or prosthetic patches, or be mycotic.

Most CAs are treated, primarily because of their potential for embolization or thrombosis in the future. The majority are treated surgically, although endovascular intervention may be the treatment of choice for a CA located near the skull base.

The choice of surgical procedure depends on the underlying cause. True atherosclerotic aneurysms tend to be associated with functional elongation of the carotid artery. It is therefore often possible to resect the aneurysm and perform an end-to-end anastomosis (**Fig. 38.16**). If this is not possible or the wall is excessively thinned or potentially infected, a bypass can be performed (**Figs 38.14 & 38.16**). It is this author's preference to use autologous vein, but polytetrafluoroethylene (PTFE) is an alternative. A final option is to transpose the distal ICA onto the proximal ECA. If no operation is possible and endovascular repair deemed inappropriate, the only option is carotid ligation. This should be used only as a last resort, as up to 50% of patients will suffer a stroke as a consequence.

Carotid dissection

Carotid artery dissection (CAD) accounts for only about 2% of all strokes. However, one-fifth of strokes in young individuals will be secondary to CAD and up to 25% of patients with unexplained stroke following trauma will have suffered a dissection.

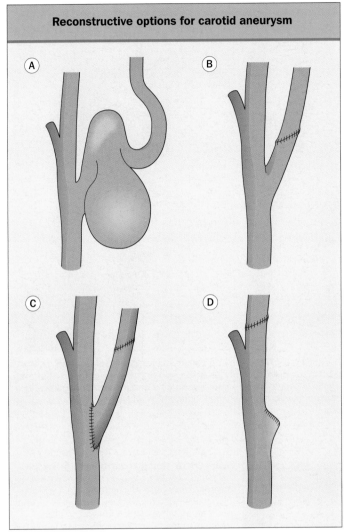

Reconstructive options for carotid aneurysm

Figure 38.16 Reconstructive options for carotid aneurysm. These include: (A) resection and (B) end-to-end anastomosis; (C) interposition vein or prosthetic bypass; (D) oversewing of internal carotid artery (ICA) origin with transposition of distal ICA onto external carotid artery.

Few surgeons have a large personal series and many cases of CAD are probably misdiagnosed. In reality, the most difficult practical aspect with regard to planning management is actually thinking about the diagnosis in the first place!

CAD can either be asymptomatic or present with one or more of headache, stroke, TIA, painful Horner's syndrome, or cranial nerve paresis (III, IV, or VI). Neurologic symptoms follow:

- ICA occlusion through compression of the true lumen by thrombus in the false lumen
- distal embolization from the mural thrombus
- formation of a symptomatic false aneurysm, especially in patients with subadventitial dissection.

Clinical suspicion should guide interpretation of preliminary investigations. Thus, the clinician should be alerted to the possibility of CAD in a young patient with duplex/MRA/angiography evidence of a carotid occlusion 2–3cm above the bifurcation, or a normal carotid bifurcation but with intimal irregularity or stenosis 2–3cm above it. Angiography is currently the standard for evaluating suspected CAD, although gadolinium-enhanced MRA may supersede this in future.

Type I dissection refers to the situation where angiography shows either minor intimal irregularity (**Fig. 38.17A**) or a stenosis less than 70%. Type II dissections show evidence of a severe stenosis >70% and/or aneurysm formation (**Fig. 38.17B**). Type III dissections classically exhibit a flame-shaped carotid occlusion 2–3cm above the bifurcation (**Fig. 38.17C**). Type I, type III, and most type II dissections should be managed by systemic heparinization followed by warfarinization. The aim is to reduce the risk of secondary dissection, thrombosis, and embolism. Surgery, and possibly endovascular intervention in the future, is reserved for complex cases with recurring symptoms despite best medical therapy and who have amenable lesions. Type II dissections extending to the skull base are particularly difficult to treat if symptoms do not settle with anticoagulation. Options include extracranial–intracranial bypass (but few centers currently offer this service). The optimal management strategy for aneurysm formation after CAD is controversial. In the past, surgery has been recommended, but recent evidence suggests that they may have a more benign prognosis.[78,79] It therefore seems appropriate to recommend conservative management and regular surveillance unless the aneurysm is associated with a severe stenosis or recurrence of symptoms.

Fibromuscular dysplasia

Fibromuscular dysplasia (FMD) predominantly affects the renal arteries of young women. However, about a quarter of all cases involve the carotid or vertebral arteries. The majority with carotid disease (60%) will be bilateral and typically the middle and upper segments of the ICA are affected. Pathologically, FMD can involve any of the three arterial layers. The commonest subtype is medial fibroplasia, which accounts for three-quarters of all cases. The arteries of patients with medial fibroplasia typically display a beaded appearance (alternating stenotic webs and dilatations). As seems typical in patients with non-atherosclerotic carotid disease, the presentation of FMD is variable, ranging from no symptoms to stroke. Stroke/TIA can be due to thrombosis, embolization, or bleeding because of the association between FMD and (i) stenosis formation, (ii) false aneurysm formation, (iii) distal dissection, and (iv) a co-association with intracranial aneurysms, thereby predisposing patients to subarachnoid hemorrhage.

Angiography currently remains the standard investigation, although newer MRA technology may take over in the future. Duplex imaging may miss high carotid lesions unless the more proximal ICA displays a beaded appearance.

Management is usually conservative. There is no evidence that anticoagulation is preferable to antiplatelet therapy. Patients who become symptomatic should be treated in the same way as if they had atherosclerotic disease. Prior to the advent of endovascular technologies, the standard treatment was either open graduated dilatation or vein bypass. Most, however, are now treated by percutaneous angioplasty, which can be combined with stenting and repeated during the course of follow-up, which should be lifelong.

Carotid body tumor

The carotid body is located within the adventitia posterior to the bifurcation of the carotid artery. Its role is to monitor blood gases and pH. Histologically, it is derived from cells originating from the neural crest ectoderm. A carotid body tumor (CBT)

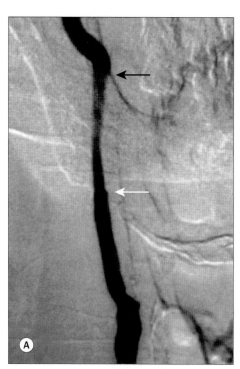

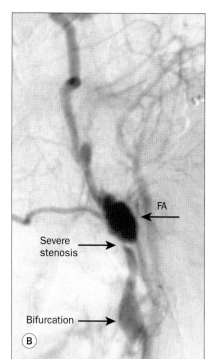

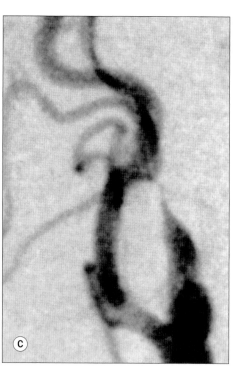

Figure 38.17 Examples of carotid dissection. (A) Type I: intimal irregularity +/− stenosis <70% seen in a patient following angioplasty of a recurrent stenosis after carotid endarterectomy. It is presumed that the guidewire caused a distal dissection (white arrow) with re-entry higher up (black arrow). (B) Type II: stenosis >70% +/− false aneurysm (FA) formation. This 40-year-old man presented with Horner's syndrome and monocular blindness and has both a severe stenosis and distal FA formation. (C) Type III: occlusion, characteristically 'flame shaped' and 2–3cm above the bifurcation. Occlusion is due to thrombus in the false channel compressing the true lumen.

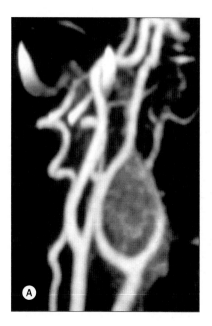

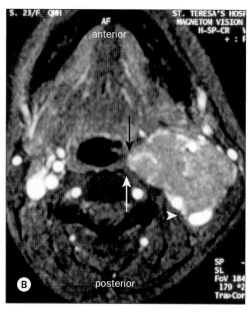

Figure 38.18 Carotid body tumor. (A) Carotid body tumor causing splaying of the bifurcation on magnetic resonance angiography. (B) Computed tomography scan showing encroachment of the tumor on the larynx (black arrow) and close proximity to the pharyngeal mucosa (white arrow). The bulk of the tumor lies anterior to the external carotid artery and internal carotid artery (arrowhead).

grows within the bifurcation and ultimately causes this to splay (**Fig. 38.18**). The CBT ultimately presents as either a painless swelling or because of pain and/or compression of adjacent cranial nerves. Stroke/TIA is rare.

Investigation begins with duplex imaging. This usually demonstrates intense vascularity with splaying of the bifurcation. Recognition of the likelihood of CBT warrants either CT or MRI to exclude bilateral tumors and provide information regarding the overall extent of the lesion. In particular it is useful to know if the ICA is encased in tumor (**Fig. 38.18B**).

A case can be made for a conservative approach in elderly patients with relatively small tumors. In the remainder, surgical excision is the mainstay of management. Some 5% of CBTs are malignant and 5% are bilateral. CBT surgery should be performed by a surgeon who is experienced at dealing with arteries, bleeding, and anastomoses. Surgery is inevitably more difficult the second time around after an inexperienced surgeon has attempted removal. Some surgeons advocate preoperative embolization of the main tumor blood supply so as to minimize operative bleeding. To date there is no consensus as to whether this alters the outcome.

The approach to the bifurcation is just as for CEA. In small tumors, it may be possible to expose each of the important cranial nerves (hypoglossal, vagus) and arteries (CCA, ICA, ECA) without difficulty. The tumor is then gradually removed via dissection that is classically described as being in the subadventitial plane. In reality, the surgeon finds the most superficial plane between artery and tumor and dissection proceeds via a combination of diathermy and a lot of ligatures. The principal blood supply to the tumor is derived from the posterior–inferior aspect of the bifurcation. Occasionally, this vessel can be inadvertently damaged during excision and brisk bleeding ensues. If the injury is small, temporary clamping will enable primary closure with interrupted 6:0 Prolene sutures (Ethicon). More extensive injuries may warrant formal arteriotomy, shunt insertion, and even vein bypass. CBT excision can be done with TCD monitoring. In the event of bleeding, TCD can guide the urgency of shunt deployment. Surgeons should also bear in mind that these patients can also have atherosclerotic disease which can embolize to the brain during injudicious dissection.

Larger CBTs require alternative strategies. First, the patient should be warned of an increased risk of permanent cranial nerve injury. Second, the surgeon should anticipate the need for high dissection. Excision of moderately large tumors is facilitated by asking the anesthetist to insert a nasolaryngeal tube as opposed to an oral tube. This opens up the angle of access between the ramus of the mandible and the mastoid process. Alternatively, the surgeon can arrange for maxillofacial colleagues to undertake a mandibular subluxation (preferable to dislocation). Note that this cannot be done once the operation is underway.

Carotid artery trauma

Most experience with carotid artery trauma (penetrating or blunt) comes from the major trauma centers in South Africa and North America or during war. Few centers in mainland Europe have significant peace-time exposure to penetrating carotid injuries. In Leicester, there is a large CEA practice, but the vascular unit has only dealt with two penetrating carotid injuries (one iatrogenic) in 10 years.

In the US, the majority (80–90%) of carotid artery injuries are penetrating. In the UK and Europe, the majority are blunt. Blunt injuries tend to follow compression or traction to the carotid arteries following rapid deceleration (road traffic accidents). This predisposes to intimal tearing and secondary thrombus formation or distal dissection. The principles of management are similar to those for carotid dissection (see above).

Penetrating carotid artery injuries are classified according to their anatomic site. Type I injuries affect the carotid artery between the clavicle and cricoid cartilage. Type II carotid injuries occur between the cricoid cartilage and the angle of the mandible. Type III injuries affect the carotid artery between the angle of the mandible and the skull base.

The management of carotid artery injuries will inevitably depend on the urgency of presentation, access to imaging and interventional modalities, and the experience of the surgeon. Patients with profuse hemorrhage require immediate exploration, but care must be taken to exclude coexistent trauma such as cervical spine injury, etc. More stable patients warrant imaging wherever possible. Duplex ultrasound has now largely replaced routine angiography in patients with a penetrating wound in the type II zone. However diagnostic intra-arterial digital subtraction angiography (IADSA) is still required in most patients with type I or III injuries because of the reduced accuracy of duplex in these regions. IADSA is also indicated in most type II injuries where duplex suggests an injury that requires surgery. Duplex can, however, be used to survey minor intimal irregularities or small false aneurysms serially, without recourse to angiography.

Individual management decisions will inevitably reflect the severity of injury, urgency of presentation, neurologic status, and the presence of coexisting trauma. As a rule, patients with occluded carotid arteries and either a dense hemiplegia or no neurologic symptoms at all should be treated conservatively. Carotid reconstruction is currently advocated in patients with less severe neurologic deficits, provided they are treated early. The aim is to improve perfusion of a hemodynamically compromised penumbra around the evolving infarct, without increasing the risk of hemorrhagic transformation.

A variety of reconstructive options are available, including primary arterial repair, vein patch, transposition of the ICA to the main ECA trunk, and reversed vein bypass. Prosthetic bypass may be necessary in proximal CCA injuries but the potential for late infection must be remembered. EC–IC bypass might be indicated in patients who would otherwise require carotid ligation. Ligation of the CCA or ICA should only ever be considered in extenuating circumstances. The most likely reason for having to perform ligation is uncontrollable distal hemorrhage in a patient where EC–IC bypass is not possible. Wherever possible, monitoring with TCD may be an invaluable aid in this difficult situation. Newer endovascular techniques now offer the potential for dealing with more of the distal, surgically inaccessible lesions of the ICA. Options include insertion of a covered stent (false aneurysms and caroticojugular fistula) or placement of a detachable balloon, which can occlude the cavernous segment of the ICA.

REFERENCES

1. European Carotid Surgery Trialists Collaborative Group. MRC European Carotid Surgery Trial: interim results for symptomatic patients with severe (70–99%) or mild (0–29%) carotid stenosis. Lancet 1991;337:1235–43.
2. North American Symptomatic Carotid Endarterectomy Trial Collaborators. Beneficial effect of carotid endarterectomy in symptomatic patients with high grade stenosis. N Engl J Med 1991;325:445–53.
3. The European Carotid Surgery Trialists Collaborative Group. Endarterectomy for moderate symptomatic carotid stenosis: interim results from the MRC European Carotid Surgery Trial. Lancet 1996;347:1591–3.
4. Barnett HJM, Taylor DW, Eliasziw M, et al., for the NASCET trial. Benefit of carotid endarterectomy in patients with symptomatic moderate or severe stenosis. N Engl J Med 1998;339:1415–25.

5. Executive Committee for the Asymptomatic Carotid Atherosclerosis Study. Endarterectomy for asymptomatic carotid artery stenosis. JAMA 1995;273:1421–8.

6. Barnett HJM, Barnes RW, Clagett GP, Ferguson GG, Robertson JT, Walker PM. Symptomatic carotid artery stenosis: a solvable problem. The NASCET trial. Stroke 1992;23:1050–3.

7. Wennberg DE, Lucas FL, Birkmeyer JD, Bredenberg CE, Fisher ES. Variation in carotid endarterectomy mortality in the Medicare population. JAMA 1998;279:1278–81.

8. Karp HR, Flanders D, Shipp CC, Taylor B, Martin D. Carotid endarterectomy among Medicare beneficiaries: a statewide evaluation of appropriateness and outcome. Stroke 1998;29:46–52.

9. Hsai DC, Krushat WM, Moscoe LM. Epidemiology of carotid endarterectomy among Medicare beneficiaries: 1985–1996 update. Stroke 1998; 29:346–50.

10. CAVATAS Investigators. Endovascular versus surgical treatment in patients with carotid stenosis in the Carotid and Vertebral Artery Transluminal Angioplasty Study (CAVATAS): a randomised trial. Lancet 2001;357:1729–37.

11. Naylor AR, Rothwell PM, Bell PRF. Overview of the principal results and secondary analyses from the European and North American randomised trials of carotid endarterectomy. Eur J Vasc Endovasc Surg (in press).

12. Barnett HJM, Eliasziw M, Meldrum HE, Taylor DW. Do the facts and figures warrant a tenfold increase in the performance of carotid endarterectomy in asymptomatic patients? Neurology 1996;466:603–8.

13. EC/IC Bypass Study Group. Failure of extracranial–intracranial arterial bypass to reduce the risk of ischaemic stroke. Results of an international randomized trial. N Engl J Med 1985;313:1191–200.

14. Sundt TM. Was the international randomized trial of extracranial–intracranial arterial bypass representative of the population at risk? N Engl J Med 1987;316:814–6.

15. Grubb RL, Derdyn CP, Fritsch S, Powers WJ. Cerebral haemodynamics and stroke risk. In: Choi D, Dacy RG, Hsu CY, Powers WJ, eds. Cerebrovascular disease: momentum at the end of the second millenium. Armonk, NY:Futura; 2002.

16. Huber TS, Wheeler KG, Cuddeback JK, Dame DA, Flynn TC, Seeger JM. Effect of the asymptomatic carotid atherosclerosis study on carotid endarterectomy in Florida. Stroke 1998;29:1099–105.

17. Hankey GJ. Asymptomatic carotid stenosis: how should it be managed? Med J Aust 1995;163:197–200.

18. Perry JR, Szalai JP, Norris JW, for the Canadian Stroke Consortium. Consensus against both endarterectomy and routine screening for asymptomatic carotid artery stenosis. Arch Neurol 1997;54:25–8.

19. Alamowitch S, Eliasziw M, Algra A, Meldrum H, Barnett HJM, for the NASCET trial. Risk, causes and prevention of ischaemic stroke in elderly patients with symptomatic internal carotid artery stenosis. Lancet 2001; 357:1154–60.

20. Morgenstern LB, Fox AJ, Sharpe BL, Eliasziw M, Barnett HJM, Grotta JC, for the NASCET trial. The risks and benefits of carotid endarterectomy in patients with near occlusion of the carotid artery. Neurology 1997; 48:911–5.

21. Rothwell PM, Warlow CP, on behalf of the ECST Collaborative Group. Low risk of ischaemic stroke in patients with reduced internal carotid artery lumen diameter distal to severe symptomatic carotid stenosis: cerebral protection due to low post-stenotic flow. Stroke 2000; 31:622–30.

22. Henderson RD, Eliasziw M, Fox AJ, Rothwell PM, Barnett HJM, for the NASCET trial. Angiographically defined collateral circulation and risk of stroke in patients with severe carotid artery stenosis. Stroke 2000;31:128–32.

23. European Carotid Surgery Trialists' Collaborative Group. Randomised trial of endarterectomy for recently symptomatic carotid stenosis: final results of the MRC European Carotid Surgery Trial (ECST). Lancet 1998;351:1379–87.

24. Blaisdell WF, Clauss RH, Gailbrath JG, Smith JR. Joint study of extracranial carotid artery occlusion: a review of surgical considerations. JAMA 1969;209:1889–95.

25. Mead GE, O'Neill PA, McCollum CN. Is there a role for carotid surgery in acute stroke? Eur J Vasc Endovasc Surg 1997;13:112–21.

26. Gasecki AP, Ferguson GG, Eliasziw M, et al. Early endarterectomy for severe carotid artery stenosis after a non-disabling stroke: results of the NASCET Trial. J Vasc Surg 1994;20:288–95.

27. Naylor AR, Mehta Z, Rothwell PM, Bell PRF. Carotid artery disease and stroke during coronary artery bypass: a critical review of the literature. Eur J Vasc Endovasc Surg 2002;23:283–94.

28. Moore WS, Barnett HJM, Beebe HG, et al. Guidelines for carotid endarterectomy. Circulation 1995;91:566–79.

29. Biller J, Feinberg WM, Castaldo JE, et al. Guidelines for carotid endarterectomy: a statement for healthcare professionals from a special writing group of the Stroke Council, American Heart Association. Stroke 1998;29:554–62.

30. Thompson JP. When is pre-operative cardiac evaluation advisable? In: Naylor AR, Mackey WC, eds. Carotid artery surgery: a problem based approach. London:WB Saunders; 2000:164–70.

31. Rodgers A, MacMahon S, Gamble G, Slattery J, Sandercock P, Warlow C, for the United Kingdom Transient Ischaemic Attack Collaborative Group. Blood pressure and risk of stroke in patients with cerebrovascular disease. BMJ 1996;313:147.

32. Neal B, Clark T, Macmahon S, Rodgers A, Baigent C, Collins R, on behalf of the Antithrombotic Trialists Collaboration. Blood pressure and the risk of recurrent vascular disease. Am J Hypertens 1998;11:25A–26A.

33. Rothwell PM, Warlow CP, on behalf of the ECST Collaborative Group. Prediction of benefit from carotid endarterectomy in individual patients: a risk modelling study. Lancet 1999;353;2105–10.

34. Johnson ES, Lanes SF, Wentworth CE, Satterfield MH, Adebe BL, Dicker LW. A meta-regression analysis of the dose–response effect of aspirin on stroke. Arch Intern Med. 1999;159:1248–53.

35. Taylor DW, Barnett HJM, Haynes RB, et al. Low dose and high dose acetylsalicylic acid for patients undergoing carotid endarterectomy: a randomised trial. Lancet 1999;353:2179–84.

36. CAPRIE Steering Committee. A randomised blinded trial of clopidogrel versus aspirin in patients at risk of ischaemic events (CAPRIE). Lancet 1996;348:1329–39.

37. Payne DA, Hayes PD, Jones CI, et al. Combined effects of aspirin and clopidogrel on platelet function in-vivo and in-vitro: implications for use in open vascular surgery. J Vasc Surg 2002;35:1204–9.

38. Wilterdink JL, Easton JD. Dipyridamole plus aspirin in cerebrovascular disease. Arch Neurol 1999;56:1087–92.

39. UK Prospective Diabetes Study Group. Effect of intensive blood glucose control with metformin on complications in overweight patients with type II diabetes. Lancet 1998;352:854–65.

40. UK Prospective Diabetes Study Group. Tight blood pressure control and risk of macrovascular and microvascular complications in type II diabetics. BMJ 1998;317:2035–8.

41. Qizilbash N, Lewington S, Duffy S, et al. Cholesterol, diastolic blood pressure and stroke: 13,000 strokes in 450,000 people in 45 prospective cohorts. Lancet 1995;346:1647–53.

42. Sudlow C, Baigent C. Cholesterol reduction. In: Clinical evidence. London:BMJ Publishing Group; 1999:116–7.

43. Goldstein LB, Adams R, Becker K, et al. Primary prevention of ischemic stroke: a statement for healthcare professionals from the Stroke Council of the American Heart Association. Stroke 2001;32:280–99.

44. Collins R, Peto R, Armitage J. The MRC/BHF Heart Protection Study: preliminary results. Int J Clin Pract 2002;56:53–6.

45. Tangkanakul C, Counsell C, Warlow CP. Local versus general anaesthesia in carotid endarterectomy: a systematic review of the evidence. Eur J Vasc Endovasc Surg 1997;13:491–9.

46. Shepard AD, Doovgan PS. What practical steps can I take if I (a) know pre-operatively that the lesion extends very high or (b) unexpectedly encounter a high lesion at operation? In: Naylor AR, Mackey WC, eds. Carotid artery surgery: a problem based approach. London:WB Saunders; 2000:224–8.

47. Counsell C, Salinas R, Warlow CP, Naylor AR. The role of carotid artery shunting during carotid endarterectomy: a systematic review of the randomised trials of routine and selective shunting and the different methods of intraoperative monitoring. In: Warlow CP, van Gijn J, Sandercock P, eds. Stroke module of the Cochrane database of

Systematic Reviews, 1996 (Issue 2). Available from BMJ Publishing Group, London.

48. Rockman CB, Riles TS. What evidence is there that regional anaesthesia confers any benefit over general anaesthesia? In: Naylor AR, Mackey WC, eds. Carotid artery surgery: a problem based approach. London:WB Saunders; 2000:199–204.

49. Ghali R, Palazzo EG, Rodriguez DI, et al. Transcranial Doppler intra-operative monitoring during carotid endarterectomy: experience with regional or general anaesthesia, with and without shunting. Ann Vasc Surg 1997;11:9–13.

50. Krul JM, van Gijn J, Ackerstaff RG, Eikelboom BC, Theodorides T, Vermeulen FE. Site and pathogenesis of infarcts associated with carotid endarterectomy. Stroke 1989;20:324–8.

51. Hayes PD, Vainas T, Hartley S, et al. The Pruitt-Inahara shunt maintains mean middle cerebral artery velocities within 10% of pre-operative values during carotid endarterectomy. J Vasc Surg 2000;32:299–306.

52. Cao P, De Rango P, Zannetti S. Eversion vs conventional carotid endarterectomy: a systematic review. Eur J Vasc Endovasc Surg 2002; 23:195–201.

53. Counsell CE, Salinas R, Naylor R, Warlow CP. A systematic review of the randomised trials of carotid patch angioplasty in carotid endarterectomy. Eur J Vasc Endovasc Surg 1997;13:345–54.

54. Riles TS, Imparato AM, Jacobowitz GR, et al. The cause of peri-operative stroke after carotid endarterectomy. J Vasc Surg 1994;19:206–14.

55. Naylor AR. Prevention of operation related stroke: are we asking the right questions? Cardiovasc Surg 1999;7:155–7.

56. Naylor AR, Mackey WC. Editorial comment: Is there any evidence that peri-operative monitoring and quality control assessment alter clinical outcome? In: Naylor AR, Mackey WC, eds. Carotid artery surgery: a problem based approach. London:WB Saunders; 2000:313–4.

57. Naylor AR, Hayes PD, Allroggen H et al. Reducing the risk of carotid surgery: a seven year audit of the role of monitoring and quality control assessment. J Vasc Surg 2000;32:750–9.

58. Lauder C, Kelly A, Thompson MM, et al. Early and late outcomes following carotid artery bypass using saphenous vein. J Vasc Surg (in press).

59. Ferguson GG, Eliasziw M, Barr HWK, et al., for the NASCET trial. The North American Symptomatic Carotid Endarterectomy Trial: surgical results in 1415 patients. Stroke 1999;30:1751–8.

60. Takolander R, Bergentz SE, Bergqvist D. Management of early neurological deficits after carotid thromboendarterectomy. Eur J Vasc Surg 1987;1:67–71.

61. Eckstein H-H, Schumacher H, Dorfler A, et al. Carotid endarterectomy and intracranial thrombolysis: simultaneous and staged procedures in ischaemic stroke. J Vasc Surg 1999;29:459–71.

62. Gaunt ME, Smith J, Martin PJ, Ratliff DA, Bell PRF, Naylor AR. On-table diagnosis of incipient carotid artery thrombosis during carotid endarterectomy using transcranial Doppler sonography. J Vasc Surg 1994;20:104–7.

63. Gaunt ME, Smith JL, Martin PJ, Ratliff DA, Bell PRF, Naylor AR. A comparison of quality control methods applied to carotid endarterectomy. Eur J Vasc Endovasc Surg 1996;11:4–11.

64. Levi CR, O'Malley HM, Fell G, et al. Transcranial Doppler detected cerebral embolism following carotid endarterectomy: high microembolic signal loads predict post-operative cerebral ischaemia. Brain 1997; 120:621–9.

65. Spencer MP. Transcranial Doppler monitoring and causes of stroke from carotid endarterectomy. Stroke 1997;28:685–91.

66. Cantelmo NL, Babikian VL, Samaraweera RN, Gordon JK, Pochay VE, Winter MR. Cerebral microembolism and ischaemia changes associated with carotid endarterectomy. J Vasc Surg 1998;27:1024–30.

67. Laman DM, Wieneke GH, van Duijn H, van Huffelen AC. High embolic rate after carotid endarterectomy is associated with early cerebrovascular complications, especially in women. J Vasc Surg 2002;36:278–84.

68. Hayes PD, Allroggen H, Steel S, et al. A randomised trial of vein versus dacron patching during carotid endarterectomy: influence of patch type on post-operative embolisation. J Vasc Surg 2001;33:994–1000.

69. Hayes PD, Patel F, Bell PRF, Naylor AR. Patients thrombo-embolic potential between bilateral carotid endarterectomies remains stable over time. Eur J Vasc Endovasc Surg 2001;22:496–8.

70. Hayes PD, Box H, Tull S, et al. The patients thrombo-embolic response following carotid endarterectomy is related to enhanced platelet sensitivity to ADP. J Vasc Surg (in press).

71. Payne DA, Hayes PD, Jones CI, Goodall AH, Bell PRF, Naylor AR. Clopidogrel reduces thromboembolism after carotid endarterectomy: a randomised trial. Lancet (in press).

72. Paciaroni M, Eliasziw M, Kappelle LJ, Finan JW, Ferguson GG, Barnett HJM, for the NASCET trial. Medical complications associated with carotid endarterectomy. Stroke 1999;30:1759–63.

73. Forsell C, Bergqvist D, Bergentz SE. Peripheral nerve injuries in carotid artery surgery. In: Greenhalgh RM, Hollier LH, eds. Surgery for stroke. London:WB Saunders; 1993:217–34.

74. Naylor AR, Payne D, Thompson MM, et al. Prosthetic patch infection after carotid endarterectomy. Eur J Vasc Endovasc Surg 2002;23:11–6.

75. Horrocks M. When should I reoperate for recurrent carotid stenosis? In: Naylor AR, Mackey WC, eds. Carotid artery surgery: a problem based approach. London:WB Saunders; 2000:371–4.

76. Moore WS, Kempczinski RF, Nelson JJ, Toole JF, for the ACAS Investigators. Recurrent carotid stenosis: results of the Asymptomatic Carotid Atherosclerosis Study. Stroke 1998;29:2018–25.

77. Houdart E, Mounayer C, Chapot R, Saint-Maurice JP, Merland JJ. Carotid stenting for radiation induced stenoses: a report of seven cases. Stroke 2001;32:118–21.

78. Guillon B, Brunereau L, Biousse V, et al. Long term follow up of aneurysms developed during extracranial internal carotid artery dissection. Neurology 1999;53:117–22.

79. Touze E, Randoux B, Meary E, et al. Aneurysmal forms of cervical artery dissection: associated factors and outcome. Stroke 2001;32:418–23.

80. Donnan GA, Davis SM, Chambers BR, Gates PC. Surgery for prevention of stroke. Lancet 1998;351:1372–3.

81. Lennard N, Smith JL, Gaunt ME, et al. A policy of quality control assessment reduces the risk of intraoperative stroke during carotid endarterectomy. Eur J Vasc Endovasc Surg 1999;17:234–40.

CHAPTER
39
Pathophysiology of Varicose Veins and Chronic Venous Insufficiency

Mark H Meissner

KEY POINTS

- Chronic venous disease includes a spectrum of clinical manifestations extending from telangiectasias and varicose veins, to lipodermatosclerosis and ulceration.

- There is no single ideal test for chronic venous disease, and a combination of physiologic and anatomic tests is often required to completely characterize the extent of disease.

- Varicose veins are present in one-quarter to one-third, and chronic venous insufficiency with skin changes and ulceration in 2% to 5%, of Western populations.

- Varicose veins have a multifactorial etiology involving the interaction of age, genetic, and environmental factors.

- Varicose veins arise in a multicentric fashion, with changes in vein wall architecture preceding the development of valvular incompetence.

- The clinical manifestations of chronic venous insufficiency are due to ambulatory venous hypertension and are mediated by chronic inflammation resulting from altered leukocyte–endothelial interactions.

- Valvular incompetence, or reflux, is the only hemodynamic derangement in primary venous disease, while secondary venous disease, usually developing after an episode of acute deep venous thrombosis, may involve a combination of reflux and obstruction.

- Reflux in asymptomatic and mildly symptomatic patients is usually isolated and segmental, while that in patients with advanced chronic venous insufficiency is usually multisegmental and frequently involves the deep, superficial, and perforating veins.

INTRODUCTION

Chronic venous disease includes a spectrum of clinical presentations ranging from uncomplicated telangiectasias and varicose veins to venous ulceration. Chronic venous insufficiency usually refers more specifically to the spectrum of skin changes associated with sustained venous hypertension. Patients with varicose veins are not classified as having chronic venous insufficiency unless they have associated skin changes or ulceration.[1] The manifestations of chronic venous disease may result from primary venous insufficiency or be secondary to other disorders, primarily acute deep venous thrombosis (DVT). Regardless of etiology, chronic venous disease has significant socioeconomic consequences and is among the most common problems encountered in surgical practice. It is estimated that chronic venous disease affects up

to 1% of the general population[2] and that as many as 164 of every 1000 people seek medical advice for venous problems.[3] In the USA, skin changes and ulceration have been estimated to affect 6 to 7 million and 400 000 to 500 000 people, respectively.[4]

The social and economic consequences of chronic venous disease are significant. Annual health care costs for venous ulceration are estimated to be £290 million in the UK and $1 billion in the USA.[5] Although the costs of wound care alone can exceed $40 000 per patient per year, the time lost from productive activity and the considerable psychological effects of ulceration are as important as the economic costs and are more difficult to measure. Feelings of fear, social isolation, anger, depression, and a negative self-image are more common in patients with venous ulcers than among those undergoing procedures such as cardiac operations.[6]

DIAGNOSTIC CRITERIA

The clinical manifestations of chronic venous disease

In order to standardize the reporting and treatment of the diverse manifestations of chronic venous disease, a comprehensive classification system (CEAP) has been proposed to allow uniform diagnosis and comparison of patient populations. The fundamentals of the CEAP classification include a description of the clinical disease class (C) based upon objective signs; the etiology (E); the anatomic (A) distribution of reflux and obstruction in the superficial, deep, and perforating veins; and the underlying pathophysiology (P), whether due to reflux or obstruction.[7] Seven clinical disease categories are recognized (Table 39.1).

Clinical classification of chronic venous disease.	
Class 0	No visible or palpable signs of venous disease
Class 1	Telangiectasias or reticular veins
Class 2	Varicose veins
Class 3	Edema
Class 4	Skin changes ascribed to venous disease (e.g. pigmentation, venous eczema, lipodermatosclerosis)
Class 5	Skin changes, as defined above, with healed ulceration
Class 6	Skin changes, as defined above, with active ulceration

Table 39.1 Clinical classification of chronic venous disease. (Adapted from Porter & Moneta.[7])

Varicose veins – diagnostic criteria.

	Telangiectasias	Reticular veins	Varicose veins
Size	0.1–1mm	1–4mm	>4mm
Color	Red to purple	Green to blue	None
Palpable	No	No	Yes

Table 39.2 Varicose veins – diagnostic criteria.

The underlying etiology can further be classified as congenital, primary, or secondary. Primary venous disorders are not associated with an identifiable mechanism of venous dysfunction. In contrast, secondary venous disorders result from an antecedent event, usually an episode of acute DVT. When developing after an episode of DVT, manifestations of pain, edema, skin changes and ulceration are commonly referred to as the post-thrombotic syndrome.

Varicose veins are the most common manifestation of primary chronic venous disease. Although various classification systems have been proposed, varicose veins are usually differentiated from reticular veins and telangiectasias (**Table 39.2**).[8] Varicose veins are usually defined as dilated, palpable tortuous veins greater than 4 mm in diameter that do not discolor the overlying skin. Their saccular, tortuous characteristics distinguish varicose veins from the prominent superficial veins that may be seen in thin, fit individuals. Reticular veins are dilated but non-palpable, blue dermal veins less than 4 mm in diameter, and are distinguished from smaller red to purple telangiectasias. The major saphenous trunks are not usually involved in patients with telangiectasias and reticular veins, but often are incompetent with varicose veins. Over 50% of patients have bilateral varicosities and there is not a particular predilection for either leg.[9,10]

The most common reasons for presentation include symptoms attributable to varicose veins (38%), cosmetic considerations (26%), and concern regarding complications.[11] Uncomplicated varicose veins have been associated with symptoms including aching, heaviness, cramps, tingling, and pruritis, the prevalence of which increase with age despite only a very limited association with the presence of trunk varicosities.[12–14] No single symptom is pathognomonic for varicose veins, and similar symptoms have been noted in 33% of men and 50% of women without varicose veins.[9] Symptoms often increase during the course of the day and with prolonged standing. Between 5% and 7% of patients will present with complications of their varicose veins, including superficial thrombophlebitis, bleeding, and, rarely, skin changes and ulceration.[3,11]

The more severe manifestations of chronic venous disease include edema, skin changes, and ulceration. Early skin changes include hyperpigmentation, corona phlebectatica, and dilated subcutaneous venules in a gaiter distribution extending from just below the malleoli to the posterior prominence of the calf muscle. Hyperpigmentation results from the accumulation of hemosiderin granules within dermal macrophages after the breakdown of extravasated red blood cells.[15] The subcutaneous tissue later becomes fibrotic and may be associated with cutaneous weeping, scaling, and erythema characteristic of venous eczema. Lipodermatosclerosis refers to the subcutaneous fibrosis and chronic inflammation that result from sustained venous hypertension. Associated physical findings may include a limited range of ankle motion and peripheral neuropathy.

Ulceration is the most advanced stage of chronic venous disease. The differential diagnosis for lower extremity ulcers includes chronic venous disease, arterial disease, collagen vascular diseases, metabolic disorders, and vasculitis. Approximately three-quarters of leg ulcers have an underlying venous cause.[16] Among venous ulcers, approximately three-quarters involve the medial aspect of the gaiter area. However, venous ulcers may also occur laterally and higher in the calf. Over 95% of medial gaiter ulcers are associated with venous disease, while fewer than 50% of calf ulcers have an underlying venous etiology.[17] Isolated lateral ulcers have been particularly associated with lesser saphenous incompetence.[18] Although features such as ulcer location and associated lipodermatosclerosis may suggest venous disease, confirmation of a venous etiology requires documentation of venous reflux.

Skin changes and ulceration may be associated with either primary or secondary venous disease, the relative frequency of which depends on the referral population. In some specialty centers, as many as 10% of patients with varicose veins have been reported to have ulcers.[19] Approximately 60% of patients with venous ulceration have no previous history of DVT.[20,21] However, DVT is frequently occult and the poor correlation between clinical history and objective evidence of DVT is well recognized.[22] Hanrahan et al. identified a history of DVT or superficial phlebitis in 33% of patients with an ulcer, with duplex evidence of such an event in 44%.[23] In contrast, Welkie et al. found that duplex imaging of patients with active or healed ulcers increased the number of patients with post-thrombotic disease from only 38% to 40%.[21]

Venous claudication warrants special consideration. As its manifestations are primarily due to proximal venous obstruction rather than valvular incompetence, it is not ordinarily considered in the spectrum of chronic venous disease. Patients with symptoms of venous claudication complain of lower extremity tightness and bursting pain on vigorous exercise.[24] In contrast to arterial claudication, pain is often less severe and affects the entire leg rather than specific muscle groups; its onset is more gradual and occurs with a higher intensity of activity; and it may require 15 to 20 minutes of rest, frequently with leg elevation, for relief. Although muscle blood flow during exercise is reduced in these patients, pain is more likely to be related to elevated intramuscular pressures than to ischemia.[25] Associated findings may include swelling of the thigh and calf, cyanosis, and prominence of the superficial veins. Patients may also have other manifestations of chronic venous disease, including varicose veins and ulceration.[25] Proposed criteria for the diagnosis of venous claudication include 1) intermittent claudication, 2) iliac vein obstruction, 3) venous hypertension at rest, and 4) increased venous pressure with exercise.[25] Venous obstruction is virtually always due to secondary causes, usually persistent stenoses or occlusions after an episode of DVT. Catheter directed thrombolysis will uncover such lesions in up to one-third of legs with iliofemoral DVT.[26] These lesions more commonly occur on the left side[24,25] and are frequently related to the May–Thurner syndrome, or compression of the left iliac vein by the overlying right common iliac artery.[27]

Venous anatomy of the leg

The nomenclature of the leg veins has been recently updated,[28] clarifying many definitions and eliminating most eponyms. The most current nomenclature is used in the following discussion. The venous system of the leg includes the deep veins, which lie beneath the muscular fascia and drain the lower extremity muscles; the superficial veins, which are above the deep fascia and drain the cutaneous microcirculation; and the perforating veins, which penetrate the muscular fascia and connect the superficial and deep veins. Communicating veins connect veins within the same system.[28] The superficial, deep, and most perforating veins contain bicuspid valves consisting of folds of endothelium supported by a thin layer of connective tissue (**Fig. 39.1**).

The superficial veins, which include the great (greater) and small (lesser) saphenous veins, drain the skin and subcutaneous tissue (**Fig. 39.2**). The great saphenous vein is duplicated in the thigh in 8%, and in the calf in 25% of individuals. There are usually two main saphenous tributaries in the calf, an anterior branch and the posterior arch (Leonardo's) vein, which begins behind the medial malleolus and joins the great saphenous vein just below the knee. A valve is present at the saphenofemoral junction in 94% to 100% of individuals and 81% have at least one valve in the external iliac–common femoral segment above the junction.[29] The great saphenous vein usually has at least six valves, while the small saphenous vein has seven to 10 closely spaced valves.[30] Varicose great saphenous veins do have slightly fewer valves (mean 6.0 ± 1.7) than normal veins (7.3 ± 2.3),[31] although the relevance of this observation is unclear.

Perforating veins may empty directly into the axial deep veins (direct perforators) or into the venous sinuses of the calf (indirect perforators). Although perforating veins are numerous and variable, four groups are of clinical significance – those of the foot, the medial and lateral calf, and the thigh. The foot perforators are unique in ordinarily directing flow toward the superficial veins.[30,32] The major perforators of the medial calf and thigh have one to three valves that direct flow from the superficial to the deep veins.[30] The medial calf perforators include the paratibial perforators joining the main great saphenous vein or its branches and the posterior tibial perforators that originate in the posterior arch vein. The perforators of the femoral canal connect the great saphenous vein with the distal superficial femoral or proximal popliteal vein.

The deep veins of the leg follow the course of the associated arteries, with the number of valves increasing from proximal to distal. The muscular venous sinuses are the principal collecting system of the calf muscle pump. Although also present in the gastrocnemius muscles, the soleal sinuses are of greatest numerical importance. There are an average of five deep venous valves between the inguinal ligament and popliteal fossa, although the number varies from two to nine.[33] Their arrangement is variable but in general the inferior vena cava and common iliac veins have no valves; the external iliac and common femoral vein above the saphenofemoral junction have one valve at most; the (superficial) femoral vein above the adductor canal has three or more valves; the distal superficial femoral and popliteal veins have one or two valves; and the tibial/peroneal veins have numerous valves spaced at approximately 2cm intervals.[30,33] Although the muscle sinusoids are valveless, they frequently empty into profusely valved, arborizing, draining veins.[33]

The hemodynamics of chronic venous disease

The accumulation of blood in the lower extremity veins while upright is limited by the physical properties of the venous wall, the function of the venous valves, and the action of the calf muscle pump. The valves function to divide the hydrostatic column of blood into segments and to ensure antegrade venous flow. Approximately 90% of the venous return in the legs is via the deep veins, through the action of the foot, calf, and thigh muscle pumps.[34] The action of these valved pumps is critically dependent on the deep fascia of the leg, which constrains the muscles during contraction and allows high pressures to be generated within the muscular compartments. Among the three pumps, the calf pump has the largest capacitance, generates the highest pressures, and is of greatest importance.[32,35] The ejection fraction of the calf muscle pump is approximately 65%, in comparison to only 15% for the thigh pump. With contraction of the calf, pressure in the posterior compartment rises to as high as 250 mmHg,[35] the veins are emptied of blood, and resting venous pressure is lowered as the valves prevent retrograde flow (**Figs 39.3A&B**). Pressure in the posterior tibial vein accordingly decreases from 80–100mmHg to less than 30mmHg (**Fig. 39.4**). A reduction in deep venous pressure during the post-contraction relaxation phase favors flow from the superficial to the deep system through the perforating veins. In the presence of competent venous valves, capillary inflow causes a slow rise in deep venous pressure during this phase of activity.

Reflux, or pathologic retrograde flow, occurs when the valves are absent or rendered incompetent either by degenerative processes (primary venous disease) or an episode of DVT (secondary venous disease). Under these circumstances, retrograde flow during calf muscle relaxation prevents the usual reduction in pressure, and rapid venous refilling occurs from the retrograde flow of blood, as well as slow capillary inflow (**Fig. 39.3C**). High venous pressure may also be transmitted from the deep to the superficial veins through incompetent perforators. The function of the calf muscle pump may also be impaired in patients with chronic venous disease, an observation that is at least partly related to a reduced range of motion at the ankle.[36]

The clinical manifestations of chronic venous insufficiency are primarily due to ambulatory venous hypertension or failure to

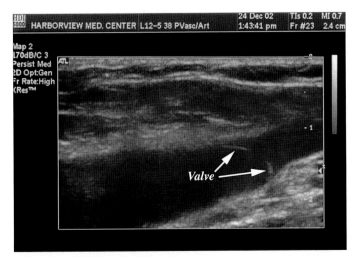

Figure 39.1 B-mode ultrasound of the great saphenous vein showing both cusps of a normal bicuspid valve.

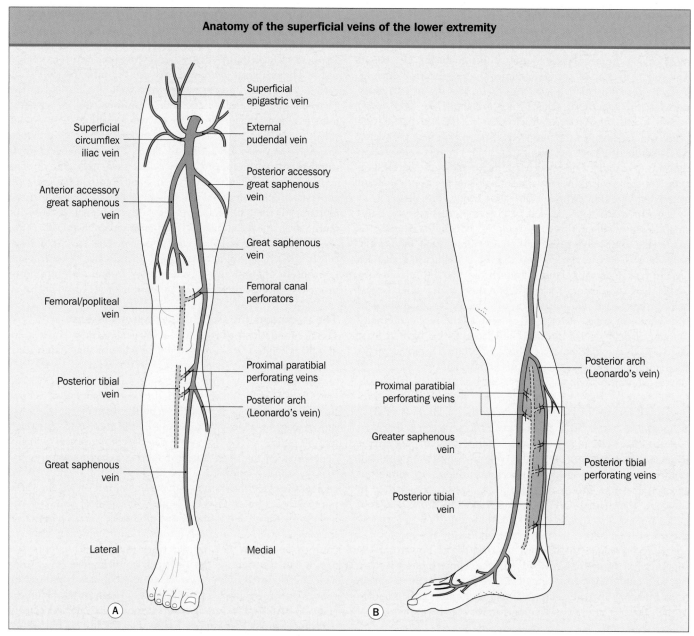

Anatomy of the superficial veins of the lower extremity

Superficial epigastric vein

Superficial circumflex iliac vein

External pudendal vein

Anterior accessory great saphenous vein

Posterior accessory great saphenous vein

Great saphenous vein

Femoral canal perforators

Femoral/popliteal vein

Proximal paratibial perforating veins

Posterior tibial vein

Posterior arch (Leonardo's vein)

Great saphenous vein

Lateral

Medial

Posterior arch (Leonardo's vein)

Proximal paratibial perforating veins

Greater saphenous vein

Posterior tibial perforating veins

Posterior tibial vein

(A)   (B)

Figure 39.2 Anatomy of the superficial veins of the lower extremity. (A) Anterior view showing the clinically important femoral canal perforators in the mid-thigh and paratibial perforators in the calf. (B) Lateral view showing the posterior tibial and paratibial perforators connecting the posterior arch and greater saphenous veins, respectively, with the posterior tibial vein.

lower venous pressure adequately with exercise. Ambulatory venous pressure (AVP) is determined using a 21-gauge needle placed in a dorsal foot vein to measure the response to ten tiptoe movements, usually at a rate of one per second. The AVP is measured as the lowest pressure achieved at the end of exercise (**Fig. 39.5**). Hemodynamically significant reflux in either the superficial or deep venous systems is associated with elevated ambulatory venous pressures, as well as short refilling times after exercise ceases. The severity of chronic venous disease is closely related to the magnitude of venous hypertension. Ulceration usually does not occur at ambulatory venous pressures of less than 30mmHg, while the incidence is 100% at pressures greater than 90mmHg.[37]

The determinants of ambulatory venous pressure are complex and include venous reflux, as well as obstruction, and calf muscle pump dysfunction.[38,39] For any degree of reflux, the ambulatory venous pressure is worsened by associated venous obstruction. Similarly, abnormal calf muscle pump function is associated with a higher incidence of ulceration and non-invasive indices of venous pressure.[36] Although the relationship with disease severity has not been consistent,[40–42] the calf muscle pump ejection fraction is lowest in legs with active ulceration (35%), followed by legs with healed ulcers (49%), and those without ulceration but with duplex evidence of reflux (53%).[43] This observation may be related to the progressive decrease in range of ankle motion with increasing severity of disease.[36] Others have

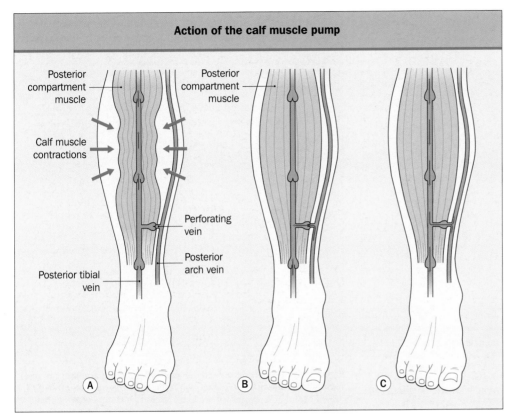

Figure 39.3 **Action of the calf muscle pump.** (A) With contraction of the calf muscle (systole), the deep veins are emptied of blood while competent distal and perforating vein valves prevent retrograde flow into the foot and the superficial system. (B) During the relaxation phase (diastole), competent proximal valves prevent retrograde flow while blood flows from the superficial to the low-pressure deep system through the perforating veins. (C) In the presence of deep venous reflux, incompetent proximal valves allow rapid venous refilling during the relaxation phase. High deep venous pressures are transmitted from the deep to superficial system through incompetent perforating veins.

Action of the calf muscle pump

Posterior compartment muscle

Posterior compartment muscle

Calf muscle contractions

Perforating vein

Posterior arch vein

Posterior tibial vein

A   B   C

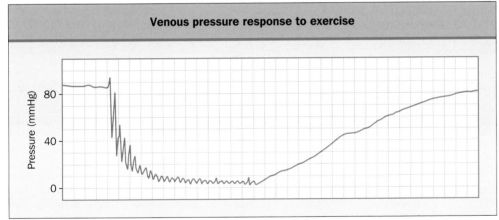

Venous pressure response to exercise

Figure 39.4 **Venous pressure response to exercise.** During treadmill walking in a patient without venous disease, the action of the calf muscle pump with each step causes a progressive reduction in venous pressure measured in a dorsal foot vein. After walking stops, arterial inflow causes a slow return to baseline (the venous refilling time).

suggested that changes in calf muscle pump function occur early in the development of chronic venous disease and do not worsen with the development of skin changes and ulceration.[21]

As there is no associated obstruction, reflux is the primary hemodynamic derangement in primary venous disease, and the severity varies with the extent and distribution of reflux. Up to 82% of legs with varicose veins show non-invasive evidence of reflux.[44,45] However, neither isolated superficial nor deep venous reflux is significantly associated with symptoms.[46] While reflux in asymptomatic and mildly symptomatic patients is usually isolated and segmental,[40] that in patients with skin changes and ulceration is usually multisegmental and frequently involves the deep, superficial, and perforating veins. Approximately two-

thirds of patients with ulcers have multisystem disease.[23] A combination of superficial and deep venous reflux, with or without documented perforator incompetence, is the most common pattern in these patients (**Table 39.3**). Reflux in the distal deep venous segments, particularly the popliteal and posterior tibial veins, appears to be particularly important in the pathogenesis of venous ulceration. Although the clinical importance remains controversial, perforator incompetence does allow transmission of elevated venous pressure from the deep to the superficial system.

The hemodynamic abnormalities associated with secondary venous disease are more complex, frequently involving both valvular reflux and venous obstruction. Post-thrombotic legs with

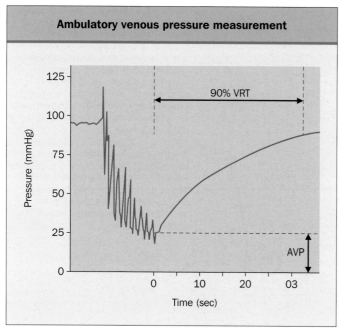

Figure 39.5 Ambulatory venous pressure measurement. In the normal leg, venous pressure as measured in a dorsal foot vein progressively declines with each plantar flexion maneuver. Ambulatory venous pressure (AVP) represents the pressure at the end of ten tiptoe maneuvers and is less than 30mmHg in normal legs. The time required for return to baseline is measured as the 90% venous refilling time (VRT). Hemodynamically significant reflux causes an elevated ambulatory venous pressure and rapid 90% VRT.

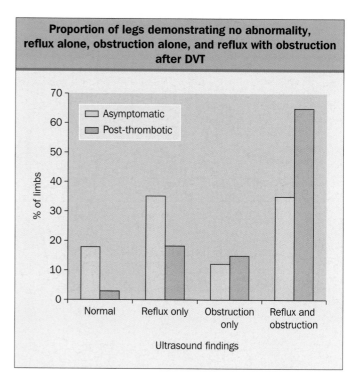

Figure 39.6 Proportion of legs demonstrating no abnormality (normal), reflux alone, obstruction alone, and reflux with obstruction after DVT. Yellow bars show asymptomatic legs; red bars indicate legs with post-thrombotic symptoms. (Adapted with permission from Johnson et al.[47])

Distribution of reflux in patients with venous ulcers.				
	Labropoulos et al.[20] n = 112	Barwell et al.[142] n = 593	Darke et al.[22]* n = 232	Hanrahan et al.[23] n = 95
Superficial (S)	23%	39%		16.8%
Perforator (P)	3%		4%	8.4%
Deep (D)	6%	8%		2.1%
S + P	21%		39%	19.0%
S + D	12%	43%		11.6%
P + D	4%			4.2%
S + P + D	28%		35%	31.6%
No reflux	4%	10%		6.3%
Occlusion/PTS		2%	22%	

*Deep venous reflux associated with any other pattern included in S + P + D; superficial incompetence, with or without perforator incompetence, included in S + P.

Table 39.3 Distribution of reflux in patients with venous ulcers. PTS, post-thrombotic syndrome.

edema, hyperpigmentation, or ulceration are more likely to have a combination of reflux and residual obstruction than either abnormality alone (**Fig. 39.6**).[47] However, despite the contribution of venous obstruction, valvular incompetence appears to be clinically more important. Post-thrombotic symptoms correlate more closely with a reduction in venous refilling time than with residual abnormalities of venous outflow.[48]

DIAGNOSTIC TESTS FOR CHRONIC VENOUS DISEASE

Tests for venous reflux

Although most patients with asymptomatic varicose veins require little more than reassurance, the appropriate management of symptomatic varicosities requires qualitative identification and localization of reflux within the superficial venous system. The surgical management of varicose veins has historically relied on a number of clinical tests for reflux. Although others have been described, the Trendelenburg test is perhaps the best recognized of these tests.[49] The lower extremity veins are drained by elevating the limb to 45 degrees, applying a tourniquet below the saphenofemoral junction, and asking the patient to stand. Rapid filling of the distal veins with the tourniquet in place suggests perforator reflux, while rapid filling after the tourniquet is released reflects saphenofemoral incompetence. Although the Trendelenburg test is 91% sensitive for the identification of superficial and perforator reflux, it has a specificity of only 15%.[49] Clinical evaluation alone will detect only 72% and 64% of incompetent saphenofemoral and saphenopopliteal junctions, respectively.[50]

Hand-held Doppler evaluation of the great and small saphenous veins has often been used as an adjuvant to the clinical tests. Doppler examination is performed in the standing position, insonating the saphenofemoral and saphenopopliteal junctions as the release of distal calf compression is used to provoke reflux.[50] Reflux that is abolished by compression of the saphenous vein above the knee and is not present in the (superficial) femoral vein is localized to the great saphenous vein. Reflux is similarly localized to the saphenopopliteal junction if it is abolished by distal compression of the lesser saphenous vein. In comparison to duplex ultrasonography, Doppler has been reported to have a sensitivity and specificity of 97% and 73%, respectively, for the identification of saphenofemoral junction reflux.[49] However, clinical examination with and without Doppler have been noted to lead to selection of inappropriate varicose vein procedures in 20% and 13% of legs, respectively.[51]

Despite the importance of clinical examination, the tourniquet tests and hand-held Doppler examination have largely been supplemented or replaced by other diagnostic tests for reflux. More detailed evaluation of the venous system may be important in establishing an etiology for non-specific complaints such as pain, swelling, or ulceration, selecting appropriate patients for ablative or reconstructive procedures, assessing hemodynamic improvement after such procedures, and establishing the natural history of chronic venous disease. The evaluation of advanced chronic venous insufficiency is usually more complicated than for simple varicose veins, as both reflux and obstruction may involve the deep, superficial, and perforating veins. The ideal diagnostic test for chronic venous disease should be capable of distinguishing primary from post-thrombotic disease, identify both venous obstruction and valvular incompetence, localize the abnormality to precise segments of the superficial and deep venous systems, and distinguish between different clinical degrees of disease. Therefore, the test should provide a quantitative measure of reflux that corresponds to the clinical stage of disease.

Of the tests available, descending venography and ambulatory venous pressure have historically been the gold standards for the anatomic localization and hemodynamic quantification of reflux. Although descending phlebography may still have a role in situations such as venous reconstruction, it does have several limitations. It is invasive, the assessment of distal valves may be impossible if proximal valves are competent, and false-positive tests can result from hyperbaric contrast streaming past normal valves. The test also provides limited assessment of the great and small saphenous veins, and the phlebographic grade of reflux correlates only loosely with the severity of disease. In contrast, ambulatory venous pressure measurements are physiologic and, to a certain extent, do correlate with the incidence of ulceration. Unfortunately, this technique also has limitations. Most notably, the test measures only global hemodynamics. It therefore requires reflux at multiple sites, may be insensitive to isolated segmental reflux, and cannot precisely localize reflux to specific venous segments. Ambulatory venous pressure is also influenced by venous obstruction, occasionally making the test difficult to interpret.

Furthermore, since these methods are invasive, they are not easily repeatable and are not appropriate screening tests for many patients with chronic venous disease. This has led to several non-invasive alternatives being developed, including photoplethys-mography (PPG), air plethysmography (APG), and duplex ultra-sonography. Global hemodynamic tests, including PPG and APG, use measurements of venous volume to reflect reflux. Measure-ment of venous refilling time with PPG was the first to be widely available and remains the simplest non-invasive test. PPG is based on transmission of infrared light into the skin and the measure-ment of backscattered light by an adjacent photoreceptor. The technique generates a recording in which there is a rapid fall from the baseline with active flexion of the ankle, followed by a gradual return with muscular relaxation. The venous refilling time (VRT) is the time required for return to baseline, and a VRT of ≤ 20 seconds has often been considered abnormal.

PPG is simple and inexpensive, although it provides little quantitative information. A normal VRT excludes significant valvular incompetence in the superficial, distal deep, and calf perforating veins. However, the specificity of an abnormal result has often been limited, and correlation of the VRT with the quantity of reflux and severity of disease has been poor. The test is probably most useful as a qualitative screening test.

Air plethysmography measures calf volume changes in response to gravity and exercise as a reflection of reflux (**Fig. 39.7**). The calf is placed in a PVC sleeve, 35cm in length, which is then inflated, connected to a pressure transducer, and calibrated with 100mL of air. After obtaining a baseline recording with the patient supine and leg elevated to 45 degrees, the patient assumes an upright position. The venous volume is recorded as the leg fills. The patient is then instructed to plantar flex on both feet to record the ejected volume, followed by 10 tiptoe movements, after which the residual volume is recorded. From this infor-mation, it is possible to calculate the venous filling index (VFI) as the ratio of the 90% filling volume and the 90% venous filling time, the ejection fraction (EF) as the ratio of the ejected volume to venous volume, and the residual volume fraction (RVF) as the ratio of residual volume to venous volume. The VFI is an index of global venous reflux, while the EF and RVF reflect calf muscle pump function and ambulatory venous pressure, respectively. The incidence of ulceration increases from 0% with a VFI of <5mL/s to 58% for a VFI >10mL/s.[52] However, as with other global tests of hemodynamics, APG cannot precisely localize segmental reflux, and the RVF correlates only loosely with the severity of disease.

Venous duplex ultrasonography has become the most widely used test in the diagnosis and management of chronic venous disease. In combining B mode imaging with pulsed Doppler, duplex is capable of accurately localizing both venous obstruc-tion and valvular reflux to specific venous segments. Duplex examination for reflux should be performed in the standing

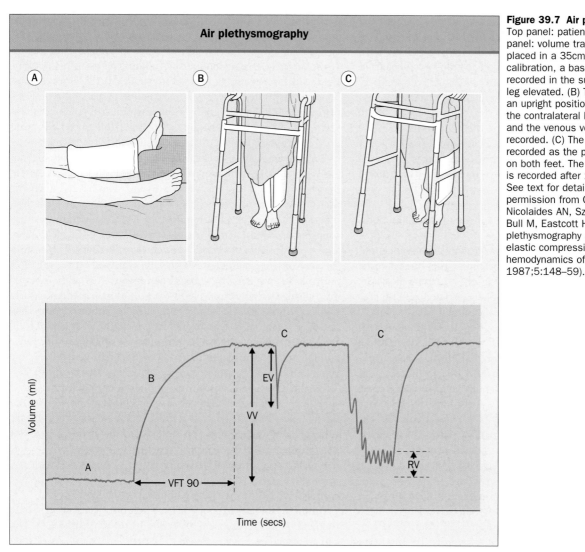

Air plethysmography

(A)   (B)   (C)

Figure 39.7 Air plethysmography.
Top panel: patient maneuvers. Bottom panel: volume tracing. (A) The calf is placed in a 35cm PVC sleeve and after calibration, a baseline tracing is recorded in the supine position with the leg elevated. (B) The patient assumes an upright position, bearing weight on the contralateral limb as the leg fills and the venous volume (VV) is recorded. (C) The ejected volume (EV) is recorded as the patient plantar flexes on both feet. The residual volume (RV) is recorded after 10 tiptoe maneuvers. See text for details. (Adapted with permission from Christopoulos DG, Nicolaides AN, Szendro G, Irvine AT, Bull M, Eastcott HGG. Air plethysmography and the effect of elastic compression on venous hemodynamics of the leg. J Vasc Surg 1987;5:148–59).

position. In addition to being physiologic, the standing position limits the occurrence of 'physiologic reflux', in which valves refluxing in the supine position are competent when upright. The duplex criteria for reflux are based upon the occurrence of reverse flow in response to a provocative maneuver. Valsalva's maneuver, proximal venous compression, and release of distal compression have been used to elicit reflux. The compression maneuvers may further be performed either manually or with standardized pneumatic cuffs. Although acceptable results can be achieved with release of manual distal compression, standardized testing using pneumatic distal cuff deflation is the most accurate and reproducible method of eliciting reflux (**Fig. 39.8**).[53] In evaluating reflux using this technique, the patient stands supported by a frame, with the leg slightly flexed and weight borne by the contralateral extremity. Pneumatic cuffs are inflated distal to the segment of interest, which is then imaged in a longitudinal plane. Doppler signals are recorded as the cuff is inflated and rapidly deflated, simulating muscular contraction and relaxation. Ninety-five percent of normal valves will close within 0.5 seconds of cuff deflation (**Fig. 39.9**).[54] Although this technique is accurate in localizing reflux to specific venous segments, attempts to incorporate this information into

a quantitative measure of reflux within a leg have met with limited success.

As with descending venography and ambulatory venous pressure measurements, most of the non-invasive tests for chronic venous disease display the fundamental dichotomy of providing either anatomic or hemodynamic information. There may thus be no ideal test for valvular incompetence and the best test may depend on the clinical indications for the study. Just as physiologic tests such as the ankle brachial index and anatomic tests such as arteriography complement one another in lower extremity arterial assessment, it may be necessary to combine the ability of duplex imaging to localize both anatomic obstruction and reflux with measurements of hemodynamic severity determined by tests such as APG. A combination of these studies may obviate the need for invasive tests in all but those requiring precise visualization of valvular anatomy in anticipation of venous reconstruction. In the simple evaluation of a patient with non-specific symptoms, any of the non-invasive tests may be sufficient for the documentation of reflux. However, in some situations, such as planning for an operative procedure, more precise anatomic localization is needed and duplex ultrasonography is the ideal diagnostic test. In contrast, in evaluating the results

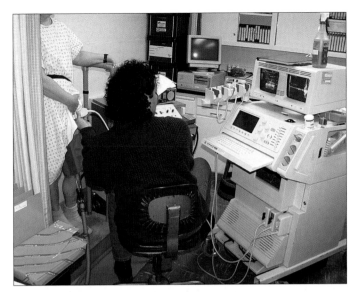

Figure 39.8 Duplex ultrasound evaluation of reflux using the standing cuff deflation technique. The patient stands, supported by a frame, with their weight borne on the contralateral leg. Pneumatic cuffs are sequentially applied to the thigh, calf, and foot with inflation pressure varied according to the hydrostatic pressure at that level. Doppler signals in the vein under investigation are recorded ≤5cm proximal to the cuff as it is deflated rapidly.

of an operative procedure, more quantitative hemodynamic information is necessary, and APG may be best.

Tests for venous obstruction

Both duplex ultrasonography and ascending venography have proved accurate in localizing infrainguinal venous obstruction. However, detailed visualization of the iliac segments may be difficult and these anatomic studies provide little information regarding the significance of an obstruction in the patient with atypical symptoms or widespread valvular incompetence. A variety of direct and indirect tests have been proposed to assess the significance of underlying venous obstruction. Most indirect

tests rely on plethysmographic techniques (strain gauge, PPG, impedance plethysmography, and APG) which, although useful in identifying acute proximal obstruction, may not adequately define the significance of chronic lesions. In comparison to legs with acute venous obstruction, legs with chronic obstruction have both a higher outflow and venous capacity or 'dead space'.[55]

Direct tests for deep venous obstruction include a number of pressure measurements. Among these, the resting arm–foot pressure differential and foot pressures after reactive hyperemia (normal <4mmHg and <6mmHg in fully compensated obstruction) are the most widely employed.[56] In combination, the arm–foot/reactive hyperemia tests have been reported to have a sensitivity and specificity of 91% and 91%, respectively.[57] Measurement of femoral vein pressures may also be useful in defining the importance of an iliac obstruction.[58] Although resting femoral pressures show considerable overlap, the femoral pressure difference (diseased versus healthy limb) after exercise provides reasonable separation between those with and without significant iliac obstruction.

Despite the contribution of these tests to the understanding of venous physiology, most have limitations in identifying the patient with clinically significant venous obstruction. Plethysmographic tests are limited by an inconsistent relationship between venous volume, outflow, and disease severity, while direct pressure measurements have not uniformly correlated with clinical symptoms. Although most demonstrate adequate specificity, the sensitivity of all tests is limited. None of the current diagnostic tests is able to identify accurately those patients with hemodynamically significant obstruction who will clearly benefit from intervention.

THE PATHOPHYSIOLOGY OF CHRONIC VENOUS DISEASE

Varicose veins

Despite improvements in understanding the epidemiology and hemodynamic derangements associated with varicose veins and chronic venous insufficiency, the underlying etiology remains

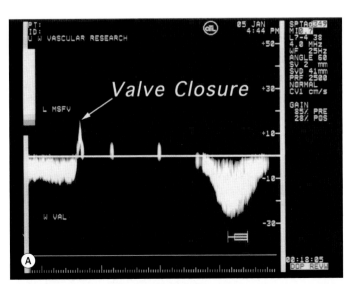

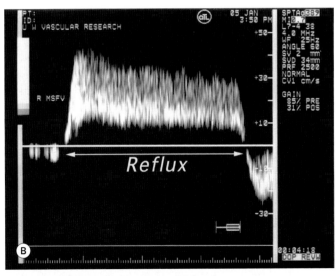

Figure 39.9 Duplex ultrasound detection of reflux in the mid-superficial femoral vein. In (A), there is no reflux and valve closure appears as a clearly demarcated period of retrograde flow (above the baseline) of less than 0.5s. In the presence of valvular incompetence, as illustrated in (B), the duration of reverse flow is greater than 0.5s.

uncertain. Treatment is accordingly based more on relief of symptoms and an attempt to correct the altered hemodynamics than on an understanding of the cause. Although the detrimental effects of prolonged standing were recognized by Hippocrates (460–377 B.C.), humoral theories relating varicose veins to the ill effects of 'gross' or 'melancholy' blood were not widely replaced by scientifically based pathophysiologic theories until the 18th and 19th centuries.[59] Early modern theories presumed that varicose veins arose from the effects of valvular incompetence and venous hypertension. Varicose veins historically were thought to arise in a descending fashion from valvular incompetence at the saphenofemoral or saphenopopliteal junction, the saphenofemoral being involved approximately four times more frequently than the saphenopopliteal junction.[50,60] Congenital absence or incompetence of ileofemoral valves was presumed to cause increased hydrostatic pressure and venous dilatation at the level of the saphenofemoral junction, with sequential failure of more distal valves.[33] Variants of this theory postulated that varicosities similarly arose from the transmission of venous pressure through incompetent perforating veins.

Unfortunately, there is little evidence of a constitutive valvular abnormality in primary venous disease and these theories are not supported by more recent observations. Descending theories of valvular incompetence cannot explain why truncal varicosities are often found below competent valves, why normal valves are often seen between those exhibiting varices, or why dilatation often precedes valvular incompetence.[31,61] Rather than being initiated at the saphenofemoral junction, detailed studies of surgical specimens suggest that varices can occur anywhere along the course of the great saphenous vein. These observations are supported by ultrasound studies similarly showing primary valvular incompetence to be a multicentric disease that develops simultaneously in discontinuous venous segments. Although the superficial, deep, and perforating veins may be involved, the below-knee great saphenous vein is the most common site of involvement. There is evidence of reflux in the below-knee great saphenous segment in 68% of patients, followed by the above-knee segment in 55%, and the saphenofemoral junction in 32%.[62] It therefore appears that, rather than developing in a descending fashion, primary venous disease is likely to begin as a local process anywhere in the lower extremity venous system.

It further appears that varicose changes precede the development of overt valvular incompetence[31,63,64] and that valvular dysfunction is a secondary phenomenon. Recent theories have focused on intrinsic structural and biochemical abnormalities of the vein wall. Such 'weak wall' theories hypothesize that varicose veins develop because of underlying connective tissue defects and altered venous tone.[29,65,66] While the histologic features may be diverse and vary in different regions of the vein, varicose veins demonstrate irregular thickening of the intima, fibrosis between the intima and adventitia, atrophy and disruption of elastic fibers, thickening of individual collagen fibers, and disorganization of the muscular layers.[34,67–71] These abnormalities are heterogeneously distributed through the great saphenous vein and its tributaries,[68] some areas appearing hypertrophic while others appear atrophic or normal. Although luminal diameter is increased, overall wall thickness is not changed.[72] That is, although localized areas of thinning may be present, dilatation is not associated with generalized atrophy of the venous wall. The saccular dilatations constituting the varices are consistently located just to the distal (upstream) side of valve cusps.[31] The configuration of the valve sinus itself is preserved in most varicose segments.

The histologic changes suggest that varicose veins have reduced contractility and compliance. Saphenous smooth muscle content, as well as total protein content, is reduced in patients with varicose veins, and effective contraction may be further compromised by fragmentation of the muscle layers.[68,72] The smooth muscle cells are also transformed from a contractile to a secretory phenotype[73] and there are corresponding changes in the extracellular matrix of both involved and uninvolved venous segments. Varicose saphenous veins show an increased collagen and reduced elastin content, with an increased collagen to elastin ratio.[63] Correspondingly, decreased venous elasticity has been demonstrated both in legs with overt varices and in those without varices but at high risk for their development.[74] Similar connective tissue defects have also been identified in the forearm veins of patients with varicosities.[65] These findings suggest that abnormalities in the vein wall architecture precede the development of both overt varicosities and valvular incompetence. Reflux is presumed to occur when the weakened vein wall dilates, causing stretching of the commissure between the valve cusps and separation of the valve leaflets.[61] Perhaps not surprisingly, these histologic alterations have been correlated with the degree of hemodynamic disturbance present on APG.[70]

It remains unclear whether the functional, biochemical, and structural changes associated with varicose veins are primary or result from other pathologic processes. Proposed mechanisms have included hypoxia-mediated endothelial changes, cell cycle dysfunction with inhibition of programmed cell death, changes in enzyme activity, and underlying defects in venous tone. Some have suggested that hypoxia-induced endothelial activation is responsible for the change in smooth muscle phenotype, leading to an increased synthesis of extracellular matrix.[73] Apoptosis, or programmed cell death, also appears to be downregulated in varicose veins, as evidenced by reduced expression of apoptosis-related proteins.[71] Increased numbers of dysfunctional cells could theoretically account for some of the observed histologic changes. A number of changes in enzyme patterns, consistent with a decline in energy metabolism and increased lysosomal activity, have also been reported.[75]

Finally, defects in venous tone associated with a loss of vascular reactivity have been postulated to have a primary role in the origin of varicose veins.[68,76] Organ chamber experiments have demonstrated reduced contractility as well as endothelium-dependent relaxation in varicose segments. In comparison to control veins, contraction in response to endothelin-1, a potent vasoconstrictor and smooth muscle mitogen, is reduced in both diseased tributaries as well as grossly uninvolved saphenous veins of patients with varicosities. This decrease in contractility may be due to both structural changes, resulting from a loss of contractile proteins, and to downregulation of the number of endothelin B receptors.[76] Patients with varicose veins also demonstrate imbalances in the humoral mediators of vasoconstriction and venodilatation. Plasma levels of endothelin-1 are increased in those with varicose veins and rise disproportionately in response to venous stasis.[77] At least some evidence suggests that such increases are mediated at the transcriptional level within the endothelial cell.[76] Plasma levels of nitric oxide, a potent mediator of vascular relaxation, have variably been found to be either reduced[78] or increased[79] in these patients.

CHRONIC VENOUS INSUFFICIENCY

Although there is little controversy that venous hypertension underlies the manifestations of chronic venous insufficiency, the pathophysiologic relationship between venous hypertension and ulceration remains unclear. The histologic findings associated with venous hypertension include atrophy and scarring of the dermis with loss of papillary structures at the dermal-epidermal junction.[80] There is associated dilatation and convolution of the dermal capillaries, fibrosis of the vein wall and dermis, and a thick amorphous perivascular cuff composed of fibrin, fibronectin, laminin, tenascin, and collagen.[80–84] It was initially presumed that these perivascular cuffs arose from the effects of increased capillary filtration, changes in venous pressure increasing filtration five to ten times more than equivalent changes in arterial pressure.[85] However, more recent data suggest that, although vascular extravasation may be important, the perivascular cuffs are assembled actively by the surrounding connective tissue. These cuffs appear to resolve with compression therapy and it has been postulated that they represent a protective measure against venous hypertension.[84] These histologic changes are associated with a dermal perivascular infiltrate consisting predominantly of lymphocytes, macrophages, and mast cells.[86–88] Scarring of the reticular dermis also leads to a lymphatic microangiopathy that is likely to impair interstitial fluid exchange.[83]

Unfortunately, investigation of the mechanisms underlying these changes has been limited by the lack of a satisfactory animal model. Early theories suggested venous stasis with slow capillary blood flow and arteriovenous shunting as causes of local cutaneous tissue hypoxia, while later theories focused on the role of venous hypertension in increasing capillary permeability. Despite increased arterial inflow, reduced oxygen extraction, and elevated lower extremity venous oxygen content in patients with chronic venous insufficiency,[74,89] there is little evidence to support arteriovenous fistulae as an important pathophysiologic mechanism.[32] Browse and Burnand focused on the role of the perivascular cuff and suggested that venous hypertension leads to the transudation of extracellular fluid and the extravasation of macromolecules such as fibrinogen.[85,90] As legs with lipodermatosclerosis have deficient fibrinolytic activity, any extravascular fibrinogen converted to fibrin is likely to accumulate. The fibrin cuff was postulated to act as a diffusion barrier leading to local tissue hypoxia and impaired cutaneous nutrition. Although extravascular fibrin may be important in the pathophysiology of chronic venous insufficiency, perhaps being chemotactic for fibroblasts and macrophages, downregulating collagen synthesis, or representing a marker for endothelial injury, most data now suggest that it does not act as a diffusion barrier.[91]

Mechanisms concentrating on skin hypoxia alone are too simplistic, and inflammatory processes are emerging as the most important factors in the pathogenesis of chronic venous insufficiency (**Fig. 39.10**). An underlying inflammatory etiology was first suggested by the observation that the ratio of white cells to red cells decreases in the dependent lower extremities, as well as the upper extremities, of patients with chronic venous insufficiency.[82,92,93] This is associated with a dermal leukocyte infiltrate that progressively increases as venous disease becomes more advanced. Leukocytes thus appear to be sequestered in the dependent lower extremities. This phenomenon appears

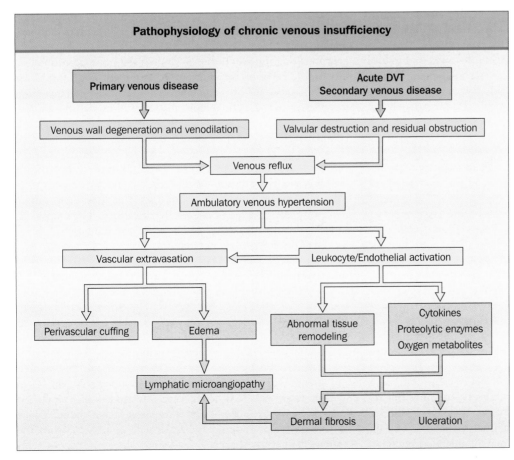

Figure 39.10 Pathophysiology of chronic venous insufficiency. Although both primary and secondary venous disease may lead to advanced chronic venous insufficiency, ambulatory venous hypertension leading to a chronic inflammatory state underlies most of the clinical sequelae.

to occur early in the course of chronic venous disease and has been observed both in limbs with varicose veins and with lipodermatosclerosis.[94-96] However, such sequestration resolves promptly on returning to the supine position in limbs with varicose veins but not in those with lipodermatosclerosis.[95]

These observations led to the 'white cell trapping' hypothesis of chronic venous insufficiency.[93] Venous hypertension is postulated to reduce flow in the post-capillary venules, leading to white blood cell margination and reversible leukocyte adhesion. Trapped leukocytes subsequently become activated, increasing endothelial permeability, migrating extravascularly, and releasing toxic oxygen metabolites, proteolytic enzymes, and cytokines. The number of dermal capillary loops is reduced as they become plugged with white cells,[93] and a perivascular infiltrate of monocytes and macrophages appears in the papillary dermis of lipodermatosclerotic skin.[81,82]

The interaction of leukocytes with the endothelium under conditions of venous hypertension appears to be critical in the pathophysiology of chronic venous disease. Leukocyte adhesion, activation, and migration are mediated by endothelial adhesion receptors, expressed in response to cytokine activation, which function as counter-ligands to those expressed on the leukocytes. Experimental venous hypertension is associated with endothelial activation and increased circulating levels of adhesion molecules, including endothelial leukocyte adhesion molecule-1, intercellular adhesion molecule-1 (ICAM-1), and vascular cell adhesion molecule-1 (VCAM-1).[82,94] Clinically, increased basal levels of adhesion molecules are likely to reflect chronic endothelial activation.[94] VCAM-1, which mediates the adhesion of monocytes and lymphocytes, shows a greater rise in response to standing among patients with lipodermatosclerosis than in those with varicose veins.[94] Endothelial expression of VCAM-1 and ICAM-1, which mediates leukocyte migration, is also increased in the dermal capillary loops of patients with venous ulcers.[86,97]

Leukocyte activation occurs concurrently with endothelial activation.[94,96,97] Leukocytes normally express adhesion molecules, such as L-selectin, which allow reversible binding to, and rolling along, the endothelium. Under pathologic conditions, L-selectin is shed as a second stage ligand, CD11b, is expressed, leading to degranulation or extravascular migration. Under conditions of venous hypertension, plasma L-selectin levels increase and circulating CD11b expression decreases as leukocytes are activated and bound to the endothelium.[96] Although primarily a chronic inflammatory process, increases in elastase levels in patients with chronic venous disease also suggest some component of neutrophil activation.[98] Neutrophil adhesion has been demonstrated in saphenous vein segments perfused under hypoxic conditions postulated to resemble those occurring in venous hypertension.[73,99]

The altered connective tissue remodeling observed in chronic venous insufficiency, which includes an imbalance between tissue degradation and repair with increased turnover of the extracellular matrix, may also be mediated by chronic inflammation.[80,81] Dermal fibrosis is a fundamental feature of lipodermatosclerosis and is associated with increased content of the cytokine transforming growth factor-β_1 (TGF-β_1).[81] TGF-beta$_1$, which is probably derived from activated leukocytes, recruits macrophages and fibroblasts into the tissue and leads to the production of extracellular matrix proteins by dermal fibroblasts. TGF-β_1 also regulates the activity of the matrix metalloproteinases

(MMP),[80,100] a group of proteases which, together with their inhibitors (tissue inhibitors of metalloproteinases; TIMP), regulate connective tissue remodeling and degradation of the extracellular matrix. Altered MMP activity, particularly decreased MMP-2 and increased TIMP-1, has been associated with the histologic changes observed in varicose veins[101] and has been implicated in the pathogenesis of lipodermatosclerosis and ulceration. Some investigators have identified increased MMP-1, MMP-2, and TIMP-1 mRNA and protein expression with corresponding increases in proteolytic activity for type I and type IV collagen in lipodermatosclerotic skin.[80] It has also been postulated that an imbalance between MMP-2 and TIMP-2 may be responsible for fragmentation of dermal elastic fibers and degradation of the epidermal basement membrane and matrix.[80,100]

The precise nature of the injury that initiates chronic inflammation remains unclear. Some authors have postulated that inflammation derives from the potent chemoattractive properties of extravasated red cells and macromolecules.[102] Others have suggested some role for hypertension-induced endothelial injury. Levels of von Willebrand factor, a marker of endothelial injury, are increased in patients with lipodermatosclerosis but not in those with uncomplicated varicose veins.[94] It has also been speculated that upregulation of endothelial adhesion molecule expression occurs in response to hydrostatic pressure-mediated changes in flow or shear.[86,103]

THE EPIDEMIOLOGY OF CHRONIC VENOUS DISEASE

Varicose veins are the most common clinical manifestation of chronic venous disease, occurring in one-quarter to one-third of Western adult populations.[46,104] However, differing terminology, diagnostic criteria, and methodology make it difficult to compare epidemiologic data from different studies and it is generally conceded that the prevalence of varicose veins is underestimated. Up to one-third of patients never seek medical attention for their varicose veins or chronic venous insufficiency.[3] Data from interviews and questionnaires may therefore be inaccurate, having a sensitivity of only 47% in men and 67% in women in comparison to physical examination.[10] However, even physical examination has limitations in the absence of clear definitions. Interobserver error in defining the presence of trunk varicosities has been as high as 85% in some studies.[105] Finally, some studies have included only clinically significant varicosities, while others have differentiated lesser degrees of disease such as prominent superficial and reticular veins. Despite these limitations, prevalence figures in Western populations have varied from 10–15% when only pronounced or medically significant varices are considered, to 30–50% when all types of disease are included.[14,105]

Most studies have documented a steep increase in the prevalence of varicose veins with age.[9,10] The prevalence increases from 1% and 8%, respectively, in men and women 20 to 29 years of age to 43% and 72%, respectively, among those in the seventh decade.[106] Others have estimated similar prevalences of less than 10% among those less than 20 years of age, 25% in men and 40% in women at age 40, and 60% in men and over 70% in women at age 80.[14] Although very few studies have reported incidence estimates, those that have suggest that the incidence of varicose veins may not increase with age. Data from the Framingham study suggest a 2-year incidence of varicose veins averaging 39.4 new cases per 1000 men and 51.9 cases per 1000 women.[107] The increase in prevalence with age may therefore simply reflect an accumulation of cases rather than an increased propensity to develop varicose veins with aging.

Data regarding gender distribution is subject to considerable methodologic and age bias. Women are more likely to seek medical attention for varicose veins and are about three times as likely to undergo treatment.[105] Most population-based studies have accordingly reported varicose veins to be two to three times more common in women. Prevalence rates have been reported to be 25% to 46% in women as compared to 7% to 19% among men.[10,108,109] A trend towards a greater prevalence of objectively documented superficial reflux has been noted in women, although deep venous reflux is more common in men.[110] At least some of these gender differences may arise from a failure to adjust for age.[1,111] Some recent studies have found no gender difference in age-adjusted prevalence. The Edinburgh Vein Study found an overall prevalence of 40% in men and 32% in women.[110] Others have suggested that although reticular veins may be more common in women, the gender distribution of more severe varicose veins is approximately equal.[14]

There do appear to be significant geographic and ethnic differences in both the incidence and prevalence of varicose veins. With respect to prevalence, rates are highest in developed countries and in industrial and working populations (**Fig. 39.11**).[3,10] Even in the same geographic region, prevalence rates are often significantly higher in industrialized areas.[112] The prevalence in the developing world has generally been very low.[113] Prevalence rates among women have varied from 0.1% in New Guinea to 60.5% in Czechoslovakia.[111,112] Population-based studies of Western women have demonstrated more consistent prevalence rates of 25% to 32%.[111] In contrast, rates among women in North and Sub-Saharan Africa are one-quarter to one-fifth of those in European women.[14] However, at least some data suggest that

ethnic and regional differences are not preserved among those emigrating at a young age.[14] The etiology of these geographic differences remains unclear. In comparison to Africans, Caucasians do have a relative deficiency of valves. Banjo reported that at least one valve was present in the external iliac–common femoral segment above the saphenofemoral junction in 81% of Caucasians in comparison to 100% of Africans.[60] However, this does not explain the similar prevalence in white and black Americans.[113] It has been suggested that cultural factors, such as diet and exercise, may be more important than genetic or geographic factors.[113]

The epidemiology of the more severe manifestations of venous insufficiency is difficult to determine. As many studies rely on self-reporting or are based upon patients receiving treatment, incidence and prevalence figures are probably underestimated. In the case of ulceration, it may also be difficult to separate chronic venous ulcers, accounting for approximately 75% of ulcers, from those due to other causes.[111] The best available data suggest that severe chronic venous insufficiency, with skin changes and ulceration, is present in 2% to 5% of Western populations.[14] The prevalence of skin changes has been reported to be 1.2% in Scotland and 3.0% (men) to 3.7% (women) in the USA.[4] Da Silva et al. reported the annual incidence of skin changes and edema to be approximately 0.8% and 1%, respectively.[114] The prevalence of active chronic venous ulcers is estimated to be about 0.3% of the adult population in Western countries, corresponding to approximately 500 000 patients in the USA. However, open ulcers constitute only 20% to 25% of the total, and the population prevalence of open and healed ulcers may be closer to 1%.[111,115]

Among patients with advanced chronic venous insufficiency, women generally predominate at all ages, with a female to male ratio of 2:1 to 3:1.[2,111,115] Skin changes and ulceration are related to the duration of venous hypertension, and the prevalence of

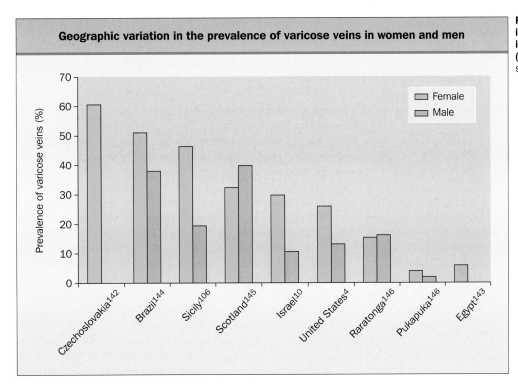

Figure 39.11 Geographic variation in the prevalence of varicose veins in women (red bars) and men (green bars). References shown in superscript.

both slowly increases after 30 years of age.[14] The prevalence of skin changes increases from 1.8% in women aged 30–39 years to 20.7% for women over 70 years of age.[4] Initial ulceration occurs after age 50 in 60% of patients.[16] Accordingly, the incidence of venous ulcer is highest in older patients and is estimated to be about 3.5 per 1000 in those over 45 years of age.[116]

RISK FACTORS FOR CHRONIC VENOUS DISEASE

Population-based studies have evaluated the risk factors associated with the development of reflux and varicose veins, often without any clear conclusions (**Table 39.4**).[4,10,107–109,117] The available data suggest that the etiology of varicose veins is multifactorial, involving various initiating, promoting, and contributing factors.[112] Age, genetic factors such as gender and family history, and environmental factors including pregnancy, obesity, and standing occupations have variously been implicated as risk factors for varicose veins. However, the data are often inconsistent and confounded by various selection biases. Age has been the most consistent and important risk factor in most epidemiologic studies.

Nulliparous women appear less likely to develop varicose veins, although there is no clear relationship to the number of pregnancies.[9,10,107] Varicose veins and telangiectasias may occur early in the first trimester of pregnancy, suggesting that hormonal factors, rather than simply the hydrostatic effects of uterine enlargement, may have a role.[106] The effects of estrogen on smooth muscle relaxation and softening of collagen fibers are well recognized, and pregnant patients, as well as those on oral contraceptives, have increased venous distensibility and decreased tone.[118] Estradiol concentrations in postmenopausal women have been related to both increased venous distensibility and the presence of truncal varicose veins.[119] However, no studies have yet suggested a relationship between oral contraceptives and varicose veins.

Some authors have found a higher prevalence of standing vocations among those with telangiectasias or varicose veins.[10,14,106] However, the data are not uniform and it is likely that standing occupations are an aggravating rather than causative factor.[111] Obesity has similarly been a variable risk factor for varicose veins, more often in women than in men.[111,112] In the absence of a consistent relationship with obesity, it has been suggested that there may be a threshold effect above which the risk of varicose veins is increased.[14] A body mass index of greater than $30 kg/m^2$ has been associated with a fivefold increased prevalence of varicose veins in postmenopausal women.[118]

Obesity was confirmed to be a risk factor in the Framingham study, although women with varicose veins also had higher systolic blood pressures, were less physically active, and reached menopause at an older age.[108] Men smoked more cigarettes and were less physically active. In addition to previous pregnancy and obesity, the Edinburgh Vein Study found that less oral contraceptive use and mobility at work in women, and height and straining at stool in men may be implicated in the development of reflux.[104] Associations with increased intra-abdominal pressure have been suggested by others and varicose veins have inconsistently been associated with constipation, tight undergarments, and inguinal hernias.[10,107] Other population-based studies have found no significant association with social class, smoking, systolic blood pressure, congestive heart failure, diabetes, serum lipids, physical exertion, or hemorrhoids.[10,112]

A hereditary component has also been implicated in the development of varicose veins. As many as 84% of women with telangiectasias or varicose veins have a positive family history.[106] Although varicose veins do appear to be more common among relatives of affected patients, the genetics of this relationship remains unclear.[9] Most data support a polygenic mode of inheritance modified by various external factors.[120] Twin studies have demonstrated concordance for varicose veins in 60% of identical twins in comparison to only 25% of non-identical twins.[75] The risk of developing varicose veins has been reported to be 90% if both parents suffered from this disease; 25% for men and 62% for women with one afflicted parent; and 20% when neither parent was affected.[121] Risk is further increased if an affected relative is male and if the onset of disease is at an early age.[120] However, others have not found a statistically significant association between family history and the development of varicose veins.[108,110,117]

THE NATURAL HISTORY OF CHRONIC VENOUS DISEASE

Primary chronic venous disease

Varicose veins and chronic venous insufficiency are slowly progressive, chronic conditions. Although varicose veins without significant valvular incompetence rarely progress to severe chronic venous insufficiency,[3] approximately 10% of patients with varicose veins presenting to specialized clinics will have ulcers.[19] Unfortunately, as most patients with symptomatic primary disease are treated early after presentation, the rate of progression from uncomplicated varicose veins to skin changes and ulceration remains very poorly defined. In one small study of 36 patients in whom varicose vein surgery was deferred for a median of 20 months, no patient developed a new ulcer. New lipodermatosclerosis developed in one of 50 legs at risk, five of 16 initially normal contralateral legs developed new varicosities, and new segmental reflux was seen in 18% of initially affected and 25% of initially normal legs.[122] However, as the authors noted, this was a select group which was felt likely to remain stable while awaiting operation. Larger studies have suggested

Risk factors for varicose veins.		
Consistent evidence	*Inconsistent but strong evidence*	*Weak or absent evidence*
Age	Female gender	Smoking
Pregnancy	Obesity	Systolic blood pressure
	Family history	Increased intra-abdominal pressure
	Industrialized populations	Physical exertion
	Standing vocation	Diabetes
		Serum lipids
		Social class

Table 39.4 Risk factors for varicose veins.

skin changes and ulceration may develop in up to 22% and 4% of patients an average of 4 years after initial presentation, respectively.[123]

There have also been few longitudinal studies evaluating the factors responsible for disease progression. Age is a major determinant of the severity of chronic venous insufficiency, and many factors such as gender and parity lose their significance when adjusted for age. Other prognostic factors that have been associated with more severe venous insufficiency include weight, a history of thrombophlebitis, the post-thrombotic syndrome, exposure to environmental heat, and occupations including being a senior citizen or housewife.[124] Some physical findings, such as corona phlebectatica, or a fan shaped cluster of dilated veins over the medial aspect of the ankle and calf, have also been suggested as early markers of progression to advanced disease.[1]

Despite vagaries in clinical prognostic indicators, the severity of chronic venous disease is clearly related to the magnitude and distribution of reflux, as well as the length of time it has been present. Among those progressing to ulceration, varicose veins have been noted to be present for a mean of 24 years prior to seeking treatment.[19] Anatomically, the quantitative extent of reflux determined by duplex better reflects the severity of disease than does standard phlebographic scoring.[125] As discussed above, most patients with advanced chronic venous insufficiency have multisystem disease with reflux in the superficial, deep, and perforating veins. From a hemodynamic perspective, the progression of chronic venous disease from mild symptoms to skin changes and ulceration is associated with venous volume expansion, increased reflux, and progressive ambulatory venous hypertension.[21] However, further hemodynamic deterioration was not noted in progression from skin changes to ulceration, perhaps reflecting the importance of microcirculatory changes rather than gross hemodynamic changes in end-stage disease.

Secondary chronic venous disease

The post-thrombotic syndrome is a common complication of acute DVT that has often been underemphasized in the medical literature. Among 224 patients followed for 5 years after venographically confirmed DVT, the post-thrombotic syndrome developed in 29.6% of those with proximal thrombosis and 30% of those with isolated calf vein thrombosis.[126] Others have reported some post-thrombotic symptoms in 29% to 79%, severe manifestations in 7% to 23%, and ulceration in 4% to 6% of patients.[126–130] As acute DVT frequently has a well-defined, symptomatic starting point, it perhaps affords a better opportunity than primary disease to study the natural history of chronic venous disease. Advances in non-invasive testing have been particularly important in relating changes occurring in the venous system to the development of clinical symptoms.

Rather than remaining static, it is now clear that venous thrombi undergo a dynamic evolution beginning soon after their formation. The processes of thrombus organization and recanalization are beyond the scope of this chapter, but also appear to be largely mediated by inflammatory cells (see chapter on Deep Vein Thrombosis and Pulmonary Embolism).[131] Approximately 55% of subjects will show complete recanalization within 6 to 9 months of thrombosis, with the greatest change in thrombus load over the first 3 to 6 months.[132–134] Reflux results from valvular damage or destruction occurring during the process of recanalization. However, reflux is not a universal consequence

of recanalization and only 33% to 59% of thrombosed venous segments ultimately become incompetent.[135] Factors contributing to the development of valvular incompetence after an episode of acute DVT may include the rate of recanalization, the degree of recanalization, and recurrent thrombotic events.

Patients with early recanalization have a lower incidence of valvular incompetence. Among 113 patients followed with serial ultrasonography, median times to complete recanalization in segments developing reflux were 2.3 to 7.3 times longer than for corresponding segments not developing reflux (**Fig. 39.12**).[136] Failure of recanalization, or persistent venous obstruction, may also contribute to development of the post-thrombotic syndrome. While the detrimental effects of venous obstruction may relate to its direct effect on ambulatory venous pressure, it may also be responsible for the development of reflux in distal segments that were not initially thrombosed. As many as 30% of segments developing reflux after an episode of DVT have not previously been thrombosed, an observation that may be related to the presence of proximal obstruction.[137] Finally, recurrent thrombotic events are highly associated with the development of both reflux and clinical symptoms. Ultrasound documented rethrombosis may occur in up to 31% of legs[138] and the incidence of reflux in such segments (36–73%) is significantly higher than in those that remain patent (5.7–18.2%). Not surprisingly, the risk of the post-thrombotic syndrome is six times greater among patients with recurrent thrombosis.[126] Others have documented recurrent thrombotic events in 45% of patients with post-thrombotic symptoms in comparison to only 17% of asymptomatic subjects.[139]

As in the case of primary venous disease, the development of clinical signs and symptoms of the post-thrombotic syndrome is

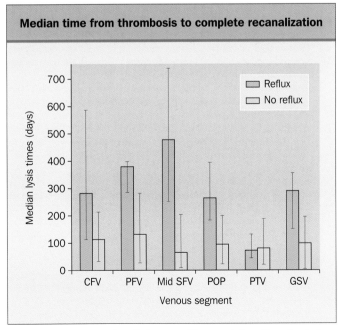

Figure 39.12 Median time (± interquartile range) from thrombosis to complete recanalization, stratified according to ultimate reflux status. Median times are 2.3 to 7.3 times longer among segments developing reflux in all but the posterior tibial veins. Segments: common femoral vein (CFV), profunda femoris vein (PFV), mid-superficial femoral vein (SFV), popliteal vein (PPV), posterior tibial vein (PTV), and greater saphenous vein (GSV). (Adapted with permission from Meissner et al.[136])

related to the global extent of reflux and anatomic distribution of reflux and obstruction.[140] Post-thrombotic skin changes are most significantly related to reflux in the popliteal and posterior tibial veins. However, superficial reflux is also commonly associated with the post-thrombotic syndrome, being present in 84% to 94% of patients with skin changes and 60% to 100% of patients with ulceration. Although concurrent superficial thrombosis is more common than appreciated, a substantial proportion of superficial reflux is not directly associated with thrombosis, develops at a rate equivalent to that in uninvolved limbs, and is likely to involve thrombus-independent degenerative processes.[141] Finally, unlike those with primary venous disease, patients with post-thrombotic disease also commonly have a component of deep venous obstruction, and obstruction of the popliteal vein appears to be clinically most important.[140]

SUMMARY

Chronic venous disease is among the most common disorders encountered by the vascular surgeon. The manifestations of chronic venous disease vary from varicose veins to venous ulceration. They may be primary in origin or secondary to other diseases such as deep venous thrombosis. Although primarily due to venous reflux, there may also be a component of venous obstruction. Among Western populations, varicose veins, skin changes, and ulceration are present in up to 33%, 1% to 3%, and 0.3% of adults, respectively. Although there does appear to be some hereditary predisposition to varicose veins, any inheritance is probably polygenic, with penetrance greatly influenced by environmental factors such as age, place of birth, pregnancy, obesity, and vocation. The factors influencing the progression of chronic venous disease are poorly characterized, but clearly include the magnitude, duration, and anatomic distribution of reflux.

Although incompletely understood, it is clear that, rather than developing in a descending fashion, varicose veins are related to intrinsic changes in the venous wall, develop multicentrically, and probably precede the development of reflux as a secondary phenomenon. Despite the variable manifestations, ambulatory venous hypertension underlies all of the clinical sequelae of chronic venous insufficiency. Furthermore, recent advances in vascular biology have identified the importance of leukocyte–endothelial interactions and chronic inflammation in the etiology of skin changes and ulceration. Although most of the manifestations of chronic venous disease are due to ambulatory venous hypertension, our ability to correct these hemodynamic derangements remains imperfect. While a surgical approach has proven to be efficacious in the treatment of varicose veins, modifications of the underlying microcirculatory disturbances and chronic inflammation hold promise as adjuncts in the management of more advanced disease.

REFERENCES

1. Ruckley CV, Evans CJ, Allan PL, et al. Chronic venous insufficiency: clinical and duplex correlations. The Edinburgh Vein Study of venous disorders in the general population. J Vasc Surg 2002;36:520–5.
2. Kurz X, Kahn SR, Abenhaim L, et al. Chronic venous disorders of the leg: epidemiology, outcomes, diagnosis and management. Summary of an evidence-based report of the VEINES task force. Venous Insufficiency Epidemiologic and Economic Studies. Int Angiol 1999;18:83–102.
3. Cesarone MR, Belcaro G, Nicolaides AN, et al. 'Real' epidemiology of varicose veins and chronic venous diseases: the San Valentino Vascular Screening Project. Angiology 2002;53:119–30.
4. Coon WW, Willis PW, Keller JB. Venous thromboembolism and other venous disease in the Tecumseh Community Health Study. Circulation 1973;48:839–46.
5. Abenhaim L, Kurz X. The VEINES study (VEnous Insufficiency Epidemiologic and Economic Study): an international cohort study on chronic venous disorders of the leg. VEINES Group. Angiology 1997;48:59–66.
6. Phillips T, Stanton B, Provan A, et al. A study of the impact of leg ulcers on quality of life: financial, social, and psychologic implications. J Am Acad Dermatol 1994;31:49–53.
7. Porter JM, Moneta GL. Reporting standards in venous disease: an update. International Consensus Committee on Chronic Venous Disease. J Vasc Surg 1995;21:635–45.
8. Bradbury A, Ruckley CV. Clinical assessment of patients with venous disease. In: Gloviczki P, Yao JST, eds. Handbook of venous disorders. Guidelines of the American Venous Forum, 2nd edn. London:Arnold; 2001:71–83.
9. Weddell JM. Varicose veins pilot survey, 1966. Br J Prev Soc Med 1969;23:179–86.
10. Abramson JH, Hopp C, Epstein LM. The epidemiology of varicose veins. A survey in western Jerusalem. J Epidemiol Community Health 1981;35:213–7.
11. O'Leary DP, Chester JF, Jones SM. Management of varicose veins according to reason for presentation. Ann R Coll Surg Engl 1996; 78:214–6.
12. Bradbury A, Evans C, Allan P, et al. What are the symptoms of varicose veins? Edinburgh vein study cross sectional population survey. BMJ 1999;318:353–6.
13. Biland L, Widmer LK. Varicose veins (VV) and chronic venous insufficiency (CVI). Medical and socioeconomic aspects, Basle study. Acta Chir Scand Suppl 1988;544:9–11.
14. Krijnen RMA, de Boer EM., Bruynzeel DP. Epidemiology of venous disorders in the general and occupational populations. Epidemiol Rev 1997;19:294–309.
15. Ackerman Z, Seidenbaum M, Loewenthal E, et al. Overload of iron in the skin of patients with varicose ulcers. Possible contributing role of iron accumulation in progression of the disease. Arch Dermatol 1988; 124:1376–8.
16. Callam MJ, Harper DR, Dale JJ, et al. Chronic ulcer of the leg: clinical history. BMJ 1987;294:1389–91.
17. Callam MJ, Ruckley CV. Chronic venous insufficiency and leg ulcer. In: Bell PRF, Jamieson CW, Ruckley CV, eds. Surgical management of vascular disease. London:W.B. Saunders Company Ltd; 1992:1267–303.
18. Bass A, Chayen D, Weinmann EE, et al. Lateral venous ulcer and short saphenous vein insufficiency. J Vasc Surg 1997;25:654–7.
19. Hoare MC, Nicolaides AN, Miles CR, et al. The role of primary varicose veins in venous ulceration. Surgery 1982;92:450–3.
20. Labropoulos N, Leon M, Geroulakos G, et al. Venous hemodynamic abnormalities in patients with leg ulceration. Am J Surg 1995; 169:572–4.
21. Welkie J, Comerota A, Katz M, et al. Hemodynamic deterioration in chronic venous disease. J Vasc Surg 1992;16:733–40.
22. Darke SG, Penfold C. Venous ulceration and saphenous ligation. Eur J Vasc Surg 1992;6:4–9.
23. Hanrahan LM, Araki CT, Rodriguez AA, et al. Distribution of valvular incompetence in patients with venous stasis ulceration. J Vasc Surg 1991;13:805–11.
24. Killewich LA, Martin R, Cramer M, et al. Pathophysiology of venous claudication. J Vasc Surg 1984;1:507–11.

25. Qvarfordt P, Eklog B, Plate G, et al. Intramuscular pressure, blood flow, and skeletal muscle metabolism in patients with venous claudication. Surgery 1984;95:191–5.

26. Mewissen MW, Seabrook GR, Meissner MH, et al. Catheter-directed thrombolysis of lower extremity deep venous thrombosis: Report of a national multicenter registry. Radiology 1999;211:39–49.

27. Hurst DR, Forauer AR, Bloom JR, et al. Diagnosis and endovascular treatment of iliocaval compression syndrome. J Vasc Surg 2001; 34:106–13.

28. Caggiati A, Bergan JJ, Gloviczki P, et al. Nomenclature of the veins of the lower limbs: an international interdisciplinary consensus statement. J Vasc Surg 2002;36:416–22.

29. Leu HJ, Vogt M, Pfrunder H. Morphological alterations of non-varicose and varicose veins. (A morphological contribution to the discussion on pathogenesis of varicose veins). Basic Res Cardiol 1979;74:435–44.

30. Mozes G, Carmichael SW, Gloviczki P. Development and anatomy of the venous system. In: Gloviczki P, Yao JST, eds. Handbook of venous disorders. Guidelines of the American Venous Forum, 2nd edn. London:Arnold; 2001:11–24.

31. Cotton LT. Varicose veins. Gross anatomy and development. Br J Surg 1961;48:589–97.

32. Burnand KG. The physiology and hemodynamics of chronic venous insufficiency of the lower limb. In: Gloviczki P, Yao JST, eds. Handbook of venous disorders. Guidelines of the American Venous Forum, 2nd edn. London:Arnold; 2001:49–57.

33. Negus D. The surgical anatomy of the veins of the lower limb. In: Dodd H, Cockett FB, eds. The pathology and surgery of the veins of the lower limb, 2nd edn. Edinburgh:Churchill Livingstone; 1976:18–49.

34. Goldman MP, Fronek A. Anatomy and pathophysiology of varicose veins. J Dermatol Surg Oncol 1989;15:138–45.

35. Ludbrook J. The musculovenous pumps of the human lower limb. Am Heart J 1966;71:635–41.

36. Back TL, Padberg FT Jr, Araki CT, et al. Limited range of motion is a significant factor in venous ulceration. J Vasc Surg 1995;22:519–23.

37. Nicolaides AN, Hussein MK, Szendro G, et al. The relationship of venous ulceration with ambulatory venous pressure measurements. J Vasc Surg 1993;17:414–9.

38. Nicolaides AN. Investigation of chronic venous insufficiency: a consensus statement (France, March 5–9, 1997). Circulation 2000;102:E126–63.

39. Hosoi Y, Zukowski A, Kakkos SK, et al. Ambulatory venous pressure measurements: new parameters derived from a mathematic hemodynamic model. J Vasc Surg 2002;36:137–42.

40. Labropoulos N, Giannoukas AD, Nicolaides AN, et al. The role of venous reflux and calf muscle pump function in nonthrombotic chronic venous insufficiency. Correlation with severity of signs and symptoms. Arch Surg 1996;131:403–6.

41. Cordts PR, Hartono C, LaMorte WW, et al. Physiologic similarities between extremities with varicose veins and with chronic venous insufficiency utilizing air plethysmography. Am J Surg 1992;164:260–4.

42. van Bemmelen PS, Mattos MA, Hodgson KJ, et al. Does air plethysmography correlate with duplex scanning in patients with chronic venous insufficiency? J Vasc Surg 1993;18:796–807.

43. Araki CT, Back TL, Padberg FT, et al. The significance of calf muscle pump function in venous ulceration. J Vasc Surg 1994;20:872–7.

44. Shami SK, Sarin S, Cheatle TR, et al. Venous ulcers and the superficial venous system. J Vasc Surg 1993;17:487–90.

45. Sakurai T, Gupta PC, Matsushita M, et al. Correlation of the anatomical distribution of venous reflux with clinical symptoms and venous haemodynamics in primary varicose veins. Br J Surg 1998;85:213–6.

46. Bradbury A, Evans CJ, Allan P, et al. The relationship between lower limb symptoms and superficial and deep venous reflux on duplex ultrasonography: The Edinburgh Vein Study. J Vasc Surg 2000;32:921–31.

47. Johnson BF, Manzo RA, Bergelin RO, et al. Relationship between changes in the deep venous system and the development of the postthrombotic syndrome after an acute episode of lower limb deep vein thrombosis: A one- to six-year follow-up. J Vasc Surg 1995;21:307–13.

48. Killewich LA, Martin R, Cramer M, et al. An objective assessment of the physiological changes in the postthrombotic syndrome. Arch Surg 1985;120:424–6.

49. Kim J, Richards S, Kent PJ. Clinical examination of varicose veins – a validation study. Ann R Coll Surg Engl 2000;82:171–5.

50. Hoare MC, Royle JP. Doppler ultrasound detection of saphenofemoral and saphenopopliteal incompetence and operative venography to ensure precise saphenopopliteal ligation. Aust NZ J Surg 1984;54:49–52.

51. Singh S, Lees TA, Donlon M, et al. Improving the preoperative assessment of varicose veins. Br J Surg 1997;84:801–2.

52. Christopoulos D, Nicolaides AN, Szendro G. Venous reflux: quantification and correlation with the clinical severity of chronic venous disease. Br J Surg 1988;75:352–6.

53. van Bemmelen PS, Beach K, Bedford G, et al. The mechanism of venous valve closure. Arch Surg 1990;125:617–9.

54. van Bemmelen PS, Bedford G, Beach K, et al. Quantitative segmental evaluation of venous valvular reflux with duplex ultrasound scanning. J Vasc Surg 1989;10:425–31.

55. Neglen P, Raju S. Detection of outflow obstruction in chronic venous insufficiency. J Vasc Surg 1993;17:583–9.

56. Labropoulos N, Volteas N, Leon M, et al. The role of venous outflow obstruction in patients with chronic venous dysfunction. Arch Surg 1997;132:46–51.

57. Raju S, Fredericks R. Venous obstruction: an analysis of one hundred thirty-seven cases with hemodynamic, venographic, and clinical correlations. J Vasc Surg 1991;14:305–13.

58. Albrechtsson U, Einarsson E, Eklof B. Femoral vein pressure measurements for evaluation of venous function in patients with postthrombotic iliac veins. Cardiovasc Intervent Radiol 1981;4:43–50.

59. Anning ST. The historical aspects. In: Dodd H, Cockett FB, eds. The pathology and surgery of the veins of the lower limb, 2nd edn. Edinburgh:Churchill Livingstone; 1976:3–17.

60. Banjo AO. Comparative study of the distribution of venous valves in the lower extremities of black Africans and Caucasians: pathogenetic correlates of prevalence of primary varicose veins in the two races. The Anatomical Record 1987;214:407–12.

61. Alexander CJ. The theoretical basis of varicose vein formation. Med J Aust 1972;1:258–61.

62. Labropoulos N, Giannoukas AD, Delis K, et al. Where does venous reflux start? J Vasc Surg 1997;26:736–42.

63. Gandhi RH, Irizarry E, Nackman GB, et al. Analysis of the connective tissue matrix and proteolytic activity of primary varicose veins. J Vasc Surg 1993;18:814–20.

64. Rose SS, Ahmed A. Some thoughts on the aetiology of varicose veins. J Cardiovasc Surg 1986;27:534–43.

65. Vanhoutte PM, Corcaud S, de Montrion C. Venous disease: from pathophysiology to quality of life. Angiology 1997;48:559–67.

66. Clarke GH, Vasdekis SN, Hobbs JT, et al. Venous wall function in the pathogenesis of varicose veins. Surgery 1992;111:402–8.

67. Bouissou H, Julian M, Pieraggi MT, et al. Vein morphology. Phlebology 1988;3(Suppl 1):1–11.

68. Lowell RC, Gloviczki P, Miller VM. In vitro evaluation of endothelial and smooth muscle function of primary varicose veins. J Vasc Surg 1992;16:679–86.

69. Porto LC, Azizi MA, Pelajo-Machado M, et al. Elastic fibers in saphenous varicose veins. Angiology 2002;53:131–40.

70. Jones GT, Solomon C, Moaveni A, et al. Venous morphology predicts class of chronic venous insufficiency. Eur J Vasc Endovasc Surg 1999; 18:349–54.

71. Ascher E, Jacob T, Hingorani A, et al. Expression of molecular mediators of apoptosis and their role in the pathogenesis of lower-extremity varicose veins. J Vasc Surg 2001;33:1080–6.

72. Travers JP, Brookes CE, Evans J, et al. Assessment of wall structure and composition of varicose veins with reference to collagen, elastin and smooth muscle content. Eur J Vasc Endovasc Surg 1996;11:230–7.

73. Michiels C, Arnould T, Thibaut-Vercruyssen R, et al. Perfused human saphenous veins for the study of the origin of varicose veins: role of the endothelium and of hypoxia. Int Angiol 1997;16:134–41.

74. Clarke GH, Vasdekis SN, Hobbs JT, et al. Venous wall function in the pathogenesis of varicose veins. Surgery 1992;111:402–8.

75. Haardt B. A comparison of the histochemical enzyme pattern in normal and varicose veins. Phleboloby 1987;2:135–58.

587

76. Barber DA, Wang X, Gloviczki P, et al. Characterization of endothelin receptors in human varicose veins. J Vasc Surg 1997;26:61–9.

77. Mangiafico RA, Malatino LS, Santonocito M, et al. Plasma endothelin-1 release in normal and varicose saphenous veins. Angiology 1997; 48:769–74.

78. Hollingsworth SJ, Tang CB, Dialynas M, et al. Varicose veins: loss of release of vascular endothelial growth factor and reduced plasma nitric oxide. Eur J Vasc Endovasc Surg 2001;22:551–6.

79. Schuller-Petrovic S, Siedler S, Kern T, et al. Imbalance between the endothelial cell-derived contracting factors prostacyclin and angiotensin II and nitric oxide/cyclic GMP in human primary varicosis. Br J Pharmacol 1997;122:772–8.

80. Herouy Y, May AE, Pornschlegel G, et al. Lipodermatosclerosis is characterized by elevated expression and activation of matrix metalloproteinases: implications for venous ulcer formation. J Invest Dermatol 1998;111:822–7.

81. Pappas PJ, You R, Rameshwar P, et al. Dermal tissue fibrosis in patients with chronic venous insufficiency is associated with increased transforming growth factor-beta1 gene expression and protein production. J Vasc Surg 1999;30:1129–45.

82. Coleridge Smith PD. Update on chronic-venous-insufficiency-induced inflammatory processes. Angiology 2001;52(Suppl 1):S35–42.

83. Scelsi R, Scelsi L, Cortinovis R, et al. Morphological changes of dermal blood and lymphatic vessels in chronic venous insufficiency of the leg. Int Angiol 1994;13:308–11.

84. Herrick SE, Sloan P, McGurk M, et al. Sequential changes in histologic pattern and extracellular matrix deposition during the healing of chronic venous ulcers. Am J Pathol 1992;141:1085–95.

85. Browse NL, Burnand KG. The cause of venous ulceration. Lancet 1982;2:243–5.

86. Hahn J, Junger M, Friedrich B, et al. Cutaneous inflammation limited to the region of the ulcer in chronic venous insufficiency. Vasa 1997; 26:277–81.

87. Pappas PJ, DeFouw DO, Venezio LM, et al. Morphometric assessment of the dermal microcirculation in patients with chronic venous insufficiency. J Vasc Surg 1997;26:784–95.

88. Wilkinson LS, Bunker C, Edwards JC, et al. Leukocytes: their role in the etiopathogenesis of skin damage in venous disease. J Vasc Surg 1993;17:669–75.

89. Hopkins NF, Spinks TJ, Rhodes CG, et al. Positron emission tomography in venous ulceration and liposclerosis: study of regional tissue function. BMJ (Clin Res Ed) 1983;286:333–6.

90. Burnand KG, Whimster I, Naidoo A, et al. Pericapillary fibrin in the ulcer-bearing skin of the leg: the cause of lipodermatosclerosis and venous ulceration. BMJ (Clin Res Ed) 1982;285:1071–2.

91. Van De Scheur M, Falanga V. Pericapillary fibrin cuffs in venous disease. Dermatol Surg 1997;23:955–9.

92. Thomas PRS, Nash GB, Dormandy JA. White cell accumulation in dependent legs of patients with venous hypertension: a possible mechanism for trophic changes in the skin. BMJ 1988;296:1693–5.

93. Coleridge Smith PD, Thomas P, Scurr JH, et al. Causes of venous ulceration: a new hypothesis. BMJ (Clin Res Ed) 1988;296:1726–7.

94. Saharay M, Shields DA, Georgiannos SN, et al. Endothelial activation in patients with chronic venous disease. Eur J Vasc Endovasc Surg 1998;15:342–9.

95. Ciuffetti G, Mannarino E, Paltriccia R, et al. Leucocyte activity in chronic venous insufficiency. Int Angiol 1994;13:312–6.

96. Saharay M, Shields DA, Porter JB, et al. Leukocyte activity in the microcirculation of the leg in patients with chronic venous disease. J Vasc Surg 1997;26:265–73.

97. Weyl A, Vanscheidt W, Weiss JM, et al. Expression of the adhesion molecules ICAM-1, VCAM-1, and E-selectin and their ligands VLA-4 and LFA-1 in chronic venous leg ulcers. J Am Acad Dermatol 1996; 34:418–23.

98. Shields DA, Andaz SK, Sarin S, et al. Plasma elastase in venous disease. Br J Surg 1994;81:1496–9.

99. Michiels C, Bouaziz N, Remacle J. Role of the endothelium and blood stasis in the appearance of varicose veins. Int Angiol 2002;21:1–8.

100. Saito S, Trovato MJ, You R, et al. Role of matrix metalloproteinases 1, 2, and 9 and tissue inhibitor of matrix metalloproteinase-1 in chronic venous insufficiency. J Vasc Surg 2001;34:930–8.

101. Parra JR, Cambria RA, Hower CD, et al. Tissue inhibitor of metalloproteinase-1 is increased in the saphenofemoral junction of patients with varices in the leg. J Vasc Surg 1998;28:669–75.

102. Pappas PJ, Duran WN, Hobson RW. Pathology and cellular physiology of chronic venous insufficiency. In: Gloviczki P, Yao JST, eds. Handbook of venous disorders. Guidelines of the American Venous Forum, 2nd edn. London:Arnold; 2001:58–67.

103. Schmid-Schonbein G, Takase S, Bergan JJ. New advances in the understanding of the pathophysiology of chronic venous insufficiency. Angiology 2001;52(Suppl 1):S27–34.

104. Fowkes FG, Lee AJ, Evans CJ, et al. Lifestyle risk factors for lower limb venous reflux in the general population: Edinburgh Vein Study. Int J Epidemiol 2001;30:846–52.

105. Madar G, Widmer LK, Zemp E, et al. Varicose veins and chronic venous insufficiency disorder or disease? A critical epidemiological review. Vasa 1986;15:126–34.

106. Sadick NS. Predisposing factors of varicose and telangiectatic leg veins. J Dermatol Surg Oncol 1992;18:883–6.

107. Brand FN, Dannenberg AL, Abbott RD, et al. The epidemiology of varicose veins: the Framingham Study. Am J Prev Med 1988;4:96–101.

108. Novo S, Avellone G, Pinto A. Prevalence of primitive varicose veins of the lower limb in a randomized population sample of western Sicily. Int Angiol 1988;7:176–81.

109. Sisto T, Reunanen A, Laurikka J, et al. Prevalence and risk factors of varicose veins in lower extremities: mini-Finland health survey. Eur J Surg 1995;161:405–14.

110. Evans CJ, Allan PL, Lee AJ, et al. Prevalence of venous reflux in the general population on duplex scanning: The Edinburgh Vein Study. J Vasc Surg 1998;28:767–76.

111. Fowkes FG, Evans CJ, Lee AJ. Prevalence and risk factors of chronic venous insufficiency. Angiology 2001;52(Suppl 1):S5–15.

112. De Backer G. Epidemiology of chronic venous insufficiency. Angiology 1997;48:569–76.

113. Geelhoed GW, Burkitt DP. Varicose veins: a reappraisal from a global perspective. South Med J 1991;84:1131–4.

114. da Silva A, Widmer LK, Martin H, et al. Varicose veins and chronic venous insufficiency. Vasa 1974;3:118–25.

115. Callam MJ, Ruckley CV, Harper DR, et al. Chronic ulceration of the leg: extent of the problem and provision of care. BMJ (Clin Res Ed) 1985;290:1855–6.

116. Lees TA, Lambert D. Prevalence of lower limb ulceration in an urban health district. Br J Surg 1992;79:1032–4.

117. Franks PJ, Wright DD, Moffatt CJ, et al. Prevalence of venous disease: a community study in west London. Eur J Surg 1992;158:143–7.

118. Goodrich SM, Wood JE. Peripheral venous distensibility and velocity of blood flow during pregancy or during oral contraceptive therapy. Am J Obstet Gynecol 1964;90:740–4.

119. Ciardullo AV, Panico S, Bellati C, et al. High endogenous estradiol is associated with increased venous distensibility and clinical evidence of varicose veins in menopausal women. J Vasc Surg 2000;32:544–9.

120. Gundersen J, Hauge M. Hereditary factors in venous insufficiency. Angiology 1969;20:346–55.

121. Cornu-Thenard A, Boivin P, Baud JM, et al. Importance of the familial factor in varicose disease. Clinical study of 134 families. J Dermatol Surg Oncol 1994;20:318–26.

122. Sarin S, Shields DA, Farrah J, et al. Does venous function deteriorate in patients waiting for varicose vein surgery? J R Soc Med 1993; 86:21–3.

123. Brewster SF, Nicholson S, Farndon JR. The varicose vein waiting list: results of a validation exercise. Ann R Coll Surg Engl 1991;73:223–6.

124. Mota-Capitao L, Menezes JD, Gouveia-Oliveira A. Clinical predictors of the severity of chronic venous insufficiency of the lower limbs: a multivariate analysis. Phlebology 1995;10:155–9.

125. Neglen P, Raju S. A comparison between descending phlebography and duplex Doppler investigation in the evaluation of reflux in chronic venous insufficiency: a challenge to phlebography as the 'gold standard'. J Vasc Surg 1992;16:687–93.

126. Prandoni P, Lensing A, Cogo A, et al. The long term clinical course of acute deep venous thrombosis. Ann Intern Med 1996;125:1–7.

127. Monreal M, Martorell A, Callejas J, et al. Venographic assessment of deep vein thrombosis and risk of developing post-thrombotic syndrome: a prospective trial. J Intern Med 1993;233:233–8.

128. Strandness DE, Langlois Y, Cramer M, et al. Long-term sequelae of acute venous thrombosis. JAMA 1983;250:1289–92.

129. Prandoni P, Villalta S, Polistena P, et al. Symptomatic deep-vein thrombosis and the post thrombotic syndrome. Haematologica 1995; 80:42–8.

130. Lindner DJ, Edwards JM, Phinney ES, et al. Long-term hemodynamic and clinical sequelae of lower extremity deep vein thrombosis. J Vasc Surg 1986;4:436–42.

131. Meissner MH, Strandness DE. Pathophysiology and natural history of deep venous thrombosis. In: Rutherford RB, ed. Vascular surgery, 5th edn. Philadelphia:W.B. Saunders Company;2000:1920–37.

132. Arcelus JI, Caprini JA, Hoffman KN, et al. Laboratory assays and duplex scanning outcomes after symptomatic deep vein thrombosis: preliminary results. J Vasc Surg 1996;23:616–21.

133. Killewich LA, Macko RF, Cox K, et al. Regression of proximal deep venous thrombosis is associated with fibrinolytic enhancement. J Vasc Surg 1997;26:861–8.

134. Rosfors S, Eriksson M, Leijd B, et al. A prospective follow-up study of acute deep venous thrombosis using colour duplex ultrasound, phlebography and venous occlusion plethysmography. Int Angiol 1997; 16:39–44.

135. Markel A, Manzo RA, Bergelin RO, et al. Valvular reflux after deep vein thrombosis: Incidence and time of occurrence. J Vasc Surg 1992; 15:377–84.

136. Meissner MH, Manzo RA, Bergelin RO, et al. Deep venous insufficiency: the relationship between lysis and subsequent reflux. J Vasc Surg 1993;18:596–608.

137. Caps MT, Manzo RA, Bergelin RO, et al. Venous valvular reflux in veins not involved at the time of acute deep vein thrombosis. J Vasc Surg 1995;22:524–31.

138. Meissner MH, Caps MT, Bergelin RO, et al. Propagation, rethrombosis, and new thrombus formation after acute deep venous thrombosis. J Vasc Surg 1995;22:558–67.

139. Beyth RJ, Cohen AM, Landefeld CS. Long-term outcome of deep-vein thrombosis. Arch Intern Med 1995;155:1031–7.

140. Meissner MH, Caps MT, Zierler BK, et al. Determinants of chronic venous disease after acute deep venous thrombosis. J Vasc Surg 1998;28:826–33.

141. Meissner MH, Caps MT, Zierler BK, et al. Deep venous thrombosis and superficial venous reflux. J Vasc Surg 2000;32:48–56.

142. Barwell JR, Taylor M, Deacon J, et al. Surgical correction of isolated superficial venous reflux reduces long-term recurrence rate in chronic venous leg ulcers. Eur J Vasc Endovasc Surg 2000;20:363–8.

143. Stvrtinova V, Kolesar J, Wimmer G. Prevalence of varicose veins of the lower limbs in the women working at a department store. Int Angiol 1991;10:2–5.

144. Mekky S, Schilling RS, Walford J. Varicose veins in women cotton workers. An epidemiological study in England and Egypt. BMJ 1969; 2:591–5.

145. Maffei FH, Magaldi C, Pinho SZ, et al. Varicose veins and chronic venous insufficiency in Brazil: prevalence among 1755 inhabitants of a country town. Int J Epidemiol 1986;15:210–7.

146. Evans CJ, Fowkes FG, Ruckley CV, et al. Prevalence of varicose veins and chronic venous insufficiency in men and women in the general population: Edinburgh Vein Study. J Epidemiol Community Health 1999;53:149–53.

147. Beaglehole R. Epidemiology of varicose veins. World J Surg 1986; 10:898–902.

CHAPTER
40

The Medical Management of Varicose Veins

Richard G J Gibbs, Soni Soumian, and Alun H Davies

KEY POINTS

- Non-surgical treatments can be used for both small and large varicose veins.

- The evidence for drug therapy for varicose veins is hampered by small, poorly designed trials and large numbers of anecdotal studies.

- Compression treatment using graduated elastic stockings can control symptoms alone.

- Sclerotherapy is used with success in the treatment of large and small varicose veins.

- Sclerotherapy for large varicose veins is associated with a higher recurrence rate than conventional surgery.

- Sclerotherapy can be enhanced by using foam preparations.

- Sclerotherapy performed with duplex ultrasound guidance may improve safety and results.

INTRODUCTION

It has always been perceived that the gold-standard treatment for varicose veins is surgical, with the intent to cure the underlying problem. However the label 'varicose veins' covers a heterogenous spectrum of venous disease; varicose veins can be small (flare veins, reticular veins) as well as large (truncal saphenous and tributaries), and ideal treatment for small veins is nonsurgical. Moreover, not all patients are suitable candidates for surgery owing to intercurrent illness, or personal choice. In this group, alternative management strategies should be used to deal with the symptoms of varicose veins. The three principal non-surgical pathways available are:

- medication;
- sclerotherapy; and
- compression.

MEDICATION

The majority of trials testing the efficacy of drug treatment in venous disorders of the leg were carried out in the 1960s and 1970s. Compared with the current gold standard of level-one evidence drawn from multicenter, randomized prospective trials, these studies are considerably weaker in design. This limits objective evidence that defines the indication and usefulness of these agents. The symptoms of varicose veins can be treated with medications. These symptoms include heaviness, discomfort along the course of the vein, itching, cramps, and swelling. Patients

Venoactive drugs.	
	Active substance/Examples
Natural products	
Flavonoids (γ-benzopyrones)	
flavones and flavanoids	Rutin
	Diosmin
flavanes and flavanones	Pyconegol
	Hesperidine
	Hesperetine
Coumarines	Coumarin
	Dicumaroids
	Esculetin
Saponins	Escin
	Ruscosides
Other plant extracts	Anthocyanosides
	Ginkgo biloba
Synthetic substances	
	Calcium dobesilate
	Naftazone
	Tribenoside

Table 40.1 Venoactive drugs.

may suffer the symptoms of venous disease in the absence of demonstrable varicose veins. Drugs used are either venoactive or non-venoactive. The non-venoactive drug category has only been used in the management of venous ulcers, and includes peripheral vasodilators and prostaglandins.[1]

Venoactive drugs act principally on the subjective symptoms of chronic venous disorders of the leg, which includes varicose veins. In Europe their use is confined to treatment of symptomatology, and they are not considered alternatives to sclerotherapy or surgery, which treat the actual condition.

There are two principal categories of venoactive drugs or 'phlebotropics': naturally occurring agents and synthetic agents (see **Table 40.1**). Their mechanism of action has not been fully elucidated, but they are thought to improve venous tone, assessed by a decrease in venous wall compliance as measured by plethysmography. Many of the studies that assessed venoactive drugs used healthy, as opposed to diseased, vein, while not establishing if the two states react in the same fashion. Increased venous pressure is associated with microcirculatory changes, namely white cell aggregation and activation with subsequent release of inflammatory mediators, increased capillary permeability, and microthrombus formation. These agents could also act to counter these responses, by decreasing white cell activation and release of inflammatory mediators, decreasing capillary fragility and permeability, and decreasing blood viscosity.

Rutin, esculetin, and dihydroergocristine have all been compared to placebo in the management of simple varicose veins. No beneficial effect was observed in any group.[2] A placebo-controlled trial of naftazone in primary uncomplicated varicose veins claimed a statistically and clinically significant improvement in reducing disability as subjectively assessed on a visual analog scale.[3]

SCLEROTHERAPY

The principal indications for sclerotherapy in the treatment of varicose veins are to relieve symptoms, and improve cosmesis by the elimination of visible varicose veins and reflux. The literature on the subject is patchy, with conflicting reports on the efficacy of sclerotherapy. The lack of a universal classification of varicose veins means comparison of different techniques is liable to misinterpretation, and different outcome measures compound this problem. There are a large number of case reports and small personal series, but only six randomized controlled studies from 1972 to date. A consensus conference on sclerotherapy of varicose veins of the leg[4] relied upon a range of expert personal opinions rather than on published results. A recent survey of practice in the UK suggested use of sclerotherapy is falling, and that most vascular surgeons reserve it for varicose veins without proximal incompetence, or residual veins.

Techniques

The basic principle of sclerotherapy is the induction of irritation in the endothelial and subendothelial layers of the wall of the vein, collapsing the walls so they lie in apposition by compression, and obliteration of the lumen by inflammation and fibrosis. The process of inflammation resolving by fibrosis takes over 6 months. Sclerosing agents can act either by osmosis, dehydrating and destroying the endothelium (e.g. hypertonic glucose) or by a detergent action on the lipid endothelial cell membrane (e.g. ethanolamine oleate).[5] The second mechanism acts faster than the first.

All methodologies described in the literature depend upon one of three different historical techniques, namely Tournay (French), Sigg (Swiss), and Fegan (Irish). Imaging modalities such as ultrasound, and new sclerosing agents have helped in modifying techniques. Sclerotherapy can be used in conjunction with surgery, either during the operation or afterwards.

Small varicose veins

Small varicose veins include telangiectasias, reticular veins, and venulectases. Intradermal venulectases (telangiectasias) are intradermal vessels visible to the human eye, measuring 0.1–2mm in diameter. Telangiectasias may be arteriole, venule or capillary. Reticular varicose veins are dilated subcutaneous veins not belonging to the main truncal veins or their major tributaries.

The unanimous recommendation of the consensus conference[3] was that sclerotherapy is the preferred treatment option for these types of veins.

Method

The technique of sclerotherapy for small veins is illustrated in **Figures 40.1–40.7**. The patient is asked to stand or sit for 5min before treatment, to fill the veins. Alternatively, a blood pressure cuff placed above the injection site is inflated to 40mmHg. The patient then sits with the leg in a horizontal position on the couch. The skin over the proposed injection site is prepared with a 70% alcohol and 0.5% acetic acid wipe. The operator can use a magnifying lamp or loupes to enhance visualization. A 3–5ml plastic or glass syringe is filled with the sclerosing agent. These include:

- chromated glycerine 25–100%*;
- polidocanol 0.2–1%*;
- sodium salicylate 6–12%*;
- hypertonic glucose*;
- sodium tetradecyl sulfate;
- dilute iodine;
- ethanolamine oleate; and
- sodium morrhhuate.

Small needles with gauges between 25 and 33G are used. A small 'test dose' on the first treatment is used to ensure there are no adverse reactions. The needle is advanced into the lumen of the vein, and aspiration of blood back into the syringe is advocated prior to injection (although this is not possible in the case of telangiectases). Some experts advise using an 'air block', in which the vein is injected with air prior to injection of the sclerosant, in order to empty it of blood.[6,7] The idea is that less sclerosant is needed, as it is relatively undiluted. Another modification to the technique is the use of a foam sclerosant. A 2cm^2 area is injected at a time, with a maximum dose of 10mL per session being used. Injection is immediately stopped if there is any evidence of extravasation. Compression can then be applied to the area, although not all experts use post-sclerotherapy compression. The interval from one session to the next should not be less than 1 week, and the same area should not be revisited within 3 weeks.

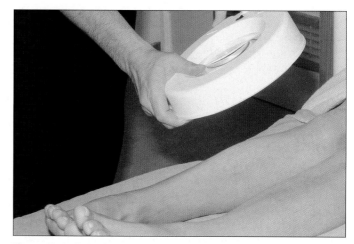

Figure 40.1 Magnification to aid sclerotherapy of small veins.

*Denotes recommendation by the consensus conference on sclerotherapy of varicose veins of the lower limb.[3]

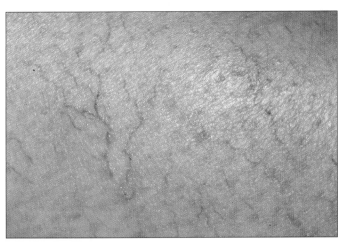

Figure 40.2 Chosen area for treatment.

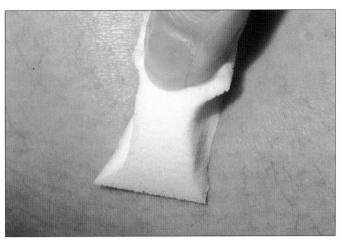

Figure 40.5 Local compression with foam-pad enhancement.

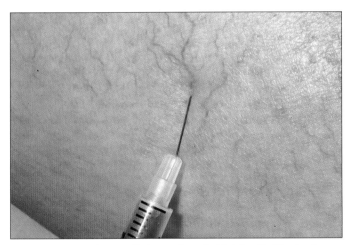

Figure 40.3 Inserting needle into vein and obtaining flashback of blood (if possible).

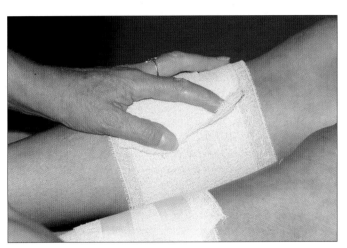

Figure 40.6 Crepe bandage over sclerotherapy site.

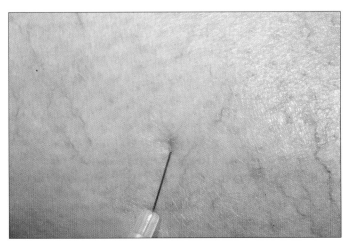

Figure 40.4 Injection of sclerosant.

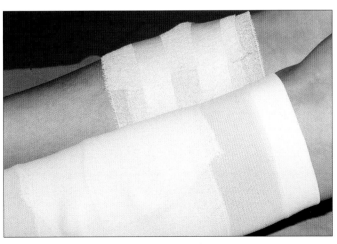

Figure 40.7 TED stocking over crepe bandage.

Large varicose veins

These include the long saphenous, short saphenous, and non-saphenous varicose veins. The consensus conference on sclerotherapy of varicose veins of the lower limb[4] failed to reach a conclusion regarding the role of sclerotherapy in the treatment of varicose long saphenous and perforating veins. It was felt sclerotherapy 'may' be indicated in the treatment of the varicose short saphenous vein, but a definitive conclusion could not be reached due to the lack of credible scientific evidence. There are three basic methods of sclerosing large varicose veins. Fegan[8,9] described sclerosing the most distal perforating veins first and moving proximally, but not injecting the trunk and saphenous junctions. Sodium tetradecyl sulfate was the sclerosing agent, and strong compression was needed (**Table 40.2**).

Tournay injected the most proximal point of reflux and worked distally, and included the saphenofemoral and saphenopopliteal junctions. Sclerosing agents included iodine, sodium tetradecyl sulfate, and sodium salicylate. Short periods of local compression were used.[10]

Sigg's technique[11] involved injecting the most distal varicose vein first and then progressing proximally until the reflux point was occluded. Iodine was the sclerosing agent, and prolonged compression was employed.

The concentration of the sclerosant should be highest at the highest point of venous reflux.

The use of compression depends upon which approach is taken, either top to bottom (Tournay) or bottom to top (Fegan and Sigg). Treatment starting distally mandates use of prolonged compression, in order to minimize inflammatory thrombophlebitis and intravascular clotting, and induce a firm fibrous cord. Bandages or compression stockings can be used, although bandaging technique is not critical as practice varies widely. Compression is not used routinely in sclerotherapy commenced proximally. When it is employed, the strength and duration of compression is less than after sclerotherapy commencing distally.

Post-sclerotherapy compression

In a review of randomized controlled trials involving injection sclerotherapy, the degree and duration of compression made no difference to recurrence rates, symptom improvement, or cosmesis.[12] The duration and strength of compression was associated with increased discomfort.

Foam sclerotherapy

The concept of using a foamy sclerosant was first described in 1950, when Orbach[13] first suggested that vigorously shaking the

sclerosant 3% sodium tetradecyl sulfate improved the thrombogenic effect. It has enjoyed a resurgence of interest since the mid-1990s. The conceptual advantage of using foam is the bioavailability. Sclerosant solutions act on venous endothelium that is reached by intravenous injection. Distribution and local concentration depend upon the volume and flow rate of blood, which vary with the size of the vein. A progressive dilution in the sclerosant will occur the further away from the point of injection the sclerosant is carried by blood. The concentration also drops off rapidly as the sclerosant fixes to red blood cell membranes, decreasing bioavailability. Microfoam is a drug delivery system that potentially prolongs the time the sclerosant is in contact with the endothelium, and achieves a more constant concentration of the sclerosant at the site of action. Foam confers the added advantage of being more easily imaged on duplex ultrasound. Foam sclerotherapy has been described in the treatment of both small and large varicose veins, including recurrent veins.

Duplex-guided sclerotherapy

Duplex-guided or echosclerotherapy was first described in 1989, and involves the injection of a vein with sclerosant under ultrasound guidance. The technique has been used in the treatment of long and short saphenous and recurrent veins. The advantages of using this technique lie in safety; intra-arterial injection is minimized, and if extravasation of sclerosant occurs, this can be seen right away and the injection stopped. The effect of the sclerosant on the vein wall can be observed immediately. Duplex imaging allows estimation of the degree of spasm, length of vein affected, and identification of tributaries, together with control of the deep veins.

COMPRESSION THERAPY

Compression can be used in the management of large varicose veins. Graduated compression stockings can be effective in symptom control, but do not treat the underlying pathology. The efficacy of compression therapy in subjective symptom improvement has been known for centuries. External compression can reduce vein diameter and decrease reflux of blood in incompetent segments. The effects on the microcirculation include the acceleration of blood flow in the capillaries, improvement of the filtration/absorption ratio in the capillary system, and reduction of tissue edema. Reduction in pain, fullness, swelling, and cramps have all been reported. There is no indication for compression in the management of small varicose veins.

Techniques

The following basic rules apply to all leg bandages:

1. A basic bandage should extend up to the head of the fibula and must have adequate number of layers with appropriate pressure decreasing continually from distal to proximal.
2. The bandage must be firm, applied without gaps, and turns must overlap by one-half to two-thirds.

There are various standard methods of bandaging. In a crossover bandage, according to Putter, the leg is bandaged in opposite directions with two bandages. In a compression crossover bandage, according to Sigg, first the foot is bandaged and then the calf up to the knee with a second bandage. The plastic walking support bandage, according to Brann, uses a combination of elastic

Recommended sclerosants for large varicose veins.			
	Saphenous veins	Perforators	Branches
Polidocanol	4–5%	2–3%	2–4%
Sodium tetradecyl sulfate	1–3%	1–3%	0.3–3%
Iodine	4–12%	2–8%	2–4%

Table 40.2 Recommended sclerosants for large varicose veins.

bandage and wet stiffened-gauze bandage, which thus exerts a constant static pressure and high dynamic pressure. This is a type of permanent bandage. In the standard method, the bandage is wound spirally in one layer with a 50% overlap up to the knee.

Types of dressings

Bandaging can be classified into two types based on the duration of usage (**Table 40.3**):

- continuous type; and
- daytime use.

Continuous-type dressings

These are indicated at the beginning of treatment for decongestion therapy. Continuous-type dressings remain on the patient's leg even during bed-rest and are changed once a week (even up to several weeks). The compression materials are either inelastic or short-stretch elastic material (**Table 40.4**). Zinc plastic bandages called Unna's boot and Circ-aid are classic examples of continuous-type dressings. As these bandages do not cling sufficiently, they cannot be applied by the patients themselves, but require specially trained personnel. Adhesive dressings belong to this group.

The advantages of these dressings are the high working pressure while walking and the uninterrupted efficacy during the night.

The disadvantages are the problems with personal hygiene and the necessity for trained personnel to change the dressings.

Daytime-use dressings

These are indicated in maintenance treatment. Bandages or graduated compression stockings can be used. Daytime elastic bandages are applied by the patients, preferably before getting up in the morning, and are removed just before going to bed at night. The materials are medium- and long-stretch bandages that cling closely to the leg and, owing to their flexibility, do not need great dexterity to apply. If applied correctly, these bandages should be so firm that it is felt to be unpleasant to sit for longer than 20–30min without moving (high resting pressures). These bandages give low working pressure as they stretch and give way to the contracting muscles.

The advantages are the relative ease of application, relatively low cost, and better hygienic conditions. The disadvantages are the potential chances of inconsistent and poor bandage application technique by patients and the decreased efficacy in deep veins due to low working pressures.

Medical elastic compression stockings are equally effective in daytime compression. They come in three lengths – short, normal, and long – and in different compression classes. While custom-made hosiery may provide better fit for some individuals, for many, ready-made stockings are available in different compression classes (**Table 40.5**).

Comparison of two types of bandaging.		
	Continuous-type dressings	*Daytime-use dressings*
Indication	Severe forms of venous congestion	Less severe forms
Technique	Sophisticated (requires trained personnel)	Ease of use (by patients)
Duration	Remains on day and night (days to weeks)	Daily change
Pressure	High working pressure	High resting pressure
Effect on deep veins	Yes	No

Table 40.3 Comparison of two types of bandaging. In general, elastic bandages and compression stockings slowly lose their elasticity and become less effective after 3 and 6 months, respectively, at which time they should be replaced.

Compression classes based on the European standard – classification for compression based on the pressures exerted at the ankle region.	
Compression class	*Absolute pressure (mmHg)*
A (light)	10–14
I (mild)	15–21
II (moderate)*	22–32
III (strong)	33–46
IV (very strong)	47 and higher
Usually, Class II compression is effective in chronic venous insufficiency, as compression pressure of more than 30–40mmHg has very minimal impact on the reduction of venous volume.	

Table 40.5 Compression classes based on the European standard – classification for compression based on the pressures exerted at the ankle region.

Categories of compression material.				
	Inelastic	*Short stretch*	*Medium stretch*	*Long stretch*
Stretch	0	<70%	70–140%	>140%
Application	Trained staff	Trained staff	Trained patient	Every patient
Duration	Continuous	Continuous	Daytime	Daytime

Table 40.4 Categories of compression material.

Compression enhancement

With the help of variously shaped rubber foam pads, the local contact pressure of a dressing can be substantially enhanced. This method is used wherever a particularly high contact pressure of the dressing appears desirable, especially in the retro-malleolar fossa and ulcer areas.

OTHER THERAPIES

Several other treatment modalities, including physiotherapy, hydrotherapy, and ultrasound therapy, are available but most of them have not been tested in controlled studies and the available data are not strong enough to draw valid conclusions about their efficacy. Physiotherapy is commonly used. Hydrotherapy provides short-term stimulation leading to venoconstriction, diuresis, and vascular–interstitial fluid shift. Ultrasound therapy may be useful as an adjunct in venous ulcer healing.

COMPLICATIONS OF NON-SURGICAL THERAPY FOR VARICOSE VEINS

Drug therapy

The most commonly reported adverse effects associated with drug therapy are nausea, headache, colicky abdominal pain, and insomnia.[14–17] Constipation, tiredness, and pruritus are seen in patients taking rutosides.[16]

Sclerotherapy

The minor side effects reported after sclerotherapy include pigmentation and local inflammatory reactions. The potential of an adverse cosmetic effect should be explained carefully to every patient before treatment, to avoid the distress associated with resulting litigation. Pruritus after injection of polidocanol was reported as often as 35–45% in the study by Norris et al.[18] Hyperpigmentation and neovascularization was concentration-dependent and seen in 50–70% of patients following use of polidocanol.

The possible risks of dangerous complications such as thrombo-embolism as well as intra-arterial injections must be avoided by careful selection of patients and meticulous technique. Other reported complications include thrombosis, superficial phlebitis, night cramps, blisters, and swollen feet.[12,19–21]

The main contraindication to use of sclerotherapy is known allergy to the agent. The procedure must be performed with caution in the following situations:

- severe systemic disease;
- recent deep vein thrombosis;
- local or general infection;
- non-ambulatory patients;
- severe arterial disorder, especially critical leg ischemia;
- allergic diathesis;
- pregnancy and breast feeding;
- hypercoagulability (protein C and S deficiency and lupus anti-coagulant); and
- recurrent deep vein thrombosis.

Compression

The main contraindication to usage is arterial insufficiency. All patients deemed at risk of peripheral arterial insufficiency should have an estimation of their ankle–brachial pressure index made prior to application of compressive hosiery or bandaging. Compression has been reported to cause phlebitis, blisters, pruritus, and foot swelling when applied too tightly.

Compared with stockings, bandages are reported to cause more ankle immobility[22] and a relatively increased risk of thrombosis. Compression of extremities should be performed with caution in patients with severe cardiac failure, owing to the effect on cardiac preload and output. In pregnancy, compression may influence maternal and fetal heart rate.

EVIDENCE OF EFFICACY OF NON-SURGICAL TREATMENTS

Drug therapy

Medications are prescribed for symptom relief in chronic venous insufficiency. The symptoms most frequently assessed in drug studies are heaviness, fullness, discomfort, cramps, itching, pain, restless legs, sensation of heat, and swelling.

Several studies have been done to assess the efficacy of medications on all of these symptoms. Treatment with coumarine rutine for 90 days improved heaviness by 61% as compared with 19% in the placebo group (p=<0.001) when the symptoms were analyzed by visual analog score.[23] Langiullat et al. studied dihydroergocristine versus placebo for 30 days.[24] Dihydro-ergocristine was significantly better at improving leg heaviness, tightness, and paresthesia compared with placebo. In another study, calcium dobesilate proved to be significantly better than placebo (p<0.005) in reducing the episodes of heaviness, restless legs, and paresthesia in a 28-day trial.[14]

Anderson et al.[17] found that rutosides had no effect on pain, aching, paresthesia, and itching. Rutosides, dihydroergocristine, and coumarine rutine were significantly more effective in relieving the frequency of cramps compared with placebo (p<0.05).[2,23,25]

Calcium dobesilate, dihydroergocristine, micronized diosmin, and coumarine rutine have significant effect (p<0.05) compared with placebo in relieving pain and aching. Although rutosides were not effective in relieving most of the symptoms, they were significantly better (p<0.05) than placebo for tiredness, fatigue, and tenderness.[25]

In some studies, the entire range of possible symptoms were examined and evaluated using a global rating score. Zuccarelli et al. studied the effect of ruscus asculeatus and found that the intensity of symptoms significantly decreased (p<0.05).[26] In a randomized placebo-controlled study, four different rutoside formulations (500mg, 300mg sustained release, 300mg regular release, and 1000mg in aqueous solution) were found to be equivalent, but superior to placebo, in reducing leg heaviness after 12-week follow-up of 100 women.[27] Diosmin, calcium dobesilate, and troxuretine were found to be effective in reducing edema.[14,16,28] A small randomized trial that compared rutosides and compression therapy found that compression therapy was more effective in reducing leg volume and increasing venous refill time over a 4-month follow-up.[29]

Compression

Most data on the effectiveness of compression therapy relate to patients with symptoms and varicose veins, or symptoms and venous ulcers. Four studies have assessed the effect of compression on varicose veins. Compression was assessed in combination with sclerotherapy in three studies and with surgery in one study.

In the study by Struckmann,[30] a reduction in symptoms (fullness, cramps, itching, swollen legs) was observed with stockings exerting compression at knee length (Sigavris), but not with compression at hip length (low-pressure stockings).[30]

A randomized controlled trial by Fraser and colleagues[12] (Tables 40.6 & 40.7) reported that there was greater reduction in symptoms in patients who used bandages for 6 weeks post-sclerotherapy. A 75% reduction in the symptom score was also observed with sclerotherapy and bandages, without any difference between the type and duration of bandaging. After sclerotherapy, stockings with ankle pressure of 30–40mmHg were effective in treating skin changes. Scurr et al.[19] found that, post sclerotherapy, high-pressure stockings were more effective than bandages (Table 40.8).

Although edema is one of the main indications for compression therapy, there are very few studies on its efficacy compared with no treatments; however, scientific evidence is available from studies that have used compression as an alternative treatment. In a randomized controlled trial to test the efficacy of rutosides,[17] all patients awaiting varicose vein surgery were assigned either

placebo alone, rutosides alone, hosiery with placebo, or hosiery with rutosides. Assessment of swelling using a visual analog scale (measured in millimeters) showed that hosiery alone had the greatest effect after 4 weeks of treatment. In a study by Travers et al.,[31] the use of stockings for 1 year after surgery dramatically reduced the rate of varicose vein recurrence from 61% to 12%.

Sclerotherapy

Although sclerotherapy is the preferred treatment in patients presenting with telangiectases, spider veins, and reticular veins, the scientific evidence is limited. A double-blind study by Norris et al.[18] examined the efficacy of different doses of polidocanol in 20 women with telangiectases. The outcomes were measured in terms of percentage of clearance of vessels and the percentage of improvement rated by clinicians based on photographs. No statistically significant differences were found, though polidocanol (0.5%) tended to achieve the highest success rate for each outcome.

Varicose veins without symptoms can be treated adequately with sclerotherapy for cosmetic reasons, irrespective of the presence or absence of reflux. No properly controlled study is available to assess the long-term results of this treatment. It is

Results of treatment with sclerotherapy and bandaging in the study by Fraser et al.

Compression treatment	Patient number	% Legs with varices at 6 weeks	% Legs with residual varices	% Reduction in symptom score at 6 months
crepe bandage x 6 weeks	53	12	18	74.2
cohesive bandage x 6 weeks	53	10	20	79.2
cohesive bandage x 3 days	52	14	22	79.5

Table 40.6 Results of treatment with sclerotherapy (scl) and bandaging in the study by Fraser et al.[12]

Side effects in patients treated with sclerotherapy and bandaging in the study by Fraser et al.

Compression treatment	Patient number	Phlebitis (%)	Pruritis (%)	Blisters (%)	Swollen foot (%)
crepe bandage x 6 weeks	53	29	17	13.2	0.0
cohesive bandage x 6 weeks	53	25	15.1	50.9	7.5
cohesive bandage x 3 days	52	24	3.8	36	7.5

Table 40.7 Side effects in patients treated with sclerotherapy (scl) and bandaging in the study by Fraser et al.[12]

Comparison of stockings and bandages in patients with varicose veins without saphenofemoral incompetence or very high perforators having sclerotherapy – Scurr.

Compression treatment	Patient number	% Legs all injections successful	% Successful injections	% Legs with >1 thrombosis	% Skin marking per site
high-pressure stockings	42	69.8	92.3	42.8	11.5
bandaging	42	50.0	79.6	64.8	30.6

Table 40.8 Comparison of stockings and bandages in patients with varicose veins without saphenofemoral incompetence or very high perforators having sclerotherapy (scl) – Scurr.[19]

Randomized trial of sclerotherapy or surgery in patients with symptomatic varicose veins – Einarrson.		
Percentage failed treatment	Sclerotherapy Fegan's method	Surgery
At 1 year	20	5
At 3 years	50	10
At 5 years	70	10

Table 40.9 Randomized trial of sclerotherapy or surgery in patients with symptomatic varicose veins – Einarrson.[21]

Randomized comparison of treatments in patients with primary varicose veins and long saphenous vein incompetence – Neglen's study.			
Percentage failed treatment	Compression sclerotherapy	Surgery	Sclerotherapy and surgery
At 1 year	18	3	5
At 2 years	31	7	10
At 2 years	51	5	20

Table 40.10 Randomized comparison of treatments in patients with primary varicose veins and long saphenous vein incompetence – Neglen's study.[34]

evident, however, that the results depend on the presence or absence of superficial venous insufficiency. Elastic compression is used following sclerotherapy. A number of studies have supported the use of compression following sclerotherapy but scientific evidence suggests that long-term treatment (more than 6 months) is no more effective than shorter treatment. Most of the scientific evidence for the effect of sclerotherapy on varicose veins is available in the form of studies using it in combination with compression,[12,19,32] and those comparing it with, or using it as an adjunct to, surgery.[15,33–35] Sclerotherapy was performed by Fegan's method in all of these studies bar one, where Sigg's method was used.

Sclerotherapy is an adequate treatment for non-saphenous varicose veins, local varicose veins, and varicose tributaries of the saphenous trunk without saphenous insufficiency. It is also an ideal choice for treatment of postoperative residual veins and recurrent varicosities. Duplex examination is helpful to exclude primary or recurrent saphenofemoral or saphenopopliteal incompetence in these patients.

Six clinical trials have compared sclerotherapy with surgery but these suffered from methodological problems, such as a lack of independent evaluation of the results, poorly defined outcomes, high dropout rates, and lack of intention-to-treat analyses (**Tables 40.9 & 40.10**). The results are probably biased in favor of surgery as only patients with venous disorders severe enough to justify surgery were enrolled. Keeping these limitations in mind, the results suggest that the recurrence or persistence rate of varicose veins after sclerotherapy is very high in the long term, ranging from 20% to 70%, significantly more than for surgery.

Comparative studies of surgery and sclerotherapy.				
Percentage rates	Piachaud study[20] (n=124)		Beresford study[15] (n=124)	
	Sclerotherapy (Fegan's)	Surgery	Sclerotherapy (Fegan's)	Surgery
No further treatment	78	86	51.3	59
Needed support stockings	11	9	18.3	12.1
Retreated	3	3	21.7	12.1

Table 41.11 Comparative studies of surgery and sclerotherapy.[15,20]

Beresford et al.[15] and Piachaud & Wedell[20] (**Table 40.11**) reported a similar rate of recurrence for sclerotherapy and surgery at 3 years (3%) but a significantly higher rate in the sclerotherapy group at 5 years (21.7% versus 12.1%). Better-defined indications like diameter of the saphenous vein, degree of reflux, and selection of patients with short or long saphenous veins might improve the result of sclerotherapy, but presently there is no scientific evidence to support precise selection criteria.

COSTS OF NON-SURGICAL TREATMENT

Venous disorders can be considered an important public health problem. Estimates per country have revealed that the management of venous disorders accounts for 1–3% of the total healthcare expenditure. The estimate of the total medical cost of venous disorders was more than £300million in the UK.[36] The costs in other European countries such as Germany and France are estimated to be even higher. The cost of injection sclerotherapy–compression was $100 according to the Beresford study.[15]

The actual financial burden is higher because societal costs and cosmetic products used by patients are not included in healthcare expenditure. Societal costs include loss of productivity due to absence from work, additional costs such as hired help for homemaking activities, and intangible costs. The direct medical costs per treatment were assessed by the Piachaud study[20] and the Beresford study.[15]

There are multiple areas of inadequate information in the field of chronic venous insufficiency that need to be evaluated by high-quality research. Studies into the epidemiology, cost-effectiveness of different strategies, validity of scoring systems, and diagnostic tests need to be conducted in order to extend the knowledge about this disorder. There is a need for randomized clinical trials with long-term follow-up to compare the existing therapies for chronic venous disease, i.e. sclerotherapy versus surgery for varicose veins, medication versus compression for symptoms, and conservative versus surgical therapy for venous ulcers.

SUMMARY

The only current indication for drug therapy in the management of varicose veins is in the treatment of isolated symptoms and edema of venous origin.

Sclerotherapy is the treatment of choice in telangiectasias, spider veins, and isolated reticular veins. Sclerotherapy is also the preferred treatment for non-saphenous varicose veins, and recurrent or residual veins after surgery without evidence of venous reflux, though retreatment is often necessary to ensure long-term benefit. The use of duplex imaging and foam-guided sclerosants has the potential to expand the use of sclerotherapy in the next decade.

Compression therapy is recommended after surgery and sclerotherapy, to maintain results and reduce recurrences, and is effective in treating skin changes caused by venous disorders.

REFERENCES

1. Rudofsky G. Intravenous prostaglandin E1 in the treatment of venous ulcers – a double blind, placebo controlled trial. Vasa Suppl 1989; 28:39–43.

2. Lambelet F. Treatment of circulatory venous diseases: double-blind study with Sandovene. Schweizerische Rundschau fur Medizin Praxis 1973;62:925–9.

3. Vayssairat M. Placebo-controlled trial of naftazone in women with primary uncomplicated symptomatic varicose veins. Phlebology 1997; 12:17–20.

4. Consensus conference on sclerotherapy of varicose veins of the lower limbs. Phlebology 1997;12:2–160.

5. Goldman MP. Sclerotherapy. Treatment of varicose and telengiectatic leg veins, 2nd edn. St Louis:Mosby Year Book; 1995.

6. Orbach EJ. Sclerotherapy of varicose veins: utilization of intravenous airblock. Am J Surg 1974;66:362.

7. Orbach EJ. Controversies and realities for therapy for varicose veins. Int Surg 1977;62:149–51.

8. Fegan WG. Varicose veins: compression sclerotherapy. London: Heinemann; 1967.

9. Fegan WG. Continuous compression technique for injecting varicose veins. Lancet 1963;2:109.

10. Tournay R. In which way is it practical to sclerose: from top to bottom? from bottom to top? Phlebologie 1976;29:203–4.

11. Sigg K. Treatment of varicose veins by injection sclerotherapy as practiced in Basle. In: Hobbs JT, ed. Treatment of venous disorders in the lower limb. Lancaster:MTP Press; 1976.

12. Fraser IA, Perry EP, Hatton M, Watkin DFL. Prolonged bandaging is not required following sclerotherapy of varicose veins. Br J Surg 1985; 72:488–90.

13. Orbach EJ. The place of injection therapy in the treatment of venous disorders of the lower extremity with comments on its technique. Angiology 1965;20:1607–12.

14. Widmer L, Biland L, Barras JP. Doxium 500 in chronic venous insufficiency: a double-blind placebo controlled multicentre study Int Angiol 1990;9:105–10.

15. Beresford SAA, Chant ADB, Jones HO, Piachaud D, Weddell JM. Varicose veins: a comparison of surgery and injection/compression sclerotherapy. Five-year follow-up. Lancet 1978;1:921–4.

16. Laurent R, Gilly R, Frileux R. Clinical evaluation of a venotropic drug in man. Example of micronized diosmin 500 mg. Int Angiol 1988; 7:39–43.

17. Anderson JH, Geraghty JG, Wilson YT, et al. Paroven and graduated compression hosiery for superficial venous insufficiency. Phlebology 1990;5:271–6.

18. Norris MJ, Cralin MC, Ratz JL. Treatment of essential telangiectasia: effects of increasing concentrations of polidocanol. J Am Acad Dermatol 1989;20:643–9.

19. Scurr JH, Coleridge-Smith P, Cutting P. Varicose veins: optimum compression following sclerotherapy. Ann R Coll Surg Engl 1985; 67:109–11.

20. Piachaud D, Weddell JM. The economics of treating varicose veins. Int J Epidemiol 1972;1:287–94.

21. Einarsson E, Eklof B, Neglen P. Sclerotherapy or surgery as treatment for varicose veins: a prospective randomized study. Phlebology 1993; 8:22–6.

22. Lentner A, Spath F, Weinert V. Limitation of movement in the ankle and talo-calcaneonavicular joints caused by compression bandages. Phlebology 1997;12:25–30.

23. Zuccarelli F. Effacite clinique et tolerance de la coumarine rutine. Etude controlee en double aveungle versus placebo. La Gazette Medicale 1987;94:1–7.

24. Languillat N, Vecchiali JF, Zuccarelli F, Bouxin A. Essai en double aveungle contre placebo des effets du Vasobral dans les troubels de la permeabilite capillaire lies a l'insuffisance veineuse par le test isotopique de Landis. Angiologie 1986;39:1–4.

25. Prerovsky I, Roztocil K, Hlavova A, et al. The effect of hydroxyethylrutosides after acute and chronic oral administration in patients with venous diseases. A double blind study. Angiologica 1972;9:408–14.

26. Zuccarelli F, Benedetti F, Houdot-Roque H, et al. Activite de Veinobiase sur les troubles fonctionnels de l'insuffisance veineuse dus a l'ortostatisme professionnel. Angiologie 1988;84:3–7.

27. Rehn D, Unkauf M, Klein P, Jost V, Lucker PW. Comparative clinical efficacy and tolerability of oxerutins and horse chestnut extract in patients with chronic venous insufficiency. Arzneimittel-Forschung 1996;46:483–7.

28. Vin F, Chabanal A, Taccoen A, Ducros J. Double-blind trial of the efficacy of troxerutin in chronic venous insufficiency. Phlebology 1994; 9:71–76.

29. Neumann H, van den Broek M. A comparative clinical trial of graduated compression stockings and O-(beta-hydroxyethyl)rutosides in the treatment of patients with chronic venous insufficiency. Phlebology 1995;24:78–81.

30. Struckmann J. Compression stockings and their effect on the venous pump – a comparative study. Phlebology 1986;1:37–45.

31. Travers JP, Makin GS. Reduction of varicose vein recurrence by use of post-operative compression stockings. Phlebology 1994;9:104–7.

32. Batch AJG, Wickeremesinghe SS, Gannon ME, Dormandy JA. Randomised trial of bandaging after sclerotherapy for varicose veins. BMJ 1980;281:423.

33. Jacobson BH. The value of different forms of treatment for varicose veins. Br J Surg 1979;66:182–4.

34. Neglen P, Einarsson E, Eklof B. The functional long term value of different types of treatment for saphenous vein incompetence. J Cardiovasc Surg 1993;34:295–301.

35. Doran FSA, White M. A clinical trial designed to discover if the primary treatment for varicose veins should be by Fegan's method or by an operation. Br J Surg 1975;62:72–6.

36. Laing W. Chronic venous diseases of the leg. London: Office of Health Economics; 1992:1–44.

CHAPTER 41

Surgical Treatment of Chronic Venous Insufficiency

Manju Kalra and Peter Gloviczki

KEY POINTS

- Chronic venous insufficiency (CVI) includes a wide variety of venous disorders, from varicose veins to venous ulceration. Primary valvular incompetence accounts for approximately 70% of cases of advanced CVI (Class 4–6), the remainder follow deep vein thrombosis.

- A complete anatomic and physiologic evaluation of the venous system is important and aids surgical intervention. Duplex ultrasound examination is sufficient in patients with varicose veins alone, plethysmography is used to evaluate patients with advanced CVI and venography is reserved for patients being considered for operative procedures on the deep venous system.

- The aim of surgery for CVI is to remove unsightly varicose veins, prevent recurrence of varicosities and treat signs and symptoms of chronic venous disease, such as venous claudication, limb swelling, eczema, pain and ulceration. Surgery is individualized, based on the results of investigation of the venous system.

- Ablation of superficial reflux is performed most effectively by high ligation and stripping of the incompetent portion of the saphenous vein, usually from the groin to the knee, using the inversion technique. Endovenous obliteration by radiofrequency/laser ablation techniques is gaining popularity due to the shorter postoperative recovery, however, long-term results are awaited.

- Subfascial endoscopic perforator vein surgery (SEPS) is now the preferred method of interrupting incompetent perforator veins. Patients with advanced CVI and perforator incompetence due to primary valvular incompetence benefit most from SEPS. Results in patients with postthrombotic syndrome are poor.

- Deep vein valve reconstructions continue to be challenging and rarely performed, however, good clinical outcome is reported in as many as 80% of patients selected for direct valve reconstruction. Results of vein transplantation or transposition are less obvious; benefit has been reported in 50% of patients.

- Endovascular treatment with venous stents is now the first option for treating deep venous obstruction, if technically feasible. The Palma procedure remains the best open surgical technique for autologous reconstruction; femoro-iliac and femoro-caval bypass grafts should be reserved for patients with severe lifestyle limiting symptoms and significant disability.

INTRODUCTION

The term chronic venous insufficiency (CVI) includes a wide variety of disorders and diseases of the venous circulation of the legs, from varicose veins to venous ulceration. Varicose veins are one of the most prevalent of medical disorders, affecting close to 40 million Americans, women almost twice as often as men.[1] CVI with advanced skin changes and ulcers affects approximately 2% (0.5–3%) of the population in Western countries, with a prevalence comparable to that of diabetes.[2] Venous ulcers are the most common form of leg ulcer, and their incidence has remained unchanged over the last 20 years. The cost to healthcare systems of chronic venous disease is massive: 5% of patients lose their jobs as a result of the disease, 4.6 million work days are missed each year in the US due to venous disease, and in the UK, 2% of the national healthcare budget (US$1 billion) is spent each year on the management of leg ulcers alone.[3]

GOALS OF SURGICAL TREATMENT

Surgical treatment of CVI is aimed at removing unsightly varicose veins, preventing recurrence of varicosities, and treating of signs and symptoms of chronic venous disease, such as venous claudication, limb swelling, eczema, pain, and ulceration (**Fig. 41.1**).

The main goal of surgical treatment of advanced disease is to correct the underlying abnormal venous physiology. Chapter 39 discussed in detail the pathophysiology of CVI. Surgical correction of the abnormal ambulatory venous pressure aims to achieve lasting relief of symptoms. The relationship between venous ulceration and ambulatory venous pressure was described by Beecher and colleagues as early as 1931. Subsequent studies have confirmed that ambulatory venous pressure has not only diagnostic but also prognostic significance in CVI.[4] Reflux caused by valvular incompetence is predominantly responsible for high ambulatory venous pressures in CVI. The CEAP classification[5,6] listed the three etiologies of CVI – congenital, primary, and secondary. Primary valvular incompetence (PVI) may involve the superficial, perforator, and deep veins, while secondary incompetence is frequently limited to the deep and perforating veins. Primary incompetence is diagnosed in the absence of documented deep venous thrombosis (DVT) by history or evidence of postthrombotic changes in the deep veins on duplex examination or incompetence on venography. Secondary incompetence occurs following one or more episodes of DVT. Deep venous obstruction secondary to DVT is a less frequent cause of advanced CVI (fewer than 10% of cases), resulting more often in leg swelling and venous claudication.[7] A rare combination of iliac vein obstruction and reflux below the common femoral vein in a

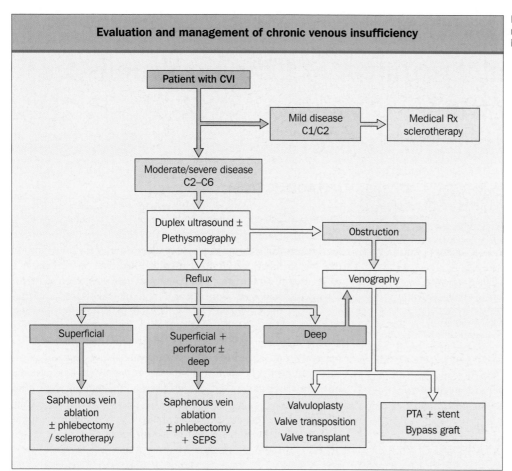

Figure 41.1 Evaluation and management of chronic venous insufficiency.

Distribution of valvular incompetence in patients with advanced chronic venous.						
Author, Year	No. of legs	Sup No. (%)	Perf No. (%)	Deep No. (%)	Sup+Perf No. (%)	Sup+Perf+Deep No. (%)
Schanzer,[99] 1982	52	3 (6)	20 (38)	4 (8)	11 (21)	14 (27)
Negus,[100] 1983	77	0 (0)	0 (0)	0 (0)	35 (46)	42 (54)
Sethia,[101] 1984	60	0 (0)	5 (8)	20 (33)	17 (28)	18 (30)
van Bemmelen,[102] 1991	25	0 (0)	0 (0)	2 (8)	3 (12)	20 (80)
Hanrahan,[103] 1991	91	16 (17)	8 (8)	2 (2)	18 (19)	47 (49)
Darke,[104] 1992	213	0 (0)	8 (4)	47 (22)	83 (39)	75 (35)
Lees,[105] 1993	25	3 (12)	0 (0)	3 (12)	10 (40)	9 (36)
Shami,[106] 1993	59	0 (0)	0 (0)	19 (32)	31 (53)	9 (15)
van Rij,[107] 1994	120	48 (40)	6 (5)	10 (8)	31 (26)	25 (21)
Myers,[13] 1995	96	15 (16)	2 (2)	7 (8)	25 (26)	47 (49)
Labropoulos,[11] 1996	120	26 (22)	1 (1)	5 (4)	23 (19)	65 (54)
Gloviczki,[8] 1999	146	0 (0)	7 (5)	0 (0)	66 (45)	73 (50)
Total no. of legs (%)	**1084**	**111 (10)**	**57 (5)**	**119 (11)**	**353 (32)**	**444 (41)**

Table 41.1 Distribution of valvular incompetence in patients with advanced chronic venous disease. Deep, deep vein incompetence; Perf, perforator incompetence; Sup, superficial incompetence.

post-thrombotic limb results in a complex lesion with severe consequences.

PVI accounts for approximately 70% of advanced CVI (class 4–6); the remainder occurs in legs following DVT.[8,9] Severe isolated incompetence of the superficial system may also lead to high ambulatory pressures and the development of ulcers, but evidence is increasing that the majority of patients with a venous ulcer have multisystem (superficial, deep, and/or perforator) incompetence, involving at least two of the three venous systems of the leg.[10,11] A duplex ultrasound study of 91 legs with venous ulceration from Boston University revealed isolated superficial vein incompetence in only 17% of legs.[12] Incompetent calf perforators, in conjunction with superficial or deep reflux, have been reported in 66% of legs with venous ulceration, and they occur more frequently in legs with advanced disease and skin changes.[13] Deep venous incompetence occurs in up to 80% of patients with a venous ulcer (**Table 41.1**).[10,13]

PREOPERATIVE EVALUATION

The initial evaluation of a patient with CVI is clinical examination supplemented by a hand-held continuous-wave Doppler examination. The extent of further investigation and treatment planning is dictated by the severity of the clinical stage of chronic venous disease as assessed by the CEAP classification and the degree to which the patient is willing to accept a change in lifestyle. In the event of spider veins or telangiectasias (Class 1) causing only cosmetic concerns, and no reflux on clinical or continuous-wave Doppler examination, no further investigation is necessary. If reflux is suspected clinically, a duplex ultrasound is warranted. Patients with varicose veins alone (Class 2) and those with moderate or advanced CVI (Class 3–6) who are potential candidates for surgery require consideration for a complete workup in the vascular laboratory. Patients who are not surgical candidates because of advanced age or multiple co-morbidities and who will only be offered conservative treatment do not require further investigation. Non-invasive investigation begins with duplex examination, which is all that is required in patients with varicose veins with no edema or skin changes (Class 2). Plethysmography may be useful to evaluate the impact of the anatomic abnormalities found on duplex on the pathophysiology of the venous system. At this stage it is possible to complete the remaining elements of the CEAP classification and provide a comprehensive description of the patient's venous problem (clinical, etiologic, anatomic, and pathophysiologic). The CEAP classification provides description of venous disease in a uniform, reproducible language, and allows an objective evaluation of the effect of treatment and comparison of treatment modalities across centers. With the level of sophistication of present-day duplex imaging, contrast venography is rarely indicated. Contrast venography is helpful in patients with suspected significant deep venous obstruction, and in those who may undergo treatment for deep vein valvular incompetence.

Duplex imaging

Duplex imaging, which combines B-mode imaging, color-flow, and pulsed Doppler, is the single most valuable test in the evaluation of venous disease. Direct visualization provides information on the patency and wall characteristics of each venous segment and the morphology of the valves. Systematic interrogation of the superficial, deep, and perforator systems provides an anatomic map of the veins of the leg. It helps determine whether obstruction, reflux, or a combination of the two is responsible for causing the symptoms and signs of CVI. In most patients it is possible to differentiate primary venous incompetence from post-thrombotic syndrome on duplex imaging. The presence and site of valvular incompetence is identified by documenting retrograde flow on the Valsalva maneuver, or release of a distal tourniquet with the patient in the standing position. Retrograde flow that lasts longer than 0.5s or the duration of antegrade flow signifies valvular incompetence.[14] Perforator veins are identified visually and incompetence confirmed by bidirectional flow on manual calf compression. Candidates for subfascial endoscopic perforator surgery (SEPS) and complex varicose vein surgery should have the sites of incompetent perforators and incompetent junctions marked on the skin the day before surgery. Duplex examination can provide qualitative information about the anatomic presence of obstruction or reflux; however, it cannot quantitate it or assess its hemodynamic significance.

Plethysmography

Duplex imaging identifies the presence and location of reflux or obstruction in the venous system, but plethysmography is required to quantify the pathophysiologic abnormality. Various plethysmographic techniques (air, strain gauge, impedence) quantify the degree of reflux, obstruction, or calf muscle dysfunction by measuring a change in calf volume on various maneuvers. Venous outflow obstruction is assessed by determining the *outflow fraction*, which is the venous outflow volume in 1s divided by the total calf volume. Valvular reflux is measured by estimating the *venous filling index*; the rate required to refill 90% of venous volume. Calf muscle pump function is assessed by measuring the *ejection fraction* and the *residual volume fraction* of calf venous volume following calf muscle contraction. However, these techniques provide global information about the hemodynamics of the entire leg without the ability to localize the abnormality. Plethysmography is especially useful in patients in whom both reflux and partial obstruction are elicited on duplex imaging, where it helps identify the dominant pathology. Repeated plethysmographic examination can be used to monitor the progression of venous disease as well as the response to surgical treatment.

Venography

Ascending venography is performed in the semi-erect, non-weight-bearing position by injecting intravenous contrast into a dorsal foot vein after placing a tourniquet at the ankle to prevent filling of the superficial veins. Anatomy of the calf and thigh veins is demonstrated accurately, obstructed segments and collaterals readily visualized, and the presence and site of incompetent perforators can be identified. It is the best available test to differentiate between PVI and post-thrombotic syndrome and remains the 'gold standard' for obtaining a visual map of the extremity veins prior to deep venous reconstruction.

Descending venography is necessary to identify the location of venous valves and evaluate their degree of incompetence prior to venous valve reconstruction. Contrast is injected into the external iliac vein via a catheter inserted through the contralateral groin and images are recorded on videotape, with and without Valsalva maneuver. The severity of venous reflux can be classified according to Kistner's grades 0 to 4 (**Table 41.2**).[15] Patients with

Kistner's grades.	
Grade	Severity of reflux
0	No incompetence
1	Reflux into the proximal femoral vein
2	Reflux limited to the thigh
3	Reflux into the popliteal vein and proximal calf
4	Reflux to the distal calf or ankle

Table 41.2 Kistner's grades of venous reflux on descending veinography.

reflux extending below the knee are suitable candidates for venous valve reconstruction or transplantation. Descending venography alone may fail to demonstrate significant femoral or popliteal reflux in the presence of a competent common femoral vein valve.

Ambulatory venous pressure measurement

Rarely performed these days in its original form, ambulatory venous pressure (AVP) measurement provides an objective assessment of venous hemodynamics and the degree of CVI. It is performed by cannulation of a dorsal foot vein and measurement of pressure in the standing position before, during, and after ten tiptoe exercises. Normal AVP ranges from 20 to 30mmHg, or a greater than 50% decrease from resting state, which is usually 80 to 90mmHg. A refill time of greater than 20s is considered normal. With the availability of non-invasive venous testing such as duplex imaging and plethysmographic techniques, the clinical application of AVP measurement, still considered by some to be the 'gold standard', has diminished.

Direct cannulation of the femoral vein to measure the pressure gradient across an iliac lesion is done routinely, however, to assess the hemodynamic significance of proximal venous occlusions. A femoral–central venous pressure gradient of 5mmHg or a twofold increase following foot exercise suggests a hemodynamically significant venous obstruction.

SURGICAL TREATMENT

Surgical treatment aims to alleviate symptoms of CVI and promote ulcer healing by reducing ambulatory venous hypertension. It needs to be individualized for each patient based on the results of non-invasive and invasive investigation of the venous system as described above. Depending on the underlying pathophysiology in a particular patient, this may be achieved by:

Ablation of superficial reflux
(a) ablation of saphenous vein reflux
(b) removal of varicose veins (phlebectomy)
Ablation of perforator vein reflux
Ablation of deep venous reflux
Treatment of deep venous obstruction.

Ablation of saphenous vein reflux
Indications
Ablation of gravitational reflux in the great/small saphenous vein is indicated in patients with varicose veins (Class 2) in whom

reflux at the saphenofemoral or saphenopopliteal junction has been identified on duplex imaging. Saphenofemoral reflux occurs in 70% of patients with varicose veins; atypical reflux at other sites or varicosities without gravitational reflux account for the remainder. Surgical or endovenous ablation of great saphenous vein (GSV) reflux is helpful in patients with advanced CVI (10%) if the deep system is patent. Ablation of superficial reflux may be performed by high ligation and stripping of the saphenous vein, high ligation alone, or by radiofrequency or laser ablation of the saphenous vein. Occlusion by coil embolization has also been reported and Chapter 40 discusses duplex-guided sclerotherapy as an option for saphenous reflux ablation.

Saphenous vein ligation and stripping
High ligation of the GSV with stripping has been practiced widely and remains the 'gold standard' against which other less invasive procedures need to be compared. Stripping of the saphenous vein in present-day practice has been limited to the thigh because this eliminates gravitational reflux which usually extends only to the knee, disconnects thigh perforators, and reduces the incidence of saphenous nerve injury associated with stripping of the below-knee segment. Below-knee calf perforators are not connected directly to the saphenous vein, so no real advantage exists in stripping the vein to the ankle. Occasionally when there is gross dilatation of the below-knee segment of the long saphenous vein with reflux on duplex, stripping may be extended to the ankle. This segment is usually stripped with the much less traumatic inversion technique. The procedure is supplemented with stab avulsion of branch varicosities.

High ligation and stripping of the great saphenous vein
High ligation of the GSV is performed through a short (2–3cm) oblique incision in the groin crease medial to the femoral pulse. The saphenofemoral junction is identified, as are all tributaries (named and unnamed). The tributaries are dissected out as far as possible and ligated, followed by flush ligation of the saphenous vein, taking care not to impinge upon the underlying femoral vein. A flexible, disposable (Codman) vein stripper is next introduced into the cut end of the vein at the groin and passed to the level of the skin crease at the knee. The saphenous vein is exposed at this level at the medial aspect of the popliteal space, the stripper is pulled through, and the distal end ligated. The vein is ligated around the stripper with a strong, non-absorbable suture which is left long and the stripper is inverted into the saphenous vein (**Fig. 41.2**). The vein is stripped from above downwards and the inverted vein is delivered through the knee incision. Hemorrhage in the tract of the stripped vein is controlled by leg elevation, external pressure, and by infiltrating the subcutaneous tissue around the saphenous vein with a tumescent solution of dilute lidocaine and epinephrine before stripping. If indicated, concomitant stab avulsion of varicosities are performed prior to stripping of the vein, so that the leg can be elevated and wrapped in an elastic bandage immediately after stripping the vein. The incisions for the stripping are closed with absorbable sutures and those for stab avulsion with Steri-Strips®. The operation is an outpatient procedure and the patient is permitted to walk the same evening.

To avoid stripping and its associated potential complications of nerve injury, pain, and hematoma, high ligation alone was proposed to remove gravitational reflux while preserving the

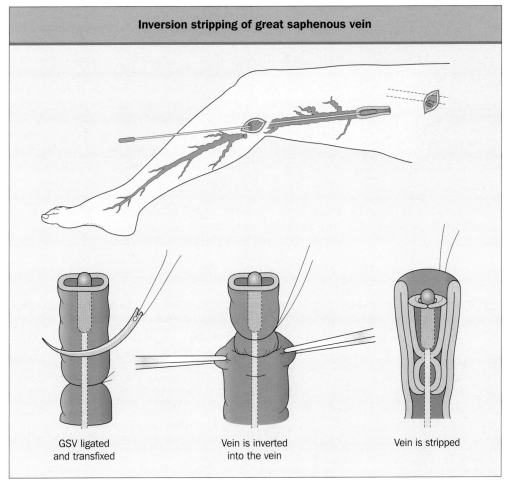

Inversion stripping of great saphenous vein

GSV ligated
and transfixed

Vein is inverted
into the vein

Vein is stripped

Figure 41.2 Inversion stripping of great saphenous vein (GSV).
Left inset: GSV is ligated with a heavy tie and a transfixing suture is placed around the vein and the stripper. Middle inset: the vein is inverted into the vein by applying tension around the outer wall of the vein. Left inset: the vein is completely inverted and stripped.

vein. However, reflux has been shown to persist following high ligation alone and recurrence of varicose veins is more frequent than that observed after high ligation with stripping.[16,17] Persistent patency of the GSV with continued reflux is frequently associated with recurrent varicose veins.[18,19]

Ligation and stripping of the small saphenous vein

Stripping of the small saphenous vein (SSV) is performed in a similar manner, keeping in mind that anatomic variations of the saphenopopliteal junction are frequent. In 42% of subjects, the vein terminates within 5cm of the knee-joint crease, this being the only termination. It may, however, terminate higher in the thigh in the femoropopliteal vein, in the vein of Giacomini (12%), or in other unnamed subcutaneous and perforator veins. This anomalous drainage may coexist with a normal saphenopopliteal junction in 50% of patients. Because of this variability in the anatomy of the SSV, it is prudent to mark the saphenopopliteal junction on the skin if the duplex ultrasound is performed immediately before the operation.

Unless otherwise marked, the procedure is performed through a small transverse incision in the middle of the popliteal fossa with the patient in the prone position. The stripper is inserted in a retrograde fashion and damage to the sural nerve is avoided by identifying the distal end of the vein with the stripper and carefully separating it from the nerve. Reflux in the SSV is commonly segmental, so the distal segment at the ankle can frequently be spared from stripping.

Radiofrequency ablation of the saphenous vein

In this era of minimally invasive surgery, it is not surprising that alternative, less traumatic methods of saphenous vein ablation are being investigated. Better cosmetic results and an earlier return to full activity make these endoluminal options more appealing to the majority of patients with Class 2 varicose veins only. The concept of vein obliteration by endoluminal means is not new: attempts at electrocoagulation of blood in the saphenous vein with subsequent occlusion of the vein were reported nearly 40 years ago. However, recanalization of thrombus with renewed patency of the vein precluded long-term success and enthusiasm for the procedure faded. The latest innovations employ either radiofrequency energy-mediated heating of the vein wall to destroy the intima and denature collagen in the media, with resulting fibrous occlusion of the vein, or laser energy for the same purpose. Considerable experience already exists with radiofrequency ablation. The Closure® radiofrequency catheter (VNUS Medical Technologies Inc., Sunnyvale, CA, USA) was studied first in Europe and approved by the Food and Drug Administration (FDA) in 1999 (**Fig. 41.3**). The vein wall temperature is chosen and set, usually at 85°C. The heating is controlled by monitoring temperature and impedance of the vein wall via a feedback system (**Fig. 41.4**). Direct heating of the vein occurs to a depth of 1mm at the site of contact with the catheter, with further heating of the deeper vein wall occurring by conduction. The catheter provides 6–8mm-wide rings of resistive heating of the vein wall.

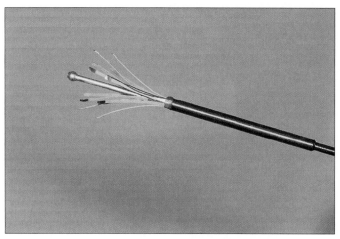

Figure 41.3 Closure catheter with electrodes unsheathed.

Procedure

The Closure® system consists of a bipolar heat generator and collapsible catheter electrodes suitable for use in veins ranging from 2 to 12mm in diameter. The procedure is usually performed under conscious sedation and local anesthesia in an outpatient setting. The catheter is usually introduced into the saphenous vein at the knee (or at the ankle) percutaneously under ultrasound guidance, or through a small incision and direct exposure of the vein. The position of the catheter at the saphenofemoral junction is confirmed by ultrasound or fluoroscopy, and obliteration proceeds in a retrograde fashion (**Fig. 41.5**). Alternatively, with groin puncture, the catheter tip is positioned at the knee and withdrawn antegradely. The vein is obliterated only to the level of the knee to avoid injury to the saphenous nerve. Local tumescent anesthetic is instilled in the subcutaneous tissues around the vein under ultrasound guidance, to prevent skin

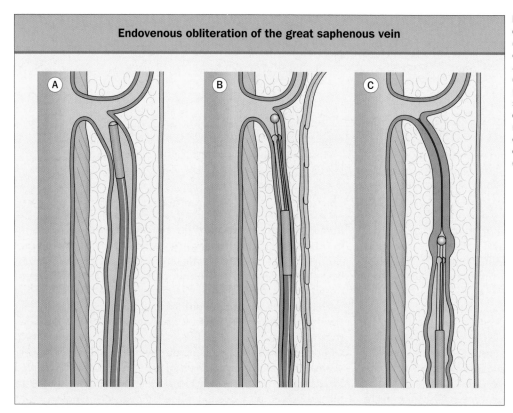

Endovenous obliteration of the great saphenous vein

Figure 41.4 Endovenous obliteration of the great saphenous vein.
(A) Closure catheter introduced with electrodes sheathed and tip positioned at the saphenofemoral junction.
(B) Electrodes unsheathed while position of catheter maintained at the saphenofemoral junction. (C) Circuit completed, temperature allowed to reach 85°C, and graduated withdrawal of the catheter as radiofrequency energy heats and contracts vein wall. (From VNUS with permission.)

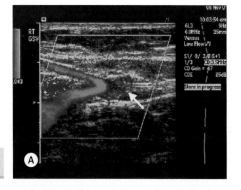

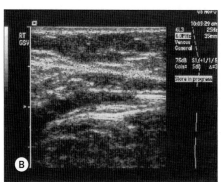

Figure 41.5 Endovenous obliteration of the great saphenous vein, under ultrasound guidance. (A) Closure catheter introduced with electrodes sheathed and tip positioned at the saphenofemoral junction (arrow). (B) Withdrawal of the catheter along length of saphenous vein begun after vein wall temperature has equilibrated at 85°C.

burns from conducted heat. The leg is elevated and wrapped with an Esmarch bandage to empty the vein and provide contact of the catheter with the vein wall. Additional compression is applied at the saphenofemoral junction to prevent reflux of blood into the vein. The electrodes are unsheathed and heparinized saline is flushed continuously through the lumen of the catheter to prevent thrombus forming on the electrodes. The vein wall temperature is allowed to equilibrate at 85°C after turning on the circuit and graduated withdrawal of the catheter is performed at a rate of 3cm/min. Vein wall impedance and the amount of energy delivered are monitored continuously. At the end of the procedure, the compression wrap is removed and obliteration of the entire length of the vein is confirmed by ultrasound. Segments not completely occluded are retreated.

Stab avulsion of varicosities (ambulatory phlebectomy)

Stab avulsions of varicosities are performed through 1–2mm incisions overlying the vein clusters marked preoperatively with the patient in the standing position. These incisions are oriented vertically to minimize injury to lymphatic channels, except at the knee or ankle, where they are placed transversely in the skin creases. The incision is deepened through the epidermis and dermis and the varicose vein is grasped with a crochet or Muller hook. It is delivered through the incision, grasped with a mosquito clamp, extracted gradually, and avulsed. As much length of vein as possible is harvested through each incision and incisions are placed as far apart as possible. Small (1–2mm) incisions are closed with Steri-Strips® and the larger ones with a single, inverted absorbable suture. A compression bandage is applied at the end of the procedure.

Power suction phlebectomy is a new, minimally invasive technique of varicosity removal that employs pulverization of the varicose vein clusters with a motorized blade and concomitant suction removal. Tumescent local anesthesia is instilled in the entire area of the varicosities. The TriVex device (Smith & Nephew, Andover, MA, USA) includes a transillumination probe inserted into a plane deep to the veins to guide accurate maneuvering of the extractor probe. This probe consists of a motorized blade with a lateral cutting edge and a distal blunt tip ensheathed within a tube. Suction draws the vein into the cutting window of the blade and removes the pulverized vein through the inner channel. The control unit allows adjustment of the level of suction and blade movement, as well as simultaneous irrigation with anesthetic solution. It is important to keep the subcutaneous space well instilled with fluid to avoid extravasation of blood with postoperative bruising. Bruising, paresthesias, and ankle swelling were seen during early experience with the technique.

Results of superficial reflux ablation

Stripping of the GSV to the level of the knee accompanied by high ligation and interruption of all tributaries in the groin is the most accepted surgical method of ablating superficial reflux. Stripping of longer segments increases morbidity, especially the incidence of saphenous neuralgia, without improving recurrence rates.[20] Compared with stripping of the GSV, high ligation alone is associated with recurrent varicose veins due to the inability of this operation to eradicate axial reflux.[16,21] In the majority of ligation procedures, the saphenous vein remains patent in its entirety or segmentally, being fed by connecting thigh perforator veins. The superior long-term outcome of stripping over high

ligation, sclerotherapy, and a combination of the two has been confirmed in prospective, randomized trials.[22–24] At a mean follow-up of 3 to 5 years, 71% to 90% of patients who had GSV stripping had functional improvement, which was also supported by improved hemodynamic parameters. The most frequent complication of saphenous vein stripping is saphenous neuralgia, which may occur in 4–8% of patients. Hematoma, cellulitis, edema, or thrombophlebitis can also occur in the residual thrombosed superficial veins. DVT or pulmonary embolism is very rare. Recurrent varicose veins develop in up to 25% of patients on long-term follow-up; the incidence increases with length of follow-up. A second, previously unrecognized saphenous system or inadequate ligation of the saphenous tributaries accounts for most failures. The significance of removing all tributaries in the groin during saphenofemoral disconnection out to primary or even secondary branches was emphasized by Ruckley's study of 128 legs with recurrent varicose veins, which identified a residual inguinal network as an important cause of recurrence.[18]

The Closure® technique of radiofrequency ablation is well tolerated, with minimal short- and long-term morbidity. Skin burns and paresthesias noted in the initial learning phase of experience with the technique are now rare. Early return to full activity is the norm and in one study 98% of patients expressed satisfaction with the procedure on a 6-month follow-up survey.[25] In the same study, which included 140 legs in 120 patients, complete obliteration of the GSV was achieved in 137 legs as documented on duplex ultrasound at 1 week, and in 19 of 21 patients followed out to 24 months. Short-term results are available from the VNUS Closure Registry.[26,27] Here, 319 legs from 286 patients with GSV trunkal reflux in veins less than 12mm diameter, enrolled from 31 centers in Europe, Australia, and the US, were treated. Partial or complete recanalization in veins initially treated successfully occurred in 14.3% of legs by 6 months, and in 12% of legs in the group of 107 patients followed out to 12 months. However, in spite of recanalization, 94% of veins had no demonstrable reflux on duplex imaging at 12 months. The Closure® technique violates one of the basic principles of the treatment of superficial reflux, namely high ligation. Early radiofrequency procedures were accompanied by high ligation; however, subsequently, users of the technique have omitted the procedure.

Neovascularization in the groin has been cited as another cause of recurrent saphenofemoral reflux. It is associated with a persistently patent GSV and occurs more frequently following high ligation (52%) than after high ligation and stripping (23%).[28] Proponents of radiofrequency ablation attribute this neovascularization to post-surgical scarring. However, the rate of saphenofemoral reflux at 6 months following radiofrequency ablation with high ligation was 2%, as compared with 8% in patients undergoing radiofrequency ablation alone in the same center.[29] A recent randomized study compared endovenous radiofrequency saphenous vein obliteration (Closure System, VNUS Medical Technologies Inc., Sunnyvale, CA, USA) with the conventional stripping operation in terms of short-term recovery and costs in 28 patients.[30] Complication rates were similar in both groups, but postoperative pain was significantly reduced after endovenous obliteration; absence from work was also shorter and physical function was restored faster. Radiofrequency ablation may be cost-saving for society because of shorter convalescence,[30] but the total number of patients treated remains small and follow-up is inadequate at present to make valid conclusions about the efficacy of this technique.

Perforator vein interruption
Anatomy of perforating veins

Perforating veins connect the superficial to the deep venous system, either directly to the main axial veins (direct perforators), or indirectly to muscular tributaries or soleal venous sinuses (indirect perforators). In calf and thigh perforators, venous valves assure unidirectional flow, from the great and small saphenous systems towards the deep veins. Perforating veins of the foot, in contrast, are valveless and flow occurs paradoxically from the deep to the superficial venous system.[31,32]

The most significant medial calf perforators, termed the Cockett perforators, do not originate from the GSV but connect the posterior arch vein (Leonardo's vein) to the paired posterior tibial veins (**Fig. 41.6**). Thus, stripping of the GSV will not affect flow through these perforators. Three groups of Cockett perforators have been identified. The Cockett I perforator is located posterior to the medial malleolus and may be difficult to reach endoscopically. The Cockett II and III perforators are located 7–9cm and 10–12cm proximal to the lower border of the medial malleolus, respectively (**Fig. 41.7**).[31] All are found in 'Linton's line', 2–4cm posterior to the medial edge of the tibia.[32] The paratibial perforators connect the GSV and its tributaries to the posterior tibial and popliteal veins. They are found in three groups – all 1–2cm posterior to the medial tibial border – located 18–22cm, 23–27cm, and 28–32cm from the inferior border of the medial malleolus, respectively. There are three additional direct perforating veins that connect the GSV to the popliteal and femoral veins: Boyd's perforator, just distal to the knee, and Dodd's and Hunterian perforators in the thigh. Boyd's perforator may be reached endoscopically, while stripping of the GSV will interrupt the drainage of Dodd's and Hunterian perforators, except in the 8% of patients with a duplicated saphenous system. Only 63% of all medial perforators are directly accessible from the superficial posterior compartment.[31] In order to interrupt all incompetent perforating veins, two additional areas require exploration; the deep posterior compartment and the inter-muscular septum in Linton's line. In the calf, anterior and lateral perforators are also found and may gain clinical significance in patients with lateral ulceration. The anterior perforators connect tributaries of the GSV and SSV directly to the anterior tibial veins. The lateral perforating veins connect the SSV to the peroneal veins (Bassi's perforator).

Indications

The contribution of incompetent perforators to the hemodynamic abnormality in legs with CVI remains a topic of debate. Skin changes and venous ulcers almost always develop in the gaiter area of the leg (the area between the distal edge of the soleus muscle and the ankle), where large incompetent medial perforating veins are located. Direct estimation of the hemodynamic significance of incompetent perforators is difficult, since isolated perforator vein incompetence in CVI is rare,[11] and because incompetent perforators have been observed in as many as 21% of normal legs. Several authors have demonstrated a correlation between the number and size of incompetent perforating veins, detected by duplex ultrasonography, and the severity of CVI.[33] Recently, Delis et al. quantified perforator incompetence based

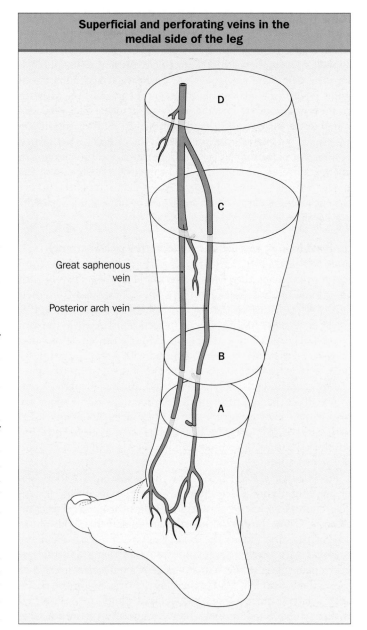

Superficial and perforating veins in the medial side of the leg

Great saphenous vein

Posterior arch vein

Figure 41.6 Superficial and perforating veins in the medial side of the leg. (From Mozes G, et al. Surgical anatomy for endoscopic subfascial division of perforating veins. J Vasc Surg 1996;24:800–8.)

on diameter, flow velocity, and volume flow. They stressed that incompetent perforators sustain further hemodynamic impairment in the presence of deep reflux.[34]

The presence of incompetent perforators in patients with advanced CVI is the indication for perforator ligation. While most authors prefer to perform open perforator ligation only after ulcers have healed, a clean, granulating open ulcer is not a contraindication for the SEPS procedure. Contraindications include morbid obesity, extensive skin change, circumferentially large ulcers, recent DVT, popliteal vein occlusion, and severe lymphedema. Diabetes, renal failure, liver failure, or ulcers in patients with rheumatoid arthritis or scleroderma are relative contraindications. Limbs with lateral ulcerations should be managed by open interruption of lateral or posterior perforators where appropriate.

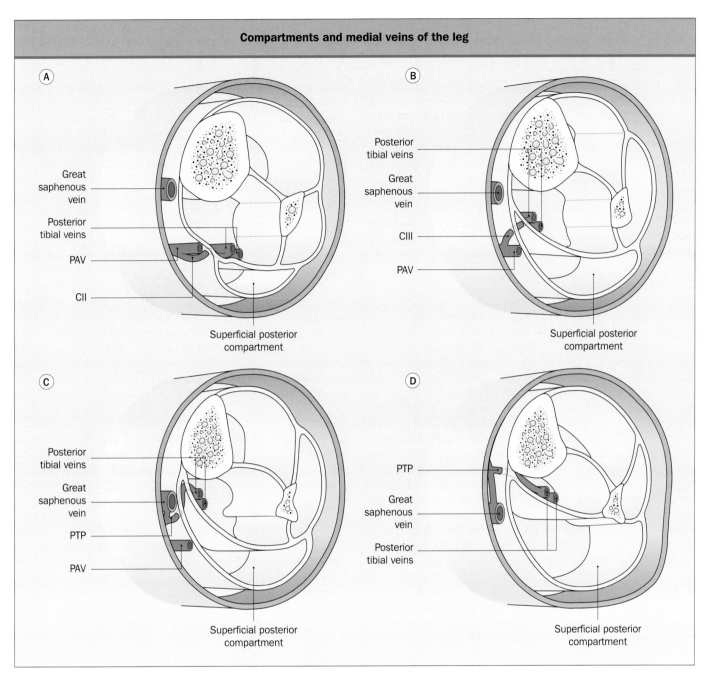

Compartments and medial veins of the leg

Figure 41.7 Compartments and medial veins of the leg. Cross-sections are at the levels of (A) Cockett II, (B) Cockett III, (C) '24cm', and (D) proximal paratibial perforating veins. CII, Cockett II; CIII, Cockett III; GSV, great saphenous vein; PAV, posterior arch vein; PTP, paratibial perforator; PTVs, posterior tibial veins; SPC, superficial posterior compartment. (From Mozes G, et al. Surgical anatomy for endoscopic subfascial division of perforating veins. J Vasc Surg 1996;24:800–8.)

Surgical technique

Open technique of perforator interruption

Linton's radical operation of subfascial ligation, reported in 1938,[35] which included long medial, anterolateral, and posterolateral calf incisions, was abandoned because of wound complications. Subsequently, in 1953, Linton advocated only a long medial incision from the ankle to the knee to interrupt all medial and posterior perforating veins. Several authors proposed modifications to Linton's open procedure, to limit wound complications. Cockett[36] advocated ligation of the perforating veins above the deep fascia. The importance of ligating the perforating veins subfascially was emphasized by Sherman,[32] as the perforating veins branch extensively once they penetrate the deep fascia. Further modifications included the use of shorter medial incisions or a more posteriorly placed stocking-seam-type incision.[37] De Palma[38] observed good results using multiple, parallel bipedicled flaps placed along skin lines to access and ligate the perforating veins above or below the fascia.

Linton[35] and Cockett[36] reported benefit from open perforator ligation, and this was supported later by data from several other investigators. In the larger series, ulcer recurrence averaged 24%, and ranged from 12% to 55%. Further controversy over the value of this operation emerged when Burnand et al.[39] reported a 55% ulcer recurrence rate in their patients, with 100% recurrence in a subset of 23 patients with post-thrombotic syndrome. Although these data are compelling evidence against perforating vein ablation, ulcer recurrence in the subset of patients without post-thrombotic syndrome was only 6%.

The concept of ablating incompetent perforating veins from a site remote from diseased skin was first introduced by Edwards in 1976.[40] He designed a device called the phlebotome, which is inserted through a medial incision just distal to the knee, deep to the fascia, and advanced to the level of the medial malleolus. Resistance is felt as perforators are engaged and subsequently disrupted with the leading edge of the phlebotome. Other alternatives include interruption of perforators through stab wounds and hook avulsion. The accuracy of this blind technique improves with preoperative duplex mapping. Sclerotherapy of perforating veins and suture ligation of perforators without making skin incisions are among other reported techniques.

Technique of SEPS

First introduced by Hauer in 1985 using endoscopic instruments, interruption of incompetent perforators may now be performed through small ports placed remotely from the active ulcer or area of skin discoloration.[41–43] Since its introduction, two main techniques for SEPS have been developed. The first, practiced mostly in Europe, is a refinement of the original work of Hauer[41] by workers including Bergan et al.[42] and Pierik et al.[44] In the early development of the 'single port' technique, available light sources such as mediastinoscopes and bronchoscopes were used. With time, a specially designed instrument was devised which uses a single scope with channels for the camera and working instruments. This sometimes makes visualization and dissection in the same plane difficult. Recent developments in instrumentation for this technique now allow for carbon dioxide insufflation into the subfascial plane.

The second technique, using instrumentation from laparoscopic surgery, was introduced in the US by O'Donnell,[45] and developed simultaneously by groups at the Mayo Clinic[46] and Conrad in Australia.[47] This 'two port' technique employs one port for the camera and a separate port for instrumentation, thereby making it easier to work in the limited subfascial space. First, the limb is exsanguinated with an Esmarque bandage and a thigh tourniquet is inflated to 300mmHg to provide a bloodless field (**Fig. 41.8A**). A 10mm endoscopic port is next placed in the medial aspect of the calf 10cm distal to the tibial tuberosity, proximal to the diseased skin. Balloon dissection is used to widen the subfascial space and facilitate access after port placement (**Fig.41.8B**). The distal 5mm port is now placed half-way between the first port and the ankle (about 10–12cm apart), under direct vision with the camera (**Fig. 41.8C**). Carbon dioxide is insufflated into the subfascial space and pressure is maintained around 30mmHg to improve visualization and access to the perforators. Using laparoscopic scissors inserted through the second port, the remaining loose connective tissue between the calf muscles and the superficial fascia is sharply divided.

The subfascial space is widely explored from the medial border of the tibia to the posterior midline, and down to the level of the ankle. All perforators encountered are divided either with the harmonic scalpel, electrocautery, or sharply between clips (**Fig. 41.8D**). A paratibial fasciotomy is next made by incising the fascia of the posterior deep compartment close to the tibia, to avoid any injury to the posterior tibial vessels and the tibial

nerve. The Cockett II and Cockett III perforators are located frequently within an intermuscular septum, and this has to be incised before identification and division of the perforators can be accomplished. The medial insertion of the soleus muscle on the tibia may also have to be exposed to visualize proximal paratibial perforators. By rotating the ports cephalad and continuing the dissection up to the level of the knee, the more proximal perforators can also be divided. While the paratibial fasciotomy can aid in distal exposure, reaching the retromalleolar Cockett I perforator endoscopically is not usually possible, and if incompetent, a separate small incision may be required over it to gain direct exposure.

After completion of the endoscopic part of the procedure, the instruments and ports are removed, the gas is expressed manually from the leg, and the tourniquet is deflated. Twenty milliliters of 0.5% marcain solution is instilled into the subfascial space for postoperative pain control. Stab avulsion of varicosities in addition to high ligation and stripping of the GSV and/or SSV, if incompetent, is performed. The wounds are closed and the limb is elevated and wrapped with an elastic bandage. Elevation is maintained at 30° postoperatively for 3 hours, after which walking is permitted. Unlike the in-hospital stay after an open Linton procedure, this is an outpatient procedure, and patients are discharged the same day or next morning (following overnight observation).

Results of SEPS

Encouraging early results with SEPS were reported by several authors,[43,48–50] with accelerated ulcer healing after ablation of the incompetent superficial and perforator systems, without intervention to the deep veins, even in patients with combined deep, perforator, and superficial incompetence (**Table 41.3**). The North American (NASEPS) registry was the first to provide uniform evaluation with the CEAP classification and reporting of results following SEPS in 146 patients with advanced CVI from 17 centers in North America.[43] Concomitant superficial venous surgery was performed in 71% of patients. The wound complication rate was 6%, and one DVT occurred 2 months after surgery. The mid-term (24 months) results from the NASEPS registry demonstrated an 88% cumulative ulcer healing rate at 1 year.[8] The median time to ulcer healing was 54 days. The cumulative rate of ulcer recurrence was significant – 16% at 1 year, 28% at 2 years – but still compared favorably with results of non-operative management.

In the largest series from a single institution, Nelzen[51] prospectively reported data from 149 SEPS procedures in 138 patients. During a median follow-up of 32 months, 32 of 36 ulcers healed, more than half within 1 month. Three ulcers recurred, one of which subsequently healed. At a median follow-up of 7 months, 91% of patients were satisfied with the results of the operation. A recent study analyzed extended results in 103 consecutive SEPS procedures performed at the Mayo Clinic.[9] The cumulative 1-year ulcer healing rate was 90% and ulcer recurrence at 5 years was 27%.

The major advantage of SEPS over traditional open surgical techniques is the lower wound complication rate.[43,44] In a non-controlled trial that compared 37 SEPS procedures to 30 antedated open perforator ligations,[52] SEPS resulted in lower calf wound morbidity, shorter hospital stay, and comparable short-term ulcer healing. A prospective, randomized study in 39 patients[53]

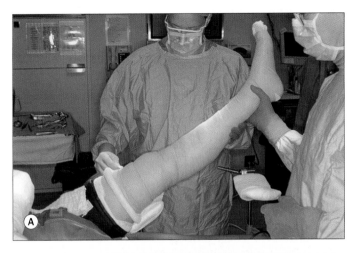

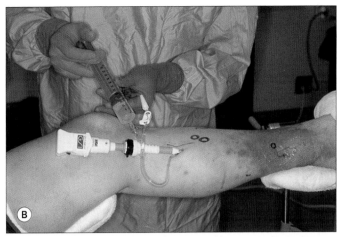

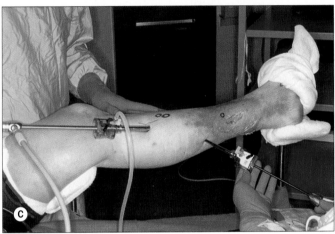

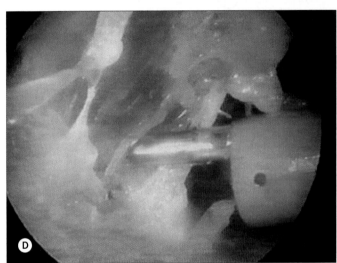

Figure 41.8 Two-port technique of subfascial endoscopic perforator surgery (SEPS). (A) A thigh tourniquet inflated to 300mmHg is used to create a bloodless field. (B) Balloon dissection is used to widen the subfascial space. (C) SEPS is performed using two ports: a 10mm camera port and a 5 or 10mm distal port inserted under video control. Carbon dioxide is insufflated through the camera port into the subfascial space to a pressure of 30mmHg to improve visualization and access to perforators. (D) The subfascial space is widely explored from the medial border of the tibia to the posterior midline and down to the level of the ankle, and all perforators are interrupted using clips or harmonic scalpel. (From Gloviczki P, Canton LG, Cambria RA, Rhee RY. Subfascial endoscopic perforator vein surgery with gas insufflation. In: Gloviczki P, Bergan JJ, eds. Atlas of endoscopic perforator vein surgery. London:Springer-Verlag; 1998:125–38.)

reported wound complications in 53% of patients undergoing open perforator ligation versus none in the SEPS group; there was no significant difference in ulcer recurrence (22% versus 12%, respectively) at 4 years. These data support the use of SEPS rather than open ligation, yet do not address the role of SEPS in the management of advanced CVI and venous ulceration.

Since the majority (more than two-thirds) of patients reported in the above studies underwent concomitant saphenous vein stripping and branch varicosity avulsion (**Table 41.3**), it is impossible to ascertain how much clinical improvement can be attributed to the addition of SEPS. Improved ulcer healing is reported in legs undergoing SEPS with saphenous vein stripping as compared with legs undergoing SEPS alone: 90% versus 49% at 90 days and 100% versus 83% at 1 year, respectively, in the NASEPS registry. Cumulative ulcer recurrence at 5 years was also higher following SEPS alone (53%) compared with SEPS with superficial reflux ablation (19%). However, the SEPS-alone group was a preselected group with failure following saphenous stripping and a relative predominance of post-thrombotic legs.

Uniformly poorer results have been reported in post-thrombotic syndrome compared with legs with PVI: cumulative ulcer recurrence in the NASEPS registry was 46% versus 20% at 2 years, respectively.[8,54] A recent study reported cumulative 5-year ulcer recurrence in post-thrombotic legs as 56% versus 15% in legs with PVI.[9] However, in spite of this, there was significant improvement in the clinical results and recurrent ulcers were small, superficial, single more often than multiple, and healed easily with conservative management.

Several investigators have studied the effect of superficial reflux ablation and perforator ligation on venous hemodynamics. However, none has been successful in attributing hemodynamic significance to perforator ligation.[55] Recent air plethysmographic studies by Padberg et al.[50] have documented persistent hemodynamic improvement up to 2 years following perforator ligation with concomitant correction of superficial reflux. Rhodes et al.[54] reported improvement in calf muscle pump function and venous incompetence following SEPS, with or without superficial reflux ablation. Akesson et al.[56] reported a significant decrease

Clinical results of subfascial endoscopic perforator surgery.							
Author, Year	No. of legs treated	No of legs with ulcer*	Concomitant saphenous ablation No. (%)	Wound complications No. (%)	Ulcer healing No. (%)	Ulcer recurrence† No. (%)	Mean follow-up (months)
Jugenheimer,[108] 1992	103	17	97 (94)	3 (3)	16 (94)	0 (0)	27
Pierek,[48] 1995	40	16	4 (10)	3 (8)	16 (100)	1 (2.5)	46
Bergan,[42] 1996	31	15	31 (100)	3 (10)	15 (100)	(0)	–
Wolters,[109] 1996	27	27	0 (0)	2 (7)	26 (96)	2 (8)	12–24
Padberg,[50] 1996	11	0	11 (100)	–	†	0 (0)	16
Pierek,[110] 1997	20	20	14 (70)	0 (0)	17 (85)	0 (0)	21
Rhodes,[54] 1998	57	22	41 (72)	3 (5)	22 (100)	5 (12)	17
Gloviczki,[8] 1999	146	101	86 (59)	9 (6)	85 (84)	26 (21)	24
Illig,[111] 1999	30	19	–	–	17 (89)	4 (15)	9
Nelzen,[51] 2000	149	36	132 (89)	11 (7)	32 (89)	3 (5)	32
Total no. of legs (%)	**614**	**273 (44)**	**416/567 (73)**	**34/556 (6)**	**246/273 (90)**	**41/392 (10)**	**–**

*Only class 6 (active ulcer) patients are included.
† Only class 5 (healed ulcer) patients were admitted in this study.
‡ Recurrence calculated for class 5 and 6 limbs only, where data available and percentage accounts for patients lost to follow-up.

Table 41.3 Clinical results of subfascial endoscopic perforator surgery (SEPS).

in ambulatory foot venous pressure following saphenous vein ligation and stripping in patients with recurrent ulcers, but there was no further hemodynamic improvement following perforator ligation performed 3 months later. Not surprisingly, patients with PVI demonstrate significantly better hemodynamic improvement than do those with post-thrombotic legs.[8,54,57]

Correction of deep venous reflux
Indications
Since the first direct venous valve reconstruction by Kistner in 1968, several techniques to repair incompetent venous valves have been developed but none has gained wide acceptance.[58] Today, several procedures exist to treat patients with advanced CVI and deep vein valve incompetence, but only a relatively small number of venous surgeons perform them. If deep venous reflux of sufficient magnitude is confirmed on non-invasive evaluation and the patient is a candidate for surgery, venography is undertaken to assist in planning the operative procedure. First, ascending venography is performed to exclude the presence of significant outflow obstruction. Next, descending venography is performed to confirm the presence, location, and magnitude of valvular reflux in the entire leg. Descending venography will also differentiate between the floppy, elongated valves and dilatation of the vein seen in PVI from the thickened, shortened valves with luminal narrowing characteristic of post-thrombotic syndrome. Patients with Kistner's grade 3 or 4 reflux down through popliteal veins into the tibial veins, in association with debilitating symptoms and signs of advanced CVI, are considered suitable candidates for correction of deep venous reflux.

Patients with PVI are usually candidates for internal or external valvuloplasty. Direct valve repair is seldom feasible with valve destruction after DVT. Options available include valve

transposition or transplantation, and attempts at de-novo valve reconstruction.

In spite of demonstrable reflux in multiple valves in the deep system, only one valve is usually repaired, most frequently the first valve of the femoral vein. If the profunda femoris vein valve is also incompetent, it also has to be repaired. An alternative is repair of an incompetent valve at the popliteal vein level, to prevent reflux into the popliteal and tibial veins.

Valvuloplasty
Internal valvuloplasty is performed most frequently for surgical correction of deep venous reflux secondary to PVI. First described by Kistner,[58] modifications to the technique have been reported by Raju and Fredericks[59] and by Sottiurai.[60] The procedure is performed through a standard groin incision with dissection of the femoral and saphenous veins. The valve attachment lines should be clearly identified on the vein wall before a venotomy is performed. In patients with a thickened, fibrotic femoral vein, adventitial dissection may be required to expose the position of the valve leaflets. Once the position of the valve is determined and it is confirmed to be incompetent on the strip test, proximal and distal control of the vein segment is obtained following systemic heparinization. Internal valvuloplasty involves plication of the valve cusps under direct vision with interrupted 7-0 Prolene sutures. Raju et al.[59] estimated that decreasing the length of the valve leaflets by approximately 20% is sufficient to restore competence. The original method described by Kistner[58] involved direct transcommissural exposure of the valve cusps via a longitudinal venotomy (**Fig. 41.9A**). A transverse venotomy situated above the valve is recommended by Raju & Fredericks[59] to avoid the potential adverse effects of a longitudinal suture line across the valve (**Fig 41.9B**). However, the position of the

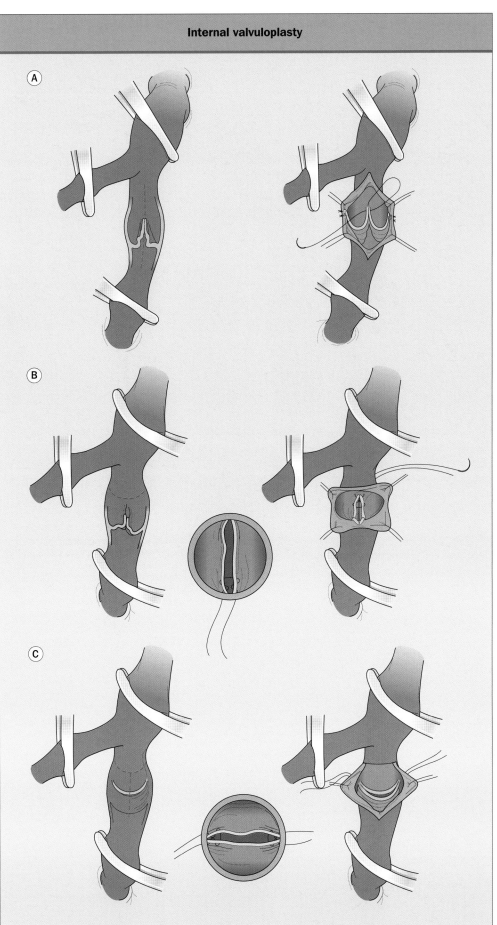

Internal valvuloplasty

Figure 41.9 Internal valvuloplasty.
(A) The Kistner transcommissural approach allows for visualization of the venous valves. Care must be taken to prevent damage to the valve cusps during the longitudinal venotomy. The transcommissural incision as well as the valve undergoing repair are pictured. (B) The Raju supracommissural approach minimizes the potential of valve cusp damage but sacrifices some of the excellent exposure afforded by the transcommissural approach. Illustrated is the valve structure during incision and valvuloplasty. (C) The Sottiurai supra-T commissural approach improves the visualization of the valve mechanism by extending the incision above the commissures parallel to the vein in a 'T' shape. (From Nachreiner RD, Bhuller AS, Dalsing MC. Surgical repair of incompetent venous valves. In: Gloviczki P, Yao JST, eds. Handbook of venous disorders, 2nd edn. London:Arnold; 2000:329–35.)

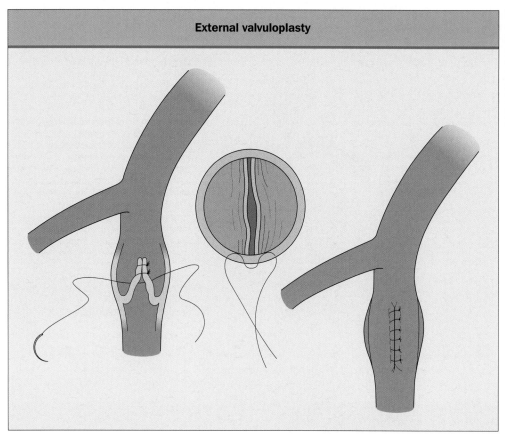

External valvuloplasty

Figure 41.10 External valvuloplasty. External valvuloplasty eliminates the need for venotomy. External suture placement is aimed at tightening the commissural angle. (From Nachreiner RD, Bhuller AS, Dalsing MC. Surgical repair of incompetent venous valves. In: Gloviczki P, Yao JST, eds. Handbook of venous disorders, 2nd edn. London:Arnold; 2000:329–35.)

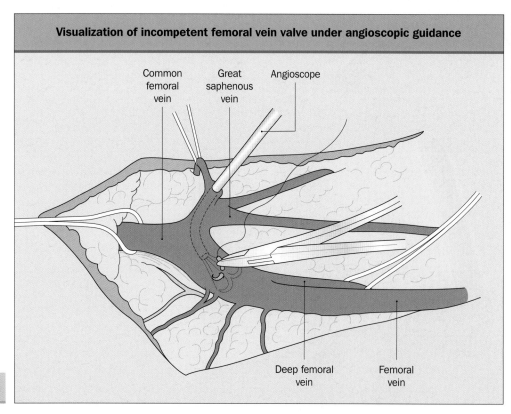

Visualization of incompetent femoral vein valve under angioscopic guidance

Common femoral vein

Great saphenous vein

Angioscope

Deep femoral vein

Femoral vein

Figure 41.11 Visualization of incompetent femoral vein valve under angioscopic guidance. (From Gloviczki P, Merrell SW, Bower TC. Femoral vein valve repair under direct vision without venotomy: a modified technique with use of angioscopy. J Vasc Surg 1991;14:645–8.)

transverse venotomy has to be very accurate to obtain an adequate view of the valve leaflets. Sottiurai[60] proposed a 'T'-shaped venotomy with addition of a longitudinal limb extending down to the level of, but not across, the valve annulus (**Fig. 41.9C**). Competence of the repaired valve is confirmed by duplex ultrasound. Anticoagulation and intermittent pneumatic compression is employed perioperatively to reduce the risk of DVT.

External valvuloplasty is a simpler technique of valve repair that avoids venotomy. It was originally suggested by Kistner. Partial-thickness transmural plicating sutures are placed from the outside to narrow the widened commissural angles (**Fig. 41.10**). Although a venotomy and full heparinization are avoided, lack of direct visualization makes this repair anatomically less precise.

Angioscope-assisted valvuloplasty was reported by Gloviczki in 1991.[61] Through and through transluminal sutures are inserted to narrow the commissures from the outside, while viewing the valve leaflets with an angioscope positioned above the valve through a tributary of the saphenous vein (**Figs 41.11 & 41.12**). Heparinization and control of the vein are required as for internal valvuloplasty. Blood is flushed out of the isolated segment and heparinized saline instilled to facilitate visualization. Competence is checked progressively during the repair by rapid flooding of the valve leaflets with heparinized saline from above. Raju & Hardy[62] prefer to insert the angioscope through a venotomy

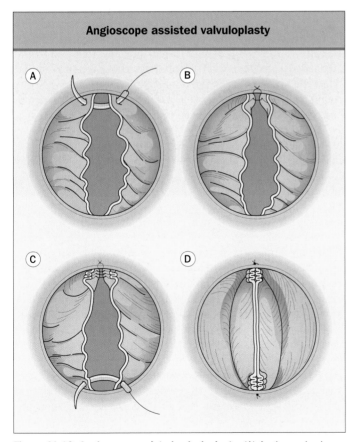

Angioscope assisted valvuloplasty

(A) (B) (C) (D)

Figure 41.12 Angioscope-assisted valvuloplasty. (A) Angioscopic view of needle passage thorough the incompetent valve leaflets.
(B) Assessment of valve redundancy after each suture placement.
(C) Suture placement on both commissures to achive complete valvular competence. (D) Angioscopic view of competent valve. (From Gloviczki P, Merrell SW, Bower TC. Femoral vein valve repair under direct vision without venotomy: a modified technique with use of angioscopy. J Vasc Surg 1991;14:645–8.)

close to the valve station and use it to visualize the valve leaflets before and after placement of full-thickness plicating sutures from the outside, but not during placement of the sutures. Dissection can be limited and operative time shortened with the use of the angioscope.

Venoplastic procedures have been employed in circumstances where extreme widening of the commissural angle raises concerns about narrowing of the vein resulting from invagination of too much tissue. A longitudinal-transverse or inverted 'Y-V' venoplasty is performed above the valve commissure after heparinization and adequate vascular control. This results in narrowing of the commissure by pulling up and tightening the valve cusps without direct placement of sutures in them. This maneuver also widens and deepens the valve sinuses somewhat, contributing to valve competence. The procedure is recommended by Raju & Hardy[62] in small veins, as well as in obese patients with compromised exposure of the valve, for standard intraluminal valvuloplasty.

De-novo valve reconstruction was first described by Durango[63] in 1993, whereby new valve cusps were created from excised saphenous vein and sutured into an appropriate host vein. The adventitia and part of the media are removed from the harvested vein segment to provide thin and supple tissue. 'U'-shaped cusps are created from this, and the corners oriented and anchored with mattress sutures tied externally to create a bicuspid valve. The rest of the edge of the leaflet is sutured in a continuous manner with 7-0 Prolene. Raju & Hardy[62] modified the technique to orient the valves with the intimal surface outward, in an effort to reduce the incidence of thrombosis in the sinus, where blood flow is relatively sluggish. They also recommended using the axillary or other deep vein or a tributary as the donor, to create thinner leaflets than is possible with saphenous vein. The technique has not been used widely so far. The complexity of the repair precludes its use except in circumstances where valvuloplasty is not feasible and no competent valve is available for transfer.

External banding with a prosthetic sleeve is an option in a small minority of valves with early reflux. It is suitable for valves with reflux secondary to vein dilatation that become competent intraoperatively on the strip test when the vein constricts in response to dissection. A 2–3cm fascial, Dacron, silastic, or polytetrafluoroethylene (PTFE) strip is wrapped around the vein segment containing the valve, to narrow the annulus slightly. It is tightened around the vein, sutured longitudinally, and then anchored to the adventitia to prevent displacement. External banding has been used to complement internal/external valvuloplasty where dilatation of the vein is suspected to contribute to incompetence.

Valve transposition

This procedure was described by Kistner in 1979 for use in patients with post-thrombotic syndrome with deep venous reflux and one competent valve at the groin – either the saphenous or profunda femoris valve.[64] The principle of valve transposition or venous segment transfer is to interpose a competent-valve-bearing venous segment into the deep venous system at the level of the groin. The simplest option is disconnection of the femoral vein and anastomosis of the distal segment end-to-end to the saphenous vein with a competent saphenofemoral valve (**Fig. 41.13**). Not infrequently, the GSV is either incompetent or has been stripped.

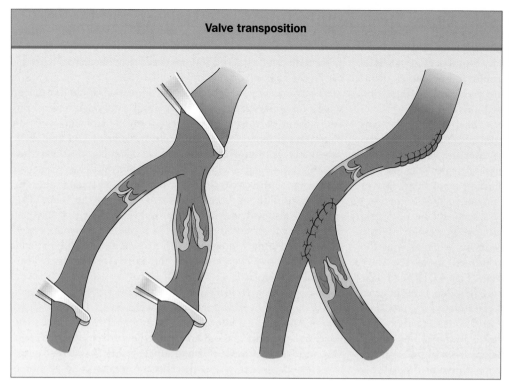

Figure 41.13 Valve transposition.
Transposition of the femoral vein after ligation distal to its junction with the common femoral vein involves implantation of the translocated femoral vein distal to a competent valve lying within the profunda femoral vein. (From Dalsing MC, Nachreiner RD, Bhuller A. Role of venous valvular surgery in chronic venous insufficiency in vascular surgery – year 2000. New York:McGraw-Hill; 2000.)

In this situation, the femoral vein may be anastomosed end-to-side to the profunda femoris vein below a competent valve. Kistner subsequently reported late fatigue of the saphenous vein with recurrence of symptoms and now preferentially uses the profunda femoris vein. Under full heparinization and appropriate vascular control, the femoral vein is divided close to its junction with the profunda vein, and the proximal end is closed with 5-0 Prolene, taking care not to narrow or distort the profunda orifice. The distal end is anastomosed end-to-side to the profunda femoris or end-to-end to its first branch, using interrupted sutures of 7-0 Prolene or the triangulation technique of Carrel. Competence of the transposed segment is confirmed by the strip test and/or duplex ultrasound.

Valve transplantation

Venous valve transplantation is the next available option in patients with post-thrombotic syndrome whose pattern and extent of disease precludes local valve reconstruction or transposition in the groin. Autogenous transplantation of a competent valve from the arm to the leg was introduced by Taheri et al. in 1982 (**Fig. 41.14**).[65] The original procedure involved transplant of a brachial vein segment containing a competent valve to replace a short segment of femoral vein. A 4–8cm segment of brachial vein is harvested through a longitudinal incision in the arm after confirming the presence of a competent valve in the segment. This may be done preoperatively with duplex ultrasound or intraoperatively with the strip test. The femoral vein is dissected as before over a length of 10–12cm, and proximal and distal control is obtained following adequate systemic heparinization. A 2–3cm segment of the femoral vein 4–5cm distal to the profunda femoris junction is excised; approximately half the length of vein segment to be implanted. The brachial vein segment is anastomosed as an interposition graft into the femoral vein.

The anastomoses are performed in a triangulated manner or with interrupted 7-0 Prolene sutures, the distal followed by the proximal. Raju & Fredericks[59] adopted the technique but preferred to use the axillary vein as the donor vein segment, citing better size match with the femoral vein. Despite the better size match, some dilatation of the transplanted vein segment still occurred, just like Taheri et al.[65] noted in the brachial vein. To circumvent this problem, they suggested an external Dacron wrap of the transplanted segment to prevent late recurrence of reflux. They also reported incompetence *in situ* in 44% of axillary vein valves explored for harvesting; 14% of patients explored had bilateral axillary vein valvular incompetence. In such a situation, they proceeded to perform bench repair of the axillary vein valve by external valvuloplasty prior to transplant, but disappointing results prompted them to change over to transcommissural repair in recent years. O'Donnell et al.[66] further adapted the technique to transplant an axillary vein segment into the popliteal vein in an effort to provide a better size match and prevent delayed dilatation of the transplanted vein segment. They also proposed that correcting reflux at the popliteal level was more critical, based on its relation to the calf muscle pump.

Results of deep vein valve reconstruction

Operative mortality of deep venous repair is negligible; the majority of series have no deaths. The considerable concern regarding the risk of DVT and pulmonary embolism following direct surgical intervention on the deep venous system has not materialized. The incidence of DVT has been reported as 0–11% in series with long-term follow-up.[59,67] Not unexpectedly, the incidence is higher following repairs in post-thrombotic limbs compared with in legs with PVI.[68] The incidence of wound hematoma is directly related to the use of heparin, and has occurred in 2–16% of patients in reported studies, with half

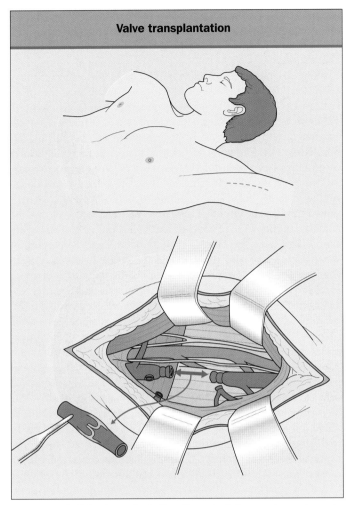

Valve transplantation

Figure 41.14 Valve transplantation. Transplantation can be performed by harvesting an axillary venous segment containing a competent valve or a valve that has been made competent by valvuloplasty. (From Dalsing MC. Chronic venous disease. In: Greenfield et al., eds. Surgery: scientific principle and practice, 3rd edn. Philadelphia:Lippincott, Williams, & Wilkins; 2001:23.)

requiring operative evacuation.[67,69,70] Early intervention on these hematomas is extremely important to avoid compression of the repair and secondary intravenous thrombosis. Wound seromas, infection, and lymphatic leak each occur in 2–4 % of patients.

Several authors have reported clinical success in 70–80% of patients on mid-term follow-up (2–4 years) following valve repair for PVI (**Table 41.4**).[62,71–73] Among patients with a good outcome, about half were asymptomatic without elastic support and the other half continued to require stockings to remain symptom-free. Masuda and Kistner[67] recently reported persistence of similar findings on longer follow-up (4–21 years), with stabilization of results in all groups of patients by 6 years. The study included 51 patients who had various deep venous reconstruction procedures: 43% with PVI, 31% with post-thrombotic syndrome, and 26% with combined disease. Cumulative clinical success was significantly superior in patients with PVI who underwent valve repair (73%) compared with patients with post-thrombotic syndrome who underwent valve transposition or transplant (43%). Patients with a mixed pattern of disease with proximal PVI and distal post-thrombotic syndrome fared somewhere in between. At 10 years, the cumulative clinical success rate of the entire group was 60%. Ulcers recurred in 15 of 29 patients with class 5 and 6 disease; five patients had multiple recurrences. In the majority of these patients, ulcers were related to neglect or trauma, were small, and healed easily.

Clinical outcome in all series has correlated closely with the eventual state of valve competence: patients with sustained competence demonstrated on duplex imaging remained asymptomatic, and patients with recurrence of symptoms invariably had failure of the reconstruction.[59,67] Modest improvement in hemodynamic parameters following valve repair has been reported by several authors.[59,66–68] In all series, hemodynamic improvement failed to reach the same levels as clinical improvement. Masuda and Kistner[67] reported significant improvement of AVPs in legs classified as class 0 or 1, but still not normalization. This is not inconceivable, as valve repair only corrects the abnormality at one level in most legs with global abnormalities. The pathophysiologic improvement may be sufficient to relieve symptoms but does not affect plethysmographic and venous pressure measurements to a significant degree.

Results of valvuloplasty.

Author, Year	No. of legs	No. of legs with ulcer	Clinical success No. (%)	Valve competency rate No. (%)	Ulcer recurrence No. (%)	Mean follow-up (months)
Eriksson,[72] 1990	27	N/A	19 (70)	19 (70)	N/A	6–108
Masuda,[67] 1994	32	0*	23 (73)	25 (77)	N/A	126
Raju,[77] 1996	258	137	N/A[†]	(62)[†]	36 (26)	12–144
Sottiurai,[73] 1997	143	N/A	N/A	107 (75)	N/A	9–168
Perrin,[75] 2000	85	35	65 (80)	67 (79)	8 (23)	12–168

*Only class 3 (96%) and class 2 (4%) legs included in study.
[†] Clinical improvement in 55% of patients with no ulcer (class 4).
[‡] Includes overall competency rate following all valve repairs.

Table 41.4 Results of valvuloplasty.

Chances of success decrease with increasing complexity of the deep venous reconstruction. Available series in the literature report a crude ulcer healing rate of 79% following valve transfer in 157 patients.[66,74,75] Cumulative ulcer-free interval at 6 years ranged from 50% to 65%. On review of series with objective evidence of clinical outcome, the overall mean occlusion rate of valve transplants in 250 legs studied with ascending venography was 5.6%, but was as high as 38% in 32 procedures in the series of Perrin et al.[66,67,74–76] Hemodynamic improvement studied variously with venous pressure measurement and air plethysmography has been equivocal. Raju et al. reported decrease in the venous filling index from 6ml/s to 4ml/s. Results of valve transposition are comparable, with ulcer recurrence rates of 35% and occlusion of the reconstruction in 10% of legs.[67,75] Only seven patients with *de-novo* valve reconstruction are reported with acceptable clinical results.[62]

Treatment of deep venous obstruction
Indications
Patients with deep venous obstruction and symptoms and signs of advanced CVI who have failed conservative treatment and all other simpler surgical procedures may be considered for intervention on the deep venous system. Deep venous obstruction is infrequent, causing less than 10% of CVI.[1] Standard hemodynamic tests are not very reliable in diagnosing deep venous outflow obstruction, having a high positive, but low negative, predictive value. Raju et al.[77] have suggested that deep venous obstruction accounts for a larger percentage of patients with CVI than generally believed; up to 40% of patients in their practice. Careful attention to the patient's symptoms and a high degree of suspicion are essential to avoid missing the diagnosis. The presence of skin changes and venous ulcers make the diagnosis easy; however, most patients present with leg swelling and disabling venous claudication.

Deep venous thrombosis is the most frequent cause of venous obstructions. In symptomatic patients, recanalization of the thrombosed veins is incomplete and collateralization inadequate. May and Thurner observed secondary changes such as an intraluminal web or 'spur' in the proximal left common iliac vein in 20% of the patients during 430 autopsies. These changes are now recognized as a predisposing factor for left iliofemoral thrombosis. Other causes include iatrogenic trauma, retroperitoneal fibrosis, radiation injury, cysts, and, rarely, arterial aneurysms. In addition to a non-invasive workup (outlined earlier), ascending venography is indicated to visualize the deep venous system of the affected leg, as well as the iliac veins and inferior vena cava. Descending venography is performed to identify the presence of concomitant reflux frequently seen in the post-thrombotic syndrome. Venous pressures are measured to assess the severity of the occlusion: a pressure difference of 5mmHg between the two femoral veins in unilateral iliac disease, or between the femoral and the central pressures, or a 5mmHg increase in femoral vein pressure after exercise indicates a hemodynamically significant lesion.

Endovascular treatment
The development of endovascular treatment of iliac vein occlusions over the last decade has significantly decreased the number of patients subjected to open surgical procedures. Initial experience was with balloon dilatation of residual stenoses following thrombolytic therapy for acute iliofemoral DVT. In recent years, the same principles have been applied to the management of chronic iliac vein stenoses and occlusion.

Procedure
Baseline diagnostic ascending venography is performed through a transfemoral route; the importance of visualizing the distal femoropopliteal and tibial segments has been emphasized. Tandem distal thromboses with compromised inflow are factors associated with early failure of iliac vein stenting. Several authors have stressed the importance of improving inflow by additional thrombolysis of the distal venous tree.[78,79] For the therapeutic procedure to disobliterate the iliac vein, the patient is positioned supine with an indwelling bladder catheter. Access is usually gained through the popliteal vein, or a tributary, under ultrasound guidance, or injection of contrast through a foot vein. This significantly decreases the incidence of puncture site hematoma. A sheath is inserted into the vein and the lesion is traversed with a guidewire. Some authors have described routine thrombolysis for 24 to 48 hours to soften chronic thrombus and facilitate the passage of wires and catheters. Others have recanalized short, subtotal occlusions without employing lytic therapy. Raju et al. have performed iliac vein stenting in over 300 patients without any pretreatment thrombolysis or post-treatment anticoagulation.[80] After completion of lytic therapy, a stiffer exchange wire is passed, following which sequential dilation of the iliac vein and vena cava is performed with 8–14mm balloons (**Fig. 41.15**). The low pressure venous system is more amenable to balloon dilatation and a previously occluded vein can be dilated to 14 to 16mm with careful attention to wall resistance. No venous ruptures have been reported. Immediate recoil is the rule in most cases and routine stenting is recommended. The flexibility and self-expansion of Wallstents makes them particularly suitable for venous stenting; however, several other stents have been employed.[79] The entire length of the lesion is stented. Stenting of the femoral vein has been recommended to improve inflow in post-thrombotic legs with stenosis. Intravascular ultrasound has been used to advantage in the accurate placement of stents. Anticoagulation is continued for 6 months in the majority and indefinitely in selected patients.

Results
The most frequent complication of venous stenting is puncture site hematoma; the incidence can be reduced with ultrasound-guided access. Major bleeding requiring transfusion is reported in 1% to 25% of patients. Early rethrombosis occurs in 10% of patients and pulmonary embolism in <1%. Death due to pulmonary embolism, intracranial and retroperitoneal hemorrhage, myocardial infarction, and/or sepsis has been reported after <1% of procedures. The large proportion of patients in most reported series consists of those with acute DVT, who, not unexpectedly, fare better than patients with chronic occlusion. The best results are in patients with short, focal lesions, where outcomes are similar to those of stenting in the arterial system. Patients with May–Thurner syndrome, with no evidence of prior DVT, have better results than those with complicating thrombosis. Initial technical success in series reporting treatment of acute and chronic lesions is >90%. Patency at 1 year ranges from 79% to 94%.[78,81,82] Nazarian et al.[83] reported 1-year primary and secondary patency rates of 50% and 81%, respectively, in a more varied group of patients, mostly with chronic occlusion. The only

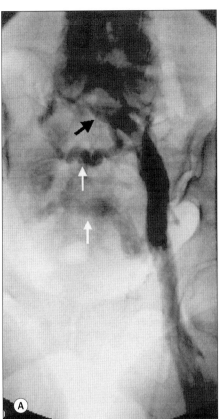

Figure 41.15 Iliac vein stenting. (A) Ascending venogram of the left leg of a 33-year-old woman with May–Thurner syndrome, showing occlusion of the common iliac vein (dark arrow) with transpelvic collaterals (white arrows) and post-thrombotic changes in the common femoral and external iliac veins. (B) Ascending venogram following insertion of two Wallstents (14mm × 40mm and 14mm × 60 mm) across the common iliac vein, extending into the inferior vena cava (arrow).

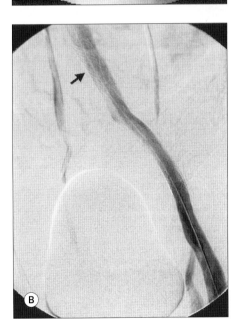

success and intermediate results are encouraging. The obvious advantages of endovascular intervention and low complication rates make iliac vein stenting an obvious first choice in most patients. Unsuccessful or failed stenting does not preclude subsequent open surgery procedures.

Surgical treatment

Surgical treatment is reserved for patients with disabling symptoms refractory to all other forms of treatment. In the infrainguinal location, autologous grafts have the best chance of long-term success. The ipsilateral/contralateral GSV, if available, is the conduit of choice, followed by arm vein. Harvesting the contralateral femoral vein in post-thrombotic patients is usually avoided unless absolutely necessary, because of possible significant added morbidity. Externally supported expanded polytetrafluoroethylene (ePTFE) grafts are currently the best choice for prosthetic replacement of large veins.

Factors responsible for poor patency in venous grafts include low flow and pressure, their susceptibility to external compression, and hypercoagulability. Some authors consider thrombophilia a contraindication to venous bypass surgery. All procedures are performed under the cover of intra- and postoperative anticoagulation and intermittent pneumatic compression. Multiple experiments have suggested that a distal arteriovenous fistula, first suggested by Kunlin in 1953, improves patency of grafts placed in the venous system. However, elevated cardiac output secondary to a large fistula may potentially accentuate the venous outflow obstruction, with worsening of symptoms until the fistula is taken down. A femoral arteriovenous fistula is recommended for prosthetic grafts anastomosed to the femoral vein and for iliocaval grafts longer than 10cm. The fistula can be closed by open or endovascular means 3 to 6 months after the operation. We maintain the fistula indefinitely in patients with no symptoms related to it. A small silastic sheet wrapped around the fistula facilitates localization at time of surgical closure. A Palma procedure can be performed in a patient with high pressure gradient (10–20mmHg) with a good chance of success, without a temporary arteriovenous fistula; but those with a lower pressure gradient and low initial flow (<100ml/min) benefit from a femoral arteriovenous fistula.

Saphenopopliteal bypass

First advocated by Warren and Thayer in 1954 and reintroduced by Husni[85] and by May,[86] saphenopopliteal bypass (May–Husni operation) is designed for patients with occlusion of the superficial femoral or proximal popliteal veins.

In the original operation, the ipsilateral saphenous vein was used for the conduit. A single distal anastomosis was performed, usually end-to-side, between the mobilized and divided saphenous vein and the distal popliteal vein, using running 6-0 or 7-0 Prolene sutures. An end-to-side arteriovenous fistula can be constructed at the ankle between the posterior tibial artery and one of the paired posterior tibial veins or the saphenous vein. Alternatively, a bypass graft may be performed with free contralateral saphenous or arm vein.

Cross-pubic venous bypass (Palma–Dale procedure)

Initially described by Palma in Uruguay and popularized by Dale in the US, the Palma–Dale procedure has remained a useful technique for venous reconstruction in patients with chronic

series reporting exclusively chronic venous occlusions was that of Raju et al.,[84] including 304 legs (142 non-thrombotic and 162 post-thrombotic). All underwent stenting without thrombolysis. Primary and secondary patency rates at 2 years were 71% and 97%, respectively; patency in legs with non-thrombotic disease was 90% versus 70% in post-thrombotic legs. In most instances, resolution of symptoms parallels patency of the stented vein. However, reported cumulative ulcer healing rates are 68%, and 2-year ulcer-free survival 62%.[84] Although long-term results of venous stenting will not be available in the near future, initial unilateral iliac vein obstruction of any etiology.[87,88] A prerequisite for the procedure is a normal contralateral iliofemoral venous system to assure venous drainage. Absence of distal deep venous obstruction or reflux is associated with superior results.

Adequate diameter of the contralateral GSV is confirmed preoperatively by duplex ultrasound or phlebography. The vein is harvested by open or endoscopic technique. All tributaries are ligated, the vein is gently distended with heparinized papaverine solution and tunneled through a suprapubic, subcutaneous route to the contralateral groin. Dissection of the femoral vein on the affected side is limited to the anterior and lateral vein wall, sufficient to place a side-biting clamp. Excision of intraluminal fibrous bands following venotomy may be needed. The anastomosis between the saphenous and femoral veins is performed end-to-side. If the vein is small, interrupted 5-0 or 6-0 sutures are preferred, to permit later dilatation of the vein and to avoid purse stringing of the venous anastomosis (**Fig. 41.16**). A small catheter placed through a tributary of the ipsilateral saphenous vein permits immediate low-dose heparinization, and postoperative phlebography.

In patients where the traditional transposition procedure results in significant kinking of the saphenous vein at the contralateral groin, it may be used as a free graft instead. Alternatively, a free graft may be performed with ipsilateral saphenous vein (with any competent valve lysed) or arm vein. Kistner[64] reported transposition of the ipsilateral iliac vein and end-to-side anastomosis to the contralateral femoral vein. The iliac vein is mobilized up to the site of occlusion and divided via a retroperitoneal approach. The internal iliac vein is disconnected to provide adequate length and the conduit is tunneled through a subcutaneous, suprapubic

route to the opposite side. When suitable autologous conduit is not available, an 8mm externally supported ePTFE graft is the best alternative.[89]

Femoro-ilio-caval reconstructions

Anatomic in-line iliac or iliocaval reconstruction is indicated for unilateral disease, when an autologous conduit for a suprapubic graft is not available, or for bilateral iliac, iliocaval, or inferior vena caval occlusion.

The femoral vessels (for the arteriovenous fistula or for the site of the distal anastomosis) are exposed at the groin through a vertical incision. The iliac vein or the distal segment of the inferior vena cava is exposed through a right oblique flank incision using the retroperitoneal approach. The iliocaval segment is usually reconstructed with a 14mm ePTFE graft and the femorocaval segment with a 10 or 12mm ePTFE graft (**Fig. 41.17**). The arteriovenous fistula is constructed first in patients who undergo a long iliocaval bypass using a tributary of the GSV. During femorocaval bypass, the proximal and distal anastomoses are performed first and the fistula is then created before opening up circulation through the graft. A small polyethylene catheter is placed to the level of the distal anastomosis to infuse low-dose heparin (500U/hour).

Results of deep venous bypass

Although the first successful venous reconstruction in a patient was reported more than 40 years ago by Warren and Thayer, results of surgical treatment for venous obstructions have been less than satisfactory for many years. Improvement in diagnosis, patient selection, and surgical technique over the last two

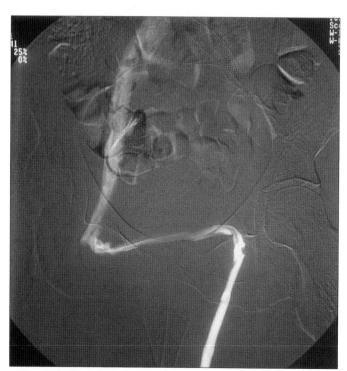

Figure 41.16 Cross-pubic venous bypass. Digital subtraction venogram of the left leg and pelvis, showing a patent left-to-right Palma graft 6 months after operation. Left iliac stent thrombosed before operation. (From Jost CJ, Gloviczki P, Cherry KJJ, et al. Surgical reconstruction of iliofemoral veins and the inferior vena cava for nonmalignant occlusive disease. J Vasc Surg 2001;33:320–7.)

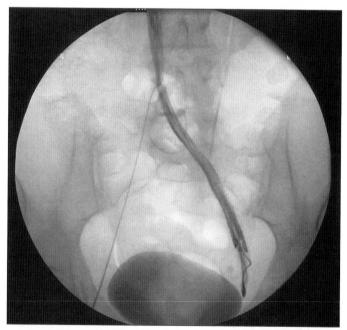

Figure 41.17 Femoro-ilio-caval reconstructions. Patent left femorocaval expanded polytetrafluoroethylene (ePTFE) bypass graft in a 54-year-old woman 11.7 years after graft placement. (From Jost CJ, Gloviczki P, Cherry KJJ, et al. Surgical reconstruction of iliofemoral veins and the inferior vena cava for nonmalignant occlusive disease. J Vasc Surg 2001;33:320–7.)

Results of femorofemoral crossover bypass.						
Author, Year	No. of legs	Follow-up (years)	Postoperative imaging (%)	Patency rate (%)	Clinical improvement (%)	Graft material
Palma,[87] 1960	8	up to 3	13	N/A	88	vein
Dale,[88] 1979	56	N/A	N/A	N/A	80	vein
May,[86] 1981	66	N/A	N/A	73	N/A	vein
Husni,[85] 1983	85	0.5–15	N/A	70	74	vein (n=83)
Halliday,[112] 1985	47	up to 18	72	75	89	vein
Danza,[93] 1991	27	N/A	N/A	N/A	81	vein
AbuRahma,[92] 1991	24	5.5	100	75	63	vein
Gruss,[90] 1997	19	N/A	N/A	71	82 overall	vein
Jost,[95] 2001	18	3.5	100	83	67 overall*	vein
*Includes outcome for all deep venous bypasses.						

Table 41.5 Results of femorofemoral crossover bypass.

Results of femorocaval/iliocaval bypass.						
Author, Year	No. of legs	Follow-up (months)	Imaging (%)	Patency rate (%)	Clinical improvement (%)	Graft material
Husfeldt,[113] 1979	4	4–30	100	100	100	ePTFE
Dale,[114] 1984	3	1–30	100	100	100	ePTFE
Alimi,[115] 1997	8	mean 19.5	100	88	88	ePTFE
Sottiurai,[73] 1997	45	11–139	100†	93*	89†	ePTFE
Jost,[95] 2001	18	42	100	56	67	13 ePTFE, 5 spiral vein
*Includes six femoroiliac, 26 femorofemoral, eight femorocaval, and five femoro-femoral-caval grafts.						
† Postoperative duplex scan, followed by annual air plethysmography and selective venography.						
‡ An additional eight patients (18%) developed recurrent ulcers during follow-up.						

Table 41.6 Results of femorocaval/iliocaval bypass. ePTFE, expanded polytetrafluoroethylene.

decades has resulted in the further development of venous bypass surgery.

The original May–Husni transposition is rarely performed and popliteo-femoral bypasses are also infrequent. In seven series, which included 218 procedures, functional improvement was reported in 77%.[76,85,88,90–93] In an earlier review of 59 operations, Smith and Trimble[94] reported clinical success in 76% of the patients. Crude patency rates at variable follow-up ranged from 5% to 100%, but only four of seven studies reported on late imaging of the grafts to ascertain patency.[76,88,91,92]

Analysis of the results of 412 Palma operations, published in nine series, revealed clinical improvement in 63% to 89% and patency rates between 70% and 83% (**Table 41.5**). However, follow-up was variable and objective graft assessment with imaging was rarely done. Husni reported patency of 47 of 67 grafts, followed from 6 months to 15 years.[85] Four-year patency of the 18 Palma grafts performed at the Mayo Clinic was 83%.[95] Expanded PTFE grafts in this location have not performed well,

with early occlusion of eight out of nine grafts reported.[95,96] However, Comerota et al.[97] reported patency in two of three grafts at 40 and 63 months. The best results with PTFE were reported by Sottiurai and associates, who observed 100% patency in 26 grafts at a follow-up ranging from 11 to 139 months.[98] Gruss et al. have the largest experience with ePTFE graft in this position. These authors reported an 85% (27/32) patency rate in a long-term follow-up study.[90] Based on his results and those of others, Gruss now recommends using an externally supported ePTFE graft with AVF for all cross-pubic venous bypasses.

An alternative is in-line femorocaval bypass for patients without suitable saphenous vein for Palma procedure. Secondary patency at 2 years of 13 ilio/femorocaval ePTFE bypasses performed at our institution was, however, only 54% (**Table 41.6**). Sottiurai et al.[98] reported patency in nine of 13 femorocaval ePTFE bypass grafts at 1 year. Overall, open venous reconstructions for iliofemoral or inferior vena caval obstruction offer 3-year patency rates of 62%.

CONCLUSION

Optimal treatment of patients with CVI and venous ulcers is not yet established. Surgical treatment focuses on correcting the cosmetic deformity by removing varicose veins in milder cases and restoring venous function to reduce ambulatory venous hypertension in patients with more advanced chronic venous disease.

Ablation of superficial reflux is performed most effectively by high ligation and stripping of the incompetent portion of the saphenous vein, usually from the groin to the knee, using the inversion technique. Endovenous saphenous vein obliteration is gaining popularity, primarily due to the shorter postoperative recovery time and faster return to work. Long-term studies are still needed to assess the rate of varicose vein recurrence and saphenous vein recanalization. Surgical or endovenous procedures will soon be compared with duplex-guided foam sclerotherapy. Stab avulsion is currently the main technique for surgical ablation of branch varicose veins.

Prospective, randomized studies comparing saphenous vein stripping versus saphenous vein stripping with SEPS are still awaited. Based on available data, patients who benefit most from SEPS are those with ulcers caused by PVI of the superficial, perforating, and deep veins. These patients derive maximum benefit in terms of accelerated ulcer healing and an estimated 80–90% chance of freedom from ulcer recurrence in the long term. SEPS continues to be controversial in patients with post-thrombotic syndrome, as only 50% of patients remain free from recurrent ulcers in the long term.

Deep vein valve reconstructions continue to be challenging and are rarely performed. Still, good clinical outcome has been reported in as many as 80% of patients undergoing direct valve reconstruction. Results of vein transplantations and transpositions are less obvious: benefit has been reported in 50% of patients.

Endovascular treatment with venous stents is used more and more frequently for iliac vein obstruction and it is the first option for treatment of symptomatic patients. For patients with unilateral iliac vein obstruction who are not suitable for or who fail endovascular treatment, the Palma procedure remains the best open surgical technique for autologous reconstruction. Patients with recurrent or persistent symptoms and significant disability should be considered for femoroiliac or femorocaval bypass grafts. Expanded PTFE continues to be the best prosthetic material for reconstruction of the vena cava, and short, large-diameter grafts have the best long-term patency. However, patients with significant infrainguinal venous disease have a poor chance of long-term success. While endovascular techniques may limit the need for surgical treatment in the future, carefully selected patients with symptomatic large vein obstruction will continue to enjoy durable benefit from open surgical venous reconstructions.

REFERENCES

1. Callam MJ. Epidemiology of varicose veins. Br J Surg 1994;81:167–73 (Review).
2. Stanley JC, Barnes RW, Ernst CB, Hertzer NR, Mannick JA, Moore WS. Vascular surgery in the United States: workforce issues. Report of the Society for Vascular Surgery and the International Society for Cardiovascular Surgery, North American Chapter, Committee on Workforce Issues. J Vasc Surg 1996;23:172–81.
3. Bosanquet N. Costs of venous ulcers: from maintenance therapy to investment programmes. Phlebology 1992;7(Suppl 1):44–6.
4. Nicolaides AN, Hussein MK, Szendro G, Christopoulos D, Vasdekis S, Clarke H. The relation of venous ulceration with ambulatory venous pressure measurements. J Vasc Surg 1993;17:414–9.
5. Nicolaides AN, Bergan JJ, Eklof B, Kistner RL, Moneta GL, and the American Venous Forum Consensus Committee. Classification and grading of chronic venous disease in the lower limbs: a consensus statement. In: Gloviczki P, Yao JST (eds). Handbook of venous disorders, 2nd Edition. London:Chapman & Hall; 2000:652–60.
6. Porter JM, Moneta GL. Reporting standards in venous disease: an update. International Consensus Committee on Chronic Venous Disease. J Vasc Surg 1995;21:635–45.
7. Raju S. Venous insufficiency of the lower limb and stasis ulceration. Changing concepts and management. Ann Surg 1983;197:688–97.
8. Gloviczki P, Bergan JJ, Rhodes JM, Canton LG, Harmsen S, Ilstrup DM. Mid-term results of endoscopic perforator vein interruption for chronic venous insufficiency: lessons learned from the North American subfascial endoscopic perforator surgery registry. The North American Study Group. J Vasc Surg 1999;29:489–502.
9. Kalra M, Gloviczki P, Noel AA, et al. Subfascial endoscopic perforator vein surgery in patients with post-thrombotic venous insufficiency – is it justified? Vasc Endovasc Surg 2002;36:41–50.
10. van Rij AM, Solomon C, Christie R. Anatomic and physiologic characteristics of venous ulceration. J Vasc Surg 1994;20:759–64.
11. Labropoulos N, Delis K, Nicolaides AN, Leon M, Ramaswami G. The role of the distribution and anatomic extent of reflux in the development of signs and symptoms in chronic venous insufficiency. J Vasc Surg 1996;23:504–10.
12. Hanrahan LM, Araki CT, Rodriguez AA, Kechejian GJ, LaMorte WW, Menzoian JO. Distribution of valvular incompetence in patients with venous stasis ulceration. J Vasc Surg 1991;13:805–12.
13. Myers KA, Ziegenbein RW, Zeng GH, Matthews PG. Duplex ultrasonography scanning for chronic venous disease: patterns of venous reflux. J Vasc Surg 1995;21:605–12.
14. van Bemmelen PS, Bedford G, Beach K, Strandness DE. Quantitative segmental evaluation of venous valvular reflux with duplex ultrasound scanning. J Vasc Surg 1989;10:425–31.
15. Kistner RL, Ferris EB, Randhawa G, Kamida C. A method of performing descending venography. J Vasc Surg 1986;4:464–8.
16. McMullin GM, Coleridge SP, Scurr JH. Objective assessment of high ligation without stripping the long saphenous vein. Br J Surg 1991;78:1139–42.
17. Munn SR, Morton JB, Macbeth WA, Mcleish AR. To strip or not to strip the long saphenous vein? A varicose veins trial. Br J Surg 1981;68:426–8.
18. Stonebridge PA, Chalmers N, Beggs I, Bradbury AW, Ruckley CV. Recurrent varicose veins: a varicographic analysis leading to a new practical classification. Br J Surg 1995;82:60–2.
19. Darke SG. The morphology of recurrent varicose veins. Eur J Vasc Surg 1992;6:512–7.
20. Bergan JJ. Saphenous vein stripping and quality of outcome. Br J Surg 1996;83:1027.
21. Fligelstone L, Carolan G, Pugh N, Shandall A, Lane I. An assessment of the long saphenous vein for potential use as a vascular conduit after varicose vein surgery. J Vasc Surg 1993;18:836–40.
22. Rutgers PH, Kitslaar PJ. Randomized trial of stripping versus high ligation combined with sclerotherapy in the treatment of the incompetent greater saphenous vein. Am J Surg 1994;168:311–5.
23. Jakobsen BH. The value of different forms of treatment for varicose veins. Br J Surg 1979;66:182–4.
24. Neglen P, Einarsson E, Eklof B. The functional long-term value of different types of treatment for saphenous vein incompetence. Cardiovasc Surg 1993;34:295–301.
25. Weiss RA, Weiss MA. Controlled radiofrequency endovenous occlusion using a unique radiofrequency catheter under duplex guidance to

eliminate saphenous varicose vein reflux: a 2-year follow-up. Dermatol Surg 2002;28:38–42.

26. Chandler JG, Pichot O, Sessa C, et al. Treatment of primary venous insufficiency by endovenous saphenous vein obliteration. Vasc Surg 2000;34:201–14.

27. Merchant RF, DePalma RG, Kabnick LS. Endovascular obliteration of saphenous reflux: a multicenter study. J Vasc Surg 2002;35:1190–6.

28. Dwerryhouse S, Davies B, Harradine K, Earnshaw JJ. Stripping the long saphenous vein reduces the rate of reoperation for recurrent varicose veins: five-year results of a randomized trial. J Vasc Surg 1999;29:589–92.

29. Chandler JG, Pichot O, Sessa C, Schuller-Petrovic S, Osse FJ, Bergan JJ. Defining the role of extended saphenofemoral junction ligation: a prospective comparative study. J Vasc Surg 2000;32:941–53.

30. Rautio T, Ohinmaa A, Perala J, et al. Endovenous obliteration versus conventional stripping operation in the treatment of primary varicose veins: a randomized controlled trial with comparison of the costs. J Vasc Surg 2002;35:958–65.

31. Mozes G, Gloviczki P, Menawat SS, Fisher DR, Carmichael SW, Kadar A. Surgical anatomy for endoscopic subfascial division of perforating veins. J Vasc Surg 1996;24:800–8.

32. Sherman RS. Varicose veins: further findings based on anatomic and surgical dissections. Ann Surg 1949;130:218–32.

33. Stuart WP, Adam DJ, Allan PL, Ruckley CV, Bradbury AW. The relationship between the number, competence, and diameter of medial calf perforating veins and the clinical status in healthy subjects and patients with lower-limb venous disease. J Vasc Surg 2000;32:138–43.

34. Delis KT, Husmann M, Kalodiki E, Wolfe JH, Nicolaides AN. In situ hemodynamics of perforating veins in chronic venous insufficiency. J Vasc Surg 2001;33:773–82.

35. Linton RR. The operative treatment of varicose veins and ulcers, based upon a classification of these lesions. Ann Surg 1938;107:582–93.

36. Cockett FB, Jones BD. The ankle blow-out syndrome: a new approach to the varicose ulcer problem. Lancet 1953;i:17–23.

37. Lim RCJ, Blaisdell FW, Zubrin J, Stallone RJ, Hall AD. Subfascial ligation of perforating veins in recurrent stasis ulceration. Am J Surg 1970;119:246–9.

38. DePalma RG. Surgical therapy for venous stasis: results of a modified Linton operation. Am J Surg 1979;137:810–3.

39. Burnand K, Thomas ML, O'Donnell T, Browse NL. Relation between postphlebitic changes in the deep veins and results of surgical treatment of venous ulcers. Lancet 1976;i:936–8.

40. Edwards JM. Shearing operation for incompetent perforating veins. Br J Surg 1976;63:885–6.

41. Hauer G. [Endoscopic subfascial discussion of perforating veins – preliminary report]. [German]. Vasa 1985;14:59–61.

42. Bergan JJ, Murray J, Greason K. Subfascial endoscopic perforator vein surgery: a preliminary report. Ann Vasc Surg 1996;10:211–9.

43. Gloviczki P, Bergan JJ, Menawat SS, et al. Safety, feasibility, and early efficacy of subfascial endoscopic perforator surgery: a preliminary report from the North American registry. J Vasc Surg 1997;25:94–105.

44. Pierik EG, van Urk H, Hop WC, Wittens CH. Endoscopic versus open subfascial division of incompetent perforating veins in the treatment of venous leg ulceration: a randomized trial. J Vasc Surg 1997; 26:1049–54.

45. O'Donnell TF. Surgical treatment of incompetent communicating veins. Atlas of venous surgery. Philadelphia:WB Saunders; 2000:111–24.

46. Gloviczki P, Cambria RA, Rhee RY, Canton LG, McKusick MA. Surgical technique and preliminary results of endoscopic subfascial division of perforating veins. J Vasc Surg 1996;23:517–23.

47. Conrad P. Endoscopic exploration of the subfascial space of the lower leg with perforator interruption using laparoscopic equipment: a preliminary report. Phlebology 1994;9:154–7.

48. Pierik EGJM, Wittens CHA, van Urk H. Subfascial endoscopic ligation in the treatment of incompetent perforator veins. Eur J Vasc Endovasc Surg 1995;5:38–41.

49. Sparks SR, Ballard JL, Bergan JJ, Killeen JD. Early benefits of subfascial endoscopic perforator surgery (SEPS) in healing venous ulcers. Ann Vasc Surg 1997;11:367–73.

50. Padberg FTJ, Pappas PJ, Araki CT, Back TL, Hobson RW. Hemodynamic and clinical improvement after superficial vein ablation in primary combined venous insufficiency with ulceration. J Vasc Surg 1996;24:711–8.

51. Nelzen O. Prospective study of safety, patient satisfaction and leg ulcer healing following saphenous and subfascial endoscopic perforator surgery. Br J Surg 2000;87:86–91.

52. Stuart WP, Adam DJ, Bradbury AW, Ruckley CV. Subfascial endoscopic perforator surgery is associated with significantly less morbidity and shorter hospital stay than open operation (Linton's procedure). Br J Surg 1997;84:1364–5.

53. Sybrandy JE, van Gent WB, Pierik EG, Wittens CH. Endoscopic versus open subfascial division of incompetent perforating veins in the treatment of venous leg ulceration: long-term follow-up. J Vasc Surg 2001;33:1028–32.

54. Rhodes JM, Gloviczki P, Canton LG, Heaser TV, Rooke T. Endoscopic perforator vein division with ablation of superficial reflux improves venous hemodynamics. J Vasc Surg 1998;28:839–47.

55. Bradbury AW, Stonebridge PA, Callam MJ, Ruckley CV, Allan PL. Foot volumetry and duplex ultrasonography after saphenous and subfascial perforating vein ligation for recurrent venous ulceration. Br J Surg 1993;80:845–8.

56. Akesson H, Brudin L, Cwikiel W, Ohlin P, Plate G. Does the correction of insufficient superficial and perforating veins improve venous function in patients with deep venous insufficiency? Phlebology 1990; 5:113–23.

57. Proebstle TM, Weisel G, Paepcke U, Gass S, Weber L. Light reflection rheography and clinical course of patients with advanced venous disease before and after endoscopic subfascial division of perforating veins. Dermatol Surg 1998;24:771–6.

58. Kistner RL. Surgical repair of a venous valve. Straub Clinical Procedures 1968;41–43.

59. Raju S, Fredericks R. Valve reconstruction procedures for non-obstructive venous insufficiency: rationale, techniques, and results in 107 procedures with two- to eight-year follow-up. J Vasc Surg 1988; 7:301–10.

60. Sottiurai VS. Technique in direct venous valvuloplasty. J Vasc Surg 1988;8:646–8.

61. Gloviczki P, Merrell SW, Bower TC. Femoral vein valve repair under direct vision without venotomy: a modified technique with use of angioscopy. J Vasc Surg 1991;14:645–8.

62. Raju S, Hardy JD. Technical options in venous valve reconstruction. Am J Surg 1997;173:301–7.

63. Durango E. Creation of new venous valves. Second Meeting of Cardiovascular Surgeons and First Ecuadorian Course on Angiology and Vascular Surgery. Quito, Ecuador, 1993.

64. Kistner RL, Sparkuhl MD. Surgery in acute and chronic venous disease. Surgery 1979;85:31–43.

65. Taheri SA, Lazar L, Elias S. Status of vein valve transplant after 12 months. Arch Surg 1982;117:1313–7.

66. Bry JD, Muto PA, O'Donnell TF, Isaacson LA. The clinical and hemodynamic results after axillary-to-popliteal vein valve transplantation. J Vasc Surg 1995;21:110–9.

67. Masuda EM, Kistner RL. Long-term results of venous valve reconstruction: a four- to twenty-one-year follow-up. J Vasc Surg 1994; 19:391–403.

68. Cheatle TR, Perrin M. Venous valve repair: early results in fifty-two cases. J Vasc Surg 1994;19:404–13.

69. Welch HJ, McLaughlin RL, O'Donnell TF Jr. Femoral vein valvuloplasty: intraoperative angioscopic evaluation and hemodynamic improvement. J Vasc Surg 1992;16:694–700.

70. Jamieson WG, Chinnick B. Clinical results of deep venous valvular repair for chronic venous insufficiency. Can J Surg 1997;40:294–9.

71. Perrin M. [Introduction: surgery of the venous valve]. [French]. J Malad Vasc 1997;22:96.

72. Eriksson I, Almgren B. Surgical reconstruction of incompetent deep vein valves. Upsala J Med Sci 1988;93:139–43.

73. Sottiurai VS. Results of deep vein reconstruction. Vasc Surg 1997; 31:276–8.

623

74. Raju S, Neglen P, Doolittle J, Meydrech EF. Axillary vein transfer in trabeculated post thrombotic veins. J Vasc Surg 1999;29:1050–62.

75. Perrin M. Reconstructive surgery for deep venous reflux: a report on 144 cases. Cardiovasc Surg 2000;8:246–55.

76. O'Donnell TFJ, Mackey WC, Shepard AD, Callow AD. Clinical, hemodynamic, and anatomic follow-up of direct venous reconstruction. Arch Surg 1987;122:474–82.

77. Raju S, Fredericks RK, Neglen PN, Bass JD. Durability of venous valve reconstruction techniques for 'primary' and post thrombotic reflux. J Vasc Surg 1996;23:357–66.

78. Thorpe PE. Endovascular therapy for chronic venous occlusion. J Endovasc Surg 1999;6:118–9.

79. Bjarnason H, Kruse JR, Asinger DA, et al. Iliofemoral deep venous thrombosis: safety and efficacy outcome during 5 years of catheter-directed thrombolytic therapy. J Vasc Intervent Radiol 1997;8:405–18.

80. Neglen P, Raju S. Balloon dilation and stenting of chronic iliac vein obstruction: technical aspects and early clinical outcome. J Endovasc Ther 2000;7:79–91.

81. O'Sullivan GJ, Semba CP, Bittner CA, et al. Endovascular management of iliac vein compression (May-Thurner) syndrome. J Vasc Intervent Radiol 2000;11:823–36.

82. Hurst DR, Forauer AR, Bloom JR, Greenfield LJ, Wakefield TW, Williams DM. Diagnosis and endovascular treatment of iliocaval compression syndrome. J Vasc Surg 2001;34:106–13.

83. Nazarian GK, Austin WR, Wegryn SA, et al. Venous recanalization by metallic stents after failure of balloon angioplasty or surgery: four-year experience. Cardiovasc Intervent Radiol 1996;19:227–33.

84. Raju S, Owen SJ, Neglen P. The clinical impact of iliac venous stents in the management of chronic venous insufficiency. J Vasc Surg 2002; 35:8–15.

85. Husni EA. Reconstruction of veins: the need for objectivity. J Cardiovasc Surg 1983;24:525–8.

86. May R. The Palma operation with Gottlob's endothelium preserving suture. In: May R, Weber J, eds. Pelvic and abdominal veins: progress in diagnosis and therapy. Amsterdam:Excerpta Medica; 1981:192–7.

87. Palma EC, Esperon R. Vein transplants and grafts in the surgical treatment of the post phlebitic syndrome. J Cardiovasc Surg 1960; 1:94–107.

88. Dale WA. Reconstructive venous surgery. Arch Surg 1979; 114:1312.

89. Lalka SG, Lash JM, Unthank JL, et al. Inadequacy of saphenous vein grafts for cross-femoral venous bypass. J Vasc Surg 1991;13:622–30.

90. Gruss JD, Hiemer W. Bypass procedures for venous obstruction: Palma and May-Husni bypasses, Raju perforator bypass, prosthetic bypasses, and primary and adjunctive arteriovenous fistulae. In: Raju S, Villavicencio JL, eds. Surgical management of venous disease. Baltimore:Williams & Wilkins; 1997:289–305.

91. Frileux C, Pillot-Bienayme P, Gillot C. Bypass of segmental obliterations of ileo–femoral venous axis by transposition of saphenous vein. J Cardiovasc Surg 1972;13:409.

92. AbuRahma AF, Robinson PA, Boland JP. Clinical, hemodynamic, and anatomic predictors of long-term outcome of lower extremity venovenous bypasses. J Vasc Surg 1991;14:635–44.

93. Danza R, Navarro T, Baldizan J. Reconstructive surgery in chronic venous obstruction of the lower limbs. J Cardiovasc Surg 1991;32:98–103.

94. Smith DE, Trimble C. Surgical management of obstructive venous disease of the lower extremity. In: Rutherford RB, ed. Vascular Surgery. Philadelphia:WB Saunders; 1977:1247–68.

95. Jost CJ, Gloviczki P, Cherry KJJ, et al. Surgical reconstruction of iliofemoral veins and the inferior vena cava for nonmalignant occlusive disease. J Vasc Surg 2001;33:320–7.

96. Eklof BG, Kistner RL, Masuda EM. Venous bypass and valve reconstruction: long-term efficacy. Vasc Med 1998;3:157–64 (Review).

97. Comerota AJ, Aldridge SC, Cohen G, Ball DS, Pliskin M, White JV. A strategy of aggressive regional therapy for acute iliofemoral venous thrombosis with contemporary venous thrombectomy or catheter-directed thrombolysis. J Vasc Surg 1994;20:244–54.

98. Sottiurai VS, Gonzales J, Cooper M, Lyon R, Ross C. A new concept of arteriovenous fistula in venous bypass requiring no fistula interruption: surgical technique and long-term results. Submitted to J Cardiovasc Surg 2002.

99. Schanzer H, Peirce EC. A rational approach to surgery of the chronic venous statis syndrome. Ann Surg 1982;195:25–9.

100. Negus D, Friedgood A. The effective management of venous ulceration. Br J Surg 1983;70:623–7.

101. Sethia KK, Darke SG. Long saphenous incompetence as a cause of venous ulceration. Br J Surg 1984;71:754–5.

102. van Bemmelen PS, Bedford G, Beach K, Strandness DE Jr. Status of the valves in the superficial and deep venous system in chronic venous disease. Surgery 1991;109:730–4.

103. Hanrahan LM, Araki CT, Rodriguez AA, Kechejian GJ, LaMorte WW, Menzoian JO. Distribution of valvular incompetence in patients with venous stasis ulceration. J Vasc Surg 1991;13:805–12.

104. Darke SG, Penfold C. Venous ulceration and saphenous ligation. Eur J Vasc Surg 1992;6:4–9.

105. Lees TA, Lambert D. Patterns of venous reflux in limbs with skin changes associated with chronic venous insufficiency. Br J Surg 1993; 80:725–8.

106. Shami SK, Sarin S, Cheatle TR, Scurr JH, Smith PD. Venous ulcers and the superficial venous system. J Vasc Surg 1993;17:487–90.

107. van Rij AM, Solomon C, Christie R. Anatomic and physiologic characteristics of venous ulceration. J Vasc Surg 1994;20:759–64.

108. Jugenheimer M, Junginger T. Endoscopic subfascial sectioning of incompetent perforating veins in treatment of primary varicosis. World J Surg 1992;16:971–5.

109. Wolters U, Schmit-Rixen T, Erasmi H, Lynch J. Endoscopic dissection of incompetent perforating veins in the treatment of chronic venous leg ulcers. Vasc Surg 1996;30:481–7.

110. Pierik EG, van Urk H, Wittens CH. Efficacy of subfascial endoscopy in eradicating perforating veins of the lower leg and its relation with venous ulcer healing. J Vasc Surg 1997;26:255–9.

111. Illig KA, Shortell CK, Ouriel K, Greenberg RK, Waldman D, Green RM. Photoplethysmography and calf muscle pump function after subfascial endoscopic perforator ligation. J Vasc Surg 1999;30:1067–76.

112. Halliday AW, Mansfield AO. Congenital arteriovenous malformations. Br J Surg 1993;80:2–3.

113. Husfeldt KJ, Gall FP, Schulz HP, Zirngibl H. [Vein substitution using PTFE prosthesis – results of animal experiments and initial clinical experiences]. [German]. Chir Forum Exp Klin Forsch 1979;11–5.

114. Dale WA, Harris J, Terry RB. Polytetrafluoroethylene reconstruction of the inferior vena cava. Surgery 1984;95:625–30.

115. Alimi YS, DiMauro P, Fabre D, Juhan C. Iliac vein reconstructions to treat acute and chronic venous occlusive disease. J Vasc Surg 1997; 25:673–81.

CHAPTER
42

Deep Vein Thrombosis and Pulmonary Embolism

Kong Teng Tan, Matthijs Oudkerk, and Edwin J R van Beek

KEY POINTS

- Deep venous thrombosis (DVT) and pulmonary embolism (PE) are a single clinicopathologic entity (venous thromboembolic disease; VTE).

- The incidence is one case of DVT and 0.5 case of PE per 1000 population/year in the western world.

- In a hospital setting, 15% of medical and 30–50% of surgical patients will develop VTE, if no thromboprophylaxis is administered.

- Clinical features are non-specific and inaccurate, resulting in misdiagnosis of VTE in many patients.

- There are serious immediate and long-term complications; untreated PE has 30–40% mortality and up to 50% of patients with DVT develop post-thrombotic syndrome.

- Several diagnostic algorithms can prove or rule out the diagnosis of VTE safely.

- Anticoagulation is the cornerstone of treatment but thrombolysis is an option for life-threatening VTE.

- Seventy percent of patients with suspected VTE do not have this condition and treatment should be withheld.

INTRODUCTION

Approximately three per 1000 population will suffer from chest symptoms suggesting pulmonary embolism (PE) every year and it is estimated that the prevalence of deep venous thrombosis (DVT) in the USA is two million cases per year.[1] About 30–50% of these patients will have concurrent PE and 10% of these die within the first hour of presentation.[2] In the USA, PE is said to cause more deaths than road traffic accidents, which in 1993 claimed 43 536 lives. Furthermore, post-thrombotic syndrome develops in 50% of patients who have ileofemoral vein thrombosis. This is a debilitating condition with major social and economic consequences.

Deep venous thrombosis and PE were considered as separate clinicopathologic entities until relatively recently. Numerous autopsy studies have demonstrated a strong association between PE and venous thrombosis.[3] In patients with proven PE, 70% also have demonstrable DVT of the leg veins. Half of all patients with proven DVT have (often silent) PE.[4] Furthermore, the clinical outcome is very similar in patients who present with DVT and those who present with PE. There is ample evidence that DVT and PE should be considered as a single medical problem, albeit at different ends of the spectrum of a disease process.

The diagnosis of PE is often difficult, and this has resulted in several (sometimes complex) diagnostic algorithms.[5] The clinical features are frequently non-specific. The disease commonly affects and complicates the course of severely ill patients, which makes interpretation of available diagnostic tests difficult. However, a speedy diagnosis is paramount as there is a 30% risk of a fatal or non-fatal recurrent PE. Autopsy studies have shown repeatedly that PE continues to be missed, especially in the elderly and those with concurrent cardiorespiratory diseases.

Thromboprophylactic measures and changes in hospital practice introduced over the last few decades have had a positive impact on the incidence of venous thromboembolic disease (VTE). A necropsy series, covering the period 1965 to 1990, from a London teaching hospital showed that the percentage of fatal PE fell progressively from 6.1% to 2.1% over the 25 years.[6] Furthermore, the incidence of postoperative DVT demonstrated by venography has halved. However, the incidence of DVT in non-surgical patients remains unchanged. These figures are supported by a recent population-based study which showed a 45% reduction in PE over the last 15 years, while the incidence of DVT remained unchanged in men of all ages, but increased in women over the age of 60 years.[7]

To date, there is no international consensus on the most effective clinical protocol for the diagnosis, prophylaxis, or treatment of venous thromboembolic disease. The clinical practices are highly variable between hospitals, with some centers advocating aggressive management (e.g. thrombolysis), where others are more conservative.[8]

EPIDEMIOLOGY

Although VTE is such a common condition, the precise incidence has not been well described. The reported figures for the incidence of DVT and PE are highly variable. Presumably this is due to many factors, including the diagnostic test used, the population studied, and whether antithrombotic prophylaxis had been used. A retrospective population-based survey found an average annual incidence of 48 primary and 36 recurrent cases of DVT, plus 23 cases of pulmonary emboli per 100 000 residents.[9] Figures from Vital Statistics and from the National Hospital Discharge Survey in the USA from 1970 to 1985 showed an age-adjusted rate for PE of 51 per 100 000 and venous thrombosis of 79 per 100 000 inhabitants.[10] A 25-year population-based study of 2218 patients in Olmsted County, Minnesota from 1966 to 1990 showed an annual incidence of VTE of 117 per 100 000 (DVT, 48 per 100 000; PE, 69 per 100 000).[7] Furthermore, the incidence of VTE was higher in men than in women (ratio 1.2:1). Reviewing the epidemiologic studies, it is a fair estimate that the annual incidence of DVT and PE in the western world is about 1 and 0.5 cases per 1000 population, respectively.

A recent study showed that the incidence of VTE demonstrated by bilateral venography or duplex ultrasonography in hospitalized, acutely ill medical patients who did not receive any anticoagulation was 14.9%.[11] In another study of postoperative neurosurgical patients who received compression stockings as the only measure of thromboprophylaxis, an incidence of 43/129 patients (33%) was demonstrated.[12]

Autopsy studies, as expected, showed higher incidences of PE (50–60%), especially when the lung specimens were examined in detail. However, it should be remembered that in the majority of cases, the emboli were small and unlikely to be the main cause of death, although they may have contributed indirectly.[13] The true incidence of PE as a cause of death is not known. Studies in the 1970s suggested that 7% of deaths in hospital were secondary to PE. This result was probably inaccurate, as subsequent investigations refuted this finding. Most recent autopsy series quote a more conservative figure of 1–3%.[14]

In conclusion, although the exact incidence of VTE is obscure, it is estimated to affect 1.5 million patients per year in the western world and, without any doubt, it is a major cause of morbidity and mortality.

PATHOPHYSIOLOGY

The pathophysiology of VTE includes the causes of thrombogenesis and the pathophysiologic consequences of DVT and PE.

Thrombogenesis

Virchow's triad (Rudolf Virchow, German pathologist 1821–1902) systematizes the understanding of intravascular thrombosis and provides a platform for a comprehensive approach to its differential diagnosis. The three components of Virchow's triad (**Fig. 42.1**) are:

- endothelial abnormality;
- stasis of blood flow; and
- hypercoagulability of the circulating blood.

A single abnormality may occasionally be sufficient to provoke thrombosis but in the majority of cases the prothrombotic states are characterized by more than one defect of Virchow's triad.

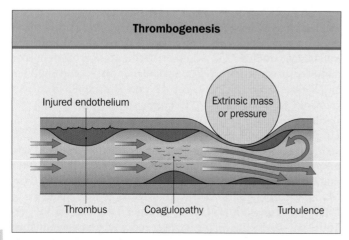

Figure 42.1 Thrombogenesis. Virchow's triad: (1) endothelial abnormalities, (2) coagulopathy, and (3) stasis of blood flow.

The most common site of DVT is the deep veins of the leg, followed, in decreasing order, by pelvic veins, vena cava, right heart chambers, and arm. Thrombosis of the veins of the arm and superior vena cava is increasing in incidence due to the use of central venous catheters for parenteral feeding and chemotherapy.[15] The rate of embolism from each specific site of thrombosis is unknown but it is suspected to be highest from central veins or right heart chambers and lowest from peripheral veins. Thrombi that are located distal to the trifurcation of the popliteal vein generally do not embolize to the lungs unless they propagate more proximally into the popliteal or femoral vein. This occurs in up to 20% of calf vein thrombi.[16] Thrombosis of the iliofemoral segment is estimated to produce emboli in 30–50% of cases and when combined with popliteal vein thrombosis, they account for over 90% of all episodes of PE.[2]

Endothelial abnormalities

The endothelial lining provides a smooth continuous surface for blood flow. It is non-thrombotic, yet it must provide a pro-thrombotic capability when protective coagulation is needed. Of the triad, endothelial injury appears to be the least important factor in the development of thrombosis.[17] Endothelial injury occurs when there is severe local trauma, for example during hip replacement[18] or venous catheterization, which can lead to adherence of platelets to the injured endothelium and activation of the coagulation cascade. Systemic illness such as autoimmune diseases or bacterial septicemia may damage the endothelium by immune complex deposition, which can lead to vasculitis and venous thrombosis.[17] The administration of traditional iodinated contrast media during venography paradoxically can itself cause venous thrombosis. The reported incidence of DVT following venography using ionic contrast media ranges from 9–30% and is thought to be due to the cytotoxic effect of the contrast medium on the endothelium.[19] The new generation low-osmolar, non-ionic contrast media are much safer, but still have a 3% incidence of DVT following venography.[20] The introduction of the dimer contrast agents (iotrolan and iodixanol) may reduce this even further.

Blood flow (stasis)

Venous stasis is the predominant factor in the development of thrombosis. The first site of thrombosis is usually in the vein valve pockets, presumably due to local stasis secondary to eddy currents (**Fig. 42.2**). Blood flow in the venous system depends on a few factors, including cardiac output, venous resistance, and compression of surrounding musculature, particularly calf muscles. Any condition that reduces cardiac output, increases venous resistance, or impairs muscular contractions predisposes to thrombus formation. Cardiac failure, an intra-abdominal mass (pregnancy or tumor), immobilization, and pressure from cast or bandage are examples encountered frequently. Intraluminal devices such as venous catheters, pacing wires, and caval filters disrupt the flow of blood and can lead to thrombus formation.[15]

Blood disorders (hypercoagulability)

In a normal person, plasma coagulation factors exist in a non-activated state. Upon activation, the intrinsic regulating system prevents excessive activation which can lead to hypercoagulation. Abnormalities in serum clotting levels, intrinsic abnormalities of their protein structure, or circulating antibodies that abnormally

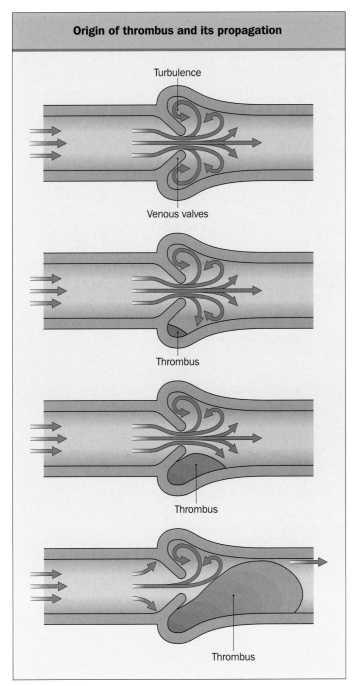

Origin of thrombus and its propagation

Turbulence

Venous valves

Thrombus

Thrombus

Thrombus

Figure 42.2 Origin of thrombus and its propagation. Thrombus forms in the valve pockets secondary to venous stasis. Subsequent deposition of fibrin-platelet layers leads to propagation of the thrombus.

Causes of hypercoagulability.
Inherited
Common Factor V Leiden Prothrombin gene mutation (G20110A) Homozygous C677T mutation in methylene tetrahydrofolate reductase gene
Rare Antithrombin deficiency Protein S deficiency Protein C deficiency Dysfibrinogenemia Homozygous homocystinuria
Acquired
Age Surgery and trauma Immobilization Malignant disease Previous venous thromboembolism Pregnancy and puerperium Oral contraceptive and hormone replacement therapy Antiphospholipid antibodies
Unknown (probably multifactorial)
Elevated levels of factor VIII, IX, XI, and fibrinogen

Table 42.1 Causes of hypercoagulability.

activate the coagulation cascade can result in hypercoagulation and thrombosis. There are many causes of hypercoagulability and they can be divided into two groups, acquired or inherited (**Table 42.1**).

Pathophysiologic consequence of deep venous thrombosis

As the thrombus enlarges, the patent lumen of the involved vein becomes smaller (see **Fig. 42.3**). This increases the resistance to blood flow, thereby diverting the blood to low resistance veins, which are the collaterals frequently seen on venography in patients with DVT. The thrombus subsequently undergoes degradation by

one or more of the following mechanisms: lysis, fragmentation, embolization, and/or organization. Thrombus that is not dissolved by the fibrinolytic process or has not dislodged to become an embolus will slowly retract and adhere to the endothelium. This instigates a local inflammatory response in the vessel wall, causing proliferation of granulation tissue, which invades the thrombus. This inflammatory response is the first step in the organization of the thrombus, a process that involves the conversion of thrombus and the affected vein into scar tissue. This process is highly variable; some patients will undergo complete recanalization while others have a permanently occluded venous segment. Furthermore, any valves involved in the thrombosis may be destroyed by the inflammatory reaction, causing the disabling post-thrombotic syndrome in some recanalized veins.

Pathophysiologic consequences of pulmonary embolism

The immediate effects of clot detaching from a peripheral vein and lodging in a pulmonary artery are:

- termination of flow distally; and
- an increase in pressure proximally.

The clinicophysiologic consequences depend on numerous factors, including the size and number of thrombi (thrombotic burden) and the cardiopulmonary status of the patient.

Pulmonary consequences

In the majority of cases, the blood supply to lung parenchyma remains normal as the perfusion is maintained by the bronchial circulation. Pulmonary artery occlusion from embolus can result

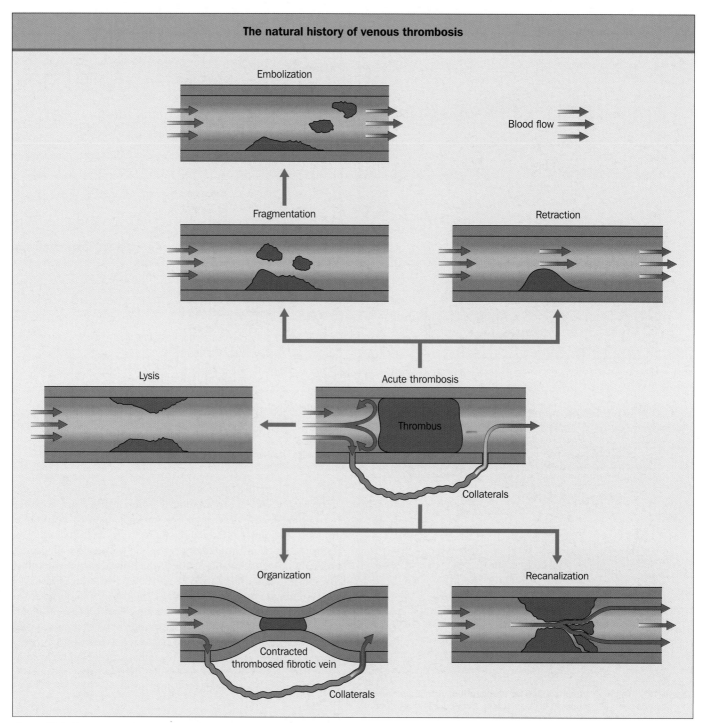

The natural history of venous thrombosis

Embolization

Blood flow

Fragmentation

Retraction

Lysis

Acute thrombosis

Thrombus

Collaterals

Organization

Recanalization

Contracted
thrombosed fibrotic vein

Collaterals

Figure 42.3 The natural history of venous thrombosis. The vein may remain occluded with venous return restored through collateral veins. If the vein recanalizes, the valves are often destroyed, leaving venous incompetence.

in ischemia and infarction of the pulmonary parenchyma, but this occurs only in occasional cases. This is more common after peripheral than central pulmonary embolization, and in patients with coexisting medical conditions such as malignancy or cardiorespiratory illness.[21] Histologically, this is manifest as hemorrhage and necrosis of the pulmonary parenchyma. Lung infarction is seen in around 10–15% of autopsy specimens of patients with PE.

Another pathophysiologic effect of acute PE is local bronchoconstriction, which is a temporary phenomenon lasting less than 4 to 6 hours. Although this is rarely detected clinically, it is present in the majority of patients on physiologic testing.[22] Serotonin and histamine released by platelets in the emboli are thought to be the chemical mediators responsible for the bronchoconstriction. Atelectasis is also a common finding in ischemic lung and this is most likely to be secondary to the combination of decreased surfactant production in non-perfused segments and bronchoconstriction.[23,24]

Although there is impairment of carbon dioxide elimination in the ischemic bronchi, compensatory hyperventilation in the normal segments usually leads to hypocapnia. Hypercapnia is only observed in patients with acute massive PE who develop right heart failure and systemic hypotension.[25] Ultimately, if sufficient lung parenchyma is affected, this will result in hypoxemia and hypercapnia. Occasionally, secondary infection of the ischemic segments may occur, resulting in pneumonia. Cavitation of the infarcted segment may be a primary process but usually it is due to superadded infection leading to abscess formation. The final outcome of the infarcted segment is fibrosis and scarring, manifest radiologically as linear bands at the periphery of the lung fields.

Hemodynamic consequences

Several factors determine the hemodynamic consequences of acute PE (**Fig. 42.4**). Most important are, firstly, the number and size of the emboli and, secondly, the cardiorespiratory health of the individual. Small emboli usually do not produce any circulatory changes unless the patient has pre-existing cardiorespiratory disease. Large emboli, in contrast, often cause cardiorespiratory signs (hypotension, tachycardia, and pulmonary

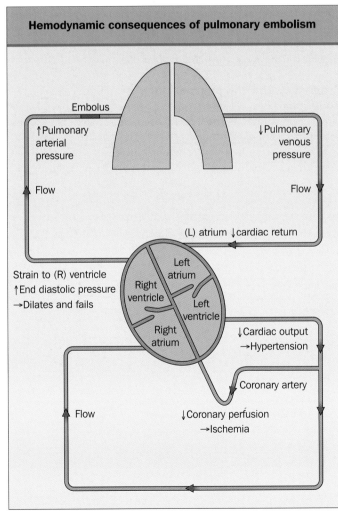

Figure 42.4 Hemodynamic consequences of pulmonary embolism. A large embolus increases pulmonary arterial pressure and therefore increases the work of the right (R) ventricle. However, the cardiac return to the left (L) atrium decreases, leading to poor cardiac output and decreased systemic and coronary perfusion, which may lead to cardiac ischemia.

hypertension). It has been estimated that at least a 50% occlusion of the vascular bed is required before there is any significant increase in pulmonary arterial pressure in a healthy individual.[26] The circulatory effect of a PE depends not only on mechanical occlusion of pulmonary arteries by the thrombus but also on reflex vasoconstriction of the vasculature mediated by local neural and humoral factors. This is demonstrated in patients who undergo pneumonectomy; cross-clamping of the pulmonary artery is usually well tolerated, with minimal increase in pulmonary arterial pressure. In contrast, a large PE obstructing a main pulmonary artery can be life-threatening, with major hemodynamic consequences. Release of vasoactive substances, such as serotonin, endothelin-1, and thromboxane A2, by endothelium and platelets is thought to mediate pulmonary artery vasoconstriction in acute PE.

Pulmonary embolism causes an increase in pulmonary wedge pressure with a consequent increase in end-diastolic pressure in the right ventricle. This stretches the right ventricular myocardium. According to the Frank–Starling mechanism in a normal heart, the stroke volume or ventricular performance will increase as the preload increases secondary to sympathetic stimulation. This mechanism works by increasing the heart rate and myocardial contractility. In acute PE, the ventricular afterload/impedance of the right ventricle increases with the pulmonary arterial pressure and this increases demand on the heart. If the right ventricle cannot cope, the end diastolic pressure rises and the ventricle dilates. A fall in systemic blood pressure due to poor cardiac return to the left heart leads to a reduction in coronary blood flow that naturally affects cardiac perfusion. This vicious cycle can lead to cardiac ischemia and death.[27] In a patient with coexisting cardiopulmonary disease, the whole process is accelerated, as there is diminished cardiac reserve.

In acute massive PE, the pulmonary arterial pressure rarely exceeds 50mmHg in a previously healthy individual. This is because the right ventricle has a small myocardial mass and therefore responds poorly to a sudden obstruction to flow. In contrast, patients with repeated episodes of submassive or small emboli (chronic thromboembolic disease) have very high pulmonary arterial pressure; it may occasionally exceed systemic pressure. In these patients, the right heart has time to respond to the stress and becomes hypertrophied, with an increase in muscle mass.

RISK FACTORS

Old age

Age is the major risk factor of VTE. The incidence of DVT and PE increase steadily with age, after adjusting for other risk factors.[7,9] Furthermore, the case-fatality index of PE is far higher in the elderly. In addition, regardless of the type of surgery, the incidence of postoperative DVT is also strongly associated with increasing age.

Previous venous thromboembolism

Although a previous history of VTE is an independent risk factor in the development of VTE, the majority of patients with recurrent DVT/PE have other persistent risk factors, for example, thrombophilia or carcinoma. A previous thromboembolic episode also places patients at a particularly high risk of recurrence should they undergo surgery, or become pregnant or immobilized.[28] Therefore, it is crucial for this group of patients to have good thromboprophylaxis to minimize the risk of recurrence.

Immobilization

Immobilization is a convincing risk factor for the development of VTE. Warlow et al., using radiolabeled fibrinogen, demonstrated this clearly in a study group of patients with hemiplegia.[29] Using the non-paralyzed leg as a control, he found that DVT was present in 60% of paralyzed legs compared with only 7% of normal legs. Long-haul economy class air travel has been implicated as a risk factor for many years, although the evidence for it was scanty until recently. Scurr et al. demonstrated a strong relationship between DVT and prolonged air travel in a randomized controlled trial.[30] Passengers over 50 years of age were randomly allocated to wear class I below-knee graduated elastic compression stockings or no stockings. Some 12/116 passengers (10%) without compression stockings developed a symptomless DVT compared with none in the control group. In the LONFLIT3 (venous thromboembolism in air travel) study, DVT was identified in 4.8% of the control group, 3.6% of subjects taking aspirin, and none of the group who received one dose of enoxaparin.[31]

Trauma and surgery

Patients who sustain major trauma or have major surgery are at high risk of VTE and the risk continues even after discharge from hospital. The incidence (**Table 42.2**) depends on numerous factors including age, previous VTE, obesity, malignancy, and type of surgical procedure. Without thromboprophylaxis, major orthopedic surgery of the legs and major abdominal or pelvic surgery has a 10–30% risk of proximal DVT, a 40–80% risk of calf DVT,

and a 1% risk of fatal PE.[32,33] The majority of thrombi develop in the deep veins in the first 5 days after operation. Following major trauma, more than 50% of patients develop a DVT, and in approximately 20% this is a iliofemoral.[34] It is therefore prudent to provide appropriate thromboprophylactic measures in this group of patients.

Malignant disease

Malignant disease per se is a risk factor for the development of venous thromboembolic complications, probably by subclinical activation of the coagulation system.[35] Moreover, patients with malignant diseases are usually less mobile and may require cytotoxic chemotherapy or surgery, which are additional risk factors. The incidence of DVT and death from PE in patients with a malignant condition are approximately twice as high as those without cancer.[36] Patients presenting with idiopathic venous thromboembolic events, i.e. no known predisposing factors, frequently have an underlying malignancy.[37] Suggested explanations include a procoagulant state as a result of the cancer, or risk factors common to both cancer and thrombosis. Extensive investigation to search for the underlying malignancy in this group of patients is not economically or clinically justifiable; up to 40% of those proven to have malignancy also have widespread metastases. A limited search by pelvic ultrasonography, mammography, chest radiography, and serum prostate specific antigen for the most common malignancies may be justified.

Pregnancy and the puerperium

Although VTE is a leading cause of maternal death, it is still rare.[38] Two studies, in the UK and Sweden, showed that the risk is minimal until close to delivery.[39,40] The relative risk of DVT or PE (in relation to a control group) increases dramatically by more than 20-fold 2 days before, and more than 50-fold 1 day

Incidence of venous thromboembolism in patients following surgery or trauma.			
	Calf DVT	Proximal DVT	Fatal PE
High risk	40–80%	10–30%	>1%
• Surgical patients with history of venous thromboembolism			
• Major pelvic/abdominal surgery for malignancy			
• Major trauma			
• Major lower limb orthopedic surgery			
Moderate risk	10–40%	1–10%	0.1–1%
• General surgery in patients >40 years			
• Patients on oral contraception			
• Neurosurgical patients			
Low risk	<10%	<1%	<0.1%
• Uncomplicated surgery in patients <40 years without any other risk factors			
• Minor surgery in patients >40 years without any other risk factors			

Table 42.2 Incidence of venous thromboembolism in patients following surgery or trauma. DVT, deep vein thrombosis; PE, pulmonary embolism.

before delivery. Most important risks factors include multiple birth, cardiac disease, previous thromboembolic events, and inherited thrombophilia. The left leg is invariably the site of the DVT, which may be explained by the anatomic position of the left iliac vein in relation to right iliac artery and compression by the enlarged uterus.

Oral contraceptives and hormone replacement therapy

Although the use of oral contraceptives (OC) is associated with a three- to sixfold increase in the risk of developing VTE, the absolute risk is minimal. A baseline risk of less than one per 10 000 person-years is increased to three to four per 10 000 person-years during the period the OC is used.[41] The risk is highest in the first year of use and persists until, but not beyond, discontinuation. Low-dose estrogen OC have small effects in reducing the risk of VTE. Third generation OC are associated with an increased risk of VTE when compared to earlier products; therefore, they should not be the first-line choice for new users.

Patients on hormone replacement therapy (HRT) have a two- to threefold increase in the risk of VTE, but the absolute risk is still minimal and confined to the first year of treatment.[42] However, in patients with a previous history of a thromboembolic event, HRT is associated with a substantially increased risk of recurrence (about tenfold) and this must be considered when the risks and benefits of therapy are being assessed.[43]

Medical conditions requiring hospitalization

The published incidence of VTE in hospitalized non-surgical patients without thromboembolic prophylaxis ranges from 9–30%.[44] Patients with cardiac failure, myocardial infarction, and neurologic diseases are at highest risk of developing VTE, with reported incidences of up to 70%, 30%, and 50%, respectively.[45] Hence, if there is no contraindication, it is essential for these patients to receive thromboprophylaxis on admission to hospital.

Varicose veins and superficial thrombophlebitis

Varicose veins, in isolation, are not an independent risk factor for VTE. However, additional factors such as prolonged immobilization, for example, following surgery, major trauma, or severe medical illness, increase the thrombotic risk. Superficial thrombophlebitis is an independent risk factor, as it can progress to DVT. It is likely that superficial thrombophlebitis and DVT have an identical pathophysiologic cause. Approximately one in 20 patients with significant untreated thrombophlebitis will develop a DVT.

Antiphospholipid antibodies

Antiphospholipid antibodies (APA) are a heterogeneous group of immunoglobulins directed against negatively charged phospholipids, protein–phospholipid complexes, or plasma proteins such as $beta_2$ glycoprotein I. APA include anticardiolipin (ACA) and lupus anticoagulant (LAC) antibodies. Although these antibodies can be present in patients with systemic lupus erythematosus (SLE), they are also frequently found in other autoimmune diseases and also in healthy persons without any underlying disease.[46] The antiphospholipid antibody syndrome (APS) consists of positive APA and clinical features of arterial and venous thrombosis, recurrent abortion, or thrombocytopenia.[47] The leg is the most common site of venous thrombosis in patients with raised APA; however, thrombosis of thoracic and abdominal

venous systems and dural venous sinuses (unusual site in the normal population) are also seen commonly.[48]

Antiphospholipid antibodies occur in approximately 2% of the population and in 30–40% of patients with SLE.[49,50] The frequency of VTE in patients with SLE and positive APA is about 40%, versus 13% in patients with no antibodies. In patients without SLE, the relationship between these antibodies and venous thrombosis is complex. There is a strong association between LAC antibody and venous thrombosis but, in contrast, the association of ACA antibody and thrombosis is less certain.

The risk of recurrent DVT in patients with positive APA following discontinuation of oral anticoagulant is about three times higher than in patients without the antibodies. Furthermore, these patients may be resistant to normal doses of anticoagulant therapy and may require higher doses to prevent recurrence of thrombosis.[51]

Other risk factors

There is no significant difference in the incidence of DVT in surgical patients who have either regional anesthesia (spinal or epidural) or general anesthesia. Smoking, chronic obstructive airway disease, and renal failure have not been shown to be independent risk factors for VTE. Surprisingly, obesity is not an independent risk factor. Patients with serious liver disease have a very low incidence of VTE, presumably due to the protective effect of a prolonged clotting time and thrombocytopenia. Tamoxifen, heparin-induced thrombocytopenia, disseminated intravascular coagulopathy, nephrotic syndrome, Buerger's disease, Behçet's disease and inflammatory bowel disease are all associated with an increased risk of venous thrombosis.

Asian communities have been observed to have a very low incidence of DVT or PE in relation to white or black communities in the USA. One possible explanation is a very low incidence of inherited thrombophilia.[52]

Inherited thrombophilia

The true prevalence of inherited thrombophilia is currently unknown, as the understanding of all the genetic abnormalities causing a tendency to venous thrombosis is in its infancy. The well-established thrombophilic syndromes include antithrombin deficiency, protein C deficiency, protein S deficiency, and resistance to activated protein C. Inherited thrombophilia should be suspected in any patient with recurrent VTE, a positive family history of venous thrombotic disease, a first event in a patient under 45 years of age, or in a patient with no obvious risk factors. The most common inherited thrombophilia is resistance to activated protein C, due to substitution of adenine for guanine at nucleotide 1691 of factor V gene, which causes the arginine in residue 506 of factor V protein to be replaced by glutamine. The resulting protein is known as factor V Leiden.[53] Mutation of prothrombin gene (G20210A) was recently discovered to be a common form of inherited thrombophilia and is due to substitution of adenine for guanine at nucleotide 20210, leading to an elevated prothrombin time.[54] Hyperhomocysteinemia causes a unique form of thrombophilia that predisposes to both arterial and venous thrombosis.[55] Hyperhomocysteinemia can be hereditary but in the majority of patients it is secondary to impairment of methionine metabolism as a result of insufficient dietary intake of folic acid and vitamins B6 or B12. The C677T mutation in the methylene tetrahydrofolate reductase gene, leading to mild hyperhomocysteinemia, is relatively common but its role in venous thrombosis is uncertain.[56] Homozygous homocystinuria is a rare form of hyperhomocysteinemia with clinical features of severe arterial and venous thrombosis presenting at a young age.

High levels of factor VIII, factor IX, factor XI, and fibrinogen are also associated with an increased risk of venous thrombosis, but the exact basis for the elevated levels is still unknown and is likely to be caused by a combination of both genetic and acquired disorders.

Epidemiological and clinical features of inherited thrombophilia

Factor V Leiden and G20210A mutation of prothrombin genes are common in the healthy Caucasian population, with an incidence of about 5% and 3%, respectively; they are very rare in the Asian and African populations. Protein C, protein S, and antithrombin deficiency are relatively rare and are transmitted in autosomal dominant fashion. In patients with VTE, the incidence of inherited thrombophilia is significantly higher than in the normal population (**Table 42.3**); up to 20% have factor V Leiden and 7% have G20210A prothrombin mutation.[57] In the majority of patients, the thromboembolic event is precipitated by surgery, immobilization, pregnancy, or the use of oral contraceptives or HRT.

Patients with either protein C, protein S, or antithrombin deficiency have a more than 50% risk of developing a thromboembolic event in their lifetime. Although these disorders are mostly inherited, they have been observed in patients with liver disease, disseminated intravascular coagulopathy, severe sepsis, or during warfarin therapy.

Patients who have the homozygous form of any inherited thrombophilia, or who have more than one type of inherited thrombophilia, are at far higher risk of developing VTE. Furthermore, they tend to present at an earlier age and have a higher recurrence rate, even with adequate anticoagulant therapy.

Women with inherited thrombophilia are at high risk of developing VTE during pregnancy or the puerperium. Up to 60% of women with antithrombin deficiency and up to 20% with either protein C or protein S deficiency develop VTE during pregnancy or postpartum.[58]

The use of OC in women with inherited thrombophilia increases the risk of venous thrombosis by up to tenfold.[59] The risk is more pronounced with third generation than second generation OC; women with an inherited thrombophilia should use an alternative method of contraception. Screening of all women for inherited thrombophilia before starting OC, however, is not recommended since it would deny this method to about 10% of white women who carry the defective gene.[57] Screening should be limited to women with a personal or family history of VTE.

Mechanisms of thrombosis in inherited thrombophilia

Regulation of thrombin activation and neutralization plays the central role in most inherited coagulopathy. In the normal coagulation pathway, prothrombin is converted to thrombin by factors Xa and Va. Thrombin hydrolyses the peptide bonds of fibrinogen, releasing fibrinopeptides A and B, which allow polymerization of fibrinogen molecules to form fibrin. The inhibitory mechanisms of coagulation are complex (**Fig. 42.5**). Antithrombin is the most potent inhibitor of coagulation. It inactivates serine proteases (thrombin, factor XIa, factor IXa, and factor Xa) by forming a stable complex with them; its action is greatly potentiated by heparin. Activated protein C is generated from its vitamin K-dependent precursor by the action of thrombin. Thrombin binds to thrombomodulin, which is an endothelium receptor, and activates protein C. Activated protein C inhibits factors Va and VIIIa in the presence of free protein S, thereby preventing the formation of thrombin. Protein C also causes inactivation of plasminogen activator inhibitor-1 (which inactivates tissue plasminogen activator) thereby promoting fibrinolysis. Furthermore, free protein S itself has an anticoagulant property. Any reduction in the activity of antithrombin, protein C, or protein S, will, therefore increase the risk of VTE (**Fig. 42.6**).

Resistance to activated protein C, caused by mutation of factor V, is the most common inherited thrombophilia. Factor Va converts prothrombin to thrombin. The mutant factor Va is resistant to the proteolytic activity of activated protein C, thus leading to uninhibited production of thrombin from prothrombin.

Investigation for suspected inherited thrombophilia

Inherited thrombophilia should be suspected in patients with unprovoked thrombotic events who have any one of the following criteria:

- age less than 45 years;
- recurrent episodes;
- family history of venous thrombosis;
- thrombosis of unusual sites such as cerebral venous sinuses; and
- three or more unexplained still births.[57]

This group of patients should be tested for the common types of inherited thrombophilias, which are G20210A prothrombin gene mutation, factor V Leiden, homocysteinemia, elevated factor VIII, and APA syndrome. Prothrombin gene mutation (G20210A) and factor V Leiden are rare in Asian or African patients. Should these tests be normal, less common forms of inherited thrombophilias should be considered; this involves testing for protein C, protein S, and antithrombin deficiency.

Incidence of inherited thrombophilia in normal subjects and patients who have venous thromboembolic disease (VTE).		
Thrombophilia	General population	Patients with VTE
Factor V Leiden	5%	20%
Prothrombin G20210A	3%	7%
Elevated factor VIII*	6–8%	10–15%
Protein C deficiency	0.2–0.5%	3%
Protein S deficiency	0.2–0.5%	3%
Antithrombin deficiency	0.02%	1%
Hyperhomocysteinemia*	5%	10%
*likely to be multifactorial		

Table 42.3 Incidence of inherited thrombophilia in normal subjects and patients who have venous thromboembolic disease (VTE).

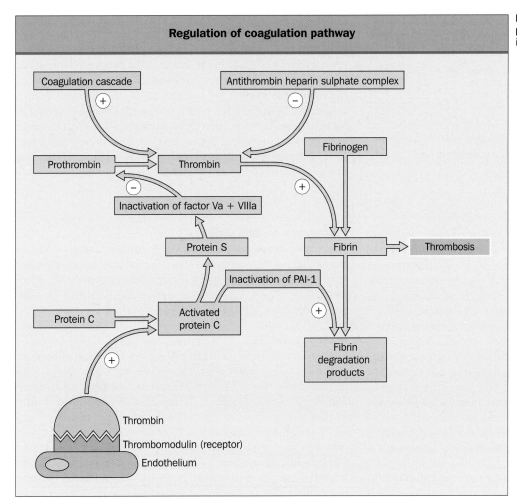

Figure 42.5 Regulation of coagulation pathway. PAI-1, plasminogen activator inhibitor-1.

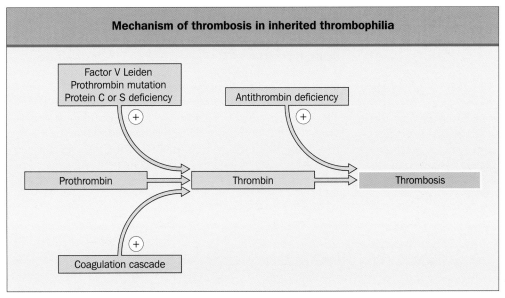

Figure 42.6 Mechanism of thrombosis in inherited thrombophilia (see Seligsohn et al.[57])

These tests should be performed before discontinuation of oral anticoagulant therapy, approximately 6 months following the thrombotic event.[57] Tests performed immediately after a thrombotic episode may not be accurate as thrombosis can affect the level of antithrombin and factor VIII. Tests for protein C and protein S activity, which are vitamin K-dependent glycoproteins (vitamin K action is inhibited by coumarins), should not be performed until 2 weeks after stopping warfarin. It is recommended that a high-risk patient should be given heparin prophylaxis during these 2 weeks, before recommencing warfarin, if required.

CLINICAL FEATURES

Deep venous thrombosis

The clinical features of DVT can be divided into local, distant, and systemic. The classic local symptoms in the leg are:

- swelling;
- pain;
- red–blue discoloration, and
- warmth.

The more proximal and severe the thrombosis, the more pronounced the symptoms and signs in the leg. Classically, Homan's sign is positive in significant calf DVT. This involves dorsiflexion of the foot, which causes calf pain by putting tension on the veins. Although taught to generations of medical students, many clinicians frown on its use, because it is uncomfortable to the patient and may risk causing embolism. Symptoms seemingly unrelated to a local subclinical DVT may occur, usually due to PE of clot material. Very rarely, DVT may present with paradoxical embolism. In a patient with a right-to-left shunt, for example in congenital arterial septal defect or pulmonary arteriovenous malformations, venous embolus can pass through the heart and lodge in the arterial tree. The most common systemic effect of DVT is pyrexia and this is often the first sign in postoperative patients; DVT should always be considered in a postoperative patient who develops a pyrexia.

Although many local signs have been associated with DVT, their sensitivity and specificity are insufficient for management purposes. The diagnostic accuracy of clinical signs of DVT is less than 40%, and many are missed. Patients with risk factors for DVT who present with non-specific leg pain, swelling, or discoloration should undergo objective diagnostic testing; DVT should not be excluded purely on clinical grounds.

Deep venous thrombosis of the arm

The upper limb veins are rarely affected by DVT (2–5%); there is generally an association with direct mechanical causes such as indwelling catheters or venous compression/obstruction due to lymphadenopathy or tumor. Following subclavian vein catheterization, approximately 30% of patients will develop (often silent) venous thrombosis.[15] Compression of the subclavian vein by an accessory rib or fibromuscular band in thoracic outlet syndrome, prolonged abduction in painters or decorators, and repetitive upper arm movements are well described as causes of venous thrombosis in the arm. Up to 20% of patients with upper limb venous thrombosis have no known risk factor and inherited thrombophilia should be considered in this group. Venous thrombosis in the arm has been considered a benign process and many patients have not been treated adequately, sometimes even without anticoagulation. Recent studies have shown that acute DVT of the arm is associated with a 10–30% risk of PE (similar to leg DVT), and a 10–15% recurrence rate after anticoagulation is stopped. Up to 50% of patients continue to have symptoms due to venous obstruction.[60]

Pulmonary embolization

The classification for PE is based on clinical features, pathophysiology, and (perhaps most importantly) therapeutic management. Thus, PE can be divided into acute massive, acute submassive, acute non-massive, and chronic thromboembolic pulmonary hypertension (**Table 42.4**).

Acute massive PE

Sudden occlusion of at least 50% of one or both pulmonary arteries causes major disturbance to both the pulmonary hemodynamic and ventilatory functions. Patients may present with severe acute dyspnea (70%), collapse, and sudden death. Within this group, 10% of fatalities occur in the first hour, and many will not reach hospital. Central angina-type chest pain may also be a feature and this is due to cardiac ischemia (see Pathophysiology section).[27] Clinical examination reveals a patient who is severely short of breath, cyanosed, with low blood pressure or circulatory shock. Raised jugular venous pressure indicates right heart failure. Changes in the heart sounds (wide splitting of the second heart sound and a loud pulmonary component of the second heart sound) are described but these are difficult to detect in a distressed patient.

Acute sub-massive PE

These patients present with a stable circulation. Often, there is underlying cardiac and/or respiratory disease. If echocardiography is performed, signs of right ventricular strain can be detected.[61,62] This group of patients is currently the subject of debate on the most appropriate therapy. Some have suggested that more active (thrombolytic) therapy is warranted, but there are currently insufficient data on which to base recommendations.

Classification of pulmonary embolism.			
Pulmonary embolism	*History*	*Pathophysiology*	*Therapy*
Acute massive	Acute	Circulatory collapse	Thrombolysis, thrombectomy
Acute sub-massive	Acute	Stable, echocardiographic signs of RV overload	Thrombolysis?, heparin
Acute non-massive	Acute	Stable	Heparin
CTEPH	Chronic	RV overload	Medical or elective thromboendarterectomy

Table 42.4 Classification of pulmonary embolism. CTEPH, chronic thromboembolic pulmonary hypertension; RV, right ventricle.

Acute non-massive PE

In a previously healthy individual, small peripheral emboli that obstruct less than 50% of the pulmonary vasculature are frequently asymptomatic. If symptoms do occur, they are due to ischemia or infarction of a small subsegment of the lung. Typical features are pleuritic chest pain (secondary to irritation of the pleura), hemoptysis, and dyspnea. Clinically, pyrexia is a common finding and can lead to the misdiagnosis of infection. The patient is often tachypneic, with rapid shallow breathing secondary to pleuritic pain. Hypoxia is not a feature, as the gas exchange is only mildly affected. Hypocapnia is frequently observed (as the CO_2 gas transfer is highly efficient) in the tachypneic patient.[63] Clinical examination is often unremarkable, but occasionally signs of pulmonary infarction, such as a pleural rub, effusion, or consolidation, are present.

Chronic thromboembolic pulmonary hypertension

There are several forms of pulmonary hypertension. Chronic thromboembolic pulmonary hypertension (CTEPH) is related either to repeated silent PE or to inadequate removal of a previous PE. Obstruction of the pulmonary arterial vasculature results in an increased resistance in the pulmonary arterial system and chronic right ventricular heart strain. Clinically, patients present with a progressive increase in dyspnea and a reduction in exercise tolerance. Signs of right heart hypertrophy, such as a parasternal heave and tricuspid regurgitation, may be present. Chest radiography may show enlarged pulmonary arteries and right heart. Right ventricular hypertrophy and strain may be detected by electrocardiography.

INVESTIGATIONS OF DEEP VENOUS THROMBOSIS

There are many tests for the diagnosis of DVT but only a few are used widely in hospital practice. These tests are either invasive or non-invasive. Some techniques visualize the thrombus directly, such as real-time compression ultrasonography, venography, computed tomography (CT), and magnetic resonance imaging (MRI), while plethysmography and Doppler ultrasonography depend on obstruction of flow by the thrombus. Radiolabeled fibrinogen was frequently used in clinical studies, but is no longer available due to possible transmission of blood-borne viruses. The D-dimer test is sensitive to degradation products of cross-linked fibrin, but unfortunately elevated blood levels of this substance are found in many other medical conditions.

Venography

This examination is still considered as the gold standard for the diagnosis of DVT, but its position is being challenged by newer, non-invasive imaging modalities. This test involves cannulation of a foot vein, followed by injection of iodinated contrast medium to outline the veins. Images are obtained at different planes for the entire limb. The most reliable criterion for the presence of thrombus is a constant filling defect seen on at least two projections (**Fig. 42.7**). Other, less reliable criteria include non-filling of the deep veins, abrupt termination of the contrast column, and abnormal venous collaterals.

The advantages of venography are that it is still considered the gold standard, and it is the only technique that has good sensitivity

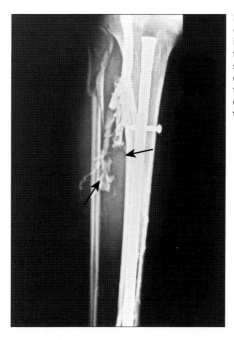

Figure 42.7 Venogram of a patient with intramedullary nail for fractured tibia, showing multiple filling defects in the calf veins consistent with deep venous thrombosis.

for calf vein thrombosis. Thus, it is the only useful technique for screening high-risk patients.

The disadvantages of venography include a failure rate of up to 20% because of difficulties with venous cannulation, and the need for ionizing radiation and iodinated contrast agents, each with their own potential complications. Furthermore, successful examination and correct interpretation are related to experience, as this is a dwindling skill following the introduction of other techniques. Finally, proximal veins, such as internal iliac, may be difficult to visualize.

It is very difficult to obtain the precise accuracy of venography in the detection of DVT because it is considered as the reference standard. An observational study following a cohort of patients with a venogram reported to be normal showed that only two out of 150 patients developed VTE.[64] Therefore, it is likely that, in experienced hands, the accuracy of venography should be over 90%.[65]

Ultrasonography

DVT can be assessed with ultrasonography, either directly or indirectly. The direct technique uses the real-time B mode setting and is easy to perform.[66] The vein is compressed under direct vision; an incompressible distended vein indicates venous thrombosis (**Fig. 42.8**). The indirect method uses the Doppler mode to assess venous blood flow. Absence of flow, lack of venous phasic flow, and absent or poor response to the Valsalva maneuver or augmentation by calf compression are features highly suggestive of venous thrombosis. Most modern ultrasound systems incorporate both settings (color Doppler and duplex ultrasonography). Ultrasonography is widely accepted as the first-line investigation for DVT in many hospitals.

The obvious advantages of ultrasonography are that it is non-invasive and widely available, no ionizing radiation or contrast agents are required, and the test is repeatable and without side effects. Alternative diagnoses, such as a Baker's cyst or popliteal artery aneurysm, can also be made. Disadvantages include the fact that it is operator-dependent, less accurate for the detection

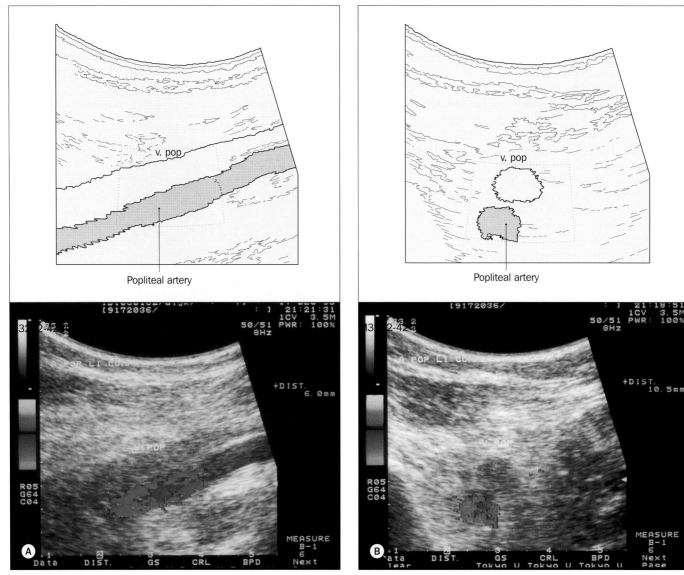

Figure 42.8 Venous thrombosis. (A) Duplex examination of the popliteal fossa in longitudinal section showing an echogenic popliteal vein with no demonstrable flow, consistent with thrombosis. (B) Transverse section of the popliteal fossa with compression, showing incompressible popliteal vein.

of thrombi in calf and pelvic veins, and it has a low sensitivity in asymptomatic patients. Furthermore, patients with recurrent symptoms are sometimes difficult to manage based on ultrasonography alone.

All ultrasonography techniques are highly effective in the diagnosis of proximal DVT, with accuracy figures exceeding 95% in many studies. The simplest, fastest, and most accurate method is the compression technique.[67] However, ultrasound examination is not sensitive for calf vein thrombosis, and repeated investigation may be required to detect proximal extension of the thrombus.

Impedance plethysmography

Impedance plethysmography (IPG) is an indirect method of investigation, as it is based on the detection of reduced venous outflow from the leg and the thrombus is not visualized directly. Although IPG has been shown to be useful, it has largely been superceded by ultrasonography. One randomized trial showed

that ultrasonography was slightly better than plethysmography.[68] IPG is cheap, reproducible, and non-invasive. It does not require ionizing radiation and can be performed by a trained technician. Disadvantages include the fact that IPG cannot diagnose isolated calf vein thrombosis, may miss non-occlusive proximal DVT, and can be falsely positive in patients with pulmonary diseases due to increased pressure in the right atrium.

Impedance plethysmography is good for detecting symptomatic proximal thrombi, with a greater than 90% sensitivity for occlusive proximal thrombosis. However, the detection rate decreases to less than 60% in isolated calf vein thrombosis.

D-dimer test

D-dimer is a degradation product of crosslinked fibrin. There are a number of different assays available but the two main types are the enzyme-linked immunosorbent assay (ELISA) and latex agglutination.[69] These tests have quite variable sensitivities and negative predictive values (80–95%), depending on the assay.

However, D-dimer testing has poor specificity and positive predictive values because elevated levels are also found in many other medical situations such as myocardial ischaemia, malignancy, sepsis, and postoperative patients. The ELISA assay is a more accurate test, with a sensitivity close to 98% (>500 micrograms per liter) but it is labor-intensive to perform.[70] A new rapid ELISA test, with similar accuracy to the classic ELISA test, has been developed.[71] The latex agglutination D-dimer test is quick to perform but of doubtful accuracy and should not be used to exclude VTE.[69,72] The D-dimer test is potentially useful as a screening tool in outpatients or accident and emergency department patients with a first presentation of clinically suspected DVT and low or intermediate clinical probability. Patients who test negative do not require other confirmatory tests such as ultrasound or plethysmography if the clinical suspicion of DVT is low. This significantly reduces workload, while maintaining safety in patient management.[73]

Magnetic resonance venography

The images acquired using this technique are displayed in a similar fashion to those of conventional venography, but with the added benefit of multiplanar or three-dimensional reconstruction (**Fig. 42.9**). A few studies have been published regarding the value and accuracy of MRI in the diagnosis of venous thrombosis. The results are promising, with sensitivity and specificity exceeding 90%,[74] but due to cost and availability, MRI is unlikely to replace ultrasonography as a first-line imaging tool. MRI is indicated in certain clinical situations such as suspected ileo-caval thrombosis in pregnant women, where ionizing radiation should be avoided.

There is a novel MRI technique that no longer requires contrast injection, as it can image thrombus directly. A large study is ongoing, and the initial results are very encouraging.[75]

Helical/spiral computed tomography

Before the introduction of slip ring technology, the peripheral venous system could not be examined well by computed tomography (CT). Spiral CT, and especially multidetector CT, currently provide efficient scan protocols that shorten the examination time and allow good quality, high resolution examinations. Initially, examinations were performed by injection of diluted contrast into a foot vein (with a tourniquet around the ankle), after which acquisition was started. This method had the advantage of good visualization of calf and proximal veins, but the same disadvantages as conventional venography, in that up to 20% of examinations were unsuccessful due to failure of venous cannulation. Lower limb CT venography (**Fig. 42.10**) can be performed following CT pulmonary angiography in patients suspected of having a PE.[76] This method has the advantage of allowing both examinations to be performed in the same visit and does not require injection of contrast medium into foot veins, although the calf veins are not seen as clearly as with the direct method.

Computed tomography has advantages, in that it is widely available and can depict the entire venous system in a single investigation. However, the disadvantages relate to the doses of radiation, the use of iodinated contrast medium, and the cost in comparison to ultrasound imaging.

Other methods

Various other methods are available, such as radioisotope tests, thermography, and light reflection rheography. None of these tests is widely accepted, due to the complexity of protocols, scarce clinical data, and lack of available equipment.

Upper limb and superior vena cava thrombosis

The upper limb venous system can be assessed easily using ultrasonography, although visibility may be difficult or impossible due to bony structures of the shoulder girdle (**Fig. 42.11**).[77] In patients with a high clinical suspicion of arm vein thrombosis, but normal ultrasonography, venography may still be indicated.

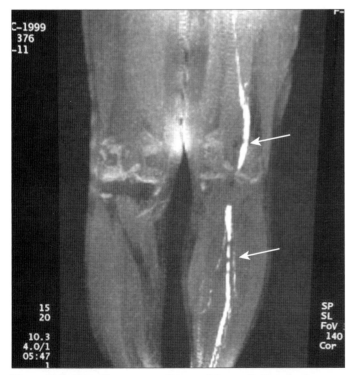

Figure 42.9 Magnetic resonance image of deep vein thrombosis.

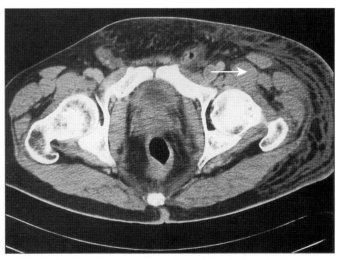

Figure 42.10 Computed tomography of a patient with deep vein thrombosis of the left femoral vein (arrow). The vein is not opacified or distended in comparison to the right femoral vein. There is also extensive subcutaneous edema on the left.

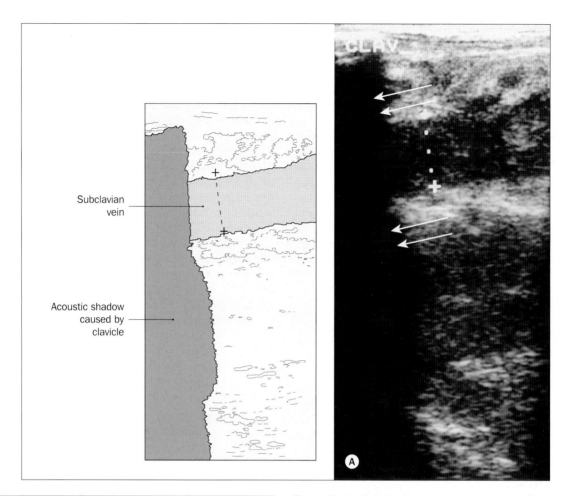

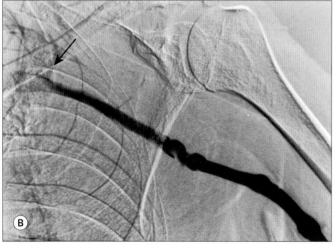

Figure 42.11 Thrombosis of the left subclavian vein. (A) Ultrasound examination showing echogenic, non-compressible subclavian vein (white dots). Examination can be difficult, due to obstruction by the bony structures. (Arrows: acoustic shadow caused by clavicle.) (B) Left subclavian vein thrombosis confirmed by venography. (Arrows: filling defects in distal subclavian vein.) Reproduced with permission from Oudkerk et al. Pulmonary embolism. © Blackwell Wissenschafts-Verlag GmbH, Berlin.

Superior vena cava and brachiocephalic veins cannot be visualized directly using ultrasonography; however, Doppler waveform analysis of flow in the veins distal to the obstruction can help to diagnose occlusion. In a non-obstructed venous system, there is a normal triphasic waveform with respiratory variation; the waveform becomes monophasic with loss of respiratory or atrial variation with venous obstruction. Other methods to diagnose proximal vein occlusions include contrast enhanced CT, MRI, or venography (**Fig. 42.12**).

DIAGNOSTIC STRATEGIES FOR DEEP VENOUS THROMBOSIS

Strategies for investigation of DVT are complex because the diagnostic tests mentioned earlier have variable accuracy depending on the clinical scenario. For example, ultrasound or plethysmography examinations have relatively poor accuracy in asymptomatic patients. Furthermore, calf vein thromboses are frequently missed by both of these tests; to counter this, serial

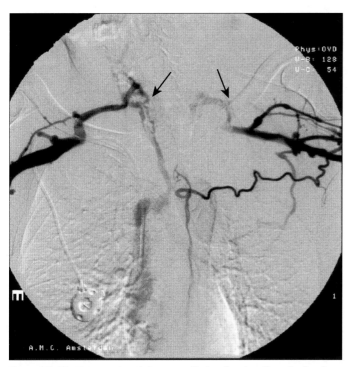

Figure 42.12 Venography of the upper limbs showing thrombosis of subclavian and brachiocephalic veins bilaterally in a patient with a right subclavian central line. Collateral veins are seen around the subclavian vein occlusion.

examinations have been employed. The principle of serial examination is that patients with calf vein thrombi that propagate proximally will be detected on a repeat investigation after approximately 7 days. Thrombus that does not extend is likely to be stable and requires no treatment.

It is best to divide the clinical presentations into three groups, as each requires a different diagnostic strategy:

- first episode of clinically suspected DVT;
- diagnosis of DVT in asymptomatic high-risk patients; and
- diagnosis of recurrent DVT.

Clinically suspected first episode DVT

These patients tend to be seen as outpatients and present in considerable numbers to emergency rooms. A strategy to deal with them should be efficient and reliable, while avoiding hospital admission if possible. Depending on equipment availability and local experience, one of the following strategies could be used.

Serial impedance plethysmography

Serial IPG has been shown to be safe.[78] Initially, up to six investigations were performed over a 2-week interval.[79] Later studies used a three-test strategy with equally good results. It is estimated that only 1–2% of patients with a normal test on two separate occasions have VTE. However, the use of IPG has now been largely superseded by serial ultrasonography.[68]

Serial ultrasonography

Repeating the ultrasound examination after 7 to 10 days following a normal first examination is a highly sensitive and specific method in the diagnosis of DVT.[80] If the first test is abnormal, anticoagulant treatment is commenced. Those with normal first

test require a repeat examination about a week later and if this is normal, they can safely be discharged. Standard treatment is given to those with an abnormal result. Follow-up studies of patients with two normal tests revealed that only 1% developed VTE.

D-dimer and ultrasound

Combining ultrasound examination and D-dimer testing has been proposed as a diagnostic strategy for the diagnosis of DVT.[81] Patients have both tests on presentation; those with normal tests are considered to have no DVT and are discharged. Those with a normal ultrasound examination but an abnormal D-dimer test have a repeat ultrasound a week later. If normal, they are discharged. Any patient with an abnormal ultrasound is considered to have a DVT and commenced on anticoagulation. With this diagnostic strategy, fewer than 1% of patients with normal tests will have VTE.

Clinical score, D-dimer and ultrasound examination

An alternative method for testing is the use of a clinical probability score in addition to D-dimer testing and ultrasonography.[73,82] This strategy is increasingly accepted as valid and safe, and applies to the vast majority of patients with suspected DVT.

Venography

Although considered the gold standard, this method is not the first-line test for DVT in most hospitals, for reasons described earlier. Follow-up of patients with a clinically suspected DVT but a normal venogram shows a 1–2% risk of developing VTE.[64]

Diagnosis of DVT in asymptomatic high risk patients

High-risk patients (after major orthopedic or pelvic surgery, or prolonged immobilization), without thromboprophylaxis, are recognized to have a very high incidence of DVT (up to 80%). A significant proportion of these patients are asymptomatic. They are frequently discharged from the hospital without any long-term anticoagulant treatment. It has been suggested that the reason the patients are asymptomatic is that the thrombus is non-occlusive. Neither ultrasonography nor IPG have sufficient sensitivity to assist in the diagnosis of these patients, and plasma D-dimer levels are invariably elevated due to recent surgery and/or underlying conditions. Venography is still the only accurate diagnostic test but it is often difficult to perform in this group of patients. MRI and CT venography are potentially useful, but costly, and therefore at this time unlikely to be widely accepted as screening tools.

Diagnosis of recurrent DVT

Recurrent symptoms are very common following DVT; two-thirds are due to post-thrombotic disease or other conditions such as Baker's cyst or musculoskeletal pain. One-third of symptoms are due to recurrent disease. Clinically, it is extremely difficult to differentiate recurrent DVT from the other conditions.

The 5-year cumulative incidence of recurrent venous thromboembolic events is up to 25% after a first DVT and 36% after a second DVT. The 5-year cumulative incidence of fatal PE is 2.6% after a first DVT.[83] These recent data suggest that recurrent disease is common and can be fatal. Unfortunately, the diagnosis of recurrent DVT is difficult because of persistent abnormalities following the first event. In 50% of patients, compression ultrasound is still abnormal 1 year after the first DVT.[84,85] Extension of thrombosis and/or an increase in the diameter of the incompressible segment of deep vein by more than 4mm have been suggested as features of new thrombosis. Hence, it is important that during ultrasound examinations, the exact anatomic segments involved and the diameter of the affected vein are carefully documented.[86] Plethysmography is only useful if the test normalized after the first DVT. Contrast venography can show new areas of involvement as filling defects, but the diagnosis is often difficult (especially in the presence of collateral vessels). The role of MRI and CT venography still needs further evaluation.

INVESTIGATIONS OF SUSPECTED PULMONARY EMBOLUS

As mentioned earlier, clinical symptoms and signs of PE are neither specific, nor sensitive and most patients will require other confirmatory tests. Physiologic tests measuring changes in cardiorespiratory function, such as blood gas analysis and electrocardiography, are disappointing as many conditions have similar physiologic outcomes. Currently, the diagnosis relies on the demonstration of a filling defect or occlusion of the pulmonary artery on angiography. However, this does not mean that these physiologic tests are unimportant, as they may reveal other conditions that could account for the symptoms, and they also assess the severity of the PE. For example, the presence of an elevated level of cardiac troponin T indicates moderate to massive PE that is causing right heart strain or ischemia; this may aid the early identification of patients in whom a more active therapy is indicated.[87]

Early investigations in the diagnosis of acute PE
Chest radiography
The chest radiograph (CXR) is frequently abnormal in acute PE. In one study, 90% of patients with proven PE had an abnormal CXR. Unfortunately, the abnormalities are not specific to PE, and the role of the CXR is to rule out other conditions that may account for the symptoms (such as pneumothorax or aortic dissection). It is also a useful adjunct to the interpretation of lung scintigraphy. The most common CXR findings in a patient with acute PE are atelectasis, consolidation, pleural effusion, and elevation of the hemidiaphragm (**Table 42.5**). Decreased

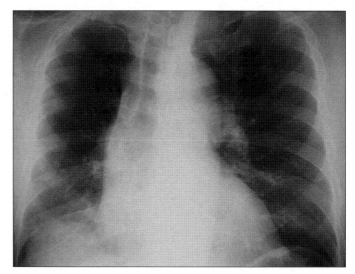

Figure 42.13 Chest X-ray: Westermark's sign. Distension of the pulmonary artery, decreased pulmonary vascularity.

pulmonary vascularity (**Fig. 42.13**), distension of the proximal pulmonary artery, or focal oligemia is rarely seen, but these features are thought to be more diagnostic of acute PE than the more common signs mentioned above.[88]

Electrocardiography
The most common abnormality in acute PE is sinus tachycardia; other tachyarrhythmias are rare. In massive PE, the electrocardiogram (EKG) is frequently abnormal, with non-specific ST wave changes. The classic findings of $S_1Q_3T_3$ (**Fig. 42.14**), T wave inversion in the right ventricular leads, and right axis deviation are rarely seen. In chronic thromboembolic disease, changes in keeping with right ventricular hypertrophy may be evident. The EKG is frequently normal (approximately 30%) in acute PE, however, and a normal result should not be used to exclude PE.[89] The main role of the EKG is to exclude other conditions such as myocardial infarction and pericarditis.

Blood gases analysis
Pulmonary embolism is generally associated with (mild) hypoxemia, but up to 25% of patients with proven PE have normal arterial oxygen pressure. In the majority of patients, the arterial carbon dioxide level is low due to hyperventilation. Although these findings are non-specific, they allow clinicians to assess the severity of the physiologic insult. Patients with a minor PE are unlikely to have an abnormal arterial oxygen pressure in comparison to those with a massive PE, but this is partly dependent on the presence of existing cardiorespiratory disease. Measuring the alveolar-arterial oxygen gradient may be more accurate than arterial oxygen pressure in the diagnosis of PE, but the results from clinical trials were disappointing.[90]

D-dimer
Similar problems are encountered with the use of D-dimer for the diagnosis of PE as in DVT, due to the variation in the tests and standards. Although D-dimer is sensitive for a large embolus, a normal test does not exclude subsegmental embolism.[91] However, the clinical significance of subsegmental embolism is uncertain and clinical outcome studies in outpatients have shown

Frequency of signs on chest radiography in patients with pulmonary embolism.	
Signs	Frequency
Atelectasis/consolidation	70%
Pleural effusion	50%
Elevation of hemidiaphragm	20%
Decreased pulmonary vasculature	20%
Distension of proximal vessels	15%

Table 42.5 Frequency of signs on chest radiography in patients with pulmonary embolism.

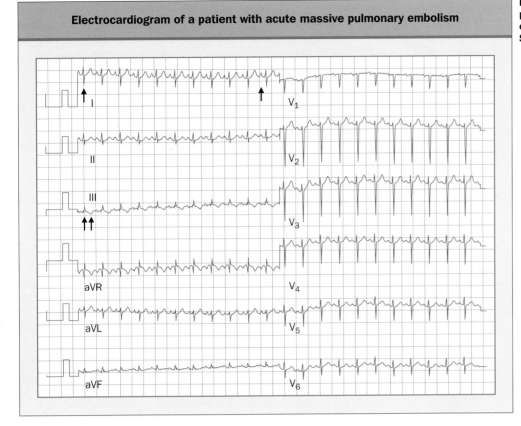

Electrocardiogram of a patient with acute massive pulmonary embolism

Figure 42.14 Electrocardiogram of a patient with acute massive pulmonary embolism showing the classic but rare $S_1Q_3T_3$ changes (arrows).

that patients with suspected PE and a negative D-dimer test can safely avoid anticoagulation therapy.[92,93]

Other diagnostic tests

As the physiologic tests are disappointing, clinicians have to rely on the direct demonstration of thrombus and its mechanical effect on flow in the pulmonary circulation to diagnose PE.

Lung scintigraphy (V/Q scan)

Until recently, this examination was the main diagnostic test in most hospitals because it is safe, non-invasive, and has been evaluated extensively. Lung scintigraphy consists of two parts: perfusion and ventilation imaging. Perfusion imaging is performed following intravenous injection of Tc-99 labeled macro-aggregates of albumin; images are obtained in six or more projections (**Fig. 42.15**). Perfusion defects appear as 'cold' areas, and may be wedge-shaped. Ventilation imaging is performed by inhalation of a radiolabeled substance. The commonly available agents are Tc-99 labeled diethylene triamine penta-acetic acid (DTPA), krypton-81, xenon-133 and Tc-99 labeled carbon particles (Technegas).

Images are acquired in the same projections as the perfusion lung scan. Mismatch between ventilation and perfusion scans is diagnostic for PE (**Fig. 42.16**). Several classifications have been proposed, the two most commonly used being the revised Prospective Investigation of Pulmonary Embolism Diagnosis (PIOPED) criteria or a simple classification of 'normal', 'high probability', or 'non-diagnostic' findings.[94,95] A recent comparative study showed that these two classifications worked equally well.[96]

Lung scintigraphy is able to either refute or confirm the diagnosis of PE with more than 85% certainty in the high probability (25% of all cases) or low probability/normal groups (25% of all cases). The remaining 50% of patients will have inconclusive scintigraphic abnormalities that are not diagnostic and require further evaluation. The advantages and disadvantages of lung scintigraphy are as follows:

Advantages

1. Well-established and evaluated.
2. Safe and non-invasive.
3. Widely available.

Disadvantages

1. Complex diagnostic criteria and classification.[97]
2. High number of non-diagnostic results, especially in patients with pre-existing respiratory disease (up to 50% of cases).
3. 30% false-negative and 10% false-positive rate in low probability and high probability scans, respectively.

Accuracy

Lung scintigraphy criteria alone should not be used to diagnose PE, as many tests are non-diagnostic, and a high number of PEs will be missed (**Table 42.6**). Including the degree of clinical suspicion of PE and the lung scintigraphy result is more accurate than scintigraphy alone.[98] For example, if both the clinical and scintigraphy probabilities of PE are high, the positive predictive value is over 90%. If there is disagreement between clinical suspicion and lung scintigraphy results, or both are of intermediate

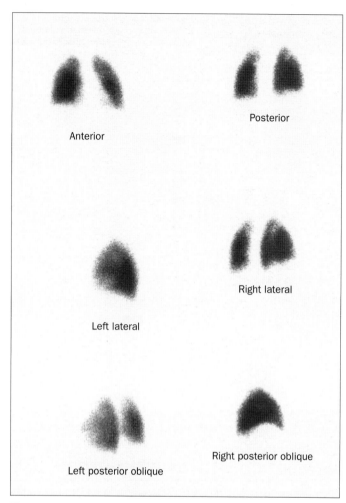

Anterior

Posterior

Left lateral

Right lateral

Left posterior oblique

Right posterior oblique

Figure 42.15 Normal perfusion lung scintigraphy.

Relation between lung scintigraphy findings and the incidence of pulmonary embolism.		
V/Q result	*% of scans*	*Incidence of pulmonary embolism in this group*
Low probability	25%	10%
Intermediate probability	50%	30%
High probability	25%	70%

Table 42.6 Relation between lung scintigraphy findings and the incidence of pulmonary embolism.

probability, other diagnostics tests are required to clarify the diagnosis.

Clinical validity

A recent meta-analysis considered the diagnostic accuracy of lung scintigraphy.[99] It was reported that it is safe to withhold anticoagulant therapy in patients with a suspected PE and a normal lung scan (the exception being a patient with high clinical suspicion of PE). In the majority of patients with a high-probability lung scan, anticoagulant therapy is warranted. The exception would be a patient with a low clinical suspicion or a patient at high risk of bleeding complications, where alternative diagnostic tests are required, such as angiography or CT.

Pulmonary angiography

Conventional contrast angiography is considered the standard of reference for the diagnosis of PE. It involves catheterization of the pulmonary artery via femoral or brachial vein puncture. A high volume of iodinated contrast (20mL/s for 2s) is injected and images are taken in at least two planes, i.e. anterior-posterior and oblique. The features of acute PE are complete obstruction of the pulmonary vessel and constant filling defects (**Fig. 42.17**).

Pulmonary angiography is valuable in patients in whom non-invasive tests are not diagnostic but there remains a reasonable suspicion of PE. In this situation, the aim of pulmonary angiography is to exclude PE, thus allowing withdrawal of anticoagulant therapy with its bleeding risk.

Pulmonary angiography should also be considered in patients with a high risk of bleeding, for instance following recent neurosurgery.

Pulmonary angiography is generally reliable, although there is some interobserver variability, especially at subsegmental artery level. An additional benefit is that pulmonary angiography can also serve as access for therapeutic intervention, such as embolectomy, thrombolysis, or insertion of a vena cava filter.

The disadvantages of pulmonary angiography are that it requires relatively expensive equipment and expertise, is invasive, and uses nephrotoxic contrast agents. Furthermore, right heart catheterization can cause cardiac arrhythmias. Nevertheless, the safety of this technique has improved over the past 10 years, and current estimates of mortality and morbidity are 0.03% and 0.47%, respectively.

Pulmonary angiography is highly sensitive and specific. It is safe to withhold anticoagulant therapy in patients with suspected PE and a normal pulmonary angiogram. This is true for patients who undergo pulmonary angiography following non-diagnostic, non-invasive tests.[100]

Helical/multi-detector computed tomography

Helical CT angiography is rapidly replacing lung scintigraphy as the initial test for suspected PE. Helical CT is not only capable of imaging PE directly (**Fig. 42.18**), but it can exclude alternative diagnoses such as aortic dissection. The introduction of multi-detector CT technology enables even more accurate visualization of thrombus down to the subsegmental level (**Fig. 42.18**).

The imaging protocol varies according to the CT system used. An iodinated contrast bolus of 130–150mL is infused, and data acquisition usually starts at the diaphragm and then moves up into the apex of the lungs. For single spiral scanners, a slice thickness of 2–3mm seems optimal, while the latest multi-detector systems are capable of sub-millimeter slices providing an isotropic resolution of $0.5mm^3$. This has repercussions on the size of emboli that can be diagnosed confidently: for single spiral scanners, imaging of subsegmental arteries is difficult and it is not usually feasible to image the entire chest, whereas this is well within the reach of multi-detector systems.

Helical CT is a fast technique and it is widely available. It can be used in most breathless patients; breath-hold times of 10s (multi-detector) and 20s (single slice) are required.

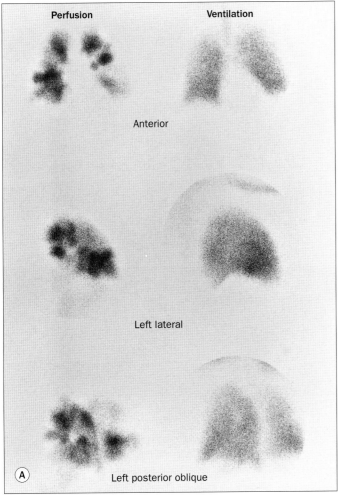

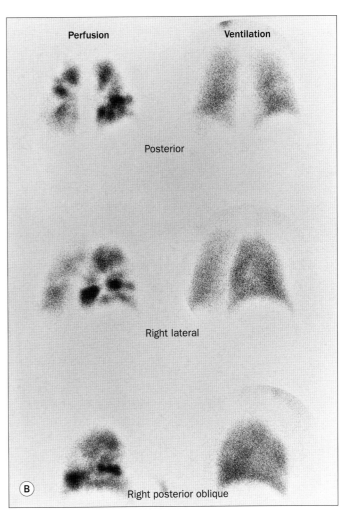

Figure 42.16 Ventilation perfusion scintigraphy showing multiple large unmatched defects between ventilation and perfusion secondary to multiple pulmonary embolism.

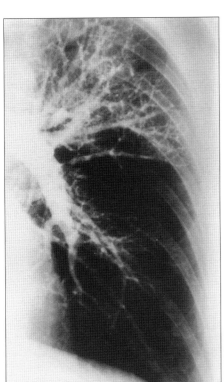

Figure 42.17 Selective left pulmonary angiogram showing marked hypoperfusion of the lower lobe secondary to multiple embolism.

Although many hospitals now use helical CT routinely, its exact role is still under discussion. Two recent reviews showed an overall sensitivity and specificity of approximately 88% and 92%, respectively.[99,101] Two management studies of PE have evaluated the clinical validity of a normal helical CT scan, and both studies had design flaws.[102,103] Thus, confirmation studies are required to show that it is safe to withhold anticoagulant therapy in patients with a normal helical CT scan.

The techniques are evolving more rapidly than is seen in the literature, and the results of ongoing studies of management based on multi-detector helical CT are awaited eagerly.

Echocardiography

Echocardiography is useful in the assessment of patients who present with cardiovascular collapse, acute dyspnea, and chest pain. Large emboli can be visualized and other conditions such as aortic dissection, myocardial infarction, and pericardial tamponade excluded. Echocardiography cannot diagnose minor PE, as typically the cardiovascular system is not affected. However, in massive PE, there are changes in right ventricular dynamics and pulmonary arterial flow. Features on echocardiography suspicious of massive PE include right ventricular dilatation and dysfunction (**Fig. 42.19**), a dilated pulmonary artery, tricuspid regurgitation, and a disturbed flow pattern in

643

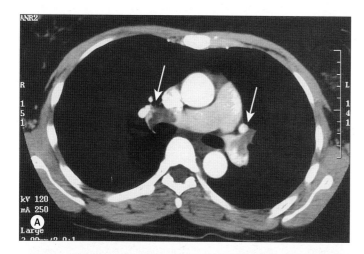

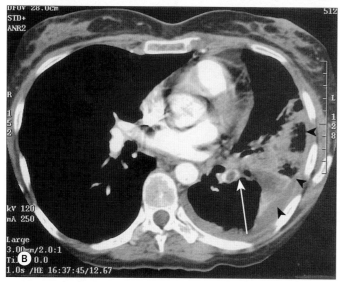

Figure 42.18 Computed tomography. (A) Large central pulmonary emboli (arrows). (B) Peripheral embolism (arrow) with secondary consolidation/infarction of the lung (arrow head).

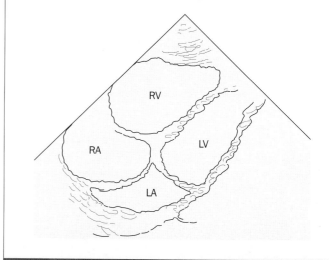

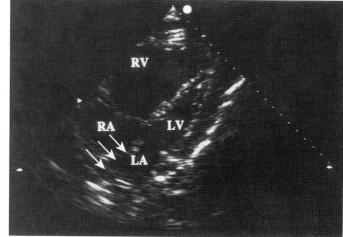

Figure 42.19 Four-chamber echocardiogram of a patient with acute massive pulmonary embolism. The interatrial septum bulges to the left (arrows) and the right ventricle is dilated in keeping with significant pulmonary outflow obstruction.

the right ventricular outflow tract. It is unlikely that a patient has a hemodynamically significant PE if their echocardiogram is normal.[104] Echocardiography is useful to identify patients with PE in whom active treatment is indicated.

There is a subgroup of patients who are hemodynamically stable, but in whom echocardiography shows signs of right heart dysfunction. There is ongoing debate as to whether these patients require thrombolytic therapy.

Other investigations

Magnetic resonance imaging (**Fig. 42.20**) has great potential for non-invasive imaging of PE. It is sensitive in diagnosing thrombi up to segmental level.[105] A recent study in more than 141 patients with an abnormal perfusion lung scan reported that magnetic resonance angiography had similar accuracy to helical CT using a single-slice system.[106] The role of MRI is currently still limited to trial patients, but with the rapid advancement in technology (shorter acquisition time and better image quality), it is expected to play a major role in the diagnosis of PE in the near future.

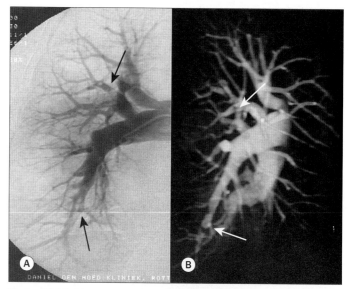

Figure 42.20 Magnetic resonance imaging of pulmonary embolism. (A) Pulmonary angiogam. (B) MR pulmonary angiogram in same patient.

DIAGNOSTIC STRATEGIES FOR PULMONARY EMBOLISM

While PE is a common clinical diagnosis, in fact only 15–30% of suspected cases actually have the disease.[92] Most patients with suspected PE do not actually have the condition; therefore, a non-invasive diagnostic approach is warranted, as the majority of tests will be negative. Furthermore, diagnostic tests that refute the diagnosis are as important as those that confirm it. Identification of patients who do or do not require anticoagulant therapy is important in view of the associated bleeding risks. Several diagnostic strategies have been examined in cost-benefit analyses.[107] They all have in common the fact that pulmonary angiography is the final diagnostic test in patients where reasonable suspicion remains and non-invasive tests do not yield a definitive diagnosis. The choice of strategy often depends on the organization of the local hospital and the availability of equipment.

Outpatient setting

D-dimer (validated assay) is a logical first test as it is non-invasive and easy to perform in this setting (**Fig. 42.21**). If the level is below 500mg/L, PE can safely be ruled out. This occurs in approximately 30–40% of patients. Those with a level greater than 500mg/L should proceed to ultrasound examination of the deep leg veins, as approximately 90% of PE originates from there. Patients with confirmed DVT should be commenced on anticoagulant treatment and lung scintigraphy is not necessary. Patients with a negative ultrasound examination of the legs but a positive D-dimer test require further investigation; 50% of patients with proven PE have a normal duplex scan. Possible reasons for the normal duplex scan of the leg veins include the fact that the clot has completely embolized (giving rise to a normal looking vein), or missed calf or pelvic vein thrombosis. This group of patients should proceed to lung scintigraphy. Patients with a normal or low probability V/Q scan do not require anticoagulant treatment, whereas those with a high probability V/Q scan should be anticoagulated. If the V/Q results are intermediate (non-diagnostic), clinical consideration is taken into account: if clinical suspicion is high, the next investigation is catheter angiography or CT pulmonary angiography. If clinical suspicion is low, the anticoagulant can be omitted safely.[108]

Patients in hospital

D-dimer test is not useful in this setting because many patients have elevated levels for reasons mentioned earlier (**Fig. 42.22**).

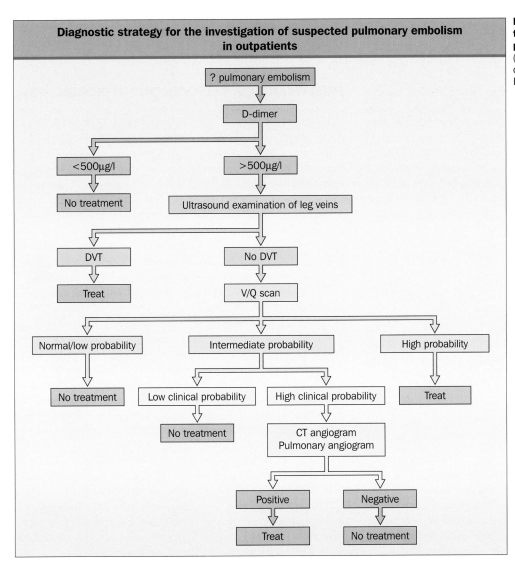

Diagnostic strategy for the investigation of suspected pulmonary embolism in outpatients

Figure 42.21 Diagnostic strategy for the investigation of suspected pulmonary embolism in outpatients. (Modified from Pevrier A. Non-invasive diagnosis of venous thromboembolism. Lancet 1999;353:190–5.)

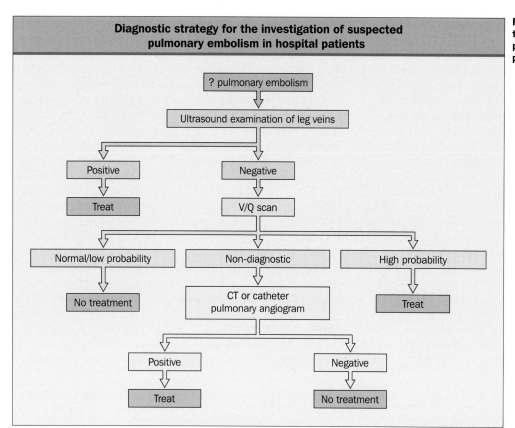

Figure 42.22 Diagnostic strategy for the investigation of suspected pulmonary embolism in hospital patients.

Ultrasound examination of the leg veins should be the first line of investigation and, if positive, anticoagulant treatment should be commenced. As before, patients with a negative duplex scan should proceed to lung scintigraphy, and if the result is normal or low probability, anticoagulation can be omitted. Patients with intermediate (non-diagnostic) results require either CT pulmonary angiography or catheter angiography, depending on local practice. Clinical probability is not helpful because most inpatients are in the intermediate or high probability group.

Suspected massive pulmonary embolism

In patients who present with shock, chest pain, and dyspnea, the differential diagnoses include massive PE, cardiogenic shock, pericardial tamponade, and aortic dissection. EKG should be the initial investigation, as it is quick and easy to perform and may reveal the cause of the symptoms. The most useful test, however, is echocardiography. Massive PE almost invariably causes right heart-strain. Furthermore, echocardiography may reveal an alternative diagnosis such as cardiac tamponade or aortic dissection.

Anticoagulant treatment should commence immediately following diagnosis, and confirmatory tests can be performed later, preferably by helical CT pulmonary angiography.

Diagnosis of recurrent pulmonary embolism

The incidence of recurrent PE is not well documented and the reported figures range from 2.5–8%. Following acute PE, the reduced perfusion seen on lung scintigraphy can be permanent or slowly revert to normal over time. New areas of ventilation/perfusion mismatch are highly suggestive of recurrent PE.

TREATMENT OF DEEP VENOUS THROMBOSIS

There are three main objectives in the treatment of DVT, and the type of intervention depends on the clinical setting. The first goal is to prevent propagation of thrombus or embolization of thrombus material. In most instances, this can be achieved by anticoagulation with heparin and then warfarin. The second aim is to reduce the risk of post-thrombotic sequelae. Warfarin reduces the risk of recurrent thrombotic events while waiting for natural lysis and thrombus organization to occur. Finally, in patients with massive PE, more active therapeutic options such as caval filter placement, venous interruption, thrombectomy, and long-term anticoagulant therapy should be considered.

The standard anticoagulants, heparins and oral vitamin K antagonists, do not actually remove thrombus. Their action is to prevent the formation of new (unstable) thrombus while the natural fibrinolytic system organizes and disposes of the thrombus. Unfortunately, valvular damage in thrombosed segments cannot be prevented after they recanalize. The incidence of post-thrombotic syndrome may be reduced by a more active approach to the management of acute thrombosis, by thrombus removal using thrombectomy or thrombolysis. However, the long-term outcome of such interventions requires further investigation.

Finally, the widely accepted belief that patients with acute DVT should have an initial period of bed rest has been refuted; early mobilization does not increase the risk of PE.[109] Most patients with DVT can be managed entirely without admission to hospital, even those with iliofemoral DVT. Ambulant treatment of acute DVT is now the norm and most hospitals have efficient processing systems that are often nurse-led.

Thrombolysis
Indications for thrombolysis

In the setting of acute DVT, there is considerable debate about the indication for thrombolysis. Current research suggests that thrombolysis may be beneficial in two main groups: patients with venous gangrene who risk limb loss and possibly young patients with recent extensive iliofemoral venous thrombosis who will almost invariably develop post-thrombotic syndrome if managed with anticoagulation alone.[110] Only fresh thrombi less than 7 days old respond to fibrinolytic therapy; old thrombi are well organized and resistant to lysis.[111] Post-thrombotic syndrome rarely complicates calf vein thrombosis, so thrombolysis is not indicated in this situation.

Contraindications to thrombolysis

Thombolysis is usually given intravenously for patients with DVT. High doses are used; this increases the risk of bleeding. Newer, catheter-directed techniques that employ lower doses may be safer.

The principal contraindication to thrombolysis is potential bleeding. Thus, the main contraindications are:[112]

- recent surgery, in particular vascular, ophthalmic and neuro-surgery; for general surgery, a minimum of 7 days after surgery is recommended;
- bleeding diatheses; patients with abnormal coagulation from any cause should not receive thrombolysis; patients on warfarin may need reversal with vitamin K before thrombolysis;
- history of previous gastrointestinal bleeding, unless the cause of the bleeding has been treated;
- recent stroke within 2 months; and
- pregnancy and severe hypertension.

Thombolytic regimens

Streptokinase is highly antigenic and, following exposure to streptococcal infection or previous administration of strepto-kinase, the immune system rapidly produces antibodies that neutralize its action. Hence, repeated administration or pro-longed use of streptokinase is ineffective and could potentially cause anaphylaxis. It is recommended that there must be at least a 6-month interval before repeat administration, but it is probably safer to use a different agent such as recombinant tissue plasminogen activator (rt-PA). Streptokinase is given intravenously, starting with a loading dose of 250 000 units over 30–60 min in order to neutralize in-situ antibodies.[113] This is followed by a maintenance dose of 100 000 units per hour for 24–48 hours or longer, depending on clinical findings and venographic appearances.

Recombinant tissue plasminogen activator is produced in abundant quantity by cultured eukaryotic cells and has identical structural and biochemical properties to native tissue plasmin-ogen activator. Many different rt-PA treatment regimens have been proposed but the original recommendation for treatment of acute myocardial infarction is the most widely used for acute DVT; 100mg of rt-PA is given intravenously over 3 hours: 60mg in the first hour, of which 10mg is given as a bolus in 2 min, followed by 20mg in the second and the third hour. This method is only suitable for rapid lysis methods; lower dose infusion rates of between 1–5mg/h can be given intravenously for 24–48 hours (see Chapter 16 for further discussion on thrombolytic therapy).

Complications of thrombolysis

Hemorrhagic complications are inevitable with thrombolytic therapy and occur in up to 60% of treatments. The majority of hemorrhage is minor, such as bruising at puncture sites and pressure areas, but serious hemorrhage occurs in approximately 10% of treatments. Intracranial hemorrhage is the most feared complication, and occurs in up to 1–2% of patients treated with high-dose intravenous thrombolysis.[114] Prior to initiation of thrombolytic treatment, it is essential to exclude any coagulopathy by performing a clotting screen. There is no need to perform coagulation tests during therapy, as they have no value in predicting complications or helping to titrate the dose. The major risk factors for intracranial hemorrhage with intravenous thrombolysis are age, hypertension, and previous cerebro-vascular disease.[115] Recently, a study showed that the incidence of PE is higher during thrombolytic treatment, in comparison to heparin alone, and this may be related to clot fragmentation by the thrombolytic agent.[116] However, the PE is seldom clinically significant. The management of major hemorrhage consists of stopping thrombolysis, transfusion, replacing coagulation factors (especially fibrinogen), and administration of antifibrinolytic agents such as tranexamic acid.

Results and outcome following thrombolysis

Studies have shown that thrombolysis produces superior clot lysis (demonstrated radiologically) in comparison to heparin. The result is best in patients with non-occlusive thrombi, where complete clot lysis was observed in 60%. In contrast, only 14% of patients with occlusive thrombus achieved complete lysis, presumably because the thrombolytic agent could not penetrate the clot in sufficient quantity.[117] A recent study showed that a higher dosage of thrombolytic agent could achieve better short- and long-term vein patency, but at the cost of higher complication rates.[116]

Catheter-directed thrombolysis

Because of the high complication rate associated with systemic thrombolysis, catheter-directed thrombolysis was introduced. This technique involves catheterization of either the popliteal or femoral vein, and the tip of the catheter is inserted into the center of the thrombus.[118] A low dose of thrombolytic agent is then administered by continuous infusion or by pulse-spray technique (0.5–1mg/h t-PA). Venography is performed every 12 hours to assess the progress of lysis and to demonstrate any stenosis that can be treated. The results published so far are encouraging, with a 1-year patency rate of 80% for iliac vein thrombosis and 50% for femoral vein thrombosis, a low compli-cation rate, and improved late quality of life. However, the long-term results of this technique, and in particular whether post thrombotic syndrome is prevented, are unknown and further studies are required.[119]

In conclusion, although thrombolysis may result in higher radiologically proven vein patency rates in comparison to anti-coagulation, the long-term result is uncertain. Given the inherent potential for serious complications associated with systemic thrombolysis, catheter-directed thrombolysis should be the first choice. It should not be used in patients with significant risks of hemorrhage, the elderly, or in patients with poor life expectancy, unless limb viability is threatened. The best results can be anticipated in patients with a first event iliofemoral DVT with fresh thrombus less than 5 days old.

Thrombolysis for upper limb venous occlusion

Patients who present with subclavian vein thrombosis are usually managed by anticoagulation and arm elevation. The late sequelae of venous claudication and the development of unsightly superficial collaterals may be reduced by catheter-directed thrombolysis. There remains a small risk of significant bleeding, which must be discussed with the patient before treatment commences. A catheter is inserted through the brachial vein and inserted into the thrombus. Low dose t-PA (0.5–1mg/h) usually dissolves occlusions less than 5 days old. The underlying cause is often seen on repeat venography, where a web is frequently seen in the subclavian vein, often on the left side. Dilatation of this area with a balloon often requires high pressures, but can result in long-term patency. Stenting should not be employed, as it will fracture on arm movement, but if significant thoracic outlet obstruction is seen as the cause, rib resection may be required.

Thrombectomy

The indications for thrombectomy are almost identical to those for thrombolytic therapy, i.e. limb-threatening thrombosis in the iliofemoral segment in a young patient with a short history of DVT.[120] Thrombectomy is not widely accepted because it is invasive, and therefore thrombolysis is the preferred choice of many clinicians who would manage DVT actively. The introduction of cleverly designed, minimally invasive percutaneous thromboembolectomy devices may cause a resurgence of thrombectomy in the management of acute DVT. Several percutaneous thrombectomy devices are under evaluation and the short-term results appear promising.[120]

As with thrombolytic therapy, the long-term result of surgical thrombectomy is uncertain but in the short term it is superior to anticoagulation alone.[121,122]

Percutaneous thrombectomy is often combined with other interventional procedures such as angioplasty or stent placement.

Technique of surgical thrombectomy

The procedure is performed under general anesthesia and can be divided into three phases.[110]

1. Exposure and prevention of embolization

A 15cm longitudinal incision is made from the inguinal ligament. The common femoral vein and its tributaries are identified, exposed, and snared. These veins should be handled carefully and not clamped, as this may cause dislodgment and embolization of thrombus. A longitudinal venotomy is made in the common femoral vein, and thrombus that extrudes is removed. If there is excessive bleeding, control can be achieved by tightening the snare loops.

Once the local thrombus is cleared, a balloon catheter large enough (2–3cm balloon) to occlude the inferior vena cava (IVC) is passed proximally into the IVC. The position of the catheter must be checked before inflation because it may be in the ascending lumbar vein. This is done by injection of contrast medium under the image intensifier. Once the position is confirmed in the IVC, the balloon is inflated and slowly pulled downwards until it lodges against the proximal end of the common iliac vein. This prevents embolization while trying to clear the iliac vein thrombus.

2. Clearance of iliac vein thrombus

A second smaller balloon is passed up until it reaches the first balloon. It is then inflated and withdrawn back to the venotomy. The procedure is repeated until the iliac vein is cleared of thrombus. Operative venography is performed and the entire procedure is repeated if residual thrombus is identified (see **Fig. 42.23**).

3. Clearance of distal vein thrombus

Thrombus in the distal vein can be removed by applying a compression bandage from the ankle upwards (which extrudes the clot) or by retrograde passage of the balloon catheter. The latter option can be difficult due to impaction on venous valves. A separate incision to expose the popliteal vein, allowing upward passage of balloon catheters has been attempted by some surgeons.

Anticoagulant regimen for acute DVT

The standard treatment for uncomplicated acute DVT is to administer heparin initially (immediate anticoagulation), followed by oral anticoagulation with warfarin. Heparin is discontinued once the oral anticoagulant has achieved a stable therapeutic level, which usually requires 3–5 days' treatment. Anticoagulants can be divided into two types, depending on the method of administration: parenteral anticoagulants (heparin-based) and oral anticoagulants.

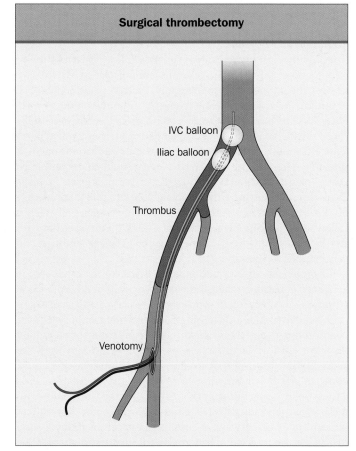

Figure 42.23 Surgical thrombectomy.

Unfractionated heparin

Heparin is present endogenously and is produced mainly by mast cells. Its main function is to inhibit the activity of thrombin. Unfractionated heparin (UFH) can be given either intravenously (bolus or continuous infusion) or subcutaneously. Continuous intravenous administration has a better pharmacokinetic profile than the bolus technique because heparin has a very short half-life of approximately 1 hour. Bolus administration every 6 hours will achieve a therapeutic level for only 4 hours and therefore patients are not anticoagulated for the other 2 hours. A number of studies have shown that continuous administration results in fewer bleeding complications.[123]

Dose

The dose of heparin depends on the accelerated partial thromboplastin time (APTT). To be effective in preventing thrombus extension, the APTT must be at least twice normal. To achieve this, a loading dose of 5000IU is given intravenously, followed by 20 000 to 40 000IU every 24 hours. The APTT should be monitored twice daily in the first few days but daily measurement is adequate once the APTT has stabilized. The dose of heparin is adjusted according to the APTT; a 'weight-based' nomogram is superior to a 'standard' nomogram for calculating the amount required.[124] It is important that therapeutic anticoagulation is achieved as soon as possible, and this may require initially measuring the APTT every 6 hours in some patients.

Complications

1. Bleeding

This is the most serious complication of heparin therapy and occurs in approximately 3–4% of patients treated.[125] There is some evidence to suggest that the risk increases with the heparin dose and increasing age (>70 years). Treatment involves stopping the heparin and, in more severe cases, administering protamine sulfate (25mg over 10 min and repeat the APTT).

2. Heparin-induced thrombocytopenia

Heparin-induced thrombocytopenia (HIT) occurs in 2% of patients on UFH and is due to the production of antiplatelet antibodies induced by heparin.[126] This usually manifests after 3–5 days of treatment, or earlier if patients have previous exposure to heparin. HIT usually causes serious bleeding but paradoxically may result in thromboembolic complications as a result of platelet aggregation. It is a serious condition, with a mortality rate of 10–30%. It is therefore prudent that patients on UFH for more than 3 days have their platelet counts monitored daily, together with APTT. Increasing requirement for heparin (decreasing APTT) and a falling platelet level suggest HIT. The heparin should be discontinued and replaced with another anticoagulant.[127] Low-molecular-weight heparins (LMWHs) should not be given to patients with established HIT, because they have a high degree of in-vitro cross-reactivity with the antibody that causes this disorder. Danaparoid sodium, which cross-reacts minimally with heparin antibodies *in vitro*, has been used successfully in this setting. Alternatively, direct thrombin inhibitors such as hirudin, bivalirudin, or argatroban can be employed.[128] The use of heparin in patients with a history of HIT should be restricted to those with a compelling indication, such as cardiac or vascular surgery; it should be considered only if heparin-dependent antibodies cannot be detected by a sensitive assay.

3. Osteoporosis

Osteoporosis is seen in patients who have undergone heparin treatment for more than 6 months. This effect is dose-related and rarely occurs below 10 000IU per day.

Low-molecular-weight heparins

Unlike UFH, which is a heterogeneous mixture of polysaccharide chains ranging in molecular weight from about 3000 to 30 000, LMWHs are fragments of UFH produced by controlled enzymatic or chemical depolymerization processes that yield chains with a mean molecular weight of about 5000. Both UFH and LMWHs exert their anticoagulant activity by activating antithrombin. LMWHs have several pharmacologic advantages over UFH, including increased bioavailability, substantially reduced protein binding, and a prolonged half-life, making once-daily dosing possible.[129] These agents also have decreased interactions with platelets, which may reduce the risk of bleeding and heparin-induced thrombocytopenia. Furthermore, outpatient treatment is safe and monitoring is generally not required, which has implications with respect to quality of life and cost. These agents are now the treatment of choice in many centers, and are the cornerstone of ambulant regimens of management for DVT.

Dose

Low-molecular-weight heparins can be given either by subcutaneous or intravenous injection. Subcutaneous injection is more widely accepted because it has a better pharmacokinetic profile. The plasma half-life of LMWHs is two to four times longer than UFH, ranging from 2 to 4 hours after intravenous injection and from 3 to 6 hours after subcutaneous injection. The dose is dependent on the type of LMWH used, the weight of the patient, and the indication for treatment. The dose of LMWH used for treating VTE is double that used for DVT prophylaxis (**Table 42.7**). As with UFH, treatment is continued until adequate oral anticoagulation is achieved.

Complications

Low-molecular-weight heparins have been shown in a number of trials to be at least as safe as UFH for the prevention and treatment of VTE. The incidence of thrombocytopenia and osteoporosis are significantly lower with LMWHs.[130,131] It should

Dose of low-molecular-weight heparins (LMWH) for venous thromboembolism.		
LMWH	*Prophylaxis*	*Treatment*
Certoparin	3000 units daily	Unlicenced
Dalteparin	2500–5000 units daily	46–56kg, 10 000 units daily 57–68kg, 12 500 units daily 69–82kg, 15 000 units daily >82kg, 18 000 units daily
Enoxaparin	2000–4000 units daily	1.5mg/kg once daily
Reviparin	1432 units daily	Unlicenced
Tinzaparin	3500–4500 units daily	175 units/kg daily

Table 42.7 Dose of low-molecular-weight heparins (LMWH) for venous thromboembolism.

also be remembered that protamine sulfate only partially reverses the anticoagulant effects of LMWHs; if serious bleeding complications occur, treatment with fresh frozen plasma may be necessary.

Clinical effectiveness in comparison to unfractionated heparin

A number of studies have suggested that LMWHs are more effective than intravenous UFH in preventing progression of VTE in patients with acute PE or DVT, with fewer complications. In addition, a study published recently showed that LMWHs are more effective in reducing thrombus size in comparison to UFH.[132] Cost–benefit analysis also favors LMWHs, with a potential 60% reduction in cost, mainly due to the option of outpatient ambulant therapy.[133]

Oral anticoagulants

The two types of oral anticoagulants are the coumarins (warfarin, dicoumarol, and nicoumalone) and the indanediones, which are rarely used due to frequent side effects. They are well absorbed in the gastrointestinal tract and highly bound to plasma albumin. These drugs are metabolized by the liver and excreted in hydroxylated form by the kidney. The half-life of warfarin is as long as 42 hours, thus leading to a more stable anticoagulant effect. These drugs inhibit the actions of vitamin K in the synthesis of procoagulant factors (factors II, VII, IX, and X) and anticoagulant factors (proteins C and S). Measuring the prothrombin time assesses the anticoagulant and is expressed as the international normalized ratio (INR), which is the ratio between the patient's prothrombin time over the laboratory control time.

Dose

The standard regimen for oral anticoagulation is to give a loading dose, which varies according to drug used, followed by a maintenance dose, depending on the INR. The INR should be measured daily from day 2 and the dose of anticoagulant is adjusted accordingly in order to achieve a therapeutic level of between 2–3. Once the INR value is stabilized, usually after 4–5 days of treatment, parenteral anticoagulation can be discontinued.

INR monitoring is performed daily until a stable therapeutic range has been achieved, then two to three times weekly for the first 2 weeks, and once weekly thereafter. For those on long-term treatment, once or twice monthly testing is adequate, depending on the stability of the INR.

Complications
1. *Hemorrhage*

This is the main complication of oral anticoagulation, with a fatal bleeding rate of approximately one per 100 treatment-years and a non-fatal serious bleeding rate of four to 16 per 100 treatment-years.[134,135] Major risk factors for bleeding include: patients over 80 years of age, INR over 2, and being in the first 3 months of therapy.[136,137] Treatment includes stopping warfarin, volume replacement, and administration of vitamin K (slow infusion of 5mg), which will return the prothrombin time to normal in 4–6 hours. In cases of severe bleeding, fresh plasma replacement may be necessary.

2. *Drug interaction*

Oral anticoagulants interact with a wide range of drugs by a variety of modes, including drug absorption, metabolism, and binding to albumin. These may result in an increase or a decrease in the anticoagulant effect. The most common drug interactions are with antibiotics, steroids, and aspirin.

3. *Skin necrosis*

This is a rare complication of warfarin therapy, with a prevalence of 0.01–0.1%. It is more common in women than in men, and may be associated with the inherited thrombophilias. It is important not to confuse this condition with venous gangrene, which can have similar clinical signs.[138]

Thrombin inhibitors

A variety of new direct thrombin inhibitors have been introduced over the last few years. Desirudin and lepirudin are recombinant derivatives of the leech enzyme hirudin, which is one of the most potent antithrombotic agents known. These drugs are more effective than heparin in the management of acute coronary syndromes but their role in the treatment of VTE is still unknown, as very few studies have been conducted in this area.[139] Fondaparinux and ximelagatran are both as effective and safe as LMWHs in preventing venous thromboembolic events in surgical patients.[140,141] Furthermore, these agents are useful in the management of patients with heparin-induced thrombocytopenia.[128]

Duration of anticoagulation

The optimal duration of oral anticoagulation depends on the balance between the risk of recurrent thrombosis if anticoagulants are stopped, and the risk of bleeding if the patient remains on treatment (see **Table 42.8**). Trials comparing short- and long-term anticoagulant treatment have suggested that long-term anticoagulation significantly reduces the incidence of recurrence of thromboembolic disease but at the cost of a higher complication rate.[142,143] The risk of recurrence is low if the DVT was precipitated by a major reversible risk factor such as surgery. Patients with an idiopathic DVT (no apparent risk factor) and those with persistent risk factors (for example, malignancy or inherited thrombophilia) have a higher risk of recurrence. Three months of anticoagulation is recommended when the risk of recurrence is low, whereas the duration of therapy should be extended to 6 months or longer when the risk is high, depending on the balance between the risk of recurrence and the risk of bleeding in each individual patient.[144,145]

Low-molecular-weight heparin preparations, at doses intermediate to those used for the acute treatment of VTE, are an alternative to oral anticoagulation during the maintenance phase of treatment. Studies have shown that they are as effective as warfarin, with similar or fewer hemorrhagic complications.[146,147] UFH given subcutaneously at a dose of 5000IU twice a day is not useful in preventing recurrent disease,[148] but is effective if given in adjusted doses (APTT twice normal).[149]

Finally, routine wearing of a below-knee graduated compression stocking for 2 years after an acute DVT has been shown to halve the risk of the post-thrombotic syndrome, although it does not influence the rate of recurrent thrombosis.[150,151]

TREATMENT OF PULMONARY EMBOLISM

The treatment is best classified according to the severity and duration of the PE; this can be grouped into:

- acute massive PE;
- acute sub-massive PE;
- acute non-massive PE; and
- chronic thromboembolic pulmonary hypertension.

Acute massive pulmonary embolism

The diagnosis of massive PE should only be entertained if the patient is hemodynamically unstable, which can range from moderate systemic hypotension to cardiac arrest. Immediate resuscitation should be provided to maximize the cardiac output, maintain systemic pressure, and improve oxygen saturation. Once the diagnosis is established, treatment needs to be commenced (sometimes during ongoing resuscitation) and this can be conservative (heparin), or involve thrombolysis or thrombectomy (surgical or percutaneous).

If the patient is easily resuscitated, it is unlikely that they have a massive PE, and heparin treatment is probably adequate. Unstable patients require urgent, more active management to remove the emboli. The first option should be thrombolytic treatment, but if this is contraindicated, surgical/percutaneous thrombectomy should be considered.

Following successful treatment, anticoagulation should be long term. The precise duration is a balance between the risk of further embolism and complications of anticoagulation therapy (**Table 42.8**).

Supportive measures
Oxygen
Oxygen saturation can easily and rapidly be improved by oxygen via mask or nasal prongs. Mechanical ventilation is rarely necessary to improve oxygenation and, if needed, ventilation pressure should be set as low as possible.[152] High positive ventilatory pressure reduces the venous return to the right heart, which is already impaired in patients with a massive PE.[27] Rapid frequency ventilation with a low tidal volume may decrease the hemodynamic effect.

Fluid resuscitation
Fluid resuscitation in patients with massive PE is a controversial issue. Experimental studies in animals that were injected with microspheres to cause massive PE and hypotension showed a negative response to fluid resuscitation. The right heart is already impaired and fluid replacement causes further dilatation of the chambers. However, a few small clinical studies contradicted the experimental results and showed that the cardiac index improved quite significantly in patients with a massive PE and poor cardiac function following 500–600mL fluid replacement.[153,154]

Inotropic agents
Dobutamine and dopamine are intravenous beta-adrenergic agonists. A small study showed a beneficial effect of these agents on cardiac index, systemic arterial pressure, and mean pulmonary arterial pressure in patients with massive PE.[155] The role of epinephrine and norepinephrine in massive PE is uncertain and the use of these agents should probably be limited to patients

Duration of anticoagulation for venous thromboembolic disease.	
Risk of recurrent DVT	*Duration*
Low	3 months
• Provoked DVT/PE (e.g. surgery or trauma)	
• Heterozygous for factor V Leiden	
• Heterozygous or homozygous for prothrombin G10120A mutation	
Intermediate	>6 months
• Unprovoked or idiopathic DVT/PE	
• First episode of recurrence (DVT/PE)	
• Persistent risk factor (malignancy, oral contraceptives, immobilization)	
• Protein C or S deficiency	
High	Indefinite
• Inherited thrombophilia – homozygous for factor V Leiden – more than one thrombophilia – antithrombin deficiency	
• Antiphospholipid antibodies	
• Recurrent DVT/PE ≥2	

Table 42.8 Duration of anticoagulation for venous thromboembolic disease. DVT, deep vein thrombosis; PE, pulmonary embolism.

with profound cardiac impairment and systemic hypotension resistant to other measures.[156]

Pulmonary vasodilators
The pathologic effect of PE depends not only on mechanical obstruction of the pulmonary arterial flow but also the release of potent vasoconstrictive agents such as thromboxane A2 and endothelin-1.[157] Antagonizing the effects of these mediators dramatically increases tolerance to experimental PE in animals.[158] Inhalation of nitric oxide, which is a selective pulmonary vasodilator, improves hemodynamics by lowering pulmonary arterial resistance and increasing cardiac output and gas exchange in patients with massive PE.[159] In the future, acute massive PE could be treated by antagonists to pulmonary vasoconstrictors, or with direct pulmonary vasodilators.

Thrombolysis
Thrombolytic treatment is reserved for patients with severe cardiorespiratory failure, hypotension (systolic pressure <90mmHg), oliguria, or hypoxia. The rationale of thrombolytic treatment is that it actively dissolves the thrombi (**Fig. 42.24**), thereby reducing pulmonary resistance and improving pulmonary circulation. Furthermore, it may lyse the primary source of thrombus, thereby preventing further embolism. Intravenous administration of a thrombolytic agent has similar efficacy to local infusion into the pulmonary artery, but it is more logical to

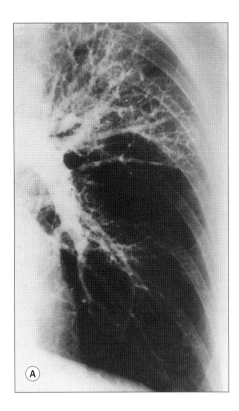
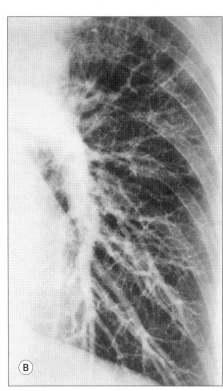

Figure 42.24 Thrombolytic treatment for pulmonary embolism. (A) Initial angiogram shows hypoperfusion of the left lower lobe. (B) Following systemic administration of streptokinase, the pulmonary circulation is restored to normal.

use catheter-directed thrombolysis in patients who are undergoing pulmonary angiography, where local agitation of the clot may improve the speed of lysis.[160] In comparison to heparin, thrombolysis improves the cardiac index and reduces the pulmonary arterial pressure much more rapidly and effectively but at the risk of hemorrhagic complications (22% versus 8%).[161] The last randomized study comparing heparin with thrombolysis in patients with massive PE and shock, was stopped for ethical reasons, after all four patients treated with heparin died, whereas four patients who received thrombolysis survived.[162]

There is no demonstrable difference in outcome between different thrombolytic agents, but some radiologists believe that rt-PA (100mg in 2 hours) acts more rapidly than streptokinase (4400IU per hour per kilogram).

Finally, thrombolytic treatment should not be used in patients with non-massive PE, but its use in patients with sub-massive PE is currently being debated.

Embolectomy

The indications for embolectomy in patients with a massive PE are: (1) contraindications to thrombolysis and (2) inadequate response to thrombolysis. Embolectomy can be performed either surgically or percutaneously using the recently developed embolectomy devices. Its use is generally reserved for only a few patients per year, even in large hospitals.

Although effective, surgical thrombectomy is associated with high perioperative morbidity and mortality rates (30–50%). However, the long-term outlook in survivors is acceptable, with 70% of patients alive after 8 years. Recent refinements in anesthesia and circulatory bypass technology should allow further improvement.[163] The surgical technique uses normothermic cardiopulmonary bypass, following which pulmonary arterial thrombectomy is performed.

The alternative to surgical embolectomy is percutaneous catheter embolectomy, which may be easier and quicker to organize. Several devices can be used, with the aim of rapid relief of central obstruction and restoration of pulmonary circulation (**Fig. 42.25**). Distal embolization of residual thrombus will still result in improved pulmonary circulation due to the relatively large size of the peripheral vascular bed (the total cross-sectional area of the distal pulmonary arterioles is more than four times than that of the central circulation). The action of thrombectomy devices is complemented by thrombolytic therapy, which helps to speed up the fragmentation and lysis of the occlusive clots. A recent review has described the various devices available.[164]

Acute sub-massive pulmonary embolism

There is debate regarding the most effective therapy in patients with sub-massive PE. These patients are hemodynamically stable, but display right ventricular dysfunction when assessed using echocardiography. Right ventricular dysfunction indicates an unfavorable prognosis and this has prompted a debate as to whether more active treatments should be employed in patients with sub-massive PE.[62,165] However, the trade-off is an increase in therapy-related complications. Further research is required to elucidate this. Meanwhile, most patients with sub-massive PE are treated conservatively.

Acute non-massive pulmonary embolism

As soon as the diagnosis of PE is suspected, heparin treatment should be started while awaiting the outcome of diagnostic tests. If UFH is used, the protocol is identical as for treatment of DVT (see Treatment of DVT section), with similar monitoring. LMWHs are now widely accepted and have replaced UFH in most centers for the treatment of PE, since two trials showed their safety and efficacy.[166,167]

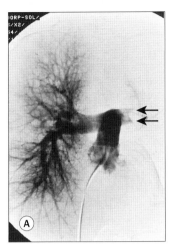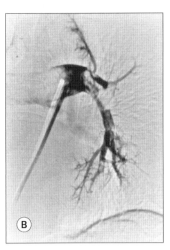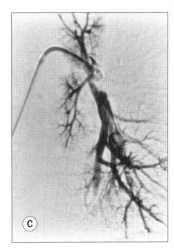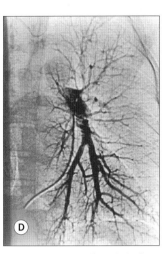

Figure 42.25 Massive pulmonary embolism treated initially by mechanical thrombectomy (Hydrolyse TM catheter) and followed by thrombolysis. (A) Catheter pulmonary angiogram showing a large left pulmonary embolus (arrows). (B) Partial fragmentation of the embolus by mechanical thrombectomy (Hydrolyse). (C) Lysis of embolus by streptokinase administered via the pigtail catheter in the left main pulmonary artery. (D) Pulmonary angiogram 2 weeks following mechanical thrombectomy and thrombolysis, with almost complete disappearance of the thrombus.

Oral anticoagulation can be commenced immediately following the confirmation of the diagnosis and, once adequate anticoagulation is achieved and stabilized (INR 2–3), heparin can be discontinued. Although treatment of PE is possible in an outpatient, this should only take place with adequate monitoring.

Anticoagulation
Long-term oral anticoagulation is the cornerstone of the management of PE, and has reduced the mortality from 25% to less than 5%.[168] The anticoagulant regimen for PE is identical to that of DVT. Heparin is commenced immediately, but as soon as the diagnosis is confirmed, oral anticoagulation therapy is begun. The duration of warfarin treatment depends on the etiology of the PE (**Table 42.8**).

Vena cava filters
Vena cava filters can be placed in the IVC to prevent emboli from the legs reaching the lungs. Vena cava filters are placed with increasing frequency; currently around 40 000 filters are deployed annually, although most are used in the USA. All filters are based on a wire mesh of different configurations, which allows blood to flow through while impeding the passage of (larger) emboli. There are many devices available on the market, varying from permanent, optional retrievable, or temporary filters (**Fig. 42.26**). The appeal of a temporary filter is that it protects the patient during a high-risk situation, but can be removed once this risk is over.[169] It does not put a patient at risk of the long-term complications that are associated with a permanent filter.

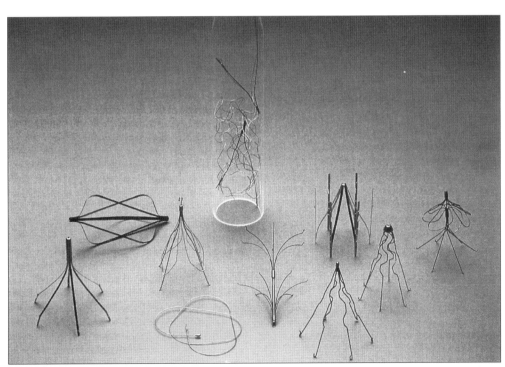

Figure 42.26 Types of vena cava filters. Back row, left to right: Antheor, Gunther tulip, Bird's nest, LGM, and Simon Nitonol. Front row, left to right: Keeper, Dil, FCP, Greenfield titanium, and Greenfield steel. With permission from Oudkerk et al. Pulmonary embolism. © 1999 Blackwell Wissenschafts-Verlag GmbH, Berlin.

Indications for filter placement

There are four absolute indications for filter placement:

- in a patient with PE and absolute contraindications to anti-coagulant therapy;
- in a patient with recurrent VTE while fully anticoagulated;
- in the case of a major bleeding complication that requires anticoagulant therapy to be stopped; and
- in a patient with DVT and right to left shunt.

Furthermore, patients who undergo surgical thrombectomy for chronic thromboembolic PE also generally receive a permanent vena cava filter. Relative indications include patients with reduced cardiopulmonary reserve or those with proven proximal free-floating thrombus.

Technique of filter placement

The preferential sites of access for insertion are the right femoral vein or right internal jugular vein, as these are the most straightforward routes to the IVC. On achieving access, the first step is to perform an inferior vena cavagram via a catheter (see **Fig. 42.27**). This will show the venous anatomy, such as the position of the renal veins, bifurcation of the IVC, and diameter of the IVC and it may demonstrate the location of the thrombus.

In patients with a caval diameter greater than 30mm, a Bird's nest filter should be used. If this filter is not available, a smaller filter in each iliac vein may be an alternative.[170]

The ideal position for the filter is just below the renal veins (**Fig. 42.28**), unless there is a thrombus in the renal veins or proximal IVC, when suprarenal filter placement will be necessary. Suprarenal placement may be an advantage in pregnancy, as otherwise the enlarging uterus may compress the filter. Superior vena cava placement can also be safely performed for VTE of the arm, but a short device such as Greenfield filter, Gunther tulip filter, or LGM-Vena Tech filter should be used.[171,172]

One anatomic abnormality that must be excluded in a patient with recurrent DVT is double IVC. Contrast enhanced CT or a venogram can demonstrate the accessory vein (**Fig. 42.29**) and a second filter will need to be deployed in this vein to prevent further embolism.

Complications of vena cava filters

Although the incidence of complications from vena cava filters is reported to be around 5–10%, death directly related to a filter is very rare.[173,174] Serious complications include the following.

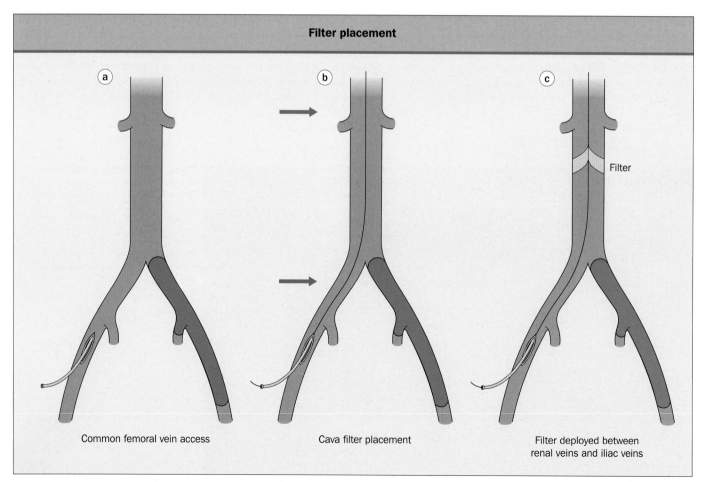

Filter placement

Common femoral vein access

Cava filter placement

Filter deployed between renal veins and iliac veins

Filter

Figure 42.27 Filter placement. (A) Common femoral vein access. A sheath is inserted and a cavagram performed. (B) Cava filter placement. The position of the renal veins and the bifurcation of the inferior vena cava are marked by metal clips on the surface of the skin. A guidewire is placed above the renal veins. (C) The filter is deployed between the renal veins and the iliac veins.

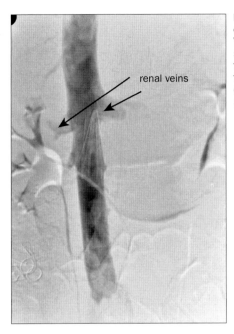

Figure 42.28 Position of a caval filter (LCM: Vena Tech). The filter should be positioned in the infrarenal section of the inferior vena cava (arrows mark the position of renal veins).

renal veins

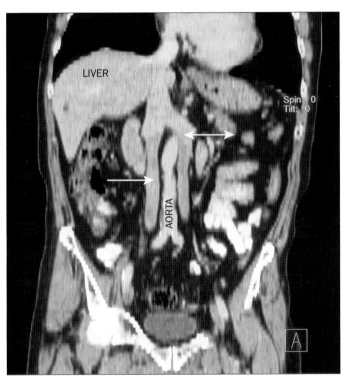

LIVER

Spin: 0
Tilt: 0

AORTA

A

Figure 42.29 Coronal reformat of computed tomography scan showing bilateral inferior vena cava (arrows).

1. Insertion site thrombosis (10%)

Before the introduction of a smaller delivery system (6–12F from the previous 24–28F), femoral vein thrombosis occurred in 30% of patients.[175]

2. Filter migration

Although this is theoretically possible, very few fatalities have been reported with any filters, other than the 23mm Mobin-Uddin umbrella, which is no longer made.

3. Caval thrombosis

The reported incidence is about 10% for the newer filter devices but the thrombosis remains asymptomatic in most patients. Although this complication may present with the post-thrombotic syndrome, it is difficult to be certain whether it is secondary to the initial DVT or is caused by the cava thrombosis.

4. Caval penetration

Perforation occurs in 20% of procedures but very rarely leads to clinical symptoms. It is due to the anchoring hooks at the end of the struts.

Effectiveness of cava filters

Following filter placement, the incidence of PE is reduced to about 2–3%. There is only one randomized study that compared cava filter plus anticoagulant with anticoagulant alone for the prevention of PE. The study involved 400 patients and it showed that the incidence of PE was significantly lower in the group with a filter (1.1% versus 4.8%) in the first 12 days, but there were no differences at 2-year follow-up.[176] Hence, the use of removable filters (without the long-term complications of permanent filters) is advocated by some clinicians.

PHLEGMASIA CERULEA DOLENS AND VENOUS GANGRENE

Introduction

Deep venous thrombosis, phlegmasia cerulea dolens (PCD), and venous gangrene are related clinical disorders. PCD is a rare condition that supervenes in fewer than 1% of patients with DVT. PCD itself is reversible, but in 50% of patients, PCD progresses to venous gangrene.[178] Both are serious medical conditions with a high mortality rate of 20–40% and an amputation rate of 30–50%.[177,178]

Pathophysiology

The fundamental process in PCD and venous gangrene is complete occlusion of the venous drainage, including the microvascular collaterals. As capillary hydrostatic pressure becomes higher than colloid oncotic pressure, fluid is driven out into the interstitium. Large amounts of fluid can be lost into the extravascular space (6–10 liters), which leads to two major clinical problems.[179] Firstly, hypovolemic shock is not unusual in PCD. Secondly, the development of the severe edema causes a marked increase in the interstitial pressure to 25–45mmHg (normal pressure 0–10mmHg), which compresses the arterioles and therefore decreases tissue perfusion, leading to ischemia. The main arterial branches, however, usually remain patent in PCD.

Aetiology

Up to 90% of patients with PCD have an underlying malignancy.[180] In half of these, the malignancy is occult and discovered later in the course of the illness. Other common risk factors are recent surgery or trauma, immobilization, and a history of inherited thrombophilia or previous VTE.

Clinical features

Venous gangrene occurs mostly in the elderly, but has been described at all ages.[181] The speed of onset and the progress of the disease is variable. Some cases are fulminant with rapid

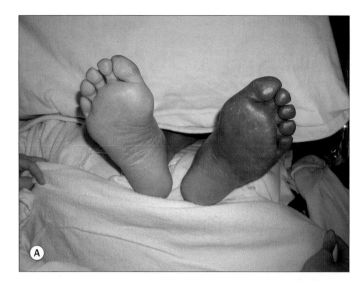

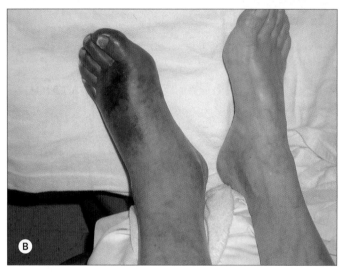

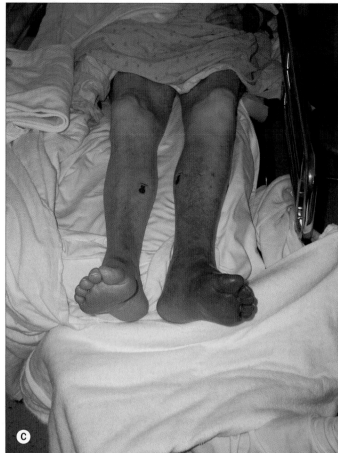

Figure 42.30 This patient had advanced metastatic lung cancer and hypercoagulability, with phlegmasia cerulea dolens and early venous gangrene. Ultrasound showed extensive obstructive, acute femoral, and popliteal vein thrombosis.

development of gangrene in 1–2 days, while others may present initially with a simple DVT that slowly progresses to venous gangrene.

The characteristic clinical features of PCD consist of pain, swelling, cold temperature, and cyanosis (**Fig. 42.30**).[182] The edema is usually severe and often causes the development of skin bullae. Cyanosis is striking and usually begins distally, progressing proximally, with trunk involvement in severe cases. Hypotension secondary to massive extravasation of intravascular fluid is another common clinical sign in PCD. Although the arterial pulses are difficult to palpate because of the gross edema, the vessels are usually patent on angiography, though they may occlude in the late stages of the illness. The diagnosis is typically based on the clinical signs and symptoms. Doppler ultrasound examination provides a rapid and accurate method of investigation and CT may reveal the cause for the thrombosis (**Fig. 42.31**).

Treatment

The aim of treatment is to prevent propagation of thrombosis, reduce the thrombus burden, preserve tissue viability, and prevent recurrence and post-thrombotic syndrome.[183] Initial treatment should consist of fluid resuscitation, heparin infusion,

and extreme leg elevation. This method of treatment alone is adequate to resolve the clinical symptoms in most patients who have not developed frank gangrene.[183] In those patients who are not responding to the initial treatment, deteriorate, or develop threatened limb viability, a more active approach is required.

Catheter-directed thrombolysis is emerging as the method of choice. Access is via jugular, femoral, or popliteal veins and the catheters are imbedded in the thrombus. Continuous infusion of thrombolytic agent is commenced and the therapeutic effect is assessed every 6–12 hours by venography, with repositioning of the catheter into residual thrombus accordingly. Simultaneous or separate infusion of thrombolytic agent into the femoral artery has also been used in severe cases.[184] The results of systemic thrombolysis and surgical thrombectomy are both poor and are no longer recommended.

The long-term treatment should consist of anticoagulation and a compression stocking to prevent recurrence and the post thrombotic syndrome.

VENOUS THROMBOEMBOLISM IN PREGNANCY

Venous thromboembolism, although uncommon, is one of the major causes of maternal mortality.[38] The incidence of PE is

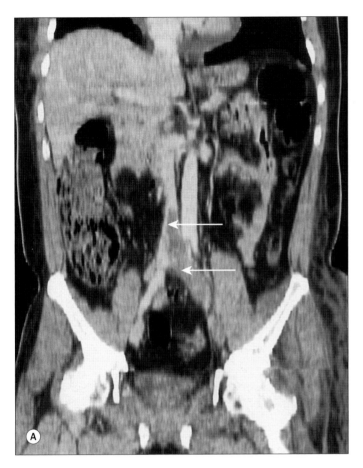

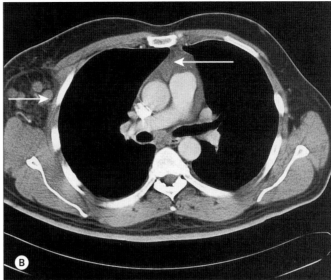

Figure 42.31 Computed tomography (CT) examination of a patient who presented with left leg venous gangrene and was subsequently found to have lymphoma. (A) Coronal reformat demonstrating extensive thrombosis of the inferior vena cava and left iliac vein (arrows). (B) CT of the thorax of the same patient showing lymphadenopathy in the right axilla and anterior mediastinum (arrows).

estimated at approximately 0.1% of all pregnancies.[185] Although the greatest risk is during the postpartum period, presentation late in pregnancy is not uncommon.[39,40] Cesarean section is associated with a slightly higher risk than normal delivery.

Diagnosis
The diagnosis of VTE can be difficult in pregnant women because of the fear of exposing the fetus to radiation. However, it is possible to diagnose DVT or PE with a radiation exposure dose less than 0.5rad (5mGy) in most women.[186] At this dose, the risk to a fetus is minimal. The first choice in the diagnosis of DVT in pregnant women is serial ultrasound imaging. For PE, the initial test should be ultrasonography of the leg veins and perfusion scintigraphy in women with a normal result. If the perfusion scan is normal, anticoagulants can be withheld, while women with segmental defects and a normal CXR should be treated with anticoagulants. When the lung scan is non-diagnostic, pulmonary angiography or CT angiography is required (**Fig. 42.32**).

Treatment
Warfarin should not be used in pregnancy because of its teratogenic effect on the developing fetus. The effect is particularly severe in the first trimester but it can also cause central nervous system abnormalities later in the pregnancy.[187] Although UFH has been the first-choice treatment, LMWHs are emerging as a good substitute because they are safe (they do not cross the placenta) and as effective as UFH, but with the added advantage of fewer complications.[187,188] Furthermore, they do not require

coagulation monitoring. Vena cava filters have been used in pregnant patients with good results, and the indications are similar to non-pregnant patients.[189]

In the postpartum period, the treatment protocol is similar to non-pregnant patients. Warfarin is not excreted in any significant amount in breast milk and can be safely given to women who are breast feeding. Vitamin K supplements can be added to milk formulas.

PREVENTION OF VENOUS THROMBOEMBOLISM

The rationale for prophylaxis is based on the high prevalence of VTE in patients in hospital, the clinically silent nature of the condition, inaccurate clinical assessment, and the potential morbidity and mortality associated with DVT/PE. Although a wide range of measures have repeatedly been shown to be effective in preventing DVT/PE, thromboprophylaxis is not implemented universally in many hospitals. The practice of routine thromboprophylaxis varies widely between hospitals, ranging from 28% to 100% of respondents.[190] A Scottish study revealed that 56% of patients who died of PE did not receive prophylaxis, despite having significant risk factors and no contraindication to anticoagulation prophylaxis.[191]

Methods of prophylaxis
Early mobilization after surgery is undoubtedly a very effective way to prevent thromboembolism but it is not always possible. In most situations, clinicians have to resort to other forms of prophylaxis which can either be mechanical or pharmacologic.

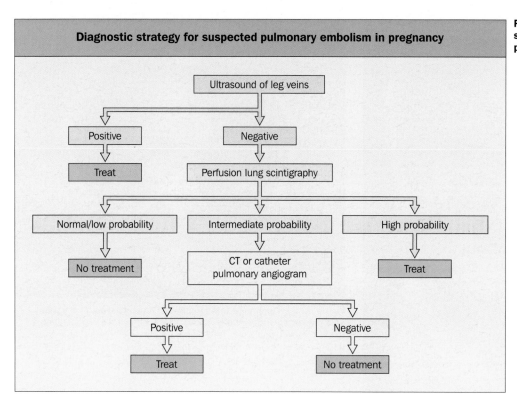

Figure 42.32 Diagnostic strategy for suspected pulmonary embolism in pregnancy.

Although these methods are effective on their own, optimum results are achieved by combining them.

Mechanical

Both graduated compression stockings and intermittent pneumatic compression have been shown to be effective in preventing venous thromboembolic events without the risks of hemorrhage.[151,192] To be most effective, they should be applied during and after surgery. They are particularly useful in patients in whom the risk of hemorrhage prohibits the use of anticoagulants (such as neurosurgical and ophthalmological patients), or where anticoagulation is contraindicated.

Pharmacologic

The three main types of antithrombotic agents used are:

- heparin (UFH or LMWHs);
- oral anticoagulant (vitamin K antagonists); and,
- aspirin.

Vitamin K antagonists

These agents are effective in preventing DVT.[193] However, they have a delayed onset of action, a long half-life and require regular monitoring, thus increasing the risk of hemorrhage. Their prolonged use in prophylaxis after discharge in patients who remain at risk due to immobilization is less contentious.

Heparin

Subcutaneous heparin (5000IU) given twice or three times daily (commencing before surgery and discontinued on mobilization) reduces the incidence of PE threefold in general surgery patients. LMWHs are as effective but with the added benefit of once daily administration and probably fewer complications. The incidence of VTE is inversely related to the dose and frequency of administration of anticoagulation.[194] However, as expected, the complication rate also increases with higher doses. The best time to start heparin (pre- or postoperation) has been the subject of many debates but unfortunately remains unresolved. Some orthopedic surgeons believe that thromboprophylaxis should be given after operation in order to minimize intraoperative hemorrhage. However, it seems more sensible to commence therapy 1–2 hours before surgery, in order to provide protection against VTE during operation, unless the risk of hemorrhage is unacceptably high. In patients having epidural anesthesia, the drug is given after the insertion of the epidural catheter.

Aspirin

Although aspirin can reduce the incidence of VTE in patients undergoing surgery,[195] it is not as effective as heparin or warfarin.[196] However, it does have the benefit of easy administration and low cost. Although it is not advisable to use aspirin on its own for thromboprophylaxis, it can supplement other treatments, especially in patients at very high risk of VTE, and in those who undergo joint replacement surgery.

Dextran

Although there is no scientific proof that dextran is effective for the prevention of VTE, there is some indication that it may be valuable.[197] It has never been widely used because of its difficult administration schedule, the risk of fluid overload, and occasional anaphylactic reactions.

Recommendations

Rather than giving standard thromboprophylaxis to all patients, it should be tailored to each patient individually, depending on the risk of developing VTE (**Tables 42.2 & 42.8**). For example, elderly patients with a history of DVT requiring pelvic surgery should receive more prophylaxis than a young patient having inguinal hernia repair. The risk can be divided into three categories (**Table 42.2**). Patients at low risk do not require prophylaxis, but early mobilization is encouraged. For the moderate risk group, either heparin (UFH or LMWH), or intermittent pneumatic compression or a graduated compression stocking is sufficient. Patients in the high-risk category need both mechanical and pharmacologic prophylaxis. Furthermore, the frequency or dose of heparin in this group should be higher than average.

In patients undergoing surgery in which minor hemorrhage may be critical to the outcome, such as neurosurgery or ophthalmic surgery, the mechanical form of prophylaxis is recommended.

SUMMARY

Venous thromboembolic disease is a common condition, especially in patients in hospital. Unfortunately, it is frequently overlooked and under-diagnosed by clinicians due to its nonspecific presentation. It is imperative that this condition is considered in patients with known risk factors. The consequences of both over- and under-diagnosing this condition are serious and may cause death or long-term disability. Although thrombo-prophylaxis does not prevent the disorder completely, it is highly effective and should be given to all patients at risk of VTE.

REFERENCES

1. Hirsh J, Hoak J. Management of deep vein thrombosis and pulmonary embolism. A statement for health professionals. Council on Thrombosis (in consultation with the Council on Cardiovascular Radiology), American Heart Association. Circulation 1996; 93: 2212–45.
2. Moser KM. Venous thromboembolism. Am Rev Respir Dis 1990; 141:235–49.
3. Salzman EW, Hirsh J. The epidemiology, pathogenesis and natural history of venous thrombosis. In: Colman RW, Hirsh J, Marder V, eds. Thrombosis and Haemostasis. Basic principles and clinical practice. Philadelphia:JB Lippincott; 1993:1275–96.
4. Huisman MV, Buller HR, ten Cate JW, et al. Unexpected high prevalence of silent pulmonary embolism in patients with deep venous thrombosis. Chest 1989;95:498–502.
5. van Erkel AR, van den Hout WB, Pattynama PM. International differences in health care costs in Europe and the United States: Do these affect the cost-effectiveness of diagnostic strategies for pulmonary embolism? Eur Radiol 1999;9:1926–31.
6. Cohen AT, Edmondson RA, Phillips MJ, et al. The changing pattern of venous thromboembolic disease. Haemostasis 1996;26:65–71.
7. Silverstein MD, Heit JA, Mohr DN, et al. Trends in the incidence of deep vein thrombosis and pulmonary embolism: a 25-year population-based study. Arch Intern Med 1998;158:585–93.
8. Turton EP, Coughlin PA, Berridge DC, Mercer KG. A survey of deep venous thrombosis management by consultant vascular surgeons in the United Kingdom and Ireland. Eur J Vasc Endovasc Surg 2001; 21:558–63.
9. Anderson FA, Wheeler HB, Goldberg RJ, et al. A population-based perspective of hospital incidence and case-fatality rates of deep venous thrombosis and pulmonary embolism. The Worcester DVT study. Arch Intern Med 1991;151:933–8.
10. Gillum RF. Pulmonary embolism and thrombophlebitis in the United States, 1970–1985. Am Heart J 1987;114:1262–4.
11. Samama MM, Cohen AT, Darmon JY, et al. A comparison of enoxaparin with placebo for the prevention of venous thromboembolism in acutely ill medical patients. Prophylaxis in Medical Patients with Enoxaparin Study Group. N Engl J Med 1999;341:793–800.
12. Agnelli G, Piovella F, Buoncristiani P, et al. Enoxaparin plus compression stockings compared with compression stockings alone in the prevention of venous thromboembolism after elective neurosurgery. N Engl J Med 1998;339:80–5.
13. Morrell MT, Dunnill MS. The post-mortem incidence of pulmonary embolism in a hospital population. Br J Surg 1968;55:347–52.
14. Karwinski B, Svendsen E. Comparison of clinical and post-mortem diagnosis of pulmonary embolism. J Clin Pathol 1989;42:135–9.
15. Horattas MC, Wright DJ, Fenton AH, et al. Changing concepts of deep venous thrombosis of the upper extremity – report of a series and review of the literature. Surgery 1988;104:561–7.
16. Lohr JM, James KV, Deshmukh RM, Hasselfeld KA. Calf vein thrombi are not a benign finding. Am J Surg 1995;170:86–90.
17. Thomas DP. Venous thrombogenesis. Ann Rev Med 1985;36:39–50.
18. Stamatakis D, Kakkar VV, Sagar S, et al. Femoral vein thrombosis and total hip replacement. BMJ 1977;2:223–5.
19. Hull R, Hirsh J, Sackett DL, et al. Cost effectiveness of clinical diagnosis, venography and non-invasive testing in patients with symptomatic deep vein thrombosis. N Engl J Med 1981;304:1561–7.
20. AbuRahma AF, Powell M, Robinson PA. Prospective study of safety of lower extremity phlebography with nonionic contrast medium. Am J Surg 1996;171:255–60.
21. Schraufnagel DE, Tsao M, Yao YT, et al. Factors associated with pulmonary infarction. A discriminant analysis study. Am J Clin Pathol 1985; 84:15–18.
22. Sasahara AA, Cannilla JE, Morse RL, et al. Clinical and physiologic studies in pulmonary thromboembolism. Am J Cardiol 1967;20:10–20.
23. Nakos G, Kitsiouli EI, Lekka ME. Bronchoalveolar lavage alterations in pulmonary embolism. Am J Respir Crit Care Med 1998;158:1504–10.
24. Gorham LW. A study of pulmonary embolism: Part 2. The mechanism of death; based on a clinicopathological investigations of 100 cases of massive and 285 cases of minor embolism of the pulmonary artery. Arch Intern Med 1961;108:189–207.
25. Soloff LA, Rodman T. Acute pulmonary embolism. Review. Am Heart J 1967;74:710–24.
26. McIntyre KM, Sasahara AA. The ratio of pulmonary arterial pressure to pulmonary vascular obstruction: Index of pre-embolic cardiopulmonary status. Chest 1977;71:692–7.
27. Ramirez-Rivera A, Gutierrez-Fajardo P, Jerjes-Sanchez C, et al. Acute right myocardial infarction without significant obstructive coronary lesions secondary to massive pulmonary embolism. Chest 1993; 104:80S.
28. Flordal PA, Bergqvist D, Burmark US, et al. Risk factors for major thromboembolism and bleeding tendency after elective general surgical operations. Eur J Surg 1996;162:783–9.
29. Warlow C, Ogston D, Douglas AS. Venous thrombosis following strokes. Lancet 1972;1:1305–6.
30. Scurr JH, Machin SJ, Bailey-King S, et al. Frequency and prevention of symptomless deep-vein thrombosis in long-haul flights: a randomised trial. Lancet 2001;357:1485–9.
31. Cesarone MR, Belcaro G, Nicolaides AN, et al. Venous thrombosis from air travel: the LONFLIT3 study – prevention with aspirin vs low molecular weight heparin (LMWH) in high-risk subjects: a randomized trial. Angiology 2002;53:1–6.
32. Turpie AGG, Levine MN, Hirsh J, et al. A randomized controlled trial of a low molecular weight heparin (enoxaparin) to prevent deep vein thrombosis in patients undergoing elective hip surgery. N Engl J Med 1986;315:925–9.
33. Clagett GP, Anderson FA, Heit J, et al. Prevention of venous thromboembolism. Chest 1995;108:312–34.
34. Geerts W, Code KL, Jay RM, et al. A prospective study of venous thromboembolism after major trauma. N Engl J Med 1994;331:1601–6.
35. Luzzatto G, Schafer AL. The prethrombotic state in cancer. Semin Oncol 1990;17:147–59.

36. Sue-Ling HM, Johnston D, McMahon MU, et al. Preoperative identification of patients at high risk of deep venous thrombosis after elective major abdominal surgery. Lancet 1986;1:1173–6.

37. Baron JA, Gridley G, Weiderpass E, et al. Venous thromboembolism and cancer. Lancet 1998;351:1077–80.

38. Rochat RW, Koorin LM, Atrash HK, et al. Maternal mortality in the United States; Report from the Maternal Mortality Collaborative. Obstet Gynecol 1988;72:91–7.

39. Simpson EL, Lawrenson RA, Nightingale AL, et al. Venous thromboembolism in pregnancy and the puerperium: incidence and additional risk factors from a London perinatal database. BJOG 2001;108:56–60.

40. Salonen Ros H, Lichtenstein P, Bellocco R, et al. Increased risks of circulatory diseases in late pregnancy and puerperium. Epidemiology 2001;12:456–60.

41. Vandenbroucke JP, Rosing J, Bloemenkamp KWM, et al. Oral contraceptives and the risk of venous thrombosis. N Engl J Med 2001; 344:1527–35.

42. Hoibraaten E, Abdelnoor M, Sandset PM. Hormone replacement therapy with estradiol and risk of venous thromboembolism – a population based case control study. Thromb Haemostas 1999;82:1218–21.

43. Lowe G, Woodward M, Vessey M, et al. Thrombotic variables and risk of idiopathic venous thromboembolism in women aged 45–64 years. Relationships to hormone replacement therapy. Thromb Haemostas 2000;83:530–5.

44. Thromboembolic Risk Factors Consensus Group: Risk of and prophylaxis for venous thromboembolism in hospital patients. Br Med J 1992;79:1–17.

45. Mismetti P, Juillard-Delsart D, Tardy B, et al. Evaluation of the risk of venous thromboembolism in the medical patients. Therapie 1998; 53:565–70.

46. Finazzi G, Brancaccio V, Moia M, et al. Natural history and risk factors for thrombosis in 360 patients with antiphospholipid antibodies: a four year prospective study from the Italian registry. Am J Med 1996; 100:530–6.

47. Ondi-Ros J, Perez-Pemaa P, Monasterio J. Clinical and therapeutic aspects associated to phospholipid binding antibodies (lupus anticoagulant and anticardiolipin antibodies). Haemostasis 1994;24:165–74.

48. Provenzale JM, Ortel TL. Anatomic distribution of venous thrombosis in patients with antiphospholipid antibody: imaging findings. Am J Roentgenol 1995;165:365–8.

49. Love PE, Santoro SA. Antiphospholipid antibodies, anticardiolipin and the lupus anticoagulant in systemic lupus erythematosus (SLE) and in non-SLE disorders. Ann Intern Med 1990;112:682–98.

50. Simioni P, Prandoni P, Zanon E, et al. Deep venous thrombosis and lupus anticoagulant. A case control study. Thromb Haemostas 1996; 76:187–9.

51. Prandoni P, Simioni P, Girolami A. Antiphospholipid antibodies, recurrent thromboembolism, and intensity of warfarin anticoagulation. Thromb Haemost 1996;75:859.

52. Klatsky AL, Armstrong MA, Poggi J. Risk of pulmonary embolism and/or deep venous thrombosis in Asian-Americans. Am J Cardiol 2000;85:1334–7.

53. Bertina RM, Koeleman BP, Koster T, et al. Mutation in blood coagulation factor V associated with resistance to activated protein C. Nature 1994;369:64–7.

54. Poort SR, Rosendaal FR, Reitsma PH, Bertina RM. A common genetic variation in the 3'-untranslated region of the prothrombin gene is associated with elevated plasma prothrombin levels and an increase in venous thrombosis. Blood 1996;88:3698–703.

55. Mudd Sh, Skovby F, Levy HL, et al. The natural history of homocystinuria due to cystathionine beta-synthase deficiency. Am J Hum Genet 1985;37:1–31.

56. Alhenc-Gelas M, Arnoud E, Nicaud V, et al. Venous thromboembolic disease and the prothrombin, methylene tetrahydrofolate reductase and factor V genes. Thromb Haemostas 1999;81:506–10.

57. Seligsohn U, Lubetsky A. Medical progress: genetic susceptibility to venous thrombosis. N Engl J Med 2001;344:1222–31.

58. Girling J, de Swiet M. Inherited thrombophilia and pregnancy. Curr Opin Obstet Gynaecol 1998;10:135–44.

59. Vandenbroucke JP, Koster T, Briet E, et al. Increased risk of venous thrombosis in oral contraceptive users who are carriers of factor V Leiden mutation. Lancet 1994;344:1453–7.

60. Monreal M, Raventos A, Lerma R, et al. Pulmonary embolism in patients with upper extremity DVT associated to venous central lines. A prospective study. Thromb Haemost 1994;72:548–50.

61. Ribeiro A, Lindmarker P, Juhlin-Dannfelt A, et al. Echocardiography Doppler in pulmonary embolism: right ventricular dysfunction as a predictor of mortality rate. Am Heart J 1997;134:479–87.

62. Ribeiro A, Lindmarker P, Johnsson H, et al. Pulmonary embolism: one-year follow-up with echocardiography Doppler and five-year survival analysis. Circulation 1999;99:1325–30.

63. Stein PD, Goldhaber SZ, Henry JW, Miller AC. Arterial blood gas analysis in the assessment of suspected acute pulmonary embolism. Chest 1996;109:78–81.

64. Hull R, Hirsch J, Sackett DL. Clinical validity of a negative venogram in patients with clinically suspected venous thrombosis. Circulation 1981;64:622–5.

65. Browse NL. Diagnosis of deep vein thrombosis. Br Med Bull 1978; 34:163–7.

66. Lensing AW, Prandoni P, Brandjes D, et al. Detection of DVT by real-time B-mode ultrasonography. N Engl J Med 1989;320:342–5.

67. Lensing AWA, Kraaijenhagen R, van Beek EJR, Buller HR. Diagnosis of venous thrombosis. In: Oudkerk M, van Beek EJR, ten Cate JW. Pulmonary embolism. Berlin:Blackwell Science; 1999:47–55.

68. Heijboer H, Büller HR, Lensing AW, et al. A comparison of real-time compression ultrasonography with impedance plethysmography for the diagnosis of DVT in symptomatic outpatients. N Engl J Med 1993; 329:1365–9.

69. Bounameaux H, de Moerloose P, Perrier A, Reber G. Plasma measurement of D-dimer as diagnostic aid in suspected venous thromboembolism: an overview. Thromb Haemostas 1994;71:1–6.

70. Goldhaber SZ, Simons GR, Elliot CG, et al. Quantitative plasma D-dimer levels among patients undergoing pulmonary angiography for suspected pulmonary embolism. JAMA 1993;270:2819–22.

71. De Moerloose P, Desmarais S, Bounameaux H, et al. Contribution of a new, rapid, individual and quantitative automated D-dimer ELISA to exclude pulmonary embolism. Thromb Haemostas 1996;75:11–13.

72. van Beek EJR, van den Ende B, Berckmans RJ, et al. A comparative analysis of D-dimer assays in patients with clinically suspected pulmonary embolism. Thromb Haemostas 1993;70:408–13.

73. Michiels JJ, Freyburger G, van der Graaf F, et al. Strategies for the safe and effective exclusion and diagnosis of deep vein thrombosis by the sequential use of clinical score, D-dimer testing, and compression ultrasonography. Semin Thromb Hemost 2000;26:657–67.

74. Montgomery KD, Potter HG, Helfet DL. Magnetic resonance venography to evaluate the deep venous system of the pelvis in patients who have an acetabular fracture. J Bone Joint Surg Am 1995; 77:1639–49.

75. Fraser DG, Moody AR, Morgan PS, et al. Diagnosis of lower-limb deep venous thrombosis: a prospective blinded study of magnetic resonance direct thrombus imaging. Ann Intern Med 2002;136:89–98.

76. Loud PA, Katz DS, Bruce DA, et al. Deep venous thrombosis with suspected pulmonary embolism: detection with combined CT venography and pulmonary angiography. Radiology 2001;219:498–502.

77. Baarslag HJ, van Beek EJR, Koopman MMW, Reekers JA. Prospective comparative study of color duplex ultrasonography and contrast venography in patients suspected of having upper extremity deep vein thrombosis. Ann Intern Med 2002;136:865–72.

78. Huisman MV, Buller HR, ten Cate JW, et al. Management of clinically suspected acute venous thrombosis in outpatients with serial impedance plethysmography in a community hospital setting. Arch Intern Med 1989;149:511–13.

79. Hull RD, Hirsh J, Carter CJ, et al. Diagnostic efficacy of impedance plethysmography for clinically suspected deep-vein thrombosis. A randomized trial. Ann Intern Med 1985;102:21–8.

80. Cogo A, Lensing AW, Koopman MM, et al. Compression ultrasonography with clinically suspected deep vein thrombosis: prospective cohort study. BMJ 1998;316:17–20.

81. Kearon C, Julian JA, Newman TE, Ginsberg JS. Noninvasive diagnosis of deep venous thrombosis. McMaster Diagnostic Imaging Practice Guidelines Initiative. Ann Intern Med 1998;128:663–77.

82. Wells PS, Anderson DR, Bormanis J, et al. Value of assessment of pretest probability of deep-vein thrombosis in clinical management. Lancet 1997;350:1795–8.

83. Hansson PO, Sorbo J, Eriksson H. Recurrent venous thromboembolism after deep vein thrombosis: incidence and risk factors. Arch Intern Med 2000;160:769–74.

84. Murphy TP. Cronan JJ. Evolution of deep venous thrombosis: a prospective evaluation with US. Radiology 1990;177:543–8.

85. Heijboer H, Jongbloets LM, Buller HR, et al. The clinical utility of real-time compression ultrasound in the diagnostic management of patients with recurrent venous thrombosis. Acta Radiol 1992;33:297–300.

86. Huisman MV. Recurrent venous thromboembolism: diagnosis and management. Curr Opin Pulm Med 2000;6:330–4.

87. Giannitsis E, Müller-Bardorff M, Kurowski V, et al. Independent prognostic value of cardiac troponin T in patients with confirmed pulmonary embolism. Circulation 2000;102:211–7.

88. Miniati M, Prediletto R, Formichi B, et al. Accuracy of clinical assessment in the diagnosis of pulmonary embolism. Am J Respir Crit Care Med 1999;159:864–71.

89. Stein PD, Henry JW. Clinical characteristics of patients with acute pulmonary embolism stratified according to their presenting syndromes. Chest 1997;112:974–9.

90. Stein PD, Goldhaber SZ, Henry JW. Alveolar-arterial oxygen gradient in the assessment of acute pulmonary embolism. Chest 1995; 107:139–43.

91. Sijens PE, van Ingen HE, van Beek EJ, et al. Rapid ELISA assay for plasma D-dimer in the diagnosis of segmental and subsegmental pulmonary embolism. A comparison with pulmonary angiography. Thromb Haemostas 2000;84:156–9.

92. Perrier A, Desmarais S, Miron MJ, et al. Noninvasive diagnosis of venous thromboembolism. Lancet 1999;353:190–5.

93. Wells PS, Anderson DR, Rodger M, et al. Excluding pulmonary embolism at the bedside without diagnostic imaging: management of patients with suspected pulmonary embolism presenting to the emergency department by using a simple clinical model and d–dimer. Ann Intern Med 2001;135:98–107.

94. Gottschalk A, Sostman HD, Coleman RE, et al. Ventilation-perfusion scintigraphy in the PIOPED study. Part II. Evaluation of the scintigraphic criteria and interpretations. J Nucl Med 1993;34:1119–26.

95. Hull RD, Raskob GE. Low-probability lung scan findings: a need for change. Ann Intern Med 1991;114:142–3.

96. Wells PS, Ginsberg JS, Anderson DR, et al. Use of a clinical model for safe management of patients with suspected pulmonary embolism. Ann Intern Med 1998;129:997–1005.

97. The PIOPED Investigators. Value of ventilation-perfusion scan in acute pulmonary embolism. JAMA 1990;263:2753–9.

98. The PISA-PED Investigators. Value of perfusion lung scan in the diagnosis of pulmonary embolism: results of the prospective study of acute pulmonary thromboembolism diagnosis (PISA-PED). Am J Respir Crit Care Med 1996; 154:1387–93.

99. van Beek EJR, Brouwers EMJ, Bongaerts AH, Oudkerk M. Lung scintigraphy and helical computed tomography in the diagnosis of pulmonary embolism: a meta-analysis. Clin Appl Thromb Hemost 2001;7:87–92.

100. van Beek EJR, Brouwers E, Song B, Stein PD, Oudkerk M. Clinical validity of a normal pulmonary angiogram in patients with suspected pulmonary embolism – a critical review. Clin Radiol 2001;56:838–42.

101. Rathbun SW, Raskob GE, Whitsett TL. Sensitivity and specificity of helical computed tomography in the diagnosis of pulmonary embolism: a systematic review. Ann Intern Med 2000;132:227–32.

102. Ferretti GR, Bosson JL, Buffaz PD, et al. Acute pulmonary embolism: role of helical CT in 164 patients with intermediate probability at ventilation-perfusion scintigraphy and normal results at duplex US of the legs. Radiology 1997;205:453–8.

103. Goodman LR, Lipchik RJ, Kuzo RS, Liu Y, McAuliffe TL, O'Brien DJ. Subsequent pulmonary embolism: risk after a negative helical CT pulmonary angiogram – prospective comparison with scintigraphy. Radiology 2000;215:535–42.

104. Task Force Report. Guidelines on the diagnosis and management of acute pulmonary embolism. Eur Heart J 2000;21:1301–36.

105. Gupta A, Frazer CK, Ferguson JM, et al. Acute pulmonary embolism: diagnosis with MR angiography. Radiology 1999;210:353–9.

106. Oudkerk M, van Beek EJR, Wielopolski P, et al. Comparison of contrast-enhanced MRA and DSA for the diagnosis of pulmonary embolism: results of a prospective study in 141 consecutive patients with an abnormal perfusion lung scan. Lancet 2002 11;359:1643–7.

107. Oudkerk M, van Beek EJ, van Putten WL, Buller HR. Cost-effectiveness analysis of various strategies in the diagnostic management of pulmonary embolism. Arch Intern Med 1993;153:947–54.

108. Perrier A, Miron MJ, Desmarais S, et al. Combining clinical probability and lung scan in suspected pulmonary embolism. Arch Intern Med 2000;160:512–6.

109. Aschwanden M, Labs KH, Engel H, et al. Acute deep vein thrombosis: early mobilization does not increase the frequency of pulmonary embolism. Thromb Haemostas 2001;85:42–6.

110. Browse NL, Burnand KG, Irvine AT, Wilson NM. Diseases of the veins. London: Arnold;1999:319–58.

111. Chavatzas D, Martin P. A study of streptokinase in deep vein thrombosis of the lower extremities. Vasa 1975;4:68–72.

112. British National Formulary March 2002; No. 43: section 2.10.2.

113. Schulman S, Lockner D, Granqvist S, et al. A comparative randomized trial of low dose versus high dose streptokinase in deep vein thrombosis of the thigh. Thromb Haemostas 1984;51:261–5.

114. Kanter DS, Mikkola KM, Patel SR, et al. Thrombolytic therapy for pulmonary embolism. Frequency of intracranial haemorrhage and associated risk factors. Chest 1997;111:1241–5.

115. Mikkola KM, Patel SR, Parker JA, et al. Increasing age is a major risk factor for haemorrhagic complications following pulmonary embolism thrombolysis. Am Heart J 1997;134:69–72.

116. Schweizer J, Kirch W, Koch R, et al. Short and long-term results after thrombolytic treatment of deep venous thrombosis. J Am Coll Cardiol 2000;36:1336–43.

117. Thery C, Bauchartt JJ, Lesenne M, et al. Predictive factors of effectiveness of streptokinase in deep venous thrombosis. Am J Cardiol 1992; 69:117–22.

118. Comerota AJ, Throm Re, Mathias SD, Haughton S, Mewissen M. Catheter-directed thrombolysis for iliofemoral deep vein thrombosis improves quality of life. J Vasc Surg 2000;32:130–7.

119. Bjarnason H, Kruse JR, Asinger DA, et al. Iliofemoral deep venous thrombosis: safety and efficacy outcome during 5 years of catheter-directed thrombolytic therapy. J Vasc Interv Radiol 1997;8:405–18.

120. Delomez M, Beregi JP, Willoteaux S, et al. Mechanical thrombectomy in patients with deep venous thrombosis. Cardiovasc Intervent Radiol 2001;24:42–8.

121. Ganger KH, Nachbur BH, Ris HB, et al. Surgical thrombectomy versus conservative treatment for deep venous thrombosis; functional comparison of long-term results. Eur J Vasc Surg 1989;3:529–38.

122. Hold M, Bull PG, Raynoschek H, Denck H. Deep venous thrombosis: results of thrombectomy versus medical therapy. Vasa 1992; 21:181–7.

123. Glazier RL, Crowell EB. Randomized prospective trial of continuous or intermittent heparin therapy. JAMA 1976;236:1365–7.

124. Raschke RA, Reilly BM, Guidry JR, et al. The weight-based heparin dosing nomogram compared with a 'standard care' nomogram: a randomized controlled trial. Ann Intern Med 1993;119:874–81.

125. Zidane M, Schram MT, Planken EW, et al. Frequency of major hemorrhage in patients treated with unfractionated intravenous heparin for deep vein thrombosis or pulmonary embolism: a study in routine clinical practice. Arch Intern Med 2000;160:2369–73.

126. Warkentin TE, Levine MN, Hirsh J, et al. Heparin-induced thrombocytopenia in patients treated with low-molecular-weight heparin or unfractionated heparin. N Engl J Med 1995;332:1330–5.

127. Walenga JM, Bick RL. Heparin-induced thrombocytopenia, paradoxical thromboembolism, and other side effects of heparin therapy. Med Clin North Am 1998;82:635–58.

128. Lewis BE, Wallis DE, Berkowitz SD, et al. Argatroban anticoagulant therapy in patients with heparin-induced thrombocytopenia. Circulation 2001;103:1838–43.

129. Weitz JI. Low-molecular-weight heparins. N Engl J Med 1997; 337:688–98.

130. Warkentin TE, Levine MN, Hirsh J, et al. Heparin-induced thrombocytopenia in patients treated with low-molecular-weight heparin or unfractionated heparin. N Engl J Med 1995;332:1330–5.

131. Monreal M, Lafoz E, Olive A, et al. Comparison of subcutaneous unfractionated heparin with a low molecular weight heparin (Fragmin) in patients with venous thromboembolism and contraindications to coumarin. Thromb Haemostas 1994;71:7–11.

132. Breddin HK, Hach-Wunderle V, Nakov R, et al. Effects of a low molecular weight heparin on thrombus regression and recurrent thromboembolism in patients with deep vein thrombosis. N Eng J Med 2001;344:626–31.

133. Bossuyt PM, Prins MH. Does low-molecular-weight heparin reduce the costs of venous thromboembolism treatment? Haemostasis 2000; 30:136–40.

134. van der Meer FJM, Rosendaal FR, Vandenbroucke JP, Briët E. Bleeding complications in oral anticoagulant therapy. An analysis of risk factors. Arch Intern Med 1993;153:1557–62.

135. Levine MN, Raskob G, Landefeld S, Hirsh J. Hemorrhagic complications of anticoagulant treatment. Chest 1995;108(Suppl 4): 276S–90S.

136. Fihn SD, McDonell M, Martin D, et al. Risk factors for complications of chronic anticoagulation. A multicenter study. Warfarin Optimized Outpatient Follow-up Study Group. Ann Intern Med 1993;118:511–20.

137. Fihn SD, Callahan CM, Martin DC, et al. The risk for and severity of bleeding complications in elderly patients treated with warfarin. The National Consortium of Anticoagulation Clinics. Ann Intern Med 1996;124:970–9.

138. Chan YC, Valenti D, Mansfield AO, Stansby G. Warfarin induced skin necrosis. Br J Surg 2000;87:266–72.

139. The Direct Thrombin Inhibitor Trialists' Collaborative Group. Direct thrombin inhibitors in acute coronary syndromes: principal results of a meta-analysis based on individual patients' data. Lancet 2002; 359:294–302.

140. Heit JA, Colwell CW, Francis CW, et al. Comparison of the oral direct thrombin inhibitor ximelagatran with enoxaparin as prophylaxis against venous thromboembolism after total knee replacement. Arch Intern Med 2001;161:2215–21.

141. Bauer KA, Eriksson BI, Lassen MR, Turpie AG. Fondaparinux compared with enoxaparin for the prevention of venous thromboembolism after elective major knee surgery. N Engl J Med 2001;345:1305–10.

142. Schulman S, Rhedin AS, Lindmarker P, et al. A comparison of six weeks with six months of oral anticoagulant therapy after a first episode of venous thrombosis. Duration of Anticoagulation Trial Study Group. N Engl J Med 1995;332:1661–5.

143. Kearon C, Gent M, Hirsh J, et al. A comparison of three months of anticoagulation with extended anticoagulation for a first episode of idiopathic venous thromboembolism. N Engl J Med 1999;340:901–7.

144. Couturaud F, Kearon C. Long-term treatment for venous thromboembolism. Curr Opin Hematol 2000;7:302–8.

145. Schulman S, Granqvist S, Holmström M, et al. The duration of oral anticoagulant therapy after a second episode of venous thromboembolism. N Engl J Med 1997;336:393–8.

146. Lopaciuk S, Bielska-Falda H, Noszczyk W, et al. Low molecular weight heparin versus acenocoumarol in the secondary prophylaxis of deep vein thrombosis. Thromb Haemost 1999;81:26–31.

147. Pini M, Aiello S, Manotti C, et al. Low molecular weight heparin versus warfarin in the prevention of recurrences after deep vein thrombosis. Thromb Haemost 1994;72:191–7.

148. Hull R, Delmore T, Genton E, et al. Warfarin sodium versus low-dose heparin in the long-term treatment of venous thrombosis. N Engl J Med 1979;301:855–8.

149. Hull R, Delmore T, Carter C, et al. Adjusted subcutaneous heparin versus warfarin sodium in the long-term treatment of venous thrombosis. N Engl J Med 1982;306:189–94.

150. Brandjes DP, Büller HR, Heijboer H, et al. Randomised trial of effect of compression stockings in patients with symptomatic proximal vein thrombosis. Lancet 1997;349:759–62.

151. Wells PS, Lensing AWA, Hirsch J. Graduated compression stockings in the prevention of postoperative VTE: a meta-analysis. Arch Intern Med 1994;154:67–72.

152. Jardin F, Gurdjian F, Desfonds P, et al. Hemodynamic factors influencing arterial hypoxemia in massive pulmonary embolism with circulatory failure. Circulation 1979;59:909–12.

153. Ozier Y, Dubourg O, Farcot JC, et al. Circulatory failure in acute pulmonary embolism. Intensive Care Med 1984;10:91–7.

154. Mercat A, Diehl JL, Meyer G, et al. Hemodynamic effects of fluid loading in acute massive pulmonary embolism. Crit Care Med 1999;27:540–4.

155. Jardin F, Genevray B, Brun-Ney D, Margairaz A. Dobutamine. A hemodynamic evaluation in pulmonary embolism shock. Crit Care Med 1985;13:1009–12.

156. Layish DT, Tapson VF. Pharmacologic hemodynamic support in massive pulmonary embolism. Chest 1997;111:218–24.

157. Smulders YM. Pathophysiology and treatment of haemodynamic instability in acute pulmonary embolism: the pivotal role of pulmonary vasoconstriction. Cardiovasc Res 2000;48 23–33.

158. Weimann J, Zink W, Gebhard MM, et al. Effects of oxygen and nitric oxide inhalation in a porcine model of recurrent microembolism. Acta Anaesthesiol Scand 2000;44:1109–15.

159. Capellier G, Jacques T, Balvay P, et al. Inhaled nitric oxide in patients with pulmonary embolism. Intensive Care Med 1997;23:1089–92.

160. Verstraete M, Miller GAH, Bounameaux H, et al. Intravenous and intrapulmonary recombinant tissue-type plasminogen activator in the treatment of acute massive pulmonary embolism. Circulation 1988; 77:353–60.

161. Goldhaber SZ, Haire WD, Feldstein ML, et al. Alteplase versus heparin in acute pulmonary embolism: randomised trial assessing right-ventricular function and pulmonary perfusion. Lancet 1993;341:507–11.

162. Jerjes-Sanchez C, Ramirez-Rivera A, De Lourdes Garcia M, et al. Streptokinase and heparin versus heparin alone in massive pulmonary embolism: a randomized controlled trial. J Thromb Thrombolys 1995; 2:227–9.

163. Jamieson SW, Auger WR, Fedullo PF, et al. Experience and results of 150 pulmonary thromboendarterectomy operations over a 29-month period. J Thorac Cardiovasc Surg 1993;106:116–27.

164. Uflacker R. Interventional therapy for pulmonary embolism. J Vasc Interv Radiol 2001;12:147–64.

165. Goldhaber SZ, Haire WD, Feldstein ML, et al. Alteplase versus heparin in acute pulmonary embolism: a randomized trial assessing right-ventricular function and pulmonary perfusion. Lancet 1993;341:507–11.

166. The Columbus Investigators. Low molecular weight heparin in the treatment of patients with venous thromboembolism. N Engl J Med 1997;337:657–62.

167. Simonneau G, Sors H, Charbonnier B, et al. A comparison of low molecular weight heparin with unfractionated heparin for acute pulmonary embolism. N Engl J Med 1997;337:663–9.

168. Barritt DW, Jordan SC. Clinical features of pulmonary embolism. Lancet 1961;1:729–32.

169. Bovyn G, Gory P, Reynaud P, et al. The tempofilter: a multicenter study of a new temporary caval filter implantable for up to six weeks. Ann Vasc Surg 1997;11:520–8.

170. Zolfaghari D, Johnson B, Weireter IJ, et al. Expanded use of inferior vena cava filters in the trauma population. Surg Annu 1995;27:99–105.

171. Spence LD, Gironta MG, Malde HM, et al. Acute upper extremity deep venous thrombosis: safety and effectiveness of superior vena caval filters. Radiology 1999;210:53–8.

172. Ascher E, Hingorani A, Tsemekhin B, et al. Lessons learned from a 6 year clinical experience with superior vena cava Greenfield filters. J Vasc Surg 2000;32:881–7.

173. Ballew KA, Philbrick JT, Becker DM. Vena cava filter devices. Clin Chest Med 1995;16:295–305.

174. Athanasoulis CA, Kaufman JA, Halpern EF, et al. Inferior vena caval filters: review of a 26 year single center clinical experience. Radiology 2000;216:54–66.

175. Greenfield LJ, Delucia A III. Endovascular therapy of venous thromboembolic disease. Surg Clin North Am 1992;72:969–89.

176. Decousus H, Leizorovicz A, Parent F, et al. A clinical trial of vena cava filters with prevention of pulmonary embolism in patients with proximal deep vein thrombosis. N Engl J Med 1998;338:409–15.

177. Brockman SK, Vasko JS. Phlegmasia cerulea dolens. Surg Gynecol Obstet 1965;121:1347–56.

178. Stallworth JM, Bradham GB, Kletke RR, Price RG Jr. Phlegmasia cerulea dolens; a 10 year review. Ann Surg 1965;161:802–11.

179. Brockman SK, Vasko JS. The pathological physiology of phlegmasia cerulea dolens. Surgery 1966;59:997–1007.

180. Anderson LA. Ischemic venous thrombosis: its hidden agenda. J Vasc Nurs 1999;17:1–5.

181. Hirschmann JV. Ischaemic forms of acute venous thrombosis. Arch Dermatol 1987;123:933–6.

182. Perkins JMT, Magee TR, Galland RB. Phlegmasia caerulea dolens and venous gangrene. Br J Surg 1996;83:19–23.

183. Hood DB, Weaver FA, Modrall JG, Yellin AE. Advances in the treatment of phlegmasia cerulea dolens. Am J Surg 1993;166:206–10.

184. Wlodarczyk ZK, Gibson M, Dick R, Hamilton G. Low dose intra-arterial thrombolytic therapy in the treatment of phlegmasia caerulea dolens. Br J Surg 1994;81:370–2.

185. Danilenko-Dixon DR, Heit JA, Silverstein MD, et al. Risk factors for deep vein thrombosis and pulmonary embolism during pregnancy or post partum: a population-based, case-control study. Am J Obstet Gynecol 2001;184:104–10.

186. Ginsberg JS, Hirsh J, Rainbow AJ, et al. Risks to fetus of radiological procedures used in the diagnosis of maternal venous thromboembolic disease. Thromb Haemostas 1989;61:189–96.

187. Burns MM. Emerging concepts in the diagnosis and management of venous thromboembolism during pregnancy. J Thromb Thrombolysis 2000;10:59–68.

188. Lepercq J, Conard J, Borel-Derlon A, et al. Venous thromboembolism during pregnancy: a retrospective study of enoxaparin safety in 624 pregnancies. BJOG 2001;108:1134–40.

189. AbuRahma AF, Boland JP. Management of deep vein thrombosis of the lower extremity in pregnancy: a challenging dilemma. Am Surg 1999;65:164–7.

190. Geerts WH, Heit JA, Clagett GP, et al. Prevention of venous thromboembolism. Chest 2001;119(Suppl):132S–75S.

191. Gillies TE, Ruckley CV, Nixon SJ. Still missing the boat with fatal pulmonary embolism. Br J Surg 1996;83:1394–5.

192. Butson ARC. Intermittent pneumatic calf compression for prevention of deep venous thrombosis in general abdominal surgery. Am J Surg 1981;142:525–7.

193. Taberner DA, Poller L, Burslem RW, et al. Oral anticoagulants controlled by the British comparative thromboplastin versus low-dose heparin in prophylaxis of deep venous thrombosis. BMJ 1978;1:272–4.

194. Koch A, Bouges S, Ziegler S, et al. Low molecular weight heparin and unfractionated heparin in thrombosis prophylaxis after major surgical intervention: update of previous meta-analyses. Br J Surg 1997;84:750–9.

195. Anonymous. Prevention of pulmonary embolism and deep vein thrombosis with low dose aspirin: Pulmonary Embolism Prevention (PEP) trial. Lancet 2000;355:1295–302.

196. Westrich GH, Haas SB, Mosca P, Peterson M. Meta-analysis of thromboembolic prophylaxis after total knee arthroplasty. J Bone Joint Surg Br 2000;82:795–800.

197. Gruber UF, Saldeen T, Brokop T, et al. Incidences of fatal postoperative pulmonary embolism with dextran-70 and low dose heparin. An International Medicine Multicentre Trial. BMJ 1980;280:69–72.

CHAPTER
43 Vascular Malformations

Vincent L Oliva, Gilles Soulez, and Josée Dubois

KEY POINTS

- Vascular malformations are congenital vascular anomalies that comprise low-flow lesions (venous, capillary, lymphatic, and mixed) and high-flow lesions (arteriovenous).

- Most vascular malformations become apparent during early adulthood.

- Common clinical presentations include the presence of a soft tissue mass, skin discoloration, pain, heaviness, bleeding, and limb ischemia.

- Doppler ultrasound and magnetic resonance imaging are the most useful diagnostic tools for characterizing and delineating these lesions.

- Percutaneous sclerotherapy or endovascular embolization, sometimes combined with surgical resection, is the preferred therapy for most symptomatic vascular malformations.

INTRODUCTION

Vascular malformations comprise a wide spectrum of lesions involving all parts of the body. In the past, the diagnosis and treatment of vascular abnormalities was hampered by considerable confusion caused by the use of complex hybrid terminology. In 1982, Mulliken & Glowacki proposed a helpful classification for vascular abnormalities based on cellular kinetics and clinical behavior.[1] Their classification includes two major categories:

- vascular tumors (lesions that arise from endothelial hyperplasia); and
- vascular malformations (lesions that arise from dysmorphogenesis and exhibit normal endothelial turnover).

Hemangioma is the most common vascular tumor, occurring in 4% to 10% of infants.[2] Typically, they grow rapidly during the first year of life, stabilize in the second year, and tend to regress slowly between 2 and 7 years of age. The term 'hemangioma' must only be applied to this pediatric entity.

Vascular malformations are the result of localized or diffuse errors of embryonic development that occur during the stage of angiogenesis. They presumably are present at birth, although they may not become evident until adolescence or adulthood, and they persist throughout life. They are the most frequently encountered vascular anomalies in adult patients.[2] Most vascular malformations are sporadic but some exhibit Mendelian autosomal dominant inheritance. Molecular studies suggest that vascular malformations are caused by a dysfunction of the

Classification of vascular malformations.	
Slow-flow malformations	Venous malformations
	Capillary malformations
	Lymphatic malformations
	Capillary and venous malformations
	Capillary, lymphatic, and venous malformations
High-flow malformations	Arteriovenous malformations

Table 43.1 Classification of vascular malformations.

signaling process that regulates proliferation, differentiation, maturation, and apoptosis of vascular cells.[3]

Classifications of vascular malformations are shown in **Table 43.1**.

CLINICAL PRESENTATIONS

Vascular malformations usually appear during childhood. Since they are often stimulated by hormonal influences during puberty or pregnancy, patients are frequently seen for the first time in the late teens or early adulthood. Depending on the type of malformation, patients can present with numerous symptoms including the development or progression of a soft tissue mass, pain, heaviness, pulsation, bleeding, distal ischemia, skin discoloration, skin atrophy, and congestive heart failure. Physical examination of a vascular malformation should assess the presence of a mass and its softness, color of the skin, the presence of a thrill or dilated veins, and variation of the mass with the Valsava maneuver. Scars from previous surgery should be noted. The examination should include inspection of the whole skin surface and mucosal membranes, searching for telangiectasia or dysplastic veins. Limb asymmetry and the presence of lymphedema should also be noted.

Syndromes associated with vascular malformations

The Klippel–Trenaunay syndrome is a capillary–lymphatic–venous malformation associated with soft tissue and skeletal hypertrophy of one or more limbs.[4] The cutaneous vascular malformation is always present at birth and is most often of the port-wine type. Varicosities occur ipsilateral to the port-wine stain and become apparent during childhood.[5] Abnormal or hypoplastic lymphatic vessels can lead to lymphedema.

Parkes–Weber syndrome combines arteriovenous fistulae, congenital varicose veins, and cutaneous capillary malformation associated with limb hypertrophy.[6] The arteriovenous fistulae are multiple, small, and confined to the affected limb.

Arteriovenous malformations (AVMs) can be associated with the Rendu–Osler–Weber syndrome, which consists of diffuse mucosal telangiectasia involving the nasopharynx, the gastrointestinal tract, and sometimes the urinary and genital mucosa. Arteriovenous fistulae and arterial aneurysms affect the pulmonary, hepatic, and digestive arteries.[7]

The blue rubber bleb nevus syndrome is a rare disorder that associates multiple dome-shaped cutaneous venous malformations of the skin with multiple gastrointestinal venous malformations and which can present with bleeding and anemia.[8] It is a sporadic disease, but familial cases have been reported. Histopathology reveals large blood-filled spaces or sinuses lined by single or multiple layers of endothelial cells.

Sturge–Weber syndrome is a non-inherited cutaneous disorder that consists of unilateral facial port-wine stain in the trigeminal area with ipsilateral leptomeningeal vascular dysplasia, atrophy and calcifications in the subjacent cerebral cortex, seizures, hemiparesis and visual field defects contralateral to the brain lesion, mental retardation of variable degree, and sometimes buphthalmos or glaucoma.[9]

Maffucci syndrome is non-hereditary syndrome considered as a mesodermal dysplasia that consists of diffuse asymmetric enchondromatosis involving preferentially phalanges of the hands as well as metacarpal and metatarsal bones in association with multiple venous and/or lymphatic malformations.[5]

Proteus syndrome associates multiple subcutaneous hamartomatous tumors, verrucous pigmented nevi with hemihypertrophy, partial gigantism involving the extremities, intraabdominal lipomatosis, pachydermia involving the palmar and plantar aspects of the hand and foot, hypertrophy of vertebral bodies, macrocrania, and venous and lymphatic malformations.[10] Its mode of inheritance is unclear.

DIAGNOSTIC TECHNIQUES

Radiography
Radiography can demonstrate the presence of phleboliths, which are typical for venous malformations. Hemihypertrophy can be seen in complex syndromes. Lytic bone changes can be seen with arteriovenous, lymphatic, or venous malformations.[11]

Doppler ultrasound
Doppler ultrasound should be performed as the initial diagnostic examination when a vascular malformation is suspected. This inexpensive and non-invasive technique allows differentiation between low-flow and high-flow lesions. Ultrasound is also useful for assessing accessibility for percutaneous injection therapy.

Magnetic resonance imaging
Magnetic resonance imaging (MRI) is the best tool to evaluate the extension of a vascular malformation and its relationship with adjacent structures.[12,13] It provides excellent contrast resolution and accurate delineation of lesions. The presence of flow void on T1- and T2-weighted sequences is typically seen in AVMs.[14] The examination should include spin-echo T1- and T2-weighted sequences with fat suppression. Gradient-echo sequences allow differentiation between low-flow and high-flow lesions.[12] Short-inversion-time inversion recovery (STIR) T2-weighted sequences are very sensitive for detecting venous malformations. T1-weighted sequences with fat suppression after gadolinium

enhancement are helpful to evaluate the circulating portion of the malformation. Finally, three-dimensional (3D) gadolinium-enhanced sequences with angiographic reconstruction are helpful to evaluate the vascular pattern of vascular malformations.[15]

Computed tomography
Computed tomography (CT) can demonstrate the extent of vascular malformations but its contrast resolution is inferior to that of MRI. It may help to evaluate skeletal involvement and to demonstrate phleboliths.

Angiography and phlebography
Catheter arteriography is indicated in high-flow malformations for demonstrating their vascular pattern and for evaluating the feasibility of trans-catheter embolization. Angiography is also useful in complex malformations to demonstrate arteriovenous fistulae or capillary components. Phlebography of venous malformations, obtained by direct puncture, is useful for evaluating their extent and their drainage pattern prior to sclerotherapy.

VENOUS MALFORMATIONS

Pathology
A venous malformation is classified as a simple malformation with slow flow and an abnormal venous network. Histopathologic examination of venous malformations shows thin-walled dilated sponge-like channels varying in size from capillary to cavernous dimensions, with sparse smooth muscle cells, adventitial fibrosis, thrombosis, and phleboliths.[3] Staining of smooth muscle actin reveals muscle in clumps instead of the normal smooth muscle architecture. The muscular abnormality present in the walls of venous malformations is thought to be responsible for their gradual expansion.[6]

Clinical presentations
Venous malformations present as soft, compressible, non-pulsatile masses. The overlying skin usually has a bluish tint (**Fig. 43.1**), but occasionally it may appear normal. The main locations are the head and neck (40%), trunk (20%), and extremities (40%). Characteristically, venous malformations expand after the Valsalva maneuver and they are easily flattened by external pressure. They tend to grow over time, proportionally to the growth of patients. They often enlarge during puberty and pregnancy, due to hormonal influences. Symptoms are related to the size and location of the lesions. Although most venous malformations are in the skin and subcutaneous tissues, they can also involve underlying muscle, bone, and abdominal viscera. Deep cutaneous or intramuscular lesions usually cause discomfort, often at the end of the day or with exertion. Intraoral venous malformations can bleed, distort the dentition, cause speech problems, or obstruct the upper airways and pharynx.[2] Thrombosis, swelling, and pain are common in venous malformations. Stagnation within large venous malformations can cause localized intravascular coagulopathy.[16] Local activation of the coagulation cascade is further facilitated by altered endothelium within vascular malformations. As such, a coagulation profile should be performed in any patient with an extensive venous malformation, especially if there is a history of bruising or bleeding. Consumptive coagulopathy should be corrected prior to initiating treatment of the venous malformation; the

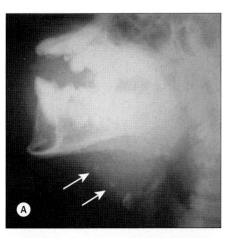

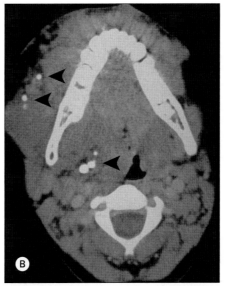

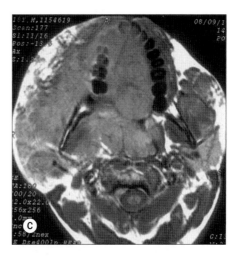

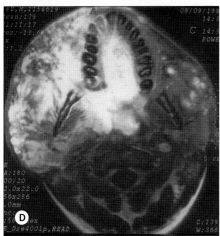

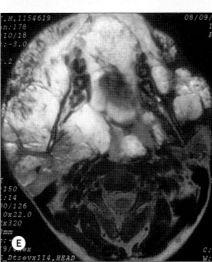

Figure 43.1 Venous malformation of the face and neck. (A) Lateral radiograph of the neck reveals a soft tissue mass around the mandible. The presence of phleboliths (arrows) is characteristic of a venous malformation. (B) Computed tomography confirms the presence of a soft tissue mass involving the cheek, lower lip, tongue, and the parapharyngeal space. Multiple phleboliths are identified (arrowheads). (C) The malformation appears isointense on axial T1-weighted spin-echo magnetic resonance (MR) imaging. Thickening of the right cheek and masseter muscle is observed. (D) The malformation appears hyperintense on T2-weighted spin-echo axial MR acquisition. Slight involvement of the contralateral cheek and masseter muscle is clearly demonstrated. (E) T1-weighted spin-echo sequence after gadolinium infusion reveals heterogeneous enhancement of the malformation, suggesting the presence of focal thrombosis.

preferred treatment for localized intravascular coagulopathy is low-molecular-weight heparin and elastic stockings to limit venous stasis.[16]

Most venous malformations are solitary, but multiple cutaneous or visceral lesions can occur. Familial forms, with multiple cutaneous and mucosal venous malformations, are inherited with an autosomal dominant pattern. In these families, a linkage to chromosome 9p21 has been established.[17] This mutation causes ligand-independent activation of an endothelial cell-specific receptor tyrosine kinase, TIE-2. In addition, familial forms of venous malformations with glomus cells (glomangioma) have been linked to chromosome 1p21–p22.[18]

Diagnostic techniques
Radiography
Plain films can reveal a soft tissue mass with phleboliths (**Fig. 43.1**). Adjacent benign skeletal erosions are sometimes present.

Doppler ultrasound
Doppler ultrasound is the best tool to differentiate venous malformations from other vascular abnormalities. Ultrasonic

examination should be performed with a high-frequency linear array transducer (5–10MHz). Imaging begins with a gray-scale examination to delineate the margins of the lesion. Venous malformations appear as compressible hypoechoic or heterogeneous lesions in 80% of patients (**Fig. 43.2**).[19,20] Anechoic channels can be demonstrated in less than 50% of the lesions. Occasionally, isoechoic thickening of the subcutaneous tissues without a solid mass or discernible channels can be the only feature. Hyperechoic foci with posterior acoustic shadowing representing phleboliths can be shown in less than 20% of cases.[19]

In most cases, spectral Doppler examination shows monophasic low-velocity flow. In 20% of the lesions, no flow can be demonstrated with a standard examination. Dynamic maneuvers such as Valsava or manual compression are sometimes necessary to induce Doppler flow (**Fig. 43.2**). Complete absence of flow may reflect thrombosis or suboptimal equipment.

CT
Computed tomography usually demonstrates the extent of a venous malformation but the contrast resolution is less than that of MRI. Venous malformations appear as hypodense or

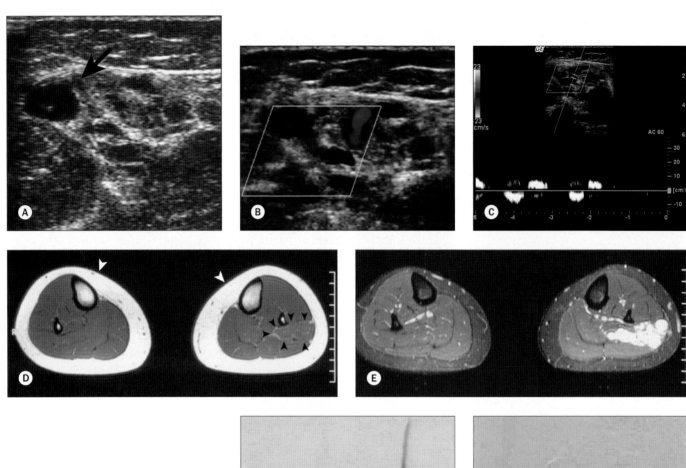

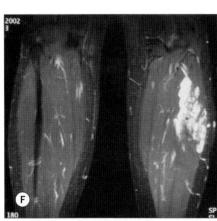

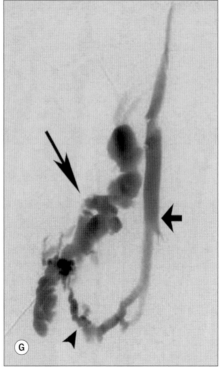

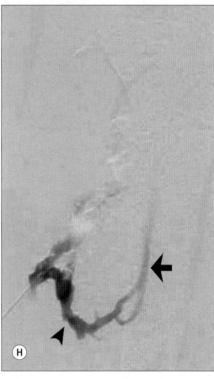

Figure 43.2 Venous malformation of the left calf. (A) Gray-scale ultrasound examination shows hypoechoic structures (arrow) in the lateral aspect of the soleus muscle. (B) Color Doppler ultrasound examination reveals slow flow inside the lesion after manual compression of the distal portion of the calf. (C) The presence of low-velocity venous flow induced by manual compression is confirmed on duplex Doppler examination. (D) Axial T1-weighted spin-echo magnetic resonance image shows infiltration of the lateral aspect of the left soleus muscle by an isointense lesion (arrowheads) that contains fatty streaks. (E) On axial T2-weighted inversion recovery acquisition, the malformation is clearly delineated. (F) Coronal T2-weighted inversion recovery acquisition shows the longitudinal extension of the lesion. (G) Percutaneous direct phlebogram. The venous malformation (long arrow) is opacified as well as the communication (arrowhead) with the deep venous system (short arrow). (H) Follow-up phlebography after sclerotherapy with 4mL of absolute ethanol reveals thrombosis of the malformation with preservation of the perforating vein (arrowhead) and deep venous system (arrow).

heterogeneous lesions that show slow peripheral enhancement after bolus injection of contrast material. Phleboliths are easily seen on CT, and fatty components can sometimes be demonstrated (**Fig. 43.1**).

MRI

Magnetic resonance imaging is the best modality to define the extent of a venous malformation and its relationship with adjacent structures. The examination protocol should begin with spin-echo or fast spin-echo T1-weighted sequences for basic anatomic evaluation. Extension of the lesion should be assessed with a T2-weighted sequence with fat suppression. STIR T2-weighted sequences with a 512 matrix are suited for this purpose (**Figs 43.1 & 43.2**). T2*-weighted gradient-echo sequences can also be used to demonstrate calcification or hemosiderin pigmentation. On gradient-echo sequences, the absence of intravascular signal suggests a slow-flow malformation.[12]

Fast spin-echo T1-weighted sequences with fat suppression should be performed after gadolinium injection, to evaluate the perfusion of the malformation (**Fig. 43.1**). The examination can be completed with a 3D FISP (Fast Imaging with Steady Precession) phlebographic sequence to evaluate the venous drainage.[21]

Usually, venous malformations are hypo- or isointense on T1-weighted sequences. When hemorrhage or thrombosis is present, the signal will become heterogeneous on T1-weighted sequences. Abnormal dilated veins can be observed in the area of the malformation. On T2-weighted sequences, venous malformations display a bright signal. Areas of hypointensity can be observed in the presence of thrombosis, phleboliths, or septation inside the malformation. On T2-weighted sequences, the extension of the malformation as well as its relationship with adjacent structures is usually clearly delineated.

After sclerotherapy, venous malformations become heterogeneous both on T1- and on T2-weighted sequences. A delay of up to several months is necessary to evaluate the therapeutic response after sclerotherapy, allowing time for the transient inflammatory reaction to resolve. In most cases, progressive shrinkage of the malformation is observed. Post-gadolinium sequences are useful to demonstrate residual perfusion of the malformation and to direct additional treatment.

Although MRI is very sensitive for identifying a venous malformation and assessing its extension, it is not very specific. Findings must be correlated with clinical and Doppler examinations to secure the diagnosis. In cases of atypical clinical or imaging findings, percutaneous phlebography is required to confirm the diagnosis. If phlebography is not conclusive, then percutaneous or surgical biopsies must be performed to rule out malignant disease.[11]

Direct percutaneous phlebography

Direct percutaneous phlebography is sometimes undertaken for diagnostic purposes in atypical venous malformations. It is more commonly performed as the initial step during sclerotherapy. Direct puncture of the malformation is achieved with a 20- or 21-gauge needle. Ultrasound can be useful for guiding the puncture, especially if the malformation is located deeply in the soft tissues. The needle is connected to a syringe through an extension tubing and is progressively withdrawn while applying slight suction. Once blood return is observed, a small amount of low-osmolarity iodinated contrast is injected in order to obtain a phlebogram. Three different phlebographic patterns can be observed with venous malformation opacification:

- a cavitary pattern without evidence of abnormal veins and late filling of the venous drainage – this is the most common appearance;
- a spongy appearance with small honeycomb cavities and late venous drainage; and
- rapid opacification of dysmorphic veins.

Peripheral phlebography

In most cases, peripheral limb phlebography is not helpful in the diagnosis of arm or leg venous malformations because most of them will not be opacified by peripheral injection. When a venous malformation is composed of dysmorphic veins, peripheral phlebography is sometimes able to demonstrate the venous drainage of the malformation.

Arteriography

Arteriography is usually not required for the diagnosis of venous malformation. It can be normal or demonstrate dysmorphic veins on the late venous phase. It can be useful in complex lesions such as capillary–venous malformations or lesions with microfistulae. Although arteriography can sometimes demonstrate microfistulae in some venous malformations, their significance remains unclear.

Management
Medical treatment

Only symptomatic malformations or lesions causing important aesthetic prejudice should be treated. Asymptomatic venous malformations should be treated conservatively. Patients must be informed of possible progression of the malformation during puberty or pregnancy, if applicable. Direct trauma to these lesions should also be avoided. Extensive arm or leg venous malformations should first be treated with elastic stockings. Low-dose aspirin seems to minimize phlebothrombotic events. Preoperative control of intravascular coagulopathy with heparin is recommended before the resection of a large venous malformation.

Sclerotherapy

Absolute ethanol and sodium tetradecyl sulfate are the most commonly used agents for treatment of venous malformations in the USA.[22] These agents are non-radiopaque but can be opacified with metrizamide powder. Absolute ethanol is the most destructive agent, and it is assumed that it is associated with the lowest recurrence rate after treatment of venous malformations.[23] Injection of ethanol produces marked tissue swelling because of intralesional thrombosis and edema. Tetradecyl sulfate is used predominantly in superficial malformations or in lesions located at the proximity of large nerves. Ethibloc (Ethicon, Hamburg, Germany), a mixture of zein (a corn protein), alcohol, and contrast medium, is a commonly used sclerosing agent in Europe.[24,25] The main drawback of using Ethibloc is its propensity to cause cutaneous fistulization with extrusion of the agent. Sclerotherapy with any agent should be performed by a skilled interventional radiologist under fluoroscopic guidance. The amount of sclerosing agent required for a given treatment is evaluated with percutaneous phlebography immediately prior to sclerotherapy (**Fig. 43.2**). It is important to avoid excessive filling of the venous drainage and normal outflow veins with the sclerosing agent. The use of a tourniquet or manual compression is sometimes useful to minimize passage of the sclerosing agent into the systemic circulation. If compression of the venous drainage is used during sclerotherapy with alcohol, it should be released progressively after injection, to avoid rapid release of alcohol in the pulmonary circulation. The main complications of sclerotherapy are cutaneous necrosis and neural toxicity, especially when alcohol is used. Cutaneous necrosis or blistering is more frequent when the malformation is bluish, indicating extension in the superficial dermis.[22] Systemic complications are rare and result from the systemic passage of alcohol; they include hemolysis with potential renal toxicity and cardiac arrest. Careful monitoring should be performed when using alcohol as a sclerosing agent, ideally in the presence of an anesthesiologist.[26] Anaphylactic reaction to sodium tetradecyl sulfate injection has also been reported.[27]

Sclerotherapy induces an inflammatory reaction that causes pain and swelling which may last several days to a week following the intervention. As such, analgesics and anti-inflammatory medication (NSAIDs or corticoids) should be given to minimize the symptoms. There should be a delay of 1 to 3 months between sclerotherapy sessions.

Venous malformations have a propensity for recanalization and recurrence,[27] and results are better for cavitary lesions after sclerotherapy. The evolution of venous malformations with dysmorphic vein pattern is variable after treatment, although results are satisfactory. Spongy patterns, especially when intramuscular, are more difficult to treat.[25]

Surgical resection

Surgery is generally contemplated for the treatment of residual lesions after sclerotherapy or when correction is required for aesthetic reasons.

Laser therapy

Laser therapy can be useful in very superficial venous malformations and in oro-mucosal lesions. Flashlamp pulsed-dye laser is effective for small superficial cutaneous lesions. The Nd-YAG laser has a deeper penetration but carries a higher risk of scarring.[28,29] For deeper lesions, laser probes can be inserted subcutaneously. Satisfactory results with minimal scarring have been reported, but recurrence and repeat treatments are common.[30]

CAPILLARY MALFORMATIONS

Pathology

Capillary malformations, also named port-wine stains, can be regarded as abnormal development of the vessels of the superficial plexus.[31] They are pink and flat at birth and become purple and nodular with irregular borders during adulthood.[5] Capillary malformations should not be confused with nevus flammus neonatorium; these pale pink macular stains composed of ectatic dermal capillaries occur in 35–50% of newborns and usually regress spontaneously.[32]

Clinical presentations

Capillary malformations commonly involve the face but can occur anywhere on the body. Cutaneous capillary malformations are often associated with hypertrophy of underlying soft tissues and skeleton as well as glaucoma.[2,5] It is also important to eliminate complex anomalies that can be associated with capillary malformations such as Sturge–Weber, Klippel–Trenaunay, Parkes–Weber, and Proteus syndromes.

Diagnostic techniques

Because capillary malformations are very superficial, imaging studies are not helpful to make the diagnosis. The role of imaging studies is to eliminate associated arteriovenous or venous malformations hidden underneath the capillary malformation. In this setting, an ultrasound examination is recommended.

Management

Capillary malformations that cause little aesthetic prejudice can be left alone. Pulsed-dye laser is the method of choice for capillary malformations that need treatment. Significant improvement is observed in 70% of patients, and results are best in facial lesions.[2] Soft tissue lesions and skeletal hypertrophy can require surgical correction.

LYMPHATIC MALFORMATIONS

Pathology

Lymphatic malformations consist of chylous fluid-filled cysts lined with endothelium.[33] Two types of lymphatic malformations exist:

- the microcystic type, which are more infiltrative, with clear or hemorrhagic cutaneous vesicles;[6] and
- the macrocystic type, sometimes misnamed cystic hygroma.

These two types can coexist in the same malformation. Combined venous–lymphatic malformations are also frequent.

Clinical presentations

Lymphatic malformations are usually present at birth but may sometimes become evident only later during childhood or adolescence. The most common locations for lymphatic malformations are the cervicofacial area, the axillary region, and the upper chest. Less common locations include the mediastinum, the retroperitoneum, the buttocks, and the anogenital region.[34,35] Lymphatic malformations can be associated with Turner syndrome.[36]

The skin color overlying lymphatic malformations can appear normal or bluish. Spontaneous shrinkage can occur, but sudden enlargement is also possible, due to infection or bleeding. Soft tissue swelling with associated skeletal overgrowth is not uncommon with lymphatic malformations located in the extremities.[2] Overgrowth of the mandible has also been described with cervicofacial malformations.[37] Effusion of chylous fluid can be observed with lymphatic malformations. Diffuse thoracic involvement can present with recurrent pleural or pericardial chylous effusions. Chronic protein-losing enteropathy with hypoalbuminemia can be observed with involvement of the gastrointestinal tract.

Diagnostic techniques
Radiography
Radiographic findings include soft tissue mass and bone distortion or hypertrophy.[38] On rare occasions, diffuse soft tissue and skeletal involvement can lead to progressive osteolysis. Also called Gorham–Stout syndrome, progressive osteolysis typically affects the clavicles.[39]

Doppler ultrasound
With Doppler ultrasound, macrocystic lymphatic malformations appear as multiloculated cystic lesions with high-resistance flow only present in septations separating the cysts (**Fig. 43.3**). The microcystic type appear hyperechoic, without flow.[38]

MRI
Lymphatic malformations appear as heterogeneous fluid-filled lesions on MRI, with a hypo- or isointense signal on T1-weighted images, and a hyperintense signal on T2-weighted images. The cysts can sometimes display a high signal on T1-weighted sequences when the cystic contents are hemorrhagic or high in protein. Pure lymphatic malformations present minimal or absent enhancement, whereas combined lymphatic–venous malformations show enhancement of fluid spaces (**Fig. 43.4**).[12]

Management
Sclerotherapy is very effective for treating macrocystic lymphatic malformations, but surgery is a good alternative option. Different sclerosing agents have been used with success: ethanol and sodium tetradecyl sulfate are used mostly in the USA; Ethibloc is popular in Europe and Canada;[40] OKT3 (picibanil), a killed strain of group A *Streptococcus pyogenes*, is commonly used in Japan.[41] Microcystic lymphatic malformations should be managed conservatively if possible. When treatment is required, surgical excision is the preferred option. Recurrence is common after surgery, with reported rates of 40% after incomplete excision and 17% after complete macroscopic excision.[42]

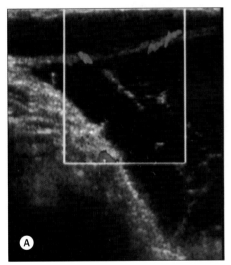
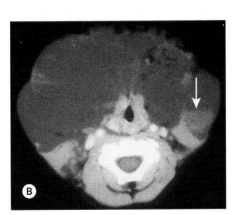
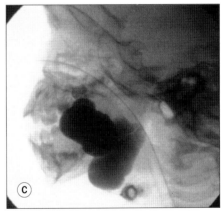

Figure 43.3 Two-year-old child with cervical macrocystic lymphatic malformation. (A) Color Doppler ultrasound of the neck shows a cystic lesion with septations. Blood flow is identified within the septations and not in the cystic portion. (B) Computed tomography of the neck confirms the presence of a large cystic lesion with septations. A fluid level seen in the left lateral portion of the malformation suggests the presence of hemorrhage (arrow). (C) Direct opacification of the malformation immediately prior to sclerotherapy reveals a multiloculated cystic pattern.

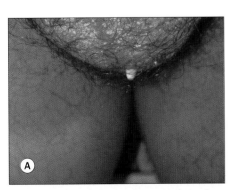
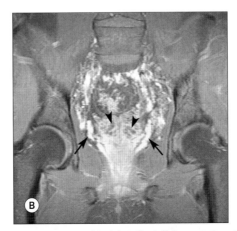
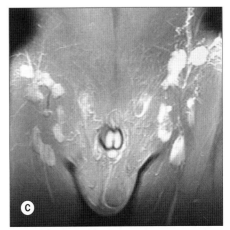

Figure 43.4 Thirty-year-old male with Klippel–Trenaunay syndrome involving the left lower extremity and pelvis, with mixed venous and lymphatic malformation. (A) Thickening of the scrotum with chylous sweating. (B) Coronal T1-weighted spin-echo acquisition of the pelvis after gadolinium injection. Hyperintense channels represent dilated veins (arrows), and centrally located hypointense channels represent lymphatic vessels (arrowheads). (C) Coronal T2-weighted inversion recovery sequence: dilated lymphatic channels and hypertrophic lymph nodes are evident.

ARTERIOVENOUS MALFORMATIONS

Pathology
Arteriovenous malformations are the result of direct connections between the arterial and venous systems.[1]

Clinical presentations
Arteriovenous malformations are usually present at birth, but they may not be evident clinically until childhood and are often exacerbated during puberty or pregnancy.[43,44] A purple or red discoloration of the overlying skin can be confused with a cutaneous port-wine stain. Closer physical examination may reveal a slightly increased skin temperature, dilated veins, and a thrill on palpation.[45] These lesions can be aggressive, with local complications such as cutaneous ischemia with ulceration or infection, and hemorrhage. Extensive AVMs can lead to high-output cardiac failure.[6] A staging system, initially introduced by Schobinger, classifies the severity of AVMs:[44]

- stage I – quiescence: pink-bluish stain, warmth, and arteriovenous shunting on Doppler ultrasound examination;
- stage II – expansion: same as stage I plus enlargement, pulsation, thrill and/or bruit, and tortuous/tense veins;
- stage III – destruction: same as stage II plus dystrophic skin changes, ulceration, bleeding, persistent pain, or tissues necrosis; and
- stage IV – decompensation: same as stage III plus cardiac failure.

Diagnostic techniques
Doppler ultrasound
Doppler ultrasound is an excellent initial technique to diagnose AVMs. These lesions are composed of multiple feeding arteries with increased diastolic flow and a high-velocity venous return with systolo-diastolic flow (**Fig. 43.5**). Power or color Doppler examination is helpful to delineate the vascular nidus of the malformation.

MRI
Magnetic resonance imaging is the best examination to evaluate the extent of an AVM and its relationship with adjacent structures, especially for bone involvement. MRI findings include dilated feeding arteries and draining veins with little tissue matrix and absence of venous lakes.[14] Signal void is typically observed in these vessels on both T1- and T2-weighted spin-echo sequences, whereas a hyperintense signal is observed on gradient-echo and angiographic sequences, indicating a high-flow lesion (**Fig. 43.6**).[12] Gadolinium-enhanced magnetic resonance

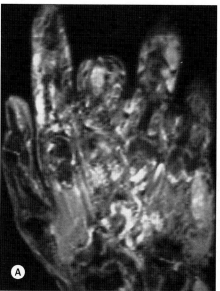

Figure 43.6 Patient with diffuse arteriovenous malformation of the right arm. (A) Coronal flash two-dimensional gradient-echo sequence of the hand shows hyperintense signal within vascular structures, suggesting a fast-flow vascular malformation. Note partial amputation of the third finger from prior ischemic event. (B) Catheter angiography of the right arm reveals diffuse enlargement of the feeding arteries with numerous arteriovenous communications.

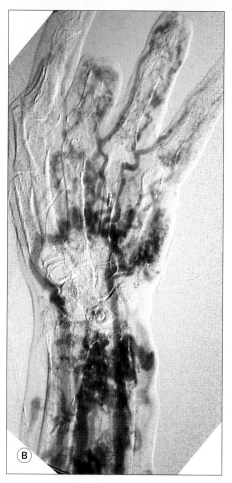

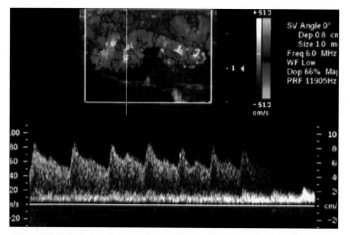

Figure 43.5 Arteriovenous malformation of right hand. Color Doppler ultrasound suggests a high-flow malformation. Duplex evaluation reveals the presence of low-resistance continuous arterial flow, thus confirming arteriovenous malformation.

angiography is helpful to evaluate feeding arteries and draining veins, although these vessels are often superimposed and difficult to differentiate.

Angiography

Angiography is strongly recommended before considering any therapeutic procedure. It allows precise evaluation of the feeding arteries and draining veins of the malformation, which is critical for evaluating the feasibility of embolization. Selective and superselective angiographic injections are often necessary to demonstrate the full extent of these high-flow lesions. The angiographic features of AVMs consist of tortuous dilatation and elongation of afferent arteries with early opacification of enlarged draining veins (**Fig. 43.7**).[46]

Management

The treatment of AVMs is complex and should be reserved for symptomatic patients. The ideal treatment is applicable only to localized lesions and combines selective embolization followed

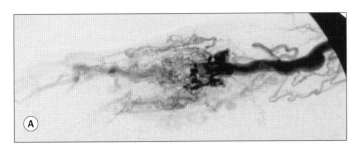

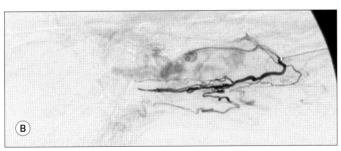

Figure 43.7 Patient with arteriovenous malformation of the right forearm causing pain due to distal ischemia and venous congestion. (A) Selective arteriogram of the interosseous artery reveals multiple arteriovenous fistulae in the carpal area with large draining veins. (B) Follow-up arteriogram performed after embolization with absolute ethanol shows occlusion of arteriovenous fistulae with absence of opacification of draining veins.

by complete resection.[44] Diffuse or extensive AVMs are more difficult to treat, and recurrence is common. Extensive stage I and II lesions can often be managed conservatively with compression garments.[44,47] Stage III and IV lesions are generally treated because of the associated symptoms and the risk of serious hemorrhage. The treatment of extensive stage III and IV lesions should aim to alleviate the symptoms rather than to obtain a complete cure. As such, the treatment must be tailored to each individual situation and should target areas of the malformation that are likely to cause ischemia or hemorrhage.

The preferred agents for embolization are absolute alcohol and N-butyl cyanoacrylate because these liquid agents can reach the nidus of AVMs. Liquid embolic agents can be injected after superselective catheterization of the feeding arteries or by direct puncture of the AVM nidus under fluoroscopic and/or ultrasound guidance.[48] Direct AVM puncture is indicated when catheterization of feeding arteries is unreasonably difficult or if selective arterial embolization carries a risk of inadvertent embolization of normal vessels.[49] Compression of the venous return either manually or with a tourniquet can prolong the transit time of liquid agents within the malformation and prevent embolization to the pulmonary circulation. Similar results can be obtained by inflating an occlusion balloon catheter on the venous side when external compression is not possible. Coils have also been used in combination with liquid agents to promote mechanical closure of arteriovenous communications prior to embolization. Complications of embolization include skin necrosis, nerve injury, distal emboli, and inadvertent embolization of coils or glue in the pulmonary circulation. Fatal cardiac arrest has also been reported with the use of alcohol.

SUMMARY

Thorough knowledge of the classification and clinical characteristics of vascular malformations is necessary to offer an appropriate investigation and treatment plan. A multidisciplinary team composed of a plastic surgeon, an interventional radiologist, and a dermatologist is an ideal combination that can offer the best therapeutic approach. It is mandatory to focus on symptoms caused by vascular malformations, in order to establish indications for treatment. Unnecessary intervention can worsen a patient's symptoms and must be avoided. A better understanding of molecular biology and genetic abnormalities related to these diseases will probably offer new therapeutic opportunities in the future.

REFERENCES

1. Mulliken JB, Glowacki J. Hemangiomas and vascular malformations in infants and children: a classification based on endothelial characteristics. Plast Reconstr Surg 1982;69:412–22.
2. Mulliken JB, Fishman SJ, Burrows PE. Vascular anomalies. Curr Probl Surg 2000;37:517–84.
3. Vikkula M, Boon LM, Mulliken JB, et al. Molecular basis of vascular anomalies. Trends Cardiovasc Med 1998;8:281–92.
4. Jacob AG, Driscoll DJ, Shoughnessy WJ, et al. Klippel-Trenaunay syndrome: spectrum and management. Mayo Clin Proc 1998; 73:28–36.
5. Esterly NB. Cutaneous hemangiomas, vascular stains and malformations, and associated syndromes. Curr Probl Pediatr 1996;26:3–39.
6. Enjolras O. Classification and management of the various superficial vascular anomalies: hemangiomas and vascular malformations. J Dermatol 1997;24:701–10.
7. Guttmacher AE, Marchuk DA, White RI Jr. Hereditary hemorrhagic telangiectasia. N Engl J Med 1995;333:918–24.
8. Moodley M, Ramdial P. Blue rubber bleb nevus syndrome: case report and review of the literature. Pediatrics 1993;92:160–2.
9. Alexander GL. Sturge-Weber syndrome. In: Vinken PJ, Bruyn GW, eds. The phakomatoses. Handbook of Clinical Neurology, Volume 14. New York:Elsevier; 1972:223–40.
10. Darmstadt GL, Lane AT. Proteus syndrome. Pediatr Dermatol 1994;11:222–6.

11. Simons ME. Peripheral vascular malformations: diagnosis and percutaneous management. Can Assoc Radiol J 2001;52:242–51.
12. Siegel MJ. Magnetic resonance of musculoskeletal soft tissue masses. Radiol Clin North Am 2001;39:701–20.
13. Disa JJ, Chung KC, Gellad FE, et al. Efficacy of magnetic resonance angiography in the evaluation of vascular malformations of the hand. Plast Reconstr Surg 1997;99:136–44.
14. Hovius SE, Borg DH, Paans PR, et al. The diagnostic value of magnetic resonance imaging in combination with angiography in patients with vascular malformations: a prospective study. Ann Plast Surg 1996; 37:278–85.
15. Dobson MJ, Hartley RW, Ashleigh R, et al. MR angiography and MR imaging of symptomatic vascular malformations. Clin Radiol 1997; 52:595–602.
16. Enjolras O, Ciabrini D, Mazoyer E, et al. Extensive pure venous malformations in the upper or lower limb: a review of 27 cases. J Am Acad Dermatol 1997;36:219–25.
17. Boon LM, Mulliken JB, Vikkula M, et al. Assignment of a locus for dominantly inherited venous malformations to chromosome 9p. Hum Mol Genet 1994;3:1583–7.
18. Boon LM, Brouillard P, Irrthum A, et al. A gene for inherited cutaneous venous anomalies ('glomangiomas') localizes to chromosome 1p21-22. Am J Hum Genet 1999;65:125–33.
19. Trop I, Dubois J, Guibaud L, et al. Soft tissue venous malformations in pediatric and young adult patients: Diagnosis with Doppler US. Radiology 1999;212:841–5.
20. Paltiel HJ, Burrows PE, Kozakewich HP, et al. Soft-tissue vascular anomalies: utility of US for diagnosis. Radiology 2000;214:747–54.
21. Li W, David V, Kaplan R, et al. Three-dimensional low dose gadolinium-enhanced peripheral MR venography. J Magn Reson Imaging 1998; 8:630–3.
22. Berenguer B, Burrows PE, Zurakowski D, et al. Sclerotherapy of craniofacial venous malformations: complications and results. Plast Reconstr Surg 1999;104:1–11.
23. Yakes WF, Luethke JM, Parker SH, et al. Ethanol embolization of vascular malformations. Radiographics 1990;10:787–96.
24. Riche MC, Hadjean E, Tran-Ba-Huy P, et al. The treatment of capillary-venous malformations using a new fibrosing agent. Plast Reconstr Surg 1983;71:607–14.
25. Dubois JM, Sebag GH, De Prost Y, et al. Soft-tissue venous malformations in children: percutaneous sclerotherapy with Ethibloc. Radiology 1991;180:195–8.
26. Yakes WF, Rossi P, Odink H. How do it? Arteriovenous malformation management. Cardiovasc Intervent Radiol 1996;19:65–71.
27. de Lorimier AA. Sclerotherapy for venous malformations. J Pediatr Surg 1995;30:188–93.
28. Rebeiz E, April MM, Bohigian RK, et al. Nd-YAG laser treatment of venous malformations of the head and neck: an update. Otolaryngol Head Neck Surg 1991;105:655–61.
29. Rosenfeld H, Sherman R. Treatment of cutaneous and deep vascular lesions with the Nd:YAG laser. Lasers Surg Med 1986;6:20–3.
30. Derby LD, Low DW. Laser treatment of facial venous vascular malformations. Ann Plast Surg 1997;38:371–8.
31. Mulliken JB, Young AE. Vascular birthmarks: hemangiomas and malformations. Philadelphia:WB Saunders; 1988.
32. Tan KL. Nevus flammeus of the nape, glabella and eyelids. Clin Pediatr 1972;11:112–8.
33. Koeller KK, Alamo L, Adair CF, et al. Congenital cystic masses of the neck: radiologic-pathologic correlation. Radiographics 1999;19:121–46.
34. Fordham LA, Chung CJ, Donnely LF. Imaging of congenital vascular and lymphatic anomalies of the head and neck. Neuroimaging Clin N Am 2000;10:117–36.
35. Brown RL, Azizkhan RG. Pediatric head and neck lesions. Pediatr Clin North Am 1998;45:889–905.
36. Chervenak FA, Isaacson G, Blakemore KJ, et al. Fetal cystic hygroma: cause and natural history. N Engl J Med 1983;309:822–5.
37. Padwa BL, Hayward PG, Ferraro NF, et al. Cervicofacial lymphatic malformation: clinical course, surgical intervention, and pathogenesis of skeletal hypertrophy. Plast Reconstr Surg 1995;95:951–60.
38. Dubois J, Garel L, Grignon A, et al. Imaging of hemangiomas and vascular malformations in children. Acad Radiol 1998;5:390–400.
39. Gohram LW, Stout AP. Massive osteolysis (acute spontaneous resorption of bone, phantom bone, disappearing bone): its relations to hemangiomatosis. J Bone Joint Surg 1955;37:985–1004.
40. Dubois J, Garel L, Abela A, et al. Lymphangiomas in children: percutaneous sclerotherapy with an alcoholic solution of zein. Radiology 1997;204:651–4.
41. Ogita S, Tsuto T, Nakamura K, et al. OK-432 therapy in 64 patients with lymphangioma. J Pediatr Surg 1994;29:784–5.
42. Alqahtani A, Nguyen LT, Flageole H, et al. 25 years' experience with lymphangiomas in children. J Pediatr Surg 1999;34:1164–8.
43. Burrows PE, Laor T, Paltiel H, et al. Diagnostic imaging in the evaluation of vascular birthmarks. Dermatol Clin 1998;16:455–8.
44. Kohout MP, Hansen M, Pribaz JJ, et al. Arteriovenous malformations of the head and neck: natural history and management. Plast Reconstr Surg 1998;102:643–54.
45. Vander Kam V, Achauer BM. Arteriovenous malformations: a team approach to management. Plast Surgic Nurs 1995;15:53–7.
46. Burrows PE, Mulliken JB, Fellows KE, et al. Childhood hemangiomas and vascular malformations: angiographic differentiation. AJR Am J Roentgenol 1983;141:483–8.
47. Upton J, Coombs CJ, Mulliken JB, et al. Vascular malformations of the upper limb: a review of 270 patients. J Hand Surg 1999;24:1019–35.
48. Yakes WF, Rossi P, Odink H. Arteriovenous malformation management. Cardiovasc Intervent Radiol 1996;19:65–71.
49. Han MH, Seong SO, Kim HD, et al. Craniofacial arteriovenous malformation: preoperative embolization with direct puncture and injection of n-butyl cyanoacrylate. Radiology 1999;211:661–6.

CHAPTER
44

Lymphedema

Catharine L McGuinness and Kevin G Burnand

KEY POINTS

- Lymphedema is swelling that occurs as a result of impaired clearance of tissue fluid by lymphatic vessels.

- Lymphedema usually affects the legs, but swelling of the arms, genitals, and face also occurs.

- Lymphedema can be primary, when it appears to be caused by genetic abnormalities, or secondary, when the lymphatic vessels have been damaged by a separate pathology.

- Primary lymphedema is associated with other congenital syndromes and abnormalities.

- The clinical onset of primary lymphedema is variable, but in most cases cause mild leg swelling.

- Mild lymphedema should be treated by compression and avoidance of skin and subcutaneous infections.

- Severe lymphedema can be treated by surgical bypass or reduction surgery.

- The rare conditions associated with megalymphatics can be treated by detailed investigation and tailored surgical operations.

- Drug treatments are not of major clinical value.

- Lymphangiosarcoma and other malignancies are a rare but important sequel of chronic lymphedema.

INTRODUCTION

Lymphedema is the term given to excessive accumulation of interstitial fluid as a consequence of defective lymphatic drainage. This results in a 'brawny' or firm edema which most commonly affects the legs, perhaps influenced by the increased hydrostatic pressure from gravity. The majority of individuals affected by lymphatic edema have a recognized cause and the lymphedema is therefore called 'secondary'.

Recent developments in genetic techniques together with mapping of the human genome have led to a major advance in the understanding of the factors responsible for lymphatic development and, as a consequence, the mechanisms responsible for some of the subtypes of 'primary' lymphedema.

ETIOLOGY

Although, by definition, the cause of primary lymphedema is not known, genetic predisposition clearly influences its development.

There are a small number of babies who have lymphedematous limbs at birth and these infants usually have 'aplastic' and truly absent lymphatics (Milroy's disease).

Milroy originally described a massive North American family who had a dominantly inherited pattern of congenital lymphedema and suggested that there was a genetic cause for this condition. Linkage studies carried out in families with Milroy's phenotypes in North America and the UK identified that the condition was mapped to the telomeric part of chromosome 5q, in the region 5q34-q35. This region contains the gene for vascular endothelial growth factor receptor-3 (VEGFR-3), which encodes a receptor, tyrosine kinase, which is specific for lymphatic vessels. Defective VEGFR-3 signaling seems to be the cause of congenital hereditary lymphedema linked to 5q34-q35.[1-5]

Vascular endothelial growth factor (VEGF) is a key regulator of blood vessel development in embryos and angiogenesis in adult tissues. Unlike VEGF, the related VEGF-C stimulates the growth of lymphatic vessels through its specific lymphatic endothelial receptor VEGFR-3. It has been shown that targeted inactivation of the gene encoding VEGFR-3 causes defective blood vessel development in early mouse embryos, leading to embryonic death.[6] Abnormalities in the *VEGFR-3* gene are therefore thought to be responsible for Milroy's disease.

Because the signaling pathway between VEGF-C and VEGF-D and their receptor, VEGFR-3, has been shown to be essential for lymphangiogenesis, it has been suggested that by using gene therapy, it may be possible to stimulate lymphatic growth and function and to treat tissue edema.[7,8] *VEGF-C* gene transfer to the skin of mice with lymphedema induced a regeneration of the cutaneous lymphatic vessel network.[7]

In the much more common Meig's disease, where mild lymphedema develops around the teenage years, numerous studies have indicated that there is about a one in three risk of inheriting the condition; three times more women are affected than men. The genetic abnormality responsible for the condition has not yet been elucidated.

Hereditary lymphedema–distichiasis (LD) is a rare autosomal dominant disorder that classically presents as primary lymphedema of the limbs, with variable age of onset, and distichiasis (extra aberrant growth of eyelashes from the meibomian gland and often abutting the conjunctiva and cornea). Photophobia, exotropia, ptosis, congenital ectropion, and congenital cataracts are additional eye findings. Fourteen families in the UK, attending Moorfield's, St Thomas', and St George's Hospitals with this syndrome, provided another important clue into the genetic origin of primary lymphedema. Confirmation of the phenotype by isotope lymphography and blood taken from affected individuals showed that the condition was mapped to the q24 position on chromosome 16. The area was subsequently identified as the

FOXC2 gene. Causative truncating mutations have now been described in FOXC2, a forkhead transcription factor gene. Numerous other clinical associations have been reported, including congenital heart disease, varicose veins, cleft palate, and spinal extradural cysts. Lymphatic imaging has confirmed the earlier suggestion that LD is associated with a normal or increased number of lymphatic vessels rather than the hypoplasia or aplasia seen in other forms of primary lymphedema.[9–12]

Lymphedema is also associated with other syndromes known to be a consequence of chromosomal abnormalities, for example, Pierre Robin syndrome (micrognathia and skeletal anomalies), Down syndrome, yellow nail syndrome (characterized by primary lymphedema, recurrent pleural effusion, and yellow discoloration of the nails), Aagenaes syndrome (cholestasis and lymphedema), and autosomal dominant microcephaly–lymphedema–chorioretinal dysplasia syndrome.[13–16] A lymphedema critical region in the X chromosome has now been identified in Turner syndrome.[17]

Another gene of interest is the homeobox gene, Prox1, which is expressed in a subpopulation of endothelial cells that by budding and sprouting give rise to the lymphatic system. The anterior cardinal veins of embryos are the initial site where the first lymphatic sacs bud off. There is a complete absence of lymphatic development in Prox1 nullizygous embryos, where budding and sprouting is arrested, although vasculogenesis and angiogenesis of the vascular system are unaffected. These findings suggest that Prox1 is a specific and crucial regulator of the development of the lymphatic system and that the vascular and lymphatic systems develop independently.[18,19]

It is still not known how and why the lymphatic system is damaged or malformed in some patients. Some degree of inheritance can be demonstrated in about one-third of all patients with primary lymphedema. Congenital abnormality or absence of the lymphatics does not explain why lymphedema develops relatively late in most patients, the most common age of onset being between 10 and 25 years.

It is possible that the constituents of the lymph draining through the lymphatics may damage the lymphangioles or lymph nodes. Lymph may contain large amounts of fibrinogen under certain circumstances, and this may coagulate and block the lymphatics; abnormal lymph may also cause nodal fibrosis, which may lead to 'die-back' or disappearance of the lymphangioles. The primary disease may therefore be in the node, and this may cause the lymphatic hypoplasia. Anticoagulant therapy has been reported to produce improvement in patients with lymphedema, lending some support to the concept that hypercoagulability of lymph may be harmful.

The benzopyrone group of drugs, which have been reported to reduce lymphedema clinically, increase proteolysis by macrophages and the number of macrophages.[20] Molecules as yet unrecognized within lymph may also be harmful to nodes and lymphatic vessels. None of these explanations accounts for the development of hyperplastic or dilated lymphatics.

It is now apparent that there are a number of genes that are responsible for the development of primary lymphedema, as they appear to control the lymphangiogenesis that occurs in the embryo and, perhaps, throughout other stages of life. A full knowledge and understanding of these genes may lead to better genetic counseling, improved diagnosis, and, possibly, genetic manipulation to improve lymphatic growth.

ANATOMY AND PHYSIOLOGY

In embryonic life, four cystic spaces appear, one on each side of the neck and one in each groin. Lymphatic vessels (lymphangioles) connect these spaces and carry lymph from the legs and abdomen to the cisterna chyli. On the left side, the thoracic duct transports lymph to the left internal jugular vein. On the right, another lymphatic trunk drains lymph from the right arm and right side of the head and neck to the right internal jugular vein. Lymph nodes develop along the course of these lymphatic pathways.

Developmental abnormalities include lymphatic aplasia, megalymphatics, cystic hygromata, lymphatic and nodal hypo- and hyperplasia, and lymphangiomas.

PATHOPHYSIOLOGY

In addition to the excessive accumulation of interstitial fluid as a result of impaired drainage, lymphedema also involves reduced transport of autologous and foreign proteins. The parenchymal and immune cells secrete cytokines, which may be responsible for the proliferation of fibroblasts and epithelial cells that cause the sclerotic changes in the skin and subcutaneous tissues.

The lymphatic system has two main functions. Firstly, it returns any large molecules and interstitial fluid that escape from the circulation to the intravascular compartment. Albumin, globulins, fibrinogen, coagulation factors, and fibrinolytic activators all pass through the lymphatics. The second major function is to return lymphocytes from the lymph back to the bloodstream. Most exogenous antigens are presented to the central lymphoid system for the first time via the lymphatics. Recognition of antigens, with subsequent proliferation of specific clones of lymphocytes, takes place in the lymph nodes. Activated lymphocytes then pass into the circulation and thus to the other lymphatic tissues throughout the body.

The interstitial space has a negative pressure and this, in combination with the hydrostatic pressure of the capillaries, encourages fluid to escape from the vascular compartment, overcoming the oncotic pressure of the intravascular plasma proteins. The intraluminal pressure of the lymph system is similar to that of the interstitial fluid, and, therefore, lymph capillaries must actively absorb proteins through their pores. The mechanism by which this is achieved is not known.

The lymphatic capillaries have large pores that allow large molecules to enter the lumen, and many valves that prevent the reflux of lymph. Lymphatics have some circular smooth muscle in their wall and are capable of contraction, and the combination of inherent contractility and valves ensure that lymph is propelled along the lymphatics and into the veins. Other factors that may influence lymphatic drainage include compression from surrounding arteries and the negative pressure in the thoracic cavity, encouraging lymph flow upwards into the thorax from the abdomen.

CLASSIFICATION AND SUBDIVISIONS

The condition may be subdivided into primary and secondary lymphedema, the latter being the most common. Secondary lymphedema is the result of some recognized pathologic process

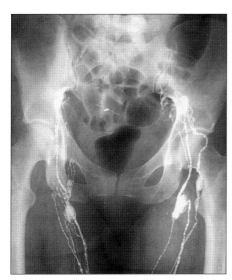

Figure 44.1 A plain X-ray after bipedal lymphangiography, demonstrating a paucity of lymphatics draining the iliac nodes in a patient with primary lower limb lymphedema.

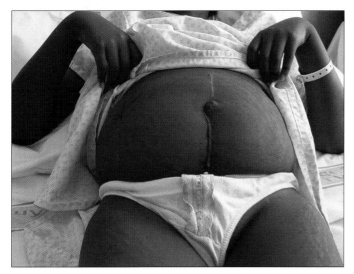

Figure 44.2 Chylous ascites in a young girl with widespread bowel lymphangiectasia, which was treated by small bowel resection of the most severe bowel segment and insertion of a Denver shunt.

disrupting the lymphatic drainage. 'Primary' or 'idiopathic' lymphedema is by comparison much rarer, although its precise prevalence/incidence is not known. Many mildly affected subjects may never attend doctors or physicians and there is, at present, a lack of good population-based studies with objective confirmatory tests. Many people with mild lymphedema develop ankle swelling after prolonged standing or sitting which does not lead them to seek medical advice.

Further subdivisions of primary lymphedema have been made on the basis of the anatomic lymphatic abnormalities. The lymphatic channels may be absent or severely hypoplastic, being few in number and disappearing more proximally (**Fig. 44.1**). They may also be excessive in number, though defective in function: such lymphatic hyperplasia is usually associated with excessive numbers of lymph nodes. The lymphatics may be dilated and ectatic (megalymphatics) and this abnormality is often associated with chylous ascites (**Fig. 44.2**), chylothorax, and lymphatic reflux. Finally, the lymphatics may be obstructed; in primary

lymphedema, this is often associated with fibrosis within the lymph nodes.

Primary lymphedema is associated with many other congenital abnormalities, including vascular deformities, gonadal dysgenesis, congenital heart disease, hypogammaglobulinemia, autoimmune hypothyroidism, nephropathy, glaucoma, xanthomatosis, esotropia, nail dystrophy, and cleft palate.[21-27]

Secondary lymphedema
All patients presenting with lymphedema must have a possible cause excluded by careful examination and special tests, where necessary.

Filariasis
This helminthic infection is the most important cause of lymphedema worldwide. There are three filarial worms which cause lymphatic filariasis: *Wuchereria bancrofti*, *Brugia malayi*, and, least often, *Brugia timori*. Infection results from a bite from an infected arthropod. The larvae mature into adult worms within the human host and the female produces microfilariae that are then transmitted to other biting insects, thus completing the life cycle. Approximately 80 million people in 76 countries are infected with filarial parasites. *Wuchereria bancrofti* accounts for about 90% of infections and *Brugia malayi* for most of the remaining cases. About two-thirds of infected people live in China, India, or Indonesia.

Worms enter the lymphatics and lodge in the lymph nodes; these become fibrotic, causing obstruction to the lymphatic pathways, which are often grossly dilated. This results in severe swelling of the limbs (usually the legs), called 'elephantiasis'.

The diagnosis is confirmed by finding microfilariae, which enter the blood in large numbers at night. A strongly positive complement fixation test suggests active or past filariasis.

Treatment with diethylcarbamazine destroys the filariae but cannot reverse established lymphedema, although progression of the disease may be slowed or prevented. Established lymphedema is treated by the same methods as those used to treat primary lymphedema.[28-30]

Non-filarial elephantiasis
Podoconiosis is a form of endemic non-filarial elephantiasis which has been reported in certain parts of East Africa and Ethiopia where filariasis does not exist. It is thought that the condition is a result of an obstructive lymphopathy caused by aluminosilicate and silica absorbed from soil through the soles of the feet. The silica causes a dense fibrotic reaction in the inguinal nodes of barefoot tribesmen.

Malignancy
Any malignant process that spreads to the lymph nodes can cause secondary lymphedema, but it is more common after surgical resection or radiotherapy directed for nodal deposits of tumor. Hodgkin's disease and the non-Hodgkin's lymphomas occasionally present with lymphedema, which may also complicate malignant melanomas and testicular seminomas (**Fig. 44.3**). The mass effect of large tumours can also obstruct lymph flow.[31]

Surgical block dissection
This operation is usually carried out to treat malignancies affecting lymph nodes, although in many cases it forms part of a staging

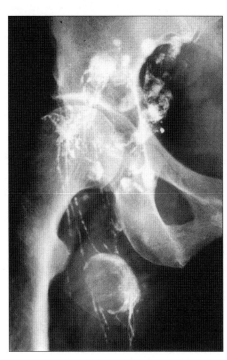

Figure 44.3 A lymphangiogram performed to investigate lymphedema of the right leg, which demonstrates malignancy in the right groin nodes. In this case, malignant melanoma deposits in the proximal nodes were the cause of secondary lymphedema.

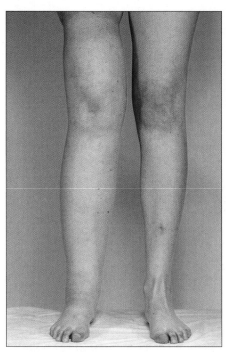

Figure 44.4 Self-induced right leg lymphedema. The indentation from the tourniquet used by the patient to effect the swelling can be seen in the upper thigh.

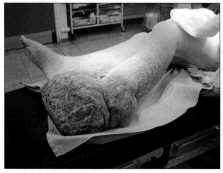

Figure 44.5 Self-induced left foot lymphedema. In this case, the swelling was produced by a combination of compression of the medial thigh by the contralateral knee, total disuse, and dependency. The patient had a through-knee amputation.

or prophylactic procedure. The carcinomas commonly treated by block dissections are those of the breast and uterus.[32] Malignant melanoma and testicular tumors are also often treated by block dissection or irradiation.

Radiotherapy

Radiotherapy was a common cause of secondary lymphedema of the arm in patients with breast carcinoma in the 1970s and 1980s, especially when given after an axillary clearance. The combination of radiotherapy and surgery carries a higher risk of lymphedema than either treatment in isolation. Radiotherapy results in nodal fibrosis, which causes obstruction of the lymphatic vessels. Recurrent tumor in an irradiated field may also be responsible for lymphedema that develops some years after treatment of the primary disease.

Trauma

Severe trauma occasionally causes tissue loss which includes lymph nodes or lymphatic channels. This is particularly common after severe degloving injuries.

Chronic infection

Although tuberculosis has often been cited as a cause of lymphedema, it is uncommon today.[33]

Chronic inflammation

Severe rheumatoid disease, psoriatic arthritis, and severe chronic eczema are recognized causes of lymphedema. Chronic stimulation of the lymph nodes in these patients results in fibrosis and mild obstruction to the lymphatic drainage.[34–37]

Acute infection

Severe cellulitis can occasionally damage the local subcutaneous lymphatics and cause mild lymphedema. Patients with subclinical primary lymphedema may also develop a secondary cellulitis: the two presentations can be difficult to distinguish.

Self-induced

This is quite a common form of Munchausen's syndrome, produced by repeated tight application of a tourniquet (**Fig. 44.4**). Total disuse of a limb can also cause swelling: this form of self-induced lymphedema should be suspected if passive movement of the limb is not possible (**Fig. 44.5**). Lymphograms are usually normal or only mildly abnormal. The cause should be suspected if there is a sharp cut-off to the lymphedema demarcated by a rut from application of the tourniquet. Patients should be informed of the doctor's suspicions and referred for psychiatric advice.

CLINICAL FEATURES

Primary lymphedema is much more common in the legs than in the arms. Although this is partly explained by the influence of gravity, anatomic abnormalities are rarely present in the lymphatics of the arm.

The swelling may affect one or both legs, the lower abdomen, the genital region, one or both arms, and, rarely, the face or chest. In the legs, swelling usually develops around the ankle and on the dorsum of the foot, and spreads proximally. In the majority of patients, the edema does not spread above the knee. Severe edema of the whole leg including the buttock suggests a proximal

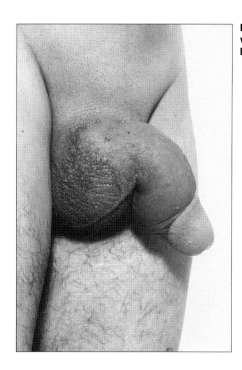

Figure 44.6 Skin vesicles seen around a lymphedematous penis.

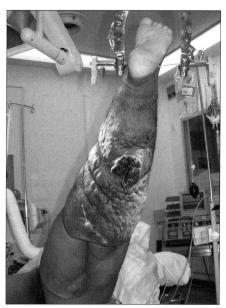

Figure 44.7 Lymphangiosarcoma in a young female with long-standing severe primary lymphedema. The area of ulceration had been present for a few months. Biopsy confirmed sarcoma, and the patient underwent amputation (a disarticulation of the hip).

nodal lymphatic occlusion. There are exceptions to this rule, however, and patients with proximal lymphatic occlusions may have no edema of the ankle or foot.

Because lymphatic edema is chronic and has often been present for many years, it stimulates a fibrotic reaction in the subcutaneous tissues, making them more resistant to deformation than does 'acute edema' associated with cardiac failure or hypoproteinemia. Prolonged digital pressure always produces a 'pit'. If pitting cannot be demonstrated, the diagnosis of lymphedema must be questioned and another cause for the swelling should be sought.

The onset of the swelling is usually insidious, and the amount of swelling may fluctuate initially. Even when lymphedema becomes fixed, the majority of patients report that the swelling decreases during sleep and is maximal at the end of the day. The onset can occasionally be sudden, and progression rapid. This is often associated with cellulitis, which can be both a cause and a result of the lymphedema. Patients with sudden severe swelling usually have a proximal lymphatic occlusion and may have an underlying cause for the condition. Patients with malignant obstruction of both the veins and lymphatics often develop a severe brawny edema of rapid onset; this can cause intractable pain, which may be very difficult to alleviate. Some patients develop marked cutaneous thickening, which can progress to lymphatic warts (condylomata) and multiple coarse papillae. Other patients are troubled by repeated attacks of cellulitis. The infecting agent may enter through the hyperkeratotic skin or through cracks in the interdigital clefts that occur in athlete's foot.

Now and then, patients develop numerous vesicles in the skin which may leak clear lymph or, occasionally, chyle. These vesicles usually indicate that megalymphatics and lymphatic reflux are present. Vesicles typically arise over the upper thighs or on the external genitalia (**Fig. 44.6**), and they may also act as a portal of entry for bacteria. Occasionally, the lymph leakage from these vesicles is severe enough to be a major source of embarrassment and irritation.

Severe edema of the male genitalia is both embarrassing and uncomfortable, interfering with work and sexual relationships. When the penis is almost hidden inside a grossly swollen scrotum, penetration may be impossible and urination may be difficult. Leaking vesicles and recurrent attacks of cellulitis often complicate the condition. Women with genital edema usually have fewer problems, but massive labial swelling can occur.

Lymph can leak into both the abdominal and pleural cavities, causing chylous ascites and pleural effusions. Patients present with abdominal distension, dyspnea, or both. These problems are usually the result of leakage from refluxing megalymphatics. Chyluria and chylous leakage from the vagina (chylometrorrhea) are rare complications. Protein-losing enteropathy can cause severe weight loss, and chylous leakage from the serosal surface of the bowel may increase the ascites.

Lymphedema may occasionally affect the arm, including the fingers, and unilateral pectoral swelling can also occur. Edema of the face usually presents as swelling of the eyelids, which are the most lax tissues in this region.

Patients with lymphedema usually seek advice because they want to know the reason for the swelling, which can cause major cosmetic embarrassment, even though it is often only of nuisance value. Severe swelling may make it impossible to buy fitting shoes, and if the leg continues to swell, its weight interferes with normal walking. Recurrent attacks of cellulitis may also be a major problem, causing the patient to lose time off school or work. Severe attacks may require admission to hospital for intravenous antibiotics and may even be life threatening.

A number of tumors are associated with lymphedema. Lymphangiosarcoma (Stewart–Treves syndrome) very rarely develops in legs following long-standing lymphedema (**Fig. 44.7**); it is more common in patients with secondary lymphedema.[38,39] Squamous cell carcinoma, cutaneous plasmacytoma, angiosarcoma, and Kaposi's sarcoma have all been reported in lymphedematous limbs.[40–45]

A detailed medical and family history should exclude secondary causes of lymphedema and should suggest a genetic cause of the primary condition. Apart from confirming the presence of pitting, physical examination excludes other causes of limb swelling and reveals any associated abnormalities. Examination of the feet may confirm the presence of 'square toes', which result from footwear preventing toe expansion. It is important to inspect the web spaces between the toes for fungal infection, which is especially common in lymphedematous legs and is an important portal of entry for bacteria that cause recurrent cellulitis.

The skin should be carefully examined for papillae and vesicles, and the circumference of the limbs should be measured at several levels, above and below fixed bony points. This allows comparison over time and the results of therapy to be evaluated. The length of the limbs should also be recorded and the presence of any abnormal veins noted. The abdomen and chest should be carefully examined for ascites or effusions. The groins, axillae, and neck should be palpated for pathologically enlarged lymph nodes. Rectal and vaginal examinations are indicated if a pelvic malignancy is suspected.

The history and physical examination should indicate whether the patient has primary or secondary lymphedema, but unequivocal confirmation of the diagnosis is desirable. Other investigations are necessary if the swelling is not considered to be the result of lymphedema.

DIFFERENTIAL DIAGNOSIS

Venous edema can sometimes be difficult to differentiate from lymphedema, especially if it is caused by the iliac vein compression syndrome, when there is often little in the way of superficial venous engorgement. The presence of dilated collateral veins, varicose veins, and lipodermatosclerosis of the calf skin suggest the likelihood of venous edema, as does a past history of deep vein thrombosis. Other causes of bilateral limb edema include cardiac disease, nephrotic syndrome, hypoproteinemia, fluid overload during intravenous therapy, and chronic liver disease. These disorders can be excluded by a careful physical examination and appropriate blood tests. Klippel–Trénaunay and Parkes–Weber syndromes also cause limb enlargement. The former is associated with bony and soft tissue overgrowth, superficial varicosities in an unusual distribution, and a large capillary nevus. Some patients with Klippel–Trénaunay have a lymphatic element to the vascular malformation, though this is usually mild.

Patients with Parkes–Weber syndrome (multiple congenital arteriovenous malformations throughout a limb) often have an oversized limb with evidence of venous hypertension (varicosities, nevi, and lipodermatosclerosis). Multiple machinery murmurs can be heard at many sites and it should be possible to elicit the Branham–Nicoladoni sign (occlusion of the arterial inflow to the fistula causes a slowing of the pulse rate).

True gigantism (Robertson's giant limb) is a rare disorder in which all the tissues (muscles and bones) are hypertrophied.

A common misdiagnosis is that of lipoidosis or 'lipodystrophy', a genetic condition that results in abnormal fat deposition, usually in proximal limbs. It can be excluded because the fat does not pit and the dorsum of the foot is unaffected and therefore not swollen (**Fig. 44.8**).

Premenstrual edema is mild and has an obvious cyclical history, and rapidly growing soft tissue tumors rarely cause diagnostic problems.

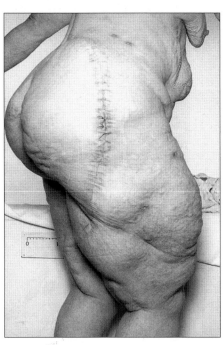

Figure 44.8 Lipodystrophy characterized by an abnormal propensity for the deposition of fat around the thighs and buttocks.

Before making a diagnosis of one of these rare conditions, for which venography, computed tomography (CT), magnetic resonance imaging (MRI), and arteriography may be required, it is often simpler to exclude lymphedema by isotope lymphography.[46]

DIAGNOSTIC TECHNIQUES

Investigations
A full blood count, erythrocyte sedimentation rate, and chest radiographs are usually requested and measurement of serum protein, blood urea, creatinine, electrolytes, and liver function tests should be obtained in all patients with bilateral edema. An electrocardiogram and echocardiogram may be helpful if cardiac edema is suspected.

Isotope lymphography
Isotope lymphography has replaced contrast lymphangiography as the primary diagnostic technique. Rhenium sulfur colloid is specifically taken up by lymphatics and allows the presence of lymphedema to be confirmed by a simple outpatient investigation with a reasonable degree of accuracy. Normally, 0.3% of the injected dose arrives in the groin within 30 min, and more than 0.6% arrives within 1 hour. In patients with venous edema, there is an excessive uptake, often above 3% at 30 min, and this test can therefore distinguish between venous and lymphatic edema, although there is a 'grey area' of overlap. Gamma-camera pictures provide information that the isotope is reaching the lymph nodes of the groin and delayed images may show a failure of progression, indicating proximal obstruction. This should be confirmed by contrast lymphography, as should any equivocal findings. Isotope lymphography is a moderately sensitive test for lymphedema, but which mistakenly classifies some normal legs as lymphedematous. It will often correctly identify patients who are suitable for lymphatic bypass surgery.[47]

Contrast lymphangiography

This is sometimes indicated to confirm the diagnosis when the isotope test is equivocal and to determine whether the lymphatic obstruction is suitable for bypass. It is also indicated in patients with chylous ascites or megalymphatics with dermal leakage to show the extent of the anomaly and indicate where leakage is occurring. Contrast is infused directly into the peripheral lymphatics of the arm or leg, which are visualized through an operative microscope after subcutaneous injection of patent blue green into the web spaces (**Fig. 44.9**). Patients are admitted to hospital for contrast lymphography, and general anesthesia is usually necessary as few patients can keep sufficiently still for the time required to obtain the radiographs. Before the test, patients often require bed rest and leg elevation in hospital for a few days to reduce foot edema and make lymphatic cannulation easier. Lymphangiography does, however, provide precise information on the presence of lymphatic hypoplasia, the extent of the megalymphatics, and the site of lymphatic obstruction. It remains the investigation against which other techniques are judged. It is still essential before lymphatic bypass is considered, and is of some value in assessing prognosis.

Magnetic resonance imaging of a limb will show dilated subcutaneous lymphatics but cannot define the site of lymphatic obstruction. MRI alone, or in combination with superparamagnetic contrast agents (lymphangiomagnetograms) or fat subtraction (suppression) has the potential to yield further information. Ultrasound imaging, CT, and MRI can all demonstrate enlarged lymph nodes, and guided biopsies of lymph nodes can be taken if malignancy is suspected. Needle or trucut biopsies are probably safer as a preliminary procedure, since removal of large solitary fibrotic nodes may worsen existing lymphedema. A calcium chloride test may be helpful when protein-losing enteropathy is suspected.

Other techniques that have been used include fluorescent microangiolymphography and intradermal brominated fluorocarbon (to identify lymph nodes). These non-invasive imaging techniques can be used to monitor and document the efficacy of treatments designed to remedy defective lymph transport in chylous reflux syndrome. They can also be used to delineate incompetent lymphangiectatic/lymphangiomatous truncal elements in order that they can be sclerosed successfully using percutaneous computer-guided catheters.[48]

MANAGEMENT

Distal hypoplasia – Meig's disease

Young women with mild lymphedema of gradual onset usually have distal lymphatic hypoplasia: there is prolongation of the time taken for the isotope to reach the groin nodes, but normal onward passage. This type of lymphedema is often inherited (around a third), and rarely becomes severe or extends above the knee. It is often bilateral, but one leg may be affected several years before the other. Rarely, the arms are also involved.[49]

Physical methods

Patients with this condition rarely require surgery. They should be given advice on leg elevation, especially in the evenings and at night. Some patients benefit from regular massage or mechanical compression, combined with wearing graduated elastic compression stockings during waking hours. Pneumatic massaging devices are available, and sequential segmental machines such as the Lymphopress™ are probably more effective than single-chamber boots (**Fig. 44.10**). These may be worn in the evenings or in bed at night, although they may interfere with sleep.[50]

Correctly fitted graduated compression stockings (30–50mmHg at the ankle, decreasing up the leg) only need to be prescribed to knee level if the lymphedema is distal in distribution. Elastic compression stockings do not cure lymphedema, but they reduce fluid accumulation during the day and often produce considerable symptomatic relief. They are poorly tolerated in warm climates, and young men and women tend to be conscious of their appearance. Many patients with mild lymphedema require little in the way of active treatment apart from reassurance and a prescription for elastic stockings. Weight reduction and physical exercise are often beneficial and never harmful. Concentrated

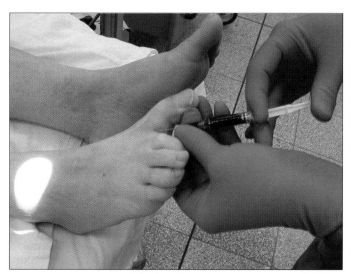

Figure 44.9 Contrast lymphangiography. Patent blue green is injected into the web spaces prior to lymphangiography.

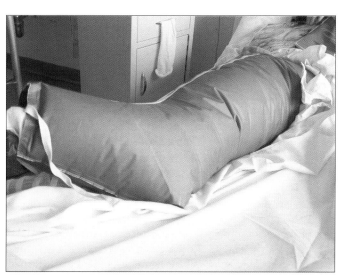

Figure 44.10 A pneumatic massaging device.

compression therapy and massage which reduces the size of lymphedematous legs can be maintained by obsessive wearing of good elastic stockings or repeated application of tight bandages.[51]

Drug therapy

Diuretics are of little value in lymphedema as they do not selectively remove fluid from the lymphedematous tissues and may cause side effects when used for prolonged intervals. Paroven (hydroxyrutosides) has some anecdotal support, as do the benzopyrones, but these compounds have not yet been tested in well-controlled clinical trials with good follow-up.[52–54]

Autologous lymphocyte infusion, which was reported to relieve swelling, has not proved to be of any long-term benefit. It was thought that cytokines produced by lymphocytes would mediate proteolysis by macrophage proteinases in the lymphedematous leg. This would remove the excess protein and relieve edema.[55,56]

Antibiotics (flucloxacillin, amoxycillin, or one of the cephalosporins) should be prescribed for cellulitis. Low-dose prophylactic antibiotics should be used if patients are troubled by repeated attacks, as prevention of cellulitis may reduce progression of the swelling.[57]

Athlete's foot must be treated by appropriate antifungal medication. Careful podiatry prevents infection and avoids an important portal of entry for virulent bacteria.

Patients with severe whole limb lymphedema (often associated with proximal obstruction)

Surgery is only indicated to treat patients with severe lymphedema where the whole limb is swollen and interferes with normal physical function or is tremendously unsightly. Most patients will have had a poor result from prolonged conservative treatment as described above.

Surgery

In a small proportion of patients, preoperative contrast lymphangiography discloses a proximal lymphatic obstruction in the ilioinguinal region, with normal distal leg lymphatics. These patients (1–3% of all those seen) can expect to benefit from some form of lymphatic bypass operation. Many patients will have been selected for investigation because the foot is 'spared' from edema and the isotope suggests that the contrast reaches the groin but fails to pass to the iliac nodes.

Lymphatic bypass

A number of methods have been used to join obstructed lymphatics to the venous system. Many of these techniques are of historical interest only, such as the omental pedicle and the skin bridge devised by Gillies, which was sutured to the obstructed lymph nodes in the groin. Direct anastomosis of lymph nodes to veins was originally performed by Niebulowitz, but fibrosis and low flow resulted in a high failure rate. Degni used a special needle to insert lymphatics into the lumen of the vein, but the imprecise nature of this procedure has prevented its widespread acceptance. The advent of the operating microscope made it possible to divide obstructed lymphatics and anastomose them directly to veins. The results, however, have generally been disappointing. At least three of four lymphatics should be attached to the femoral vein in the groin in the hope that one or two anastomoses will remain patent. Although there are centers throughout the world that advocate microvascular techniques for the treatment of lymphedema, lack of evidence of long-term efficacy has resulted in little interest in the UK.[58–64]

Kinmonth and his associates developed the mesenteric bridge procedure as an alternative to direct lymphovenous anastomosis. This operation uses the copious submucosal lymphatic plexus and the mesenteric lymphatics to drain lymph from obstructed nodes in the ilioinguinal region. About 5cm of the terminal ileum is resected on its mesenteric pedicle, as for an ileal conduit, taking great care to maintain the mesenteric lymphatic drainage. The small bowel is reanastomosed behind the pedicle. The isolated segment is then opened along its antimesenteric border and the mucosa stripped off the submucosa by a combination of sharp and blunt dissection after a submucosal injection of a solution of adrenaline in saline (1:400 000). The isolated pedicle is then brought down to the first normal group of lymph nodes below the level of the obstruction, and sutured over them after they have been bivalved. Connections develop between the divided nodes and the submucosal plexus so lymph from the legs drains up the pedicle into the mesenteric lymph nodes, and eventually into the thoracic duct.

This operation has been performed on over 40 patients at St Thomas' Hospital, London, and has produced good results in approximately half of them. Unfortunately, there is no means of predicting which patients will benefit from the procedure. Young patients appear to fare better, and the distal leg lymphatics must still be functioning if a successful result is to be achieved. Resolution is poor if legs are too swollen, but the swelling must be severe enough to justify major abdominal surgery. Perhaps for this reason, lymphatic bypass surgery is appropriate for relatively few patients.

Reduction operations

Absence of any functioning lymphatics in the leg precludes bypass, and limb 'reduction' is the only other surgical option.

Four types of excisional operation have been described to reduce the size of lymphedematous legs. The Sistrunk operation consists of the excision of a large wedge or ellipse of skin and subcutaneous tissue, which is then closed by skin sutures. In Homan's reduction, skin flaps are elevated from the subcutaneous fat, excising the underlying subcutaneous tissue and redundant skin. The skin flaps are then sutured back in place (**Fig. 44.11**).

Thompson modified the Homan's operation by suturing one of the skin flaps to the deep fascia. Denudation of the superficial layers of the flap stops hair growth and prevents pilonidal sinus formation. The second flap is then sewn over the top of the denuded skin. This operation has now largely been abandoned: it leaves unsightly scars, it is often complicated by pilonidal sinus formation, and the results appear to be no better than those of the simpler Homan's procedure. The theoretical benefit that cutaneous lymphatics could connect to the deep lymphatics through the buried flap has not been realized in practice.

Both Homan's and Thompson's operations can be complicated by skin flap necrosis and poor healing, particularly at the corners of the flaps. Great care needs to be taken to maintain the blood supply of the flaps, which must not be cut too thin. Flap reduction of the calf and foot is normally combined with a Sistrunk operation on the thigh if the whole leg is to be reduced in size.

Charles invented an operation to remove the severely thickened skin in patients with filariasis in India. He excised all

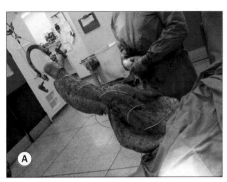

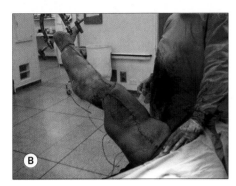

**Figure 44.11
Homan's reduction.**
(A) Intraoperative Homan's procedure, showing the extent of dissection used to elevate the skin and subcutaneous flaps. (B) The same patient, at the end of the procedure.

especially in a grossly enlarged leg with very abnormal calf skin (**Figs 44.13 & 44.14**).

Liposuction

It should be possible to remove large quantities of edematous fat from the subcutaneous tissue by this technique, but it has proved disappointing in patients with severely swollen legs from primary lymphedema. Brorson has reported excellent long-term results in patients with secondary edema of the arm after mastectomy.[65] These results must be confirmed by others.

LYMPHEDEMA OF OTHER SITES

Genital lymphedema

Minor scrotal and penile lymphedema can be tolerated without specific treatment, although support garments may be helpful. Severe scrotal edema is best treated by excisional reduction surgery in which a large central segment is excised from the scrotum, preserving the spermatic cords and testicles. The flaps are then primarily sutured using an absorbable material and the scrotum is drained. Mobilization of the testes with gentle abrasion of their surfaces may encourage adhesions to form, allowing lymph to drain via the testicular lymphatics, aiding the scrotal reduction (**Fig. 44.15**).

The penis may be reduced by simple excisional procedures, combined with circumcision if necessary. Alternatively, surgical excision of the affected tissue and split-skin grafting (a Charles' reduction) is effective for severe lymphedema of the scrotum and penis. Both scrotal and penile reduction operations produce gratifying results for the patient.[66–68]

Massive labial swelling can also be treated by simple excision.

Eyelids and upper limb

Eyelid swelling can be treated by lid reduction,[69,70] but management of lymphedema of the head and neck is usually by manual lymphatic drainage.[71]

Arm swelling can be treated by liposuction or a Homan's type of limb reduction. This can be performed on both the inner and outer sides of the arm. Patients with postmastectomy edema must be assessed carefully to ensure that the venous drainage is satisfactory and to be certain that there is no evidence of recurrent axillary nodal disease. Both venous obstruction and recurrent malignancy are contraindications to arm reduction.

the diseased skin and the waterlogged subcutaneous tissue down to, and often including, the deep fascia, from just above the ankle to just below the knee. The periosteum over the tibia was left intact and split skin grafts were then taken from normal donor skin (the opposite normal leg, or the abdomen, back, and buttocks) and used to cover the deep fascia or muscle. This operation produces the best reduction in leg size, but often at the expense of cosmesis (**Fig. 44.12**). The ankle and knee area have to be tailored carefully to avoid a pantaloon effect, and thigh reduction is also often necessary. Some patients have a poor acceptance of split skin grafts and require multiple operations to achieve complete healing. Other patients develop severe hyperkeratotic scars with warty excrescences, which produce severe deformity in the operated leg. These can be treated by shaving off the warty nodules and thickened scars with a scalpel or skin graft knife; additional skin grafts are then occasionally needed to cover denuded areas. Final results are often very satisfactory,

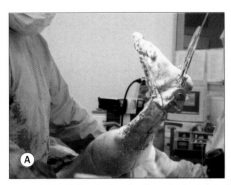

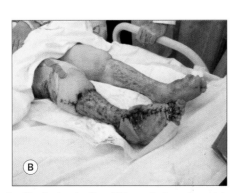

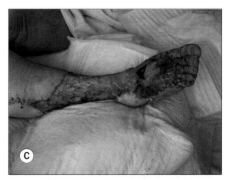

Figure 44.12 Charles' reduction. (A) At the end of a Charles' reduction. Skin grafts have been taken from the ipsilateral thigh, and the foot has been reduced by a Homan's-type procedure. (B) The appearance of a Charles' procedure on the fifth postoperative day, when the dressings are removed. The patient previously had her left leg reduced by a Charles' operation. (C) This patient has had a Charles' operation and skin grafting to the dorsum of the foot.

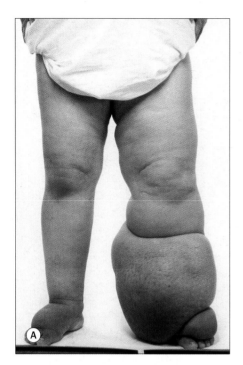

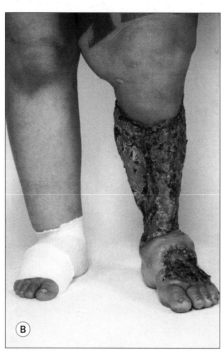

Figure 44.13 Before and 2 weeks after a Charles' reduction of the lower leg and foot.

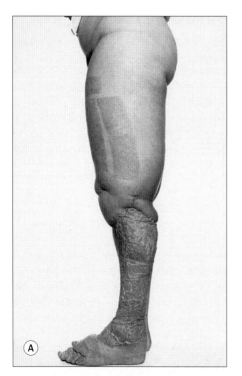

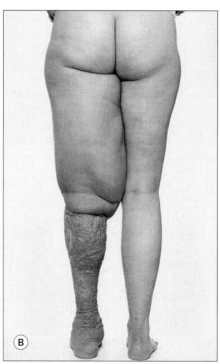

Figure 44.14 Results of a Charles' reduction at 6 months.

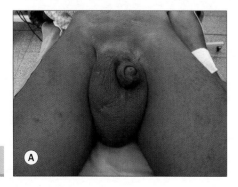

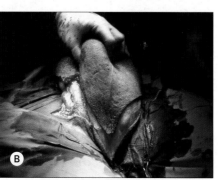

Figure 44.15 Genital lymphedema. (A) Genital lymphedema. (B) Scrotal reduction.

Postoperatively, an elasticated sleeve should be worn to try to prevent recurrent swelling.

Chylous reflux

Some patients have dilated valveless megalymphatics that allow the reflux of lymph (often chyle) against the expected direction of flow. These dilated lymphatics often end in cutaneous vesicles which are visible in the skin or which may rupture into body cavities such as the pleura, peritoneum, kidney, bladder, uterus, or vagina. Rupture results in the accumulation of lymph or chyle in the relevant cavity (chylothorax, hydrothorax, chylous ascites, chyluria), and chylous discharge onto the skin surface or mucosa is also common. Accumulation of chyle in the pleural and peritoneal cavities produces severe symptoms, and patients often become dyspneic and very distended. Some patients have a more generalized lymphatic abnormality associated with lymphedema of the limbs. Patients with megalymphatics often also have leakage of lymph from the mucosal or serosal surfaces of the bowel, leading to hypoproteinemia and ascites, respectively. Primary intestinal lymphangiectasia is characterized by widespread dilation of the small bowel lymphatics, a protein-losing enteropathy with loss of lymph into the bowel lumen, which can cause weight loss and hypoproteinemia, which further exacerbates accumulation of fluid in the body cavities and tissues.[72]

The diagnosis of chylous ascites or chylothorax must first be confirmed by aspiration of the fluid, which is then tested for chylomicrons, although the milky appearance is usually obvious. The condition may be suspected if there is pre-existing lymphedema of the extremities and it is especially likely if vesicles with lymphatic leakage are present. In quite a few patients, the condition develops *de novo*. Chylothorax and chylous ascites must be distinguished from malignant ascites or a malignant effusion: cytologic examination of the aspirate may help to exclude or confirm the presence of malignant cells. CT and ultrasound can demonstrate or rule out enlargement of the abdominal or mediastinal lymph nodes. Enlarged nodes suggest the possibility of a lymphoma or secondary malignant spread. Guided biopsy, laparoscopy, or laparotomy may be necessary to confirm these diagnoses. Contrast lymphography demonstrates lymphadenopathy, filling defects, or the presence of megalymphatics. It is only indicated if the diagnosis remains in doubt. Contrast lymphography may also demonstrate and localize a lymphatic leak, which can be sealed surgically.[73,74]

Lymphedema associated with megalymphatics rarely requires reduction surgery, but the complications of lymphatic vesicles, recurrent infections, lymphatic discharge onto the skin, chylous ascites, chyluria, and chylothorax often demand intervention. Leakage of chyle or lymph may be prevented by ligating or underrunning the dilated lymphatic channels, but this carries the risk of causing lymphatic obstruction, which will worsen the leg swelling. Despite this, many patients benefit from ligation of dilated lymphatics, and sealing off of any obvious site of fistulation.

Chromium chloride studies and a small bowel enema may provide useful information before a laparotomy is performed, if a patient with chylous ascites or chylothorax has no obvious leak on the lymphangiogram. At laparotomy, the posterior abdominal wall over the main lymphatic pathways must be inspected carefully for the presence of leakage, and the whole of the intestine should be examined. If the surface of the small bowel is grossly abnormal and leaking lymph, the involved or most abnormal segment should be resected. If this fails, the ascites can be returned back into the venous system using a Denver shunt. Although these shunts work well in patients with other types of ascites, chyle often blocks the tubing or the valve, and produces an early occlusion of the shunt. Many patients improve with simple avoidance of fat and prescription of medium-chain triglycerides combined with diuretics.

Chylothorax may respond to aspiration but often recurs and is best prevented by surgical pleurodesis involving pleural stripping. There is a small mortality associated with this procedure and some patients die from fluid- or lymph-overloaded lungs as the lymphatics draining the lung become obstructed when they are no longer able to empty into the pleural cavity.

The prognosis of many patients with severe problems from their megalymphatics can be helped by some of the procedures outlined above. Cutaneous vesicles may simply be excised or touched with diathermy or cautery, but they tend to recur. Recurrent infections should be treated by a prolonged course of broad-spectrum antibiotics.

Lymphangioma circumscriptum

These cutaneous vesicles and associated subcutaneous swellings are considered to be hamartomas or localized abnormalities of the cutaneous lymphatic drainage. They present as a number of clear or slightly hemorrhagic cutaneous vesicles, often associated with subcutaneous thickening in the underlying fat. Whimster thought that lymphangioma circumscriptum was the result of defective lymphatic drainage from the subcutaneous tissue, where a number of cisterns 'pump' lymph back into the overlying skin. These areas should be excised if they are unsightly or painful. They often occur on the trunk and it is important to excise a generous amount of subcutaneous tissue well beyond the ellipse of skin bearing the vesicles, in order to remove the subcutaneous bladders described by Whimster. It is often quite difficult to excise all the skin lesions and they have a propensity to recur: excisional surgery is only required if they are symptomatic.[75]

Cystic hygroma

In this developmental abnormality of the lymphatic system, lymphatic fluid collects in a cystic space which is frequently multilocular and situated at the base of the neck, often extending into the axillae. It commonly appears in childhood and presents as a soft, brilliantly translucent swelling in the base of the neck. Aspiration and injection of sclerosant may be attempted, but the multiloculated swellings often recur and may require surgical excision. Cystic hygromas must be dissected with great care as a number of important structures lie adjacent to them.

Mesenteric cysts

These localized lymphatic cysts within the mesentery appear as well-circumscribed mobile lumps within the abdomen. The diagnosis can be confirmed by ultrasound or CT. They are treated by resection, often in association with the overlying area of small bowel. Although harmless, they may reach a considerable size if left untreated.

PROGNOSIS

The majority of patients with lymphatic disorders can be managed conservatively. Few patients are suitable for bypass surgery: when surgery is indicated, an enteromesenteric bridge is probably the best form of bypass, having an excellent result in about half of the patients. Bypass surgery should be reserved for patients with severe leg swelling that interferes with limb function. Patients with really gross leg swelling and severe skin changes are best treated by a Charles' reduction, combined with a local excision of thigh tissue. Homan's operation should be reserved for those with a moderate-to-severe degree of swelling interfering with limb function after a prolonged course of conservative treatment. Patients with secondary lymphedema caused by malignancy often have associated venous edema. The results of reduction surgery under these circumstances are extremely poor.

REFERENCES

1. Karkkainen MJ, Ferrell RE, Lawrence EC, et al. Missense mutations interfere with VEGFR-3 signalling in primary lymphoedema. Nat Genet 2000;25:153–9.
2. Karkkainen MJ, Saaristo A, Jussila L, et al. A model for gene therapy of human hereditary lymphedema. Proc Natl Acad Sci USA 2001; 98:12677–82.
3. Irrthum A, Karkkainen MJ, Devriendt K, Alitalo K, Vikkula M. Congenital hereditary lymphedema caused by a mutation that inactivates VEGFR3 tyrosine kinase. Am J Hum Genet 2000;67:295–301.
4. Holberg CJ, Erickson RP, Bernas MJ, et al. Segregation analyses and a genome-wide linkage search confirm genetic heterogeneity and suggest oligogenic inheritance in some Milroy congenital primary lymphedema families. Am J Med Genet 2001;98:303–12.
5. Evans AL, Brice G, Sotirova V, et al. Mapping of primary congenital lymphoedema to the 5q35.3 region. Am J Hum Genet 1999;64:547–55.
6. Dumont DJ, Jussila L, Taipale J, et al. Cardiovascular failure in mouse embryos deficient in VEGF receptor-3. Science 1998;282:946–9.
7. Saaristo A, Veikkola T, Tammela T, et al. Lymphangiogenic gene therapy with minimal blood vascular side effects. J Exp Med 2002;196:719–30.
8. Karkkainen MJ, Jussila L, Ferrell RE, Finegold DN, Alitalo K. Molecular regulation of lymphangiogenesis and targets for tissue oedema. Trends Mol Med 2001;7:18–22.
9. Brice G, Mansour S, Bell R, et al. Analysis of the phenotypic abnormalities in lymphoedema-distichiasis syndrome in 74 patients with FOXC2 mutations or linkage to 16q24. J Med Genet 2002;39:478–83.
10. Erickson RP, Dagenais SL, Caulder MS, et al. Clinical heterogeneity in lymphoedema-distichiasis with FOXC2 truncating mutations. J Med Genet 2001;38:761–6.
11. Bell R, Brice G, Child AH, et al. Analysis of lymphoedema-distichiasis families for FOXC2 mutations reveals small insertions and deletions throughout the gene. Hum Genet 2001;108:546–51.
12. Rosbotham JL, Brice GW, Child AH, Nunan TO, Mortimer PS, Burnand KG. Distichiasis-lymphoedema: clinical features, venous function and lymphoscintigraphy. Br J Dermatol 2000;142:148–52.
13. Casteels I, Devriendt K, Van Cleynenbreugel H, Demaerel P, De Tavernier F, Fryns JP. Autosomal dominant microcephaly-lymphoedema-chorioretinal dysplasia syndrome. Br J Ophthalmol 2001;85:499–500.
14. D'Alessandro A, Muzi G, Monaco A, Filiberto S, Barboni A, Abbritti G. Yellow nail syndrome: does protein leakage play a role? Eur Respir J 2001;17:149–52.
15. Hashem FK, Ahmed S. Idiopathic scrotal lymphedema in Down's syndrome. Aust NZ J Surg 1999;69:75–7.
16. Aagenaes O. Hereditary cholestasis with lymphedema. New cases and follow-up from infancy to adult age. Scand J Gastroenterol 1998; 33:335–45.
17. Boucher CA, Sargent CA, Ogata T, Affara NA. Breakpoint analysis of Turner patients with partial Xp deletions: implications for the lymphoedema gene location. J Med Genet 2001;38:591–8.
18. Wigle JT, Oliver G. Prox1 function is required for the development of the murine lymphatic system. Cell 1999;98:769–78.
19. Wigle JT, Harvey N, Detmar M, et al. An essential role for Prox1 in the induction of the lymphatic endothelial cell phenotype. EMBO J 2002; 21:1505–13.
20. Casley-Smith JR, Casley-Smith JR. The effects of O-(beta-hydroxyethyl)-rutosides (HR) on acute lymphoedema in rats' thighs, with and without macrophages. Microcirc Endothelium Lymphatics 1990; 6:457–63.
21. Jones AL, Webb DJ. Selective IgA deficiency, hypothyroidism and congenital lymphoedema. Scott Med J 1996;41:22–3.
22. Usta M, Dilek K, Ersoy A, et al. A family with IgA nephropathy and hereditary lymphedema praecox. J Intern Med 2002;251:447–51.
23. Karg E, Bereczki C, Kovacs J, et al. Primary lymphoedema associated with xanthomatosis, vaginal lymphorrhoea and intestinal lymphangiectasia. Br J Dermatol 2002;146:134–7.
24. Fatinni Y, Asindi A, Al Falki Y, Al Harthi A, Al Fifi S, Al-Daama S. Possible new autosomal recessive syndrome of congenital lymphoedema, nail dystrophy and esotropia in a Saudi family. Acta Paediatr 2001; 90:151–3.
25. Benson PF, Taylor AI, Gough MH. Chromosome anomalies in primary lymphoedema. Lancet 1967;1:461–2.
26. Haugen OH, Krohn J. Bilateral congenital glaucoma in a child with hydrops fetalis, congenital pulmonary lymphangiectasia, and lymph-oedema. J Pediatr Ophthalmol Strabismus 2000;37:44–6.
27. Tatnall FM, Sarkany I. Primary facial lymphoedema with xanthomas. J R Soc Med 1988;81:113–4.
28. Bockarie MJ, Tavul L, Kastens W, Michael E, Kazura JW. Impact of untreated bednets on prevalence of *Wuchereria bancrofti* transmitted by *Anopheles farauti* in Papua New Guinea. Med Vet Entomol 2002; 16:116–9.
29. Ngwira BM, Jabu CH, Kanyongoloka H, et al. Lymphatic filariasis in the Karonga district of northern Malawi: a prevalence survey. Ann Trop Med Parasitol 2002;96:137–44.
30. Molyneux DH, Taylor MJ. Current status and future prospects of the Global Lymphatic Filariasis Programme. Curr Opin Infect Dis 2001; 14:155–9.
31. Mogulkoc N, Onal B, Okyay N, Gunel O, Bayindir U. Chylothorax, chylopericardium and lymphoedema – the presenting features of signet-ring cell carcinoma. Eur Respir J 1999;13:1489–91.
32. Sparaco A, Fentiman IS. Arm lymphoedema following breast cancer treatment. Int J Clin Pract 2002;56:107–10.
33. Ramesh V, Ramesh V. Lymphedema of the genitalia secondary to skin tuberculosis: report of three cases. Genitourin Med 1997;73:226–7.
34. Schmit P, Prieur AM, Brunelle F. Juvenile rheumatoid arthritis and lymphedema: lymphangiographic aspects. Pediatr Radiol 1999;29:364–6.
35. Bohm M, Riemann B, Luger TA, Bonsmann G. Bilateral upper limb lymphoedema associated with psoriatic arthritis: a case report and review of the literature. Br J Dermatol 2000;143:1297–301.
36. Gach JE, King CM. Constitutional pompholyx eczema complicated by secondary lymphoedema. Acta Derm Venereol 2001;81:437–8.
37. Fitzgerald DA, English JS. Lymphoedema of the hands as a complication of chronic allergic contact dermatitis. Contact Dermatitis 1994;30:310.
38. Stewart FW, Treves N. Lymphangiosarcoma in post mastectomy lymphoedema: a report of six cases in elephantiasis chirurgica. Cancer 1948;1:64–81.
39. Aygit AC, Yildirim AM, Dervisoglu S. Lymphangiosarcoma in chronic lymphoedema. Stewart-Treves syndrome. J Hand Surg [Br] 1999; 24:135–7.
40. Lister RK, Black MM, Calonje E, Burnand KG. Squamous cell carcinoma arising in chronic lymphoedema. Br J Dermatol 1997;136:384–7.
41. Echenique-Elizondo M, Elorza J. Squamous-cell carcinoma on long-lasting lymphoedema. Lancet Oncol 2002;3:319.
42. Corazza M, Lombardi A, Strumia R, Cuneo A, Virgili A. Primary cutaneous plasmacytoma on chronic lymphoedema. Eur J Dermatol 2002;12:191–3.

43. Atillasoy ES, Santoro A, Weinberg JM. Lymphedema associated with Kaposi's sarcoma. J Eur Acad Dermatol Venereol 2001;15:364–5.

44. Schwartz RA, Cohen JB, Watson RA, et al. Penile Kaposi's sarcoma preceded by chronic penile lymphoedema. Br J Dermatol 2000; 142:153–6.

45. Azurdia RM, Guerin DM, Verbov JL. Chronic lymphedema and angiosarcoma. Clin Exp Dermatol 1999;24:270–2.

46. Parkes-Weber F. Angioma formation in connection with hypertrophy of limbs and hemihypertrophy. Br J Dermatol 1907;19:231.

47. Burnand KG, McGuinness CL, Lagattolla NR, Browse NL, El-Aradi A, Nunan T. Value of isotope lymphography in the diagnosis of lymphoedema of the leg. Br J Surg 2002;89:74–8.

48. Witte CL, Witte MH. Diagnostic and interventional imaging of lymphatic disorders. Int Angiol 1999;18:25–30.

49. Mortimer PS. Managing lymphedema. Clin Exp Dermatol 1995; 20:98–106.

50. Chen AH, Frangos SG, Kilaru S, Sumpio BE. Intermittent pneumatic compression devices – physiological mechanisms of action. Eur J Vasc Endovasc Surg 2001;21:383–92.

51. Mason M. Bandaging and subsequent elastic hosiery is more effective than elastic hosiery alone in reducing lymphedema. Aust J Physiother 2001;47:153.

52. Casley-Smith JR. Changes in the microcirculation at the superficial and deeper levels in lymphoedema: the effects and results of massage, compression, exercise and benzopyrones on these levels during treatment. Clin Hemorheol Microcirc 2000;23:335–43.

53. Casley-Smith JR. Benzo-pyrones in the treatment of lymphoedema. Int Angiol 1999;18:31–41.

54. Piller NB, Morgan RG, Casley-Smith JR. A double-blind, cross-over trial of O-(beta-hydroxyethyl)-rutosides (benzo-pyrones) in the treatment of lymphoedema of the arms and legs. Br J Plast Surg 1988;41:20–7.

55. Nagata Y, Murata R, Mitsumori M, et al. Intraarterial infusion of autologous lymphocytes for the treatment of refractory lymphedema. Preliminary report. Eur J Surg 1994;160:105–9.

56. Knight KR, Ritz M, Lepore DA, Booth R, Octigan K, O'Brien BM. Autologous lymphocyte therapy for experimental canine lymphedema: a pilot study. Aust NZ J Surg 1994;64:332–7.

57. Woo PC, Lum PN, Wong SS, Cheng VC, Yuen KY. Cellulitis complicating lymphedema. Eur J Clin Microbiol Infect Dis 2000;19:294–7.

58. Campisi C, Boccardo F. Role of microsurgery in the management of lymphedema. Int Angiol 1999;18:47–51.

59. Campisi C, Boccardo F. Frontiers in lymphatic microsurgery. Microsurgery 1998;18:462–71.

60. Binoy C, Rao YG, Ananthakrishnan N, Kate V, Yuvaraj J, Pani SP. Omentoplasty in the management of filarial lymphedema. Trans R Soc Trop Med Hyg 1998;92:317–9.

61. Chen HC, O'Brien BM, Rogers IW, Pribaz JJ, Eaton CJ. Lymph node transfer for the treatment of obstructive lymphoedema in the canine model. Br J Plast Surg 1990;43:578–86.

62. Ipsen T, Pless J, Frederiksen PB. Experience with microlymphaticovenous anastomoses for congenital and acquired lymphedema. Scand J Plast Reconstr Surg Hand Surg 1988;22:233–6.

63. Dimakakos PB, Arkadopoulos N. E Kondoleon: the man behind the procedure. Int Angiol 2000;19:84–8.

64. Rao YG, Ananthakrishnan N, Pani SP, Kate V, Yuvaraj J, Krishnamoorthy K. Factors influencing response to lymphonodovenous shunt in filarial lymphedema. Natl Med J India 1999;12:55–8.

65. Brorson H. Liposuction gives complete reduction of chronic large arm lymphoedema after breast cancer. Acta Oncol 2000;39:407–20.

66. Bolt RJ, Peelen W, Nikkels PG, de Jong TP. Congenital lymphoedema of the genitalia. Eur J Pediatr 1998;157:943–6.

67. Ollapallil JJ, Watters DA. Surgical management of elephantiasis of male genitalia. Br J Urol 1995;76:213–5.

68. Hegemann B, Helmbold P, Marsch WC. Genital inflammatory lymphoedema: peculiar microvascular long-distance metastasis of gastric carcinoma. Br J Dermatol 2001;144:419–20.

69. Kabir SM, Raurell A, Ramakrishnan V. Lymphoedema of the eyelids. Br J Plast Surg 2002;55:153–4.

70. Austin MW, Patterson A, Bates RA. Conjunctival lymphoedema in Turner's syndrome. Eye 1992;6(Pt 3):335–6.

71. Withey S, Pracy P, Wood S, Rhys-Evans P. The use of a lymphatic bridge in the management of head and neck lymphoedema. Br J Plast Surg 2001;54:716–9.

72. Ballinger AB, Farthing MJ. Octreotide in the treatment of intestinal lymphangiectasia. Eur J Gastroenterol Hepatol 1998;10:699–702.

73. Browse NL, Wilson NM, Russo F, al-Hassan H, Allen DR. Aetiology and treatment of chylous ascites. Br J Surg 1992;79:1145–50.

74. O'Driscoll JB, Chalmers RJ, Warnes TW. Chylous reflux into abdominal skin simulating lymphangioma circumscriptum in a patient with primary intestinal lymphangiectasia. Clin Exp Dermatol 1991;16:124–6.

75. Konen O, Rathaus V, Dlugy E, et al. Childhood abdominal cystic lymphangioma. Pediatr Radiol 2002;32:88–94.

Index